High
Performance
Biomaterials

HOW TO ORDER THIS BOOK

BY PHONE: 800-233-9936 or 717-291-5609, 8AM–5PM Eastern Time

BY FAX: 717-295-4538

BY MAIL: Order Department
Technomic Publishing Company, Inc.
851 New Holland Avenue, Box 3535
Lancaster, PA 17604, U.S.A.

BY CREDIT CARD: American Express, VISA, MasterCard

High Performance Biomaterials

A COMPREHENSIVE GUIDE TO MEDICAL AND PHARMACEUTICAL APPLICATIONS

Edited by **Michael Szycher, Ph.D.**

POLYMEDICA INDUSTRIES, INC.

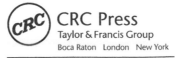

CRC Press
Taylor & Francis Group
Boca Raton London New York

CRC Press is an imprint of the
Taylor & Francis Group, an **informa** business

High Performance Biomaterials
a **TECHNOMIC** publication

Published in the Western Hemisphere by
Technomic Publishing Company, Inc.
851 New Holland Avenue
Box 3535
Lancaster, Pennsylvania 17604 U.S.A.

Distributed in the Rest of the World by
Technomic Publishing AG

10 9 8 7 6 5 4 3 2 1

Main entry under title:
  High Performance Biomaterials: A Comprehensive Guide to Medical and
     Pharmaceutical Applications

A Technomic Publishing Company book
Bibliography: p.

Library of Congress Card No. 91-58007
ISBN No. 87762-775-4

To my wife, Laurie, who actually put the book together

my sons, Mark and Scott, who some day will author their own books

*and to my faithful companion, Spicky, who silently watched the proceedings
with a wagging tail and a good disposition.*

Contents

Preface

Medical and pharmaceutical applications of synthetic polymers contribute significantly to the quality and effectiveness of the world's health care system. These applications range from catheters to vascular grafts, from semiocclusive dressings to mammary implants, and from transdermal drug delivery systems to medicated patches.

Current activities of device designers, manufacturers and research physicians indicate that devices manufactured from synthetic polymers are being increasingly accepted as the biomaterial of choice in most applications requiring compliance with soft tissue, cardiovascular tissue, or being non-irritating to the skin for transdermal applications.

The Food and Drug Administration estimates there are now 2,700 kinds of medical devices and another 2,500 diagnostic products. The majority of these devices utilize a synthetic biomaterial as its principal component; a biomaterial is a nondrug substance for inclusion in a physiological system that augments or replaces the functions of a bodily tissue or organ.

A biomaterial must be mechanically adaptable for its designated function, and have the required shear, stress, strain, modulus, compliance, tensile strength, and temperature-related properties to fit the application. It must be compatible and inert; that is, it must interact with the assorted tissues and organs in a nontoxic manner and not destroy the cellular constituents of the body fluids with which it interfaces.

The Pharmaceutical Manufacturers Association estimated sales of medical devices and diagnostic products in 1989 at over $24 billion, a gain of 400 percent since 1972. Even when the impact of inflation is taken into account, it is clear that a major new industry has emerged. Yet, many product managers and designers are unaware of the technical revolution brought about by the utilization of medical-grade synthetic polymers, and how these polymers are helping physicians diagnose disease and lower morbidity and mortality of millions of patients.

This book, composed of 46 chapters authored by a distinguished group of international scientists, bridges the gap between a "medical device" and a "drug". We have attempted to bring into clearer focus the fundamental similarities between biomaterials which are intended for devices, and those which are intended for drug delivery, for in the final analysis, they may be one and the same.

Michael Szycher, Ph.D.
Boston, Massachusetts
Spring, 1991

Part 1

MARKETS

Medical/Pharmaceutical Markets for Medical Plastics

MICHAEL SZYCHER, Ph.D.*

ABSTRACT: America spent $425 billion on health care in 1985 an amount equal to 10.7 percent of the gross national product. In 1991 health care expenditures are expected to rise to nearly 12 percent of the gross national product.

Pressures to contain health care costs and improve product performance are spurring new product development and creating new opportunities for medical plastics. Plastics are found in implants and components, medical instruments and equipment, packaging materials and a wide variety of disposable products.

The advent of synthetic polymers has changed the entire character of health care delivery. Polymers originally developed for commercial use are now qualified for implantable prostheses, thus opening the way for pacemakers, vascular grafts, artificial skin and artificial hearts. This chapter summarizes those medical devices in which synthetic biomaterials play a dominant role.

INTRODUCTION

In the past decade, plastics have assumed a major role in a variety of medical/pharmaceutical applications, making the medical market into the fourth largest area of plastics application [1]. Plastics are now found in implants and components for reconstructive surgery, as components in medical instruments and equipment, as packaging materials, and finally in a wide variety of disposable products.

Plastics currently account for over 1.8 billion pounds in medical devices as shown in Table 1. PVC, PS, PE and PP find the greatest usage since they are the lowest priced, however a significant fraction of polymers are of the "high performance" variety where

they replace traditional materials in those applications requiring outstanding mechanical properties, environmental resistance, sterilizability, biocompatibility, etc.

Pressures to contain health care costs and improve product performance are spurring new product development and creating new opportunities for plastics, according to market analysts at Dow Chemical [2]. Medical devices, consumables, and their packaging are estimated to use 2.3 billion lbs of plastics in 1992. Growth in clinical laboratory products will come from increased testing for AIDS, abused substances, and cholesterol. According to the Dow report, packaging which now accounts for half of medical plastics usage must be redeveloped to meet changes from ethylene oxide to gamma sterilization, concern about disposability of medical wastes, and product integrity.

HEALTH CARE COSTS

Americans spent $425 billion on health care in 1985, an amount equal to 10.7 percent of the gross national product. Medical costs are climbing faster than prices in the rest of the economy, although medical inflation dropped below double-digit levels for the second consecutive year.

Of these expenditures, an estimated $36 billion were spent on drugs and medical devices, as shown in Figure 1. Medical devices and medical disposables accounted for $11 billion, while drugs (and related products) consumed the other $25 billion.

Medical devices and medical disposables contribute significantly to the quality and effectiveness of the American health care system. These products range from the relatively unsophisticated tongue depressor, to the state-of-the-art artificial heart, designed to support life in many end-stage cardiac patients. The Food and Drug Administration estimates that we use some 2700 medical devices, plus 2000 diagnostic products (with sales of about $7 billion), and over 1500 medical disposables (with sales of $4 billion).

*PolyMedica Industries, Inc., Woburn, MA 01801

Table 1. Usage of plastics in medical/ pharmaceutical applications.

Polymer Family	Usage, mm lbs, 1989
Polyvinyl Chloride (PVC)	480
Polystyrene (PS)	340
LD Polyethylene (LDPE)	320
HD Polyethylene (HDPE)	250
Polypropylene (PP)	175
Polycarbonate (PC)	60
Thermoplastic Polyesters	45
Acrylics	40
Silicones	25
Nylon	20
Acrylonitrile Butadiene Styrene (ABS)	15
Thermoplastic Urethanes (TPU)	10
All others	50
Total	1830

With total sales in the $11 billion range, the medical devices industry has clearly emerged as a major new industry. Biomaterials represent the fundamental reason for this impressive performance; in the early 1930s the only "medical materials" available were wood, glass and metals. These materials were used mostly as paracorporeal and disposable products, not designed for long-term body contact or implantable devices.

The advent of synthetic polymers changed the entire character of health care delivery. Polymers originally developed for commercial products were qualified for implantable prostheses, thus opening the way for pacemakers, vascular grafts, artificial skin, and artificial hearts.

This chapter summarizes those medical devices in which synthetic biomaterials play a dominant role. The data presented were gleaned from annual reports, company promotional literature, investment banking firms, market reports and personal industry contacts. We hope this information will provide our readership with a comprehensive overview of biomaterials applications.

DEFINITIONS AND MARKET SEGMENTS

A biomaterial is a material used for, or suitable for use in, prostheses designed for contact with the living body. This may seem a straightforward definition, but we must also account for both the intended period of use, as well as the intended method of application. We may thus classify biomaterials, as shown in Table 1.

Although biomaterials (or medical grade polymers) play such a crucial role in medical devices, medical grade polymers are not an officially recognized grade of polymers. The U.S. Department of Commerce, which normally provides statistics regarding plastics consumption for such diverse uses as construction, aerospace, and footwear industries, does not list biomaterials or medical applications. Plastics trade associations, such as the Society of Plastics Engineers (SPE) and the Society of Plastics Industry (SPI) do not classify biomaterials or list medical applications. Ironically, the SPE has a very active "Medical Plastics Division", in which this author twice served as divisional chairman.

At present, all we have are voluntary industry standards about what constitutes a "medical grade" polymer, or "biomaterial". In an attempt to more clearly delineate specialized grades of silicones, Dow Corning recently promulgated the steps necessary to qualify silicones as implantable/medical grade, as shown in Table 2. This supplier also distinguishes two other grades, namely clean/industrial grades of silicones. While some of the steps are specific to silicones, this is nonetheless an excellent example of corporate foresight that is years ahead of our vaunted regulatory agencies.

The term "device" as defined by the 1976 amend-

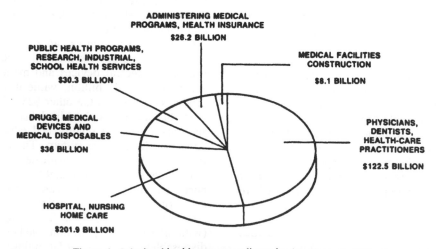

Figure 1. Calculated health care expenditures by Americans in 1985.

Table 2. Definitions of biomaterials (implant/medical grades) versus clean/commercial grades.

	Implant Grade	Medical Grade	Clean Grade	Commercial Grade
Bio-Testing				
Two-year implant data available				
Meet or exceed USP XX, Class VI Plastics Test				
Pyrogen				
Skin sensitization				
Tissue cell culture				
90-day implant with histopathology on all major organs				
Quality Controls				
Lot testing for 24 trace metals*				
FDA Registered plant using GMPs				
Lot quality control				
Lot traceability				
Product certification				
Physical properties audited on a regular basis				
Four-year sample retention				
90-day sample retention				
All multi-component materials are lot matched				
Packaging				
Units separately wrapped, sealed and labeled				
Each 25 lb unit wrapped separately				
Strained through 200 mesh				
50 lb boxes strained through 120 mesh				
1,000 lb boxes screened through 120 mesh				
Tech. Service & Samples				
Free samples				
Test results on request				

ment to the Food, Drug and Cosmetic Act is, in abbreviated form, "an apparatus, implant or other similar article which is intended for the diagnosis, cure or prevention of disease which does not achieve any of its principal intended purposes through chemical action within the body of man, and which is not dependent upon being metabolized for achievement of any of its intended purposes". This definition makes clear the fundamental difference between a device and a drug, in that drugs are dependent on chemical action and/or metabolism for therapeutic effects.

We must also define another word of Greek origin, prosthesis. Dorland's Medical Dictionary defines prosthesis as "the replacement of an absent part by an artificial substitute. An artificial substitute for a missing part, such as an eye, leg, or denture; the term is also applied to any device by which performance of a natural function is aided or augmented, such as a hearing aid or eyeglasses".

The overall usage of prostheses and medical devices in the U.S. is shown in Table 3. We will explore these markets in greater detail in subsequent sections.

REGULATORY ASPECTS

All biomaterials must meet certain regulatory requirements before they can be qualified for use in a medical product. These requirements are unprecedented in the polymer industry; depending on the intended end-use, a biomaterial may be subjected to a combination of the tests presented below.

Requirements of Medical-Grade Polymers [3]

Test	Purpose
Biodegradation	Loss of functional properties
Blood Compatibility	Absence of unwarranted reactions
Carcinogens	No detectable amounts
Cytotoxicity	Sensitive cell culture tests for elutables
EtO Residuals	Must meet regulatory requirements
Flexure Endurance	Determination of flexure life
Heavy Metals Content	Must meet regulatory requirements
Implant Toxicity	Response to long-term implant
Tissue Compatibility	Eliminate pathological response

All products used in the medical market must fall within one of three areas regulated by the Food and Drug Administration, as shown on the following page.

Table 3. U.S. usage of prostheses and medical devices (1987 E).

	No. of Patients
Cardiovascular	
Heart valves	42,000
Pacemakers	120,000
Peripheral vascular grafts	200,000
Artificial hearts	80
Coronary angioplasty	140,000
Angiographic studies	935,000
Peripheral angioplasty	70,000
Extracorporeal	
Blood oxygenation	200,000
IV Lines	75,000,000
Over the needle catheters	90,000,000
Cardiopulmonary bypass	160,000
Colostomy bags	42,000,000
Ileostomy bags	31,000,000
Urostomy bags	17,000,000
Neurosurgical	
Hydrocephalus shunts	30,000
Opthalmology	
Intraocular lenses	1,200,000
Orthopedic Applications	
Finger joints	22,500
—Metacarpal phalangeal	21,300
—Interphalangeal	1,200
Plastic and Reconstructive Surgery	
Mammary prostheses	100,000
Penile prostheses	40,000
Nose, chin	10,000

Class I	Requires general control methods as to labelling and good manufacturing practices. These products are not life supporting, and do not pose a potential risk of injury.
Class II	Must conform to performance standards as to materials, testing methods, specifications and design.
Class III	Requires pre-market notification and FDA consent, predicated on the safety and effectiveness of the device, which is life sustaining.

Table 4. Cardiovascular disease in the U.S.

Disease	Prevalence (Patients)	Deaths per Year
Heart attack	5,000,000	559,000
Stroke	2,000,000	164,000
Hypertension	60,000,000	32,000
Rheumatic heart disease	2,000,000	6,500

THE CARDIOVASCULAR MARKET

Cardiovascular disease remains the leading cause of death in the United States. According to the American Heart Association, during 1981 approximately 1,500,000 people in the United States experienced a heart attack, and 559,000 of those people did not survive. An additional 500,000 people experienced a stroke during 1981, 164,000 of whom did not survive. The most common cause of cardiovascular disease is atherosclerosis, the accumulation of cholesterol and blood products on the inner wall of an artery. In a coronary artery, which carries oxygenated blood to the heart muscle itself, this process is referred to as coronary heart disease. More than four million Americans have been diagnosed as having coronary heart disease.

The aging of the general population is increasing the number of people worldwide in need of cardiovascular care. Since heart disease remains the major cause of death around the world, global demand for cardiovascular devices will continue to rise. Currently, the estimated worldwide market for cardiovascular therapeutic devices is about $1.9 billion annually and is expected to rise to $2.5 billion by 1990.

Treatments that enable patients to resume normal, productive lives are the therapies of choice. Breakthroughs such as rate-responsive pacing, steroid eluting pacing leads, tachyarrhythmia devices, vascular grafts, ventricular assist devices, and angioplasty are leading the way to a new era in cardiovascular medicine. The breakdown of these markets is shown in Figure 2. Cardiovascular devices are aimed at the number one killer in American society, as shown in Table 4.

Heart attacks are frequently caused by atherosclerosis, which clogs coronary arteries, leading to myocardial infarctions. Atherosclerosis is also implicated in hypertension by stiffening blood vessels. Strokes may be due to embolized fragments originating from atherosclerotic plaques; therefore, atherosclerosis is a major risk factor in cardiovascular disease.

The treatment of cardiovascular disease can be subdivided from a physiological standpoint into four main categories: (1) arrhythmias, (2) afterload reduction, (3) increase cardiac output, and (4) increase vascularity. These treatment modalities are presented in Table 5.

The Pacemaker Market

Pacemakers are devices prescribed by physicians for patients who have suffered an impairment of the natural electrical conduction system of the heart which renders the heart incapable of pumping blood throughout the body at a rate and rhythm proper for the body's needs. The pacemaker treats the condition by electrically stimulating the heart to restore proper rhythmic contractions of the heart muscle.

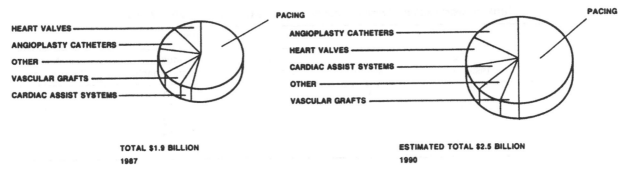

Figure 2. Worldwide markets for cardiovascular devices.

A pacemaker is a battery-powered electronic circuit encased in material compatible with the body's tissue. It is usually implanted in the upper area of the patient's chest just beneath the skin. The pacemaker's electrical stimulus is conveyed to the heart by means of a lead which is either affixed to the exterior of the heart or inserted through a vein into the interior of the heart.

In 1986, approximately 250,000 pacemakers were implanted worldwide, an increase of 2 percent over 1985. Over one million pacemaker patients are currently active. The worldwide market for pacing systems—pulse generators and pacing leads—is estimated at approximately $1 billion, comprising $550 million domestic, and about $450 million overseas. The market is expected to grow to $1.5 billion by 1995. Among the catalysts for future market expansion are greater replacement demand, an increase in the population susceptible to heart disease, and the impact of technological advances.

Rate-responsive pacing has forever changed cardiac pacing by creating a single-chamber unit that automatically adjusts its rate to meet the needs of the patient. It soon will be the standard of single-chamber applications. Dual-chamber physiologic pacemakers currently make up approximately 20 to 30 percent of total sales in the United States and over 15 percent of worldwide sales. Domestically, pacemakers are sold to hospitals at prices ranging from $1800 to $5000, depending on the complexity of the units.

Among the latest innovations in pacemaker systems are multiprogrammable units that allow changes in

Table 5. Treatment of cardiovascular disease.

Physiological Function	Devices	U.S. Market (1986)	Leading Supplier
(1) Regulation of arrhythmias	Pacemakers Implantable Defibrillation	$1 billion	Medtronic Intermedics Cordis, CPI Cook Pacemakers
(2) Afterload reduction, workload reduction	Heart valves	$175 million	Shiley, St. Jude Medtronic Extracorporeal Edwards Labs
(3) Increase cardiac output	Intraaortic balloon	$80 million	Datascope Kontron Smec, Aries Medical
	Artificial hearts Ventricular assist	$4 million	Symbion, Thermedics, Novacor, BioMedicers Abiomed
(4) Increase vascularity	Coronary angioplasty	$100 million Schneider Medintag ACS	C. R. Bard
	Peripheral angioplasty	$20 million	Cook Industries MediTech
	Vascular grafts	$125 million	W. L. Gore Meadox Impra C. R. Bard

Table 6. World sales of major American pacemaker manufacturers (1986).

Company	Sales (estimated)	Percent			
		Market	Dual Chamber	Multi-Programmable	Non-Programmable
Medtronic	308	44	22	63	15
Intermedics	154	22	25	58	17
Cordis	126	18	27	60	13
Pacesetter	77	11	32	49	19
CPI	35	5	4	73	23

rate, pulse, width, sensitivity, and operating modes noninvasively, by means of transcutaneous transformers, thereby avoiding surgery. These pacemakers can be programmed to more than 3000 prescribed combinations. Some models include a telemetry system enabling the pacemaker to communicate vital operational information directly to the physician via telephone lines.

The newest types of multiprogrammable pacemakers are specifically designed to treat various forms of excessively rapid heart rates, or tachyarrhythmias. At the present time, the only way of treating this life-threatening condition is drug therapy. These pacemakers are classified as investigational devices and are currently undergoing clinical trials.

Table 6 compares the competitive ranking of American pacemaker manufacturers in their worldwide sales. These estimates include new pacemaker implants as well as replacements.

Projections for the pacemaker industry show a 6 percent compounded annual rate, since this is considered a mature market. Table 7 presents a summary of market projections to 1990.

The Heart Valve Market

Physicians select mechanical valves, tissue valves, or occasionally, human homografts, to replace diseased or deteriorated human heart valves. After implantation, a prosthetic valve greatly increases the flow of freshly oxygenated blood to the body, allowing the patient active life again.

Table 7. Pacemaker market projections.

	1986	1990 (E)
Units		
U.S.	110,000	135,000
Overseas	140,000	180,000
Totals	250,000	315,000
Sales (millions)		
U.S.	$ 550	$ 825
Overseas	450	675
Totals	$1,000	$1,500

Mechanical valves, made from titanium and a pyrolitic carbon disc, can last a lifetime, but patients require anticoagulant therapy to avoid possible blood clots. Soft, flexible tissue valves generally do not require anticoagulant therapy, but may stiffen or deteriorate after six to ten years in the heart.

The size of the prosthetic valve market is about $220 million worldwide, growing at an annual rate of 3 percent to 5 percent in industrialized countries and close to 15 percent in developing nations. Approximately 120,000 prosthetic heart valves were implanted worldwide in 1986, divided almost equally between mechanical and tissue valves. Among physicians there is currently a shift in favor of mechanical valves.

Table 8 profiles market segments held by American manufacturers of mechanical heart valves. Tissue valve statistics are not included since these valves are obtained from animal sources and are thus not fabricated from biomaterials.

The Cardiovascular Catheter Market

Atherosclerosis can be diagnosed using cardiovascular catheters in a procedure referred to as angiography. After insertion of the catheter into a peripheral artery (often the femoral artery of the leg), the catheter is delicately maneuvered with a guidewire to the desired site using fluoroscopic guidance. After removal of the guidewire, a radiopaque contrast material is injected through the catheter into the designated vessel and a recording, called an angiogram, is made on X-ray film. Angiography enables the physician to study the heart, blood vessels, and other organs that are composed of soft tissue and that cannot otherwise be seen on an ordinary X ray. A common type of angiography is coronary angiography, which is used to evaluate suspected obstructions in the coronary arteries to determine the patient's suitability for coronary bypass surgery and to monitor the results of bypass surgery. Other types of angiography include cerebral angiography, used to view arteries and veins in the head; visceral angiography, used to view arteries and veins in the abdomen; and peripheral angiography, used to view arteries and veins in the arms and legs.

Coronary angioplasty catheters address the growing

market demand for treatment of cardiac arteries occluded with atherosclerotic plaque. They are cost-efficient, only moderately invasive, and increasingly exhibit long-term benefits. These technologies are expected to evolve and develop rapidly. Some experts anticipate a 35 percent annual growth rate in the worldwide market through 1990. Estimates for the size of the 1990 global market range from $400 million to $600 million.

Coronary angioplasty, using balloon dilatation catheters, is projected to be the fastest growing area in the cardiovascular market over the next five years.

Restenosis, or reclosing of the vessels, is sometimes called the "Achilles heel of angioplasty". Up to 30 percent of the vessels opened initially by angioplasty reclose during the first six months after surgery. New mechanical and laser technologies that would inhibit this process are in the early stages of development.

A related cardiac procedure, valvuloplasty, is gaining increased acceptance in the cardiovascular community. Valvuloplasty is the balloon dilatation of severely stenosed, and often calcific, incompetent heart valves seen in the very old and the very young with congenital heart defects. Percutaneous introduction of the valvuloplasty catheter into a peripheral artery, followed by sequential balloon dilatation, restores stenosed valves to more acceptable physiological function. Table 9 presents the U.S. market for selected cardiovascular catheters.

The Vascular Graft Market

Vascular disease, such as atherosclerosis, is usually progressive. A fatty streak in the vessel can develop rapidly into fibrous plaque deposits and ultimately to a complex material that impedes blood flow. Some patients eventually need vascular grafts to bypass severely obstructed arteries. Vascular disease resulting in an arterial aneurysm, a balloon-like dilation of an artery, may also require a graft replacement.

The 1987 international market for vascular grafts exceeds $150 million, with an annual growth rate of 5 to 7 percent. The current market is restricted to large-diameter and medium-diameter grafts.

To date, no organization is marketing arterial grafts suitable for the replacement of the coronary arteries. Each year, there are 320,000 coronary bypass surgeries. Surgeons still harvest saphenous vein grafts from the patient and are interested in a viable off-the-shelf arterial substitute. Thus, a major new market opportunity exists in the development of an improved small diameter (4 mm or less) vascular prosthesis. If that product could be used for both peripheral and coronary applications, the vascular graft market could grow to $500 million annually.

Two biomaterials dominate the vascular graft market: dacron and PTFE (polytetrafluoroethylene). Dacron (polyethylene terephthalate) monofilaments are woven into various intricate designs to form the grafts; these grafts are generally used in the large-

Table 8. Unit sales of major American manufacturers of heart valves (1986).

Company	U.S.	International	Total
St. Jude	10,000	14,000	24,000
Shiley Labs	6,000	9,500	15,500
Medtronic	3,500	6,000	9,500
American Edwards	1,200	2,000	3,200

diameter category, i.e., 12 to 22 mm diameter. Blown PTFE grafts are generally used in the intermediate-diameter category, i.e., 6 to 12 mm diameter. Table 10 presents the usage of vascular grafts in 1986, the most recent year for which complete statistics are available.

PTFE is a fully fluorinated polymer with the structural formula $(-CF_2-CF_2)_n$. It was discovered accidentally in 1938 by DuPont researcher R. J. Plunkett. PTFE, with an unusually high crystalline melting point of 342°C and a melt viscosity of 10^{11} P at 380°C, rendered the polymer intractable to conventional processing.

In 1963, Shinsaburo Oshiga of Sumitomo Industries in Japan discovered a process for expanding PTFE during extrusion. This opened the way for the production of expanded PTFE vascular grafts as we know them today. These expanded grafts consist of nodes and fiber; nodes are open channels perpendicular to the graft axis, while fibers are open channels parallel to the graft axis.

The porosity of these PTFE grafts encourages the formation of a biological lining on the lumenal surface, variously known as a neointimal or pseudointimal lining. A strict biological definition classifies a neointimal lining as a cellular lining, whereas a pseudointimal lining refers to a mostly acellular lining, composed of various fibrous proteins, such as fibrin and/or collagen. In humans, the linings seen in PTFE grafts are pseudointimal linings since they are essentially acellular.

Dacron and PTFE grafts are clinically acceptable

Table 9. U.S. market for selected cardiovascular catheters (1986).

Procedure	Yearly Incidence	Sales (E) (million)	Major Manufacturers
(1) Coronary			
Angiography	875,000	$ 65	C. R. Bard
Angioplasty	110,000	$100	Scimed
			Medtronic
			Cordis
(2) Peripheral			
Angiography	1,300,000	$ 60	Mansfield
Angioplasty	75,000	$ 20	
(3) Valvuloplasty	Experimental 70,000 cases by 1990 (E)		Mansfield C. R. Bard

Table 10. Vascular graft market (1986).

Surgical Procedure	Yearly Incidence	U.S. Sales (million)	World Sales (million)	Major Suppliers
Peripheral/vascular	350,000	$50	$25	C. R. Bard, Meadox,
Arteriovenous shunts	150,000	15	10	W. L. Gore, Impra,
Miscellaneous	95,000	25	15	(and others)
Totals		$90	$50	

for peripheral vascular surgery, arteriovenous shunts, and aneurysm repairs where the internal diameter exceeds 6 mm. The current worldwide market for vascular grafts is shown in Table 11.

The Cardiac Support Market

When the heart fails in its pumping function because of ventricular hypokinesis, the patient is said to be in cardiogenic shock. Cardiogenic shock is a primary emergency, since low cardiac output can be fatal in a very short time. Cardiogenic shock can occur under several circumstances, which include acute myocardial infarction, in patients awaiting heart surgery, and in patients unable to be weaned from cardiopulmonary bypass.

At present, there are two clinical modalities capable of supporting the failing ventricle during cardiogenic shock: (1) the intraaortic balloon pump and (2) artificial hearts (which include total artificial hearts and ventricular assist devices). In this section we report these modalities separately.

Intraaortic Balloon (IAB) Market

IAB pump was clinically introduced in 1967 by Avco Corporation, to provide cardiac output without the need for open-chest surgery. The IAB is a polyurethane-based catheter that is implanted within the thoracic aorta via a percutaneous incision through the femoral artery. The polyurethane balloon at the end of the catheter is rhythmically inflated and deflated synchronously with the heart, thus helping to support the failed left ventricle. The IAB can only provide a moderate level of support to the heart (2 liters per minute of cardiac output), in comparison to ventricular assist devices and artificial hearts, which can develop 6 to 10 liters per minute of cardiac output.

The IAB provides cardiac suppport by increasing cardiac output, thus improving the balance between the heart's capability of pumping blood (supply of oxygen), and the body's need for blood (demand for oxygen). Under electronic control provided by a bedside console, the balloon within the aorta is inflated during diastole, and deflated during cardiac systole, thus doing most of the pumping work normally done by the left ventricle.

The IAB is clinically useful in stabilizing patients prior to open-heart surgery, and for patients unable to be weaned from cardiopulmonary bypass. In some cases, the IAB has been used to stabilize patients being transferred to the hospital following myocardial infarction or accidents.

Table 12 summarizes the total revenue of companies involved in the manufacture of IAB pumps. The figures represent the total revenues due to sales of bedside consoles, as well as all disposable items.

Artificial Hearts (AH) and Cardiac Assist Devices (CAD)

Cardiovascular disease is, as we have seen, the most significant medical problem in the United States. As illustrated in Table 13, cardiovascular disease is still the leading cause of death, responsible for almost as many deaths as all other causes combined. Consequently, its diagnosis, monitoring, and treatment is a national concern. According to American Heart Association estimates, Americans will spend over $50 billion this year for drugs, physician and nursing services, and hospital and nursing home services, to diagnose, monitor and treat cardiovascular disease.

It is estimated that the U.S. spent $4.8 billion in 1983 for diagnostic, monitoring and therapeutic products. When analyzing the societal costs of cardiovascular disease, it is important to note that therapeutic drugs represented 72 percent of these expenditures. Therapeutic drugs are often prescribed to treat coronary artery disease, hypertension and arrhythmias, since these are the diseases that are most amenable to pharmacological support.

Further examination of cardiovascular disease discloses two other major causes of mortality and morbidity: congestive heart failure (CHF) and vascular disorders. Table 14 presents a breakdown of the major causes of cardiovascular disease in the U.S. Coronary artery disease, hypertension and arrhythmias respond reasonably well to medications; valvular disorders are treated surgically; but CHF remains the last of the major heart complications for which appropriate therapy is still unavailable.

While the number of deaths from coronary artery and cardiovascular disease is clearly decreasing in the U.S., the prevalence of CHF is increasing. Congestive heart failure accounts for almost 400,000 deaths each year in the U.S. alone. Approximately half of these deaths are sudden, and presumably related to the particularly high incidence of ventricular arrhythmias in patients with congestive heart failure. In 1971, the Framingham study found that, for those who have acquired CHF, the probability of dying within five years was 62 percent for men and 42 percent for women. The investigators stated, "despite early recognition and increasingly sophisticated and potent treatment of CHF, its clinical cause and prognosis remains surprisingly grim and not much better than those for cancer in general". Unfortunately, this statement remains true 16 years later.

Congestive heart failure is a condition in which the heart pumping function is inadequate to supply the metabolic need of the body; in other words, CHF is present when the heart fails in its function as a pump. When cardiac pumping is inadequate, congestion (or pooling of blood) is observed in the lungs, legs, and stomach, depending upon which side of the heart is affected.

The heart's prime mechanical function is to generate sufficient force to propel blood throughout the peripheral vasculature. Within its ventricular chambers the normal heart generates enough driving pressure to perfuse downstream components of the vasculature where the blood pressure is lower. One fundamental measure of mechanical function is cardiac output, which is a clinical expression of the heart's performance as a pump. Whenever cardiac output is inadequate on a chronic basis, we say the patient suffers from CHF.

Since failures can be traced to the left ventricle, the right ventricle, or both, CHF is classified into three forms: left-sided failure, right-sided failure, or biventricular failure, as listed below.

- left-sided heart failure
  Left-sided heart failure, usually due to a damaged or diseased left ventricle—as with acute myocardial infarction, hypertension, cardiomyopathy, bacterial endocarditis—causes:
  — pulmonary congestion and as a result, exertional dyspnea and rales; nocturnal dyspnea; orthopnea.
  — reduced tissue perfusion and as a result, fatigue, alteration in behavior, reduced activity and tachycardia, and hypotension.
- right-sided heart failure
  Right-sided heart failure may result from left-sided failure or occur independently, usually due to pulmonary vascular disease or pulmonary or tricuspid valve disease. Symptoms are due to systemic congestion: weight gain, abdominal pain, dependent edema, ascites, etc.
- biventricular heart failure
  Biventricular failure occurs when the right ventricle fails as a consequence of left-ventricular failure, or in myocarditis or cardiomyopathy (primary or secondary).

Table 11. Usage of vascular grafts by procedure.

	Peripheral	Shunts	Coronary Artery Bypass
Dacron	30,000	—	—
PTFE	80,000	75,000	—
Biograft	7,000	1,000	—
Saphenous vein	233,000	—	320,000
Other	—	74,000	—
Total	350,000	150,000	320,000

Table 12. U.S. market for IAB (1986).

Manufacturer	Revenues ($ millions)	Market Share (percent)
Datascope	25	58
Kontron	10	23
Smec	5	12
Aries Medical	3	7

Table 13. Leading causes of death in the U.S.

Cause	Number of Deaths	Percent of Total
Disease of heart and blood vessels	989,600	50
Cancer	422,700	21
Accidents	102,100	5
Chronic obstructive pulmonary disease	59,900	3
Pneumonia and influenza	54,400	3
All other causes	358,300	18
Total	1,987,000	100

Table 14. Breakdown of cardiovascular expenditures by disease.

Disease	1983 Expenditures ($ millions)	Percent of Total
Coronary artery disease	1708	37
Hypertension	1311	28
Arrhythmias	871	19
Congestive heart failure	488	11
Valvular disorders	225	5
Total	4603	100

— Causes other than disease of the left ventricle include mitral stenosis, left atrial mlyxoma, ruptured chordae, acute bacterial endocarditis, and cor triatriatum (rare). Symptoms are associated with systemic hypoperfusion, pulmonary congestion and systemic congestion.

The clinician treating cardiogenic failure patients has little hope of saving these desperately ill patients. Drug therapy is the only choice available at this time other than a biologic heart transplant. Drug therapy is effective, initially, but limited in many ways because the disease state progresses to a point where the natural heart cannot provide the necessary energy level to maintain life. At that point, biologic heart transplant is the only other choice. Significant progress has been made on this front, although the lack of sufficient donor hearts has greatly limited this activity. It is estimated that between 1500 and 2000 donor hearts are available yearly while there are approximately 40,000 patients a year in CHF who need them. Obviously, there is a significant clinical need to provide an alternative for those patients in CHF who require cardiac support.

At present, the only hope for patients with CHF is twofold: (1) biological heart transplants, or (2) artificial hearts. Since only a maximum of 2000 donor hearts become available per year, the only logical alternative is the development and widespread clinical availability of artificial hearts. Artificial hearts are best utilized in those patients who have developed cardiogenic shock, a condition resulting from sudden decline in cardiac output secondary to CHF, usually a myocardial infarction.

The societal need for artificial hearts is large. We estimate that of 400,000 deaths caused by CHF, approximately 84,000 occur as a result of cardiogenic shock. This is the primary patient population which could benefit from either biologic heart transplants or artificial hearts. We further subdivide artificial hearts into total heart (where the natural heart is surgically excised) and ventricular assist devices (where the natural heart remains in place, and the assist device is surgically connnected in parallel between the left ventricle and the aorta). This relationship is shown in Figure 3.

We base our estimates on a widely cited study, performed by the Congressional Office of Technology (OTA) in 1982, which estimated a total of 84,000 deaths below the age of 80, and 33,600 deaths occurring below the age of 65, as shown below:

<80 years	84,000
<75 years	64,400
<70 years	47,000
<65 years	33,600

Of these 33,600 patients in CHF below age 65, 31,000 are survivors of heart attacks with deteriorating cardiac symptoms, 2400 are patients with severe chronic heart disease, and 300 are patients with cardiomyopathies unable to sustain life following open-heart surgery.

Thus the OTA estimated that there would be 33,600 artificial heart candidates under the age of 65. This is our primary patient population, since it is our goal to implant our assist device in young patients and return these patients to society as productive and normal individuals.

At present, the market for artificial hearts is very small, estimated at only $4 million in 1986. This does not include the support provided by the NIH to several R&D companies and their clinical affiliations (shown in Table 15).

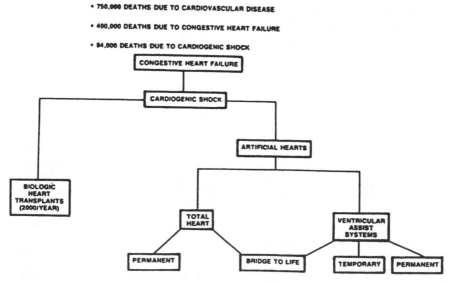

Figure 3. Artificial hearts—clinical needs.

Table 15. Investigators and clinical affiliations.

Investigators	Type	Energy Converter	Clinical Affiliation
ABIOMED (AVCO) Danvers, MA	Ventricular assist	Electrohydraulic	Mass General
Cleveland, Clinic Cleveland, OH	Total Heart	Pneumatic	Cleveland Clinic Foundation
Gould Inc. Oxnard, CA	Ventricular assist	Electromechanical (torque motor)	Texas Heart Institute
Nimbus (Aerojet) Rancho Cordova, CA	Ventricular assist	Electrohydraulic and thermo compressor	Cleveland Clinic Foundation
Novacor (Andros) Oakland, CA	Ventricular assist	Electromechanical (solenoid)	Stanford Medical Center
Hershey Medical Center (Sarns Inc.) Ann Arbor, MI	Total ventricular assist	Electromechanical torque motor (pneumatic temporary)	Hershey Medical Center Penn State University
Symbion (Kolff) Salt Lake City, UT	Total heart	Pneumatic	U. Utah Medical Center Baylor College of Med. Hospital Corp. of America Humana
Thermedics Inc. (thermo electron) Woburn, MA	Ventricular assist	Electromechanical torque motor and pneumatic temp.	Children's Hospital Mass General Beth Israel Peter Bent Brigham Veteran's Administration University Hospital
Thoratec Berkeley, CA	Ventricular biventricular total	Pneumatic	Hershey Medical Center Pacific Medical Center
University of Washington (McDonnell Douglas) Richland, WA	Ventricular assist	Thermohydraulic	Cleveland Clinic Foundation

THE DISPOSABLES MARKET

In this chapter we define "disposable" as any device fabricated of biomaterials which is not intended for permanent implantation in the human body by surgical methods. Obviously this category includes hospital products, patient use supplies, and physician office products.

Many of the disposable items are single-use devices, which are classified as Class I or Class II devices by the FDA. Pursuant to the Medical Device Amendments of 1976 to the Federal Food, Drug and Cosmetic Act, medical devices intended for human use are classified into three categories depending upon the degree of regulatory controls to which the device will be subject. Class I and Class II products are subject to the least stringent regulatory controls.

While there are many disposable products used in hospitals, such as hypodermic needles, towels, gowns, and absorbent materials, these are not included in this paper since they are not made of biomaterials. Table 16 shows the explosive growth of the hospital disposable market.

We will next focus our attention on the catheter market. As shown in the previous table, the catheter market is estimated to total $450 million per year. We

need to further divide this complex group as follows: urology, intravenous, cardiovascular, and others. Table 17 presents the catheter market by groups.

THE OBSTETRICS AND GYNECOLOGY MARKET

More than 860,000 cesarean sections are performed annually in the U.S., along with 730,000 hysterec-

Table 16. Growth of the hospital disposables market.

Products	Units (millions) 1979	1986	$ Millions 1979	1986
Blood collectors	160	200	85	165
Catheters (all)	60	120	100	450
Bags	150	195	370	725
Tubing	115	150	80	150
Tray kits	215	325	110	250
Hypodermics	2000	4700	115	210
Gloves	1000	1255	110	175
Petri dishes/pipettes	610	980	65	125
Prepackaged lab tests	780	1100	790	800
Prepackaged kits	160	300	525	950
Total			$2350	$4000

Table 17. U.S. catheter market (1986).

Classification	Sales ($ millions)
Urology	165
IV	115
Cardiovascular	110
Other	60
Total	450

tomies and 490,000 tubal ligations. Obstetrics and gynecological procedures, which include biopsy procedures, represent the largest segment of major surgery both in the U.S. and abroad, as shown in Table 18.

Use of resorbable sutures made of polylactic acid/polyglycolic acid provides important advantages over traditional methods of cesarean section closures. C-sections require tearing or cutting the uterus, causing profuse bleeding. In manual C-sections, the multiple layers of the uterine wall retract unevenly when torn or cut, making precise closure difficult and resulting in a weakened uterine wall after healing. Consequently, the possibility of a vaginal birth in future pregnancies is reduced.

The new automatic stapler enables the surgeon to perform a rapid, more controlled entry with essentially no blood loss. Milliseconds before the instrument creates an incision to open the uterus, a double row of absorbable staples is placed, sealing the blood vessels and securing all uterine layers in the correct position for subsequent closure. As a result, blood loss and tissue trauma are reduced dramatically, postoperative complications such as anemia are minimized, and delivery of the newborn is easier and less traumatic. Because all uterine layers are properly realigned, the uterine wall is stronger after healing, facilitating subsequent vaginal delivery. Fewer postoperative complications can reduce the length of stay, providing economic benefits to patients, insurers, and hospitals.

Table 18. Most frequent operations (1986) (AHA).

Surgical Procedure	Number	Rate per 1000 Population (percent)
1. Biopsy (all)	1,500,000	6.1
2. Cesarean	860,000	3.8
3. Hysterectomy	730,000	2.9
4. Skin excision	595,000	2.5
5. Obstetric laceration	550,000	2.3
6. Spinal injuries	530,000	2.2
7. Oophorectomy and salpingo-oophorectomy	525,000	2.2
8. Arthroplasty	505,000	2.1
9. Fractures	500,000	2.1
10. Cholecystectomy	475,000	2.0

The current total market for polymeric-based absorbable staples is estimated at $15 million annually, and is growing at a 25 percent rate.

THE OPHTHALMOLOGY MARKET

Ophthalmology represents one of the largest markets in terms of patient potential and devices. In the U.S. alone, an estimated 135 million persons wear some device designed to correct impaired vision. One in every 19 suffers from a vision impairment that cannot be totally corrected with eyeglasses or contact lenses. About 1.5 million are unable to read ordinary newsprint even with the aid of glasses or contact lenses; another half million are classified as legally blind. The costs of visual disorders were estimated at $7 billion in 1984 (U.S. figures). An estimated 36 million office visits were made for medical eye care in 1985. In 1986 some 800,000 persons required hospitalization for an eye disorder, over 1.0 million eye surgeries were performed (this includes patients with multiple operations); and some 350,000 eye injuries were treated in hospital emergency departments.

Purchasing power within this industry rests with approximately 12,000 active ophthalmologists, about 75 percent solo/group practice-based and, to a significantly lesser extent, with 25,000 optometrists. The latter, nearly all office-based, determine patient refraction problems and fit contact lenses. The outlook for ophthalmic products and services is bright. Growth is spurred on by an increasing elderly population and the "information age" (more reading and CRT viewing) which, together with patients' overall refusal to accept reduced vision, will sustain above average market growth.

Although polymers are used in the production of eyeglass casings, plastic lenses and ophthalmic solutions, we will focus only on two ophthalmic applications, contact lenses and intraocular lenses.

Soft Contact Lens Market

It is estimated that the total potential market for contact lens wearers is 25 percent of the patient base that requires vision correction, or about 35 million people today. To derive this figure, we assumed that 20 percent of the 138 million people who need vision correction do not wear glasses enough of the time to justify contacts, 20 percent believe they look better in glasses, 15 percent are presbyopes who cannot wear currently available bifocals, 10 percent have astigmatism that cannot be managed with current contact lenses, and 10 percent will not try contact lenses or have tried contact lenses and did not like them. In order to penetrate this potential base of 35 million people further, lenses will become even more comfortable, require less time to clean, and correct a greater number of vision problems. Soft contact lenses—especially flexible wearing cycle, or extended wear lenses—will be worn by at least 65 percent of contact lens wearers. The remainder will be fitted with hard gas-permeable lenses. Hard PMMA contact lenses will be relegated to a minor position in the market. Annual sales of soft lenses make up 80 percent of the total unit sales of contact lenses, an even higher share than soft lenses as a percentage of all fits. This is caused by the fact that soft lenses are replaced more often than hard lenses. Table 19 shows the breakdown of total wearers using contact lenses.

Contact lenses first became available in the early 1950s, when hard polymethyl methacrylate (PMMA) lenses were introduced commercially. These lenses are generally difficult to adapt to because they are thick and therefore uncomfortable for most wearers; in addition, they do not allow the transmission of water or oxygen through the lens to refresh and maintain the health of the cornea. Because of this latter characteristic, wearers must rely on the tear-pump action of the eye to provide oxygen to that part of the cornea covered by the contact lens. As the wearer blinks, tear interchange occurs from outside the lens to beneath it, providing needed oxygen to the cornea. As a result of the discomfort caused by PMMA lenses' impermeability, only about half of the people fitted with this type of lens become long-term wearers.

Soft lenses, developed in the 1960s by Otto Wichterle, a Czechoslovakian chemist, are made of hydrophilic (water-absorbing) plastic materials called hydrogels. These plastics can absorb water up to as much as 85 to 90 percent of their weight and are soft and flexible in proportion to their water absorbency. In 1964, Wichterle granted National Patent Development Corporation exclusive Western Hemisphere rights to the hydrogel materials and also to a manufacturing process called spin casting. National Patent in turn licensed Bausch & Lomb to use the product and process patents, and in 1971 Bausch & Lomb obtained FDA approval to sell soft contact lenses in the United States.

Because of their water content, soft lenses are generally gas permeable, and oxygen passes through easily to keep the cornea healthy. Because the lenses are soft and thin (thicknesses range from 0.03 mm to 0.20 mm compared with 0.30 to 0.60 mm for PMMA lenses), they are considerably more comfortable for most wearers. Soft lenses have disadvantages, however: because of what is called their bag-of-water character, the lenses have a refractive effect, resulting in less clear images than with hard lenses; in addition, the lenses are more fragile than hard lenses, necessitating replacement every twelve to eighteen months on average, compared with a two and a half year replacement cycle for PMMA lenses; finally, the potential exists for the accumulation of surface deposits and bacteria, thus requiring regular cleaning, a compliance chore difficult for some wearers.

In the early 1970s, a British optometrist, John DeCarle, experimented with making soft lenses that could be worn for extended periods of time. In 1971, Cooper Labs bought the patent from DeCarle and in 1979 CooperVision (then a wholly owned subsidiary of Cooper Labs) received FDA approval for aphakic use of extended wear lenses. (Aphakics are people whose natural lenses have been removed during cataract surgery.) In 1981, extended wear lenses were approved for traditional vision correction.

The final type of contact lens on the market today (first approved by the FDA in 1978) are hard gas-permeable (HFP) lenses made of cellulose acetate butyrate (CAB), PMMA/silicone combinations, or pure silicone. These lenses provide the same optical properties as hard PMMA lenses (that is, vision is not distorted by the bag-of-water effect), and they approach the comfort of soft lenses because they allow oxygen transmission through the lens. Because they are rigid, they can be produced more easily into shapes that correct more complex vision problems. However, they are as thick as PMMA lenses.

Table 20 presents our estimates of contact lens sales by major manufacturers. Bausch & Lomb clearly dominates the soft daily wear lens market; Bausch & Lomb had practically no competition until 1981 when Hydrocurve, Johnson & Johnson, Schering-Plough and Ciba-Geigy entered the market, rapidly cutting Bausch & Lomb's share.

Intraocular Lens Market

Few segments of the medical technology industry have grown as fast, or as consistently, as intraocular lenses. These products are now routinely implanted as a replacement for natural lenses removed due to cataracts. More than 750,000 cataract procedures are performed annually in the U.S., a growing proportion of which are done on an outpatient basis, and about one-third that number are now being done in foreign countries. In the U.S., cataract procedures are growing at about a 12 percent rate, propelled by the increasing average age of the population, the remarkable relative ease of this once-complex surgical procedure, and the treatment of the problem—the gradual clouding of the natural lens—at earlier stages.

Table 19. Total wearers of contact lenses.

	(Millions of People)				
	1983	1984	1985	1986	1987E
Soft contact lenses					
Daily wear	8.9	10.6	12.1	13.3	14.0
Extended wear	1.6	2.3	3.2	4.3	5.5
Subtotal	10.5	13.0	15.3	17.5	19.5
Hard PMMA lenses	4.0	2.5	1.5	1.0	0.5
HGP lenses	2.5	3.1	3.9	4.8	6.0
Total	17.0	18.6	20.7	23.4	26.0

Table 20. Domestic contact lens shipments by manufacturer ($ in millions).

Soft Daily Wear						
	1982	1983	1984	1985	1986	1987
Bausch & Lomb	81	79	77	77	78	79
Hydron	15	25	30	35	39	42
Ciba-Geigy	19	21	24	30	34	36
Wesley Jessen	14	16	19	22	24	26
Hydrocurve	13	14	15	16	17	18
CooperVision	10	12	18	18	19	20
Syntex	9	10	12	11	10	10
Others	28	17	15	10	7	5
Total	189	194	210	219	228	236

Soft Extended Wear						
	1982	1983	1984	1985	1986	1987
CooperVision	26	38	46	47	53	60
Hydrocurve	36	42	44	47	49	53
Bausch & Lomb	0	12	18	26	37	49
Wesley Jessen	0	2	4	9	14	19
Hydron	0	0	0	5	14	18
Syntex	0	2	4	7	8	9
Others	0	6	8	10	11	12
Total	62	102	124	151	186	220

Gas Permeable						
	1982	1983	1984	1985	1986	1987
Syntex	25	30	32	34	37	40
Paragon Optical	5	9	12	15	18	21
Bausch & Lomb	0	2	11	15	23	31
CooperVision	0	0	3	4	6	12
Hydrocurve	0	1	1	3	6	9
Others	9	11	11	14	17	19
Total	39	53	70	85	107	132

Intraocular lens implants are growing at an even faster rate than cataract procedures, as fewer of these procedures result in vision correction with high-powered, bulky spectacles and more are corrected by the surgical insertion of a small 6 mm plastic lens. Intraocular lenses reached a total market size of $207 million in 1982, and are expected to grow to $496 million by 1988, as shown in Table 21.

THE DRUG DELIVERY MARKET

The global market for drug delivery through transdermal patches is approaching $1 billion and is projected to expand to $6.5 billion by 1995. Transdermal drug delivery is now limited to drugs for which passive administration is adequate. Through the use of iontophoresis, the propelling of charged drug molecules through the skin via an external electrical current, this application is expected to expand to larger molecule drugs.

Currently, there is a concerted effort in the pharmaceutical industry to enhance and/or change the route of administration of many older drugs in the pharmacopeia, although only 10 percent of drugs can be expected to be delivered by the newer modalities.

Table 22 presents a compilation of clinical conditions most likely to benefit from continuous drug therapy. Table 23 shows some categories of potential uses of continuous nasal drug delivery products in the U.S.

Although nitroglycerine patches are the best known of the continuous transdermal delivery systems, in the U.S. no fewer than 15 drugs are currently being offered in various controlled delivery formulations, as shown in Table 24.

Since the advent of Diagnostic Related Groups (DRGs), or predetermined payments for medical treatments, an important new market has evolved: the home enteral delivery industry. This fast-rising segment of the health care market is discussed in the next section.

The ongoing trend toward out-of-hospital drug treatment continues to accelerate, due to DRG pressures. A patient's drug therapy treatment in a hospital costs on the average $200/day, compared to only $55/day at home (a cost which includes the services of a skilled nurse).

When a patient cannot be treated at home, nursing homes become the logical alternative. There are currently 21,000 nursing homes in the U.S., totalling 1.6 million beds. These institutions deliver a variety of health care services, which include enteral nutrition and continuous drug therapy. The current domestic market for enteral pumps and tubing is estimated at about $100 million annually, and the nutritional products' market is estimated at an additional $150 million. Leading suppliers of enteral feeding products are shown in Table 25.

The importance of good nutrition, particularly in the elderly population, is underscored by the fact that 5 percent of all hospitalized patients die of malnutrition, a death toll of 200,000 annually. In addition, medical complications related to malnutrition account for an additional 350,000 hospital deaths annually.

The continuous drug delivery market, traditionally dominated by hospitals, is undergoing one of the most radical changes experienced in the health care industry. Serious efforts to contain costs are moving patients out of hospitals and toward home drug delivery methodologies.

In 1986 this market reached $850 million in revenues; by 1990 we predict that revenues will reach about $2.8 billion, an astonishing 34 percent growth rate, as shown in Table 26.

Although the home infusion therapy industry is almost nine years old, the explosion in both its medical acceptance and its revenue growth began in

Table 21. Domestic IOL market (dollar share—$ in millions).

	1983	1984	1985	1986	1987	1988	Comp. Annual Growth Rate
Cilco	41	52	66	81	95	110	21.8%
Iolab	45	46	50	59	68	77	12.3
Optical Radiation	17	33	43	53	64	74	34.2
Intermedics	28	31	31	34	37	40	7.4
Amer. Med. Optics	23	28	32	38	45	51	17.3
Precision Cosmet	21	22	24	27	28	31	8.1
Ioptex	6	14	20	23	25	24	31.9
CooperVision	2	9	13	19	26	35	77.3
STAAR Surgical	0	1	7	15	28	41	NM
Surgidev	12	6	4	2	1	0	NM
Medical Workshop	0	1	2	4	6	8	NM
Coburn	6	4	4	4	3	2	NM
Others	6	3	4	3	3	3	NM
Total	207	250	302	364	429	496	19.1
Yr/Yr % Change		20.8%	20.8%	20.5%	17.8%	15.6%	
Percentage Share							
Cilco	19.8%	20.8%	21.9%	22.3%	22.1%	22.2%	
Iolab	21.7	18.4	17.2	16.3	15.9	15.5	
Optical Radiation	8.2	13.2	14.3	14.6	14.9	14.9	
Intermedics	13.5	12.4	10.6	9.4	8.6	8.1	
Amer. Med. Optics	11.1	11.2	10.9	10.7	10.5	10.3	
Precision Cosmet	10.1	8.8	7.9	7.4	6.5	6.3	
Ioptex	2.9	5.6	6.6	6.3	5.8	4.8	
CooperVision	1.0	3.6	4.3	5.2	6.1	7.1	
STAAR Surgical	0.0	0.4	2.3	4.1	6.5	8.3	
Surgidev	5.8	2.4	1.3	0.6	0.2	0.0	
Medical Workshop	0.0	0.4	0.7	1.1	1.4	1.6	
Coburn	2.9	1.6	1.3	1.1	0.7	0.4	
Others	2.9	1.2	2.3	0.8	0.7	0.6	
Total	100.0%	100.0%	100.0%	100.0%	100.0%	100.0%	

1983. In that year, the industry generated an estimated $265 million in revenues; today, revenues have more than tripled to an estimated $868 million. Strong growth in the industry has been propelled by four significant factors: (a) changes in the economic environment for health care delivery, (b) more disease states becoming treatable by home infusion therapy, (c) growth in Medicare reimbursement revenues, and (d) the entrance of entrepreneurial companies into a former cottage industry. We discuss each of these factors briefly below.

First, changes in the economic structure of health care delivery have been instrumental in setting the stage for explosive revenue growth. The factor with probably the strongest impact on the economics of health care delivery was the implementation of DRGs by the Medicare administration in the fall of 1983. This new federal prospective payment system, which preestablished reimbursement payments by individual procedure, collided with corporate America's response to rising health care costs in the form of higher deductions and copayments. As a result of the combined impact of these two forces, health care delivery changed from a system that seldom considered the cost of treatment to one that is tracking expenses carefully. New financial incentives—infusion therapy is 50 to 60 percent cheaper delivered in the home—began to force patients out of the hospital sooner than they would have left in the past. This movement of patients

Table 22. Potential continuous drug therapy market (U.S.).

Clinical Indication	Drug	Patient Population
Hypertension	Antihypertensives	35,000,000
Alcoholism	Antabuse	10,000,000
Thrombosis	Heparin	5,500,000
Epilepsy	Dilantin	2,000,000
Intractable pain	Analgesics	1,750,000
Ulcerative colitis	Azulfidine	1,250,000
Diabetes (insulin-dependent)	Insulin	1,000,000
Cancer	Chemotherapy	1,000,000

Table 23. Potential markets worldwide for nasally delivered products.

Pharmaceutical Product	1986 Sales ($ millions)
Insulin	456
Progesterone	100
Metoclopramide	75
Propranolol (for migraine)	40
Vitamin B$_{12}$	162
Antihistamines	307
Antiobesity	245
Narcotic analgesics	513

away from the hospital has been crucial to the recent high revenue levels being experienced by almost all home infusion therapy providers.

The second element contributing to the growth of the industry is the increasing number of disease states being treated with home infusion therapy, a list that is growing for two related reasons: financial incentives coupled with increased awareness among physicians. The most conspicuous of the therapies now being delivered in the home are antibiotic treatments for nosocomial infections (infections acquired in the hospital) and total parenteral nutrition (TPN) for ovarian and breast cancers, but these are just the beginning. Over time, more and more patients will be identified as appropriate for home drug delivery treatment plans as the medical community increases its understanding of disease states. In particular, the for-profit home infusion therapy companies increasingly will work with academic medical hospitals to develop drug deliveries that reach untapped markets. Expanding indications for home drug delivery have been an important component of recent revenue growth for the industry, and

will probably be an even stronger component in future revenue growth.

The third factor contributing to recent growth in the home infusion therapy market is the increase in Medicare revenues available for home treatments. It is estimated that 1984 Medicare reimbursement contributed 50 percent of the total revenues generated by providers of parenteral nutrition and enteral nutrition (EN). Today, in spite of a decreased proportional contribution from Medicare to these therapies—an estimated 30 percent to the TPN revenue base and an estimated 40 percent to the EN revenue base—the total Medicare contribution in terms of dollars has increased from 1984's $120 million to 1986's $220 million. This increase reflects mainly an increase in the number of patients receiving TPN and EN therapies; Medicare's reimbursement schedule has not changed over the past few years.

Finally, over the past few years the home infusion therapy industry has been changing from a fragmented cottage industry to one serviced by small, aggressive entrepreneurial companies, the majority of which were funded by venture capitalists in the early 1980s. Before the advent of these ventures, only a few companies were actively pursuing the home infusion market, and most TPN patients were serviced either by hospitals' in-house pharmacies or by mom-and-pop operations. In 1986, entrepreneurial companies with sales of less than $10 million per year claimed about 40 percent of the industrywide $868 million in estimated revenues. The other 60 percent of the industry's revenues came mainly from hospital-based programs and from mom-and-pop operations. However, these small concerns cannot provide care for critically ill patients that need more complex treatment plans, nor can they enjoy the economies of scale of a larger company.

The industry that once provided infused nutrients

Table 24. Controlled drug delivery formulations.

Name	Drug	Uses	Developer
Accutrim	Phenylpropanolamine	Oral dose for long lasting appetite suppression	Alza
Gradumet	Ferrous Sulfate	Oral delivery of iron in anemic patients	Abbott
Lacrisert	Hydroxypropyl Cellulose	Stabilization of corneal tear film	Merck
Modas	Indomethacin	Oral dosage for arthritis, pain relief and gout	Elan
NitroDisc	Nitroglycerine	Transdermal dosage for angina pectoris	Searle
Nitro Dur I and II	Nitroglycerine	Transdermal dosage for angina pectoris	Key
Norplant	Levonorgestrel	5 year anti-contraceptive	Endocon
Ocusert	Pilocarpine	Ocular system for glaucoma	Alza
Oros	Indomethacin	Arthritis, gout, pain relief	Alza
PennKinetic	Dextromethorphan	12 hour antihistaminic	Pennwalt
Progestasert	Progesterone	Intrauterine contraceptive	Alza
Slow K	Potassium	K$^+$ deficiency from diuretics, cortisone drugs or digitalis	Ciba Geigy
Soluprin	Aspirin	Instantly dissolving aspirin	Pharma Control
Synchron	Nitroglycerin	Transdermal dosage for angina	Forest
Tetracycline Hollow Fibers	Tetracycline	Periodontal disease	Alza
Theo Dur	Theophylline	Bronchial Asthma	Key
Transderm Nitro	Nitroglycerine	Transdermal dosage for angina	Ciba Geigy (Alza)
Transderm Scop	Scopolamine	Transdermal system for motion sickness	Alza

and antibiotics to patients in the home is fast expanding to become a home drug delivery industry. The outlines of the newer market are just beginning to take shape. Over the next four years, the home drug delivery industry could easily grow to $2.8 billion in revenues because the hospital's inpatient infusion market will be eroded at an accelerated rate, especially in antibiotic infusion therapy; new markets as well as more treatable disease states will open up; and, finally, managed care and the continuing rise of the self-insured market will change the way a patient is routed through the medical delivery system. All three of these market forces are interrelated to each other.

Hospitals' Inpatient Market Erosion

The most dramatic growth in the home infusion therapy industry is expected to occur in the antibiotic/anti-infection drug market segment. In 1986, approximately 29,000 patients received infused antibiotics in the home rather than in the hospital, and this figure could grow to a staggering 189,000 by 1990. We base these estimates not only on an increased percentage of patients being treated in the home instead of the hospital, but on the anticipated rapid growth of the progressively debilitating and thus-far fatal disease, AIDS.

Improved technology will be a significant driving force in the home antibiotic market because new pump technologies will allow more patients to be discharged from the hospital for treatment in the home. Currently, almost all antibiotic infusion therapy is delivered with gravity. New pump technologies will stop runaways, administer the antibiotics at more accurate rates and doses, and allow the patient to be ambulatory.

Currently, a patient receiving home infusion therapy is usually referred to a home infusion provider by either a hospital discharge planner or a physician. Physicians route approximately 70 percent of all the patients referred to the home infusion market. The hospital discharge planner controls approximately 20 percent of the market, and the prepaid health care insurer directs the remaining 5 to 10 percent of home therapy patients. In particular, private insurers and self-insured employers are becoming more experienced in managing critically ill patients, and soon the hospital discharge planner will no longer control the exit patterns of these individuals. Instead, insurers will assume more control over patient discharges based on hospital days and costs, which are easy to monitor.

Therapies Delivered in the Home

Total Parenteral Nutrition Therapy

Patients unable to ingest or digest food via their gastrointestinal tract are sustained by an intravenous

Table 25. Suppliers of enteral feeding products.

Company	Pumps	Feeding Tubes	Bags, Nutritional Fluids
Biosearch	X	X	X
Chesebrough Pond's	X	*	*
Corpak (Thermedics)	X	X	*
IVAC	X	X	X
Ross (Abbott)	*	*	X
Baxter Travenol	X	X	X

Key: X = manufactures
     * = distributes

therapy known as total parenteral nutrition, or TPN. In this therapy, a host of life-sustaining nutrients is supplied to the patient via a catheter that delivers the fluids directly into the bloodstream. These nutrients are generally infused over an eight- to ten-hour period on a daily basis. Since 1984 more patients have become appropriate for treatment in the home. These include patients with breast cancer, ovarian cancer, Crohn's disease, and Hirschprung's disease.

Approximately 7,441 patients received TPN in the home in 1986, generating $532 million in revenues. Although the cost savings of treating a TPN patient in the home versus the hospital is considerable (50 to 60 percent), home TPN therapy is very expensive: we estimate that a private patient pays $70,000 per year for it. Based on revenues, Medicare represents an estimated 30 percent of the total TPN market, with the government paying approximately $60,000 per year for each Medicare recipient treated with TPN.

Enteral Nutrition Therapy

Enteral nutrition therapy provides nutrients to patients who cannot eat either because of an obstruction to the gastrointestinal tract or because they simply are unable to feed themselves. Most commonly, nutritional formulas are tube-fed to the patient through the nose. This type of therapy does not bypass the gastrointestinal tract, as does TPN therapy, but delivers nutrients directly into the stomach or small intestine.

In 1986, 11,572 patients were treated with enteral therapy in the home, contributing approximately $154 million to the home infusion therapy market. These estimates are based on an annual cost per treatment of $11,439 for a private patient and $5,223 for a Medicare patient.

Growth in the enteral therapy market has been steady, in part, we believe, because it is gaining market share from the parenteral patient base. In some cases, EN is as effective as TPN when the gastrointestinal tract allows complete absorption of nutrients. Enteral therapy is less than 20 percent the cost of parenteral therapy and is a simpler, lower-risk technique. In today's cost-saving environment, enteral

Table 26. Home drug delivery market.

	No. of Patients Discharged or Diagnosed with the Disease	1986				
		Est. No. of Patients Treated in Home	% Patients Discharged from Hosp. to Home	Medicare ($ mil)	Private Pay ($ mil)	Annual Market ($ mil)
Total Parenteral Nutrition						
Abdominal cancer	300,000	1,200	0.4	24.8	58.8	83.6
Colitis	48,000	1,214	2.5	25.0	59.5	84.5
Short bowel and ischemic syndromes	37,000	851	2.3	19.8	41.7	61.5
Malabsorption syndrome	9,000	180	2.0	3.4	8.8	12.3
Breast cancer	231,000	820	0.4	19.3	40.2	59.5
Ovarian cancer	98,000	980	1.0	21.8	48.5	70.3
Hirschsprung's disease	5,000	250	5.0	0	17.5	17.5
Crohn's disease	25,000	625	2.5	19.4	30.6	50.0
AIDS	26,000	200	0.8	0	14.0	14.0
Others	35,000	1,120	3.2	28.8	49.7	78.5
Total	814,000	7,441	0.9	162.2	369.4	531.6
Enteral Nutrition						
Head and neck cancer	42,000	1,491	3.6	10.9	11.9	22.9
Abdominal and esophageal cancer	314,000	3,737	1.2	14.5	29.9	44.4
Esophageal stricture	41,000	1,472	3.6	10.9	11.8	22.7
Central nervous system disease	405,000	2,714	0.7	12.9	21.7	34.6
Others	84,000	2,159	2.6	12.0	17.3	29.3
Total	886,000	11,572	1.3	61.1	92.7	153.8
Antibiotic/anti-infective						
Osteomyelitis	93,000	10,137	10.9	—	40.6	40.6
Pyelonephritis/urinary tract infection	53,000	1,113	2.1	—	4.5	4.5
Cystic fibrosis	19,000	950	5.0	—	3.8	3.8
Septic arthritis	12,000	1,104	9.2	—	4.4	4.4
Endocarditis	19,000	1,653	8.7	—	6.6	6.6
Pelvic inflammation	93,000	558	0.6	—	2.2	2.2
Respiratory infections	97,000	582	0.6	—	2.3	2.3
Cellulitis	257,000	5,783	2.3	—	23.1	23.1
Septicemia	159,000	159	0.1	—	63.6	63.6
Nosocomial infections	612,000	5,943	1.0	—	23.8	23.6
AIDS	26,000	1,001	3.9	—	10.0	10.0
Total	828,000	28,983	3.5	—	121.9	121.9
Pain Management						
Terminally ill cancer patients	472,000	1,982	0.4	—	10.1	10.1
Cancer Chemotherapy	1,402,000	8,005	0.6	—	32.0	32.0
Congestive Heart Failure	200,000	50	0.0	—	1.4	1.4
Biotechnology						
Interleukin-2						0
Tissue plasminogen activator						0
Atrial natriuretic factor						0
Human growth hormone						60,000
Total						60,000
Total home drug delivery market	5,214,000	58,033	1.3	223.4	627.5	868.0

Table 26. (continued).

	No. of Patients Discharged or Diagnosed with the Disease	1990E				
		Est. No. of Patients Treated in Home	% Patients Discharged from Hosp. to Home	Medicare ($ mil)	Private Pay ($ mil)	Annual Market ($ mil)
Total Parenteral Nutrition						
Abdominal cancer	300,000	1,800	0.6	332.1	88.2	120.3
Colitis	48,000	1,762	3.7	31.5	86.3	117.9
Short bowel and ischemic syndromes	37,000	1,055	2.9	21.4	51.7	73.0
Malabsorption syndrome	9,000	198	2.2	9.0	9.7	18.7
Breast cancer	231,000	1,155	0.5	22.8	56.6	79.4
Ovarian cancer	98,000	1,274	1.3	24.5	62.4	86.9
Hirschsprung's disease	5,000	500	10.0	0	35.0	35.0
Crohn's disease	25,000	700	2.8	16.2	34.3	50.6
AIDS	26,000	3,500	2.3	0	245.0	245.0
Others	35,000	1,645	4.7	29.9	80.6	110.5
Total	814,000	13,588	4.5	188.0	749.8	937.3
Enteral Nutrition						
Head and neck cancer	42,000	4,032	9.6	21.6	32.3	53.9
Abdominal and esophageal cancer	314,000	4,710	1.5	22.7	37.7	60.4
Esophageal stricture	41,000	3,239	7.9	20.4	25.9	46.3
Central nervous system disease	405,000	4,455	1.1	22.3	35.7	57.9
Others	84,000	3,864	4.6	21.4	30.9	52.3
Total	886,000	20,300	2.3	108.4	162.6	270.9
Antibiotic/anti-infective						
Osteomyelitis	93,000	37,200	40.0	—	148.8	148.8
Pyelonephritis/urinary tract infection	53,000	10,600	20.0	—	42.4	42.4
Cystic fibrosis	19,000	5,700	30.0	—	22.8	22.8
Septic arthritis	12,000	3,600	30.0	—	14.4	14.4
Endocarditis	19,000	3,800	20.0	—	15.2	15.2
Pelvic inflammation	93,000	13,950	15.0	—	55.8	55.8
Respiratory infections	97,000	24,250	25.0	—	97.0	97.0
Cellulitis	257,000	28,527	11.1	—	114.1	114.1
Septicemia	159,000	1,590	1.0	—	6.4	6.4
Nosocomial infections	612,000	15,000	2.5	—	60.0	60.0
AIDS	26,000	45,000	60.0	—	675.0	675.0
Total	828,000	189,217		—	1,251.7	1,251.9
Pain Management						
Terminally ill cancer patients	472,000	23,600	5.0	—	120.4	120.4
Cancer Chemotherapy	1,402,000	12,001	0.9	—	48.0	48.0
Congestive Heart Failure	200,000	2,000	0.5	—	55.0	55.0
Biotechnology						
Interleukin-2						100.0
Tissue plasminogen activator						800.0
Atrial natriuretic factor						130.0
Human growth hormone						300.0
Total						1,330.0
Total home drug delivery market	5,214,000	260,706	5.7	295.8	2,387.6	2,816.0

therapy has become and will continue to be the modality of choice whenever possible.

Antibiotic/Anti-Infective Therapies

Antibiotic infusion therapy was developed to treat stubborn infections because, when antibiotics are infused directly into the bloodstream, they are at least six times more effective than when orally ingested. In addition, intravenous antibiotics are used to treat infections in the areas of the body that do not receive an abundant blood supply. Anti-infective drugs are chemically derived and have been used for the treatment of AIDS patients. The length of treatment for both therapies in the home is generally six to eight weeks, at an average cost of $4,000 per treatment.

The IV antibiotic therapy market is the fastest growing segment of the home drug delivery market. Revenues generated by this market are expected to grow from $122 million today to $1.3 billion in 1990. In particular, this growth will be driven by the increasing number of AIDS patients treated in the home. More generally, however, physicians are detecting infections more readily and are becoming more educated about the comfort and convenience of treating a number of disease states in the home.

Osteomyelitis, an infection resulting in inflammation of the bone, is one of the first disease states to be treated in the home. Once stabilized in the hospital, patients with this infection are ideal candidates for home care. Although osteomyelitis is difficult to diagnose, over the past several years there has been a 21 percent increase in patients discharged from the hospital with this disease. We believe that physicians' growing ability to diagnose this disease accounts for the increase, which reflects a larger patient base. Osteomyelitis has taught physicians that infections can safely be treated in the home. We believe we will see the same pattern of treatment growth for other such disease states.

Anti-Infective Drugs and TPN for AIDS Therapy

Acquired immune deficiency syndrome, or AIDS, is one of the most devastating health issues that mankind has ever faced. Not only is it spreading extremely rapidly; it is relentlessly affecting a relatively young population. AIDS has no definitive diagnostic test, no effective treatment, no vaccine, and no cure. Moreover, despite breakthroughs in isolating the cause of the disease, the development of a workable treatment and a preventative vaccine appears to be some years away. In fact, we still know relatively little about AIDS beyond that the immune system is gradually destroyed by a newly described and probably newly evolved virus. The disease is progressively debilitating, and so far it is fatal.

Because the AIDS virus compromises the immune system, its victims are vulnerable to one of several infections and malignancies. AIDS-related infections are usually recalcitrant and difficult to control with oral drugs; in these cases, delivering active pharmaceutical agents to combat infections intravenously is the treatment of choice. In addition, some AIDS patients are treated with pain analgesics and TPN therapy. These modalities, coupled with the fact that the increasing number of patients will limit the ability of hospitals to care for them, make AIDS victims appropriate candidates for home infusion therapy.

In 1985, the home anti-infective infusion market for AIDS patients generated approximately $15 million in revenues and grew to $24 million in 1986. Infusion therapy to fight infections in AIDS patients will be the fastest growing market segment of the home infusion industry, reaching an estimated $675 million by 1990. These projections are based on medical estimates of a staggering 150,000 diagnosed cases by that year. We believe that 50 percent of these cases will have enough insurance to afford therapy in the home. Of insured patients, approximately 60 percent, in our opinion, will have three to four home infusion treatments—one six-week treatment costs approximately $4,000—at an average of $15,000 per year by 1990.

Revenue growth in the fast-growing home anti-infective infusion market will be driven by incredible growth in the AIDS patient base. In addition, insurers will be attracted by the cost savings and the improved quality of care that home drug delivery brings to the AIDS patient. Most companies servicing this market are still in the learning stages and will increase market revenues through volume, not pricing. In fact, the cost of the service will increase only slightly over the next few years.

Despite the current trend toward moving patients into the home for TPN treatment, the home TPN market will slow to a 15 percent growth rate from its historic rate of 46 percent in 1983 to 1986 for two reasons: (a) the length of time required by this treatment is decreasing, and (b) hospitals are treating fewer TPN patients in general; therefore, the home industry's penetration into the hospital base is moderate. The home enteral market will treat some patients that historically were parenteral patients because the cost of enteral therapy is almost one-fifth the cost of parenteral therapy. Also for cost reasons, insurers are more receptive to the enteral treatment plan. Both enteral and parenteral therapies will continue to penetrate the hospital inpatient market and will contribute an estimated 40 percent to the total market by 1990.

New Markets and Expanded Indications to More Disease States

As the home drug delivery companies blanket the country with service centers, new drug delivery therapies will be accepted by the industry with greater ease than TPN and EN therapies were in the early 1980s for two reasons: insurance carriers are better educated about home infusion therapy, and physicians are more accepting of alternative health care services. In addition, growing patient exposure to the cost of care and the increasing use of historical clinical data by both the public and private insurers are trends started in the early 1980s that will continue to direct the health care consumer to less costly treatment plans, in many cases with improved quality of care as a result.

By 1990, the largest of the new home infusion therapy markets are expected to deliver TPN therapy and anti-infective drugs to AIDS patients. This growth will be driven by the base number of patients, by improved home drug delivery devices, and by the fact that AIDS patients increasingly will be privately insured. The second largest new market will probably be the delivery of biotechnology products, which will find their way into the home infusion system because they call for precision doses delivered at accurate rates. Another significant new market, pain management, could grow out of recently developed new pump devices that may radically increase the number of patients receiving pain analgesics. And finally, two classes of drugs in advanced clinical trials, enkephalins for pain management and prostaglandins for protection against ulcers, are appropriate for home infusion therapy.

By 1990, infusion therapy should treat disease states that are not currently being served or that have just begun to be treated in the home today. For example, dobutamine home infusion for the management of congestive heart failure could reach an annual market value of $50 to 100 million by 1990. Pain management could reach an annual market value of $120 million by 1990, affecting 23,600 sufferers. Finally, nosocomial infections could be treated more frequently in the home.

The Rise of Managed Care

Managed care—the routing of a patient through a cost-effective and high-quality treatment plan—is just beginning to take hold in the health insurance delivery market. Private insurers have discovered that they have a wealth of historical information about their insurees in the medical claims they have already paid. Although currently these databases are somewhat crude, we believe that in the near term improved individual tracking procedures, both retrospective and concurrent, will allow private insurers to exert a stronger influence on the course of a patient's health care treatment. As this trend in patient charting develops, several elements will change the way patients are referred to home treatment: (a) the rapidly growing self-insured market will begin to target and track its critically ill employees and become a patient router in addition to a referral source, thereby weakening the referral power of the hospital and physician, and (b) capitated Medicare programs will begin to reimburse for home antibiotic infusion therapy.

Pain Management

Pain management is an emerging therapy that is being nourished by improved infusion pumps, by increasing interest in the technique, and, most important, by the issue of quality of life for the terminally ill patient. Infusion pumps currently in clinical trials combine the technologies of chemotherapy pumps and patient-controlled analgesic pumps, which enable patients previously incapacitated by pain to lead more comfortable lives in their terminal condition. These pumps could allow pain management for the terminally ill to become a very acceptable treatment modality.

Both cancer patients and patients with chronic pain are candidates for pain management therapies. Approximately 2,000 of these patients were treated in the home in 1986. Assuming a 30-day treatment plan at $170 per day, today's pain management market is estimated to be $10 million. If technology develops this therapy it is possible that 23,000 people could be treated in the home, generating $120 million in revenues by 1990.

Cancer Chemotherapy

Many see the physician as the barrier to treating chemotherapy in the home setting. Oncologists depend on chemotherapy for 65 percent of their revenues and as a result are very protective of this revenue stream. Although home drug delivery companies currently administer this therapy in the home, it is not a sizable market. However, some home infusion companies believe that opportunity exists in mixing toxic chemotherapy drugs for physicians.

Chemotherapy is administered in two ways: by intermittent bolus, which is a series of direct, periodic injections, and by continuous infusion. Only 10 percent of all chemotherapy patients receive continuous infusions. There is evidence that continuous infusion results in reduced side effects; however, there is no evidence of improved clinical results. Until this debate is settled, chemotherapy should not be a significant contributor to the home drug delivery market.

Drug Infusion for Congestive Heart Failure

Congestive heart failure is deterioration of the heart muscle and is a terminal disease. Treating congestive heart failure in the home, a methodology in its infancy, is a controversial issue among cardiologists, who differ in their opinions of its efficacy and appropriateness. Currently, oral drugs are used to treat congestive heart failure patients; however, when their condition becomes refractory, they must be hospitalized for stabilization. Dobutamine is the drug of choice for the condition and is infused on a short-term basis in the hospital; additional infusions are usually required within one to three months. This process continues until the patient dies.

The controversy surrounding caring for congestive heart patients in the home is twofold. The first issue concerns the effectiveness of dobutamine. Dobutamine has been used on a short-term basis because over the long term it loses its effectiveness. However, recent studies show that when the drug is infused on an intermittent basis, the patient is more responsive to the drug, and several home infusion therapy companies are successfully using this technique. The second issue reflects the fact that patients suffering from congestive heart failure suffer from a life-threatening condition. Some physicians feel that these patients are too seriously ill to be released from the hospital under any circumstances.

Treating congestive heart failure with dobutamine is an example of the way research and development can create a new infusion market. Other markets for home drug delivery could be identified in the same manner.

THE UROGENITAL MARKET

In this section we discuss two urogenital treatment modalities which depend on the use of biomaterials: penile implants and urinary incontinence.

Penile Implants

Epidemiological studies indicate that impotence afflicts 8 to 15 percent of adult males (particularly diabetic men), increasing with age from 21 percent of 60-year-olds to 55 percent at age 75. Besides diabetes, the most common causes appear to be endocrine imbalances, excessive alcohol intake and certain drugs. Almost 8 percent of the top 200 prescription drugs in the U.S. have been directly implicated in impotence cases, and may account for 20 percent of all reported cases.

In 1986 approximately 25,000 penile prostheses were surgically implanted, generating $43 million in revenues. Penile prostheses are available in a variety of types, as shown in Table 27.

Urinary Incontinence

Urinary incontinence is an embarrassing, potentially disabling, and costly health problem. Defined as an involuntary loss of urine sufficient in quantity and/or frequency to be a social or health problem, this condition disrupts the lives of 5 to 10 million Americans, their families, friends, and caregivers. The severity of incontinence ranges from occasional dribbling to total loss of control over excretory functions with incontinence of both urine and stool. It has adverse effects on physical health, psychological well-being, social functioning, and the cost of health care. When inadequately or inappropriately managed, it can lead to skin breakdown and recurrent urinary infections. Incontinent individuals often withdraw from their usual social activities and may subsequently become isolated and depressed. Because it is difficult for affected individuals and their families to manage at home, incontinence often plays a pivotal role in an individual's decision to enter a long-term care institution.

Despite the availability of many effective forms of treatment, incontinent persons are rarely evaluated thoroughly to determine the precise causes of the condition and are therefore often not treated optimally. This deficiency in the care of incontinent persons results from a number of factors, including:

- lack of knowledge on the part of health-care professionals about the underlying causes of incontinence, appropriate methods of diagnostic evaluation, and treatment options available (in some instances, health-care professionals even consider incontinence a normal condition in elderly patients and therefore do not evaluate or attempt to treat it)
- reluctance on the part of affected individuals to discuss the problem with a health-care professional because of embarrassment and the misconception that it cannot be treated
- the relatively small number of experts (urologists, gynecologists, neurologists, geriatricians, nurse clinicians, etc.) available to treat these patients, train other health-care professionals, and carry out well-designed research on the management of this important health problem

Table 27. Types of penile prostheses (1986).

Type	Number Implanted	Percent	Leading Manufacturers
Inflatable	7800	31	American Medical Systems Mentor
Malleable	7280	29	American Medical Systems Mentor, Medical Eng.
Self-Contained	7280	29	American Medical Systems Medical Eng.
Rigid Rod	2080	8	Mentor C. R. Bard
Mechanical	560	2	Dacomed

Prevalence of Incontinence

Because little accurate data on the extent of urinary incontinence have been consistently maintained, estimates of its prevalence and change over time are difficult to make. Current data indicate that risk of urinary incontinence is strongly associated with age. From 10 to 20 percent of the community-dwelling elderly, whose median age is 72, are incontinent to some degree. But approximately 50 percent of all elderly persons in nursing homes, whose median age is 83, are incontinent. Not only is the prevalence much greater among the latter group, but the type of incontinence is also likely to be more severe. Although these population subgroups are not directly comparable, the differences in prevalence indicate the increased risk of urinary incontinence for persons 65 to 74 and 85 and over. Risk of institutionalization is increased because of urinary incontinence. Thus, the very old (persons 85 and over) are most likely to suffer from incontinence and to be at risk of institutionalization.

Types and Causes

Incontinence can be classified into several types, which have clinical and therapeutic differences. Acute incontinence refers to the sudden onset of episodes of involuntary loss of urine; it is usually associated with an acute illness or environmental factors that impair the mental or physical ability of the patient to reach a toilet or toilet substitute in time.

Established or persistent incontinence (i.e., repeated episodes of involuntary loss of urine not associated with an acute condition) can be divided into four types. Stress incontinence implies leakage of urine, either in small or large amounts, as intra-abdominal pressure increases. Urge incontinence involves leakage of varying amounts of urine because of the inability to delay voiding long enough to reach a toilet or toilet substitute; it can be caused by a variety of genitourinary and neurologic disorders. Overflow incontinence is caused by anatomic obstruction to bladder emptying and/or inability of the bladder to contract, with subsequent leakage of small amounts of urine. Functional incontinence occurs in those individuals who have chronic impairments of either mobility or mental function, are unable to toilet themselves independently and do not have sufficient help with this task, or who, because of psychological disturbances, are unwilling to maintain continence. Table 28 summarizes the types, causes and populations affected by incontinence.

Treatments for Incontinence

Devices for incontinence can be divided into those that attempt to prevent or delay urine flow and those that collect urine before or after it leaves the bladder. Devices such as the pessary, a donut-shaped piece of inert material inserted into the vagina to support the bladder outlet in women with stress incontinence, and the external penile clamp are used relatively infrequently at the present time. Newer techniques such as the artificial sphincter, which is an inflatable cuff surgically implanted around the urethra, and electrical stimulators, which contract muscles of the pelvic floor in stress incontinence and inhibit bladder contraction in urge incontinence, have been used increasingly over the last 10 to 15 years.

Catheters are commonly used to manage incontinence, despite the well-known risks (e.g., infection) associated with their use. Probably the most actively marketed products used to manage incontinence are undergarments and bedpads. In general, these products are designed with a layer of highly absorbent material sandwiched between layers designed to keep the patient and the bed or clothing dry. A wide variety of techniques, which we have labeled training procedures, have also been described in the management of incontinence. These training procedures have been categorized into five basic techniques: pelvic floor (Kegel) exercises, biofeedback, bladder retraining, habit training, and behavioral modification.

The treatment options currently available for urinary incontinence are summarized in Figure 4.

Costs of Incontinence

If one assumes that there are approximately 600,000 nursing home patients with some degree of urinary incontinence and that in three-quarters of these patients the incontinence is sufficiently severe that catheters or other specific management techniques are used, the yearly costs of incontinence in U.S. nursing homes can be estimated at between $0.5 and $1.5 billion (first-order costs only). This cost range represents between 3 and 8 percent of the total expenditure on nursing home care in this country. The costs of incontinence in the community are much more difficult to estimate. No studies have addressed these costs in any detail. Table 29 presents the current costs of treatment in the U.S.

Ostomy Devices

An artificial stoma, or opening, into the gastrointestinal tract is called an ostomy. An ostomy device generally consists of a bag attached to the skin by an adhesive material, intended for use as a receptacle for the collection of urine or feces following an ileostomy, colostomy or ureterostomy operation.

Ostomy devices and accessories include the ostomy pouch, ostomy adhesive, disposable colostomy appliance, ostomy collector, pouch, bag and ostomy size selectors.

Table 28. Types of incontinence.

Type	Definition	Causes	Population(s) Affected
Acute	Incontinence of sudden onset associated with an acute illness (and/or other factors) that subsides once the acute condition has been resolved or other factors have been removed	Acute illnesses associated with one or more of the following: (a) immobility and/or environmental factors that diminish the ability to get to and use a toilet; (b) impaired mental function that diminishes toileting ability; (c) fecal impaction. Acute urinary tract infections Drugs: (a) those that increase urine flow (e.g., diuretics); (b) those that inhibit bladder contractions and cause urinary retention and overflow (e.g., anticholinergics); (c) those that decrease mental awareness (e.g., sedatives, hypnotics) Metabolic—increased urine flow (polyuria) associated with poorly controlled diabetes	Elderly, usually in acute hospitals
Established *			
Stress	Leakage of small amounts of urine with increases of intraabdominal pressure (e.g., coughing, sneezing, laughing, exercise)	Weakened supporting tissue surrounding bladder outlet and urethra associated with: (a) lack of estrogen in postmenopausal women; (b) previous vaginal deliveries; (c) previous pelvic surgery (e.g., hysterectomy)	Women, especially those over age 40
Urge	Leakage of urine caused by inability to delay voiding long enough to reach the toilet after urge to void is felt	Neurological diseases such as stroke, dementia, Parkinsonism, multiple sclerosis, spinal cord diseases Genitourinary disorders such as unstable bladder ("detrusor instability"), bladder stones, diverticuli of urethra and bladder, atrophic urethritis, vaginitis (females), chronic cystitis, mild outflow obstruction (usually males)	Men and women of any age; most common in the elderly
Overflow	Leakage of small amounts of urine associated with obstruction to urine flow	Hypotonic or acontractile bladder associated with diabetic neuropathy; spinal cord injury; or drugs such as anticholinergics (which inhibit bladder contractions), smooth muscle relaxants, narcotics, and alcohol Anatomic obstruction associated with prostatic enlargement of urethral stricture	Older men with prostatic enlargement Diabetics
Functional	Inability or unwillingness to reach a toilet in time	Impaired mobility Impaired mental function Inaccessible toilets (or caregivers) Psychological disorders such as depression, psychosis, anger, or hostility	Elderly in acute hospitals and nursing homes and those with acute or severe psychiatric illness

*Incontinence is persistent and unrelated to an acute illness.

Table 29. Incontinence treatment costs (1986).

Treatment	Cost ($ thousands)
Artificial Sphincters	4000
Silicone gel prostheses	3900
Disposable pads	2700
Indwelling catheter	2000
Periurethral Teflon injection	1500

Table 30. U.S. usage of ostomy devices.

Device	1985 (millions)	1986 (millions)	1986 Retail Price ($)
Colostomy caps	24	15	1.00
Colostomy pouches	24	15	1.40
Colostomy bags	65	40	2.50
Ileostomy bags	50	30	2.00
Urostomy bags	25	15	2.50

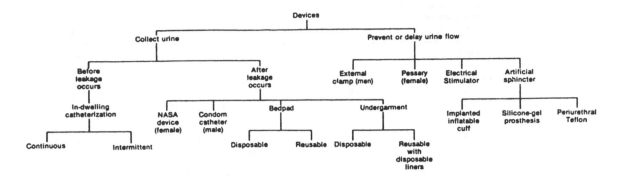

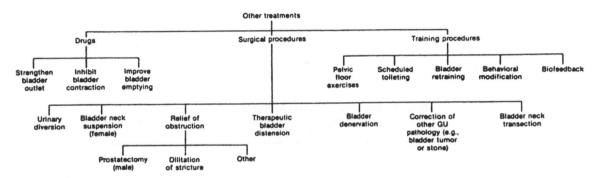

Figure 4. Treatment options for urinary incontinence.

New surgical procedures, new synthetic sphincter valves, and improved appliance are significantly lowering the usage of ostomy devices as shown in Table 30.

THE HEMODIALYSIS MARKET

The kidneys are vital organs traditionally associated with the excretion of waste products. These paired complex organs, lying along the first through third lumbar vertebrae and weighing only 150 grams each, have numerous other functions. They are primarily concerned with maintaining volume and composition of body fluids, regulation of blood pressure and maintenance of red blood cells.

The kidneys are divided into functional units termed nephrons, with over 1 million nephrons per kidney. Whenever the kidneys chronically fail in their function (as a result of nephron-associated disease), the patient is said to be in end-stage kidney disease. End-stage renal disease (ESRD), a terminal condition, is currently treated through artificial hemodialysis and/or kidney transplantation. Hemodialyses are techniques designed to purify the blood when the kidneys are incapable of performing their normal function.

There are four basic principles for blood purification therapies: dialysis, ultrafiltration, adsorption, and exchange. Eight treatment modalities are available as an outgrowth of these basic principles: inter-

mittent peritoneal dialysis (IPD), continuous ambulatory peritoneal dialysis (CAPD), hemodialysis (HD), hemofiltration (HF), hemodiafiltration (HDF), direct hemoadsorption (DHA), plasma exchange (PE), and combined uses of hemodialyzers (HDA) or hemofiltration with hemoadsorption (HFA). Materials or methods used for each treatment along with short comments on their advantages and disadvantages are summarized in Table 31.

For each treatment it is necessary to circulate the blood extracorporeally or else to infuse dialysate fluid into the peritoneal cavity. If we group the components of devices from a functional viewpoint, the dialyzers, filters, and sorbents are the essential parts.

Dialyzers: Dialyzers can be grouped into three groups based on their difference in membrane assembly. They are called coil, plate, and hollow fiber types.

In the coil type, wide tubular membranes are wound together with plastic mesh to make a coil that is placed in a plastic case so as to prevent overexpansion. As for the plate type, membranes and grooved plastic plates are laminated in alternate layers similar to a sandwich. The hollow fiber type is a newly developed configuration that uses hollow fiber membranes with inner diameters from 200 to 300 microns.

Approximately 10,000 fibers, 250 mm in length, are necessary to provide 1.5 square meters of surface; that is, an area sufficient to treat an adult patient. Every dialyzer type has the dialysate channels placed external to the membrane assembly.

Table 31. Principles and therapeutic modalities of blood purification.

Principles	Materials or Methods Used	Therapeutic Modalities	Advantages	Disadvantages
Dialysis	Peritoneum	IPD	Long experience	Peritonitis
		CAPD	Homeostasis	Peritonitis
	Semipermeable membrane	HD	Long experience	
		HDF	Efficient for SMS* and MMS** short time dialysis	Limited experience
Ultrafiltration	Ultrafiltration	HF	Efficient for MMS removal	Limited experience
Adsorption	Activated charcoal ion exchange resins Nonionic resins	HF + HP	Selective removal	Limited experience
		HP	Selective removal	No water and electrolytes removal
Exchange	Centrifugal separation membrane	PP or PE	Effective removal for protein conjugated substances	Plasma for substitution necessary

*SMS = small molecular substance.
**MMS = middle molecular substance.

Table 32. Membranes used for blood purification.

Purpose	Materials	Molecular Structure
Dialysis	Regenerated cellulose	
	Cellulose diacetate	
	Cellulose triacetate	
Filtration	Polyacrylonitrile	
	Polymethyl methacrylate	
	Polyethersulfone	
	Ethylene-Vinyl alcohol copolymer	
	Carbonate-Ethylene Oxide Copolymer	
	Polyamide	
Sorbent Microcapsulation	Collodion/albumin	See above
	Regenerated cellulose	
	Polyhydroxyethylmethacrylate	
	Nitrocellulose (collodion)	
Plasmapheresis	Cellulose acetate	See above
	Polyvinyl alcohol	

Table 33. Total deaths related to kidney-urinary tract diseases in the U.S. (1986).

Diagnosis	Number of Deaths
Nephritis and nephrosis	14,500
Infections of the kidney	13,500
Malignant neoplasms	26,100
Hypertensive heart and kidney disease	10,700
Hypertensive renal disease	9,400
Other renal disease	5,300
Other diseases of urinary tract	3,500
Congenital anomalies of urinary system (over ½ of deaths are caused by cystic disease of the kidney)	2,000
Total	85,000

Filters and Separators: Filters for hemofiltration have an appearance and structure similar to hollow fiber or plate dialyzers. Separation membranes used for cell separation are incorporated into a unit similar to a hollow fiber dialyzer, although the pore size and surface area are different.

Sorbent Columns: A majority of sorbent columns commercially available are filled with activated charcoal granules derived from petroleum or shells of coconuts. The granules are encapsulated by blood compatible semipermeable membranes, for example, polyhydroxyethylmethacrylate (Poly HEMA) or cellulose nitrate. The total amount of sorbent filling is generally between 100 to 300 g depending on the proposed use. Amberlite XAD-2 (styrene divinyl benzene) and XAD-7 (acryl ester) are nonionic resins available for hemoadsorption applications. No coating is required for these resins sorbents.

From a biomaterials viewpoint, the greatest challenge arises from the need to produce membranes capable of cleansing the blood of a bewildering array of impurities. The materials found most useful in hemodialysis membranes are shown in Table 32.

End-Stage Renal Disease

End-stage renal failure is a major cause of morbidity and mortality in the U.S. and abroad. It is estimated that there are 8 million Americans suffering from diseases of the kidney and urinary tract. This figure is very large because it includes mild urinary tract related disorders, such as cystitis and urethritis that are easily treated and rarely assume life-threatening proportions. However, about 85,000 patients die annually from kidney-related disease as illustrated in Table 33, based on data collected in 1980. Today this number has been reduced to about 45,000 because of the ESRD treatment program instituted in 1973.

Normally, renal disease is chronic in nature and end-stage renal failure occurs when the disease has progressed beyond the stage when drugs or other nonmechanical maintenance approaches can help the patient.

Naturally, the ideal approach to combating renal disease is through prevention or early treatment and arrest. Early treatment of high blood pressure, for instance, could be critical in preventing renal failure caused by hypertension. About 60 million Americans suffer from hypertension, however, but only 4 to 5 million are being adequately treated. Better treatment programs should reduce the incidence of ESRD caused by hypertension. Another cause of renal failure is analgesic abuse, which can also be prevented.

Other causes of ESRD, however, are difficult to overcome. There is no method to prevent or arrest the course of glomerulonephritis, diabetic nephropathy, systemic lupus erythematosus, etc. Actually, aggressive treatment of juvenile diabetics has increased the incidence of ESRD, as these patients live longer and eventually become victims to diabetic nephropathy. The NIH spends about $150 million annually in funding research in the kidney disease area and similar amounts for diabetes and arthritis-related research.

The two major treatment options for ESRD are transplantation and dialysis. At present transplantation is a solution for a small minority of patients, but with major advances of the recent past in transplantation techniques and immunosuppressive drugs, its use may grow in the future. Nevertheless, at present the vast majority of patients undergo regular dialysis treatment, during which the patient's blood is cleansed of accumulated waste products.

In 1986, 88 percent of all dialysis patients (175,000 patients) chose a form of dialysis known as hemo-

Table 34. U.S. chronic dialysis market size (1986).

Equipment	Outpatient ($ million)	Inpatient ($ million)	Total ($ million)
Dialyzers	70	10	80
Blood tubing	30	3	33
Miscellaneous disposables	8	4	12
Totals	108.	17	125

Table 35. Patients undergoing dialysis (1986).

Location	Treatment Modality	
	Hemodialysis	CAPD
North America	64,000	9,000
Europe	65,000	4,000
Japan	44,000	1,500
All others	2,000	500
Totals	175,000	15,000

dialysis. In this modality the patient's blood is pumped from the body by a machine, subjected to dialysis, and then returned to the body in a continuous extracorporeal blood loop. Dialysis occurs as the blood passes through a dialyzer, or artificial kidney. Patients must undergo this treatment about three times per week in sessions running about 3 1/2 to 5 hours each. This can be accomplished in a hospital-based center, in a free-standing facility, or at home.

A major alternative form of dialysis, chosen by 12 percent (15,000 patients) of ESRD patients in 1983, is continuous ambulatory peritoneal dialysis (CAPD). In CAPD, dialysis occurs within the patient's body across the peritoneal membrane. CAPD requires a manual exchange of fluid every 4 to 6 hours, but it can be done at home and it frees the patient from dependency on a dialysis machine. Although patients experience some risk of developing peritonitis, the

modality has been growing in popularity. Peritonitis accounts for 60 percent of complications, followed by terminal infection at 30 percent, and catheter replacement at 10 percent.

The estimated market for chronic dialysis which utilizes biomaterials is shown in Table 34.

A summary of patients requiring dialysis is shown in Table 35.

REFERENCES

1. Lantos, P. R. 1988. "Plastics in Medical Applications", *JBA*, 2:359.
2. 1989. "Medical Uses of Plastics to Grow 6% Annually", *C&E News* (July):10.
3. Williams, J. L. 1988. "TPE Technology Unfolds a New Biomedical Market Frontier", *Elastomerics*, 120:11, p. 35.

Medical Markets for Radiation Sterilizable Plastics

JEFFREY R. ELLIS, Ph.D., MBA*

ABSTRACT: Sterilization of medical devices and products by ionizing radiation is rapidly becoming a mature technology. More healthcare product manufacturers are perceiving the savings caused by greater rapidity of processing; and Environmental Protection Agency (EPA) based restrictions on exposure to the traditional chemical sterilant, ethylene oxide, have been enough of an incentive to many other companies to switch their processing either to in-house sterilizing or to the use of outside radiation sterilizing facilities. However, as the more dilatory companies catch up regarding this technology, others are pioneering in new methods of sterilizing. Alternative chemicals—for example, chlorine dioxide—are being evaluated and other methods of sterilizing, such as plasma exposure, are being developed.

APPLICATIONS OF RADIATION STERILIZATION AND RADIOACTIVE SOURCES

Radiation sterilization in the United States is used almost exclusively for the production of medical items. While some personal care products such as baby bottle nipples and sanitary napkins are radiation-sterilized, these are at most 5–10% of the volume of devices so sterilized. The most likely future growth area for radiation sterilization is in the processing of foods. Food ingredients, especially spices, are already being irradiated at levels sufficient to kill harmful pathogens. In the future, fruits, vegetables, and meat products may also be irradiated to control infestation and ripening. Although irradiation of foods has seen only limited application in the U.S., it is used extensively in other countries.

Two types of radiation are used for sterilizing. One is a high-energy beam of electrons—a variant of beta radiation. The second is gamma radiation from a source such as Cobalt 60, generating photons which are then transformed into electrons with an even higher energy content. The electron beams obtain their energy either from a linear accelerator such as is used by Radiation Dynamics, Inc. (Edgewood, NY) or from a microwave energy acceleration as is used by Varian Associates, Inc. (Palo Alto, CA). The capital costs of putting in an electron beam sterilizing facility are almost equivalent to that of putting in a gamma sterilizing facility (c. $2 million). The costs of sites, permits, and other items not directly associated with putting up the processing facility and making certain it is properly shielded are extra.

Although both forms of radiation sterilizing are quite safe, the gamma sources are dangerous and must be handled by properly trained personnel. There is also the problem of eventually disposing of spent but still potentially harmful nucleotides. Gamma radiation does have the advantage of greater penetrating power and can be applied effectively to all types of constructions. Electron beam radiation is effective in sterilizing surfaces and thin-walled materials, but attenuation greatly diminishes the sterilizing power even after passing through a few thousandths of an inch. Companies specializing in electron beam sterilizing capability maintain, however, that such sterilization is more than adequate for thin-walled hollow constructions.

Radioactive sources, especially Cobalt 60, are also used in cancer treatment, in the sterilization of infectious and biological wastes, and occasionally to cross-link plastic and cellulosic products such as flooring materials.

Of the Cobalt 60 that is used as a gamma radiation source, over 80% is provided by Nordion International (formerly Atomic Energy of Canada Limited Radiochemical Company) of Kanata, Ontario. An additional source in the U.S. is Neutron Products (Dickerson, MD). Another gamma source isotope that is being used for radiation sterilization is Cesium 137,

---

*President, J. R. Ellis, Inc., Technical and Economic Services, 35 Teaberry Lane, Newtown, PA 18940

Table 1. Estimates of volumes of plastics radiation-sterilized for healthcare use (1988).

Table 1. Estimates of volumes of plastics radiation-sterilized for healthcare use (1988).

Plastic	Volume (millions of pounds)
Polystyrene	90
Polypropylene	52
High-density polyethylene	50
Thermoplastic polyesters	28
Acrylonitrile-butadiene-styrene copolymers (ABS)	15
Polyvinyl chloride	14
Low-density polyethylene	13
Polycarbonates	12
Acrylics	4
Others	3
Total:	279

Source: Private industry estimates.

which has been provided by U.S. Dept. of Defense and Department of Energy sources at the Hanford, Washington and Oak Ridge, Tennessee nuclear processing facilities. In practice, however, the energy obtained from the cesium nucleotide is "hotter" than that from Cobalt 60, and there have been leakage problems necessitating costly clean-ups.

SCOPE OF PLASTICS IRRADIATION

Approximately 280 million pounds of plastics are radiation-sterilized annually. Estimates of the annual volume of each plastic sterilized by ionizing radiation are given in Table 1. It is also estimated that among the six largest manufacturers of medical devices, 50–60% of such products are currently being radiation-sterilized. Most of the plastics sterilized are commodity plastics such as polystyrene and various grades of polyethylene which, because of their molecular structure, have a very high resistance to gamma radiation. Products sterilized include medical devices, laboratory apparatus, pharmaceutical containers, and protective clothing and handwear. Much of this total (c. 35%) is represented by packaging.

Companies using radiation sterilization extensively now design their new products and are changing existing product lines to be radiation-sterilized if at all possible. Not all products, however, can be radiation-sterilized. Many therapeutic formulations are degraded by ionizing radiation. Aqueous systems such as intravenous fluids and blood fraction components are susceptible to formation of hydroxyl radicals, which can cause damaging reactions. Another problem is that the FDA considers irradiated therapeutic agents to be new drugs. Consequently, the approval procedure for the product will have to be repeated. Some plastics cannot withstand ionizing radiation at levels required by healthcare industry. Therefore, other sterilization methods must be employed.

Concerns have also been raised about long-term implants such as pacemakers and pacemaker accessories. The healthcare industry currently is of the opinion that ionizing radiation might significantly decrease the useful life of these long-term use products. Thick materials such as prostheses are also of concern although gamma radiation is generally an effective penetrant. Polypropylene-based dialysis membranes, even though based on new "resistant" grades of polymer, are still degraded significantly by ionizing radiation exposures.

COMPETING STERILIZATION METHODS

Chemical Sterilization with Ethylene Oxide

Ethylene oxide (EtO) has long been the traditional method of chemical sterilization of healthcare devices and therapeutic materials. It has been safe, effective, and of reasonable cost especially regarding capital expenditures. Disadvantages of this technique are (1) the flammability of the gas, (2) the slow rate of desorption and potential chemical reactivity, and (3) the toxicity of the chemical prompting more restrictive EPA criteria of human exposure levels. The flammability problem has largely been overcome either by ensuring appropriate care and equipment in facilities using 100% EtO, or by using a blend of 12% ethylene oxide with a chlorofluorocarbon (usually CFC-12) to make a nonflammable gas mixture. However, restrictions regarding the chlorofluorocarbons traditionally used will necessitate reformulation, because of the damage done to the environment due to depletion of the upper-atmosphere ozone layer. As of now it is not known if potential substitutes are likely to be as efficient.

The slow rate of desorption of ethylene oxide and its potential chemical reactivity to form ethylene glycol under various conditions adds inventory costs to the price of medical products. Exposure to reactive chemicals must be limited and in some cases meeting residual ethylene oxide guidelines can mean having products stay in inventory for one week or more.

The most pressing reason to switch from ethylene oxide sterilization is that the EPA has placed restrictions on exposure to ethylene oxide because of suspected human oncogenicity. As a result, some of the older sterilizing facilities have been shut down, and others have been modified to meet new EPA standards. Many companies have assessed their future needs for sterilization and have decided either to use outside ionizing radiation facilities or to build their own, as analysis shows radiation processing to be more advantageous to adopt once faster throughput factors have been considered.

Steam and Dry Heat Sterilization

The other sterilization method usually involves pressurized steam at 121°C. Occasionally dry heat sterilization can also be used. Steam, however, is not suitable for plastics such as many grades of polyethylene which have melting points or glass transition temperatures well below the sterilizing processing level. Steam can also hydrolyze or degrade certain plastics. Consequently its use is limited to heat resistant plastics, or to plasticized materials especially polyvinyl chloride which are not affected significantly in their physical properties under steam exposure.

EFFECTS OF GAMMA RADIATION ON PLASTICS AND OTHER MATERIALS

Most other structural materials, namely metals, most glasses and ceramics are impervious to electron beam or gamma sterilization. Some ceramics, and most glasses will discolor, but rarely if ever will these have lower physical performance properties or different chemical properties from unirradiated materials. If discoloring in glass products is objectionable, Cerium (IV) oxides can be formulated into the glass in parts per million quantities based on the concentration of radiation sensitive ingredients such as Fe (III) and Nd (III) oxides. Plastics, however, vary markedly in their resistance. Also, it must be recognized that sterilization processability is not the only criterion for plastics selection.

Some plastics have a very high sensitivity to radiation. Fluorocarbons, which are inert to almost all chemicals, are especially vulnerable. So far, nothing has been discovered which can improve the radiation resistance of such plastics. Other plastics, such as acrylics and polycarbonates, tend to discolor, usually to an unaesthetic greenish or grayish-yellow. This discoloring is often masked by addition of a blue dye, giving the plastic a bluish-gray tint and as a result compromising the clarity of these particular plastics. Major commodity plastics such as polypropylene and polyvinyl chloride have a very poor intrinsic resistance to ionizing radiation, and are made serviceable only by compounding in additives that enable the plastic to withstand the radiation sterilization process. As was previously mentioned, most grades of polyethylene and polystyrene withstand extremely high doses of radiation (c. 10 Mrads) without undergoing any harm. Filled ABS resins, most acrylonitrile copolymers, and most engineering polymers such as polysulfones are also impervious to ionizing radiation.

CRITERIA FOR PLASTICS SELECTION AND RADIATION STERILIZATION

Sterilization processing performance is not the only criterion by which a plastic is selected as a component of a medical device or of packaging. Industrywide sterilization criteria, which were originally drawn up with EtO sterilization as the preferred method of processing, are given primarily in terms of standards set by the Association for the Advancement of Medical Instrumentation (AAMI), although individual manufacturers and products often set even stricter guidelines. Standards are set in terms of "bioburden," a residual pathogen count in the parts-per-thousand range for non-invasive devices or in the parts-per-million range for invasive medical products. Usually, the lower the residual "bioburden" required, the greater the level of ionizing radiation to which the device must be exposed.

A medical device industry guideline of 2.5 Mrads cumulative exposure is usually enough to achieve the lower "bioburden" count. However, because of certain manufacturing and packaging practices, actual cumulative exposure for some devices has sometimes exceeded 4.0 Mrads. Consequently, specifying engineers are now requiring plastics with a radiation imperviousness at the 5.0 Mrad cumulative level for their company's products. Such specifications, particularly concerning the affected commodity plastics, can add two to five cents to the cost-per-pound of such products to pay for the higher levels of additive needed.

Another problem is that plastics, especially those used for packaging and for disposable items, have economic constraints. These cost factors often dictate the use of a plastic which may lose some of its desirable properties while undergoing radiation sterilization. Other factors, such as impact resistance, appearance or clarity, and tensile and burst strengths are also, depending upon the application, significant criteria, and are often more important than radiation resistance. For example, radiation-resistant high-density polyethylene must be set aside if the specification is for a clear plastic. Similarly, crystal grades of polystyrene must be set aside if high impact resistance and toughness are important properties.

A further concern is what might happen if bonded dissimilar materials (e.g., metal and plastic) are radiation-sterilized. Exposure to either electron beam or gamma radiation will cause a heat buildup. Consequently, devices made with bonded materials of differing heat capacities and different coefficients of thermal expansion can suffer unacceptable stress levels.

CURRENT CONCERNS OF HEALTHCARE COMPANIES REGARDING RADIATION STERILIZATION

As healthcare companies increasingly adopt radiation sterilization, they have concerns that the current products used for devices and packaging will be able to withstand the sterilization process. In most cases, little switching is needed, but occasionally a radiation-resistant grade of material must be substituted.

Concerns are beginning to be raised about the future of radiation sterilization, especially in the U.S. Almost all sources of gamma-emitting Cobalt 60 come from Canada. Therefore, almost everything associated with the source and the facility must be imported. The privatization of Atomic Energy of Canada, Ltd. into the profit-oriented company, Nordion, is causing concern among major customers about price rises because of the near-monopoly positions in sales and service currently held by Nordion. Transportation restrictions can also hamper end-users from obtaining radionucleotides, and environmental concerns have been occasionally raised, particularly about facility siting, although almost all radiation sterilization facilities have had excellent safety records.

Although research is just beginning, alternative chemicals such as chlorine dioxide are being studied to see if they are safe and non-damaging to the environment. Chlorine dioxide may be acceptable environmentally because radical formation takes place on the oxygen atom. Oxygen radicals are much less damaging to the atmosphere than are halogen- or halocarbon-based radicals.

An alternative radiation process that is beginning to be evaluated is plasma-induced sterilization. Plasma discharge ionizes gas molecules and these ions can then form sterilizing molecules. It is not known what levels of capital investment would be required, but it is likely to be less costly than using ionizing radiation if found suitable. An alternative possibility might be to use highly oxygenated chemicals such as peroxides, superoxides, and ozonides. Washing with 15–35% hydrogen peroxide solution is an accepted method of sterilizing aseptic packaging materials. It has not been fully explored at this point to see if such a chemistry can be employed to meet AAMI and internal manufacturing "bioburden" standards. It is also speculated by healthcare manufacturer sterilization engineers that even higher energy electron beam or highly efficient X-ray devices could be used in the future. Most engineers with knowledge of the various medical product sterilization processes believe that none of the new techniques has the breadth of application of gamma radiation, and that new techniques at most will only take over certain niches.

CHANGES IN STERILIZING SERVICES AND THE POTENTIAL CUSTOMER BASE

Until very recently, only the largest U.S. manufacturers of medical products have opted to construct their own in-house radiation-processing facilities. It is possible that as ethylene oxide is phased out, more will build their own facilities. Many however, will employ outside radiation sterilization services, and delay commitment of the many millions of dollars that would be necessary to construct an in-house facility, whether it would use electron beam or gamma radiation.

Potential customers for radiation sterilization services would include, in addition to original equipment manufacturers, hospitals and medical equipment service companies. Hospitals, like other generators of wastes, are finding it increasingly expensive to dispose of waste products. Also, it might be less costly to sterilize a used product rather than manufacture a new one. Although hospitals and medical equipment service companies are unlikely to build their own on-site facilities, it is quite possible that they might opt for radiation sterilization. Medical equipment service companies are even able to offer further savings. Much of the equipment or apparel bought by hospitals is reusable, but for sanitary reasons is discarded after only a single use. Service companies now exist which purchase such medical devices and apparel, launder and/or disinfect after each use, and then resterilize—usually through a radiation sterilization processing facility. Surgical instruments, bedding, and gowns are now being designed to be reusable as well as disposable. It must be remembered, however, that for some plastics, high cumulative doses of radiation will harm the physical performance properties of the products.

SUMMARY

Ionizing radiation has achieved most of its potential market share for the sterilization of medical devices. Electron beam and gamma radiation processes will compete for any new facilities being constructed. Despite the need to find alternative methods to ethylene oxide processes, and the fact that many sensitive materials such as most plastics and glass can be made more stable to ionizing radiation by the incorporation of suitable additives, ionizing radiation cannot be used on all medical products because of the damage it will do. For such sensitive products as electronics, long-term implants and microsurgical equipment, ethylene oxide use must continue until alternative chemical or other less taxing sterilizing methods are developed.

ACKNOWLEDGEMENTS AND REFERENCE NOTES

The information obtained for this chapter was compiled from telephone interviewing of (1) sterilization processing directors, engineers, and quality control personnel at major healthcare manufacturing facilities, (2) directors of marketing for radiation sterilization service companies, (3) marketing managers from suppliers of gamma radiation source isotopes, (4) personnel from FDA, and (5) medical market managers at companies supplying resins and chemicals to the healthcare industries. The author thanks his wife, Nancy, for reviewing the manuscript.

Part 2

FUNDAMENTAL PROPERTIES AND TEST METHODS

Part 2

FUNDAMENTAL PROPERTIES AND TEST METHODS

3

An Assessment of Elastomers for Biomedical Applications

CARL R. McMILLIN, Ph.D.*

ABSTRACT: There are many commercially available elastomers that are used in biomedical applications, generally in *in vitro* situations. As could be expected, the lower cost of commercial elastomers dictates that they be used whenever the special attributes of medical-grade elastomers is not required. Some of these elastomers include acrylic elastomers such as poly (ethylene methylmethacrylate), butadiene rubber, butyl rubber, along with brominated and chlorinated butyl rubbers, epichlorohydrin rubber, ethylene–propylene, ethylene–propylene–diene (EPDM), and other olefinic thermoplastic elastomers including chlorinated and chlorosulfonated polyethylene, ethylene vinylacetate (EVA), fluorocarbon rubbers such as vinylidene fluoride chlorotrifluoroethylene copolymer, natural rubber, nitrile rubber, polychloroprene, polyisoprene, polysulfide rubbers, plasticized polyvinyl chloride, silicone rubber, styrene–butadiene rubber (SBR), and urethane elastomers and copolymers.

The polyurethanes and silicone rubbers are the most common elastomers in use in medical settings, although medical grades of many of the commercial elastomers are also available. Much of the current biomedical elastomer research is focused on the causes of environmental stress cracking sometimes seen with the polyurethanes in applications such as cardiac pacemaker leads, and on the ways to make elastomers more compatible with blood, e.g., the worldwide race to achieve a successful 4 mm vascular graft.

INTRODUCTION

Elastomers used in biomedical applications can be roughly divided into three groups: (1) those that are made commercially for other purposes and used in the biomedical field, (2) biomedical grades of commercially available elastomers, and (3) elastomers that have been specifically designed for biomedical use.

The commercial elastomers are generally used in external biomedical applications where no biological contact is made, such as in biomedical disposables, packaging, and biomedical instrumentation, equipment and supplies. The biomedical grades of elastomers are generally used in less-critical applications, while specifically designed elastomers have been optimized for properties such as blood compatibility, extraordinary fatigue strength, or controlled biodegradability. Modifications to existing elastomers would either fall into the biomedical grades of elastomers or the custom-designed group of elastomers.

COMMERCIALLY AVAILABLE ELASTOMERS

By far the largest volume of elastomers used in biomedical applications are the relatively low cost, commercially available elastomers [1–3]. Descriptions of the more common elastomers follow.

Acrylic elastomers [e.g., poly(ethylene methylmethacrylate)] are useful over a wide temperature range ($-40°$ to $+212°C$) and are used for O-rings, seals, and packings.

Butadiene rubber generally has a tensile strength and tear strength lower than natural rubber and SBR, but has high abrasion resistance, high resilience, good resistance to flex-cracking and low heat build-up. It is often blended with other elastomers because of its high abrasion resistance and is used in golf balls because of its resilience.

Butyl rubber [poly(isobutylene) copolymerized with 1.5–4.5% isoprene for vulcanization unsaturation] has a very low air and moisture permeability and is used for inner tubes. It has moderate tensile strength, a good resistance to ozone, and a poor resistance to aromatic hydrocarbon solvents. Brominated

*Director of R&D, AcroMed Corporation, 3033 Carnegie Avenue, Cleveland, OH 44115

and chlorinated butyl rubbers are also commercially available and can be vulcanized by additional cure systems.

Epichlorohydrin rubber (and copolymers of epichlorohydrin and ethylene oxide) have a very low permeability to gases (the homopolymer has half the permeability of butyl rubber), a high resistance to solvents and ozone, high resilience, and good low-temperature performance. Epichlorohydrin is attacked by ketones, esters, aldehydes, chlorinated and nitro hydrocarbons. The chlorine in the polymer is somewhat labile and can cause corrosion problems with metals unless compounded with appropriate acid acceptors.

Ethylene–propylene–diene (EPDM) elastomers have the termonomer (such as ethylidene norbornene) added to provide unsaturation for vulcanization. It has a high resistance to ozone, steam, and gas permeability; but it has poor resistance to oil and other hydrocarbon solvents. Varieties of ethylene–propylene rubber are made without the termonomer, which are fully saturated and usually require peroxide catalysts for vulcanization. When olefin rubbers are intensively mixed while they are being vulcanized, olefinic thermoplastic elastomers can be produced.

Other forms of modified polyethylene elastomers include chlorinated and chlorosulfonated polyethylene. These elastomers have low flammability, and a high resistance to abrasion, ozone, and oil. They have a low resistance to esters and ketones, as well as to chlorinated, aromatic, and nitro hydrocarbons; they are not recommended for immersion in water.

Ethylene vinylacetate (EVA) is generally synthesized with the vinyl acetate being the minor component (e.g., 20%). The resulting polymer is a thermoplastic elastomer and as such needs no vulcanization. It is generally tough, has good flexibility, and good low temperature properties.

Fluorocarbon rubbers (e.g., vinylidene fluoride-chlorotrifluoroethylene copolymers) have a high resistance to aliphatic, aromatic, and halogenated hydrocarbons, as well as to strong acids, strong bases, oils, solvents, and ozone. They have a wide temperature range (e.g., up to 240°C), and a good toughness. They are attacked by ketones, esters, and nitro-containing compounds.

Natural rubber, primarily cis-polyisoprene, undergoes strain crystallization upon stretching which gives it a high tensile strength. Natural rubber has a good blend of properties including high resilience, good tear resistance and good compression set; but it has low heat, oil, solvent and ozone resistance.

Nitrile rubber (a copolymer of acrylonitrile and 20–50% butadiene) has good tensile strength, is resistant to abrasion and compression set, and is highly resistant to petroleum-based materials. It is not as good as polychloroprene in oxidation resistance and weathering, and it should not be used with chlorinated hydrocarbons or highly polar solvents such as acetone.

Polychloroprene is the oldest of the synthetic rubber; it was first made available in 1931 as Neoprene from DuPont. It is resistant to oxygen, ozone, oil, many solvents and inorganic chemicals; it has a high resilience and is flame resistant. Latex polychloroprenes have high elongations similar to natural rubber. Polychloroprene is attacked by strong oxidizing acids, esters, ketones, chlorinated aromatic, and nitro hydrocarbons.

Polyisoprene has a natural rubber-like structure, but it has a lower tensile strength than natural rubber. However, it is much more reproducible and contains none of the non-rubber (mostly protein) components of natural rubber.

Polysulfide rubbers are prepared by the reaction of sodium polysulfide with ethylene dichloride and bis (2-ethyl) formal. These rubbers have a high resistance to sunlight, ozone, aromatic hydrocarbons, esters, ketones, and weathering. They have a good low temperature flexibility, and a low permeability. However, they are not resistant to chlorinated hydrocarbons, esters, amines, or heterocyclics. They have poor physical properties, a low resilience, high creep, and a characteristic sulfurous odor.

Polyvinyl chloride (PVC or vinyl) is actually a plastic (glass transition temperature below ambient), but is often compounded with plasticizers which make it flexible. PVCs are generally inexpensive, tough, strong, and can be transparent.

Silicone rubber has a wide temperature capability and is resistant to oxidation, ozone, compression set, and many chemicals. In general, it has a somewhat low tensile strength and is attacked by oils, concentrated acids, and dilute sodium hydroxide. Fluorosilicones have a good temperature service range and improved solvent resistance to oxidizing chemicals, aromatic and chlorinated solvents. They are attacked by brake fluids and ketones.

Styrene–butadiene rubber (SBR) can be made using a wide variety of ratios of the styrene and the butadiene, with the most common formulation containing 23.5% styrene. Because of its low cost, SBR is one of the most widely used synthetic elastomers. SBR has good water and organic acid resistance, but poor resistance to oil, ozone, strong acids, and hydrocarbons. Styrene and butadiene can also be polymerized with termonomers to make elastomers such as butadiene/styrene/vinyl pyridiene terpolymer, which has good adhesive qualities.

Urethane rubbers are formed by reactions involving the isocyanate functional group. This reactive functionality can combine with a wide variety of groups including hydroxy-terminated polyethers and polyesters, alcohols and glycols, amines and ureas. The urethane group is only a small part of any resulting polymer, such that the final properties are determined by the other components of the elastomer. Polyurethanes generally have a high tensile strength, tear strength, abrasion, oil and ozone resistance. However, they usually have a poor solvent resistance (concentrated acids, ketones, esters, chlorinated and nitro hydrocarbons), and some urethanes degrade in high-humidity environments.

BIOMEDICAL GRADES OF ELASTOMERS

In order to market a biomedical grade of an elastomer, more quality control, higher purity, and additional paperwork (for traceability) is maintained. Most of the more stringent requirements are codified in a group of written procedures which are called Good Manufacturing Practices (GMP).

Biomedical grades of elastomers should not produce adverse reactions when they come in contact with biological materials. Actually, very few polymers cause adverse reactions (e.g., cytotoxicity) in and of themselves. It is most often either additives or polymer degradation products that migrate from the polymer which cause most adverse reactions. Therefore, medical-grade elastomers usually consist of a base polymer that is biologically stable. Any required plasticizers, fillers, or other additives are selected to be non-toxic and non-leaching.

Before medical devices can be sold, they must be proven to be both safe and effective in order to obtain approval from the Food and Drug Administration (FDA). Note that the FDA only approves materials as they are used in specific applications, not the materials themselves.

Some manufacturers establish a "Master File" on their medical-grade elastomers at the FDA. This establishes the properties of the materials and the processing controls under which the elastomer is produced. The availability of a Master File on a material assists a device manufacturer in the biomedical use of that material. During the device approval process, the FDA can review the Master File documentation to assure that appropriate GMP is in place and is being followed for the materials that are used in the device under consideration.

Many commercial elastomers are available in medical grades that have been manufactured under GMP. The applications for medical grades of these elastomers range from butyl rubber used in chewing gum to latex polychloroprenes used in gastric balloons and polyvinyl chloride formulations used in blood pumps. The following sections describe some elastomers that are available in biomedical grades, along with some of the elastomers that have been specifically designed for biomedical use.

BIOMEDICAL POLYURETHANES

The term "polyurethane" refers to a broad variety of elastomers which are usually formed by the addition of a polyglycol to an isocyanate. Typically, the isocyanate is part of an aromatic molecule which gives rigidity and hardness to this portion of the polymer chain, while the polyglycol portions form less rigid or softer portions of the polymer chain. Additional aliphatic segments are added as "chain extenders" to give more of the soft segments on the polymer chain. Most polyurethanes therefore have hard and soft segments and are called segmented polyurethanes.

Polyurethanes can be readily tailored for many applications either by changing the chemical used in any of the components or by changing the length of the prepolymer of extender chains used to make the polyurethane. Thus, polyurethanes are in themselves a wide class of materials. Ether-based polyurethanes are known to be less susceptible to hydrolytic cleavage than ester-based polyurethanes and have therefore been used for most biomedical applications.

The wide variety of polyurethanes and urethane copolymers which have been synthesized and in many cases made available for biomedical applications are usually strong, flexible, transparent or translucent, tissue-compatible and reasonably blood-compatible. They have been used for a variety of applications requiring these properties, such as peristaltic pump tubing, parenteral solution tubing, mammary augmentation, dialysis membranes, balloon pumps, and catheters. Polyurethane foams have also been used in many biomedical applications, mostly *in vitro* such as sponges to promote adhesions and surgical sponges.

Much of the research on biomedical polyurethanes focuses on relatively few commercial elastomers. For competitive reasons, the chemical composition of these polyurethanes are sometimes kept as trade secrets. The composition of some of the polyurethanes which have been published are shown in Table 1.

The DuPont Company, Wilmington, DE, invented a linear segmented aromatic ether polyurethane called Lycra™ and uses this elastomer to make the elastic fiber Spandex™. Ethicon Inc. of Somerville, NJ, a Johnson & Johnson Company, manufactures a slightly modified and biomedical-grade version of this elastomer under the tradename of Biomer™ under license from DuPont. Biomer has an excellent balance of physical, mechanical, chemical, and biological properties and has become one of the most widely researched polyurethanes in the biomedical field. I have used it extensively as a control material in fatigue testing.

Biomer is made by combining polytetramethylene ether glycol (PTMEG) with methylene diisocyanate (MDI) to produce an isocyanate-terminated prepolymer. Ethylenediamine (ED) is used as the chain extender, which gives the final polymer urethane and substituted urea linkages. The decomposition temperature of Biomer is within two degrees C of its melting temperature so that it can only be formed by techniques such as film casting or spinning from solution. Biomer is generally supplied as a 30% by weight solution in a dimethylacetamide solution and is easily processed in a low relative humidity environment.

Because of its exceptionally good fatigue endurance and biostability, Biomer has been used to make both

Table 1. Composition of some polyurethane biomedical elastomers.

Trade Name	Urethane Components*						
	PTMEG	MDI	ED	BD	PD	HMDI	PDMS
Biomer	X	X	X				
Surethane	X	X	X				X
Pellethane	X	X		X			
Corplex	X	X		X			(X) (post-treatment)
Toyobo TM5	X	X			X		
Tecoflex HR	X			X		X	
Cardiothane-51	X	X		X			X

*PTMEG—polytetramethylene ether glycol
 MDI—methylene diisocyanate or
 ED—ethylenediamine
 BD—1,4-butanediol
 PD—propylenediamine
 HMDI—hydrogenated MDI
 PDMS—polydimethylsiloxane

the pumping diaphragm and semi-rigid housing (fabric reinforced) of the highly publicized Symbion Jarvik-7™ artificial hearts. Ethicon has been reluctant to sell Biomer to most device manufacturers where it would be used in clinical (i.e., human) applications, apparently because of potential legal liability. Because of the potential unavailability of Biomer, other manufacturers have made polyurethanes similar to Biomer both for their own internal use and for sale commercially.

One of the polyurethanes with properties similar to Biomer is Mitrathane™, from Mitral Medical Ltd., Wheat Ridge, CO. Specimens of Mitrathane that I have tested have had tensile strength, elongation, modulus of elasticity, and fatigue endurance properties virtually identical to those of my Biomer controls.

Cardiac Control Systems, Inc. of Palm Coast, FL, uses and also sells a biomedical-grade polyurethane similar to Biomer that is called Surethane™. Cardiac Control Systems buys Spandex fiber from DuPont. After incoming quality control tests, they remove the surface lubricants from the Spandex and redissolve the fiber in dimethylacetamide. Whereas Biomer is a pure polyurethane, Spandex and the resulting Surethane has about 3–5% polydimethylsiloxane that is blended with and partially covalently bonded to the polyurethane.

Scanning electron micrographs of a Surethane-coated pacemaker sent to me from Cardiac Control Systems look promising, as do the written quality control procedures that are followed, the results of fatigue testing, cytotoxicity testing, rat and rabbit biocompatibility testing, and preliminary pacemaker tests in animals and humans. A number of other urethane–silicone blends and urethane–silicone copolymers are discussed in a later section.

Another polyurethane designed to substitute for Biomer is BPS-215M from Mercor Inc., Berkeley, CA. It has been validated as a substitute elastomer for Biomer in the Pierce–Donachy ventricular assist pump [4]. It is being made available commercially for other clinical applications, but only under very constrained conditions.

Unithane 80F from the National Institute for the Control of Pharmaceutical and Biological Products, Temple of Heaven, Beijing, China, has been reported in the literature [5] to be made using polytetramethylene ether glycol, methylene diisocyanate, and ethylenediamine, closely following the Biomer composition.

Biomedical Polyurethanes with Different Compositions

A series of medical-grade elastomers of varying types and hardness are sold by Dow Chemical U.S.A., Plastics Department, Polyurethanes Group, Midland, MI, under the tradename Pellethane™ (sold previously by Upjohn Corp., New Haven, CT, with the same name). Pellethane 2363™ is a medical-grade linear segmented aromatic ether polyurethane. Like Biomer, it is made using a prepolymer of MDI and PTMEG, but it is chain-extended with 1,4-butanediol (BD) instead of ethylenediamine.

Pellethanes are used both for normal commercial products as well as for biomedical applications. Pellethanes can be processed by most thermoplastic techniques including extrusion, injection molding, thermoforming and solution casting. The use of Pellethane is attractive because of its processability and lower cost due to high-volume non-medical production. Pellethane is clear, smooth, and has been found to be biocompatible with tissues as well as hydrolytically stable. I have found it to be non-cytotoxic, non-mutagenic, and reasonably fatigue resistant.

Pellethane 2363 is presently being used for many biomedical applications including balloon catheters, coatings on blood-contact catheters, medical tubing, and for the construction of artificial heart valves, blood pump housings and pumping diaphragms. However, Dow Chemical has recently indicated that Pellethane will be withdrawn from the general biomedical market in 1992 because of liability and litigation concerns.

Another series of related medical-grade polyurethanes are the Tecoflexs from Thermedics Inc., Woburn, MA. Tecoflex HR™ is synthesized using PTMEG with the BD extender but uses the cyclohexane analog of MDI (replaces the aromatic ring) for the diisocyanate. This produces an aliphatic polyurethane with a lower processing temperature and melting point [6]. Because of the lower melting point, Tecoflex can not be steam-sterilized. Tecoflex has the ability to be processed by extrusion, injection molding, or solution casting.

Thermedics uses Tecoflex internally and also markets it. Several types of Tecoflex have been designed for different applications. Sales literature focuses on its biocompatibility, narrow molecular weight distribution, high purity, uniform pellet size, availability in a wide array of colors and durometers in clear and radiopaque grades. Tecoflex has been successfully used for such applications as tubing, extrusions, and blood pumping diaphragms, and is being evaluated for controlled release of lidocaine for treatment of tachycardia [7].

Angioflex™ from Applied Biomedical Corporation (ABIOMED), Danvers, MA, is another medical-grade ether-type segmented polyurethane. Angioflex is solution cast from a mixture of tetrahydrofuran and dioxane to make an elastomer that I have found easy to process, clear, tough, and highly fatigue-resistant. There is a wider range of acceptable processing conditions for Angioflex than for some of the other solution cast polyurethanes. ABIOMED uses Angioflex for applications including trileaflet heart valves and artificial heart blood pumping diaphragms. Unfortunately, it is intended primarily for internal use at ABIOMED.

Corvita, Miami, FL has developed an ether polyurethane called Corplex™ that is being used for vascular prostheses [8]. Parts are manufactured from the base polyurethane and then polydimethylsiloxane is covalently bonded to them as a post-treatment. Corvita intends to make Corplex available to manufacturers of medical devices.

Corvita has also developed a urethane-like elastomer called Corethane that is substantially devoid of ether and ester linkages. Porous filamentous tubes of Corethane implanted for six months stretched 400% showed no surface cracking.

Isoplast™ is a clear, rigid thermoplastic polyurethane from Dow Chemical Company, Dow Plastics Medical Group, Midland, MI, that is used for tubing, syringes, IV components, and catheter hubs.

Teleflex Medical Inc., Woburn, MA, has announced a variety of ultrapure polyurethanes designed for medical applications. J.P. Stevens & Co., Inc., Urethane Products Division, Easthampton, MA, has several types of ether and ester polyurethane films, some of which are proposed for medical and food-contact use.

Another medical-grade polyurethane intended to be used for applications such as the pumping diaphragm of artificial hearts is Hemothane™, from the Sarnes Division of 3M in Ann Arbor, MI. I have been told, however, that this material is primarily intended for internal use at 3M and is most likely not available commercially. Also for captive use only is Tygothane™, a plasticizer-free polyurethane from Norton Performance Plastics, Akron, OH, that is used to make medical-grade polyurethane tubing.

Toyobo TM5™ from Toyobo Co., Osaka, Japan, uses MDI and PTMEG for the soft segment, and MDI and propylene diamine (PD) for the hard segment. It has generally been prepared as a 15% by weight solution in dimethylformamide. The published data suggests that the properties of this material are similar to those of Biomer. Several years ago, however, Toyobo was unwilling to provide samples of this material to me for comparative fatigue test evaluation. I do not know whether it is still unavailable to researchers and medical device manufacturers.

Internationally, there are many other polyurethanes that are being used for biomedical applications, such as the commercial polyurethane Czech PU™ made in the U.S.S.R. using a complex oligoester, MDI, and hydrazine hydrate [9]. Cust-II™ is said to be similar to Biomer and is made at The National Institute for the Control of Pharmaceutical and Biological Products, Temple of Heaven, Beijing, China, using polyoxycetramethylene glycol instead of PTMEG. Unithane OUE™, Unithane PU-80B, Unithane PU-90B, Unithane TPE-80B, and Unithane TPE-95B are segmented ether polyurethanes made either by the Tianjin Institute of Synthetic Materials, Beijing, China, or The National Institute for the Control of Pharmaceutical and Biological Products, Beijing [10].

Less similar to Biomer are some other biomedical polyurethanes being sold such as Biothane™, a two part polyurethane casting system from CasChem Inc., Bayonne, NJ, and Medadhere 2110™, an ether-free polyurethane from Medtronic, Inc., Brooklyn Center, MN.

Additional research polyurethanes include those synthesized in the Dept. of Chimica Industriale e Ingegneria Chimica, Politecnico, Milano, Italy, using either polytetramethylene ether glycol (PTMEG) or polypropyleneoxide along with methylene diisocyanate (MDI) and propylenediamine (PD). An ether-based polyurethane containing polybutadiene and polyethylene oxide segments has been synthesized in the Sophia University, Tokyo, Japan.

A wide variety of commercial polyurethanes are available which might be useful in some biomedical applications [1-3]. Some of these are shown in Table 2.

Table 2. Commercially available polyurethanes.

Trade Name	Manufacturer
Bayflex 150 DOI Bayflex 120	Polyurea urethanes from Mobay Corp., Pittsburgh, PA
Cyanaprene	American Cyanamid, Wayne, NJ
Desmopan	Bayer AG, Pittsburgh, PA
Elastolan	BASF Corp., Wyandotte, MI
Elastolit R 4500	Polyurea amide urethane elastomer from BASF Corp., Parsippany, NJ
Estane TPR	Uniroyal-Goodrich, Akron, OH
Geolite Hyperlite Ultracell-CM	Polyurethane foams from Union Carbide Corp., Danbury, CT
Hypol	Polyurethane rich with polyoxyethylene from W.R. Grace & Co., CT
Isoplast	Clear polyurethane from Dow Chemical Co., Midland, MI
Lycra 126 Lycra 420	Ether polyurethane Ether plus urea polyurethane from DuPont Corp., Wilmington, DE
Orthane	Ohio Rubber, Denton, TX
Polycast UR-2970	Minor Rubber Company Inc., Bloomfield, NJ
RIMline	Urea urethanes for reaction injection molding from I.C.I. Polyurethanes Group, Deptford, NJ
Texin	Mobay Chemical Corp., NY, NY
Polyurethanes	K. J. Quinn & Co., Malden, MA

Environmental Stress Cracking of Polyurethanes

Almost all of the polyurethanes used for *in vitro* biomedical applications are of the ether type and not of the ester type. This is because the ester-based polyurethanes are generally not as hydrolytically stable in the aqueous *in vivo* environments. Segmented ether polyurethanes have been used as the coating of cardiac pacemaker leads. Although supe-

Table 3. Potential causes of pacemaker lead failures.

Autooxidative processes involving metal-catalyzed peroxide
   decomposition
Cellular–polymer interactions
Enzymatic chain cleavage
Extraction of low molecular weight material leading to
   surface defects
Lipid adsorption
Metal ion-catalyzed chain cleavage (especially cobalt and
   silver)
Oxidative chain cleavage
Residual processing stresses
Stress crazing
Swelling of the polyurethane

rior to silicone-coated pacing leads in several respects, there has been some environmental stress cracking of the polyurethane pacing leads reported.

For example, Medtronic has reported 240 cases of cracked insulation in the 185,000 polyether urethane insulated cardiac pacing leads distributed between 1977 and 1983, with 104 of these (a small but significant number) affecting the device performance. The polymer cracking allows moisture to penetrate to the metal core, and sometimes results in the lead becoming shorted. Some of the potential causes of polyurethane cardiac pacing lead insulation failure are listed in Table 3 and discussed in the following.

The effect of enzymes on environmental stress cracking of polyurethanes has been investigated. In one series of tests, papain and urease were found to degrade Biomer [11]. In another report, papain, chymotrypsin, and leucine aminopeptidase were all found to degrade some polyurethanes [12]. In a third report, papain, esterase, bromelain, ficin, chymotrypsin, trypsin, and cathepsin C, but not collagenase or the oxidative enzymes xanthine oxidase and cytochrome C oxidase, were found to degrade a radiolabeled polyurethane [13]. The mixed enzymes found in rabbit liver homogenate also affected the polyurethane in this study. Yet another study found papain and bacterial protease to cause crack growth in stressed Pellethane 2363-80A [14].

Applied voltage as a cause of Pellethane coated pacemaker lead environmental stress cracking has been evaluated by *in vitro* studies in a Hank's balanced salt solution [15]. After exposure to the solution for 14 months with a 5 to 20 volt potential, it was found that current leakage occurred in only a few areas of the pacing lead. The checkerboard-type cracking reported in *in vivo* studies was not observed in this static *in vitro* test, although there were some cracks observed on the outer surface of the leads.

Metal ions have been implicated in the degradation of polyurethane pacemaker leads. Polyurethane-insulated Co-Ni-Cr-Mo (MP35N alloy) leads have been used for cardiac pacing since 1977. Tests were conducted to determine if the failures that have occurred with these leads were due in part to a metal catalyzed degradation of the polyurethane insulation.

In one study, 0.1 M silver nitrate at 90°C for 35 days oxidized the ether linkages of polyurethanes in increasing severity for Pellethane, Tecoflex EF, Biomer and Cardiothane-51 [16]. In another study, cobalt was found to cause bulk degradation of Pellethane by what was described as an autooxidative mechanism [17]. Indications from additional studies are that the chloride anion may be significant in the degradation of polyurethanes, and that the chloride anion has more effect on polyurethane degradation than does the acetate anion [18]. Although no cracks were observed in explanted Jarvik-7 Biomer polyurethane diaphragms, metal ion complexes were detected [19].

Cholesterol and lipids may contribute to polyurethane degradation as evidenced by the decrease in fatigue life of polyurethanes when tested in solutions of these chemicals [20].

The effect of cell–polymer interactions on environmental stress cracking of Pellethane 2363-80A has been investigated. Polyurethane was placed in the Anderson stainless steel cage system in rats. It was found that cell–polymer interactions are required for stress cracking to occur. When effective cellular interactions with the polymer were destroyed by co-implantation of cytotoxic agents or suppressed by anti-inflammatory drugs, the deterioration of the polyurethane was minimized [21,22].

The relative contributions of all of the above mentioned factors has not been determined. It is likely that relative significances of each of these factors will vary with different polyurethanes in differing environments. However, the problem of environmental stress cracking of polyurethanes is a continuing research topic.

BIOMEDICAL POLYURETHANES MODIFIED WITH SILICONES

Many other modifications have been made to polyurethanes in attempts to improve on the properties of the elastomer. Incorporation of polydimethylsiloxane into polyurethanes has been used by several groups in attempts to improve blood compatibility. This improved hemocompatibility is particularly important in the development of vascular grafts of 4 mm diameter and smaller which are needed for cardiac bypass surgery. No presently available 4 mm synthetic grafts have demonstrated long-term patency, although many groups around the world are racing to achieve this goal.

Many of the modified polyurethanes have incorporated silicones, as shown in Table 4. Most of these polymers have been reported in the literature to have improved hemocompatibility, improved physical properties, and/or improved biostability.

Cardiothane-51™ from Kontron Instruments, Everett, MA, (formerly Avocothane-51™ from Avco Everett, Everett, MA) was one of the first commercially available biomedical elastomers to couple polyurethane with polydimethylsiloxane (silicon rubber). Cardiothane-51 uses the same backbone as Pellethane (PTMEG, MDI, & BD). Then, about 10 percent acetoxy-terminated polydimethylsiloxane is grafted onto the base polyurethane polymer. Optimal properties for Cardiothane-51 can only be obtained by solution casting from a 2:1 mixture of tetrahydrofuran (THF) and 1,4-dioxane under precisely controlled temperature, humidity, and rate of solvent evaporation.

Recent research has shown that Cardiothane-51 may be more of a polyblend with only part of the polydimethylsiloxane grafted onto the polyurethane chain. A variable amount of the silicone component has been

Table 4. Urethane–silicone elastomers.

Polymer	Manufacturer
Cardiothane-51	Kontron
CUST-I	Chengdu University of Science and Technology
Rimplast	Petrarch
ZH-III	Zhongshan Medical University
Research	Mercor
Research	Kanegafuchi Chemical Industry Co.
Research	Hokkaido University
Research	Government Industrial Research Institute

found on the surface of Cardiothane-51 samples depending on the technique used to prepare the samples [23].

High-quality sheets of this material that I have tested have had extremely good mechanical properties and fatigue endurance. Because of its good blood compatibility and mechanical properties, Cardiothane-51 is used in such demanding applications as intra-aortic balloon pumps.

Rimplast™ of Petrarch, Bristol, PA, is a reactive silicone-urethane interpenetrating network system. An interpenetrating network is an arrangement of two discrete superimposed polymer networks. The Rimplast system is said to be processable by either extrusion or molding.

Mercor Incorporated, a Thoratec Company, Berkeley, CA, has produced a thermoplastic block copolymer of polydimethylsiloxane and polyurethane using BD and hexamethylene diisocyanate urethane blocks [24]. Additional siloxane–urethane copolymers reported include ZH-III™ and CUST-I™ being studied by Zhongshan Medical University and Chengdu University of Science and Technology, Beijing, People's Republic of China, and biomedical siloxane–urethane copolymers synthesized in the U.S.S.R.

A polyethylene oxide–polydimethyl siloxane–polyethylene oxide block copolymer with 13% by weight siloxane, made by the Kanegafuchi Chemical Industry Company, Kobe, Japan, in conjunction with the Institute of Physical and Chemical Research, Wako, Saitama, has been used to evaluate more compliant (elastic) vascular grafts [25].

Compliant vascular grafts were also made by the Hokkaido University, Sapporo, Japan, from another polyurethane block copolymer with PTMEG, MDI, ethylene glycol, coupled with a polyethylene oxide-polydimethylsiloxane–polyethylene oxide block [26].

Modifications to Polyurethanes for Improved Hemocompatibility

Many attempts have been made to improve the blood compatibility of polyurethanes as shown in Table 5. Modifying polyurethanes by substituting propyl sulfonate groups for urethane hydrogens to produce ionic polyurethanes [27,28] and octadecyl groups

Table 5. Modifications to polyurethanes for hemocompatibility.

Modification	Institution
Enzyme immobilization of urokinase	Kumamoto University School of Medicine
Fluorination	Asahi Glass Company
Fluorination	Becton Dickinson Polymer Research
Grafting for heparin bonding:	
with poly(amido-amine)	Centro Didattico Nuovo Policlinico
with polyethylene glycol	Korea Advanced Institute of Science and Technology
with polyethylene oxide	University of Utah
Propyl sulfonate	University of Wisconsin

to produce alkyl derivatives of the polyurethanes [29] have been conducted at the University of Wisconsin, Madison, WI.

Fluorinated polyurethanes were synthesized using PTMEG, ethylenediamine (ED), and octafluorodiisocyanatohexane at Asahi Glass Company, Yokohama, Japan [30]. Additional fluorinated polyurethanes were synthesized using PTMEG, MDI, and a fluoropolyether glycol, with either BD or 1,6-hexanediol at Becton Dickinson Polymer Research, Dayton, OH [31].

Pellethane was grafted with a heparin-bonding poly(amidoamine) which had been previously treated with hexamethylenediisocyanate by the Centro Didattico Nuovo Policlinico, Siena, Italy [32]. The same reactants were used to attach polyethylene glycol to Pellethane to achieve heparin bonding by the Korea Advanced Institute of Science and Technology, Seoul, Korea [33]. Similarly, Biomer has been grafted with heparin-bonding polyethylene oxide which had been previously treated with toluene 2,4-diisocyanate at the University of Utah, Salt Lake City, UT [34].

The plasminogen activator urokinase was immobilized onto polyurethane by the Kumamoto University School of Medicine, Kumamoto, Japan [35]. Urokinase converts plasminogen into the active enzyme plasmin, which digests fibrin of blood clots. A C-18 alkyl group has been attached to polyurethanes to enhance albumin adsorption onto the polyurethane in an attempt to improve the polyurethane blood compatibility [36,37].

BIOMEDICAL SILICONE RUBBERS

Another class of rubbers used extensively in biomedical applications are the silicone rubbers, which are best known in the form of polydimethylsiloxanes. They were first made available in a medical grade in 1962. Siloxane polymers can usually be steam-sterilized to 250°F, are resistant to ozone, have reasonably high strength, and are for the most part biologically inert. Generally, silicone rubbers are reinforced with silica filler and vulcanized in order to develop their optimum properties.

Silicone rubbers have been successfully used in a wide variety of applications including tubing, cannulas, catheters, drainage tubes, biomedical balloons, artificial finger joint hinges, wire coating for pacemaker leads, drug delivery systems, denture liners, artificial heart compliance chamber diaphragms, breast implants, and arthroplasty. They are widely used in reconstructive plastic surgery [38,39].

Early in the development of artificial heart valves, a problem occurred with some silicone rubber ball heart valves. After implant, caged poppet balls made from silicone rubber were occasionally found to absorb lipids from the blood. When this happened, serious problems would develop. The balls would swell and fail either by sticking in an open or a closed position or by cracking, with some of the resulting pieces of silicone rubber going into the bloodstream to cause downstream blood vessel blockages. After much research, it was found that this problem resulted from sporadically under-cured silicone rubber balls. Better cure systems and a practice of post-curing the silicone rubber have virtually eliminated this silicone rubber problem.

There are still some concerns, however, about the use of silicone rubber in applications where fragmentation and migration of the implant into local tissues has been seen. This situation is most likely to occur in implants where there are higher stresses and/or abrasion of the implant, such as in temporomandibular joint meniscal replacements [40]. In these cases, morphological studies of the tissue surrounding long-term implants have found foreign body reactions, synovitis, dystrophic calcification, fibrocartilaginous metaplasia, hyalinization, and scarring.

Because of the common biomedical use of silicone rubber, it has been selected to be one of the standard reference materials made available to researchers by the National Institutes of Health (NIH). Under contract to NIH, Thoratec Company, Berkeley, CA, has manufactured standard reference material silicone rubber tubing. The 4 mm tubing is made from silica-filled silicone rubber with a silica-free silicone rubber inner surface and is available in 0.5, 1.0, and 1.5 m lengths. I had no problem obtaining some of this material for a blood/materials interaction study I was conducting [41].

The Medical Products Division of Dow Corning Corporation, Midland, MI, markets Silastic™, the most common medical-grade silicone rubbers. Medical-grade Silastics with either platinum or peroxide cure systems are available as sheet, tubing, or a wide variety of molding compounds. Silastics with specific properties such as extra high tear strength are also available. For example, Silastic GP-30, GP-45, and GP-70 are FDA-approved for food contact; Silastic NPC-40 and NPC-80 require no post-cure and are approved for food contact; and biomedical-grade Silastic 1125U is listed as having FDA approval for making molded, extruded and calendered goods [1]. Samples of Silastic HP-100, a grade of Silastic used at Dow for artificial finger joints, was highly fatigue-resistant in accelerated fatigue tests I conducted. Unfortunately, Dow has been unwilling to sell this polymer externally for orthopedic applications.

General Electric, Silicone Products Department, Waterford, NY, lists GE Silicones SE 435™, SE 475, SE478, and SE 479 for food contact applications [1].

McGhan Nusil Corporation, Carpinteria, CA, has a broad silicone product line including MED-6382™, a two component medical-grade silicone elastomer, MED-6210/MED-6230, a silicone intraocular lens elastomer, and MED-6640, a medical-grade high tear silicone dispersion [42].

Rhodia Inc., Manmouth Junction, NJ, lists Rhodorsil Base 5™, Rhodorsil K-1045, K-1046 and K-1047 for food contact applications and Rhodorsil RE-85 and RE-87 as special food-grade silicone rubbers [1].

Sil-Med Corporation, Taunton, MA, sells SM-1100™, SM-2100, and SM-7700 series of medical grade silicone rubber compounds that are said to be biocompatible and suitable for catheters, tubing, wound-drainage systems, vascular ties, and short- and long-term implants.

Petrarch Systems Silanes, Bristol, PA, sells many types of medical-grade silicone rubbers and products including a high tear strength and low-friction silicone rubber tubing. Silicone Technology, Carpinteria, CA, sells specialty biomedical silicone rubbers.

Other silicones are manufactured internationally, such as Silaplen and Silaplen AC that I have fatigue tested which were produced in the U.S.S.R.

Biomedical Silicone Copolymers

Siloxanes have not only been copolymerized with urethanes, but have also been blended and copolymerized with other monomers and polymers. C-Flex™ is a family of medical-grade thermoplastic elastomers made by blending polysiloxanes with styrene–ethylene/butylene–styrene block copolymers by Concept Polymer Technologies, Inc., Clearwater, FL [43,44]. The blends are tailored for individual biomedical applications. C-Flex is relatively inexpensive, transparent, biocompatible, and can easily be extruded and molded. Samples I have tested have had moderately good mechanical properties. C-Flex is both sold to device manufacturers and is used internally for tubing, catheters, stents, and other molded parts.

SMA-400™ is a family of triblock caprolactone-siloxane–caprolactone copolymers which have passed most of the toxicity tests and are available as experimental materials from Mercor [45]. A similar ABA triblock polymer with (2-ethyl-2-oxazoline) and siloxane is also available from Mercor as SMA-500™. Norton Performance Plastics, Wayne, NJ,

makes a PVC/silicone blend that they use in the manufacture of medical tubing.

There are several research reports on siloxane-containing copolymers. Polydimethylsiloxane has been grafted onto polystyrene at the Technological University of Nagaoka, Nagaoka, Japan, for anti-thrombogenicity [46]. A siloxane–polyethylene oxide copolymer synthesized at Harvard and The Massachusetts Institute of Technology, Cambridge, MA, has been evaluated for use as a drug-releasing polymer [47]. Similarly, AB and ABC copolymers of polydimethylsiloxane–polyethylene oxide–heparin have been synthesized by the University of Utah, Salt Lake City, UT, with the University of Washington, Seattle, WA, in attempts to achieve better blood compatibility [48].

Although urethanes and siloxanes appear to dominate the biomedical field, there are many other polymer systems that have also found use in biomedical situations.

OLEFIN-BASED BIOMEDICAL ELASTOMERS

Olefin is the term used for straight-chain hydrocarbons. One olefin-based rubber is Hexsyn™, patented by Goodyear Tire and Rubber Company, Akron, OH. Hexsyn is synthesized from 95% 1-hexene and 3–5% methylhexadiene (which provides cross-linking sites) using a Ziegler-Natta polymerization. The gum rubber is compounded with carbon black and an accelerated sulfur cure system prior to compression molding. The vulcanizate must be solvent extracted prior to *in vivo* use with solvents such as an acetone/toluene or methanol/toluene mixture to remove cytotoxic vulcanization chemicals.

After extraction the rubber is an almost entirely hydrocarbon vulcanizate that is amorphous, biocompatible, and extremely fatigue-resistant. This polyolefin rubber has previously been used in finger joint hinges by Lord Corporation under the tradename of Bion™ and is presently now being used for artificial heart pump diaphragms and artificial heart variable-volume chamber diaphragms at the Cleveland Clinic and the University of Washington because of its high flex fatigue resistance.

It is presently licensed for biomedical uses to the Cleveland Clinic Foundation, Cleveland, OH, The University of Akron, Akron, OH, and AcroMed Corporation, Cleveland, OH. The AcroMed rubber, under the tradename AcroFlex™, is being used in the development of an intervertebral disk prosthesis.

I have conducted extensive testing of this rubber and have found it to have a very low tear strength, high gas permeability, low water permeability, extremely high fatigue resistance, good ozone resistance, and excellent biostability. I recently published an extensive compilation of data on the characterization of this rubber [49].

Another olefin-based elastomer, is the commercially available thermoplastic elastomer Santoprene™

from Monsanto Company, Akron, OH. Santoprene does not require vulcanization and is processed like a thermoplastic, e.g., extruded and injection-molded. Santoprene is available in both commerical and in medical grades (grades 271 and 273) of differing hardness. I have found Santoprene to be non-cytotoxic, non-mutagenic, resistant to ozone, and relatively good in fatigue. Its olefin nature should make Santoprene resistant to biodegradation. Because of their relatively low cost, easy processing, biocompatibility, and ability to be reprocessed, thermoplastic elastomers such as Santoprene should find many uses in biomedical applications.

Ethylene–propylene rubbers for applications such as closures with sealing gaskets for food containers and packaging materials for use in radiation preservation of prepackaged foods are available from Exxon Chemical Company, Buffalo Grove, IL, under the tradename Vistalon EPM™.

BIOMEDICAL GRADES OF POLYVINYL CHLORIDE

Pure polyvinyl chloride (PVC) is a hard and rigid plastic used to make items such as pipe. However, when plasticized, PVC becomes flexible and has the characteristics of an elastomer. PVCs can be tough, strong, transparent, abrasion resistant, chemical resistant, smooth, low-friction, sterilizable, and most important, inexpensive. In order to make it flexible, plasticizers are incorporated. Fillers give PVC added strength and generally lower its cost. Stabilizers, antioxidants, colorants and other ingredients are often incorporated into PVC formulations such that often the polymer represents less than half of the volume of the elastic plastic. For biomedical applications, these additives need to be "non-toxic" and may not migrate or leach out of the plastic.

For example, PVC plasticized with di(2-ethylhexyl) phthalate (also called dioctyl phthalate or DOP) is the most common material from which blood storage bags have been manufactured. Recently, much concern has been expressed that plasticizers leaching into the blood from the PVC bags could have an adverse effect on the patients, particularly those receiving large quantities of blood. The leaching of the plasticizers from PVC is even more important for *in vivo* (inside the body) applications where the plasticizers can be a cause of adverse tissue reactions or where their loss can make the plastic brittle.

Note that most polymers, including PVC, do not cause adverse tissue reactions while they are still polymers. Any cytotoxicity (cell toxicity) observed is generally due either to low molecular weight degradation products of the polymers or to components that migrate from the polymers such as plasticizers, fillers, lubricants, processing aids, dyes, antioxidants, stabilizers, and so forth.

Extraction-resistant PVC medical compounds are therefore being developed which use non-toxic non-leaching additives for long-term contact with blood and human tissue.

PVC is used for a wide range of biomedical applications including medical tubing and catheters, blood collection and administration sets, endotracheal tubes, surgical drapes, aprons, disposable gloves, diapers, mattress covers, and wound-drainage tubes.

Medical grades of plasticized PVC are available from suppliers which maintain an FDA masterfile and/or manufacture in compliance with GMP. Goodtouch 250 × 100™ is a vinyl resin from BFGoodrich, Cleveland, OH, that is sold for applications such as vinyl medical gloves. BFGoodrich also has a complete line of medical-grade rigid and flexible vinyl compounds that it sells under the name Geon RX™.

In a few applications, the leaching of substances from polymers is beneficial. The controlled leaching of substances is one method of controlled release of drugs. In these devices, substances are released at predetermined rates from the devices. Controlled release of heparin as a method of achieving blood compatibility has recently been attempted by binding heparin onto silica which was then incorporated into the PVC [50].

PVC has also been blended with other polymers such as in the PVC/polyurethane blend used by Norton Performance Plastics, Wayne, NJ, in their production of tubing.

BIOMEDICAL GRADES OF OTHER ELASTOMERS

There are a myriad of other elastomers that have found use in biomedical applications. Many of these are being produced by manufacturers in biomedical grades. Some information on a few of these follows.

Ethylene vinylacetate is being made in the biomedical grade EVA 3120™ by E. I. du Pont de Nemours and Company, Wilmington, DE, for use in food contact applications. U.S. Industrial Chemicals Company, a divison of National Distillers and Chemical Corporation, New York, NY, sells Ultrathene UE 630™ for use in surgical and pharmaceutical supplies.

Acrylonitrile-butadiene is being marketed by Polysar Inc., Akron, OH, under the name KRYNAC 803™ for pharmaceutical seals.

Butadiene sold by I.S.R. Company Ltd., Southampton 509 3AT, England, for food containers carries the name Intene 50A™.

Fluoroelastomers and fluorochloroelastomers have excellent thermal and chemical stability. The Commercial Chemicals Division of 3M, St. Paul, MN, sells Fluorel FC™ fluoroelastomer and provides compounding recommendations for formulations to be used in FDA-controlled food contact applications. Samples of Fluorel that I have tested have had good mechanical properties and are resistant to a wide variety of solvents.

Allied-Signal Engineered Plastics, Morristown, NJ, retails Aclar 22A™ and Aclar 88A copolymer (primarily chlorotrifluoroethylene) and Aclar 33C terpolymer films for pharmaceutical packaging. Saran HB™ films are sold by Dow Chemical Co., Midland MI, for applications such as blood bags and packaging of drugs, instruments, and supplies. TN-80™ fluoroelastomer terpolymer is available from Ausimont, Morristown, NJ.

Ethyl Corporation, Baton Rouge, LA, has a polyphosphazine fluoroelastomer, Eypal F that is being evaluated as a dental liner material [51].

Isobutylene/isoprene copolymers are commonly called butyl rubber. Polysar Inc., Akron, OH, lists Butyl 101-3™ for use with pharmaceuticals, Butyl 402 for food and drug applications, and Butyl 111 for other food contact applications. These polymers have differing degrees of unsaturation, from 0.7 to 2.2%. Polysar Bromobutyl X2 is faster-curing and suitable for use in pharmaceutical closures.

Polysar also sells Butyl 101-3 as a stabilizer-free isoprene/isobutylene copolymer that is used as a chewing gum base and other food and drug applications. I have successfully used it in the manufacture of artificial heart compliance chamber diaphragms.

Natural rubber and synthetic polyisoprenes are available from companies. For example, Exxon Chemical Company, Buffalo Grove, IL, also has an assortment of isobutylene and isobutylene-based butyl and chlorobutyl rubbers which comply with FDA regulations for diverse end-use applications. Goodyear Tire and Rubber Company, Akron, OH, sells Natsyn™ (polyisoprene) which can be used for biomedical applications such as urinary drainage catheters, tourniquets, rubber gloves, and stethoscope tubing.

Polychloroprene latex can be formulated to have properties superior to natural rubber. DuPont Neoprene™ latex has been used in biomedical applications such as gastric balloons.

Polyester/polyadipate copolymer named Pellethane 2355™ is said to meet FDA and USDA requirements by Dow Chemical Company, Midland, MI.

PVC/nitrile butadiene blends are marketed by B.F. Goodrich, Chemical Group, Cleveland, OH under the name Hycar 503-H™ for food packaging.

Styrene butadiene rubber (SBR) medical grades are sold by a variety of suppliers. The Goodyear Tire and Chemical Company, Akron, OH sells Plioflex 1027™ and Plioflex 1028 for a chewing gum base. Shell Chemical Company, Houston, TX sells Kraton 1101™ for some food contact applications, and Texas-U.S. Chemical Company, Greenwich, CT sells Synpol 1061™ with an FDA-approved stabilizer.

POLYPEPTIDE ELASTOMERS FOR BIOMEDICAL APPLICATIONS

Poly-alpha-L-amino acids are the building blocks of proteins. When the primary structure (sequence of amino acid residues), secondary structure (conformation or 3-dimensional structure) and tertiary structure (arrangement or organization of multiple molecules to form a structure) of the poly amino acids are suitable, an elastomeric macromolecule is formed that can have biomedical application. These can either be produced naturally or they can be custom synthesized. The naturally occurring polypeptides or proteins can be modified or post-treated to change desired properties.

Collagen is the structural protein that provides strength to both skin and bones. The primary structure of collagen has glycine as every third amino acid residue along the approximately 1050 amino acid chain, with the exception of the short teleopeptide end region. This allows the collagen molecule to form a 3_1 helix as the secondary structure, with the glycines in the center of the helix. The tertiary structure of collagen is an overlapping quarter stagger arrangement with some supercoiling. When collagen is heated, the 3_1 helixes fall apart, forming a random organization called gelatin.

Biomedically, collagen is used in the form of intact tissues such as the pericardium (the sac around the heart), for items such as artificial heart valves. Most often, these natural tissues are post-treated with either formaldehyde or glutaraldehyde to retard *in vivo* degradation and to diminish the antigenicity of the materials.

The most common pericardium used for heart valves is bovine (that of the cow). Bovine pericardium has also been evaluated as a ligament substitute at the University of Arizona, Tucson, AZ [52] and an evaluation of its tensile strength after differing treatments has been conducted at the University of Sheffield, Sheffield, United Kingdom [53]. Porcine (pig), ovine (sheep), and caprine (goat) pericardia have been used, along with pericardia from some less common sources, such as that of the yak used at the Chengdu University of Science and Technology, Chengdu, Peoples Republic of China [54].

Human dura mater, the tough coating that protects the brain from the skull, is mostly collagen and is routinely used for construction of the artificial heart valves used in artificial hearts and left ventricular assist systems at the Cleveland Clinic Foundation, Cleveland, OH, and as a meniscus replacement at Loma Linda, CA [55]. Gelatin is used as a blood-compatible surface on artificial heart pump diaphragms at the Cleveland Clinic Foundation, Cleveland, OH, after cross-linking with glutaraldehyde.

Elastin is an amorphous, elastic protein that is the primary elastic component of arteries and skin. Elastin has been used at the Université de Bordeaux, Bordeaux, Cedex, France [56], and the Université Louis Pasteur, Strasbourg, France [57] in combination with fibrin, fibronectin, and collagen to produce an artificial connective tissue matrix. The University of Arizona has experimented with primarily elastin vascular prostheses.

Random copolymers synthesized with specifically

selected ratios of amino acids can give polymers with a wide range of mechanical properties and elasticities from stiff to flexible. Synthetic sequential polypeptides that mimic the peptide sequence of natural elastomers have also been evaluated for biomedical uses. Researchers at locations such as Case Western Reserve University, Cleveland, OH, for example, have made small quantities of sequential polypeptides since the early 1970s. These polypeptides can mimic natural functions and can be designed to be either relatively biostable or biodegradable. When they degrade, they form for the most part only their component amino acids. A review of some of this field focusing on elastomeric polypeptides has recently been published [58].

Polyamino acids can also be copolymerized with other synthetic polymers, as evidenced by the work at Chonnam National University of Korea on poly (benzyl-L-glutamate)/poly(propylene glycol) block copolymers [59] and the work at Konan University, Kobe, Japan, on poly(L-leucine)/poly(ethylene oxide)/poly(L-leucine) triblock copolymers [60].

Research continues, and the range of biomedical elastomers available for selection continues to increase at a rapid pace.

REFERENCES

1. Howard, Michael J., ed. 1980. *Elastomers, Edition #2*. San Diego, CA: Cordura Publications, Inc.

2. "An Engineering Guide to Elastomer Selection and Manufacturing Standards", Minor Rubber Company Inc., Bloomfield, NJ.

3. Martino, R. 1990. *Modern Plastics*, 67(1):53–109.

4. Ward, R., P. Litwak, K. White, J. Robinson, I. Yilgor and J. Riffle. 1987. *Trans. of 13th Annual Meeting of the Society for Biomaterials*. Society for Biomaterials, p. 259.

5. Tingfei, X., W. Chunren, T. Wenhua and L. Xuehui. 1988. *Trans. 3rd World Biomaterials Congress 1988, Volume XI*. Kyoto, Japan: Business Center for Academic Societies Japan, p. 426.

6. Szycher, M., W. Clay, D. Gernes and C. Sherman. 1986. *J. Biomaterials Applications*, 1:39.

7. Sintov, A., W. Scott, K. Beckel, R. Siden and R. J. Levy. 1989. *Trans. of 15th Annual Meeting of the Society for Biomaterials*. Society for Biomaterials, p. 140.

8. Pinchuk, L., D. C. MacGregor, G. J. Wilson, J. B. Martin Jr., P. Klement, M. C. Esquivel and S.P. Halbert. 1989. *Trans. of 15th Annual Meeting of the Society for Biomaterials*. Society for Biomaterials, p. 136.

9. Sevastianov, V. I. and V. M. Parfev. 1987. *Artificial Organs*, 11(1):20–25.

10. Ting-Fei, X., W. Chun-Ren, T. Wen-Hua and L. Xue-Hui. 1989. *Trans. of 15th Annual Meeting of the Society for Biomaterials*. Society for Biomaterials, p. 11.

11. Ratner, B. D., K. W. Gladhill and T. A. Horbett. 1988. *J. Biomed. Mater. Res.*. 22:509–527.

12. Phua, S. K., E. Castillo, J. M. Anderson and A. Hiltner. 1987. *J. Biomed. Mater. Res.*, 21:231–246.

13. Smith, R., D. F. Williams and C. Oliver. 1987. *J. Biomed. Mater. Res.*, 21:1149–1166.

14. Brown, S. A., J. Milman, J. Piontkowski, J. Mason, A. Moet and K. Merritt. 1989. *Trans. of 15th Annual Meeting of the Society for Biomaterials*. Society for Biomaterials, p. 202.

15. Sung, P. and A. C. Fraker. 1987. *J. Biomed. Mater. Res.*, 21(3A):287–297.

16. Coury, A., P. Cahalan, E. Halverson, P. Slaikeu and K. Stokes. 1988. *Trans. 3rd World Biomaterials Congress 1988, Volume XI*. Kyoto, Japan: Business Center for Academic Societies Japan, Tokyo, p. 432.

17. Stokes, K., P. Urbanski and A. Coury. 1988. *Trans. 3rd World Biomaterials Congress 1988, Volume XI*. Kyoto, Japan: Business Center for Academic Societies Japan, Tokyo, p. 434.

18. Thoma, R. J., R. E. Phillips and F. R. Tan. 1988. *Trans. 3rd World Biomaterials Congress 1988, Volume XI*. Kyoto, Japan: Business Center for Academic Societies Japan, Tokyo, p. 430.

19. Benson, R. S. and R. P. Wong. 1988. *Trans. 3rd World Biomaterials Congress 1988, Volume XI*. Kyoto, Japan: Business Center for Academic Societies Japan, Tokyo, p. 124.

20. Hayashi, K. 1988. *Trans. 3rd World Biomaterials Congress 1988, Volume XI*. Kyoto, Japan: Business Center for Academic Societies Japan, Tokyo, p. 123.

21. Zhao, Q., M. P. Agger, M. Fitzpatrick, J.M. Anderson, A Hiltner, K. Stokes and P. Urbanski. "Cellular Interactions with Biomaterials: *In vivo* Cracking of Prestressed Pellethane 2363-80A", pre-publication manuscript.

22. Zhao, Q., M. P. Agger, M. Fitzpatrick, J. M. Anderson, K. Stokes and P. Urbanski. 1989. *Trans. of 15th Annual Meeting of the Society for Biomaterials*. Society for Biomaterials, p. 203.

23. Iwamoto, R., K. Ohta, T. Matsuda and K. Imachi. 1986. *J. Biomed. Mater. Res.*, 20:507–520.

24. Ward, R. S., K. A. White and I. Yilgor. 1988. *Trans 3rd World Biomaterials Congress 1988, Volume XI*. Kyoto, Japan: Business Center for Academic Societies Japan, Tokyo, p. 433.

25. Takamatsu, T., Y. Tanaka, H. Sasabe and K. Kira. 1988. *Trans. 3rd World Biomaterials Congress 1988, Volume XI*. Kyoto, Japan: Business Center for Academic Societies Japan, Tokyo, p. 427.

26. Hayashi, K., K. Takamizawa, K. Kira, K. Hiramatsu and H. Matsumoto. 1988. *Trans. 3rd World Biomaterials Congress 1988, Volume XI*. Kyoto, Japan: Business Center for Academic Societies Japan, Tokyo, p. 132.

27. Grasel, T. G., A. P. Hart and S. L. Cooper. 1988. *Trans. 3rd World Biomaterials Congress 1988, Volume XI*. Kyoto, Japan: Business Center for Academic Societies Japan, Tokyo, p. 424.

28. Okkema, A. T., T. J. McCoy, Q. J. Lai, R. W. Hergenrotter and S.L. Cooper. 1989. *Trans. of 15th Annual Meeting of the Society for Biomaterials*. Society for Biomaterials, p. 6.

29. Cooper, S. L., T. G. Grasel, W. G. Pitt, A. T. Okkema

and A. D. Peterson. 1988. *Trans. 3rd World Biomaterials Congress 1988, Volume XI.* Kyoto, Japan: Business Center For Academic Societies Japan, Tokyo, p. 30.

30. Takakura, T., M. Kato, H. Nishimura, K. Kataoka, T. Okano and Y. Sakural. 1988. *Trans. 3rd World Biomaterials Congress 1988, Volume XI.* Kyoto, Japan: Business Center for Academic Societies Japan, Tokyo, p. 423.

31. Zdrahala, R. J., M. A. Strand and E. Pechhold. 1988. *Trans. 3rd World Biomaterials Congress 1988, Volume XI.* Kyoto, Japan: Business Center for Academic Societies Japan, Tokyo, p. 425.

32. Barbucci, R., M. Benvenute, G. Dal Maso, M. Nocentini and F. Tempesti. 1988. *Trans. 3rd World Biomaterials Congress 1988, Volume XI.* Kyoto, Japan: Business Center for Academic Societies Japan, Tokyo, p. 286.

33. Kim, Y. H., K. D. Ahn, S. Y. Jeong, U. Y. Kim, D. K. Han, J. Park, H. I. Cho and Y. S. Hwang. 1988. *Trans. 3rd World Biomaterials Congress 1988, Volume XI.* Kyoto, Japan: Business Center for Academic Societies Japan, Tokyo, p. 288.

34. Park, K. D., T. Okano, C. Nojiri and S. W. Kim. 1988. *Trans. 3rd World Biomaterials Congress 1988, Volume XI.* Kyoto, Japan: Business Center for Academic Societies Japan, Tokyo, p. 287.

35. Kitamoto, Y., H. Sugai, H. Takahashi, Y. Yabushita, M. Nakayama, T. Sato and K. Mori. 1988. *Trans. 3rd World Biomaterials Congress 1988, Volume XI.* Kyoto, Japan: Business Center for Academic Societies Japan, Tokyo, p. 321.

36. Pitt, W. G and S. L. Cooper. 1988. *J. Biomed. Mater. Res.*, 22:359-382.

37. Frautschi, J. R., G. P. Clagett, P. V. Kulkarni and R. C. Eberhart. 1988. *Trans. 3rd World Biomaterials Congress 1988, Volume XI.* Kyoto, Japan: Business Center for Academic Societies Japan, Tokyo, p. 318.

38. Alexandrou, B., R. Read and S. K. Li. 1978. *J. Med. Eng. Technol.* 2:75-76.

39. DeChamplain, R. W., C. S. Gallagher Jr. and E. T. Marshall Jr. 1988. *J. Oral Maxillofac. Surg. (U.S.A.),* 522-525.

40. Hartman, L, R. W. Bessette, R. E. Baier, A. E. Meyer and J. Wirth. 1988. *J. Biomed. Mater. Res.*, 22:475-484.

41. McMillin, C. R., M. R. Malladi, D. W. Ott, M. M. Evancho and S. P. Schmidt. 1988. *J. Biomed. Mater. Res.*, 22:339.

42. 1988. "High Technology Silicones from McGhan NuSil", McGhan NuSil Corporation, Carpinteria, CA, (February).

43. Deisler, R., E. Perrin, R. Carew and E. P. Goldberg. 1988. *Trans. 3rd World Biomaterials Congress 1988, Volume XI.* Kyoto, Japan: Business Center for Academic Societies Japan, Tokyo, p. 429.

44. Carew, R. 1988 Winter Meeting Technical Papers. Akron, OH: Akron Rubber Group, Inc., pp. 55-58.

45. 1987. "Catalog of Biomaterials, Specialty Polymers and Reactive Intermediates", Mercor Incorporated, A Thoratec Company (February).

46. Miyake, H. and T. Fujimoto. 1988. *Trans. 3rd World Biomaterials Congress 1988, Volume XI.* Kyoto, Japan: Business Center for Academic Societies Japan, Tokyo, p. 100.

47. Sung, C., M. R. Sobarzo, J. E. Raeder and E. W. Merrill. 1988. *Trans. 3rd World Biomaterials Congress 1988, Volume XI.* Kyoto, Japan: Business Center for Academic Societies Japan, Tokyo, p. 237.

48. Grainger, D. W., S. W. Kim and J. Feijen. 1988. *J. Biomed. Mater. Res.*, 22:231-249.

49. McMillin, C. R. 1987. *J. Biomaterials Applications*, 2:3-100.

50. Yamashita, I., N. Yamamoto, K. Hayashi and K. Iwata. 1988. *Trans. 3rd World Biomaterials Congress 1988, Volume XI.* Kyoto, Japan: Business Center for Academic Societies Japan, Tokyo, p. 289.

51. Gettleman, L., L. R. Guerra, I. M. Finger, G. T. McDonald, L.M. Jameson, M. M. Salib, A. K. Agarwal, J. M. Vargo and K. C. Coist. 1988. *Trans. World Biomaterials Congress 1988, Volume XI.* Kyoto, Japan: Business Center for Academic Societies Japan, Tokyo, p. 162.

52. Chvapil, M., D. Gebeault and T. F. Wang. 1987. *J. Biomed. Mater. Res.*, 21:1383-1393.

53. Crofts, C. E. and E. A. Trowbridge. 1988. *J. Biomed. Mater. Res.*, 22:89-98.

54. Yi-lun, Y. and Z. Sheng-ping. 1988. *Trans. 3rd World Biomaterials Congress 1988, Volume XI.* Kyoto, Japan: Business Center for Academic Societies Japan, Tokyo, p. 77.

55. Stringer, D. E., P. J. Boyne and P. M. Scheer. 1988. *Trans. 3rd World Biomaterials Congress 1988, Volume XI.* Kyoto, Japan: Business Center for Academic Societies Japan, Tokyo, p. 90.

56. Rabaud, M., M. T. Martin, R. Schmittheausler, F. Lefebvre and M. Aprahamian. 1988. *Trans. 3rd World Biomaterials Congress 1988, Volume XI.* Kyoto, Japan: Business Center for Academic Societies Japan, Tokyo, p. 79.

57. Marescaux, J., M. Aprahamian, M. Wilhelm, M. Rabaud, E. Loza and R. Schmitthauesler. 1988. *Trans. 3rd World Biomaterials Congress 1988, Volume XI.* Kyoto, Japan: Business Center for Academic Societies Japan, Tokyo, p. 81.

58. Urry, D. W. 1988. *Research and Development*, 30:(8)57.

59. Cho, C. S., S. C. Song, Y. O. Kim, S. S. Kim, S. P. Suh, K. Y. Kim and Y. K. Sung. 1989. *Trans. of 15th Annual Meeting of the Society for Biomaterials.* Society for Biomaterials, p. 8.

60. Kugo, K., T. Kitaura, J. Nishino, H. Matsuda, M. Iwatsuki, M. Kayama and M. Honma. 1989. *Trans. of 15th Annual Meeting of the Society for Biomaterials.* Society for Biomaterials, p. 27.

4

Structure-Property Relations in Polyurethanes

RUDOLPH D. DEANIN, Ph.D.*

ABSTRACT: Polyurethanes enjoy outstanding versatility in their range of monomers, polymerization reactions, processing, structures, properties, and applications. This versatility has contributed greatly to our understanding of polymer structure-property relations in general and to the production of high-performance elastomers, plastics, fibers, foams, coatings, and adhesives. Structure-property relations are best analyzed stepwise from the smallest submolecular structural features, up through molecular weight and flexibility, intermolecular order and bonding, and supermolecular structural features.

INTRODUCTION: MONOMERS, REACTIONS, AND STRUCTURES [1]

Polyol + Polyisocyanate → Polyurethane

Organic polymer researchers can synthesize polyurethanes in many interesting ways. Commercial manufacture is based primarily on the addition reactions of polyols with polyisocyanates:

$$ROH + R'NCO \rightarrow RO\overset{\overset{\displaystyle O}{\|}}{C}-\overset{\overset{\displaystyle H}{|}}{N}R'$$

Diols + diisocyanates produce linear polymers. Triols, triisocyanates, and/or monomers of still higher functionality produce branched and cross-linked polymers. These reactions generally proceed readily at room temperature, particularly with the help of amine and/or organo-tin catalysts. This is the most general reaction for the production of polyurethanes.

*University of Lowell, Plastics Engineering Department, Lowell, MA 01854

Polyols

Three families of structures are commonly used to provide the polyols for manufacture of polyurethanes: polyethers, polyesters, and hydrocarbon backbones.

Polyethers

The most common polyether polyol is poly(oxypropylene) glycol:

$$HO(CH_2\overset{\overset{\displaystyle |}{CH}}{\underset{\underset{\displaystyle CH_3}{|}}{}}O)_nH$$

made by alkaline polymerization of propylene oxide; this provides good flexibility and low cost. For higher strength, poly(oxytetramethylene) glycol:

$$HO(CH_2CH_2CH_2CH_2O)_nH$$

is made by acid polymerization of tetrahydrofuran. Other polyether structures are sometimes used for specialty purposes.

Polyesters

Linear aliphatic polyesters are commonly structures such as poly(ethylene adipate):

$$HO(CH_2CH_2O\overset{\overset{\displaystyle O}{\|}}{C}CH_2CH_2CH_2CH_2\overset{\overset{\displaystyle O}{\|}}{C}O)_nCH_2CH_2OH$$

and are used to provide higher strength. For improved resistance to hydrolysis, polyester polyols are sometimes based on polycaprolactone:

$$HO\left[(CH_2)_5\overset{\overset{\displaystyle O}{\|}}{C}O\right]_n(CH_2)_6\left[\overset{\overset{\displaystyle O}{\|}}{O}C(CH_2)_5\right]_nOH$$

or polycarbonate:

$$HO(CH_2)_6 \left[O\overset{O}{\overset{\|}{C}}O(CH_2)_6 \right]_n OH$$

A naturally-occurring polyester polyol often used in polyurethanes is castor oil:

$$CH_2O\overset{O}{\overset{\|}{C}}(CH_2)_7CH{=}CH{-}CH_2\overset{OH}{\overset{|}{C}H}(CH_2)_5CH_3$$
$$CH{-}O\overset{O}{\overset{\|}{C}}(CH_2)_7CH{=}CH{-}CH_2\overset{OH}{\overset{|}{C}H}(CH_2)_5CH_3$$
$$CH_2O\overset{O}{\overset{\|}{C}}(CH_2)_7CH{=}CH{-}CH_2\overset{OH}{\overset{|}{C}H}(CH_2)_5CH_3$$

Again, other polyester structures are sometimes used for specialty purposes.

Hydrocarbons

For lower polarity, better electrical insulation, and higher resistance to hydrolysis, aliphatic hydrocarbon polyols are sometimes synthesized in structures such as hydroxy-terminated polybutadiene oligomers:

$$HO(CH_2CH{=}CHCH_2)_nOH$$

and their hydrogenated derivatives:

$$HO(CH_2CH_2CH_2CH_2)_nOH$$

These structures are seen more often in research and development than in commercial use [2].

Triols and Higher-Functionality Polyols

Branching and cross-linking are most commonly accomplished by use of higher-functionality polyols. These are most conveniently grown upon a triol or hexol backbone:

$$CH_3CH_2\overset{CH_2OROH}{\underset{CH_2OROH}{\overset{|}{C}}}CH_2OROH$$

$$\begin{array}{c} CH_2OROH \\ | \\ CH{-}OROH \\ | \\ CH{-}OROH \\ | \\ CH{-}OROH \\ | \\ CH{-}OROH \\ | \\ CH_2OROH \end{array}$$

Polyisocyanates

The most common polyisocyanates are toluene diisocyanate (TDI):

2,4-TDI   2,6-TDI

and methylene diphenylisocyanate (MDI):

plus higher oligomers of MDI for higher functionality and cross-linking:

Other aromatic isocyanates, such as naphthalene diisocyanate, are mentioned occasionally.

For resistance to ultraviolet light and outdoor weathering in general, manufacturers usually turn to aliphatic isocyanates such as hexamethylene diisocyanate (HDI):

$$OCN(CH_2)_6NCO$$

and hydrogenated MDI (HMDI):

even though they involve lower polymerization reactivity and higher cost.

Prepolymers

Mixing all the reactants at once—a "one-shot" process—provides the fastest, simplest, and most economical manufacturing technique, and is most often favored in highly competitive commodity fields such as flexible foam. On the other hand, two-step or three-step processes give the manufacturer much greater control over toxicity, reactivity, structure, properties, processability, and finished product quality. In a typical two-step process, the first step is production of a prepolymer:

$$2\ OCNRNCO + HOR'OH \rightarrow OCNR\overset{H\ O}{\overset{|\ \|}{N{-}C}}OR'O\overset{O\ H}{\overset{\|\ |}{C{-}N}}RNCO$$

The second step is then reaction of the prepolymer with a "chain extender", such as a diol or a diamine:

```
OCN-Prepolymer-NCO + HXRXH →
                O H              H O
                ‖ |              | ‖
        ∼∼∼C-N-Prepolymer-N-COXRX∼∼∼
```

to produce growth to high molecular weight. In many cases, controlled cross-linking is introduced as the second or third step.

Cross-Linking (Curing) Agents

For stepwise cross-linking (cure) reactions, the three most common additives are 1,4-butanediol, diamines, and water:

```
OCN-Prepolymer-NCO + HOCH₂CH₂CH₂CH₂OH →
              O H              H O
              ‖ |              | ‖
    ∼∼∼OC-N-Prepolymer-N-COCH₂CH₂CH₂CH₂∼∼∼

OCN-Prepolymer-NCO + H₂N-Diamine-NH₂ →
            H O H            H O H
            | ‖ |            | ‖ |
   ∼∼∼N-C-N-Prepolymer-N-C-N-Diamine∼∼∼

OCN-Prepolymer-NCO + H₂O →
        CO₂↑ + OCN-Prepolymer-NH₂ →
                  H O H
                  | ‖ |
          ∼∼ N-C-N-Prepolymer∼∼∼
```

Thus these additives function as chain-extenders and/or cross-linking agents, depending on the functionality of the prepolymer and the overall stoichiometry of the reaction.

In vulcanization of polyurethane elastomers, rubber compounders also use conventional sulfur cure, producing sulfide and polysulfide links between polyurethane chains, and sometimes peroxide cure, producing direct $C-C$ links between polyurethane chains.

Indigenous Cross-Linking Reactions

Aside from higher-functionality polyols, polyisocyanates, and/or polyamines, there are several other reactions which can contribute significant cross-linking during polymerization and cure of polyurethanes.

Allophanate

When polyurethane is formed in the presence of excess polyisocyanate, the urethane group can supply active hydrogen to react with the isocyanate:

```
        O                      O
        ‖                      ‖
∼∼RNCO   + OCNR'∼∼  →  ∼∼RNCO
    |                      |
    H                      C-NR'∼∼
                           ‖
                           O H
```

thus forming a branch point. Obviously a diisocyanate could similarly form a cross-link between two polyurethane chains. These cross-links are not as stable as the conventional cross-links formed from polyfunctional polyols and polyisocyanates; they are thermally labile and open quite easily at higher temperatures.

Biuret

When polyurea is formed in the presence of excess polyisocyanate, the urea group can supply active hydrogen to react with the isocyanate:

```
      O H                              O H
      ‖ |                              ‖ |
∼∼RNC-N∼∼  + OCNR'∼∼   →   ∼∼RNC-N∼∼
      |                              |
      H                              C-NR'∼∼
                                     ‖
                                     O H
```

thus forming a branch point. Obviously a diisocyanate could similarly form a cross-link between two polyurea chains. These cross-links form more readily than allophanates and are somewhat stabler than allophanates, but are still thermally labile and open fairly easily at higher temperatures.

Isocyanurate

Under proper conditions, excess isocyanate forms cyclic trimers which are isocyanurates:

```
                              O
                              ‖
                              C
                       R-N        N-R
       3 RNCO →
                      O=C        C=O
                           N
                           |
                           R
```

When the isocyanate is a diisocyanate or higher polyisocyanate, these isocyanurate rings act as extremely stable cross-links in the polyurethane network. They are used to produce polyurethanes of high heat stability and flame retardance.

Block Copolymers

When small comonomer units are assembled randomly into a polymer molecule:

```
∼∼∼-ABAABABBBABBAAABABBAB-∼∼∼
```

the resulting random copolymer has an overall average structure which is fairly uniform, and forms a single homogeneous phase containing this average composition and structure. When the growth of a copolymer molecule produces fairly large areas (blocks) of one monomer structure, alternating with fairly large areas (blocks) of another monomer structure:

~~~~ -AAAAAAAAAABBBBBBBBBB- ~~~~

these blocks will tend to separate into microphases or "domains", and each type of domain will contribute independently to the properties of the block copolymer. In polyurethanes, the polyol generally forms fairly large blocks even before they are reacted with the polyisocyanate. Furthermore, in stepwise synthesis of polyurethanes, the first-stage prepolymer forms one type of block (often called the "soft" block), while the reaction of short chain-extender with isocyanate forms another type of block (often called the "hard" block). Thus polyurethanes are block copolymers. In many cases, the separation of these blocks into domains has major synergistic effects on their properties.

Hetero-Block Copolymers

The stepwise synthesis of polyurethanes, with active hydroxyl, amine, and/or isocyanate end-groups remaining after each intermediate step, provides the organic polymer chemist with the additional possibility of combining these polyurethane blocks with blocks of other polymer structures, to combine the best properties of polyurethanes with the best properties of the other polymers as well. Some of the most common may be described briefly as follows.

Acrylic Esters

Acrylic esters which contain hydroxyl groups are readily combined with polyurethanes which contain isocyanate groups, to produce acrylic-urethane block copolymers.

Epoxy Resins

Some epoxy resins contain hydroxyl groups, and most of them form hydroxyl groups during cure. These react readily with excess isocyanate groups of polyurethanes, to form block copolymers. Conversely, polyurethanes containing terminal hydroxyl or amine groups can act as curing agents for epoxy resins, again forming block copolymers.

Drying Oils

Drying oils are often transesterified with glycerol to form mono- and di-glycerides, containing both drying oil groups and hydroxyl groups. These copolymerize readily with excess isocyanate groups in polyurethanes, to form drying-oil-urethanes, the most common form of polyurethane coatings.

Silicones

Cure of silicone elastomers and resins goes through a transient intermediate silanol stage. At this point, the silanol can react with the hydroxyl and isocyanate end-groups of polyurethanes to form silicone-urethanes which combine some of the best properties of each.

Structure-Property Relationships

All of this polyurethane chemistry produces a broad spectrum of polymer structures which contribute many interesting and useful properties for many fields of technology. On the one hand, study of polyurethane structure and properties has contributed greatly to our understanding of polymer structure-property relationships in general [3,4]. On the other hand, systematic organization of our understanding of polymer structure-property relationships in general [5] can contribute to a sounder understanding of the specific practical relationships in polyurethane polymers and end-products. These are best reviewed from smallest to largest structural features, starting with Sub-Molecular Structure, and continuing on to larger and larger structural features: Molecular Weight, Molecular Flexibility, Intermolecular Order, Intermolecular Bonding, and finally Supermolecular Structures.

SUB-MOLECULAR STRUCTURE: ATOMS AND FUNCTIONAL GROUPS

Polyurethanes may contain aliphatic, ether, ester, aromatic, hydroxyl, amine, isocyanate, urethane, urea, allophanate, biuret, and isocyanurate groups during processing and/or use of the finished product. They may also contain plasticizers and other additives, along with variable amounts of water and other impurities. All of these contribute individually to many properties. A brief review of some of the more important effects is instructive.

Processability

Polyurethanes are the leading example of reactive processing, including all their foams and reaction injection molding (RIM), along with most of their elastomers, castings, coatings, and adhesives. These are high-speed processes based on the high reactivity of aromatic isocyanates. Reactions are fastest with aliphatic amines, slower with aromatic amines. Reactions with polyols and water are fairly competitive, depending on choice of catalyst (amines favor water, organo-tins favor polyols). Primary hydroxyl groups are more reactive than secondary, while aromatic hydroxyls (phenols) are slower and more likely to revert on heating. Reactions with urea and urethane groups are more difficult, but they can form biuret and allophanate cross-links at higher temperatures. Use of aliphatic isocyanates in place of aromatic, for UV- and weather-resistance, generally requires considerably more time and forcing.

Moisture is a ubiquitous impurity which causes hydrolytic waste of isocyanate, unbalanced stoichi-

Table 1. Isodecyl pelargonate plasticizer in polyether urethane elastomer [3].

IDP, wt.%	Glass Transition Temperature, °C
0	−52.5
5	−57.5
10	−61.5
15	−63.5
20	−66.5

ometry, and poor properties in end products. Thus all ingredients and process conditions must be scrupulously dry, and most processors routinely add several percent excess isocyanate to account for all wasteful side-reactions.

Thermal reversion is most noticeable when urethane groups are formed from phenols, somewhat less with allophanate, still less with biuret, but significant in all these structures. Even normal urethane groups can open at higher process temperatures. Such reversion can actually be useful when the rubber processor wants to recycle lightly thermoset scrap.

The N−H groups in urethane and urea structures are still reactive enough for derivatization, grafting, and cross-linking reactions. These are used in allophanate and biuret cross-linking, epoxy copolymerization, heparinization for anti-thrombotic *in vivo* plastics, and controlled release of drugs.

Mechanical Properties

Mechanical properties are most often controlled by molecular flexibility, crystallinity, and cross-linking, which will be discussed later. It is possible to soften polyurethane elastomers by addition of plasticizers such as isodecyl pelargonate (Table 1), similarly to conventional PVC technology; but such techniques have not been of commercial importance. It is also possible that water absorption provides plasticization here as it does in nylons; but since most polyurethanes are already flexible, the added plasticization is not usually significant.

Thermal Properties

Thermal stability of polyurethanes depends primarily on the polymerization ⇌ depolymerization equilibria of the functional groups in the polymer molecule. Urethane groups made from phenols revert quite readily at higher temperatures. Allophanate and biuret cross-links also reopen quite readily on heating. Conventional urethane and urea links decompose at considerably higher temperatures, and isocyanurate rings are stablest of all.

Residual catalysts would be expected to promote such thermal reversion processes. It is not common practice to remove catalysts after polyurethane production, and such a development would certainly be very difficult, but it might be worth the effort in specialized applications.

Flammability of polyurethanes is a frequent concern, particularly in flexible foam bedding and upholstery and in rigid foam insulation. Burning is very effectively retarded either by reactive flame retardants such as polyols containing phosphorus and/or chlorine or bromine, which are built right into the polyurethane molecule during polymerization; or by additive flame retardants such as phosphate esters, halogenated phosphates, and halogenated hydrocarbons, either liquid (plasticizers) or solid (fillers). When halogen is used, either in reactive or additive flame retardants, addition of antimony oxide produces excellent synergism [6].

Electrical Properties

Polyurethanes contain many polar groups which tend to orient in an electrical field, and most polyurethane molecules have enough flexibility to permit their polar groups to orient in this way, producing high dielectric constants. On the other hand, molecular flexibility, and the resulting polar group mobility, are very sensitive to frequency and temperature, so that dielectric "constants" are far from constant, and electrical-mechanical hysteresis produces considerable and variable dielectric loss. Thus polyurethanes are not generally used as high-performance electrical insulation. They are, however, often used as outer sheathing to protect electrical insulation from abrasion and attack by fuel and oil.

Optical Stability

Aromatic polyurethanes absorb ultraviolet light from the sun, but are unable to cope with the excess energy, and degrade to quinoid structures which discolor and often suffer loss of mechanical properties as well. Where weather resistance is important, particularly in coatings, most manufacturers replace aromatic isocyanates by aliphatic isocyanates to solve this problem.

Chemical Properties

Strong polarity and hydrogen-bonding make polyurethanes highly resistant to hydrocarbon fuel and oil, a major advantage for polyurethane elastomers over conventional hydrocarbon rubbers. They also enjoy another major advantage because their saturated structure is resistant to ozone and oxidative aging, whereas most diene-based rubbers have serious problems in this respect.

On the other hand, polarity and hydrogen-bonding make linear polyurethanes dissolve, and cross-linked polyurethanes swell, in polar organic solvents. This is useful in solution processing of fibers, coatings, and adhesives, but a limitation in chemically-resistant products.

Water absorption and hydrolysis, particularly at higher temperatures, cause aging problems in polyurethanes, particularly polyester urethanes. In poly-

Table 2. Hydrolytic stability of polyurethane elastomers [4].

Polyol Used in Making the Elastomer	Hydrolytic Stability
Poly(diethylene glycol adipate)	Poor
Poly(ethylene adipate)	Fair
Poly(butylene-1,4-adipate)	Good
Polycaprolactone	Good
Poly(hexanediol-1,6-carbonate)	Very good
Poly(oxytetramethylene)	Very good

esters, hydrolytic resistance can be improved by use of polycaprolactone and hexamethylene polycarbonate polyols (Table 2). More often the problem is minimized by changing from polyester to polyether polyols, and occasionally even to hydrocarbon-based polyols.

Biodegradation can attack the aliphatic polyester segments of polyurethanes, degrading them to much smaller molecular units. This is a problem in long-life products, but useful in controlled release of drugs, and a possible solution to solid waste disposal problems. Biostability is greatly increased by changing to polyether polyols and by addition of biocides and biostats. Biodegradation can be promoted by use of short straight-chain aliphatic polyester units, and by inocculation, humidity, and temperature control in solid waste disposal units.

MOLECULAR WEIGHT

High molecular weight is the most distinctive structural feature that differentiates between polymer molecules and all other types of materials. The effects of molecular weight on polymer properties are commonly generalized by the rule that "Lower molecular weight is easier to process, but higher molecular weight gives better end-use properties". Many properties change from low to medium molecular weight, but then approach an asymptote and become fairly constant from high to very high molecular weight. In the polyurethane field, it is generally assumed that final molecular weights are in this high to very high range, and that therefore molecular weight is not a significant variable affecting polyurethane properties.

While this may be true in respect to many properties, there are some properties which depend significantly on molecular weight. These deserve careful consideration.

Processability

Most polyurethane processing is based on the use of low-molecular-weight liquid prepolymers, which are easily handled at atmospheric or low pressure in lightweight equipment, before rapid reactions convert them into solid end products. Liquid viscosities are a direct function of prepolymer molecular weight, so specific process techniques dictate the optimum molecular weight that can be used.

Solution processing of fibers, coatings, and adhesives depends on optimum solution viscosity, which is controlled by polyurethane molecular weight and solution concentration. Generally it is desirable to work at maximum concentration, to minimize solvent problems such as flammability, toxicity, recovery, and cost. Thus lower molecular weights are generally desirable. Often these are achieved by use of reactive prepolymers.

Melt processing viscosities depend on polymer molecular weight. This is important in extrusion of fibers, and in extrusion and injection molding of thermoplastic elastomers. Sometimes the lower molecular weight required for easy melt processing conflicts with the higher molecular weight required for best end-use properties. Some "thermoplastic" elastomers are designed with some residual reactivity, which permits them to be melt processed at lower molecular weight and then polymerized or cross-linked up to higher molecular weight to improve end-use properties. Reaction injection molding takes the extreme position, mixing and injecting low-molecular-weight prepolymers, and then polymerizing and cross-linking them rapidly in the mold to produce the best end-use properties.

The largest usage of polyurethanes is in production of flexible and rigid foams by reactive processing. Here low-molecular-weight reactive prepolymers are mixed and poured, with polymerizing, foaming, and curing happening in rapid overlapping succession. The dynamic balance between increasing viscosity and gas bubble formation is very critical for optimum foam formation [7]. If gas bubbles form at too low a viscosity, they grow irregularly, burst, and collapse. If they form at too high a viscosity, the gas pressure is insufficient to produce full expansion, and the foam is too dense. The optimum dynamic balance is achieved in flexible foam by balancing catalysis of the isocyanate-polyol reaction vs. the isocyanate-water reaction. In rigid foams it is achieved by balancing polymerization rate and exotherm against volatility of the physical blowing agent.

Mechanical Properties

Modulus, strength, extensibility, creep resistance, lubricity, and abrasion resistance generally increase with increasing molecular weight. This is particularly true in thermoplastic polymers, so these effects should be observable in thermoplastic polyurethanes, particularly elastomers. In thermoset polymers of infinite molecular weight, they would tend to approach high level values which would then become a function of cross-linking rather than of molecular weight itself. This will be discussed later.

Thermal Stability

Thermal stability is generally greater at higher molecular weight, because higher molecular weights have less mobility and reach asymptotic properties which are less sensitive to scission. Such effects might be observed in thermoplastic polyurethanes; but in cross-linked polymers, stability would probably depend primarily on cross-link concentration rather than on the molecular weight itself.

Solubility

In many linear polymers, low molecular weights are soluble in a fairly broad range of solvents; as molecular weight increases, choice of solvents becomes more restricted (as predicted from thermodynamic theory), and solution viscosity rises rapidly. This is undoubtedly true in solution processing of thermoplastic polyurethanes. Since most polyurethanes are cross-linked, solubility becomes irrelevant; if they are attracted to solvents of similar polarity and hydrogen bonding, degree of swelling is limited precisely by the degree of cross-linking, which will be discussed later.

MOLECULAR FLEXIBILITY

The inherent flexibility of the individual polymer molecule is an important theoretical concept, and it has many consequences in practical properties. The subject is best divided into these two separate aspects.

Effect of Structure on Molecular Flexibility

The structure of the individual polymer molecule determines its inherent flexibility. In the absence of crystallinity, intermolecular attractions, or cross-linking, the polymer molecule is free to exhibit its inherent flexibility, and has major effects on polymer properties. Even in the presence of such conflicting factors, the inherent flexibility of the polymer molecule is still very important, but the evidence for it is more obscure, and the practical effects are more complex. Those conflicting factors will be discussed later. For the present, let us consider the simple concept of the inherent flexibility of the individual polymer molecule.

Molecular flexibility depends upon freedom of rotation about the single bonds in the main chain of the polymer molecule; restriction of rotation reduces molecular flexibility. A linear aliphatic chain:

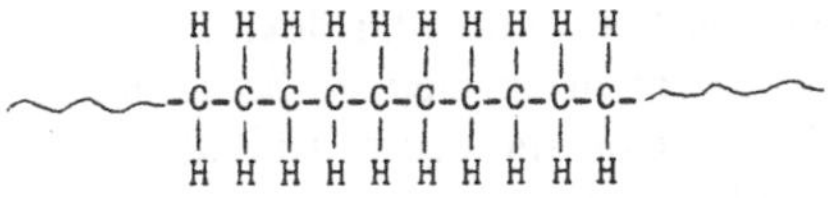

is fairly free to rotate about its $C-C$ bonds, but is restricted by (a) the 109° angle between $C-C-C$ bonds

Table 3. Molecular flexibility of ether groups [3].

Glycol Reacted with Hexamethylene Diisocyanate	Polyurethane Melting Point
HO(CH$_2$)$_5$OH	151°C
HO(CH$_2$)$_2$O(CH$_2$)$_2$OH	120°C
HO(CH$_2$)$_2$S(CH$_2$)$_2$OH	132°C

Table 4. Aromatic stiffening of polyester urethane foams [3].

Aromatic Structure	Tensile Strength	Ultimate Elongation
21.8%	55 PSI	10%
16.6	35	60
15.9	27	160
14.7	26	270
12.6	25	350

and (b) the electropositive repulsion between adjacent H atoms, requiring a certain amount of energy to rotate them past each other. When a $-CH_2-$ is replaced by an oxygen:

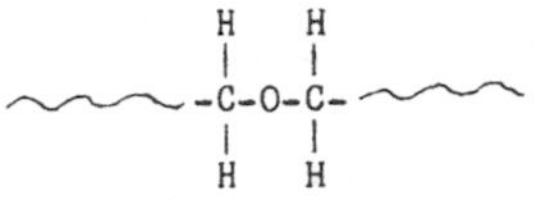

rotation around the $C-O$ bond does not bring H atoms into conflict with each other, so rotation is easier and the molecule is more flexible; this occurs in polyethers (Table 3), polyesters, and even polyurethanes. Sulfide links:

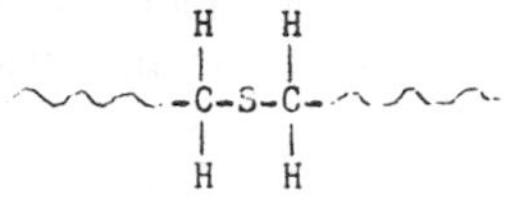

although less common, have a similar effect. When methyl side groups are attached to the aliphatic main chain

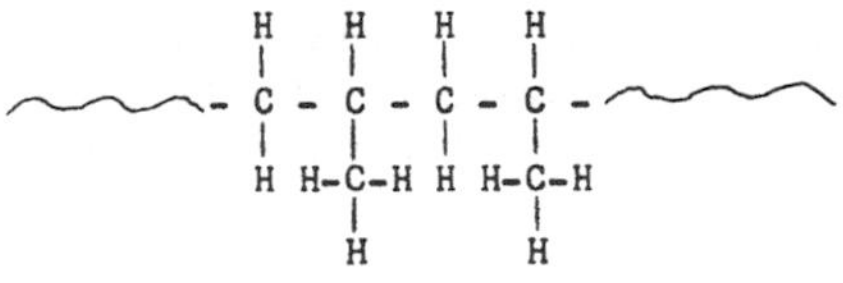

in an amorphous polymer, steric hindrance restricts rotation around the main chain, and the molecule becomes stiffer. (It will be noted later that, in crystalline polymers, random methyl side groups reduce regularity and crystallinity, and thus make the solid *mass* of polymer molecules more flexible.) When aro-

Table 5. Polyaromatic stiffening of polyester urethane elastomer [3].

Diisocyanate Used in Making Polyurethane	Tensile Strength
2,4-Toluene diisocyanate	3200 PSI
1,5-Naphthalene diisocyanate	4400
2,7-Fluorene diisocyanate	6200

matic groups are present, particularly in the main chain:

they introduce large flat rigid units which greatly reduce molecular flexibility (Table 4). When the aromatic rings are conjugated with adjacent unsaturated groups in the main chain, the entire conjugated resonating unit becomes much larger:

and the stiffening effect is much greater. Likewise, in polyaromatic systems such as naphthalene units:

the stiffening effect extends further and becomes much greater (Table 5). To repeat, these effects are most clearly seen in amorphous polymers of low intermolecular attraction and no cross-linking; when these complications occur, they interact with molecular flexibility, and often overpower it so that its effects are no longer clearly seen. This will be discussed later.

Processability

In liquid and melt processing, flexible polymer molecules coil and uncoil and disentangle more easily, and give lower viscosity and easier processing. Similarly, in solution processing, flexible polymer molecules form a random coil of small diameter, low viscosity, and easy processing; whereas stiff polymer molecules remain extended in solution, presenting much larger end-to-end dimensions, higher viscosity, and more difficult processing. Thus molecular flexibility generally brings easier processing.

Mechanical Properties

Without the complications of crystallinity, intermolecular attraction, and cross-linking, molecular flexibility generally permits the polymer molecules to disentangle and flow more easily when mechanical stress is applied. This generally gives lower hardness, modulus, strength, creep resistance, and lubricity, along with higher extensibility and friction (Tables 6–7).

Thermal Properties

For any given molecular structure, increasing temperature means increasing atomic and molecular motion, greater free volume, higher energy to overcome electronic repulsion and steric hindrance, and thus greater molecular flexibility. Thus, practical molecular flexibility is the summation of (a) inherent molecular flexibility plus (b) thermal mobility. Conversely, polymers with inherent molecular flexibility retain this flexibility down to lower temperatures, giving lower glass transition temperature, retaining flexibility or toughness down to lower temperature, but suffering lower heat deflection temperature, and greater loss of strength and creep deformation at high temperatures.

Thermal stability tends to correlate with molecular rigidity, because chemical reaction and degradation depend on molecules moving and meeting each other, and these become more difficult when the molecules have less flexibility.

Electrical Properties

As noted earlier, molecular flexibility permits polar groups to orient in an electric field, producing high dielectric constant; molecular rigidity prevents orientation, producing low dielectric constant. Since practical molecular flexibility/rigidity depends not only on molecular structure, but also on temperature and frequency, polyurethanes do not have constant dielectric "constant"; and in the transition region they have considerable dielectric loss, so they are not generally used in demanding electrical insulation applications.

It is probably also true that molecular flexibility gives lower electrical resistivity, but these data are not usually available.

Table 6. Poly(oxypropylene) flexibility in polyurethane elastomers [3].

Poly(oxypropylene) MW:	1000	1250	1500	2000
Hardness, shore A	88	77	67	60
300% Secant modulus, PSI	2100	1000	600	400
Tensile strength, PSI	5050	4500	3500	1200
Graves tear strength, lb/in	310	240	225	125
Bashore resilience, %	24	20	22	38
Taber abrasion loss, Mg/1000 cycles	85	60	25	8
Tinius Olsen brittle point, °C	−40	−50	−55	−56

Table 7. Molecular flexibility in polyurethane elastomers [8].

	Poly(oxytetramethylene)			Poly(ethylene adipate)		
	650 (MW)	1000 (MW)	2000 (MW)	1000 (MW)	2000 (MW)	3000 (MW)
Hardness, shore A	78	76	75	74	73	71
100% Secant modulus, PSI	605	521	446	462	376	341
Tensile strength, PSI	3500	2980	2530	2320	1620	1350
Tear strength, PI	385	361	344	330	315	306
Ultimate elongation, %	488	640	710	643	735	856
Rebound, %	33	51	55	21	39	45
Coeff. kinetic friction	0.57	0.63	0.59	0.47	0.58	0.52
Abrasion loss, Mg/5000 C	13	9	8	9	9	6

Infrared Spectroscopy

Bending, stretching, and rotation about bonds in the polymer molecule occur at frequencies and energies primarily found in the infrared region of the electromagnetic spectrum. Since each bond absorbs energy at very specific frequencies, this provides sensitive analytical techniques to characterize the structure of polyurethanes. Conversely, for rapid preheating during processing, radiation with these specific frequencies provides a very convenient technique for bringing polyurethanes up to processing temperatures.

Some of these properties depend only on the inherent flexibility of the individual polymer molecule. Other structural features, however, particularly crystallinity, intermolecular attraction, and cross-linking, can immobilize polymer molecules and thus exert controlling effects on many practical properties. These will now be considered.

INTERMOLECULAR ORDER: CRYSTALLINITY

Factors Affecting Crystallinity of Polyurethanes

In the melt and in solution, polymer molecules tend to form random coils, more or less entangled with each other, but relatively free to disentangle, uncoil, recoil, and exhibit more or less liquid flow. On cooling from the melt, or evaporation or coagulation of the solution, irregular molecular structures, such as poly(oxypropylene):

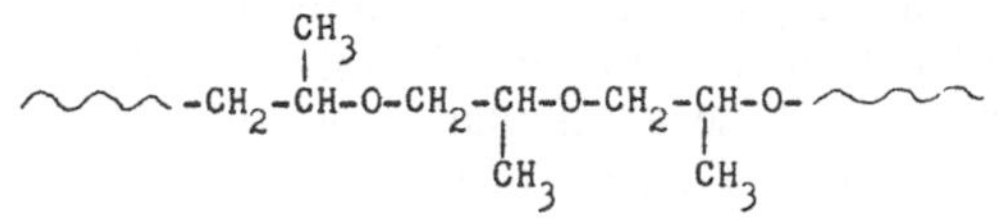

and urethanes from 2,4-toluene diisocyanate:

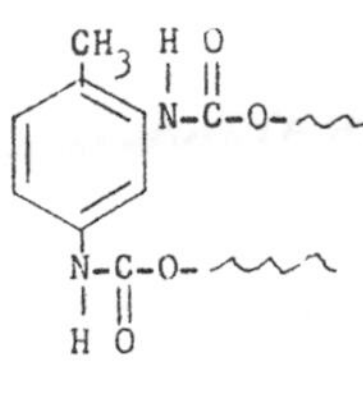

remain in the form of random entangled amorphous coils, and come closer together, with less free volume and less mobility, gradually becoming rubbery and then glassy in properties.

On the other hand, regular molecular structures of reasonable flexibility, such as poly(oxytetramethylene):

polyesters, and urethanes from diphenyl methane-4,4'-diisocyanate (MDI):

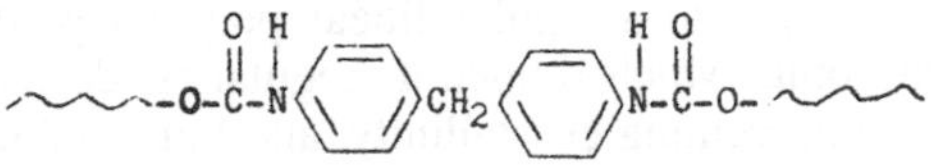

on cooling from the melt or coming out of solution, tend to organize and pack into regular dense crystalline lattice structures, which immobilize the polymer molecules and greatly restrict their "inherent" flexibility, producing much harder, stronger, chemically resistant products. Even in elastomeric polyurethanes, such crystallization may become very apparent in low-temperature stiffening and embrittlement. Thus crystallinity plays a major role in practical properties, often overpowering the significance of inherent molecular flexibility.

Several types of structural features affect the ability of regular polymer structures to fit and pack into the tight regular lattice required for crystallization. On the positive side, (1) a reasonable degree of molecular flexibility makes it possible for polymer molecules to disentangle from random coils and conform and fit into the precise positions required for lattice formation. (2) Intermolecular attractions, which will be discussed later, help to bind the polymer molecules into the crystal lattice, making it stronger and more resistant to mechanical, thermal, and chemical stresses. (3) Monomer units with an even number of atoms in the main chain tend to pack and fit more neatly and densely than those with an odd number, giving stronger crystalline structures (Figure 1).

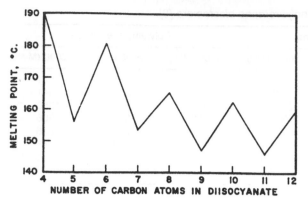

Figure 1. Melting points of polyurethanes from 1,4-butane-diol + Aliphatic isocyanates [3].

Several other types of structural features have negative effects on the ability of polyurethanes to fit and pack into the crystal lattice: (1) Short side groups such as CH_3- make it more difficult for polymer backbones to fit neatly and tightly into the crystal lattice, and thus reduce or prevent crystallinity. (2) When side groups become much longer, they may tend to form little crystallites among themselves, generally referred to as "side-chain crystallization", which restrict molecular mobility and usually give stiffer, more waxy type of properties. (3) Introduction of cross-linking into a regular linear polymer produces branch points which reduce its regularity, decreasing and even preventing crystallinity, and thus "softening" mechanical, thermal, and chemical properties at first; as the degree of cross-linking is increased further and further, it eventually immobilizes the polymer molecules so effectively that properties revert and become "harder" again. The effects of high cross-linking will be discussed separately later.

Effects of Crystallinity on Properties

Processability

Crystalline polymers are held together by a high accumulation of intermolecular attractions, which require more energy to separate the polymer molecules and permit them to flow during processing. In melt processing this means higher temperatures. In solution processing it means much more difficulty in dissolving the polymer molecules into the solvent and keeping them there. In highly crystalline polyurethanes, this can make processing difficult to impossible, thus placing limits on the enthusiasm of the synthetic organic polymer chemist. On the other hand, fast crystallization from the melt can solidify molded and extruded products much faster than the gradual stiffening of amorphous polymers, and thus help to shorten processing cycles handsomely.

Mechanical Properties

Crystallization packs and immobilizes even very flexible polymer molecules, making them much more resistant to mechanical stress. This produces higher hardness, modulus, strength, lubricity, and resistance to creep. All these are desirable in rigid products, but loss of softness and flexibility can be a major concern in flexible foams and elastomers.

Thermal Properties

The attractive forces between polymer molecules tend to hold them into the crystal lattice. Temperature represents the vibrations of atoms and molecules which tend to free them from the crystal lattice and into the mobility of the random coil. Thus the balance of these factors determines the melting point of the crystal structure,

$$T = \frac{\Delta H}{\Delta S}$$

and the contrast between properties above and below this point.

Molecules with high inherent flexibility tend to remain amorphous, soft, and flexible at ambient temperatures. If they are regular in structure, cooling reduces vibrations and encourages crystallization, producing serious stiffening and embrittlement of flexible elastomeric products; whereas random uncrystallizable structures can retain their soft rubbery properties down to much lower temperatures.

Molecules with high intermolecular attractions tend to form more stable crystals, and resist thermal vibrations up to higher temperatures, retaining higher hardness, modulus, strength, and creep resistance, before they eventually melt. In fact, melting point is often accepted as direct evidence of intermolecular attraction, as will be seen later.

Chemical Resistance

Polar solvents are attracted to polar polyurethane molecules. In random amorphous coils, these solvents can easily penetrate the free volume in the random coils, separate them from each other, and dissolve them. In a tightly packed crystalline lattice, on the other hand, there is no room for solvent molecules to penetrate; and the accumulation of attractive forces between polymer chains in the crystal lattice is too great for solvent molecules to compete with it. Thus crystalline polymers have much greater solvent resistance.

INTERMOLECULAR ATTRACTION

In a solid product made of linear polymer molecules, the ability to resist mechanical, thermal, electrical, and chemical stress depends on the attractive forces between the polymer molecules, which transfer these stresses from one molecule to another throughout the solid mass. These secondary attractive forces cover a spectrum from weak long-distance attractions up to fairly strong close-range forces (Table 8), which may be arranged in order as follows.

Order of Intermolecular Attractions

London Dispersion Forces

London dispersion forces are due to the interaction between non-polar electron cloud bonds, typically the $C-C$ and $C-H$ bonds in the hydrocarbon portions of polymer molecules. They are generally 1–2 kcal/mol in strength and 3–5 Å in length.

Permanent Dipoles

Permanent dipoles exist in polyurethane bonds such as $C-O$, $C=O$, $C-N$, $O-H$, and $N-H$. Attractions between such dipoles are typically about 3 kcal/mol in strength and 3 Å in length.

Hydrogen Bonds

Hydrogen bonds form when an electronegative atom in one molecule pulls electrons away from a hydrogen, leaving the hydrogen relatively electropositive and electron-deficient; and an electronegative atom in another molecule shares its extra electrons with the electropositive hydrogen atom:

Such hydrogen bonds are very important in polyurethanes, and are typically 1.5–6 kcal/mol in strength and about 3 Å in length.

Ionic Bonds

Ionic bonds may occur occasionally in polyurethanes:

Table 8. Molar cohesive energies of functional groups in polyurethanes [3].

Group	Cohesive energy, kcal./mole
—CH_2— (Hydrocarbon)	0.68
—O— (Ether)	1.00
—COO— (Ester)	2.90
—C_6H_4— (Aromatic)	3.90
—$CONH$— (Amide)	8.50
—$OCONH$— (Urethane)	8.74

and are typically 10–20 kcal/mol in strength and 2–3 Å in length.

Total Intermolecular Attraction

Total intermolecular attraction is the critical concept, and may be expressed in the form:

$$I = S \times C \times M \times F$$

where I is the total intermolecular attraction per unit volume; S is the strength of a single intermolecular attraction as given above; C is the concentration of such groups in the polymer molecule (the size of the repeat unit); M is the molecular weight of the polymer, which determines the number of such groups in the molecule; and F is the frequency with which such potential intermolecular attractions come close enough to each other to actually form. Thus, for example, London dispersion forces individually have low strength S, but their concentration C is so ubiquitous that they add up to a major portion of the total intermolecular attraction in all polymer molecules; in fact, in hydrocarbon polymers, they alone account for the useful properties of such widely-used polymers as polyethylene, polypropylene, and polystyrene. For another example, in polyurethanes the strength S of polar and hydrogen bonding attractions is great enough to accumulate and give useful properties even at rather modest molecular weight M; whereas in polyolefins, the lower strength S of London dispersion forces requires much higher molecular weights M before they can accumulate to produce useful properties. Additionally, in the random coils of amorphous polyurethanes, the polar and hydrogen-bonding groups (S) of adjacent polymer molecules only rarely come close enough to function (low F), leaving such polymers soft and flexible; whereas in the neatly packed areas of crystalline polyurethanes, the same groups (S) occur close to each other with high frequency (F), producing much greater total attraction and much greater strength and heat resistance.

In general, it is the total intermolecular attraction which best explains effects on practical properties.

Table 9. Intermolecular attraction of urethane groups in elastomers [3].

Urethane Wt. %:	8.4	9.3	10.9	13.6	17.0
Tensile strength, PSI	110	110	140	250	2000
Ultimate elongation, %	190	180	220	340	720
Glass transition, °C	−51	−48	−43	−34	−24
Swelling in benzene, %	524	492	450	368	300

General Effects on Properties

In general, increasing intermolecular attraction makes processing more difficult, requiring higher melt temperatures and more-polar higher-boiling solvents to overcome these attractions and produce good flow. As intermolecular attractions increase, they bring increasing hardness, modulus, strength, and creep resistance. They decrease low-temperature flexibility, but increase hot strength and melting point. They also increase resistance to non-polar fuels and oils, a major advantage over conventional hydrocarbon elastomers and foams (Tables 9 and 10).

Typical Effects

A few examples from polyurethane structure-property relations can serve to illustrate some of these principles.

Polyesters alone have oxygens to serve as electron donors, but only meager amounts of electropositive hydrogens to serve as electron acceptors; for this reason, aliphatic polyesters tend to be weak and low-melting. When aliphatic polyesters are used in polyols to make polyurethanes, however, the N−H groups provide electropositive hydrogens which act as electron acceptors; the resulting hydrogen-bonding in polyester urethanes makes them the optimum choice for high-strength elastomers.

Hydrogen-bonding in polyurethanes is sufficient to provide good properties, but hydrogen-bonding in polyureas is much stronger, and gives much higher strength and melting points. Thus, in making high-performance polyurethane elastomers, use of diamines to create urea groups contributes even more to performance than the urethane groups which take total credit in conventional nomenclature. Even in flexible polyurethane foams, use of water + diisocyanate to produce CO_2 for foaming also incidentally produces diamine, which then reacts to introduce polyurea units into the foam and contributes greatly to its strength.

Introducing ionic bonding between polyurethane chains has been observed to increase hardness, modulus, strength, and glass transition temperature, along with decrease in elongation (Table 11) [9]. All of these effects are evidence that ionic bonding serves to immobilize the polymer molecules and make them more resistant to mechanical and thermal stress.

CROSS-LINKING

The ultimate intermolecular force is a primary covalent cross-link, and these are generally used in the vast majority of polyurethane products.

Cross-Linking Reactions

Most often, cross-links are introduced by use of trifunctional or higher-functional polyols:

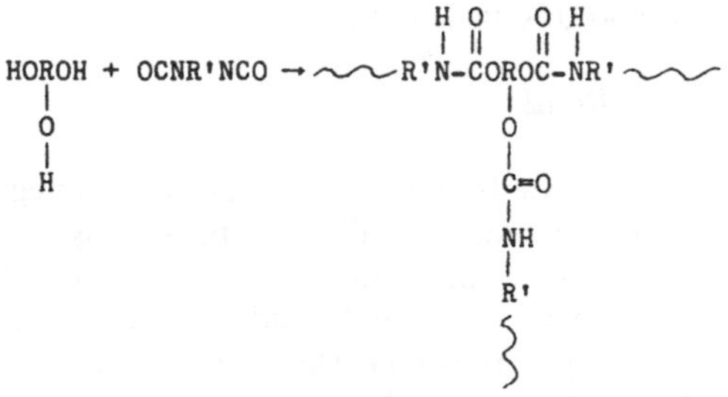

In flexible urethane foams and cast elastomers, the polyol is a long linear Y-shaped triol. In rigid urethane foams, it may be a short-chain polysaccharide hexol. Here the cross-links have the same chemical composition and stability as the main chains.

Second in importance is the use of low-molecular-weight polyisocyanates made from aniline-formaldehyde oligomers:

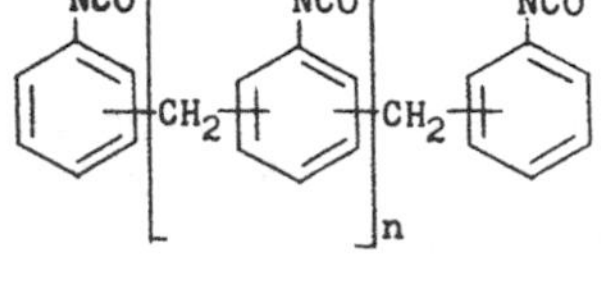

Table 10. Intermolecular attraction of urethane groups in flexible foams [3].

Urethane Wt. %:	10.5	8.3	5.3	4.5	3.4	2.7
100% Secant modulus, PSI	30	16	12	10	7	6
Tensile strength, PSI	30	21	18	20	22	15
Ultimate elongation, %	100	130	155	200	295	340
Compression load at 75%, PSI	8.3	4.3	2.1	1.9	1.6	0.9
Rebound, %	16	15	44	49	42	—
Swelling in dimethyl acetamide, %	145	170	237	240	350	—

These are used primarily in production of rigid foams. Here again the cross-links have the same chemical composition and stability as the main chains.

Often the cross-links are produced by using excess isocyanate in the formulation, and allowing it to react with urethane groups already formed, to produce allophanate cross-links:

or with urea groups already formed, to produce biuret cross-links:

Here the cross-links form somewhat reluctantly, and are less heat-stable than the main chains, tending to open and revert on heating.

The stablest cross-links are formed by using excess isocyanate in the formulation and causing it to form cyclic trimers called isocyanurates:

These are by far the stablest types of cross-links, and are used to produce maximum heat- and flame-resistance.

Cross-linking may be induced by peroxides, either by abstraction of hydrogen, which is quite difficult; or by introduction of vinyl groups into the polyurethane, which requires extra synthetic effort. Either way, the cross-links formed are C−C bonds, which are as stable as the main chain itself.

Rubber processors sometimes buy thermoplastic polyurethane elastomer gums and compound them as they would conventional rubber, using sulfur and accelerators. Such sulfur cross-linking is difficult using saturated elastomers; it can be improved by synthesizing the polyurethane with some vinyl groups to permit conventional sulfur vulcanization reactions. Such sulfur cross-links appear to be less heat-stable than the more common conventional polyurethane cross-linking systems.

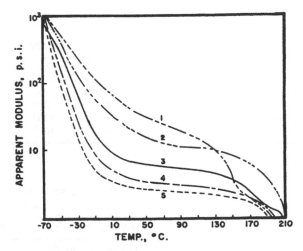

Figure 2. Effect of cross-linking on the modulus vs. temperature curves of polyether urethane foams [3].

Curve	MW between cross-links
1	680
2	1100
3	1350
4	1600
5	2000

Mechanical Properties

The introduction of cross-links between polyurethane molecules produces a definite quantitative restriction of molecular mobility. At low degrees of cross-linking, where long segments of the backbone molecule are still free to move, there is little loss of soft flexible rubbery behavior; and there are distinct improvements in strength and creep resistance (Tables 12,13). In crystalline polymers, low cross-linking de-

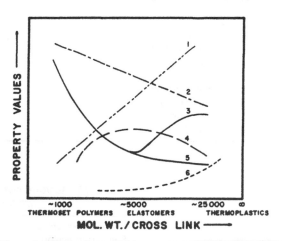

Figure 3. Effects of cross-linking on properties of polyurethanes [3]. Curve 1: solvent swelling, elongation, and tear strength, Curve 2: glass transition temperature and melting point, Curve 3: modulus and hardness for polymers with high intermolecular attractions, Curve 4: elasticity, Curve 5: modulus and hardness for polymers with relatively low intermolecular attractions, Curve 6: creep and compression set.

Table 11. Intermolecular attraction of quaternary ammonium ions [9].

Degree of quaternization, %:	10	20	30	40	60	80	100
Shore A hardness	48	57	65	67	73	78	82
100% Secant modulus, PSI	110	270	320	380	730	780	940
Tensile strength, PSI	670	1080	2800	2980	3170	3620	4250
Ultimate elongation, %	1280	1080	1000	840	790	770	710

Table 12. Low cross-linking of polyether urethane elastomers [3].

MW between cross-links:	2500	4500	8500	12,500
Tensile strength, PSI	200	220	130	160
Ultimate elongation, %	110	190	160	310
Glass transition, °C	−59	−59	−59	−59
Swelling in benzene, %	294	342	384	467

Table 13. Low cross-linking of polyester urethane elastomers [3].

MW between cross-links:	2100	3100	4300	5300	7100	10900	21000	∞
Shore B hardness	57	53	49	46	51	55	56	61
100% Secant modulus, PSI	570	420	300	270	330	460	500	630
Tensile strength, PSI	1800	1750	1450	2800	4500	5600	5500	6750
Ultimate elongation, %	170	200	280	350	410	490	510	640
Tear strength, PI	30	25	30	30	40	60	140	300
Compression set, %	2	16	10	5	25	40	45	55

Table 14. High cross-linking produces rigid thermoset polyurethane plastics [10].

Hexol/diol ratio:	80/20	90/10	100/0
Shore D hardness	77	85	91
Barcol hardness	61	73	83
Tensile modulus, PSI	170,000	410,000	600,000
Ultimate tensile strength, PSI	4,300	8,800	13,250
Ultimate elongation, %	4	2	2
Flexural strength, PSI	7,000	16,700	18,000
Izod notched impact strength, FPI	2.7	0.8	0.5
Abrasion loss, Mg/1000 cycles	32	32	25
Heat deflection temperature, °C	52	78	87
Swelling in acetone, %	27.4	17.9	0.3

Table 15. Acetone-swelling of cross-linked polyether urethane foams [3].

MW between cross-links	1630	1070	690
Swelling in acetone	116	90	83

stroys regularity and reduces crystallinity, and thus actually produces softer properties. With increasing degree of cross-linking, modulus increases and extensibility decreases, giving tough flexible products (Figure 2). At still higher degrees of cross-linking, the polymer molecules are thoroughly immobilized, and become rigid thermoset plastics (Table 14) [10]. Thus cross-linking alone can develop a broad spectrum of polyurethane properties and products (Figure 3).

Thermal Properties

Increasing cross-linking draws polymer backbones closer together, reduces molecular mobility, and thus raises glass transition temperature. Thus, flexible elastomers begin to stiffen at low temperatures. On the other hand, where secondary attractions permit weakening and creep at high temperatures, these are both controlled by the introduction of permanent cross-links.

At higher temperatures the weaker, less-stable types of cross-links tend to reopen and revert back to linear structures. This is noticed first in allophanates, then in biurets. Sulfur vulcanization cross-links are less stable than conventional polyol and polyisocyanate cross-links. When direct $C-C$ cross-links can be formed, these have very good stability. Generally, the stablest are those formed by isocyanate cyclic trimerization into isocyanurate rings. This last is most commonly used for heat- and flame-resistance.

Chemical Resistance

Even the lightest degree of cross-linking will prevent individual polymer molecules from dissolving in solvent. Since there is still strong attraction between polyurethanes and polar solvents, lightly cross-linked polymers will absorb large amounts of solvent and swell to soft gels. Increasing degree of cross-linking produces less free volume for absorption of solvent molecules, and less freedom for polymer chains to move apart to accept them. Thus there is a precise quantitative relationship between swelling and cross-linking (Table 15), which can actually be used to calculate the concentration of cross-links in the polymer. High degrees of cross-linking can even produce considerable improvement in resistance to polar solvents.

Water absorption should similarly be reduced by cross-linking. Furthermore, the degrading effects of hydrolysis upon molecular weight and properties should be retarded by the presence of cross-links to maintain the molecular weight above the critical level needed for useful properties. The extent of such improvement in individual products must however be determined experimentally.

SUPERMOLECULAR STRUCTURE

A number of larger structural features are of major practical importance in the properties and uses of polyurethanes, and some of these are also fairly well understood at the theoretical level as well.

Latex

Polyurethane coatings, adhesives, and fibers are frequently processed by conventional organic solution techniques. Such use of solvents introduces growing problems, of cost, toxicity, flammability, disposal, and recycling, creating growing pressure to reduce or eliminate the use of organic solvents. One attractive alternative is to disperse the polyurethane in aqueous latex, put it in place, and remove the water to deposit the solid polyurethane product. A variety of techniques have been studied to accomplish this.

Finished thermoplastic polyurethanes can be emulsified and used in latex form. Fatty isocyanates of low polarity can be emulsified in water without suffering hydrolysis, and then formulated into reactive systems. Isocyanates can be temporarily blocked to make them stable in water; then the blocking reaction is reversed to liberate the isocyanate for the cure reaction. Such techniques have been described theoretically and sometimes demonstrated experimentally, but practical use is not common.

Table 16. Copolymers of urethane elastomer with epoxy resin [12].

Urethane/ Epoxy	Shore D Hardness	Flexural Modulus	Flexural Strength	Bashore Rebound	Vol. Res.	Diel. Const.	Diss. Factor
100/0	39	4,230 PSI	393 PSI	31%	4×10^{11} oc	7.2	0.048
90/10	41	2,460	224	23	4×10^{11}	6.6	0.047
80/20	50	2,850	270	22	7×10^{11}	5.7	0.036
70/30	64	15,500	480	20	1×10^{12}	4.7	0.024
60/40	72	51,200	2,270	18	7×10^{12}	4.4	0.019
50/50	81	165,000	6,320	17	6×10^{13}	4.1	0.014
40/60	84	238,000	10,300	14	9×10^{13}	3.9	0.012
30/70	87	326,000	13,000	12	2×10^{14}	4.2	0.011
20/80	87	338,000	13,300	9	4×10^{14}	4.4	0.013
10/90	88	361,000	14,000	14	6×10^{14}	4.5	0.015
0/100	90	380,000	15,600	15	2×10^{15}	4.6	0.015

Table 17. Block copolymers of polyester urethane elastomers with poly(ethylene terephthalate) [3].

Second Polyester	15 mole % PET			35 mole % PET			50 mole % PET		
	Tensile Str., p.s.i.	Elong., %	T_g, °C	Tensile Str., p.s.i.	Elong., %	T_g, °C	Tensile Str., p.s.i.	Elong., %	T_g, °C
Poly(ethylene succinate)	1560	6.7	5			27			35.5
Poly(ethylene adipate)	3400	700	−60	4050	500	−41	5300	100	−20
Poly(diethylene adipate)	1700	200		1900	113		4000	90	
Poly(ethylene azelate)	1650	400	−34	1280	13	−30			−6
Poly(ethylene sebacate)			−24	2400	27	−15	2850	10	0

Copolymers

The versatile reactivity of polyols and polyiso-cyanates invites the preparation of copolymers with various other polymer systems to combine the best properties of each. Thus, there are occasional reports of polyurethane copolymers with other common polymer systems. Most important are probably the polyurethane drying oils, which combine conventional drying oil processability with the high performance of polyurethanes [11]. Also popular are acrylic polyurethanes, which combine the easy radiation-cure of the acrylics with the end-use performance of the polyurethanes. More specialized are copolymers with epoxy resins (Table 16) [12], polyesters (Table 17), and silicones. Most of these systems are fairly homogeneous one-phase copolymers, and thus not truly supermolecular structures.

Block Copolymers

Polyurethanes are generally made up of polyol segments of lower polarity, plus polyurethane and/or polyurea segments of higher polarity. When the segments are fairly short, the polymer may have a fairly random homogeneous structure. When the segments are longer, the resulting block copolymer will tend to separate into microphases. The phase present in larger amount will tend to form the continuous matrix and control most of the properties, while the phase present in smaller amount will tend to segregate as discrete domains and contribute specific properties to the composite structure.

Generally the polyol blocks are lower polarity, long and flexible, frequently referred to as "soft segments"; they form the continuous matrix, and make the majority of polyurethanes soft, flexible, and rubbery. In some cases, very regular polyols such as poly(oxytetramethylene) and poly(ethylene adipate) will tend to crystallize, giving higher-strength elastomers, but stiffening when cooled to lower temperatures.

The polyurethane and polyurea blocks are generally higher in polarity and hydrogen-bonding, short and bulky, frequently referred to as "hard segments"; they form the dispersed domains, and contribute strength and creep resistance, and retain these to higher temperatures. Irregular structures such as 2,4-toluene diisocyanate and polymethylene polyphenyl isocyanates generally give glassy hard segments, held together by steric hindrance, polar attraction, and hydrogen-bonding; while regular structures such as diphenylmethane-4,4′-diisocyanate tend to give crystalline hard segments, also held together by steric hindrance, polar attraction, and hydrogen-bonding.

Thus, block copolymer structure and microphase separation permit polyurethanes to combine the best properties of both the "soft" polyol continuous matrix and the "hard" urethane and/or urea dispersed domains. This supermolecular structure is a major reason for their high performance and versatility.

Polyblends and Interpenetrating Polymer Networks

When two polymers are mixed, the requirement for thermodynamic miscibility at equilibrium is a decrease in free energy ΔG:

$$\Delta G = \Delta H - T\Delta S$$

where ΔH is the enthalpy of mixing (attraction be-

Table 18. Flame-retardation of polyester urethane elastomer by addition of polyvinyl chloride and antimony oxide [16].

PUR	PVC	Sb_2O_3	Oxygen Index
100	0	0	22.0%
100	10	0	22.0
100	5	5	29.1
100	0	10	23.5
100	20	0	21.4
100	15	5	31.0
100	10	10	31.3
100	5	15	29.4
100	0	20	23.5
100	40	0	22.1
100	35	5	27.9
100	30	10	32.6
100	25	15	32.2
100	20	20	29.8
100	15	25	31.5
100	10	30	27.5
100	5	35	26.8
100	0	40	22.3

Table 19. Polyblends of polyurethane elastomer with phenoxy resin [17].

PUR/Phenoxy Ratio:	100/0	90/10	80/20	70/30	60/40	50/50	40/60	30/70	20/80	10/90	0/100
Melt index, Gm/10′	10.4	2.3	0.7	0.4	0.2	0.3	0.5	0.6	0.9	1.5	1.7
Shore A hardness	79	79	79	85	90	92	92	93	93	93	93
Tensile modulus, PSI	310	300	340	590	1,100	1,200	20,000	92,000	101,000	131,000	85,000
Tensile strength, PSI	2,300	2,130	1,800	2,840	3,680	3,230	5,080	6,780	8,230	7,930	8,440
Ultimate elongation, %	754	706	526	480	354	256	25	8	8	6	10
Notched Izod impact strength, FPI							1.7	1.2	1.3	1.6	1.9
Rebound, %	37	14	10	14	23	24	25	26	25	23	22
Flex temperature, °C	−48	−34	−27	−10	0	+17					
Heat deflection temperature, °C							36	47	54	64	67

tween the two polymers) and ΔS is the entropy of mixing (gain in statistical randomness). Two unlike polymers will generally repel each other, making ΔH unfavorable, unless there is some specific group attraction between them such as hydrogen-bonding. Mixing of large polymer molecules does not produce much gain in randomness ΔS, because all the atoms in a polymer molecule remain attached to each other during the process. Thus, most polymer blends are not miscible at the molecular level, and tend to separate into microphases. If the interface between these microphases is strongly bonded, each phase may be free to contribute some of its best properties to the blend, and such two-phase blends can benefit from synergistic balance of properties. This has made polymer blending one of the fastest-growing segments of the polymer industries.

Polyurethanes contain aliphatic, aromatic, ether, ester, urethane, and urea groups, offering a wide range of polarities and hydrogen-bonding possibilities, which should promote miscibility, or at least strong interfacial bonding, with a wide variety of other polymers [13,14]. Blends with ABS combine the melt processability, rigidity, and heat deflection temperature of the ABS with the elastic recovery and abrasion resistance of the polyurethane [15]. Blends with PVC combine the rigidity and flame-retardance of the PVC with the impact resistance of the polyurethane (Table 18) [16]; in more miscible blends, the polyurethane acts as a permanent polymeric plasticizer [13]. Blends with epoxy resins combine the rigidity and heat and chemical resistance of the epoxy with the ductility and impact resistance of the polyurethane (Table 19) [17]. Research studies have occasionally mentioned other interesting and useful polyurethane polyblends [4,13], but extent of serious commercial practice is not clear.

When a polymer is lightly cross-linked, swollen with a second monomer, and the second monomer is then polymerized in the swollen network, the resulting interpenetrating polymer network (IPN) contains the two polymer phases in a controlled degree of dispersion [18]. IPN synthesis benefits from the use of two distinctly different polymerization mechanisms. Since polyurethanes are formed by a unique chemical reaction, they can conveniently form one of the two polymer phases in IPNs and have proved to be one of the most popular polymer systems in IPN research. Surprisingly, many polyurethane IPNs, particularly with acrylics and polyesters, have shown remarkable synergistic improvement of tensile strength, as compared with the individual polymers involved. Much IPN research has been directed toward broad spectrum damping of noise and mechanical vibration.

Reinforcing Fillers

The use of fibers to produce high-performance reinforced composites has been developed primarily in epoxy resins and thermoset polyesters. In reaction injection molding (RIM), addition of short glass fibers produces reinforced RIM (RRIM), with much improved rigidity and strength (Table 20) [19]. Similarly, addition of short glass fibers to rigid urethane foam produces major improvements in modulus and strength (Table 21) [20]. The most extreme reinforcement is of course observed when flexible poly-

Table 20. Reinforced reaction injection molding (RRIM) [19].

Type of RIM	Glass Fiber	Flexural Modulus	Coefficient of Thermal Expansion, In./In./°F × 10⁶
Semi-high modulus	None	60 KPSI	78
Semi-high modulus	17%	120	24
High-modulus	None	275	70
High-modulus	17%	400	19
Rigid foam	None	50	60
Rigid foam	17%	110	32

Table 21. Reinforcement of rigid low-density polyurethane foam [20].

1/4″ Glass Fiber	Compressive Modulus	Compressive Strength	Flexural Modulus	Flexural Strength
0	537 PSI	31 PSI	1327 PSI	55 PSI
10	713	33	2376	76
20	761	35	2947	90
30	856	39	3296	94
40	1349	54	3837	111
50	1697	72	6136	148

urethane foam is coated onto cloth, for upholstery and clothing, combining the high planar modulus, strength, and dimensional stability of the cloth with the high transverse flexibility, softness, and thermal insulation of the foam.

Foams

When gas bubbles are dispersed in a solid polymer to form a foam, it is possible to combine some of the best properties of each phase, and to produce some synergistic benefits as well [21]. In polyurethanes in general [7], the gas contributes light weight, thermal and electrical insulation. The thermal insulation is used in rigid foams for refrigeration and freezer applications, in flexible foams for winter outerwear clothing. In closed-cell foams, the gas contributes flotation, rigidity and strength (!) and impact absorption; while in open-cell foams, the fluidity of the gas contributes softness, elastic recovery, impact absorption, noise damping, filtration, and sponge performance. Thus the gas phase, negligible in weight but most prominent in volume, contributes many useful properties and uses the polyurethane alone did not have.

Coatings

Thin surface films of polyurethanes contribute useful properties far beyond their several mils dimensions. They are easy to apply by a variety of techniques. They can have a wide range of modulus as desired. They have strong adhesion to many substrates. They are strong, impact-resistant, extremely abrasion-resistant, and resistant to hot aging, aqueous solutions, fuels, oils, and many other chemicals. When aliphatic isocyanates are used, they are also very resistant to weathering. They find increasing use in corrosion-preventive maintenance coatings.

Adhesives

Polyurethanes combine the fluidity needed to wet irregular substrates, the cure reactions needed to con-

vert them into high-molecular-weight materials of strong cohesion, and the range of polarities and hydrogen-bonding needed to form strong adhesive bonds with many types of surfaces. For these reasons, they have proved useful in a wide range of specialty adhesives [22].

SUMMARY

Polyurethanes offer a range of versatility in monomer structures and reactivities, process techniques, molecular flexibility, crystallinity, intermolecular attraction, cross-linking, copolymers, polyblends, and compounding additives, which make them useful in an extremely wide and rapidly growing variety of applications.

REFERENCES

1. Saunders, J. H. and K. C. Frisch. 1962. *Polyurethanes: Chemistry and Technology*. New York: Interscience Publishers, Ch. 3,4.
2. Ashida, K., I. F. Raza and C.-J. Chang. 1989. *SPI 32nd Annual Polyurethane Technical/Marketing Conf.*, October 1–4, p. 379.
3. Saunders, J. H. and K. C. Frisch. Op. Cit., Ch. 6,9,12.
4. Meckel, W., W. Goyert and W. Wieder. 1987. Ch. 2 in Legge, N. R., G. Holden, and H. E. Schroeder, 1987. *Thermoplastic Elastomers*. Munich: Hanser Publishers.
5. Deanin, R. D. 1972. *Polymer Structure, Properties, and Applications*. Boston: Cahners.
6. Lyons, J. W. 1970. *The Chemistry and Uses of Fire Retardants*. New York: Wiley-Interscience, Ch. 8.
7. Benning, C. J. 1969. *Plastic Foams*. New York: Wiley-Interscience, Ch. 2.
8. Deanin, R. D., M. R. Murarka and V. C. Kapasi. 1985. *SPE ANTEC*, 31:1297.
9. Xiao, H. X., K. C. Frisch, G. S. L. Hsu and H. A. Al-Salah. 1989. *SPI 32nd Annual Polyurethane Technical/Marketing Conf.*, October 1–4, p. 398.
10. Deanin, R. D., E. J. Ellis, T. A. Briere and M. R. Dunn. 1972. *SPE J*, 28(4):56.
11. Saunders, J. H. and K. C. Frisch. Op. Cit., Ch. 10.
12. Deanin, R. D. and J. A. Zgrebnak. 1974. *SPE ANTEC*, 20:654.
13. Deanin, R. D., S. B. Driscoll and J. T. Krowchun. 1979. *ACS Org. Coatings and Plastics Chem.*, 40:664.
14. Deanin, R. D. 1988. in Seymour, R. B. and H. F. Mark. *Applications of Polymers*. New York: Plenum Press, pp. 53–64.
15. Deanin, R. D., A. Manochehri, and C. J. Kanakia. 1987. *SPE EPS RETEC*, Chicago, Sept. 23, p. 179.
16. Deanin, R. D. and R. P. Gendron. 1988. *SPE ANTEC*, 34:1419.
17. Deanin, R. D., M. L.-F. Lin and J. A. Zgrebnak. 1989.

in Culbertson, B. M., *Multiphase Macromolecular Systems*, New York: Plenum Press, p. 561.

18. Manson, J. A. and L. H. Sperling. 1976. *Polymer Blends and Composites*. New York: Plenum Press, Ch. 8.

19. Krutchkoff, L., and R. D. Deanin. 1981. *SPE ANTEC*, 27:371.

20. Deanin, R. D. and V. A. Bourgault. *SPI RP/C, 40th Ann. Conf., 20-A, Jan. 28–Feb. 1, 1985.*

21. Deanin, R. D. 1985. Ch. 20 in R. W. Tess, and G. W. Poehlein. *Applied Polymer Science*. Washington: ACS.

22. Schollenberger, C. S. 1990. Ch. 20 in I. Skeist. *Handbook of Adhesives*. New York: Van Nostrand Reinhold.

5

Polyurethanes

N. HASIRCI*

ABSTRACT: Polyurethanes are the polymers most widely used in the construction of blood-contacting products and devices. This chapter begins with a general look at polyurethanes, including a discussion of how the properties of polyurethanes vary with respect to applied stress and temperature. Infrared spectrophotometry is applied to surface analysis—one of the most important parameters to consider, since it is the surface of the polyurethane material that contacts the blood. Biomedical applications are then studied, particularly with respect to the use of polyether urethanes in the cardiovascular field. Finally, the problems of blood compatibility are discussed, and various methods of altering surface characteristics to decrease thrombogenicity are presented.

FORMATION AND CHEMICAL PROPERTIES

Polyurethanes were discovered in 1937 and the research on the synthesis of polyurethanes has gained impetus especially since World War II [1,2]. Since they could be synthesized in very different forms and with widely varying properties, they have found many areas of application, including foams, adhesives, coatings, fibers, resins and elastomers.

Polyurethanes are polymers which contain urethane groups ($-\overset{\text{H}}{\underset{}{\text{N}}}-\overset{\text{O}}{\underset{}{\text{C}}}-\text{O}-$) in their structure. They are generally obtained by the reactions of polyisocyanates with polyhydroxy compounds. The general reaction for polyurethane formation can be given as:

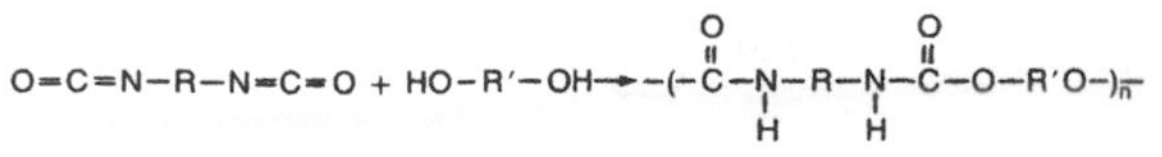

$$O=C=N-R-N=C=O + HO-R'-OH \rightarrow -(\overset{O}{\underset{H}{C}}-\overset{}{\underset{H}{N}}-R-\overset{}{\underset{H}{N}}-\overset{O}{C}-O-R'O-)_{\overline{n}}$$

In the preparation of polyurethanes, the compounds containing amino or carboxyl groups may also be used. These reactions can be summarized as:

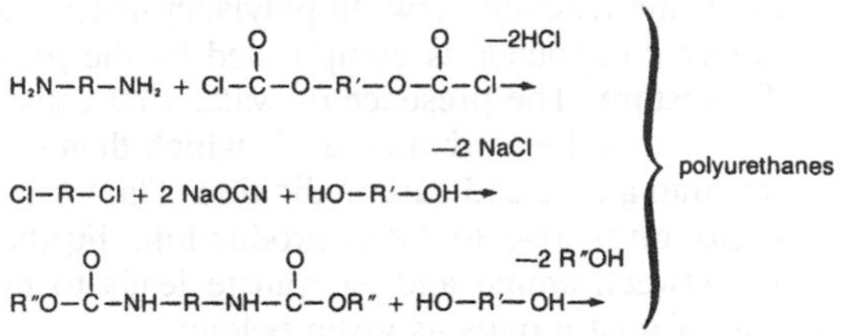

$$\left. \begin{array}{l} H_2N-R-NH_2 + Cl-\overset{O}{C}-O-R'-O-\overset{O}{C}-Cl \xrightarrow{-2HCl} \\ Cl-R-Cl + 2\,NaOCN + HO-R'-OH \xrightarrow{-2\,NaCl} \\ R''O-\overset{O}{C}-NH-R-NH-\overset{O}{C}-OR'' + HO-R'-OH \xrightarrow{-2\,R''OH} \end{array} \right\} \text{polyurethanes}$$

Isocyanates, which are the starting materials of polyurethanes, contain very reactive $-N=C=O$ groups. These groups can react with a large number of compounds and even with themselves. The addition reaction takes place at the carbon–nitrogen double bond. For example, the hydrogen bound to the nitrogen of a urethane, or urea, or amide linkage, can react further with isocyanate and lead to the formation of allophanate, biuret, or acylurea groups:

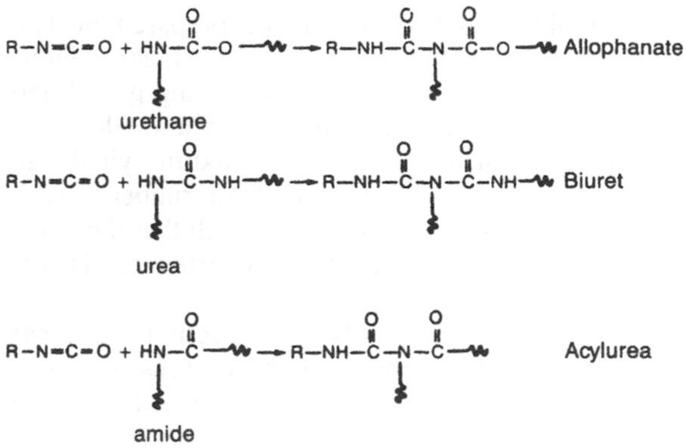

$$R-N=C=O + HN-\overset{O}{C}-O-\text{\Large\char`~} \rightarrow R-NH-\overset{O}{C}-\overset{}{N}-\overset{O}{C}-O-\text{\Large\char`~} \quad \text{Allophanate}$$
urethane

$$R-N=C=O + HN-\overset{O}{C}-NH-\text{\Large\char`~} \rightarrow R-NH-\overset{O}{C}-\overset{}{N}-\overset{O}{C}-NH-\text{\Large\char`~} \quad \text{Biuret}$$
urea

$$R-N=C=O + HN-\overset{O}{C}-\text{\Large\char`~} \rightarrow R-NH-\overset{O}{C}-\overset{}{N}-\overset{O}{C}-\text{\Large\char`~} \quad \text{Acylurea}$$
amide

Under certain conditions isocyanates trimerize and form isocyanurates:

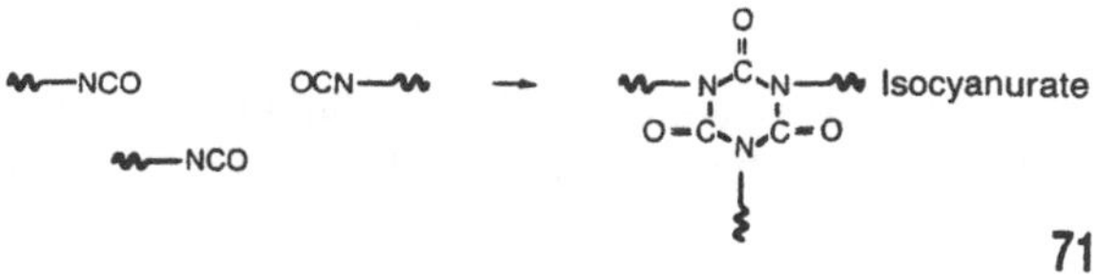

$$\text{\Large\char`~}-NCO \quad OCN-\text{\Large\char`~} \rightarrow \text{Isocyanurate}$$
$$\text{\Large\char`~}-NCO$$

---

*Associate Professor, Middle East Technical University, Faculty of Arts and Sciences, Department of Chemistry, Ankara, Turkey

At ordinary temperatures (up to 50°C), reactions of isocyanates with hydroxyl groups produce urethanes, while with amine and with water they will produce urea. At higher temperatures (up to 150°C) further reactions to give allophanates, biurets, and isocyanurates occur at a significant rate. Polyurethanes can be viewed as mixed amide esters of carbamic acids, and thus their properties are between polyesters and polyamides [3,4].

The primary reactions of isocyanates with active hydrogen compounds occur with remarkable ease at ordinary temperatures with the evolution of heat. If a linear polyurethane is desired, then the application of the lowest temperature is required. If high cross-linking and branching through secondary reactions is desired, then higher temperatures (50–150°C) are needed. At about 150°C phenolic polyurethanes start to decompose. For aliphatic polyurethanes this process takes place at around 220°C. Decomposition yields free isocyanates, alcohols, free amines, olefins and carbon dioxide [5].

Polyisocyanates are also very reactive substances. As a result, the reaction between polyisocyanates and polyhydroxy compounds is complicated by the presence of moisture. The presence of water first causes formation of unstable carbamic acid, which then disintegrates into amine and carbon dioxide. The formation of gas gives rise to foam production. Further reaction between amine and isocyanate leads to the formation of urea groups as given below:

$$OCN-R-NCO+2H_2O \rightarrow HO-\overset{O}{\overset{\|}{C}}-HN-R-NH-\overset{O}{\overset{\|}{C}}-OH \rightarrow H_2N-R-NH_2+2CO_2$$

carbamic acid   amine

$$H_2N-R-NH_2 + OCN-R-NCO \rightarrow -(HN-R-NH-\overset{O}{\overset{\|}{C}}-NH-R-NH-\overset{O}{\overset{\|}{C}}-)_n-$$

polyurea

Polyurethane elastomers can be prepared by two basic processes. The simplest and most obvious method is to mix a liquid or low-melting glycol and polyisocyanate, and cast the mixture in a mould while still liquid. Curing of the cast mixture yields an elastomeric product. In order to obtain rubber elasticity, the reactants should be chosen such that they produce a lightly cross-linked network structure. This is called the "one shot" process.

The second method involves the reaction of a linear hydroxy-terminated polymer with an excess of diisocyanate to form an isocyanate-terminated polymer called "prepolymer".

$$2OCN-R-NCO+HO-R'-OH \rightarrow OCN-R-NH-\overset{O}{\overset{\|}{C}}-O-R'-O-\overset{O}{\overset{\|}{C}}-NH-R-CO$$

prepolymer

Prepolymer is either a viscous liquid or a low-melting solid. The next step is chain extension and network formation with a small molecular weight polyol or amine called "chain extender". This step is usually accompanied by allophanate or biuret branch point formation.

The development of necessary cross-linking in elastomers also depends on the reaction of some isocyanate groups with atmospheric moisture to form urea groups, which then react with other isocyanate groups to form biuret cross-links. In order to obtain the required amount of cross-linking, a more useful procedure is the use of formulations with at least one component having more than two reactive end groups.

Relatively simple linear polymers may be obtained by using compounds with two active groups such as diisocyanates and diols. In each polymerization reaction, however, secondary reactions take place to a certain extent. Polyurethanes contain urea, ester and ether groups, and aromatic rings, in addition to urethane groups. These groups affect the properties of the resultant polymer.

The reactions between a diisocyanate, a linear long chain diol, and a low molecular weight chain extender lead to the production of elastomers. The properties of the elastomers are determined mainly by the chain structure, the degree of branching of the polymeric intermediate, and the stoichiometric balance of the components. The ratio of NCO to OH for optimum mechanical strength is usually 1.0 to 1.1. As the ratio falls below 1.0 the mechanical strength, hardness and resilience decrease and elongation and compression increase very sharply.

The isocyanates commonly used in the manufacture of polyurethanes are not many. Some important ones are illustrated below:

Hexamethylene diisocyanate (HDI)

$$OCN-(CH_2)_6-NCO$$

Toluene 2,4-diisocyanate (TDI)

Toluene 2,6-diisocyanate (TDI)

Diphenylmethane 4,4'-diisocyanate (MDI)

p-Phenylene diisocyanate (p-PDI)

HDI gives products which, unlike aromatic compounds, are not discolored in light and in air. TDI is almost always used as a mixture of 2,4 and 2,6 isomers, usually as a 80:20 mixture. MDI is generally used in elastomer and in rigid foam production.

There are some other isocyanates which are used in relatively small quantities. These are:

Naphthylene 1,5-diisocyanate (NDI)

p-Xylene diisocyanate (XDI)
or
m-Xylene diisocyanate (XDI)

3,3′-Dimethyl 4,4′-diphenylmethane diisocyanate (DMDI)

3,3′-Dimethyl 4,4′-diphenyl diisocyanate (TODI)

4,4′-diphenylisopropylidene diisocyanate (DPDI)

Dicyclohexylmethane diisocyanate (PICM)

NDI is commonly used in the production of high-grade elastomers. XDI and PICM are important in the production of non-discoloring polyurethanes, used in industry for such things as surface coating.

Reactivity of isocyanates depends on their chemical structures. Aromatic isocyanates are generally more reactive than aliphatic ones. The presence of electron-withdrawing substituents on the isocyanate molecule increases the partial positive charge on the isocyanate carbon and moves the negative charge farther away from the site of reaction. This makes the transfer of the electron from the donor substance to the carbon easier, thus causing a faster reaction. On the other hand, the presence of electron-donating substituents on isocyanate compounds can cause slower reactions. Bulky groups in the ortho positions of aromatic isocyanates, and bulky and branched groups in aliphatic isocyanates retard the reaction because of steric hindrance. In the reactions of diisocyanates, the reactivity of the second isocyanate decreases significantly after the first has been reacted. The difference in the

reactivities is less if the two isocyanates belong to different aromatic rings or are separated with an aliphatic chain.

Diol compounds used in polyurethane production are generally polyether- or polyester-based compounds with molecular weights in the range of 400–5000. Depending on the chain length of these diols or glycols the properties of the polyurethane changes. If the glycol has a low molecular weight it creates hard plastics and if it has a high molecular weight it creates flexible elastomers. The reactivities are not the same for all hydroxyl groups. Primary alcohols react readily at 25–50°C, while the secondary and tertiary alcohols are about 0.3 and 0.005 times less reactive than the primary ones.

The reaction between an alcohol and an isocyanate is catalyzed by mild and strong bases, by many metals and by acids. Bases such as sodium hydroxide, sodium acetate, tertiary amines, and certain metal compounds (especially tin compounds such as dibutyltin dilaurate and stannous octoate) are the most commonly used catalysts.

The type of diisocyanate, glycol, and solvent used may affect the rate and the type of the reaction as well as the properties of the product. Polyols give the high flexibility to the backbone of the network chains and therefore are called soft domains or soft segments. On the other hand, isocyanate and chain-extender components give rigidity to the chains and are called hard domains or rigid segments. Physical and mechanical properties of polyurethanes which contain these types of segments can be explained in terms of morphological structure, i.e, rigid domains dispersed in a flexible segment matrix. Because the hard and soft blocks are partly incompatible with each other the elastomers show a two-phase morphology, although there is a significant level of mixing of the hard and soft blocks. At low temperatures, the soft matrix having a low T_g influences the properties. Hard segments in the domains act as cross-link points as well as reinforcing filler entities, and these govern the performance of the material at elevated temperatures.

The general principles of the property–structure relationship can be summarized as:

(1) Molecular weight: As the molecular weight increases some properties such as tensile strength, melting point, elongation, elasticity, glass transition temperature, etc. increase up to a limiting value and then remain constant.

(2) Intermolecular forces: The weaker bonds such as hydrogen bonding, polarizability, dipole moments, van der Waals forces may form in addition to the primary chemical bonds, and these weaker bonds are affected by temperature and stress. If there is repulsion between like charges or bulky chains, or if there is high cross-link density, the effect of intermolecular forces will be reduced.

(3) Stiffness of chain: Presence of aromatic rings stiffens the polymer chains and causes a high

Table 1. Effect of isocyanate structure on the properties of polyester urethanes.

Diisocyanate	Tensile Strength (psi)	Elongation		Modulus at 300% (psi)	Tear Strength lb/in	Hardness (Shore B)
		%	Set %			
NDI	4300	500	85	3000	200	80
p-PDI	6400	600	25	2300	300	72
TDI	4600	600	1	350	150	40
MDI	7900	600	10	1600	270	61
TODI	4000	400	10	2300	180	70
DMDI	5300	500	0	600	40	47
DPDI	3500	700	10	300	90	56

melting point, hardness and a decrease in elasticity. On the other hand, the presence of flexible bonds (such as ether bonds) favors softness, low melting point, low glass transition temperature and elasticity.

(4) Crystallization: Linearity and close fit or polymer chains favor crystallinity, which leads to reductions in solubility, elasticity, elongation and flexibility, and increase in tensile strength, melting point and hardness.

(5) Cross-linking: Increase in the degree of cross-linking cause an increase in rigidity, softening point, and modulus of elasticity for amorphous polymers, and reduces elongation and swelling by solvents.

It is possible to use more than one polyol component in order to vary the formulation and hence the processing characteristics and the properties of the product. This affects the degree of branching and also the order of interaction of the polyols with the diisocyanates. It is also possible to vary processing factors such as temperature, viscosity, rate of set-up, cure of the casting mix, or incorporation of fillers. Addition of low molecular weight polyols such as glycerol or trimethylol propane may introduce branching.

Generally, in the preparation of polyurethanes, the excess diisocyanate may first react with polyol to form isocyanate-terminated prepolymer, which is stable in the absence of moisture and catalyst. This prepolymer reacts with more polyol at the casting stage. Therefore, by varying the polyol component added in this stage, it is possible to change the properties of the resulting elastomer. Depending on the chemical com-

position and the amount of cross-linking and branching, it is possible to obtain products ranging from soft elastomers to hard resinous materials.

The chain structure of the polymeric intermediate determines the level of mechanical properties. Fillers, if used may increase hardness and modulus of elasticity and reduce elongation, but they do not have a very substantial effect on strength.

For a given set of diols and triols and a given NCO/OH ratio, the molecular weight per branch point may be altered by varying the proportions of diols and triols. The molecular weight per branch point may be varied while retaining the same proportion of polyisocyanate, either by using polyols which are the same equivalent weight or by simultaneously varying the equivalent weights of the polyols to give a combination of the same average equivalent weight. An increase in the proportion of polyisocyanates results in a decrease in the molecular weight per branch point, and thus to an increase in tensile strength, modulus of elasticity, and hardness, while decreasing elongation.

Besides the triols, cross-linkage and branching will also take place at the urethane and the urea groups. When the NCO/OH ratio is low, the branching will occur at the urethane linkage. At higher NCO/OH ratios the probability for the formation of urea linkages will be high and thus branching will occur at the urea linkages. The presence of higher atmospheric pressure and relative humidity, assures the presence of cross-linkage and branching at the urea groups, and the percentage of urea to urethane will be higher than at lower NCO/OH ratios.

The effect of secondary valence interchain bonding through polar interchains and hydrogen bonding is

Table 2. Effect of polyester structure on the properties of polyester urethanes.

Polyester	Tensile Strength (psi)	Elongation		Modulus at 300% (psi)	Tear Strength lb/in	Hardness (Shore B)
		%	Set %			
Poly(ethylene adipate)	6900	590	15	1550	240	60
Poly(1,4-butylene adipate)	6000	510	15	1900	280	70
Poly(1,5-pentylene adipate)	6300	450	10	1800	60	60
Poly(1,3-butylene adipate)	3200	520	15	1100	100	58
Poly(ethylene succinate)	6800	420	40	3200	200	75
Poly(2,3-butylene succinate)	3500	380	105	—	—	85

Table 3. Effect of curing agent on the properties.

Diamine	Tensile Strength (psi)		Elongation (%)	Graves Tear Strength lb/in	Hardness (Shore A)
	Ultimate	100% Modulus			
4,4'-Diaminodiphenylmethane	4420	1150	520	535	86
3,3'-Dichloro-4,4'-diamino-diphenylmethane	5000	925	450	475	91
Benzidine	4340	1190	470	565	86
3,3'-Dimethylbenzidine	7000	1845	550	675	95
3,3'-Dimethoxybenzidine	2470	745	550	415	93
3,3'-Dichlorobenzidine	5450	1700	390	625	94
p-Phenylenediamine	2320	1560	300	645	91

also manifested in the modulus of elasticity and hardness of the cured product, which increase markedly with increases in the proportion of diisocyanate to glycol. Although this increase is accompanied by some loss in resilience it is possible to obtain very hard products which still retain elastomeric character. In the production of high-grade, high-modulus elastomers, symmetrical diisocyanates such as naphthylene 1,5-diisocyanate, phenylene 1,4-diisocyanate and diphenylmethane 4,4'-diisocyanate, and symmetrical glycols such as 1,4-butanediol, 1,6-hexanediol, p-bis-(β-hydroxy ethoxy)-benzene, 1,5-bis-(β-hydroxy ethoxy)-naphthalene are useful.

Unsymmetrical diisocyanates and glycols result in very different processing characteristics and physical properties. Low proportions of the diisocyanate-glycol urethane segment yield elastomers which are substantially softer and of lower modulus than analogous compositions based on symmetrical diisocyanates. Interchain attractive forces between rigid segments are very high because the urethane group is highly polar and exhibits a strong tendency to hydrogen bonding between the $-NH-$ and the $-COO-$ parts of the group. Consequently, it has a strong tendency toward association and a high energy of cohesion. Regular polyurethanes are generally similar in character to other polymers containing regularly occurring groups with high energy of cohesion.

Polyurethanes are separated into two classes according to their hydroxy-containing compounds. They can be either polyester urethanes or polyether urethanes. Aliphatic polyethers and polyesters are the most commercially important materials. They have low glass transition temperatures (below room temperature) and are generally amorphous or have low melting points. Polyurethanes made from lightly branched poly(oxypropylene) polyols and TDI may be formulated to give property ranges as shown below [6]:

Tensile strength (psi)	100–500
Elongation (%)	100– >1000
Modulus at 100% extension (psi)	50–500
Hardness (Shore A)	5–70

In the preparation of elastomers with high mechanical strength and of a wide range of hardness, the process consists essentially of reacting the hydroxy-terminated polymer with an excess of diisocyanate to produce an intermediate prepolymer which is in effect a mixture of isocyanate-terminated polymer and free unreacted diisocyanate. This prepolymer is then mixed with a difunctional agent such as a glycol or diamine to give a rapid-setting liquid mixture, which is cast into a mould while still liquid. This mixture then sets and is cured, usually in an oven at a temperature up to about 110°C. The amount of glycol or diamine used is slightly less than that required to react with the isocyanate groups in the prepolymer. The glycol or diamine is usually referred to as the chain-extending agent.

Polyester urethanes: Their thermal behaviors are dependent upon the concentration of ester groups on the polyester. An increase in ester group concentration leads to reduced flexibility at low temperatures, to higher hardness, higher modulus, and a marked increase in permanent elongation. Conversely, reducing the ester group concentration improves the low-temperature flexibility and reduces the tear strength. Glass-transition temperatures of polymers prepared with poly(1,4-butylene adipate) and poly(1,5-pentylene adipate) are significantly lower than that of the poly(ethylene adipate) elastomer.

Effect of isocyanate structure on the properties of polyester urethanes which are prepared by using 0.1 equivalents polyethylene adipate (mol wt 2000), 0.32 equivalents diisocyanate, and 0.2 equivalents, 1,4-butanediol chain extender, is shown in Table 1 [7].

Polyester structure also affects the properties of product. For a special polyurethane series prepared from diphenylmethane diisocyanate, 1,4-butanediol (as chain extender) and different polyesters, the properties could be summarized as shown in Table 2 [8].

Polyether urethanes: In the preparation of this type of polymers, polyether-based glycols are used. If they are cured with aromatic diamines then their structure–property relationships will be very similar to those of polyester urethanes. At high NCO/NH$_2$ ratios the excess isocyanate forms biuret branch points. Thus, an increase in cross-linking causes a reduction in modulus, elongation, compression set, and tear strength. The effects of various aromatic diamines are shown in Table 3 [9].

The secondary reactions occur to a much less extent

than the primary reactions but their importance must not be underestimated. Formation of allophanates or biurets is responsible for some of the cross-linking and branching and therefore has an important influence on the properties of the polyurethane product.

MECHANICAL PROPERTIES

The mechanical properties of a material are concerned with the effects of stress on the material. Materials can react in a number of various ways to an applied stress.

Laboratory tests for measuring mechanical properties generally are:

(1) Static tests, in which the loads are applied slowly enough that quasi-static equilibrium of forces is maintained

(2) Cyclic tests, in which loads are applied and then (a) partly or wholly removed or (b) reversed a sufficient number of times to cause the material to behave differently than under static loading

(3) Impact tests, in which loading is applied so rapidly that the material must absorb energy rather than resist a force

The simplest mechanical test is the tensile test, generally carried out with an Instron tensile tester, in which the specimen is gradually elongated under an applied stress and the resulting changes in length are recorded. The stress is the force applied per unit cross-sectional area of specimen. The strain is the fractional change in the length of the specimen. It can be measured as linear strain, ϵ, which is the change of length per unit length, or as shearing strain, γ, which measures the change in angle from the original right angle. In a tensile test, a specimen is subjected to a progressively increasing tensile force until it fractures. At the beginning the test material extends elastically. The strain is directly proportional to the stress and the specimen returns to its original length immediately on the removal of the stress. In this region, loads are not great enough to cause permanent shifting between the atoms. Beyond the elastic limit the applied stress produces plastic deformation, so a permanent extension remains after the removal of the applied load. The material either fractures or undergoes some change in shape due to flow of the material. In the elastic region the stress and strain are linearly proportional to each other. Stress is called normal stress, σ, when it acts perpendicular to a given area and the slope, E, of the line defined as $E = \sigma/\epsilon$ where E is named as Young's modulus. When a shear stress which acts in a plane rather than normal to the plane is applied, the relation between the shear stress, τ, and shear strain, γ, is given as $G = \tau/\gamma$ where G is named as shear modulus [10,11].

The amount of deformation in any direction depends on the magnitude and direction of the loading, and on the condition of the material. When the stress

reaches a critical value, the atomic bonds fail across an atomic plane. The relation between stress and strain departs from linearity, and plastic deformation begins accompanied by a reduction in the cross section known as necking. As deformation continues, the applied load increases until the tensile strength or ultimate strength is reached. This strength is the maximum point shown on the stress–strain curve. Polymers have a wide spectrum of mechanical properties ranging from hard brittle materials to gel-like structures, from flexible elastomers to tough materials, from porous foam structures to nonporous rigid materials. The general tensile properties can be classified as shown in Figure 1.

The applied force may cause fractures on the material. The fractures form either under constant-stress (creep) or fluctuating-stress (fatigue) conditions.

Creep tests are carried under certain combinations of stress and temperature. All materials, when subjected to a constant stress, will exhibit an increase of strain with time. This phenomenon is called creep. Most materials creep to a certain extent at all temperatures. High temperatures lead to a rapid creep which is often accompanied by microstructural changes. A typical creep curve is shown in Figure 2.

Fatigue test is the measurement of the failure of a structure under the repeated application of a constant stress smaller than that required to cause failure in one application. The material initially suffers some microstructural damage. Eventually the cyclic application of load leads to the formation of cracks which grow larger with every application of load. A series of specimens of the material are tested to failure by application of different values of stress. Properties such as fatigue life time, number of cycles to failure after crack initiation, permanent set, and total elongation are also measured. Generally, logarithms of the stress are plotted versus the logarithms of the number of cycles to failure. This type of a curve is called a S–N curve and is shown in Figure 3.

Impact test measures the brittleness of the material. In this test, a standard notch is cut in a standard test specimen, which is then struck under impact conditions by a heavy weight forming the end of a pendulum. The notch serves to introduce triaxial tensile stresses into the specimen, encouraging brittle failure to occur. The weight is released from a known height

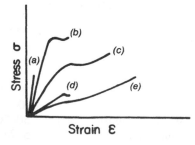

Figure 1. (a) Hard and brittle; (b) hard and strong; (c) hard and tough; (d) soft and weak; (e) soft and tough.

so as to strike the specimen on the side opposite the notch and to induce tensile stresses in it. After breaking the specimen the pendulum swings on and the height to which it rises on the other side is measured. Thus the energy absorbed in breaking the material under high-speed loading can be determined, and if this is low the specimen is called brittle.

The techniques of continuous and intermittent stress relaxation measurement have been used successfully for studying the thermal behaviour of elastomers [12,13]. In these tests, with continuous stress relaxation, a strip specimen of an elastomer is held at a fixed extension while it is being exposed to a constant elevated temperature. Meanwhile, the tensile force or stress at constant extension and temperature is monitored continuously. If the temperature is high enough to induce random thermal scission of the elastomers' network chains, the measured force of stress will decrease with time at a rate which is proportional to the rate of chain scission. Such a stress decay process is often referred to as a chemorheological or simply a chemical stress relaxation [14].

The continuous stress relaxation data are often fitted to a simple exponential Maxwell model, expressed as:

$$f_t = f_0 e^{(-t/\tau)}$$

$$E_t = E_0 e^{(-t/\tau)}$$

where f_0 is the initial tensile force measured at constant extension and constant temperature, and f_t is the tensile force measured after some relaxation time t. In the second expression, E_0 and E_t are relaxation modulus values initially and at time t. τ is a characteristic relaxation time constant. Stress relaxation technique measures the rate of network chain scission, but does not give information about the rate of reversible reactions. Recombination of thermally cleaved chains might occur in a relaxed condition. Therefore, continuous relaxation measurements are often supplemented by intermittent relaxation measurements. The specimen is maintained in stretched position at widely spaced intervals of time, and the resulting stress is rapidly measured, after which the strip is immediately returned to its unstretched state.

Mechanical properties of polyurethanes can be controlled by using components of different chemical structure at appropriate molar ratios. The final deformational properties of segmented polyurethane rubbers result from the combination of segment flexibility, cross-linking, chain entanglement, orientation of segments, rigidity of aromatic units, hydrogen bonding and other van der Waals forces. These parameters affect the applied force and lead to different types of deformations [15]. There is a correlation between morphological structure and stress–strain behavior. The modulus decreases with decreasing hard segment content in poly(ethylene oxide)-based elastomers extended with either ethylenediamine or phenylenediamine. Such trends are explained in terms of greater

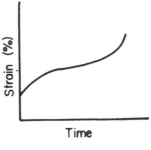

Figure 2.

degree of domain-formation with increasing hard segment content. Decrease in hard segment content cause a decrease in modulus, but in some cases where the hard content value is less than 10% crystallization of soft segments may occur and create an unexpectedly high modulus.

Temperature affects the tensile properties and demonstrates a decrease of stress at a given strain with increasing temperature. This negative temperature coefficient of stress can be explained in terms of the viscoelastic softening of hard segment domains resulting in a decrease in effective physical cross-links.

Due to dissimilarity in chemical structure of the hard and soft segments, there is a thermodynamic incompatibility between these segments. There is a driving force which causes them to form separate phases. This effect is, however, limited due to the presence of covalent links. It therefore forms domains or leads to microphase separation.

The experiments carried out with small-angle X-ray scattering showed that microphase separation for segmented poly(urethane urea) is improved with an increase of average molecular weight of poly(tetramethylene glycol) [16]. Some processing parameters of the casting method also affect the morphology. The temperature of the prepolymer synthesis as well as the temperature of the mold, strongly influence the phase segregation. Generally, the spherulites are bigger if the temperature of the mold is higher [17].

Polyurethanes, especially the linear segmented polyurethanes show significant time-dependent changes in their physical properties. Time dependency is observed in stress–strain behavior. For the samples annealed at certain temperature and then rapidly cooled, it was observed that the Young's modulus value was much lower than before annealing. With in-

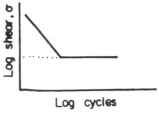

Figure 3.

Table 4. Effect of different backbone polyols on properties of polyurethanes.

Polyol	Tensile Strength (psi)	Modulus 100% (psi)	Modulus 300% (psi)	Ultimate Elongation (%)	Set-up Rupture (%)	Hardness (Shore A)	Melt Temp. (°C)
Polyethylenepropylene adipate(9:1), MW:1040	5650	705	1150	1035	50	81	200
Polycaprolactone MW:1050	6410	655	1050	1000	45	81	197
Polytetramethylene glycol, MW:808	5840	765	1270	930	45	82	172
Polytrimethylene glycol, MW:658	3875	780	—	830	45	83	140

crease in time after annealing, Young's modulus increases but complete recovery is not observed [18].

In *in vitro* experiments, it was observed that some elastomers, including segmented polyurethanes, lose their strength after immersion in whole blood [19]. It was also observed that, for polyether urethane samples reacted with lipids, the absorption of lipids cause a decrease in the fatigue lifetime. Examination of the surface with SEM revealed microcracks [20].

Stress–relaxation measurement is an easy method for the examination of viscoelasticity of the polymer. Processes of breaking and rebuilding polymer network as well as changes occurring in molecular structures can be examined by this method. In stress-relaxation processes, many reactions may happen. Breaking of urethane or allophanate type relatively weak linkages, disruption of hydrogen bonds or other secondary bonds, and decrease in the number of free entanglements are some of these reactions. During stress-relaxation, it has been observed that cleavage of polymer chain occurs most readily in groups having nitrogen atoms. When the length of the diols increase it is observed that relaxation speed increases. When cross-linking density and stiff-segment content increase, relative relaxation speed decreases with a parallel influence on the disappearance of viscoelastic properties [21].

The molecular weight of polyglycol is another parameter that affects the properties of the polyurethane. For example, for a sample prepared with polyoxyeth-

Table 5. Effect of molecular weight and structure of diol on MOCA-MDI elastomers.

Diol	Tensile Strength (psi)	Modulus 100% (psi)	Elongation (%)	Hardness (Shore A)
Polypropylene glycol				
MW:2000	148	650	560	83
MW:1500	2400	1060	690	88
Polyethylene adipate				
MW:2000	5050	880	930	88

yleneglycol, MDI and 1,5-pentanediol, the molecular weight of polyether was changed between 600 and 2000. With longer polyether chains, the system was more flexible and more hydrophilic, and had lower elastic modulus. Percent water absorption was increased from 9.9 to 62.4 with an increase in the molecular weight of polyether from 600 to 2000. For the same polyurethanes, experiments to measure shear modulus were carried out in saline solution at 37°C, and relaxed and unrelaxed moduli showed an increase from 0.33 MPa to 0.92 MPa and 0.57 MPa to 2.58 MPa, respectively. An increase in shear modulus values with a decrease in the molecular weight of the polymers was observed [22,23].

Like the isocyanates, polyols have an important effect on the properties of the polyurethanes. The mechanical properties of polyurethanes prepared from different polyols as the backbone for polyurethanes are given in Table 5. The preparation mixture consisted of two mols of DMI, 1 mol backbone diol, and 1.02 mols of either 1,3-propane diol or 1,4-butane diol as chain extender [24] (see Table 4).

The formation of the backbone from polyester or polyether glycols lead to considerably different properties. Such differences are shown in Table 5 for polyethylene adipate and polypropyleneglycol urethane [25,26].

For the given set, it is observed that polyester urethane is far superior to its polyether counterpart of the same molecular weight. However, reducing the molecular weight of the polypropylene glycol improved the properties, although the tensile strength was still greatly inferior to the polyester compound.

A more detailed study on the effect of the polyether polyurethane molecular weight on the mechanical properties involved polyurethanes prepared from a range of polypropylene glycols of different molecular weights, 2,4-tolylene diisocyanate and 4,4′-methylene bis(o-chloroaniline) [MOCA] [27]. As observed in the previous example, a decrease in the molecular weight leads to increases in the tensile and tear strengths, and in the modulus. The results are tabulated in Table 6.

In polyurethanes, cross-linking can occur by use of trifunctional chain extenders, by allophanate formation or by biuret formation. It is assumed that cross-linking by isocyanurate formation is of little importance.

Increasing the amount of cross-linking by decreasing the molar ratio of chain extenders results in hysteresis loss, lower heat build-up, and lower flex–fatigue resistance. The molecular weights between branch points (Mc) and modulus has been found to vary in opposite directions for some polyurethanes [28] as shown in Table 7.

Chemical cross-linking can be controlled by varying the proportion of diol to triol. The data in Table 8, obtained by substituting trimethylol propane for butanediol, shows the effect of increasing average molecular weight per cross-link unit.

The number of repetitions and the length of the chains of the hydrocarbon, ether, and ester groups appear to control the properties. Table 9 summarizes few known effects of the various groups. In order to control properties, we must not only have the means to correctly and accurately identify qualitatively and quantitatively these groups in the end polymer, but we also must be able to evaluate them as they form in the polymerizing mass. The table is given as a guideline only, but unfortunately there is no way to chart all the effects and side effects of the various reactions, nor the sequence in which they occur.

THERMAL ANALYSIS

Thermal analysis comprises a group of techniques in which a physical property of a substance is measured as a function of temperature while the substance is subjected to a controlled-temperature program.

A complete modern thermal analysis instrument measures temperature and energy of transitions, weight loss, dimensional changes, and viscoelastic properties.

In differential thermal analysis (DTA), the temperatures of the sample and a thermally inert reference material are measured as a function of temperature. Any transition which the sample undergoes will result in liberation or absorption of energy by the sample, with a corresponding deviation of its temperature from that of the reference. This tells us whether the transition is endothermic or exothermic.

In differential scanning calorimetry (DSC), the sample and a reference material are subjected to a closely controlled, programmed temperature variation. In case of a transition in the sample, thermal energy is added or subtracted from the sample or reference container in order to keep both at the same temperature. Recording of this balancing energy yields a direct calorimetric measurement of the transition energy.

Thermogravimetric analysis (TGA), provides a quantitative measurement of any weight change associated with a transition.

Thermomechanical analysis (TMA), provides measurements of penetration, expansion, contraction, and extension of materials as a function of temperature.

Table 6. Effect of molecular weight on the mechanical properties of MOCA-MDI polyurethanes.

| Properties | Molecular Weight | | | |
	1000	1250	1500	2000
Tensile strength (psi)	5050	4500	3500	1200
Elongation at break (%)	—	860	—	—
Modulus at 300% (psi)	2100	1000	600	400
Tear strength, Graves (lb/in)	310	240	225	125
Hardness (Shore A)	88	77	67	60

Dynamic mechanical analysis (DMA), detects transitions associated with movement of polymer chains. The technique involves measuring the resonant frequency and mechanical damping of a material forced to flex at a selected amplitude. Mechanical damping is the amount of energy dissipated by the sample as it oscillates, while the resonant frequency defines Young's modulus of stiffness. Loss modulus and the ratio of loss modulus to elastic modulus can be calculated from the raw frequency and damping data. In general, modulus and frequency, as well as damping, change more dramatically than heat capacity of thermal expansion during secondary transitions. For example, dynamic mechanical analysis is helpful in determining the effectiveness of reinforcing agents and fillers used in thermoset resins.

Since polyurethanes are made up of three types of ingredients (isocyanates, polyhydroxy compounds and chain extenders) which can be selected from a wide variety of chemicals, generalization of their thermal properties is not a simple task. Still, three endothermic peaks, one for the glass transition temperature of the soft segments and two for the dissociation of the short- and long-range order of the hard segments can be observed in most polyurethanes. For a two-phase block copolymer the width of the soft-phase glass transition zone provides a qualitative measure of soft-phase homogeneity. At higher temperatures melting of the hard-segment microcrystallites may also be observed. In the DSC of a MDI, 1,4-butanediol and polytetramethyleneoxide (mol wt 1000) polyurethane these four peaks were observed at −35°C, 71°C, 176°C and 193°C, respectively [30]. However, the lack of high temperature endotherms related to hard segment ordering are commonly reported for MDI-based polyurethane block copolymers, especially when asymmetric chain-extender diols are used [31].

The chemical structure and the linkages present in polyurethanes have a significant effect on thermal behavior. If diamines are used as chain extender, urea linkages will form rather than urethane linkages, which leads to an increase in hydrogen bonding resulting in stronger resistance to thermal disruption. The hydrogen bonding promotes greater cohesiveness of the hard-segment domains. In DMA analysis of polyurethaneimides an increase in the storage modulus E was observed with an increase in the fraction of the hard phase [32].

Table 7. Effect of the degree of chemical cross-linking on the physical properties of some polyurethanes.

Curing Agents	Equivalents Used	Mc	Tensile Strength (psi)	Elongation (%)	Modulus 100% (psi)	Hardness (Shore A)	Tear Strength, Graves, lb/in
Hexanetriol	1.0	2090	475	235	250	55	45
Polypropylenetriol MW:700	1.0	3700	555	380	170	43	40
Polypropylenetriol + pentanediol	0.6 0.4	5800	1340	645	105	38	85
Polypropylenetriol + polypropylenediol (MW:425)	0.6 0.4	6150	945	625	80	37	65

Table 8. Effect of M_c on the mechanical properties.

M_c	Tensile Strength (psi)	Elongation %	Set %	Modulus at 100% (psi)	Tear Strength lb/in	Hardness (Shore B)	Compression Set %
2100	1800	170	0	570	30	57	1.5
3100	1750	200	0	420	25	53	16
4300	1450	280	0	300	30	49	10
5300	2800	350	0	270	30	46	5
7100	4500	410	0	330	40	51	25
10900	5600	490	5	460	60	55	40
21000	5500	510	10	500	140	56	45
∞	6750	640	15	630	300	61	55

Table 9. Effects of different groups on properties.

Group	Hardness	Elongation	Tensile Strength	Tear Strength	Resistance to: Abrasion	Chemical	Heat
Hydrocarbon CH_2	G	NK	NK	NK	NK	G	G
Aromatic C_6H_4	E	F	E	F–G	E	G	G
Urea (carbamide)	E	P	G	G	F	G	G
Urethane (carbamate)	NK	NK	E	E	E	G	G
Disubstituted urea	E	P	G	G	F	G	G
Allophanate	F	G	P	P	G	F	P
Biuret	F	F	F	F	G	F	P
Substituted biuret	F	F	F	F	G	F	P
Substituted urea	E	P	G	G	F	G	G
Acyl urea	G	P	G	G	G	G	G
Ester	P	E	E	E	NE	F	P
Ether	P	G	F	F	NE	NK	P
Amide	G	G	G	G	G	F	F

NE = No effect.
NK = No known effect.
 E = Excellent.

G = Good.
F = Fair.
P = Poor.

SURFACE ANALYSIS

A surface is, theoretically, an infinitely thin layer separating two phases. Surface is generally examined with spectroscopy which involves probing a sample target with a flux of energetic particles and detecting characteristic particles emitted from the surface after interaction. Activation may be achieved by electro-magnetic radiation, as in electron spectroscopy for chemical analysis (ESCA), by a beam of incident ions, as in secondary ion mass spectrometry (SIMS) and ion scattering spectroscopy (ISS), or by an incident electron beam as in Auger electron spectroscopy (AES), or by electron microprobe (X-ray fluorescence) analysis.

Infrared spectrophotometry (IR) measures the energies involved in the twisting, bending, rotating and vibrating motions of asymmetrical chemical bonds in a molecule. Upon interaction with infrared radiation, portions of the incident radiation are absorbed at particular wavelengths. These wavelengths correspond to particular vibrations of the bonds, and thus yield information about the chemical structure of the absorbing species. Fourier transform infrared spectrophotometry (FTIR) makes use of computer technology and yields much higher resolution through processing of very large amounts of data obtained through numerous runs. IR and FTIR give information about the chemical bonds present in the bulk structure. On the other hand, attenuated total reflectance infrared spectrophotometry (AT-IR or AT-FTIR) gives information about the chemical bonds present on the surface.

Adsorption and segregation depend on surface chemistry as well as on surface free energy. Determination of contact angles (advancing, receding, or critical) by the use of goniometers is a convenient and simple method of measuring the surface free energies of the polymeric samples.

Polyurethanes have very widely varying structures, depending on the components used in the formulation. The aromatic isocyanates will give more urea groups in the finished structure than will the aliphatic diisocyanates. Excess NCO in the formulation will react with atmospheric moisture, to form urea and biuret groups in the structure. Aromatic diamines will produce a great amount of urea groups in the structure of the polymer, with some amide groups and aromatic rings. Polyester components will give far more urethane groups, along with a few ester groups in some cases, and the urethane linkages will be predominant. Polyether components give a very large number of allophanate groups in the polymer, with a few ether groups and, in some cases, a few ester groups. The amount of these groups in comparison with the urethane linkages can be varied easily by choice of the individual polyether. Other groups such as urea and biuret can be decreased by reacting these hydroxyl components with an aliphatic diisocyanate at very near to the stoichiometric 1:1 ratio by avoiding any further reaction with atmospheric moisture, and by using completely anhydrous components.

Structure of the diisocyanate and the structure of the hydrogen donors have a great influence on the final properties. NCO/OH ratios, the manner in which they are reacted, the presence of catalyst, and the cure conditions all have large degree of influence on the end product.

Although the types of ingredients are much more varied in polyurethanes than other polymers, the methods mentioned above make a quantitative analysis of a polyurethane surface quite feasible.

In the IR (or ATIR or FTIR), the wavelengths of the absorption bands for some groups can be summarized as [33]:

$-N{=}C{=}O$ (diisocyanate): 2275 cm^{-1} $- 2250$ cm^{-1}, 1350 cm^{-1}

$$-NH-\overset{\overset{\textstyle O}{\|}}{C}-O-$$ (urethane): 1640 cm^{-1} $- 1610$ cm^{-1}, 1650 cm^{-1} $- 1680$ cm^{-1}

$C{=}C$ (in benzene): 1600 cm^{-1} $- 1610$ cm^{-1}

Aromatics: 3030 cm^{-1}, 1600 cm^{-1} $- 1500$ cm^{-1}

Substitution to aromatics: below 900 cm^{-1}, between 2000 cm^{-1} $- 1660$ cm^{-1}

$-OH$ (hydroxyl): 3200 cm^{-1} $- 3400$ cm^{-1}

$C-O-C$ (ether): 1150 cm^{-1} $- 1070$ cm^{-1}

$ArNH_2$ (aromatic): 1350 cm^{-1} $- 1250$ cm^{-1}

$COOH$ (carboxyl): 3000 cm^{-1} $- 2500$ cm^{-1}, 1760 cm^{-1} $- 1710$ cm^{-1}

$AlNH_2$ (aliphatic): 1280 cm^{-1} $- 1180$ cm^{-1}

However, interferences and shifts caused by the neighboring groups may be encountered. In large polymers like polyurethanes, the characteristic spectra become diffuse and identification of small amounts of any given functionality becomes increasingly difficult.

BIOMEDICAL APPLICATIONS

The first generation of polyurethanes used for implant studies was the commercially available Estane® (BFGoodrich), a polyester urethane, but it was found that Estane® degrades rapidly when implanted in the muscle of dogs or when used as valvular prostheses [34,35]. Therefore, attention shifted to polyether urethanes and biomedical-grade polyether urethanes were synthesized [36,37].

Segmented polyurethane polymers are widely used as artificial heart [38], vascular grafts [39], catheter [40], diaphragm of blood pump for artificial heart systems [41], intraaortic balloon pump [42], pacemaker wire insulation [43,44], heart valves [45,46], cardiac-assist devices [47], components of hemodialysis units [48,49], skin grafts [50,51] and blood filters [52]. Since the segmented polyurethanes exhibit high flexure endurance, high strength, nonthrombogenic characteristics, the most important applications appear to be in the cardiovascular area. Some polyurethane elastomers synthesized from polycaprolactones can be used as medical, solvent-activated, pressure-sensitive adhesives since they have higher hydrolytic resistance and better properties at low temperatures. The structures of polyurethanes prepared from lactones are more regular. Due to their quick crystallization they can be used as medical, solvent-activated, pressure-sensitive adhesives [53].

Some current biomedical applications of polyurethanes can be tabulated as:

- blood bags, clausers, fittings
- blood oxygenation tubing
- breast prosthesis
- cardiac assist pump bladders, tubing, housing, coatings
- catheters
- dental cavity liners
- endotracheal tubes
- heart pacemaker connectors, coatings, lead insulators, fixation devices
- hemodialysis tubing, membranes, connectors
- leaflet heart valves
- mechanical heart valve coatings
- orthopedic splints, bone adhesives
- percutaneous shunts
- reconstructive surgery materials
- skin dressing and tapes
- surgical drapes
- suture materials
- synthetic bile ducts
- vascular grafts and patches

Some commercially available biomedical polyurethanes can be listed as shown in Table 10.

High molecular weight polymers are generally very inert and insoluble in physiological fluids. Therefore, such polymers are assumed to have minimal toxicity [54]. Catalysts, diluents, plasticizers, solvents, fillers, pigments etc. may leach out from an uncured structure and cause severe allergic contact dermatitis. Contact with the fully cured resin, however, is unlikely to result in any hypersensitivity response [55].

BLOOD COMPATIBILITY OF POLYURETHANES

Blood clots when fibrinogen, a plasma protein, changes from its normal soluble state to a mass of tiny fibrils. These fibrils trap blood cells and foreign material at the injury site. A series of enzymatic reac-

Table 10. Some commercially available biomedical polyurethanes.

Name	Supplier	Material	Processing
Biomer (solution grade)	Ethicon, Inc.	MDI, poly(tetramethylene ether glycol), diamine extended, Linear	Solution casting from 60% dimethylacetamide solution
Biomer (extrusion grade)	Ethicon, Inc.	MDI, poly(tetramethylene ether glycol) (MW 650–2000), water cured, Linear	Can be processed by thermal methods
Pellethane	The UpJohn Chemical Co.	MDI, poly(tetramethylene ether glycol), butanediol extended	Extrusion, injection molding, solution casting
Cardiothane	Kontron, Inc.	MDI, polyether based, cross-linked with silicone	Solution casting
Tecoflex	Thermoelectron Corp.	Linear segmented, HMDI, poly(tetramethylene ether glycol), butanediol extended	Extrusion, injection molding, solution casting
Elastomeric adhesive 1-MP	Thermedics, Inc.	Linear segmented, aromatic polycaprolactone based	Single component pressure sensitive adhesive
Hypol plus FHP 4000 FHP 5000	W.R. Grace	Aromatic prepolymers, polyethers with high amounts of ethylene oxide	Two-component reactive hydrophilic foams
Rimplast PTUA 102	Petrarch Systems	Interpenetrating polymer network of polyurethane and silicone	Extrusion, injection molding
Avcothane	Avco-Everet Corp.	Copolymer of polyurethane and polydimethylsiloxane	A multi-coating system

tions are responsible for this process. Prothrombin and fibrinogen are found in the blood at all times. Prothrombin can be converted to thrombin by the enzyme thrombokinase (released from disintegrating platelets) in the presence of calcium ions. Thrombin then catalyzes the conversion of soluble fibrinogen to insoluble fibrin. The whole series of reactions is triggered by damage to a tissue. In the final stage, the platelets clump together and stick to the blood vessel wall at the injury site as a thrombus.

When a biomaterial is implanted at a blood-contacting site, the injury inflicted by the implantation procedure is only one of the causes of thrombosis. Besides, thrombus formation is only one of the several adverse effects that a biomaterial can cause. Among the other damages, decrease in plasma proteins, decrease in (or damage to) blood cells such as platelets, retention, and shape change in platelets or variation in their consumption should be considered. For a biomaterial to be accepted as hemocompatible, all these damages have to be assessed and must be negligible.

Biomaterials intended for use in contact with blood are subjected to a series of tests. These can be classified as *in situ*, *in vitro*, *ex vivo*, and *in vivo* tests. As the test system approaches simulating the biological environment, the results become more relevant for the intended future use but simultaneously become more costly and more time consuming [56].

In situ Tests

These involve the determination of the basic chemical and mechanical properties through the use of conventional techniques such as spectroscopic surface and bulk chemistry analysis (IR, FTIR, UV, ESCA, XPS, SSIMS, etc.), surface energy determination through contact angles, stress–strain relations, impact and repeated loading tests, as well as detection of leachables or degradability by extraction in various solvents, accelerated aging, determination of permeability towards various solutes, and microscopic (light microscopy, SEM or TEM) examination. These preliminary tests characterize the material to a fair degree, but yield only clues as to the behavior of the substance in contact with blood.

In vitro Tests

Data from *in vitro* tests are useful before expanding to more expensive *in vivo* testing. They also are very useful for quality control purposes. In order for a good correlation between *in vitro* and *in vivo* tests blood from the species for which implantation is to be carried out must be used. Some of the tests, commonly used to determine the *in vitro* behaviour of the biomaterials (tests to determine the properties of the material and to determine the effect of the material on blood) are given below in two categories.

a. Examination of the Test Material

- gravimetric analysis (mainly for the determination of the thrombus weight)
- light microscopy, scanning and transmission electron microscopies (for adhered platelets, erythrocytes, leukocytes, etc.)
- XPS (X-ray photoelectron spectroscopy)
- autoradiography (for labeled adsorbates)

b. Examination of the Anticoagulated Blood

- cell count (erythrocyte, leukocyte)
- platelet count and aggregation
- erythrocyte morphology
- recalcified whole blood clotting, partial thromboplastin, prothrombin, and thrombin times
- plasma free hemoglobin determination

Ex vivo Tests

This term is applied to test systems that shunt blood directly from the test animal into a test chamber located outside the body and may either be shunted directly back to the animal (recirculating) or collected into test tubes (single pass). It is advantageous because flowing native blood is used and the measured parameters are monitored in real time. They, however, are of relatively short term duration and do not allow an accurate prediction of long-term use. These tests can be carried as acute (minutes to hours) or as chronic (days to weeks).

a. Acute Tests

- cannula and shunts (platelet adhesion and activation)
- stagnation point flow test (platelet and leukocyte adhesion)
- annular axial test (thrombus deposition)

b. Chronic Tests

- arteriovenous shunt (platelet consumption and activation, coagulation activation, radiographic analysis, gamma imaging)

In vivo Tests

These tests do not allow blood to flow outside the body and thus are quite good in simulating actual use. The major limitation of this test system is the use of experimental animals as models for humans. *In vivo* test results depend more on flow parameters, compliance, porosity, and implant design than the blood compatibility of the material. *In vivo* tests are also carried out in two categories; acute (hours to days) and chronic (weeks to months).

a. Acute Tests

- intravascular catheters
- vena cava ring test

b. Chronic Tests

- vena cava ring test
- renal embolus test

Blood compatibility of a biomaterial is affected by many parameters, some of which are its surface properties [57], bulk chemistry [58], and morphology [59].

The surface of the blood-contacting biomaterials is the major area of contact with blood. Thus, the surface properties, and especially its chemical structure, are very important in deciding its thrombogenicity. However, it is not a simple matter to decide how the surface chemistry influences blood compatibility because other factors (i.e., surface roughness, porosity, design, surface free energy etc.) also have an effect [60]. As a result, it is not surprising to find different views and contradictory results in the literature.

A variety of biomedical drawbacks of polyurethanes are associated with the hydrophobic character of their surfaces. Hydrophilic property of polymers can be measured by the percent moisture absorption of the dry polymer film. Generally, films of uniform size and thickness are dried under vacuum to a constant weight and then exposed to certain relative humidity or immersed in water. The amount of adsorbed water can be found by weighing [61]. Hydrophilicity depends on the chemical composition of the polyurethane. Polymers prepared from TDI and poly(ethylene-propylene oxide) demonstrated increasing hydrophilicity as the ratio of glycol to TDI was increased from 0.018 to 0.363 [62]. On the other hand, increasing hydrophilicity was reported for the samples in which the molecular weight of glycol increased from 600 to 2000 without changing the molar ratios of components [63]. Obviously such an alteration in the composition also affects the mechanical properties of the polymer.

It is known that accumulation of the platelets onto the implant surface can cause clotting. On the other hand, it is also known that the sizes of proteins are much lower than any kind of blood cells and therefore their diffusion to the implanted material surface will be faster than that of the blood cells. The nature, the degree of denaturation, and the molar ratio of these plasma proteins adsorbed to the polymer material have an influence on the activation and adhesion of platelets [64]. It was found that if the first adsorbed protein is albumin the surface becomes more antithrombogenic compared to the fibrinogen or γ-globulin adsorbed surfaces [65]. Presence of an albumin layer on the surface greatly or totally reduces thrombosis. Polyurethanes are thromboresistant materials. Their apparent thromboresistance is thought to reside in their ability or preferentially adsorb serum albumin [66].

Generally, the initial result of blood material interaction is protein adsorption by the material, which yields a protein-coated sample. This initial rapid protein adsorption is strongly dependent on the chemical and physical surface properties of the material. Many attempts have been made to correlate surface parameters, such as surface charge, critical surface tension, work of adhesion, interfacial free energy with the adsorption of proteins or platelet adhesion [67,68]. Hydrogels, the hydrophilic insoluble network materials, have lower interfacial free energy than hydrophobic ones and as this energy gets lower, the adsorption of plasma proteins is reduced [69].

It is also stated that polyurethanes with higher contribution from the hydrogen-bonding property in the surface free energy, would have better antithrombogenicity [70]. According to a study on polyurethanes, an inverse correlation exists between baboon platelet consumption per unit area and the fraction of carbon atoms forming $C-H$ chemical bonds on the surface [71].

As seen from these reports higher hydrogen-bonding ability (higher hydrophilicity, lower surface free energy) leads to more antithrombogenic polyurethanes. The surface free energy introduces a selectivity to the polyurethane surfaces towards the type of blood protein it adsorbs. When the samples of polyurethanes which have different surfaces were incubated with solutions of ^{125}I labeled albumin, γ-globulin or fibrinogen, it was observed that the presence of a hydrophilic coat caused an increase in albumin adsorption, while in fibrinogen and γ-globulin a slight increase was observed [72,73].

The surface free energy also affects the accumulation or shape change and organization of platelets. The accumulation of labeled homologous ^{32}P platelets was measured in a polyurethane graft in the carotid arteries of sheep and thrombus was found slightly higher compared to polytetrafluoroethylene grafts [74]. In another study, the surfaces which have different chemistry but similar surface-water energetic properties to that of polyurethanes showed different results in platelet shape change and cytoskeletal reorganization. Therefore, it was concluded that properties other than surface-water energetics must be involved in determining platelet responses [75].

The type of proteins adsorbed on the surface affects the adsorption of lipids. In order to examine this effect, the film specimens were immersed in aqueous solution of lipids for various time intervals. The samples were extracted with CS_2, and extracts were examined with IR spectrophotometry. Peaks belonging to cholesterol and lecithin were observed in these samples. But if the surface was previously treated with bovine serum albumin the sorption of lipids was remarkably reduced [76]. Biomer extracts did not show any lipid adsorption even after 35 weeks of implantation [77] and were found more successful when artificial hearts made from Biomer and Silastic were compared in calves [78].

The surface properties are markedly affected by the method of fabrication [79]. For example, the casting process affects the surface properties and therefore thrombogenicity. It has been shown that some poly-ether urethanes which have been cast from N,N-dimethyl acetamide are more thrombogenic than the same polyurethane cast from tetrahydrofurane [80].

The microphase separation of polyurethanes is another parameter that was shown to have an influence on blood compatibility [81,82]. In several *ex vivo* [83] and *in vitro* [84,85] studies it has been shown that the concentration of soft segments correlates with blood compatibility. A decrease in platelet adhesion or surface-induced spreading with an increase in the relative concentration of polyether soft segment was reported [86,87]. However, it was also reported that the changes in the amount of polyether soft segment were not found to significantly affect platelet adhesion from anticoagulated human blood [88].

The chemical structure of glycol is one parameter in the polyurethanes' blood compatibility. Polyurethanes containing a poly(ethylene oxide) soft segment exhib-ited less platelet adhesion or shape change than corre-sponding polyurethanes containing poly(propylene oxide) or poly(tetramethylene oxide) *in vitro*. They were examined in an acute canine *ex vivo* shunt, and it was shown that poly(ethylene oxide)-based urethane was more thrombogenic than poly(tetramethylene oxide)- or poly(propylene oxide)-containing elasto-mers [89]. On the other hand, some researchers found that a minimum amount of platelet shape change oc-curred *in vitro*, when an intermediate molecular weight of soft segment was used [90]. In all, it can be stated that the relation between the type or the con-centration of the polyurethane soft segment and its hemocompatibility is still controversial, due to the contradictory results reported.

It was decided in most laboratories that, since the surface is so important in blood compatibility, the properties of the surface of the original biomaterial can be improved by coating with a hydrophilic com-pound, a blood protein (e.g., albumin), or heparin. In one such study, artificial blood vessels using albumin-ated Dacron fabrics were devised and a decrease in platelet adhesion on these albuminated surfaces was observed [91]. In other studies, quaternization and further heparinization of polyetherurethaneureas showed a decrease in platelet adhesion [92,93].

However, not all coating procedures yielded suc-cessful results. For example, in one study polyure-thane tubings inserted as arteriovenous shunts in dogs demonstrated occlusion in the case of heparinization [94].

Grafting of hydrophilic monomers onto segmented polyurethanes offers an attractive technique for im-proving the biocompatibility properties of these materials while maintaining some of the properties of the backbone polymer and the side chain graft

polymer. In order to achieve this, hydrophilic monomers such as N-vinyl pyrrolidone [95], 2-hy-droxyethyl methacrylate [96], 2,3-epoxypropyl meth-acrylate, 2,3-dihydroxypropyl methacrylate, and acrylamide [97] were grafted onto segmented poly-urethanes by γ-irradiation.

Another method involves copolymerization with such monomers, but this has the disadvantage of alter-ing the chemical structure and mechanical properties of the bulk. The most important copolymerization of polyurethanes was carried out with siloxanes [98]. Silicone–urethane copolymers can be thrombogenic or nonthrombogenic depending on whether the blood comes into contact with the side that was against the mold or the side exposed to air during casting. Air facing surface of Avcothane 51® was examined with ESCA and FTIR and found to be covered with poly-dimethyl siloxane. This surface was more nonthrom-bogenic than the other [99]. The casting at different temperatures and different evaporation rates of sol-vents can cause anisotropic distribution of the silicon component and alter the compatibility properties [100].

Obviously, not only the initial properties of a polyurethane are influential on its behavior in bio-medical applications. The biological medium is a very adverse medium for implanted materials due to the presence of various ions, enzymes, cells and cell frag-ments besides water. As a result of interaction with these, the behavior of the polyurethanes *in situ* and *in vivo* are very different. Upon implantation, the pro-cesses which can take place are production of leach-ables (i.e., low molecular weight substances such as fillers, monomers, solvents, catalysts, etc.), adsorp-tion and absorption of biological molecules (such as platelets, lipids and proteins), cross-linking and degradation. As a result of any of these processes, modifications in the polyurethane properties take place. For example, polyurethane elastomers used for artificial heart systems end up with altered cyclic elastomeric properties upon absorption of body fluids [101,102].

The action of the biological environment on poly-urethanes can lead to varying results. Some polyure-thanes undergo an extensive degradation within a few weeks while others stand long term implantation with-out any noticable change in their properties. The major difference in degradability is shown by poly-ester urethanes. Polyether urethanes, generally are known to be quite stable [103–105] although there are few reports about their rapid degradation *in vivo* [106,107].

Under *in vivo* conditions, polyester urethanes were almost completely degraded in four months while polyether urethanes showed only a 5–10% decrease in weight, 10% decrease in molecular weight and 10% reduction in tensile strength in two months. When the same samples were immersed in phosphate buffer for one year, polyester urethanes had a 5% decrease in weight and a 10% decrease in molecular weight while polyether urethanes did not show any reduction in weight and molecular weight [108].

Estane, a polyester urethane, has been reported to have a greater susceptibility for hydrolytic degradation [109] than polyether urethanes. However, it was also reported that some polyester urethanes were more stable than some polyether urethanes [110]. It is clear from these data that polyester urethanes are more susceptible to degradation than the polyether urethanes.

In vitro and *in vivo* experiments are not correlated to each other properly. *In vivo* conditions are more severe than a simple immersion in buffer, due to the contributions of the enzymes as well as other biological molecules on the degradation process. Although hydrolytic microporous polyurethane vascular prostheses showed good mechanical properties and excellent behaviour *in vitro*, they were disappointing *in vivo* [111]. Mitrathane grafts became occluded by thrombosis after 24 h implantation [112].

One method of examining the degradative effect of enzymes involves using radio-labeled biomaterials and analyzing the medium for released radioactivity. In a study, ^{14}C-labeled polyether urethanes consisting of TDI, MDI, polytetramethyleneoxide and ^{14}C ethylenediamine were brought in contact with different types of enzymes (e.g., hydrolytic, oxidative, or a mixture). The molecular weight of the polyether urethane was found to be important in the degradation process. Polymers prepared from a polyether with a molecular weight of 1000 were found to be affected by many different enzymes such as esterase, papain, bromelain, ficin, chymotrypsin, trypsin, cathepsin C, while were stable against collagenase, xanthine oxidase, cytochrome C oxidase [113]. Polymers prepared from polyethers having molecular weights of 650 and 2000 were, however, unaffected by any of the above enzymes. In other studies, papain caused a decrease in fracture stresses of poly(ether urethane ureas) and on Biomer® in a month. Fatigue lifetimes for the treated samples were found to be lower than those of the untreated controls [114].

GPC chromotography was also employed in the determination of the effects of various enzymes on polyether urethanes. The *Mw* and *Mn* of the samples treated with papain showed a decrease while urease had almost no effect. The explanation of the activity of papain and the inactivity of urease can be based on the enzyme size. Since the molecular weight of urease is about 20-fold higher than that of papain, diffusion of papain into the polymer bulk would be easier and thus more sample would be exposed to enzyme. ATR-FTIR analysis showed that papain degrades the polymer by hydrolysing urethane and urea linkages producing free amines while urease hydrolyses only the urea linkages [115]. This larger number of target bonds for papain must also contribute to its higher activity. When the blank solutions were tested, an increase in molecular weight of the polyurethane was observed. This was explained by the free isocyanate

groups undergoing chain extension reactions with water. With polyurethanes cast in metal and glass molds, and treated with papain, α-chymotrypsin and leucine aminopeptidase, it was found that leucine caused a 120% increase in molecular weight of Pellethane that was prepared on gold surface [116].

In vivo, the appearance of a bright yellow stain on the prostheses occurs due to the absorption of bilirubin, a pigment formed from degradation of hemoglobin. In order to test the role of polyetherurethane on the degradation of hemoglobin, freshly withdrawn heparinized blood was circulated in polyether urethane tubings. No hemolitic activity and no yellow color was observed [117].

The changes in mechanical properties or the changes in the number of the cycles to failure in fatigue are very sensitive ways to measure the degradation. Comprehensive flexure endurance tests were carried out for polyurethanes synthesized for artificial heart assist pump bladders. They were tested for 80–160 beats per minute against a pressure head of 100 mmHg and some of them withstood 80 million cycles for 2 years in cardiac assist pumps [118].

Sterilization is another process which might influence the properties of a biomaterial, leading to changes in its behavior in a biological medium. Most polymers soften or degrade at elevated temperatures, therefore for such polymers autoclaving is not an appropriate method of sterilization. Sterilization by gamma irradiation may also cause varying degrees of structural changes. On the other hand, during the ethylene oxide sterilization the gas may be absorbed by the material and subsequently released into the tissue after implantation [119]. For PVC, polyurethanes, and silicone rubbers complete desorption of ethylene oxide can occur within 24 hours if aeration of the plastic device is carried out for this period [120]. With polyurethanes steam autoclaving, gamma irradiation, and ethylene oxide sterilization all were shown to cause molecular weight reduction, most probably due to the instability of the ether bonds in the structure [121].

It is, therefore, not possible to recommend a specific method of sterilization for polyurethanes although ethylene oxide sterilization is the most frequently preferred one. It would be most appropriate to select a sterilization method for an individual product after careful testing.

CONCLUSION

Polyurethanes, among all polymers, have a special place in blood-contacting products and devices. The reason for this lies in the inherent, relative nonthrombogenicity of their surfaces, their simple design for obtaining widely varying viscoelastic properties, the large array of physical forms in which they can be produced, and their controllable degradability. Due to their excellent mechanical and flexure properties they are used especially in cardiovascular devices. The current research on polyurethanes is concentrated on understanding the mechanism of plasma cell, cell fragment and macromolecule adsorption on their surfaces with the aim of obtaining ultimate hemocompatibility.

REFERENCES

1. Bayer, O., H. Rinke, L. Siefken, L. Orthner and H. Schild. 1942. German patent 728,981.

2. Bayer, O. 1947. *Angew. Chem*, 59:275.

3. Bruins, P. F. 1969. *Polyurethane Technology*. Interscience Pub. New York: John Wiley and Sons.

4. Buist, J. M., and H. Gudgeon. 1968. *Advances in Polyurethane Technology*. London: MacLaren and Sons Ltd.

5. Lyman, D. J. 1960. *J. Polym. Sci.*, 45:49.

6. Wright, P., and A. P. C. Cumming. 1969. *Solid Polyurethane Elastomers*. New York: Gordon and Breach Sci. Pub.

7. Pigott, K. A, "Polyurethanes", in *Encyclopedia of Polymer Science and Technology*. 11:506–563.

8. Pigot, K. A., B. F. Frye, K. R. Allen, S. Steingiser, W. C. Darr, J. H. Saunders, and E. E. Hardy. 1960. *J. Chem. Eng. Data.*, 5:391.

9. Blaich, C. F., Jr. and A. J. Sampson. 1961. *Rubber Age*, 89:263.

10. Anderson, J. C., K. D. Leaver, J. M Alexander, and R. D. Rawlings. 1974. *Materials Science*, 2nd ed. Middlesex: Thomas Nelson and Sons Ltd.

11. Smith, C. O. 1977. *The Science of Engineering Materials*. New Jersey: Prentice-Hall Inc.

12. Andrews, R. D., A. V. Tobolsky, and E. E. Hanson. 1946. *J. Appl. Phys.*, 17:352.

13. Tobolsky, A. V., and A. Mercurio. 1959. *J. Polym. Sci.*, 36:467.

14. Singh, A. 1971. "Effect of Chemical Structure on the Thermal Stability of Cross-linked Urethane Elastomers", in *Advances in Urethane Science and Technology, Volume 1*. K. C. Frich and S. L. Reegen, eds. Lancaster, PA: Technomic Pub. Co. Inc.

15. Smith, T. L. 1977. "Strength of Elastomers. A Perspective", *Polym. Eng. Sci.*, 17:114–129.

16. Van Bogart, J. W. C., P. E. Gibson, and S. L. Cooper. 1983. "Structure-Property Relationships in Polycaprolactone-Polyurethanes", *J. Polym. Sci., Polym. Phys. Ed.*, 21:65–96.

17. Foks, J., H. Janik, R. Russo and S. Winiecki. 1989. "Morphology and Thermal Properties of Polyurethanes Prepared under Different Conditions", *Eur. Polym. J.*, 25:31–37.

18. Wilkes, G. L., T. S. Dziemianowicz, Z. H. Ophir, E. Artz, and R. Wildnauer. 1979. "Thermally Induced Time Dependence of Mechanical Properties in Biomedical Grade Polyurethanes", *J. Biomed. Mater. Res.*, 13:189–206.

19. Lemm, W. 1985. "Biodegradation of Polyurethanes", in *Polyurethanes in Biomedical Engineering*. H.

Planck, G. Egbers, and I, Syre, ed. Amsterdam: Elsevier Sci. Pub. pp. 103–108.

20. Zartnack, F., W. Dunkel, K. Affeld, and E. S. Bucherl 1978. "Fatigue Problems in Artificial Blood Pumps", *Trans. Am. Soc. Artif. Intern. Organs*, 24:600–605.

21. Dzierza, W. 1982. "Stress-Relaxation Properties of Segmented Polyurethane Rubbers", *J. Appl. Polm. Sci.*, 27:1487–1499.

22. Wong, E. W. C. 1981. "Development of a Biomedical Polyurethane", in *Urethane Chemistry and Applications, ACS Series*, pp. 489–504.

23. Parsons, J. R. and J. Black. 1977. "The Viscoelastic Shear Behaviour of Normal Rabbit Cartilage", *J. Biomechanics,* 10:21.

24. Rausch, K. W. and A. A. R. Sayigh. 1965. *Ind. Eng. Chem. Prd. Res. Dev.*, 4(2):92.

25. Rausch, K. W., R. F. Martel and A. A. R. Sayigh. 1964. *Ind. Eng. Chem. Prd. Res. Dev.*, 3(2):125.

26. Cooper, S. L. and J. C. West. "Polyurethane Block Polymers", *Encyclopedia of Polymer Science and Technology*. 16:521–543.

27. Axelrood, S. L. and K. C. Frisch. 1960. *Rubber Age*, 88(3):465.

28. Saunders, J. H. and K. C. Frisch. 1962, 1964. *Polyurethanes, Chemistry and Technology Parts I and II*. New York: Interscience Pub. Inc.

29. Willard, H. H., L. L. Merritt, J. A. Dean, F. A. Settle. 1981. *Instrumental Methods of Analysis, 6th ed.* New York: D. Van Nostrand Co.

30. Okkema, A. Z., D. J. Fabrizius, T. G. Grasel, S. L. Cooper, and R. J. Zdrahala. 1989. "Bulk, Surface, and Blood Contacting Properties of Polyether Polyurethanes Modified with Polydimethysiloxane Macroglycols", *Biomaterials*, 10:23–32.

31. Speckhard, T. A., K. K. S. Hwang, C. Z. Yang, W. R. Laupan and S. L. Cooper. 1984. "Properties of Segmented Polyurethane Zwittemonomor Elastomers", *J. Macromol. Sci. Phys. B.*, 23(2):175–199.

32. Masiulanis, B., J. Hrouz, J. Baldrian, M. Jlavsky and K. Dusek. 1987. "Dynamic Mechanical Behavior and Structure of Polyurethaneimides", *J. Appl. Polym. Sci.*, 34:1941–1951.

33. Doyne, E. N. 1971. *The Development and Use of Polyurethane Products*. New York: MacGraw Hill Co.

34. Mitkovitch, V., T. Akutsu and W. J. Kolff. 1962. "Polyurethane Aortas in Dogs. Three Year Results", *Trans. Am. Soc. Artif. Intern. Organs*, 8:79.

35. Sharp, W. V., D. L. Gardner and G. J. Andersen. 1966. "A Bioelectric Polyurethane Elastomer for Intravascular Replacement", *Trans. Am. Soc. Artif. Intern. Organs*, 12:1979.

36. Boretos, J. W. and W. S. Pierce. 1966. "A Polyether Polymer", *J. Biomed. Mat. Res.*, 2:121–130.

37. Lyman, D. J., J. L. Brash and K. G. Klein. 1969. "The Effect of Chemical Structure and Surface Properties of Synthetic Polymers on Coagulation of Blood", *Proceedings Artificial Heart Program USGPO*, R. J. Hegyeli, ed. Washington, DC, p. 113.

38. Lawson, J. H., D. B. Olsen, E. Hershgold, J. Kolff, K. Hadfield and W. J. Kolff. 1975. "A Comparison of Polyurethane and Silastic Artificial Hearts in 10 Long

Survival Experiments in Calves", *Trans. Am. Soc. Artif. Intern. Organs*, 21:368–373.

39. Lyman, D. J., F. J. Fazzio, H. Voorhees, G. Robinson and D. Albo, Jr. 1978. "Compliance as a Factor Affecting the Patency of a Copolyurethane Vascular Graft", *J. Biomed. Mater. Res.*, 12:337–345.

40. Durst, S., J. Leslie, R. Moore and K. Amplatz. 1974. "A Comparison of the Thrombogenicity of Commercially Available Catheters", *Radiology*, 113:599–600.

42. Brash, J. L., B. K. Fritzinger and S. D. Bruck. 1973. "Development of Block Copolyether Urethane Intra Aortic Balloons and Other Medical Devices", *Biomed. Mater. Res.*, 7:313–334.

43. Devanathan, T., J. E. Sluetz and K. A. Young. 1980. "*In vivo* Thrombogenicity of Implantable Cardiac Pacing Leads", *Biomat. Med. Dev. Artif. Organs*, 8:369–379.

44. Szycher, M., D. Dempsey and V. L. Poirier. 1984. "Surface Fissuring of Polyurethane Based Pacemaker Leads", *Trans. Soc. Biomat.*, 7:24.

45. Tsutsui, T., E. Imamura, H. Koyanagi, Y. Tsuda and K. Tsuchida. 1981. "The Development of Non-Stended Trileaflet Valve Prostheses", *Artif. Organs* (Japan), 10:590–593.

46. Wisman, C. B., W. S. Pierce, J. H. Donachy, W. E. Pae, J. L. Myers and G. A. Prophet. 1982. "A Polyurethane Trileaflet Cardiac Valve Prothesis: *In vitro* and *in vivo* Studies", *Trans. Am. Soc. Artif. Intern. Organs*, 28:164–168.

47. Snow, J., H. Harasaki, J. Kasick, R. Whalen, R. Kiraly and Y. Nose. 1981. "Promising Results with a New Textured Surface Intrathoracic Variable Volume Device for LVAS", *Trans. Am. Soc. Artif. Intern. Organs*, 27:485–489.

48. Lyman, D. J., W. C. Seare, Jr., D. Albo, Jr., S. Bergman, J. Lamb., L. C. Metcalf and K. Richards. 1977. "Polyurethane Elastomers in Surgery", *Int. J. Polymeric Mater.*, 5:211–229.

49. Wong, E. W. 1969. "Urethane-Polyether Block Copolymer Membranes for Reverse Osmosis, Ultrafiltration and Other Membrane Processes", ORF Record of Invention No. 335.

50. Queen, D., J. H. Evans, J. D. S. Gaylor, J. M. Courtney and W. H. Reid. 1987. *Biomaterials*, 8:372–376.

51. Woodroof, E. A. 1984. *Biobrane®, A Synthetic Skin Prosthesis in Burn Wound Coverings*, Vol. 2. D. L. Wise, ed. Boca Raton: CRC Press Inc.

52. Guidon, R., D. Domurado, S. Poignant, C. Grosselin and J. Awad. 1977. "Stored Blood Microfiltration-Evaluation of Micro-Aggregate Filter Composed of Polyurethane Foam and Nylon Wool", *Res. Exper. Med.*, 171:129–139.

53. Balas, A., G. Palka, J. Foks and H. Janik. 1984. "Properties of Cast Urethane Elastomers Prepared from Poly(E-caprolactone)s", *J. Appl. Polym. Sci.*, 29:2261–2270.

54. Williams, D. F. 1981. "Introduction to the Toxicology of Polymer-Based Materials", in *Systemic Aspects of Biocompatibility, Volume 2*. D. F. Williams, ed. Boca Raton: CRC Press Inc.

55. Fisher, A. A. 1967. *Contact Dermatisis*. London: Kimpton.

56. 1985. *Guidelines for Blood-Material Interactions*. Report of the National Heart, Lung and Blood Institute Working Group, NIH Publication.

57. Lyman, D. J., K. Knutson, B. McNeil and K. Shibatani. 1975. "The Effects of Chemical Structure and Surface Properties of Synthetic Polymers on the Coagulation of Blood. IV. The Relation Between Polymer Morphology and Protein Absorption", *Trans. Am. Soc. Artif. Intern. Org.*, 21:49–54.

58. Ratner, B. D. and R. W. Paynter. 1984. "Polyurethane Surfaces: The Importance of Molecular Weight Distribution, Bulk Chemistry and Casting Conditions", in *Polyurethanes in Biomedical Engineering*. H. Planck, G. Egbers and I. Syre, eds. Amsterdam: Elsevier Sci. Pub.

59. Picha, G. J. and D. F. Gibbons. 1978. "Effect of Polyurethane Morphology on Blood Coagulation", *J. Bioeng.*, 2:301–311.

60. Andrade, J. D., L. M. Smith and D. E. Gregonis. 1985. *Surface and Interphase Aspect of Biomedical Polymers*, Vol. 1. J. D. Andrade, ed. New York: Plenum Press, pp. 249–292.

61. Burke, A., V. N. Hasirci and N. Hasirci. 1988. "Polyurethane Membranes", *J. Bioactive and Compatible Polymers*, 3:232–242.

62. Hasirci, N. and A. Burke. 1987. "A Novel Polyurethane Film for Biomedical Use", *J. Bioactive and Compatible Polymers*, 2:131–141.

63. Boretos, J. W. 1981. "The Chemistry and Biocompatibility of Specific Polyurethane Systems for Medical Use", *Biocompatibility of Clinical Implant Materials*. D. F. Williams, ed. Boca Raton: CRC Press.

64. Stupp, S. I., J. W. Kaufmann and S. H. Carr. 1977. "Interactions Between Segmented Polyurethane Surfaces and the Plasma Protein Fibrinogen", *J. Biomed. Mater. Res.*, 11:237–250.

65. Grasel, T. G. and S. L. Cooper. 1986. "Surface Properties and Blood Compatibility of Polyurethane Ureas", *Biomaterials*, 7:315–328.

66. Songuine, A. 1982. "Future for Biomaterials", *Science*, 217:1125.

67. Lyman, D. J., W. M. Muir and I. J. Lee. 1965. "The Effect of Chemical Structure and Surface Properties of Polymers on the Coagulation of Blood, I. Surface Free Energy Effects", *Trans. Am. Soc. Artif. Intern. Organs*, 11:301–306.

68. Bischoff, K. B. 1968. "Discussion of Correlations of Blood Coagulation with Surface Properties of Materials", *J. Biomed. Mater. Res.*, 2:89–93.

69. Andrade, J. D. 1973. "International Phenomena and Biomaterials", *Med. Instrum.*, 7(2):110–120.

70. Shibuta, R., T. Tanaka, M. Sisido and Y. Imanishi. 1986. "Synthesis of Novel Polyaminoether Urethaneureas and Development of Antithrombogenic Materials by Their Modifications", *J. Biomed. Mater. Res.*, 20:971–987.

71. Hanson, S. R., L. A. Harker, B. D. Ratner and A. S. Hoffman. 1980. "*In vivo* Evaluation of Artificial Surfaces with a Non-Human Primate Model of Arterial Thrombosis", *J. Lab. Clin. Med.*, 95:289–304.

72. Greenwood, F. C., W. M. Hunter and S. S. Glover. 1963. "The Preparation of ^{131}I-Labeled Human Growth

Hormone of High Specific Radioactivity", *Biochem. J.*, 89:114–119.

73. Murphy, P. V., A. La Croix, S. Merchant and W. Benhard. 1971. "Development of Blood Compatible Polymers Using the Electret Effect", in *Medical Applications of Plastics*. H. P. Gregor, ed. NY: John Wiley & Sons, Inc., pp. 59–74.

74. Lannerstad, O., D. Bergqvist, P. Dougan, B. F. Ericsson and B. Nilsson. 1987. "Acute Thrombogenicity of a Compliant Polyurethane Urea Graft Compared with Polytetrafluoroethylene: An Experimental Study in Sheep", *Eur. Surg. Res.*, 19:6–10.

75. Ruckenstein, E. and S. V. Gourisankar. 1984. "A Surface Energetic Criterion of Blood Compatibility of Foreign Surfaces", *J. Colloid Interface Sci.*, 101:436–451.

76. Takahara, A., J. Tashita, T. Kajiyama and M. Takayanagi. 1985. "Effect of Aggregation State of Hard Segment in Segmented Poly(urethaneureas) on Their Fatigue Behaviour After Interaction with Blood Components", *J. Biomed. Mater. Res.*, 19:13–34.

77. Boretos, J. W., W. S. Pierce, R. E. Baier, A. F. LeRoy and H. J. Donachy. 1975. "Surface and Bulk Characteristics of a Polyether Urethane for Artificial Hearts", *J. Biomed. Mater. Res.*, 9:327.

78. Lawson, J. H., D. B. Olsen, E. Hershgold, J. Kolff, K. Hadfield and J. A. Kolff. 1975. "A Comparison of Polyurethane and Silastic Artificial Hearts in 10 Long Survival Experiments in Calves", *Trans. Am. Soc. Artif. Intern. Organs*, 221:368.

79. Lelah, M. D., L. K. Lambrecht, B. R. Young and S. L. Cooper. 1983. "Physicochemical Characterization and *in vivo* Blood Tolerability of Cast and Extruded Biomer", *J. Biomed. Mater. Res.*, 17:1–22.

80. Lelah, M. D., T. G. Grasel, J. A. Pierce and S. L. Cooper. 1986. "*Ex vivo* Interactions and Surface Property Relationship of Polyether Urethanes", *J. Biomed. Mater. Res.*, 20:433–468.

81. Smith, T. L. 1977. "Strength of Elastomers. A Perspective", *Polym. Eng. Sci.*, 17:114–129.

82. Takahara, A., J. Tashita, T. Kajiyama, M. Takayanagi and W. J. MacKnight. 1985. "Microphase Separated Structure, Surface Composition and Blood Compatibility of Segmented Poly(urethaneureas) with Various Soft Segment Components", *Polymer,* 26:987–996.

83. Lelah, M. D., J. A. Pierce, L. K. Lambrecht and S. L. Cooper. 1985. "Polyether Urethane Ionomers. Surface Property/*ex vivo* Blood Compatibility Relationship," *J. Colloid Interface Sci.*, 104:422–439.

84. Sa da Costa, V., D. B. Russell, E. W. Salzman and E. W. Merrill. 1981. "ESCA Studies of Polyurethanes: Blood Platelet Activation in Relation to Surface Composition", *J. Colloid Interface Sci.*, 80:445–452.

85. Merrill, E. W., V. Sa da Costa, E. W. Salzman, D. B. Russell, L. Kuchner, D. F. Waugh, G. Trugel, S. Stopper and V. Vitale. "A Critical Study of Segmented Polyurethanes, in Biomaterials: Interfacial Phenomena and Applications", S. L. Cooper and N. A. Peppas, eds. *ACS Adv. Chem. Ser.*, 199:95–107.

86. Whicher, S. J. and J. L. Brash. 1978. "Platelet Foreign Surface Interactions: Release of Granule Constituents from Adhered Platelets", *J. Biomed. Mater. Res.*, 12:181–201.

87. Lyman, D. J., L. C. Metcalf, D. Albo, Jr., K. F. Richards and J. Lamb. 1978. "The Effect of Polyurethane Morphology on Blood Coagulation", *J. Bioeng.*, 2:301–311.

88. Picha, G. J., D. F. Gibbons and R. A. Auerbach. 1978. "Effect of Polyurethane Morphology on Blood Coagulation", *J. Bioeng.*, 2:301–311.

89. Michael, D. L., T. G. Grasel, J. A. Pierce and S. L. Cooper. 1984. "*Ex vivo* Interactions and Surface Property Relationships of Polyetherurethanes", *J. Biomed. Mater. Res.*, 18:1059–1072.

90. Takahara, A., J. Tashita, T. Kajiyama and M. Takayanagi. 1982. "Blood Compatibility and Microphase Separated Structure of Segmented Poly(urethaneureas) with Various Soft Segment Components", *Rept. Progr. Polym. Phys.*, Japan. 25:841–844.

91. Guidoin, R., L. Martin, M. Marcis, C. Gosselin, M. King, K. Gunasekera, D. Domurado, M. F. Sigot-Luizard, M. Sigot and P. Blais. 1984. "Polyester Prostheses as Substitutes in the Thoracic Aorta of Dogs. II. Evaluation of Albuminated Polyester Grafts Stored in Ethanol", *J. Biomed. Mater. Res.*, 18:1059–1072.

92. Ito, Y., M. Sisido and Y. Imanishi. 1989. "Platelet Adhesion onto Protein Coated and Uncoated Polyether Urethaneurea Having Tertiary Amino Groups in the Substituents and its Derivatives", *J. Biomed. Mater. Res.*, 23:191–206.

93. Ito, Y., M. Sisido and Y. Imanishi. 1986. "Synthesis and Antithrombogenity of Polyetherurethaneurea Containing Quaternary Ammonium Groups in the Side Chains and of the Polymer-Heparin Complex", *J. Biomed. Mater. Res.*, 20:1017–1033.

94. Arnander, C. 1989. "Enhanced Patency of Small-Diameter Tubing after Surface Immobilization of Heparin Fragments. A Study in the Dogs", *J. Biomed. Mater. Res.*, 23:285–294.

95. Egboh, S. H., M. H. George and J. A. Barrie. 1984. "The γ-Radiation Induced Grafting of Unsaturated Segmented Polyurethanes with N-Vinylpyrrolidone Polymer", *Polymer*, 25:1157–1160.

96. Lee, H. B., H. S. Shim and J. D. Andrade. 1972. "Radiation Grafting of Synthetic Hydrogels to Inert Polymer Surfaces I. Hydroxyethylmethacrylate", *Am. Chem. Soc., Div. Polym. Chem. Polym. Prepr.*, 13(2):729–735.

97. Jansen, B. and G. Ellinghorst. 1984. "Modification of Polyether Urethane for Biomedical Application by Radiation Induced Grafting II. Water Sorption, Surface Properties, and Protein Adsorption of Grafted Films", *J. Biomed. Mater. Res.*, 18:655–669.

98. Nyilas, E. 1970. "Development of Blood Compatible Elastomers, Theory Practice and *in vivo* Performance", *23rd Conference on Engineering in Medicine and Biology*, 12:147.

99. Paik, Sung, C. S., C. B. Hu, E. W. Merrill and E. W. Salzman. 1978. "Surface Chemistry Analysis of Avcothane and Biomer by Fourier Transform IR Internal Reflection Spectroscopy", *J. Biomed. Mater. Res.*, 12:791.

100. Nyilas, E. and R. S. Ward, Jr. 1974. "Development of Blood Compatible Elastomers. V. Surface Structure and Blood Compatibility of Avcothane Elastomers", *J. Biomed. Mater. Res.*, 8:69.

101. Akutsu, T. and A. Kantrowitz. 1987. "Problems of Materials in Mechanical Heart Systems", *J. Biomed. Mater. Res.*, 1:33–54.

102. Lelah, M. D. and S. L. Cooper. 1986. *Polyurethanes in Medicine*. CRC Press: Boca Raton, FL.

103. Hunter, S. K., D. E. Gregonis, D. L. Coleman, J. D. Andrade and T. Kessler. 1982. "Molecular Weight Characterization of Pre and Post Implant Artificial Heart Polyurethane Materials", *Trans. Am. Soc. Artif. Intern. Organs*, 28:473–477.

104. Pierce, W. S., J. H. Donachy and W. M. Philips. 1978. "A Ten Year Experience Using Segmented Polyurethane for Cardiac", *AAMI 13th Ann. Meet.*, March, Washington, DC

105. Lemm, W. and E. S. Bucherl. 1983. "The Degradation of Some Polyurethanes *in vitro* and *in vivo*", in *Biomaterials and Biomechanics*. P. Ducheyne, G. Van der Perre and A. E. Aubert, eds. Amsterdam: Elsevier.

106. Lemm, W., G. R. Trukenberg, K. Gerlach and E. S. Bucherl. 1981. "Biodegradation of Some Biomaterials after Subcutaneous Implantation", *Proc. Eur. Soc. Artif. Org.*, 8:71–75.

107. Marchant, R. E., J. M. Anderson, E. Castillo and A. Hiltner. 1986. "The Effects of an Enhanced Inflammatory Reaction on the Surface Properties of Cast Biomer", *J. Biomed. Mater. Res.*, 20:153–168.

108. Gogolewski, S., G. Galletti and G. Ussia. 1987. "Polyurethane Vascular Prostheses in Pigs", *Colloid and Polymer Sci.*, 265:774–778.

109. Szycher, M., V. Poirier and J. Keiser. 1977. "Selection of Materials for Ventricular Assist Pump Development and Fabrication", *Trans. Am. Soc. Artif. Intern. Organs*, 23:116.

110. Ratner, B. D., K. W. Gladhill and T. A. Horbett. 1988. "Analysis of *in vitro* Enzymatic and Oxidative Degradation of Polyurethanes", *J. Biomed. Mater. Res.*, 22:509–527.

111. Teijeira, F. J., G. Lamoureux, J. P. Tetreault, R. Bauset, R. Guidoin, Y. Marais, R. Paynter and F. Assayed. 1989. "Hydrophilic Polyurethane Versus Autologous Femoral Vein as Substitutes in the Femoral Arteries of Dogs: Quantification of Platelets and Fibrin Deposits", *Biomaterials*, 10:80–84.

112. Martz, H., R. Paynter, J. C. Forest, A. Downs and R. Guidoin. 1987. "Microporous Hydrophilic Polyurethane Vascular Grafts as Substitutes in the Abdominal Aorta of Dogs", *Biomaterials*, 8:3–11.

113. Smith, R., D. F. Williams and C. Oliver. 1987. "The Biodegradation of Poly(etherurethanes)", *J. Biomed. Mater. Res.*, 21:1149–1166.

114. Zhao, Q., R. E. Marchant, J. M. Anderson and A. Hiltner. 1987. "Long Term Biodegradation *in vitro* of Poly(etherurethaneurea): A Mechanical Property Study", *Polymer*, 28:2040–2046.

115. Phua, K., E. Castillo, J. M. Anderson and A. J. Hiltner. 1987. "Biodegradation of Polyurethane *in vitro*", *J. Biomed. Mater. Res.*, 21:231–246.

116. Ratner, B. D., K. W. Gladhill and T. A. Horbett. 1988. "Analysis of *in vitro* Enzymatic and Oxidative Degradation of Polyurethanes", *J. Biomed. Mater. Res.*, 22:509–527.

117. Martz, H., R. Paynter, M. Loiser, D. Domurado, J. C. Forest and R. Guidoin. 1987. "Blood Hemolysis by PTFE and Polyurethane Vascular Prostheses in an *in vivo* Circuit", *J. Biomed. Mater. Res.*, 21:1187–1196.

118. Poirier, V., D. Germes and M. Szycher. 1977. "Advances in Electric Assist Devices", *Trans. Am. Soc. Artif. Intern. Organs*, 23:72.

119. Gilding, D. K. and A. M. Reed. 1979. "Systematic Development of Polyurethanes for Biomedical Applications. I. Synthesis, Structure and Properties", *Trans. 11th Int. Biomat. Symp.*, p. 3.

120. McGunnigle, R. G., J. A. Renner, S. J. Romano and R. A. Abodealy. 1975. "Residual Ethylene Oxide: Results in Medical Grade Tubing and Effects on an *in vitro* Biological System", *J. Biomed. Mater. Res.*, 9:273.

120. Gilding, D. K. 1981. "Degradation of Polymers: Mechanisms and Implications for Biomedical Applications", in *Fundamental Aspects of Biocompatibility*. D. F. Williams, ed. Boca Raton: CRC Press Inc., pp. 43–65.

6

Advanced Testing Methods for Biomaterials

LECON WOO, Ph.D.*
MICHAEL T. K. LING*
WILSON CHEUNG*

ABSTRACT: One engages in testing of biomaterials with a simple common objective: ensuring the best possible clinical outcome when the biomaterial is finally used in an *in vivo* situation. A number of more advanced techniques are covered in this chapter. Since molecular weight plays such a critical role in polymeric materials' performance, rheological techniques and instrumentations capable of direct measurement of polymer's molecular weight and molecular weight distribution are discussed. Also, since molecular relaxations frequently govern engineering properties of biological responses, both the dynamic mechanical analysis (DMA) and dielectric spectroscopy are presented. In this regard, the widely used thermal analysis technique, primarily that of the differential scanning calorimetry (DSC), provides a wealth of fundamental information on the polymer system at hand. In many cases the reliability of devices often depends on fracture and failure phenomenon. A thorough and vigorous discussion on fracture mechanics, fatigue phenomenon and reliability prediction provides some basic tools that can be applied in this area. Finally, a brief discussion on the shelf life aspect of product performance is given.

INTRODUCTION

Numerous publications [1–3] have addressed the very important issue of biomaterial testing. Invariably a testing method is selected to measure material responses, and to compare differences among compositional or other variables; finally, an attempt is made to relate the measured properties to performance, before drawing conclusions on the possible structural basis of performance.

Due to the immense complexity of human physiology, the relationship between various test results and *in vivo* product performance has frequently been very difficult to establish. This area is where we will concentrate our efforts.

The total performance of the product depends on a triad of factors: biocompatibility, physical properties, and processing. These three factors can frequently interact to greatly alter the total performance. For example, sterilization by gamma radiation can alter the molecular weight and molecular weight distribution to render the physical properties unacceptable, especially after a prolonged shelf life storage time. Likewise, ethylene oxide, a common sterilant, can leave significant residues that alter the biocompatibility very dramatically.

Product performance, the ultimate goal of all biomaterial efforts, came about through carefully designed and executed clinical trials. However, long before the clinical stage, numerous *in vitro* or *ex vivo* tests can be carried out on the device. If appropriate care is taken to mimic the critical controlling factors, *in vitro* material testing can frequently predict accurately the clinical outcome. We will examine several of the more relevant testing techniques in their ability to relate to product efficacy.

For polymeric biomaterials, the molecular weight is the controlling factor for most physical properties, although the chemical properties are not very different from the monomeric units making up the polymer. The average molecular weight, or the degree of polymerization (DP), and the associated breadth of the molecular weight distribution, determines to a large extent, the mechanical strength, ultimate elongation, and frequently the resistance to chemical and biological stress cracking agents. Determination of molecular weight is traditionally a difficult and time-consuming procedure. Solution viscosity determinations require meticulous care in the cleaning and maintenance of the glasswares, with good experimental techniques. Gel permeation chromatography (GPC) or size exclusion chromatography (SEC) also require demanding techniques in sample preparation and actual experimental practices.

*Baxter Healthcare Corporation, Applied Sciences, Round Lake, IL 60073

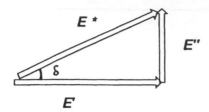

Figure 1. Dynamic moduli definition.

Recently, rheology-based molecular weight determinations have advanced both theoretically and experimentally. We will introduce this powerful technique to the reader.

A closely related rheological technique is dynamic mechanical analysis (DMA), normally carried out in the solid state. The relaxation spectrum thus obtained contains all the identifiable assignments related to motions and relaxations of all the sub-units on the polymer chain. In the multiphase polymer system frequently used in biomaterials, the interface between domains often plays a dominant role in the physiological response. As we shall demonstrate, these types of morphological data are very frequently and easily interpreted on the dynamic mechanical spectra.

Dielectric spectroscopy complements dynamic mechanical analysis in probing polymer relaxation spectra through coulombic and dispersive electrical coupling to the sample material. In this regard, the relationship between the external experimental field and the sample is not as direct as the mechanical stress field in the dynamic mechanical analysis. However, with dielectric analysis, the span of frequency is much greater. It is not uncommon to obtain dielectric spectra covering over six decades of frequencies or more in a single experimental run. Recently, there have been reports that the dielectric response of hard tissue implants greatly influenced the remodeling and repair of bones.

Differential scanning calorimetry by either the heat flow method or the power balance method, has advanced to a high level of sophistication where even the most subtle transitions in biomaterials are observable. In DSC, the biomaterial's thermodynamic state is observed as a function of temperature or time. In first order transitions, the material undergoes a net exchange of heat with its surroundings. Phase transitions such as melting point, boiling point, and solid phase transitions are obvious examples. However, for biomaterials, the second order transitions are more relevant. Second order transitions are located where a discontinuity occurs on the heat capacity function. The glass transition temperature, T_g, is the most prominent example. T_g marks the boundary between glassy and liquid behavior while on the molecular level, it represents the onset of large scale segmental motion along the biopolymer's main chain. Needless to say, from the point of view of both mechanical properties and biocompatibility, the T_g of the material is of paramount importance.

In numerous biomaterial applications, the component is subjected to repetitive stress cycles. Fatigue testing is an invaluable tool in predicting product performance, recognizing again that *in vitro* testing covers only one aspect of durability. That is, in the complexities of human physiology, other factors may come into play to influence the ultimate *in vivo* service life. However, it is generally recognized that an acceptable set of *in vitro* data is the minimum requirement for product performance. Needless to say, if more accurate simulation is performed, and a closer approximation to *in vivo* conditions covered, there is a greater likelihood that data will accurately predict the *in vivo* outcome.

Recently, the science of fatigue testing and lifetime prediction has advanced significantly both in analytical description of the process and in experimental techniques. A rather thorough theoretical introduction will be given to familiarize the reader with the physical basis of prediction. Also, the most up-to-date testing techniques will be covered.

Finally, the question of post-fabrication shelf life will be addressed. Here, one must remember that before reaching the final user, the device must be sterilized, either by ionizing radiation or ethylene oxide, stored, shipped through widely varying environmental conditions, and frequently stored again at the user's site. The product's efficacy is the final outcome after these processes. We need to understand and take into consideration, all possible reactions and degradations possible to ensure the product's success. With all these complexities, there have been good examples of shelf life prediction. We will cite the basis for success and outline some of the approaches for the reader.

DYNAMIC MECHANICAL ANALYSIS (DMA)

DMA is perhaps the single most powerful tool in probing a polymer's relaxation processes while complementary data on the material's mechanical modulus is obtained over a wide temperature range. The basic concept of DMA is very simple: a sinusoidal strain is imposed on the sample, and the resultant stress is measured. Since virtually all materials are viscoelastic in nature, that is, the material's response is both elastic (in-phase with excitation) and viscous (out-of-phase), the total response will lag behind the excitation by a phase angle δ. By vector decomposition of the response into in-phase and out-of-phase components, one obtains the quantity E' and E'' (Figure 1).

Definitions:

E = Stress/Strain

$$E^* = E' + E'' \qquad \tan \delta = E''/E'$$

where

E^* = complex Young's modulus
E' = elastic (storage) modulus

E'' = loss (viscous) modulus

tan δ = loss tangent

Similarly, if the sample were deformed in shear, G, the shear modulus would replace E.

The DMA measurement can be carried out either in a resonant mode, where the sample's rigidity determines the resonant frequency (torsion pendulums, DuPont DMA), or in a forced driven mode at a fixed frequency (Rheovibron, DuPont DMA, Seiko DMS, Rheometrics DTMA etc.). Generally, the resonant instruments offer superior tan δ resolutions while the fix frequency instruments allow more rigorous data analysis on frequency or time superposition.

In a typical DMA experiment, one can in principle scan either temperature or frequency to bring the polymer's relaxation process into the measurement window. However, experimentally, it is much simpler to scan temperature over a wide range. Therefore, the great majority of DMA data are presented as a function of temperature. Schematically, for a semicrystalline polymer one observes the following spectra (Figure 2).

At the highest temperature, one encounters the melting point, where the polymer solid becomes liquid. Second highest on the temperature scale is the T_g, the glass transition temperature, where main chain segments in the amorphous phase begin to take place on a long range basis. It is not uncommon for amorphous polymers to see the modulus drop by more than two orders of magnitude (several hundred fold) during the glass transition process. Also, the glass transition temperature defines for amorphous polymers the onset of thermoplastic behavior for material processing. Further down the temperature scale, one sees a multitude of the so-called secondary relaxation peaks, conventionally labelled as β-, γ-, and δ-transitions, with the T_g as the α process. These secondary relaxation processes are associated with the motion of a specific functional group or a supramolecular structure. Concurrent with the loss modulus relaxation peaks, the elastic modulus exhibits a stepwise change at each of the relaxation processes. In principle, the two spectra can be transformed into one another by the so-called Kramers-Kroning relationship. In practice, both spectra are directly measured simultaneously in a given experiment.

From multi-frequency experiments one can plot the peak temperature of these relaxation processes against frequency to construct a "relaxation map", typically with temperature represented as $1/T$, the absolute temperature. The slope of the line for each relaxation process is the Arrhenius activation energy of the process and is very useful in helping to assign the origin of the process. The complete assignment for a well known polymer, polymethylmethacrylate (PMMA), at a frequency of about 1 Hz, is given in Figure 3.

The glass transition at about 110°C indicates the strong stiffening effect due to the methyl group on the main chain. The corresponding acrylate polymer has

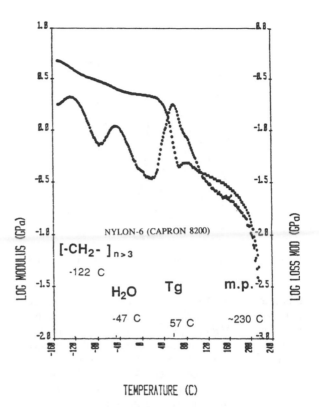

Figure 2. DMA spectrum of nylon-6 at ca. 10 Hz.

a T_g of only about 5°C. The next highest transition is due to the onset of the motion of the entire ester side chain. If water were present in the glassy matrix, sometimes one would see a weak transition below the ester peak. Further down the temperature scale, the motion of the main chain methyl group is encountered, and at the very low cryogenic temperatures, the motion of the side chain methyl group is seen.

At once, one recognizes the power of the DMA as a spectroscopic tool: each of the functional groups is uniquely represented by a relaxation maximum. In

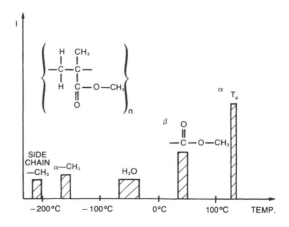

Figure 3. Schematic DMA spectrum of PMMA at ca. 1 Hz.

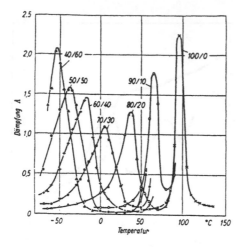

Figure 4. Dynamic loss spectra of PVC-DOP system from Ref. [4].

this way the DMA rivals other spectroscopic techniques such as infrared and nuclear magnetic resonance (NMR) for providing details of a polymer's molecular structural information. In the following section, we will present examples where the structural information presented by DMA is applied to many of the important issues in biomaterial design and performance evaluation. Among the most important applications are:

- T_g, modulus determinations
- structure–property relationship in phase-separated systems
- impact–property correlations
- rheochemical reaction (thermosetting) kinetics
- inorganic, ceramic systems

The glass transition temperature or T_g is of central importance for all biomaterials. DMA offers the most

sensitive, accurate determination among all techniques. For example, the T_g's as indicated as damping peaks of the PVC/DOP system was depicted in a classic paper in 1951 (Figure 4) [4]. Also, silicone rubber or polydimethyl siloxane, posseses one of the most flexible main chains known, accounting for its extremely low T_g of about $-120°C$ (Figure 5). The glass transitions of a selected list of polymers are listed in Table 1. It can be seen that the location of T_g depends on the flexibility of the polymer chain backbone, and the existence of stiffening side groups or bulky side groups which tend to induce main chain motion and to lower T_g.

In their studies of chemistry, structural–property relationship, and biocompatibility of polyurethanes, S. L. Cooper and his collaborators make heavy use of DMA as one of the principal tools of investigation. For example, in a series of homologous polyurethanes with the same soft segment content but different MDI contents, as a result of the increasing hard segment diisocyanate contributions, the T_g, softening temperatures are increased. Concurrently, the modulus also increases (Figure 6) [5]. In another series where the soft segment molecular weight was varied while the soft/hard segment ratio was kept constant, the increased soft segment molecular weight led to a greater tendency to crystallize and more complete phase separation. This resulted in higher modulus and separate relaxation process during the softening process near T_g [6] (Figure 7). Needless to say, all these phenomena have immense consequences in the material's biocompatibility.

Likewise, Reichert and Barenberg studied the DMA behavior of polyphosphazenes under UV irradiation and correlated the results to blood compatibility [7].

Heijboar [8] was the first to hypothesize that there existed a relationship between polymers' relaxation

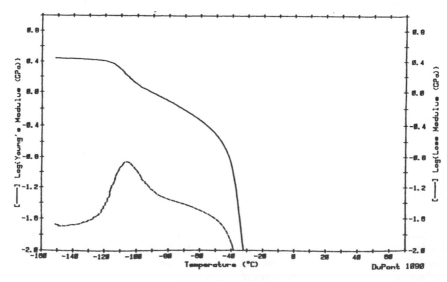

Figure 5. DMA spectrum of silicone rubber.

behaviors and their impact resistances. He theorized on the basis of mode of energy dissipation: if a polymer is subjected to a sudden mechanical shock or deformation, in order to dissipate this potential energy initially stored in the bulk along the main chains of the polymer, there must exist high-frequency dissipative modes along the main chain to convert the energy into heat and to avoid fracture. Of course, the high-frequency modes appear at lower DMA frequencies as subambient secondary relaxations. Thus the hypothesis can be restated as: if there exist subambient secondary relaxations originating from the main chain, the polymer may have good impact performance. Despite the fact that DMA primarily probes a polymer's linear, small-strain behavior, while impact is a highly nonlinear, large-strain event, the correlation has been impressive. For example, PMMA cited earlier possesses no subambient loss peaks arising from the main chain, therefore brittle behavior is predicted. Polyethylenes have a so-called gamma transition around $-120°C$ at low frequencies, derived from the so-called "crank shaft" motion of the methylene units along the main chain. As is usually known, polyethylenes are tough materials (Figure 8).

Likewise, for polypropylene an addition of a methyl group on every other methylene unit on the backbone can greatly inhibit the main chain motion. As a consequence, the low temperature transition is absent and the polymer quite brittle (Figure 9).

Recently, several investigations were directed toward the origin of the superior impact properties of polycarbonates. From both monomer modification experiments and nuclear magnetic resonance experiments [9], it was positively identified that the subam-

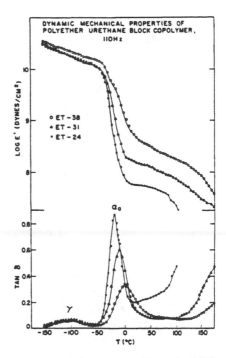

Figure 6. Polyether polyurethanes with varying MDI contents.

bient relaxation at about $-60°C$ due to benzene ring flips on the main chain bisphenol units was primarily responsible for the toughness.

Sometimes, it was reported that even for multiphase systems, the magnitude of the rubber impact modifier loss peak be correlated to impact behavior [10] (Figure 10).

Thermosetting systems constitute a major class of

Table 1. Glass transition temperatures of common polymers.

Polymer	T_g (°C)
Methacrylic acid	106
Methylacrylate	3
Ethylacrylate	−22
n-Propylacryl	−44
n-Butylacrylate	−56
Methyl methacrylate	110
Ethyl methacrylate	65
n-Propyl methacrylate	35
n-Butyl methacrylate	21
PTFE (tetrafluoroethylene)	−10
Polyethylene	−120
PDMS (dimethyl siloxane)	−120
Polypropylene	0
Polystyrene	100
Polyamides (nylon)	75
Polyethylene terephthalate	82
PVC (rigid)	90
Polybutadiene (1-4 addition)	−90
Polybutadiene (1-2 addition)	−5

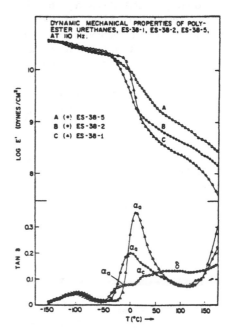

Figure 7. Polyurethanes with different soft segment molecular weights.

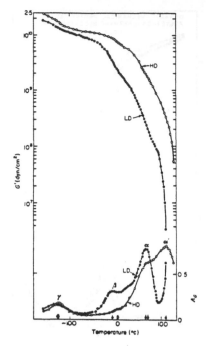

Figure 8. Comparisons of polyethylenes of high density with low density.

biomaterials. It is well known that the cross-linking reaction pathway can greatly influence the resulting structure and thereby the properties. Macosko [11] has studied in detail the kinetics of polyurethane formation using a variety of rheological tools, including DMA. Gillham and his collaborators [12] have been using a torsional braid analyzer to study cure. This technique has the unique capability of operating over the entire liquid, gel, and glassy regions while offering excellent resolution. Many of today's understandings on the phase behavior of cross-linking systems were carried out on the braid apparatus.

For hard tissue replacement and augmentation, a variety of ceramic, glassy, and carbon materials have been used. These materials frequently consisted of complex mixtures of crystals of oxides, glasses of supercooled liquids, and microcrystallites. The com-

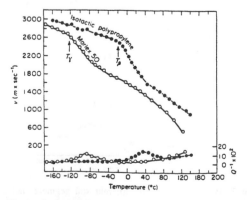

Figure 9. Comparison of PP with PE, at ca. 10 KHz.

plexity of these systems often makes the bioresponse difficult to reproduce. Therefore, one must have the most complete material characterization available before attempting to reproduce an experiment or to attribute results to a given structural factor. It is surprising, that one of the earliest applications of dynamic mechanical analysis was to metals and inorganic systems. In contrast to motions and relaxations of polymer chain segments, one examines relaxations due to grain boundaries, interstitial solute atoms etc. [13]. In direct analogy with the polymer systems, information learned can be applied to better structures and fabrication techniques, and ultimately, to better *in vivo* performance.

CRACK PROPAGATION, RELIABILITY, LIFETIME PREDICTION, AND PROOF TESTING

Ceramics belong to a unique class of biomaterials, due to their biocompatibility with bone, soft tissue and blood [14–15]. Moreover, ceramics possess mechanically stable, abrasion-resistant, low-friction properties. Ceramic materials, such as graphite and pyrolytic carbon, have been used in the prosthetic mechanical heart valves [15–17] to regulate blood flow continuously in physiological environments for a patient's lifetime. However, the structural integrity can be limited by the reliability and durability of material and the design.

The durability of a ceramic's structure is often limited by the initiation and subsequent growth of cracks. Cracks could result in a performance reduction or even a total failure of the structure during service. Since it is very difficult or even impossible to prevent the cracks from occurring in service it is necessary to have a means of assessing and minimizing their effects.

Fracture mechanics provides the foundation necessary for assessing failure prediction to assure the reliability and durability under various loading conditions in operational environments. The parameters necessary for making operational lifetime predictions may be obtained directly from crack velocity measurement and indirectly from static or dynamic strength experiments. This section reviews the basic fracture mechanics concept and subcritical crack growth theory in ceramic materials which are used for making lifetime prediction, and examines the proof testing techniques developed to ensure the reliability of ceramics structure uses in service.

Basic Principles of Fracture Mechanics

Fracture mechanics allows calculation of the resistance of a material to crack growth due to the many possible stresses imposed on a flaw. Fracture mechanics also provides the basic understandings of the fracture processes. In general, fractures may be divided into four convenient classes as depicted in

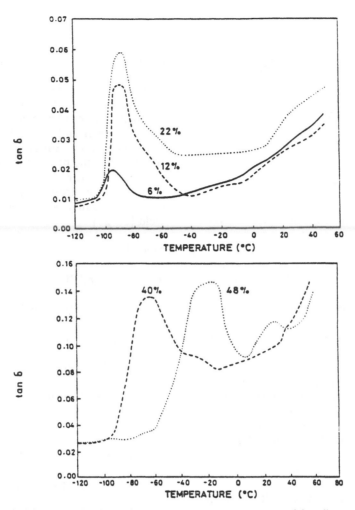

Figure 10. Loss spectra curves of HIPS, containing constant polybutadiene (6%), but with different volume contents of rubber particles (Ref. [10]).

Figure 11. The classification of the fracture is based on the size scale for yielding, δ. If $\delta \ll a, w, b$, then we have a class 1 situation which is called elastic fracture mechanics, where a, b, w are the crack length, thickness and width of the plate, respectively. If $\delta < w-a$, the ligament length, but is significant compared with a or b, then we have class 2 called contained yield. In class 3, $\delta > w-a$, the whole ligament contains yield and the deformation is controlled by the plastic collapse situation. Class 4 involves diffuse dissipation throughout the entire body.

All materials, except for some of the most brittle solids (e.g., ceramics), undergo yield process at a certain stress level, σ_y. Such deformations are irreversible and lead to energy dissipation. The stress level at which yield will occur is commonly defined in terms of Levy-Von Mises yield criterion which may be expressed in terms of the three principle stresses (σ_1, σ_2, σ_3) at a point as [18]:

$$2\sigma_y^2 = (\sigma_1 - \sigma_2)^2 + (\sigma_2 - \sigma_3)^2 + (\sigma_3 - \sigma_1)^2 \quad (1)$$

For a plane strain condition, $\sigma_3 = \nu(\sigma_1 + \sigma_2)$, where ν is the Poisson ratio of the material.

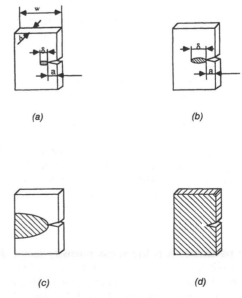

Figure 11. Types of fracture. (a) Class 1, $\delta \ll a$, w, b (elastic deformation; (b) class 2, $\delta < w-a$ (contained yield); (c) class 3, $\delta > w-a$ (fully yield); (d) class 4 (diffuse dissipation).

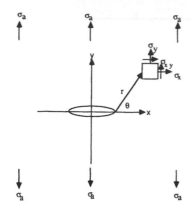

Figure 12. Sharp crack in a uniformly stressed, infinite lamina.

If we now define a constraint factor M to describe the elevation of the applied stress at yield, we have

$$M = \sigma_1/\sigma_y = [(1 + \sigma_2/\sigma_1)^2(1 - \nu + \nu^2) - 3\sigma_2/\sigma_1]^{-1/2}$$

where σ_1 is assumed to be greater than σ_2 and σ_3 since in general, the applied stress, σ_1, may be elevated to any value by σ_2 and σ_3.

In the crack tip region along the crack line, $\sigma_2 = \sigma_1$. The stress state is controlled by the elastic field for small-scale yielding, and we have $M = (1 - 2\nu)^{-1/2}$. The size scale for the yielded zone at the crack tip for the linear elastic case (class 1) is estimated as [19]:

$$\delta = K_{IC}^2/(2\pi M^2 \sigma_y^2) \quad (2)$$

Detailed derivation of Equation (2) will follow in a latter section.

Stress States in a Crack

Westergaard [20] developed a stress function solution which relates the applied stress σ_a to the local concentration of stresses at the crack tip for a sharp crack in a uniformly stressed infinite lamina. The stress fields in the vicinity of a crack tip have the solution of the form

$$\sigma_{ij} = \sigma_a(a/2r)^{1/2}f_{ij}(\theta) \quad (3)$$

where σ_{ij}, r and θ are the components of a stress tensor and polar coordinates at a point, respectively. Crack tip is chosen as the origin as shown in Figure 12.

Irwin [21] modified this equation to give

$$\sigma_{ij} = K/(2\pi r)^{1/2}f_{ij}(\theta) \quad (4)$$

The parameter K is the stress-intensity factor. K is a factor which characterizes the intensity of the stress field ahead of a crack, and it is this factor that drives the crack opening. K is a function of the applied loading, the geometry of the structure, and the size and shape of the crack.

A crack in a structure may be stressed in three different modes, denoted I, II, and III as illustrated in Figure 13. Each mode associated with a local mode of deformation and stress-intensity factor K_I, K_{II}, and K_{III}. The superposition of the three modes constitutes the general 3-D case of local crack tip stress fields and deformation. Mode I refers to a tensile opening mode in which the opening crack surfaces move directly apart. Mode II and mode III are fundamental shear modes of fracture. Stresses and deformation of mode II stay within the plane of the plate while mode III is out of plane shear.

The crack tip stresses (σ_x, σ_y, τ_{xy}) and displacement (u, v, w) field may be developed from Equation (4) to yield [20–23]

Mode I:

$$\sigma_x = [K_I/(2\pi r)^{1/2}] \cos(\theta/2)[1 - \sin(\theta/2)\sin(3\theta/2)]$$

$$\sigma_y = [K_I/(2\pi r)^{1/2}] \cos(\theta/2)[1 + \sin(\theta/2)\sin(3\theta/2)]$$

$$\tau_{xy} = [K_I/(2\pi r)^{1/2}] \cos(\theta/2)[\sin(\theta/2)\sin(3\theta/2)] \quad (5)$$

$$u = K_I(r/2\pi)^{1/2} \cos\theta/2(\beta - \cos^2\theta/2)(1/G)$$

$$v = K_I(r/2\pi)^{1/2} \sin\theta/2(\beta - \cos^2\theta/2)(1/G)$$

Mode II:

$$\sigma_x = [K_{II}/(2\pi r)^{1/2}](-\sin\theta/2)(2 + \cos\theta/2\cos 3\theta/2)$$

$$\sigma_y = [K_{II}/(2\pi r)^{1/2}] \sin\theta/2\cos\theta/2\cos 3\theta/2$$

$$\tau_{xy} = [K_{II}/(2\pi r)^{1/2}] \cos\theta/2(1 - \sin\theta/2\sin 3\theta/2) \quad (6)$$

$$u = K_{II}(r/2\pi)^{1/2} \sin\theta/2(\beta + \cos^2\theta/2)(1/G)$$

$$v = K_{II}(r/2\pi)^{1/2}(-\cos\theta/2)(\beta - 2 + \cos^2\theta/2)(1/G)$$

Mode III:

$$\tau_{xz} = -[K_{III}/(2\pi r)^{1/2}] \sin\theta/2$$

$$\tau_{yz} = K_{III}/(2\pi r)^{1/2} \cos\theta/2$$

$$\sigma_x = \sigma_y = \sigma_z = \tau_{xy} = 0 \quad (7)$$

$$u,v = 0$$

$$w = K_{III}(2r/\pi)^{1/2} \sin\theta/2(1/G)$$

where G is the shear modulus equal to $2(1 + \nu)/E$, E is the Young's modulus and ν is the Poisson ratio of the material and $\beta = 2/(1 + \nu)$. In the case of plane strain condition $\sigma_z = \nu(\sigma_x + \sigma_y)$, $\tau_{xz} = \tau_{yz} = 0$, $w = 0$, and $\beta = 2(1 - \nu)$.

Figure 14 shows the displacement field of mode I and II. The distortion of the circle illustrates clearly the symmetrical deformation and crack opening of mode I; and antisymmetrical deformation and the crack surface slide relative to each other for mode II.

Small Scale Yielding (Class 1)

An approximation to yielding behavior around the crack tip may be obtained by determining where the elastic stress field reaches the yield criterion. The principal stresses near the crack tip are expressed as:

$$\sigma_1 = [(\sigma_x + \sigma_y)/2] + \{[(\sigma_x - \sigma_y)/2]^2 + \tau_{xy}^2\}^{1/2}$$
$$\sigma_2 = [(\sigma_x + \sigma_y)/2] - \{[(\sigma_x - \sigma_y)/2]^2 + \tau_{xy}^2\}^{1/2} \tag{8}$$

By substituting Equation (5) into this equation for mode I loading condition yields:

$$\sigma_1 = [K_I/(2\pi r)^{1/2}] \cos \theta/2 \, (1 + \sin \theta/2)$$
$$\sigma_2 = [K_I/(2\pi r)^{1/2}] \cos \theta/2 \, (1 - \sin \theta/2) \tag{9}$$

For the plane strain condition at the crack tip, we have

$$\sigma_z = \sigma_3 = \nu(\sigma_1 + \sigma_2)$$

By using this in conjunction with Equations (1) and (9), an expression for the size and shape of the plastic zone is obtained.

$$r_p = (1/2\pi)(K_I/\sigma_y)^2 \cos^2 \theta/2$$
$$\times [4(1 - \nu + \nu^2) - 3\cos^2 \theta/2)] \tag{10}$$

Figure 15 shows the shape of the plastic zone for both plane strain and plane stress condition. The plane stress zone is clearly larger than those achieved in the plane strain because of the higher constraint in the plane strain situation. There is also a distinct change in form from the double lobes of plane strain to the almost circular for plane stress. The index of size scale, δ, for yielding as mentioned earlier in Equation (2) is directly deduced from Equation (10) with $\theta = 0$.

$$\delta = (1/2\pi)(K_{IC}/\sigma_y)^2(1 \times 2\nu)^2 \tag{11}$$

Effect of Thickness

In general, increasing the thickness of the part leads to a decrease in the critical stress-intensity factor, K_{IC}, and this increase will ultimately reach a plateau. The value of K_{IC} approaches an asymptotic minimum value with increasing thickness because deformation in the thickness direction at the crack tip is constrained by the surrounding elastic material so that most of the strain occurs in the two directions that lie in the plane of the plate. The asymptotic value is called the plane strain critical stress-intensity fac-

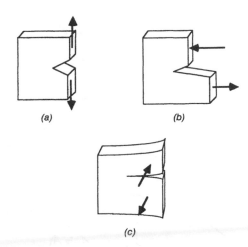

Figure 13. Modes of loading. (a) Mode I: tensile opening mode; (b) Mode II: inplane shear mode; (c) Mode III: outplane shear.

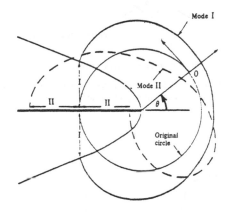

Figure 14. Displacement around a crack tip: Modes I and II (Refs. [19], p. 45).

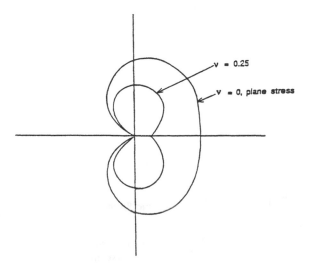

Figure 15. Plastic zone shapes.

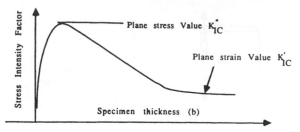

Figure 16. Variation of the measured critical stress-intensity factor as a function of specimen thickness.

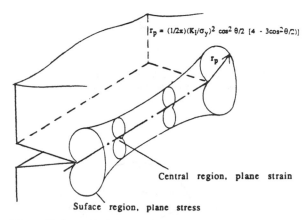

$$r_p = (1/2\pi)(K_I/\sigma_y)^2 \cos^2 \theta/2 \; [4 - 3\cos^2 \theta/2)]$$

Central region, plane strain

Surface region, plane stress

Figure 17. Shape of plastic zone at crack tip as a function of specimen thickness, b. Von Mises yield criterion.

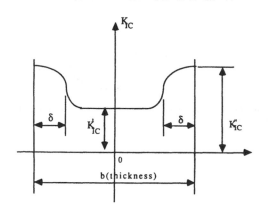

Figure 18. K_{IC} distribution across a crack front.

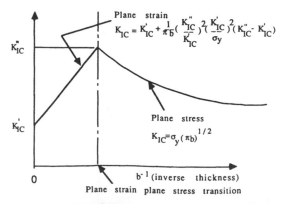

Plane strain

$$K_{IC} = K'_{IC} + \frac{1}{\pi b} \left(\frac{K''_{IC}}{K'_{IC}}\right)^2 \left(\frac{K'_{IC}}{\sigma_y}\right)^2 (K''_{IC} - K'_{IC})$$

Plane stress

$$K_{IC} = \sigma_y (\pi b)^{1/2}$$

Plane strain plane stress transition

Figure 19. Variation of measured value with specimen thickness: plane strain–plane stress effect.

tor, and represents a lower bound to the material toughness. A typical form of K_{IC} and the specimen thickness, b, relationship is shown in Figure 16, where K'_{IC} is the value for fracture under plane strain condition and K''_{IC} is for full plane stress condition. It should be noted that K_{IC} is often referred to as plane strain fracture critical stress-intensity factor of mode I. The thickness effect arises because the state of stress near the crack tip varies from plane stress in the surface region ($\sigma_3 = 0$), to the plane strain in the center region as illustrated in Figure 17. This results in a distribution of K_{IC} values across the thickness as shown in Figure 18. Any measured value obtained will be an average and is given by the following integral

$$K_{IC} = (2/b) \int_0^{b/2} K_{IC} \, dX \tag{12}$$

Now consider the plane stress, plane strain transition occurs at a distance of L from the surface zones and assumed to be equal to the size scale of yielding δ [Equation (11)], a useful approximation to the distribution based on a bimodal distribution is obtained as

$$K_{IC \, (average)} = (2/b)[K''_{IC} * L + K'_{IC}(b/2 - L)] \tag{13}$$

Substituting $L = \delta$ into Equation (13) gives

$$K_{IC \, (average)} = K'_{IC} + (1/\pi b)(K''_{IC}/K'_{IC})^2$$
$$\times [K'_{IC}/\sigma_y)^2 (K''_{IC} - K'_{IC}) \tag{14}$$

where K'_{IC} and K''_{IC} are referred to plane strain and plane stress critical stress-intensity factor; respectively. Therefore, the measured K_{IC} value is inversely proportional to the plate thickness, b, and tends to K'_{IC} (plane strain condition) for large thickness. When $b = (1/\pi)(K''_{IC}/K'_{IC})^2(K'_{IC}/\sigma_y)^2 = [1/\pi(1 - 2\nu)^2]*$ $(K'_{IC}/\sigma_y)^2$; $K_{IC} \propto \delta(\theta = 0)$, a transition plane strain to plane stress occurs, and when $b = 2L$, the fracture will be entirely plane stress and the K_{IC} value is equal to $\sigma_y(\pi b)^{1/2}$. K_{IC} versus b^{-1} relationship is best described in Figure 19.

Crack Propagation

The major objective of studying crack growth is to develop a framework for failure prediction. Generally, three regions of crack growth as shown in Figure 20 are observed. Crack growth for ceramic materials such as glasses, oxides, etc. is greatly enhanced by the environment. The primary environmental constituent that enhances crack growth is water, although other molecular species can also be effective. Region I and II result from a stress corrosion reaction involving attack by water. Chemical reaction rate theory has been employed to describe chemically enhanced crack growth [24,25,28].

$$\lambda = \lambda_0 a(H_2O) e^{(-E^* + bK_I)/RT} \qquad (15)$$

where λ_0 is a proportionality constant, $a(H_2O)$ is the activity of water in the environment, E^* is an activation energy for surface corrosion at a stress-free surface, b is a parameter proportional to the stress dependence of the chemical reaction and is directly proportional to the slope of V–K_I curve, where V is the crack velocity. R is the gas constant, and T is the temperature. It is apparent from Equation (15) that the crack growth is directly proportional to the activity of the H_2O in the environment and involves no details of the actual chemical reaction. Such details are often needed to aid in the material's selection. Michalske and Freiman [26] have used vitreous silica as a model system to study the chemical environment's effect on the crack growth. They put forth a specific chemical mechanical mechanism by which the strained $Si-O$ bonds at the crack tip in the vitreous silica react with the water molecule. The reaction mechanism between H_2O and SiO_2 at the crack tip may be depicted in Figure 21 as a three step process. Step 1 involves formation of a hydrogen bond between the oxygen of the silicon and the hydrogen of the water, and the alignment of O_{H_2O} electron pair toward the silicon atom. In step 2 an actual chemical reaction takes place on the strained $Si-O-Si$ bond bridging the crack tip. Electron transfer from O_{water} to the silicon and proton transfer to the O_{silica} occurs simultaneously. Two new bonds of $Si-O_{water}$ and $H-O_{silica}$ are formed. A consequence of the chemical reaction is the rupture of the weak hydrogen bond between O_{water} and the transferred hydrogen to yield a $Si-OH$ group on the fracture surfaces.

Michalske and Freiman [26] have also demonstrated that other molecules such as methanol (CH_3OH), ammonia (NH_3), hydrazine (N_2H_4), and formamide ($HCONH_2$) can also enhance crack growth in silica. Penetrants such as acetonitril (CH_3CN), which can donate electrons but not protons, are ineffective in promoting crack growth. Therefore, based on the above model it is reasonable to conclude that if a molecule can donate both electrons and protons and is small enough to reach the crack tip, it is effective in accelerating the crack growth rates. The rate of crack growth in region II is controlled by the rate of diffusion of the corrosion reagents to the crack tip. The crack velocity at which this plateau occurs depends only on the corroding media, not on the material itself. Crack growth in region III is quite steep and is independent of the corroding substance, but it was found to be affected by the dielectric properties of the bulk liquid [25,27].

For most ceramic systems, regions II and III usually occur at a sufficiently high crack velocity that the crack propagation time is controlled almost exclusively by crack growth in region I. Therefore, for engineering design and failure prediction purposes,

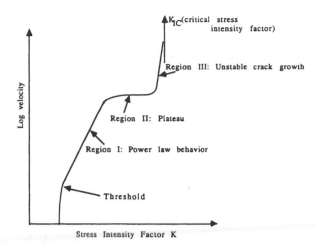

Figure 20a. Schematic of crack growth behavior for a material subjected to a stress corrosive environment.

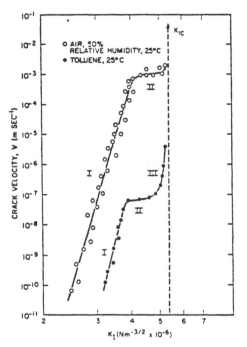

Figure 20b. Crack velocity versus stress-intensity factor data for polycrystalline alumina in moist air, 50% relative humidity, and in toluene. Regions I, II, and III are apparent (Ref. [52]).

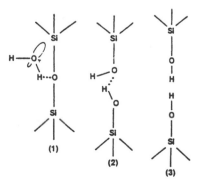

Figure 21. Reaction sequence of a water molecule with strained $Si-O$ bond at a crack tip in SiO_2 vitreous (Ref. [28]).

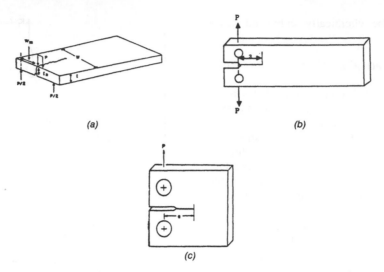

Figure 22. Various types of fracture mechanic specimens. (a) Double torsion specimen; (b) double cantilever specimen; (c) compact tensile specimen.

crack growth can be assumed to be dominated by region I. The crack velocity in region I can generally be expressed as a power function of the stress-intensity factor as [30].

$$da/dt = V = AK_I^n \qquad (16)$$

where A and n are system constants which depend on the environment and the temperature. When cyclic loading is imposed, an independent source of crack growth may occur. This mode of crack propagation depends primarily on the amplitude of the cycle, ΔK_I. The crack growth per cycle, da/dN, is expressed as

$$da/dN = A'(\Delta K_I)^m \qquad (17)$$

where A' and m are system empirical constants.

Experimental Techniques for Obtaining Crack Propagation Parameters

Crack propagation parameters may be obtained in two different ways: direct and indirect methods. The direct method measures the crack velocities as a function of the stress-intensity factor by using fracture mechanics specimens, while the indirect method derives the crack propagation parameters from strength measurements on specimens that represent structural components.

Both methods have their advantages. The direct method provides all detailed information of fracture behavior that can not be obtained when indirect methods are used, because only the overall average crack behavior is measured. However, the indirect method could be advantageous because specimens are used that more closely resemble real structural parts than do specimens containing artificial cracks.

DIRECT METHOD

Crack propagation behaviors for ceramic materials have been studied by various investigators [29–45,52] by using different specimen geometries. Figure 22 presents schematics of double torsion (DT), double cantilever beam (DCB), and compact tensile (CT) geometries. Of these, the double torsion and double cantilever beam geometries are most frequently used on ceramic material because they provide stable crack growth, which facilitates data acquisition. Moreover, due to the simplicity and many advantages of the DT specimen, this technique for crack growth study will be critically examined.

Double torsion technique was first designed by Outwater [46,47], and developed by Kies and Clark [48]. William and Evans [49,50] have described this method in detail, including the development of the

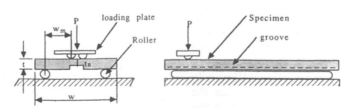

Figure 23. Double torsion test device.

final mathematical expression relating load and specimen dimension to the stress-intensity factor and the strain energy release rate, for studying slow crack growth in brittle materials. The specimen is a simple rectangular plate supported on two parallel rollers as shown in Figure 23. The specimen is usually side-grooved along the lower surface to ensure that the crack propagates along the specimen axis during the crack growth study. The stress-intensity for this configuration is independent of the crack length and is given by [49,52,54]:

$$K_{\mathrm{I}} = PW_m[3(1 + \nu)/(wt^3t_n)]^{1/2} \qquad (18)$$

where P is the load, w_m is the moment arm, w is the specimen width, t is the sample thickness, t_n is the sample thickness at the groove and ν is the Poisson's ratio. The crack velocities [49] can be obtained directly from the rate of load relaxation experiment at constant displacement and the initial or final crack length by using the equation [49,52]:

$$V = da/dt = -\phi[P_i/P^2][a_i + D/B][dP/dt]_y$$
$$= -\phi[P_f/P^2][a_f + D/B][dP/dt]_y \qquad (19)$$

where a_i and P_i are the initial crack length and load, and a_f and P_f are the corresponding values at the end of the relaxation. $B = dC/da = [6w_m^2(1 + \nu)]/wt^3 E$ is the slope of the compliance calibration; $y/p = (Ba + D) = C$, D is the intercept of the compliance plot, y is the specimen deflection, and $\phi = t/(\Delta a^2 + t^2)^{1/2}$ is the geometrical factor [52] of the crack propagation profile as shown in Figure 24.

Generally, except for small initial crack lengths, $C/B \ll a_i$, V of Equation (19) can be reduced to

$$V = da/dt = -\phi[a_iP_i/P^2][dP/dt]_y$$
$$= -\phi[a_fP_f/P^2][dP/dt]_y \qquad (20)$$

A general description of the load relaxation technique is as follows. A precracked specimen is rapidly loaded to a preselected load P, somewhat less than the critical load P_{IC}, at a controlled displacement rate. The load is then monitored as a function of time to obtain the rate of relaxation. Usually, when the load has decreased to a plateau value so that no further crack growth can be detected, the load relaxation test is considered complete. After the test is completed, the specimen is removed from the loading fixing and the final crack length may be determined by using a dye penetrant. By measuring the P and the corresponding dP/dt at time t, K and V are calculated from Equations (18) and (20), respectively. In a load relaxation experiment, it is important to ensure that there are no extraneous relaxation effects from the loading fixing and the testing machine. Background relaxation will increase the total load drop observed and lead to an invalid n value calculation. Background relaxation could be minimized by preloading the fixture using a "dummy" specimen to about twice or more of the anticipated peak load and holding until the relaxation stops.

Like any other fracture mechanic specimen geometries, precracking for a DT specimen is necessary before any crack propagation studies, otherwise erroneously high stress-intensity factors are obtained [33]. Several potential precracking techniques including fatigue loading, thermal shock, and wedge loading may be used for precracking. For a DT type specimen, a constant displacement rate can be used for precracking the specimen. In this method, the specimen is loaded at a slow crosshead speed until a crack is initiated as noted by a rapid decrease in the load.

DT specimens have been used by many investigators [40,48–55] to obtain subcritical crack growth data for several materials. The popularity of the DT technique could be attributed to the following reasons.

- The simple loading configuration allows one to measure the K–V curve in high temperature as well as in hostile physiological environments.

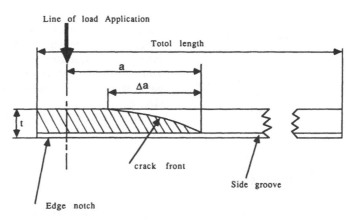

Figure 24. The crack front in the test specimen, showing that crack extends more at the lower face.

- The DT specimen is a constant K specimen, that is, K is independent of crack length, and does not require crack length monitoring during the test for K and V calculation. This advantage allows crack growth data to be obtained on an opaque specimen and under a physiological environment.
- The simple geometry facilitates easy specimen preparation.
- In a single load relaxation experiment, a range of K–V data is obtained.

The DT specimen may also be used by applying a constant displacement rate [56]. In this mode, a plateau load occurs when crack propagation commences. The crack growth equation is given by:

$$V = y'/BP \qquad (21)$$

In this way the crack velocity is measured from the constant load, P, and the crosshead speed, y', of the testing machine. The constant B can be determined either empirically from experimental compliance calibration [49] or analytically [56]. The analytical form is given by

$$B = 3w_m^2/wt^3G \qquad (22)$$

where G is the shear modulus. Constant displacement rate mode provides valid slow crack growth rate measurements when gross plasticity of linear viscoelastic deformation is occurring. Equation (21) may also be used by fixing the load. V is obtained by measuring the displacement rate y'; y' will be constant if crack growth is not accompanied by gross plastic flow. The limitation of the constant load and constant displacement rate techniques is that only a few measurements can be made on each specimen. This is because an extensive crack growth will occur for each level of y' or P. On the other hand constant displacement techniques can provide a V-K curve by just using one specimen. This method is effective only when crack growth is not accompanied by gross plasticity.

INDIRECT METHOD

Under the assumption that the power function law of Equation (16) can be used to describe the propagation of the microscopic cracks present in ceramic material, the parameters A and n can be obtained also from the static or dynamic strength (constant stress rate, $d\sigma/dt$, or constant strain rate, $d\epsilon/dt$) measurements. Under static conditions, the parameters are obtained by measuring the time to failure of a sufficiently large number of samples at several constantly applied stresses. Substituting Equation (35) into Equation (28) and rewriting in the logarithmic form yields

$$\ln t_s = \ln B + (n - 2) \ln \sigma_{IC} - n \ln \sigma_a \qquad (23)$$

where $B = 2/[A(n - 2)Y^2K_{IC}^{n-2}]$. The value of n is

determined from the slope of $\ln t_s$ versus the $\ln \sigma_a$ plot, and B (therefore A) is determined from the $\ln t_s$ axis intercept. The fracture strength, σ_{IC}, can be determined from another identical group of samples. Similarly, parameters A and n can also be obtained by measuring the fracture strength as a function of stressing rate $d\sigma/dt$. The relationship between median values of σ_f and σ_{IC} in a logarithmic form is given by [57]:

$$\ln \sigma_f = [1/(1 + n)][\ln B + \ln (1 + n) + (n - 2)$$

$$\times \ln \sigma_{IC} + \ln d\sigma/dt] \qquad (24)$$

n is determined from the straight line plot of $\ln \sigma_f$ versus $\ln d\sigma/dt$, and A from the $\ln \sigma_f$ axis intercept. The slope is equal to $(1 + n)^{-1}$. For a constant strain rate experiment, n and A are determined from the above equation by replacing $d\sigma/dt$ by $E\ d\epsilon/dt$ based on the equality $\sigma = E\epsilon$.

Failure Prediction [58–64]

The failure time of a component due to crack growth under stresses can be predicted from the slow crack growth data by combination of the K, V relation of Equation (16) with the fracture mechanics relation, $K = Y\sigma(a)^{1/2}$, to give

$$da/dt = V = AK_I^n = A(Y\sigma a^{1/2})^n \qquad (25)$$

where σ is the applied stress, a is the flaw size, and Y is a geometric factor which depends on the shape and location of the flaw as well as the mode of the applied stress. By rearranging and integrating Equation (25), the crack growth in time t, is obtained as:

$$\int_0^t \sigma^n(t)dt = [2/(n - 2)AY^n]$$

$$\times [(1/a_i)^{(n-2)/2} - (1/a)^{(n-2)/2}] \qquad (26)$$

where a_i is the initial crack length and is related to the initial stress-intensity factor and initial stress σ_i through the fracture mechanic relationship, $K = Y\sigma a^{1/2}$. Failure occurs only when a crack is propagated from an initial subcritical size, a_i, to a critical size, a_c.

For a constant loading, $\sigma(t) = \sigma_s$, Equation (26) becomes

$$t_s = [2/(n - 2)AY^2\sigma_s^2K_{Ii}^{n-2}][1 - (K_{Ii}/K_{IC})^{n-2}] \qquad (27)$$

where K_{Ii} is the maximum initial stress-intensity factor in the component on initial loading, and is related to the maximum initial crack length, a_i, by $K_{Ii} = $

$Y\sigma_s(a_i)^{1/2}$ [59]. K_{IC} is the critical crack length for rapid fracture in an inert environment with no subcritical crack growth prior to fracture. For most ceramic materials, n is typically a large number greater than 9, and $K_{Ii} < 0.9 K_{IC}$ for the usual range of service stresses. Thus $(K_{Ii}/K_{IC})^{n-2} \ll 1$, except in the case of short times to failure and to a good approximation, the failure time of Equation (27) becomes

$$t_s = [2/(n-2)AY^2\sigma_s^2 K_{Ii}^{n-2}] \quad (28)$$

It is apparent from Equation (28) that the time required for the initial maximum flaw size to grow to a critical size for catastrophic failure decreases with increasing applying stress, σ_s, and with increasing initial stress-intensity factor or initial crack length, a_i. It is also apparent from Equation (27) that the critical crack length, a_c, or critical stress-intensity factor, K_{IC}, at rapid fracture in an inert environment does not significantly affect the time to failure. For large K_{IC} or a_c, the ratio of $(K_{Ii}/K_{IC})^{n-2}$ approaches zero; therefore the t_s in Equation (27) reduces to the t_s in Equation (28). Hence the simple relation for failure time given by Equation (28) can be used for failure prediction at constant stress without incurring significant error.

For a variable stress, $\sigma(t)$, condition, if there is no enhanced cycling effect, the failure time, t_c, for any periodic loading can be correlated directly with that obtained under quasi-static conditions. The left hand integral of Equation (26) may be solved by using series solution for various $\sigma(t)$ [58] and the results can be expressed as

$$t_c = g^{-1}(\sigma_s/\sigma_{ave})^n t_s \quad (29)$$

where t_s is the static time to failure at the quasi-static stress, σ_{ave} is the average cyclic stress and, g^{-1} is a dimensionless proportionality factor that depends on the type of stress cycle, the amplitude of the cycle and also n. Thus, if there is no enhanced cyclic effect on the crack growth rate, the time to failure is frequently independent and amplitude dependent on the ratio $(\sigma_s/\sigma_{ave})^n$. For instant, $\sigma_s = \sigma_{ave} + \sigma_o = \sigma_a(1 + \zeta)$; $\zeta = \sigma_o/\sigma_{ave}$, $\sigma_o = $ amplitude, the g^{-1} values for various waveforms such as sinusoidal wave, square wave, and saw-tooth type loading have been evaluated and the solutions are available [58] both in graphical and analytical form. For the sinusoidal stress

$$g(n,\zeta) = \sum_{K=0}^{n/2} [n!/(n-2K)!(K!)^2][\zeta/2]^{2K} \quad (30)$$

The results for the square wave stress are

$$g(n,\zeta) = \sum_{K=0}^{n/2} [n!/(n-2K)!(2K)!][\zeta]^{2K} \quad (31)$$

and for the saw-tooth stress wave

$$g(n,\zeta) = \sum_{K=0}^{n/2} [n!/(n-2K)!(2K+1)!][\zeta]^{2K} \quad (32)$$

where ζ is restricted to the range $0 \le \zeta \le 1$.

The correlation between static and cyclic behavior has been verified experimentally by measuring the slow crack growth rates under static and cyclic loading for a number of ceramic materials. For example, Evans [58] has compared crack velocities for two kinds of ceramic materials of porcelain and soda-lime glass under static and cyclic loading conditions by using double torsion specimen techniques. The data obtained are plotted in Figures 25 and 26. There is no significant difference between the measured crack velocities and predictions from the static slow crack growth. This finding implied no enhanced cyclic effect on the rate of slow crack growth for this particular type of ceramic material. Equations (28) and (29) can be used directly for failure prediction by inserting the values of initial stress-intensity factor, K_{Ii}. This method requires an estimate of maximum initial flaw size. Flaws in most ceramic materials are usually 10 to 50 μm in size and their dimensions are not easily measured by currently available nondestructive test methods such as x-ray radiography, ultrasonic, dye penetrant, etc.; therefore, indirect methods must be employed to estimate the initial stress-intensity factor in the component. There exist at least two indirect methods, namely, statistic and proof testing, which

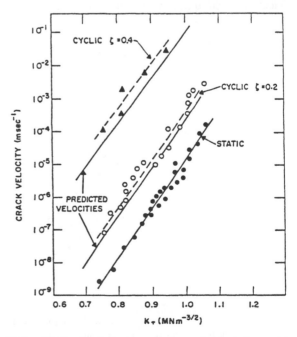

Figure 25. Crack velocity measurements of electrical porcelain under static and cyclic loading conditions, including cyclic velocities predicted from static measurements. Using double torsion specimen (Ref. [58]).

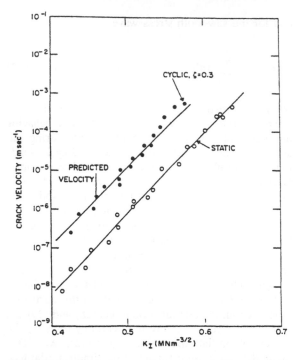

Figure 26. Crack velocity measurements of soda-lime glass under static and cyclic loading conditions. Predicted cyclic velocity from status data is compared with experimental data. Using double torsion specimen (Ref. [58]).

can be used to determine the largest initial flaw size in the component. One method uses statistics to characterize the strength of the ceramic material as a function of cumulative probability for failure. The second method, which is one of the most effective flaw-detection techniques for ceramic materials, is the

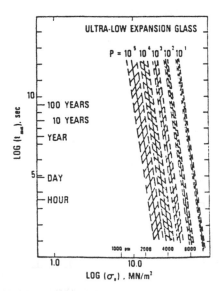

Figure 27. Statistically based design diagram for ultra-low expansion glass. Each line on this diagram relates the minimum failure time to the applied stress. The position of the line depends on the failure probability. The cross-hatched area represents 95% confidence limits.

overload proof testing. Once the initial largest flaw size, a_i, is available, the initial largest stress-intensity factor is determined from the relationship $K_{Ii} = Y\sigma a_i^{1/2}$, and the expected service life of the structure component is estimated by substituting K_{Ii} into Equations (28) and (29).

Statistical Approach [65–68,76]

Weibull [65] developed the relationship between the cumulative failure probability, a fraction of specimens that will break at a given stress level, and the strength σ_{IC}. The Weibull distribution function takes the form

$$\mathbf{P} = 1 - e^{-[(\sigma_{IC}-\sigma_\lambda)/\sigma_o]^m}$$

$$(33)$$

$$\ln\{\ln 1/(1-\mathbf{P})\} = m \ln(\sigma_{IC}-\sigma_\lambda) - m \ln(\sigma_o)$$

where m is the shape parameter for the distribution, σ_o is a scaling parameter, σ_λ is the lowest possible strength and is usually set equal to zero, $\mathbf{P}$ is the fracture probability and σ_{IC} is the strength measured in an inert environment where no subcritical crack growth occurs prior to failure. By arranging the inert fracture strength of all the tested samples in an ascending order, $\mathbf{P}$ may be determined from the following equation

$$\mathbf{P} = n/(1 + N) \qquad (34)$$

where n is the position of the nth strength measurement in the ordered set of strengths and N is the total number of measurements. The m and σ_o are determined from $\ln\{\ln 1/(1-\mathbf{P})\}$ versus $\ln \sigma_{IC}$ plot by fitting a straight line to the strength data. The slope is m and the $\ln\{\ln 1/(1-\mathbf{P})\}$ axis intercept is $m \ln(\sigma_o)$ with σ_λ assumed to be zero. A time-dependent variable can be easily introduced into the Weibull strength distribution function by expressing K_{Ii} in terms of the failure probability. At failure, K_{IC} is related to the fracture strength and the crack length by $K_{IC} = Y\sigma_{IC}a_i^{1/2}$. The initial crack length a_i is used because K_{IC} is determined at rapid loading rate with no subcritical crack growth prior to fracture. At the service load K_{Ii} is related to the service stress, σ_a, and the crack length by $K_{Ii} = Y\sigma_a(a_i)^{1/2}$. From these equations, the initial stress-intensity factor K_{Ii} may be expressed in terms of K_{IC} by [31].

$$K_{Ii} = (\sigma_a/\sigma_{IC})K_{IC} \qquad (35)$$

With the introduction of the Weibull equation into Equation (35), a relationship between K_{Ii} and the cumulation failure probability is established.

$$K_{Ii} = (\sigma_a/\sigma_o)K_{IC}\{\ln[1/(1-\mathbf{P})]\}^{-1/m} \qquad (36)$$

By substituting this equation into Equation (28), the

failure time as a function of cumulative probability for failure is obtained and takes the form

$$t = \sigma_a^{-n} f(\mathbf{P}) \qquad (37)$$

$$\ln t = -n \ln (\sigma_a) + \ln f(\mathbf{P}) \qquad (38)$$

The failure time is a power function of the applied stress for each value of **P**. A series of straight lines of slope $-n$ is obtained from a logarithmic plot of t versus $\ln \sigma_a$ as shown in Figure 27. This type of diagram completely describes the failure characteristics of a material on a statistical basis and is very useful for design purposes. A statistical approach in the determination of crack propagation parameters A and n based on static or dynamic strength measurements could be advantageous, because the testing specimens more resemble real structural parts than do specimens containing artificial cracks that are used in the fracture mechanics study. When the Weibull function is used to characterize the strength distribution of the material some precautions must be followed.

This is true especially if only a small number of strength measurements are used to determine m and σ_o, since the statistical uncertainty of these parameters can cause substantial errors in the estimates of the strength at low failure probability. Even if m and σ_o can be measured accurately, error may still occur in the strength because strength usually depends on component size. The larger the component is, the greater probability of larger flaws. In these cases, scaling equations must be used to account for size effects. It is important to verify the accuracy of the scaling equation before it is used for failure prediction by using laboratory test specimens of varying shape and size, because of the uncertainty regarding the flaw location and whether the crucial flaws lie at the surface or in the volume of the component.

Proof Testing [31,62,69–77]

Proof testing overcomes many of the difficulties present in the statistical approach to failure prediction. The principal idea of proof testing is to limit the maximum flaw size remaining in the component after the proof test. During the proof testing all specimens containing flaws larger than the critical value would have failed because the flaw tip stress-intensity factor exceeds the critical value. On the other hand, flaws that are less than the critical size will survive the proof test. Therefore, $K_p < K_{IC} (K_p = \sigma_p Y a_i^{1/2})$ if failure doesn't occur during a proof testing, where K_p and σ_p are the stress-intensity factors at the largest flaw and the applied stress during the proof test, respectively. From $K_{Ii} = \sigma_a Y a_i^{1/2}$ and $K_p < K_{IC}$ relationship, the initial stress-intensity is estimated to be

$$K_{Ii} < K_{IC} (\sigma_a/\sigma_p) \qquad (39)$$

where σ_a is the applied stress in service and σ_p is the

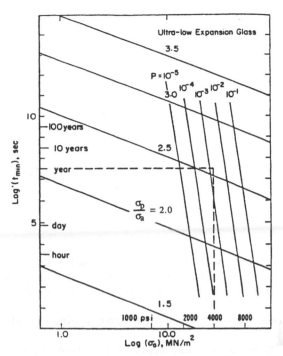

Figure 28. A proof test diagram for ultra-low expansion glass. The minimum time to failure after proof test and the time to failure without proof test (included here for comparison, from Figure 27) are shown for various applied stress and proof test ratios (Ref. [31]).

applied stress in the proof test. Based on this, the minimum time to failure for the static fatigue is estimated by substituting $K_{Ii} = K_{IC}(\sigma_a/\sigma_p)$ into Equation (28) to obtain [77]:

$$t_{min} = (B/\sigma_a^2)(\sigma_p/\sigma_a)^{n-2} \qquad (40)$$

where $B = 2/AY^2(n-2)K_{IC}^{n-2}$. From this equation it appears that the minimum time to failure depends on the ratio of the proof stress to the applied stress, and is inversely proportional to the square of the applied stress. By rewriting Equation (40) in the logarithmic form,

$$\ln t_{min} = -2 \ln \sigma_a + \ln B + (n-2) \ln \sigma_p/\sigma_a$$

$$(41)$$

a series of parallel straight lines with a slope of -2 can be drawn on the $\ln t_{min}$ versus $\ln \sigma_a$ coordinates. The position of the line depends only on the σ_p/σ_a ratio. An example for ultra-low expansion glass is shown in Figure 28. Equation (38), which is based on the statistical approach, is also included in this diagram for comparison. This type of diagram is particularly important for material selection for certain application. For example, if one year survival time at a service stress of 4,000 psi is required, a proof test stress of about 11,000 psi is required to assure zero probability failure. It is apparent from Equation (38) that the failure probability is 2×10^{-3} at the same

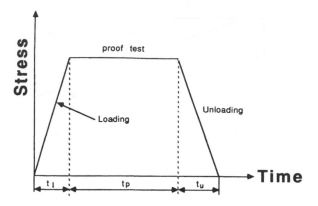

Figure 29. Proof testing stress profile.

stress levels without proof test. During the proof test at 11,000 psi, only one specimen in a thousand will fail according to the Weibull diagram in Equation (38).

Probability of Failure after Proof Testing [31,74]

In the proof testing approach as described above, the minimum time to failure was estimated based on the assumptions that the crack growth did not occur during the proof test, and failure will occur instantaneously if a flaw in the component exceeds the critical stress-intensity factor. These assumptions have been found valid for silicon carbide, silica, silicon nitride, chemical Pyrex, space shuttle glass [31]. Also, the probability of failure under this assumption is zero for all periods of time less than the predicted minimum failure time. On the other hand, if crack growth occurs during a proof test, the probability of failure is no longer zero, but finite, and is determined by the proof test condition as well as the proof test environment.

Evans and Fuller [74] have developed a theoretical basis for calculating the amount of crack growth during the proof test, and the failure probability after a proof test by assuming a stressing profile consisting of constant rates of loading, $d\sigma_l/dt$, and unloading, $d\sigma_u/dt$, in the proof test and that the proof test load σ_p was held on the test component for t_p period of time as depicted in Figure 29. The amount of crack growth during the proof test due to the loading time of $t_l = \sigma_p/(d\sigma_l/dt)$, proof testing time of t_p, and the unloading time of $t_u = \sigma_p(d\sigma_u/dt)$ may be calculated from Equation (26) by integrating the stress profile of Figure 29 to obtain:

$$a_f = a_i[1 - \alpha a_i^{(n*-2)/2}]^{-2/(n*-2)} \quad (42)$$

where a_i and a_f are the crack length before and after the proof test. $A*$ and $n*$ are the crack propagation parameters representing the proof test environment and α is given by:

$$\alpha = [A*\sigma_p^{n*}Y^{n*}(n* - 2)/2][t_p + (t_l + t_u)/(1 + n*)] \quad (43)$$

Now, if we assume that there exists an initial crack length of $(a_i)_{max}$ that will just grow to failure at the end of the unloading process during the proof test, and that $(a_i)_{max} + \delta a$ is much larger than a_i, we have

$$(a_i)_{max} = \alpha^{-2/(n*-2)} \quad (44)$$

Combining Equations (42) and (44) gives:

$$a_f = a_i\{1 - [a_i/(a_i)_{max}]^{(n*-2)/2}\}^{-2/(n*-2)} \quad (45)$$

Since a_f in Equation (45) is the crack length after the proof test (loading, proof load and unloading), it is also the initial crack length when the component is placed in service. By substituting Equation (45) as an initial crack length and $K_{Ii} = \sigma_a Y a_f^{1/2}$ into Equation (28), the time to failure after the proof test is:

$$t/t_{min} = (K_{IC}/\sigma_p Y)^{n-2}[a_i^{-(n*-2)/2} - (a_i)_{max}^{-(n*-2)/2}]^{(n-2)/(n*-2)} \quad (46)$$

and where t_{min} is the minimum time to failure that was used to compute the proof test diagram [Equation (40)].

The failure probability in the proof test (P_p) by using the Weibull distribution function [Equation (33)] is given by:

$$P_p = 1 - \exp[-(\sigma_{min}/\sigma_o)^m] \quad (47)$$

where σ_{min} is the minimum initial strength of the material that will just result in fracture by the end of the unloading process in the proof test. Components with an initial strength greater than σ_{min} will survive the proof test, and this variable is related to $(a_i)_{max}$ by $\sigma_{min} = K_{IC}/Y(a_i)_{max}^{1/2}$.

After the proof test, the strength distribution must be truncated at σ_{min} and the failure probability, P_a is given by [62]:

$$P_a = (P - P_p)/(1 - P_p) \quad (48)$$

where P_p is the fraction of specimens broken during the proof test and P is the initial flaw distribution. Substituting for P_p from Equation (47) gives:

$$\sigma_{min}/\sigma_{IC} = [1 - \ln(1 - P_a)/\ln(1 - P)]^{1/m} \quad (49)$$

where $\sigma_{IC} = K_{IC}/Y\sqrt{a_i}$ is the initial fracture strength distribution of the components. Replacing σ_{min}/σ_{IC} of Equation (49) by the failure time from Equation (46) gives:

$$\{1 + [t/t_{min}]^{(n*-2)/(n-2)}[\sigma_p/\sigma_{min}]^{n*-2}\}^{-m/(n*-2)}$$

$$= [1 - \ln(1 - P_a)/\ln(1 - P)] \quad (50)$$

Since the crack length, a_i and $(a_i)_{max}$, is related to the strength, σ_{IC} and σ_{min}, by the fracture mechanic relationship $\sigma_{IC} = K_{IC}/Y\sqrt{a_i}$ and $\sigma_{min} = K_{IC}/Y\sqrt{a_{imax}}$. For sufficiently small values of probabilities ($p < 0.1$) and $t < t_{min}$, Equation (50) [74] may be reduced to

$$\mathbf{P}_a/\mathbf{P} = [m/(n^* - 2)][t/t_{min}]^{(n^*-2)/(n-2)}[\sigma_p/\sigma_{min}]^{n^*-2}$$

(51)

where m is a Weibull parameter, n is the crack propagation parameter in the service environment, n^* is the crack propagation parameter in the proof test environment, t_{min} is the minimum failure time calculated from Equation (40) which is based on a no-crack-growth assumption during the proof test and $\sigma_{min} = K_{IC}/Y\sqrt{a_{imax}}$.

The result represented by Equation (50) shows that the failure probability, $\mathbf{P}_a$, after proof testing can be made many orders of magnitude less than failure probability without proof testing for the same lifetime chosen as $t < t_{min}$. Since n^* is usually much larger than n, the failure probability is very sensitive to the t/t_{min} ratio. Therefore, the value of $\mathbf{P}_a$ can be reduced to a very small value by proper selection of a service time less than t_{min}.

Precautions in Proof Testing

It has been shown that both statistic and proof testing methods can be used to predict the reliability of the ceramic structural uses in service environment, and that proof testing approaches are preferred over statistical approaches. This is because lifetime prediction based on statistical approaches can be greatly affected by the crucial flaw distribution contained in the component, the accuracy of the scaling equation, and uncertainty in the Weibull parameter m and σ_o, whereas prediction obtained by the proof testing approach is not affected by the crucial flaws distribution contained within the component. The lifetime prediction depends more on the material properties, such as critical stress-intensity factor, K_{IC}, crack growth parameters A and $n(n^*)$, etc. and these parameters can usually be obtained with high precision. Therefore, lifetime prediction after proof testing will be much more reliable.

Although proof testing is a valuable and reliable method for making lifetime prediction, however, some precautions must be taken into consideration in the application of proof testing. First, the proof tests must duplicate the expected service stress distribution as closely as possible. It is also very important to ensure that every point in the component is subjected to the required proof stresses, otherwise some portions will remain untested and an incorrect assessment of the lifetime prediction will result. Next, the crack propagation data used to construct the design diagrams for the overload proof test must be measured in

an environment that represents the failure mechanisms that occur in service. More importantly, one has to be certain that the crack tip environment between the crack propagation measurement and the component in service is the same because the crack tip environment may differ from the bulk environment as a result of the chemical reaction at the crack tip [24–27]. Third, one must avoid specimen damage that may be caused by the proof test apparatus in the overload proof testing. Finally, the proof test should be conducted in an inert environment to minimize the subcritical crack growth during the proof test, since crack growth could result in premature failure.

MELT RHEOLOGY AND MOLECULAR WEIGHT DEPENDENCE

For polymeric biomaterials, molecular weight is of the central importance in determining most physical properties. It has been well established that most of the materials follow an asymptotic functional approach. That is, at low molecular weights, properties increase nearly linearly with molecular weight, and at some molecular weight specific to a given polymer, properties begin to level off toward a limiting value. Figure 30 is a graphical representation of this property dependence. In addition, most polymers are a collection of fractions each with different molecular weights. Or, more accurately described, as a distribution of molecular weights. Figure 31 shows the typical molecular weight distribution and the location of the weight average molecular weight, M_w, and the number average molecular weight. M_w and M_n and their ratio M_w/M_n or MWD are defined below:

$$M_n = \Sigma n_i W_i / \Sigma n_i$$

$$M_w = \Sigma n_i (W_i)^2 / \Sigma n_i W_i$$

From these definitions, one notices that the M_w is heavily influenced by high molecular weight fractions

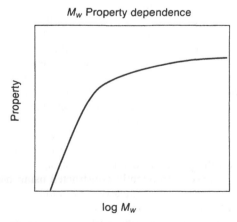

Figure 30. Molecular weight property dependence for polymeric materials.

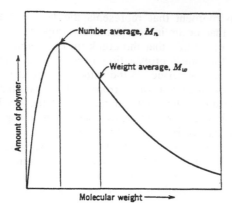

Figure 31. Molecular weight average definitions.

while low molecular weight species contribute more heavily to M_n. M_w is found to be the main determinant for mechanical properties while M_n determines many of the colligative properties such as vapor pressure of polymer solutions.

Despite the historical importance, accurate molecular weight determinations have not been simple. From dilute solutions, the so-called intrinsic viscosity or limiting viscosity number is obtained by measuring the efflux time of dilute polymer solutions versus the pure solvent, and extrapolating this ratio to zero concentration. By the Mark Houwink equation:

$$[n] = K(M_v)^a$$

Where, M_v is the viscosity average molecular weight and the exponent a, is usually between 0.5 and 0.8. The M_v as defined normally lies between M_n and M_w, but is typically 10 to 20% lower than M_w. To achieve good accuracy and reproducibility, one must maintain temperature accurately to 0.02 degree C, ensure absolute cleanliness of the glasswares, and apply the best techniques in dilution and flow time measurements.

Molecular weight determination by gel permeation chromatography (GPC) or size exclusion chromatography (SEC) has come into widespread use due to recent advances in column technology and instrumentation. Again, polymer solutions are prepared. For samples that are semicrystalline such as polyethylene or nylon, solvents at high temperatures near the melting point of the material must be employed throughout the analysis. The principle of the molecular weight determination is by steric exclusion into pores of various dimensions on the stationary phase on the columns. Since it is the hydrodynamic volumes of the polymer chains that have been separated, and they depend on the polymer solvent pair, an "apparent" calibration curve is frequently constructed using narrow MWD polystyrene standards. In addition to this difficulty in obtaining absolute calibration, instrumental factors such as baseline drift, and lack of total dissolution of the sample, frequently reduce the overall accuracy.

Membrane osmometry and light scattering methods [79] can determine absolute M_n and M_w, respectively. However, the lack of reliable, easy-to-use instrumentation has limited their widespread application. Here again, difficulties with solution techniques apply, with the additional constraint that in light scattering experiments, samples need to be meticulously free of dust contamination.

By intuition, one would expect that the polymer's melt viscosity must be related to its molecular weight. Indeed, in a classic study by Berry and Fox [80] for a variety of linear polymers, all systems beyond a critical molecular weight (entanglement limit or M_e) exhibited zero shear viscosities, that is, 3.4 power of the M_w. Zero shear viscosity is the low shear limiting plateau viscosity where no shear rate dependence is observed. The strong molecular weight dependence is attributed to temporary cross-links created by polymer chain entanglements. Theoretical works by Doi, Edwards, and by Graessley and others [81] applied the reptation model originally proposed by de-Gennes [82] have established a solid foundation for this molecular weight dependence.

This powerful relationship allows M_w determinations to be made very rapidly and accurately. Also, due to the high power dependence, errors in viscosity determinations result in much smaller errors in molecular weight.

In a modern melt rheometer, one can carry out, in addition to steady shear experiments, dynamic experiments spanning many decades of frequencies. One obtains, in direct analogy with DMA, described in previous sections,

$$G' = \text{the elastic shear modulus}$$
$$G'' = \text{the viscous shear modulus}$$
$$\omega = \text{angular frequency}$$
$$\tan \delta = G'/G'$$

and

$$n^* = (|G'| + |G''|)/\omega : \text{the dynamic viscosity}$$

A typical dynamic viscosity spectrum is presented in Figure 32.

Recently, several authors have studied the molecular weight information one can extract from the dynamic spectrum [83]. It is apparent that in addition to M_w, the average molecular weight, one can also get a fairly good measure of molecular weight distribution. The significant advantage of melt rheology based molecular weight determination is that no sample preparation is necessary, and high accuracy data can frequently be obtained in just a few minutes of experimental time.

For example, Zeichner and Patel [84] determined M_w for commercial polypropylenes and used the modulus at the crossing point of G' and G'' on a frequency scan to determine MWD (Figures 33, 34). Their success was duplicated in many laboratories pursuing a similar goal. Also, numerous other cor-

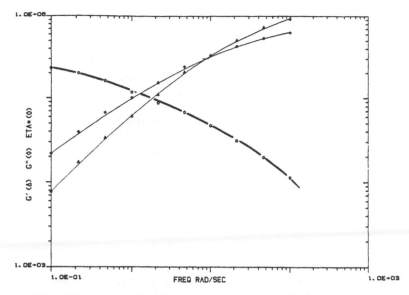

Figure 32. Dynamic viscosity scan of a 1.5 melt flow polypropylene at 200°C.

relations were reported on the relationship of molecular weight parameters with dynamic viscosity determinations. Among the most successful are Wu and Tuminello's methodology to calculate the entire molecular weight distribution from melt rheology data [85] of monodisperse polystyrenes and their blends.

It is evident that the correlation of M_w and rheological functions is under rapid development. In the near future, many other polymer systems will be examined, and a truly universal, rapid (Figure 35) technique will appear to allow reliable determination of these important parameters.

DIFFERENTIAL SCANNING CALORIMETRY (DSC)

Differential scanning calorimetry (DSC) is probably the most versatile thermo-analytical tool available for materials characterization. Various material properties like first order and second order thermo-dynamic transitions, crystallinity, and heat capacity can be precisely determined by monitoring the differential heat flow between a reference and a sample as a function of temperature at a prescribed heating or cooling rate. Kinetic parameters including reaction rate constant and reaction order are easily obtained by analyzing the reaction exotherms. Avrami analysis [86] which monitors the growth or the evolution of the crystallization exotherm is often employed to measure the kinetics of crystallization and to characterize the modes of nucleation and crystal morphologies.

The primary components of a DSC usually consist of a DSC cell, furnace, differential temperature detector, amplifier, temperature programmer, and a recorder [87]. There are primarily two types of DSC, namely, heat-flux (Dupont and Mettler), and power-compensational (Perkin-Elmer). The power-compensational DSC measures the amount of heat required to maintain isothermal conditions between the reference and sample as a function of time or temperature. The

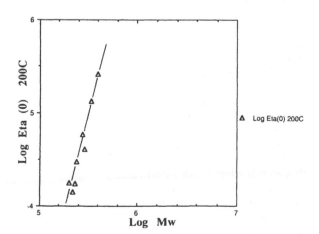

Figure 33. Polypropylene viscosity molecular weight dependence.

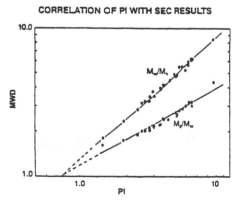

Figure 34. Polypropylene MWD correlation from rheology data (from Ref. [84]).

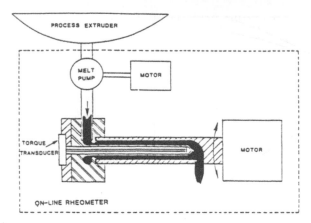

Figure 35. Process rheometer for on-line molecular weight, MWD control.

heat-flux DSC monitors the differential heat flow or the differential temperature between the reference and sample. Since the heat-flux DSC constitutes more than 60% of the market, we will confine our discussion to this differential heat flow system.

The single most important component of a DSC system is the DSC cell [88] which is composed of a thermoelectric disc made of constantan as depicted in Figure 36. The constantan disc provides a means of heat transfer to and from the sample and reference and also serves as one element of the thermoelectric junctions. The sample and reference platforms are situated above this constantan disc which is in turn attached to a silver programming surface. The underside of each platform is connected to chromel and alumel wires thereby forming a chromel–constantan differential monitoring system. Purge gas is introduced from the cell base and circulates through the heating block and enters the DSC cell at the block temperature. Temperature control is normally achieved with a thermocouple imbedded in the silver block via a feedback loop coupled with proportional, derivative and integral control. For most DSC, the heat flow sensitivity is about 0.01 mW-cm^{-1} with heating rates ranging from 0.1 to 100°C-min^{-1} operating from −180°C to 700°C. For pressure sensitive samples, calorimetry may be performed at extreme pressures covering from a few torrs to tens of atmospheres.

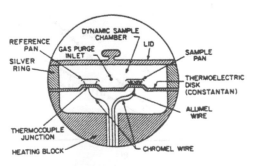

Figure 36. Schematics of a DSC cell (from Ref. [88]).

Many models [89,90] have been proposed to describe the heat conduction phenomena occurring in the DSC. The governing principle of these models is based on the Fourier heat conduction equation where the rate of heat transfer is proportional to the thermal gradient. To model the dynamics of the calorimeter, Baxter [89] assumes that the DSC is symmetric, that is, the thermal resistances are identical on the reference and sample sides. There is no thermal gradient across the reference and sample containers, thus zero heat flow. The temperature difference between the reference and sample holders or the instrument response is given by the following equation:

$$\Delta T = T_{SH} - T_{RH} = [R_D/(R_D + R_C)](T_S - T_R)$$

$$(52)$$

where T_{SH} and T_{RH} are the sample and reference container temperature, R_D is the constantan disc resistance, R_C is the contact resistance, T_S and T_R are the sample and reference temperatures. Employing the heat balance and thermal Ohm's law, Baxter concluded that the rate of heat evolution is composed of three terms:

(1) The instrument response, $T_{SH} - T_{RH}$, divided by the disc resistance R_D
(2) Product of the difference between the sample and reference heat capacity and the heating rate
(3) Product of the sample heat capacity and the rate of change of the instrument signal

It is evident from Equation (52) that the instrument sensitivity is a strong function of both the disc and contact resistance. Moreover, the onset slope of a rapidly melting transition is given by:

$$SLOPE = \{DT/Dt\}_{onset} = (DT_R/Dt)[R_D/(R_D + R_C)]$$

$$(53)$$

where T is the measured signal, (DT_R/Dt) is the heating rate. This relationship indicates that the steepest onset slope, often used as a criterion to determine the accuracy of a calibration run, is achieved by maximizing the ratio of R_D/R_C, which would yield optimized response sensitivity as demonstrated by Equation (52). This model readily reveals that the disc resistance or the thermal conductivity of the constantan disc is the single most important operating parameter for the DSC. Furthermore, the contact resistance, which is determined by the contact of the sample with container and container with detector, is always a source of variation in the DSC measurement, although this effect is not significant. This analysis also accounts for the observation that the measured thermal response is heating/cooling rate-dependent.

As stated earlier, differential scanning calorimetry can be applied to a wide spectrum of areas ranging from thermodynamic miscibility to clustered water analysis. To demonstrate the utility of this technique, several applications will be critically examined. The phenomena to be discussed include microphase separation in block copolymers, physical aging of amorphous polymers, clustered water analysis in thermoplastics, crystallization kinetics based on Avrami analysis, and oxidation induction time or temperature measurement.

One of the central problems in the study of multiphase polymer structure–property relationships is to elucidate polymer blend morphology and thermodynamic miscibility [91–93]. Polyurethane block copolymers, which are very common synthetic biomaterials used for many blood contact applications, derive their elastomeric properties from the microphase separation between the rubbery soft-segment and glassy hard-segment. Three endotherms have been observed in the DSC thermograms for these materials [94,95]. It has been generally accepted that the low-temperature endotherm observed 20–40°C above the annealing temperature originates from the short-range reorganization within the hard domains. The intermediate endotherm observed below 200°C is believed to arise from the disruption of long-range order. The high temperature endotherm found above 200°C is attributed to the melting of microcrystalline regions of hard domains.

Koberstein has conducted extensive study, through DSC and small angle x-ray scattering (SAXS), on the microphase separation and multiple endothermic behavior of a series of polyether polyurethane copolymers [96–98]. This series of segmented polyurethanes contains hard segments of 4,4′-methylenediphenyl diisocyanate and soft segments of poly(oxy-propylene), with a varying degree of hard segment contents subjected to DSC study. Based on the annealing experiments, the peak temperature of the low-temperature endotherm is found to increase with an increase in the hard segment content. The intermediate endotherm arises from the disruption of microdomain structure that occurs at the microphase separation transition (MST) temperature, often defined as the temperature at which phase separation from the homogeneous phase occurs. The MST temperature is found to increase with the hard segment content. Three distinct regimes of the DSC endotherm's dependence on the annealing temperature were identified. For annealing temperatures above MST, crystallization of the hard segment is achieved from the homogeneous solution of hard and soft segments. The degree of crystallinity is governed by the undercooling. The other two regimes occur at annealing temperatures below the MST. At temperatures far above the hard-domain glass transition temperature T_g, crystallization appears to be diffusion controlled where the endotherm enthalpy increases with the annealing period. The third region is found at temperatures close to the hard segment domain T_g. Since molecular motions are highly restricted at these temperatures, the high tem-

perature endotherm virtually disappears, indicating that crystallization is greatly retarded.

Amorphous polymers occupy a unique position in the hierarchy of medical plastics because they are fairly low-cost, rigid, transparent and often steam-sterilizable. However, these materials undergo physical aging at temperatures below their glass transition temperatures where degradation in physical properties, including modulus and ultimate elongation, occurs [99–101]. As a material ages, the excess thermodynamic properties like the enthalpy and entropy relax back to the lower equilibrium state. Physical aging can therefore easily be monitored by measuring the kinetics and degree of enthalpy relaxation as manifested by the presence of an endotherm occurring around the glass transition region. DSC studies [102–105] have unequivocally demonstrated that the endotherm increases with aging time and approaches an equilibrium value that is strongly dependent on the deviation from equilibrium or $T_g - T_a$, where T_a is the aging temperature.

Residual water present in polymers could greatly affect the mechanical integrity of the processed products. It has been known that water in polycarbonate during extrusion would lead to hydrolytic degradation [106]. Total water absorbed in a polymer is generally classified into two types: (1) clustered (crystallizable), and (2) bound. One major distinction between the two is that bound water will depress the glass transition temperature of the polymer while clustered water has no effect on the T_g. Bair [107,108] has employed DSC to measure clustered water by monitoring the fusion endotherm found in the vicinity of 0°C. In this scheme, a polymer sample is cooled below -40°C to ensure complete crystallization of the clustered water, and then heated to 50°C. This large undercooling is required because of the microscopic size of the water clusters and the absence of heterogeneities to accelerate nucleation. In the polycarbonate study, Bair [108] found that the endotherm is time-dependent at undercooling above -40°C thus indicating incomplete crystallization. Figure 37 shows the DSC plots for the cooling and heating curve. The concentration of clustered water in parts per million (ppm) is given by

$$C = (10^6 \Delta H_{tr})/(\Delta H_f) \qquad (54)$$

where ΔH_{tr} is the heat of fusion of sample, and ΔH_f is the heat of fusion of water or 79.7 cal/g. The bound water content is just simply equal to the difference between the total water, which can be determined by coulometric technique [87], and the clustered water.

Crystallinity is one of the most important determinants in controlling the physical properties of semicrystalline polymers like polyolefins. Isothermal crystallization kinetics is often modelled by the Avrami equation in which the crystal growth from centers, nucleated either homogeneously or heterogeneously, is assumed to proceed in a given number

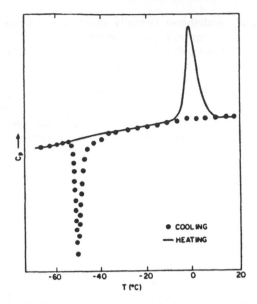

Figure 37. Heating and cooling curves for polycarbonate after 800 hours in 97°C water (from Ref. [107]).

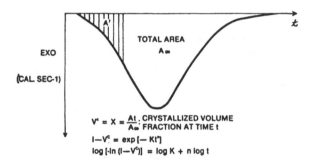

Figure 38. Crystallization kinetics based on Avrami analysis.

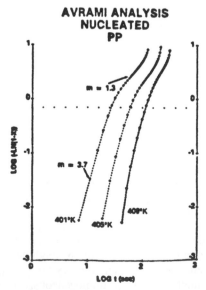

Figure 39. Crystallization isotherms for nucleated polypropylene.

of dimensions until impingement. The following equations, depicted by Figure 38, form the basis of this analysis [86]

$$V^c = X(t) = A(t)/A \qquad (55)$$

$$1 - V^c = \exp(-kt^n) \qquad (56)$$

where V^c is the crystallized volume fraction at time t, $A(t)$ is the crystallization exotherm at time t, A is the total crystallization exotherm, k is a constant, and n is the Avrami exponent which is a function of the growth conditions and the modes of transport. The Avrami exponent takes on either integral or half-integral value. Table 2 displays the Avrami exponents along with the crystal morphologies. According to this table, an Avrami exponent of 4 indicates that crystal growth is characterized by spherulites nucleated sporadically in time with growing fronts propagating in three dimensions. The isothermal curves for nucleated polypropylene are shown in Figure 39. It is apparent that these curves deviate from the theoretical isotherms at the later states of crystallization. The onset of nonlinearity exhibited by these isotherms signifies the transition from primary to secondary crystallization. In the secondary crystallization stage, spherulites have impinged and growth is accompanied either by subsidiary lamellae or increase in crystallinity associated with isothermal thickening.

Thermal oxidative stability [109] of polymers including vinyls and polyolefins is generally assessed by monitoring either the time or the temperature at which an abrupt departure from the baseline occurs as indicated by Figure 40. In the oxidation induction time (OIT) measurement, time scan is performed at isothermal temperature under oxygen atmosphere in which the onset of the oxidative reaction exotherm is recorded as the OIT. In the continuous temperature scanning method, the oxidative induction temperature is measured. Oxidative induction time measured at various temperatures can be used to construct an Arrhenius plot, often expressed as log (OIT) versus ($1/T$), in which the activation energy is extracted from

Table 2. Tabulation of Avrami exponents (from Ref. [86]).

Type of Morphology	Nucleation	n
Fibrillar	Athermal	≤ 1
Fibrillar	Thermal	≤ 2
Circular Lamellar	Athermal	≤ 2
Circular Lamellar	Thermal	≤ 3
Spherical	Athermal	3
Spherical	Thermal	4
Solid Sheaf	Athermal	≥ 5
Solid Sheaf	Thermal	≥ 6

Ref.: Wunderlich. 1976. *Macromolecular Physics, Vol. 2.* NY: Academic Press, p. 149.

the slope of this line. As expected, OIT is dependent on the base polymer stability (molecular weight effect), stabilizer system, and shear and thermal history.

DIELECTRIC SPECTROSCOPY

Dielectric spectroscopy is often defined as the study of dipole polarization or re-orientation, in response to an alternating electromagnetic field, in polar polymers as a function of frequency and/or temperature [110–112]. When a sinusoidal electric field is applied to a polymer placed between two parallel plates, the resulting current is out-of-phase with the applied voltage by a phase angle between 0 to 90°C. By examining this current–voltage relationship as a function of frequency and/or temperature, the complex dielectric permittivity or constant can be calculated. Similar to the complex modulus, ϵ' is the real component representing storage and ϵ'' is the imaginary component representing dissipation. Molecular relaxations and rheological (flow) behaviors of polymers, kinetics and state of cure of thermosets can easily be monitored by examining the dielectric responses. Probably the most unique feature of the dielectric technique is that measurements can be performed almost continuously over frequency range from 10^{-4} to 10^{10} Hz (cycle/sec) and temperature range from $-180°C$ to $500°C$. Multifrequency measurement is often employed to deconvolute overlapped transitions. For example, the α and β transition in poly(methyl methacrylate) or PMMA becomes increasingly distinct as the test frequency is reduced [111]. Moreover, the transition temperature dependence on the frequency can be used to calculate the activation energy for molecular motions.

It is not surprising that no one method can be applied over fourteen decades of frequency range. Table 3 summarizes the methods which are commonly used for measuring the dielectric responses in particular frequency regions. However, we will concentrate our discussion on the frequency bridge method because most of the dielectric work of polymers is performed in this frequency regime. These methods are mainly

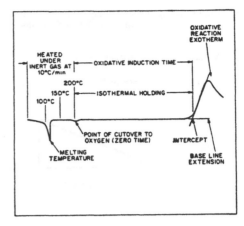

Figure 40. Oxidation induction time scan for polyethylene (from Ref. [87]).

divided into two general groups [111] "lumped circuit" and "distributed circuit" methods. The "lumped circuit" technique covers frequency from about 10^{-4} to 10^8 Hz while the "distributed" method is applicable in the frequency range from 10^8 to 10^{10} Hz. The "low" frequency technique is based on the measurement of equivalent capacitance and resistance at a given frequency whereas the "high" frequency method is designed to measure the attenuation factor α and the phase factor β at a given frequency.

As stated above, dielectric spectroscopy of polymers is normally confined to the frequency range 10^1 to 10^6 Hz or MHz therefore the "lumped circuit" method is widely used for the dielectric work. In this technique, a polymer sample is placed between two parallel electrodes and regarded as being electrically equivalent to a capacitance C_x in parallel with a resistance R_x, at a given frequency. The capacitance of a vacuum-filled parallel plate capacitor is given by

$$C_o = (A\epsilon_o)/d \qquad (57)$$

where A is the plate area, d is the plate separation, ϵ_o is the absolute permittivity of free space or

Table 3. Experimental methods for measuring ϵ^* in various frequency regimes (from Ref. [111]).

Frequency Range	Method	Remarks
10^{-4} to 10^{-1}	d.c. Transient measurements	Analogous to creep effect
10^{-2} to 10^2	Ultra-low frequency bridge	Precise determination of $\epsilon' - i\epsilon''$
10 to 10^7	Schering bridge Transformer bridge	Precise determination of $\epsilon' - i\epsilon''$
10^5 to 10^8	Resonance circuits	Upper limit of lumped circuit methods
10^8 to 10^9	Coaxial line	Good only for medium and large ϵ''
	Re-entrant cavity	Good only for low ϵ'' values; poor for temperature variation
10^9 to 3×10^{10}	H_{oln} cavity resonator Coaxial lines and waveguides	Same as above Good for medium and high ϵ'' only

Lumped Circuit Analysis-Parallel Equivalent Circuit of a Dielectric Filled Capacitor

Periodic Voltage: $V(t) = V_0 \exp(i\omega t)$

Resulting Current: $I(t) = \omega C_0 \epsilon^* V(t)$

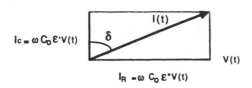

Figure 41. Vectorial representation of the current–voltage relationship in a sample-filled parallel plate capacitor.

8.85×10^{-12} F/m. The polymer-filled capacitor exhibits a complex capacitance C^*

$$C^* = \epsilon^* C_o \qquad (58)$$

where ϵ^* is defined as the complex permittivity or constant. If a sinusoidal voltage $V(t) = V_o \exp(i\omega t)$ is applied to the polymer-filled capacitor, the resulting current $I(t)$ flowing across the capacitor is

$$I(t) = dq(t)/dt = d[C^* V(t)]/dt \qquad (59)$$

where $q(t)$ is the charge on the capacitor plates at time t. Differentiating Equation (59) yields the following equalities

$$I(t) = i\omega C_o \epsilon^* V_o \exp(i\omega t) =$$

$$[i\omega\epsilon' + \omega\epsilon'']C_o V(t) = iI_c(t) + I_R(t) \qquad (60)$$

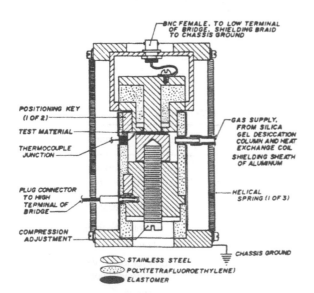

Figure 42. Cross section of a dielectric test fixture (from Ref. [113]).

It is apparent that the total current $I(t)$ is divided into two components, namely, the capacitive (storage) component $I_c(t)$ and the resistive (dissipative) component $I_R(t)$. Figure 41 depicts the vectorial diagram of current $I(t)$ in relation to voltage $V(t)$. The capacitive current component is orthogonal to the applied voltage while the resistive component is in phase with the applied voltage and a power loss will occur in the medium. Similar to $I(t)$, the complex dielectric constant ϵ^* may be defined as

$$\epsilon^*(\omega, T) = \epsilon' - i\epsilon'' \qquad (61)$$

where ϵ^* is a function of frequency ω and temperature T. The dielectric loss tangent $\tan \delta$ is given by

$$\tan \delta = \epsilon''/\epsilon' \qquad (62)$$

The permittivity ϵ' measures the alignment of dipoles while the loss factor ϵ'' represents the energy required to align dipoles and move ions. As a material undergoes a dielectric relaxation or transition, the loss factor will experience a maximum where the peak temperature increases with increasing frequency.

An equivalent circuit consisting of a capacitance C_x in parallel with a resistance R_x is employed to model the above current–voltage relationship. The electrical admittance Y_x for such a simple circuit is

$$Y_x = (1/R_x) + i\omega C_x \qquad (63)$$

The current $I(t)$ is given by

$$I(t) = Y_x V(t) \qquad (64)$$

Equating (60) to (64) and substituting (63) into (64) yields

$$\epsilon' = C_x/C_o \qquad (65a)$$

$$\epsilon'' = 1/(R_x \omega C_o) \qquad (65b)$$

$$\tan \delta = 1/(R_x C_x \omega) \qquad (65c)$$

Obviously, determination of ϵ^* reduces to measuring the equivalent capacitance C_x and resistance R_x of a polymer-filled parallel plate capacitor. These electrical quantities can be easily obtained with any impedance analyzers (Hewlett Packard) or frequency bridges (General Radio).

At frequencies above 10^8 Hz, the parallel plate method fails to yield accurate measurements due to the increasing importance of residual inductance. The "distributed circuit" technique, which is based on the concepts of wave propagation through a dielectric medium, is preferred. Both the transmission line and cavity resonator techniques are extensively reviewed by McCrum [111]. As stated earlier, the distributed technique relates the attenuation and phase factor, determined by an experimental quantity known as the propagation factor γ of dielectric, to the complex dielectric constant. It should be emphasized that this technique is seldom applied to the study of dielectric responses of polymers because the time scales corresponding to these high frequencies are usually too short compared to the relaxation time span for molecular relaxations.

There are presently two commercial dielectric systems on the market, namely, Polymer Labs, and Dupont. Frequency ranges for these systems span from 10 Hz to about 100 KHz. The heart of a dielectric spectrometer is the dielectric cell in which the equivalent capacitance and resistance (*C-D*) of the sample-filled capacitor is measured. Basic designs of a dielectric test fixture included a spring-loaded mechanism and force monitoring device to ensure intimate and reproducible contact, and a guarded electrode to eliminate edge effects or fringing fields [111]. Figure 42 shows a schematics of a typical dielectric cell. For high-frequency (up to 15 MHz) measurement, the Hewlett Packard (HP) 16451B dielectric test fixture is preferred. This dielectric cell is based on a four terminal (high/low voltage and current) configuration equipped with a guarded electrode. Unlike the common spring-loaded fixture, this HP cell contains a micrometer electrode adjustable down to 10 μm spacing.

Dielectric responses of many polymeric systems have been investigated [113–116]. In their poly(ethylene terephthalate) or PET dielectric relaxation study, Coburn and Boyd [116] prepared PET samples with crystallinities ranging from the amorphous state to 62%. The dielectric loss curves for a 26% crystalline sample is shown in Figure 43. Both the α and β transitions are clearly visible in these spectra. Based on a very extensive analysis of these curves, they concluded that the β process originates in the amorphous state and the distribution of relaxation times for the α process is strongly dependent on crystallinity.

Another application of dielectric spectroscopy is monitoring of the rheological changes accompanying curing of an epoxy or amine [110,112]. The bulk ionic conductivity, σ is defined as

$$\sigma = \epsilon'' \omega \epsilon_o \qquad (66)$$

where σ is directly correlated with viscosity. The changes in the dielectric loss reflect the changes in fluidity which are a measure of the ease with which ionic impurities can migrate through the polymer. As a material becomes fully cured, the dielectric loss will undergo a precipitous drop. It has also been demonstrated that the dielectric technique is more sensitive than DSC for analyzing the later stages of cure.

Dielectric spectroscopy also offers valuable information on the radio frequency sealability of materials. Dielectric or radio frequency (*rf*) heating of polymers is based on the energy dissipated by fast oriented dipoles in response to a high frequency, generally of the order of MHz, electric field as depicted in Figure

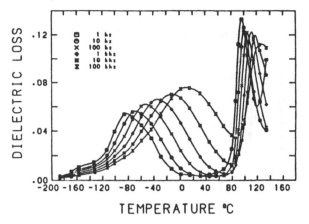

Figure 43. Dielectric loss curves for 26% crystalline PET (from Ref. [117]).

44. This mode of heat seal is commonly used in the medical industry due to the complex geometry that could be imparted to the final container and also the exceptionally strong seal strength. The power generated by a polymer placed between two electrodes is given by

$$P = \pi f \epsilon_o \epsilon'' E_0^2 \qquad (67)$$

where

P = energy dissipation per unit time per unit volume, W/cm^3
f = frequency of the generator in Hz
E_0 = amplitude of field strength between the electrode (*V*/cm)
ϵ_o = 8.854 × 10⁻¹⁰ F/cm, permﾞ ﾞity of vacuum
ϵ'' = dielectric loss of the polyr

For most materials, *rf* heating is ﾞ selfﾞ limiting process where the heating power drﾞ ﾞs as the temperature reaches above the dielectric loss peak temperature.

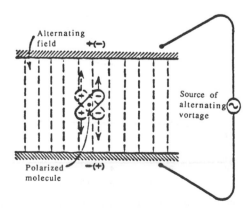

Figure 44. Dipole reorientation in response to a high-frequency electric field.

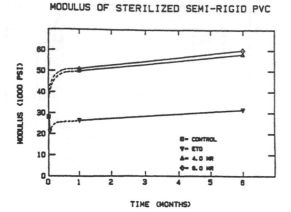

Figure 45. PVC post-radiation modulus change as function of time.

SHELF LIFE TESTING AND PREDICTION

Frequently, the manufacturing and distribution aspects of biomaterial-based medical devices receives little attention. Here, one must remember that after the product is successfully fabricated, it must first be sterilized, put into warehouse storage, shipped to customers through various routes and conditions, and expected to function as designed sometimes even after additional shelf storage at the user's location.

Sterilization by ionizing radiation is becoming increasingly popular as the mode of choice, because it is clean, efficient, environmentally preferred, and has easily controlled worker exposure conditions compared to ethylene oxide. However, radiation-sterilization does generate some undesirable side effects which must be understood and carefully controlled before full advantage can be realized. Among these side effects on biomaterials are:

- changes in color or clarity
- embrittlement, loss of elongation
- exudation, increases in extractables
- changes in modulus

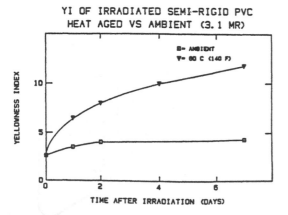

Figure 46. PVC post-radiation color development as function of time.

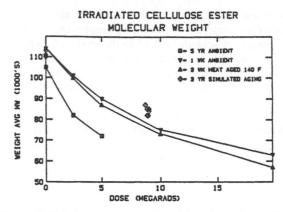

Figure 47. Cellulose ester molecular weight under various radiation dose and aging conditions.

- decreased resistance to flexural fatigue
- reduced adhesive bond strengths

In this section we will discuss shelf life prediction in general, but with particular emphasis on post-radiation shelf life. It was noted that commonly employed multiple temperature accelerated aging techniques based on the assumption that the Arrhenius relationship holds were not applicable to many of the shelf life situations. Among the well-known examples that do not follow the Arrhenius relationship are the modulus and color changes upon post-radiation aging (Figures 45, 46). Also, the physical properties of polypropylenes can undergo disastrous degradations especially after gamma irradiation, likewise for cellulose esters.

In formulating a predictive strategy, one may need to identify the controlling intrinsic material parameters that relate aging degradation to performance. Some of the independent variables may include:

- molecular weight and MWD
- loss of stabilizers, antioxidants
- free radical concentration buildup
- peroxide buildup
- changes in morphology

If possible, the predicted results should be compared with real-time aging experience to increase the confidence of the predictions. For less satisfactory results, additional factors that may contribute must be identified.

For example, in 1988 Woo and Sanford discovered that for a series of cellulose copolyesters, the dominant factor for product performance is molecular weight, regardless of radiation dose or storage conditions or age (Figure 47) [118]. In this case, a high radiation dose (or any other method of degradation) can be used to simulate real time aging with predictive results. Similarly, a method based on physical acceleration rather than chemical means was used to simulate post-radiation shelf life aging for polypropylenes. When compared with real time data, excellent correlation was achieved (Figure 48) [119].

Most polymeric biomaterials rely on antioxidants to retard the degradation. As expected, if the device is fabricated through a melt process, most degradation would occur at this stage. However, over shelf life storage, diffusion of oxygen will lead to a gradual reduction of antioxidant throughout the shelf life. If the morphology of the material is relatively simple (homogeneous distribution of antioxidants and reaction products), then an assay of the antioxidant content over time may serve as a good indicator of property reduction.

Another very important and yet seldom recognized phenomenon is the so-called physical aging, or free volume relaxation process. Briefly stated, all glassy materials when quenched from the liquid state possess a specific volume higher than that of the equilibrium glass, and thus have a tendency to slowly relax and consolidate toward the equilibrium volume. The kinetics of this relaxation process is governed by the material type, and the proximity to the glass transition temperature T_g.

At first glance, such processes seem to have little to do with the product performance. However, many of the post-fabrication processing steps involve temperatures reaching very close to T_g. For example, the precondition step for ethylene oxide sterilization frequently calls for temperatures as high as 65°C, and the drying step following aqueous cleaning could be as high as 75°C. When compared with PET and nylon's T_g of about 80°C, and PMMA's T_g of about 110°C, significant physical aging can and does take place.

Upon aging, the physical properties of material could be drastically degraded. In one of the studies carried out at the author's laboratories, a commonly used amorphous PET was found to reduce its ultimate elongation from more than 150% to less than 6%, a drastic embrittlement indeed [120] (Figures 49, 50).

A simplified diagram of the free volume relaxation process is shown in Figure 51 and numerous studies have documented the property losses in a wide variety of materials [121].

One of the most convenient methods to quantify the degree of the aging process is DSC. Using a modified specific heat procedure, Woo and Cheung demonstrated precision data generation quite routinely [122].

Since the mechanical properties are related to the degree of aging, and aging kinetics can be quantified from accelerated aging experiments conducted at elevated temperatures, this method allows a relatively rigorous determination and prediction of long-term shelf life and expected degradations during post-fabrication processing, transport and storage.

By systematically varying the T_g using plasticizer incorporation, Woo and Cheung determined the physical aging kinetics for the amorphous PET system to have an activation energy of about 24 KCal/Mole

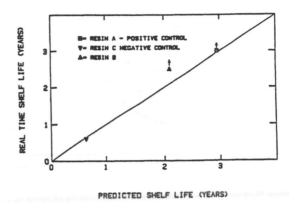

RADIATION STERILIZED POLYPROPYLENE SHELF LIFE PREDICTION

Figure 48. Irradiated polypropylene shelf life prediction versus real shelf life data.

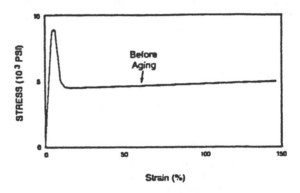

Stress-strain curve recorded at 1 in/min for unaged PETG.

Figure 49. Amorphous PET mechanical property before aging.

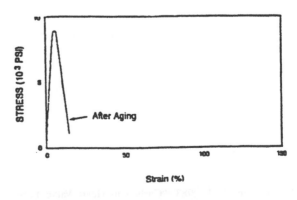

Stress-strain curve recorded at 1 in/min for aged PETG.

Figure 50. Amorphous PET mechanical property post-aging.

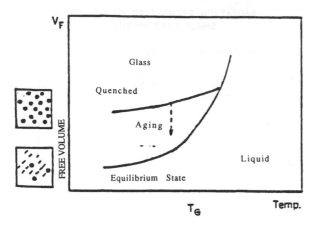

Figure 51. Free volume temperature behavior during physical aging.

covering a temperature range from T_g to approximately 50°C below T_g. It should be noted that this activation energy indicated a nearly tripling of the aging rate per each 10°C rise in temperature, in contrast to the conventional Arrhenius rule of doubling per 10°C for chemical reactions.

REFERENCES

1. Lee, S., ed. 1987. *Advances in Biomaterials*. Lancaster, PA: Technomic Publishing Company.

2. Hench, L. L. and Ethridge, E. C. 1982. *Biomaterials, an Interfacial Approach*. New York: Academic Press.

3. Szycher, M., ed. 1983. *Biocompatible Polymers, Metals, and Composites*. Lancaster, PA: Technomic Publishing Company.

4. Wolf, K. 1951. *Kunstoffe*, 41:89.

5. Huh, D. S. and S. L. Cooper. 1971. *Poly. Eng. Sci.*, 11:369.

6. Ibid.

7. Reichert, M., Ph.D. Thesis, Univ. of Michigan (1982).

8. Heijboar, J., 1977. *Intl. Poly. Matl.*, 6:11.

9. Yee, A. F. 1981. *Polymer Preprints*, 22(2):285.

10. Bucknall, C. B. 1977. *Toughened Plastics*, London: Applied Science Publishers, p. 113.

11. Macosko, C. W. 1983. *Soc. of Plas. Eng. Antec.*, p. 525.

12. Gillham, J. K. 1974. *Polymer Preprints*, 15(1):241.

13. Zener, C. 1948. *Elasticity and Anelasticity of Metals*, Chicago: Univ. of Chicago Press, p. 151.

14. Ducheyne, P. and J. E. Lemons, ed. 1988. *Bioceramics: Material Characteristics versus in vivo Behavior*, The New York Academy of Sciences, Vol. 523.

15. Schoen, F. J. 1983. "Carbon in Heart Valve Prostheses: Foundations and Clinical Performance", in *Biocompatible Polymers, Metals and Composites*. M. Szycher, ed. Lancaster, PA: Technomic Publishing Co., pp. 239–261.

16. Gentle, C. R. 1980. "A Porous Ceramic Mitral Valve Prosthesis", in *Mechanical Properties of Biomaterials*. G. W. Hastings and D. F. Williams, eds. NY: John Wiley & Sons, Ltd., p. 557.

17. Yoganathan, A. P., Y. R. Woo and H. W. Sung. 1988. "Advances in Prosthetic Heart Valves: Fluid Mechanics of Aortic Valve Design", in *J. of Biomaterials Applications*, Vol. 2 (April).

18. Shigley, J. E. and L. D. Mitchell. *Mechanical Engineering Design*. McGraw-Hill Book Company, 4th Ed., p. 234.

19. Williams, J. G. 1984. *Fracture Mechanics of Polymers*. NY: Ellis Horwood Limited, John Wiley & Sons.

20. Westergaard, H. M. 1939. *J. Appl. Mech.*, p. 46 (June).

21. Irwin, G. R. 1964. *Appl. Mats. Res.*, 3:65.

22. Rice, J. R. 1968. In *Fracture, an Advance Treatise, Vol. 2*. H. Liebowitz, ed. NY: Academic Press, p. 192.

23. Tada, H., P. C. Paris and G. R. Irwin. 1985. *The Stress Analysis of Cracks Handbook, 2nd Ed.* Missouri: Paris Productions Incorp. and Del. Research Corp.

24. Wiederhorn, S. M. 1967. "Influence of Water Vapor on Crack Propagation in Soda-Lime Glass", *J. Am. Ceram. Soc.*, 50(8):407–414.

25. Wiederhorn, S. M., S. W. Freiman, E. R. Fuller, Jr. and C. J. Simmons. 1982. "Effect of Water and Other Dielectrics on Crack Growth", *J. of Materials Science*, 17:3460–3478.

26. Michalske, T. A. and S. W. Freiman. 1983. "A Molecular Mechanism for Stress Corrosion in Vitreous Silica", *J. Am. Ceram. Soc.*, 66(4):284–288.

27. Freiman, S. W. 1974. "Effect of Alcohols on Crack Propagation in Glass", *J. Am. Ceram. Soc.*, 57(8): 350–353.

28. Freiman, S. W. 1988. "Brittle Fracture Behavior of Ceramics", *A. Cer. Soc., Ceramic Bulletin*, 67(2).

29. Wiederhorn, S. M. 1974. In *Fracture Mechanics of Ceramics, Vol. 2*. R. C. Bradt, D. P. H. Hasselman and F. F. Lange. NY: Plenum Press, pp. 613–646.

30. Evans, A. G. and S. M. Wiederhorn. 1974. "Proof Testing of Ceramic Materials—An Analysis Basis for Failure Prediction", *International Journal of Fracture*, 10(3):379–392.

31. Wiederhorn, S. M. 1975. "Reliability, Lift Prediction, and Proof Testing of Ceramic", in *Ceramics for High Performance Applications*. J. J. Burke, A. E. Gorum and R. N. Katz, eds. Chestnut Hills, MA: Brook Hill Publishing Company, pp. 633–663.

32. Fuller, E. R., Jr. 1979. "An Evaluation of Double-Torsion Testing-Analysis", in *Fracture Mechanics Applied to Brittle Materials*. S. W. Freiman, eds. ASTM STP 678, American Soc. for Testing and Materials, Philadelphia, p. 3.

33. Pletka, B. J., E. R. Fuller and B. G. Koepke. 1979. "An Evaluation of Double-Torsion Testing-Experimental", in *Fracture Mechanics Applied to Brittle Materials*. S. W. Freiman, ed. STP 678, American Soc. for Testing and Materials, Philadelphia, p. 19.

34. Fourney, W. L. and T. Kobayashi. 1979. "Influence of Loading System on Crack Propagation and Arrest Be-

haviour in a Double-Cantilever Beam Specimen", in *Fracture Mechanics Applied to Brittle Materials*. S. W. Freiman, ed. STP 678, American Soc. for Testing and Materials, Philadelphia, p. 47.

35. Schoen, F. J. 1973. "On the Fatigue Behavior of Pyrolytic Carbon", *Carbon*, 11:413–414.

36. Shim, H. S. 1974. "The Behavior of Isotropic Pyrolytic Carbons under Cyclic Loading", *Biomaterials and Medical Devices: Artificial Organs*, 2:55–64.

37. Dauskardt, R. H. and R. O. Ritchie. 1989. "Cyclic Fatigue-Crack Growth Behavior in Ceramics", *Closed Loop*, Vol. 17.

38. Ewart, L. and S. Suresh. 1986. "Dynamic Fatigue Crack Growth in Polycrystalline Alumina under Cycle Compression", *Journal of Materials Science Letters*, 5:774–778.

39. Ritchie, R. O. 1979. "Near-Threshold Fatigue Crack Propagation in Steels", *International Metal Reviews*, 20:205–230.

40. Minnear, W. P., T. M. Hollenbeck, R. C. Bradt and P. L. Walker. 1976. "Subcritical Crack Growth of Glassy Carbon in Water", *Journal of Non-Crystalline Solids*, 21:107–115.

41. Hodkinson, P. H. and J. S. Nadeau. 1975. "Slow Crack Growth in Graphite", *Journal of Material Science*, 10:846–856.

42. Pelloux, P. M. N. 1970. "Crack Extension by Alternating Shear", *Engineering Fracture Mechanics*, 1:697–704.

43. Ritchie, R. O. 1988. "Mechanism of Fatigue Crack Propagation", in *Metals Composites and Ceramics: Role of Crack-Tip Shielding*, Materials Science and Engineering, 103A:15–28.

44. Kawakubo, T. and K. Komeya. 1987. "Static and Cyclic Fatigue Behavior of a Sintered Silicon Nitride at Room Temperature", *Journal of American Ceramics Society*, 70:400–405.

45. Swain, M. V., V. Zelizko, S. Lam and M. Marmach. 1989. "Comparison of the Static and Cyclic Fatigue Behavior of Mg-PSZ and Alumina in Ringer's Solution", in *Biomaterials, MRS International Meeting on Advanced Materials Proceedings, Vol. 1*. Pittsburgh, PA: Materials Research Society.

46. Outwater, J. O. and D. J. Gerry. 1967. "On the Fracture Energy, Rehealing Velocity and Refracture Energy of Cast Epoxy Resin", *22nd Society of Plastic Industry Conference*, Paper 13-D, also *J. of Adhesion*, 1:290–298 (1969).

47. Outwater, J. O. and D. J. Gerry. 1966. "On the Fracture Energy of Glass", *NRL Interim Contract Report*, Contract NONR 3219(01)(X), AD640848, University of Vermont, Burlington, VT (Aug.).

48. Kies, J. A. and A. B. J. Clark. 1969. In *Fracture 1969 (Proceedings, 2nd International Conference on Fracture, Brighton, April 1969)*. P. L. Pratt, ed. London: Chapman and Hall, pp. 483–491.

49. William, D. P. and A. G. Evans. 1973. "A Simple Method for Studying Slow Crack Growth", *Journal of Testing and Evaluation*, 1(4):264–270.

50. Evans, A. G. 1972. *Journal of Material Science*, 7(10):1137–1146.

51. Champomier, F. P. 1979. "Crack Propagation Measurements on Glass: A Comparison between Double Torsion and Double Cantilever Beam Specimens", *Fracture Mechanics Applied to Brittle Materials*, ASTM STP 678. S. W. Freiman, ed. American Society for Testing and Materials, pp. 60–72.

52. Evans, A. G. 1973. "A Simple Method for Evaluating Slow Crack Growth in Brittle Materials", *International Journal of Fracture*, 9(3):267–275.

53. Outwater, J. O., M. C. Murphy, R. G. Kumble and J. T. Berry. 1974. "Double Torsion Technique as a Universal Fracture Toughness Test Method", *Fracture Toughness and Slow-Stable Cracking*, ASTM STP 559, American Society for Testing and Materials, pp. 127–138.

54. Hodkinson, P. H. and J. S. Nadeau. 1975. "Slow Crack Growth in Graphite", *Journal of Material Science*, 10:846–856.

55. Wiederhorn, S. M. "Subcritical Crack Growth in Ceramics", in *Fracture Mechanics of Ceramics*, 2:613–646.

56. Evans, A. G. and S. M. Wiederhorn. 1974. "Crack Propagation in Silicon Nitride at Elevated Temperatures", *Journal of Material Science*, 9:270–278.

57. Evans, A. G. 1974. "Slow Crack Growth in Brittle Materials under Dynamic Loading Conditions", *International Journal of Fracture*, 10:251–259.

58. Evans, A. G. and E. R. Fuller. 1974. "Crack Propagation in Ceramic Materials under Cyclic Loading Conditions", *Met. Trans*, 5:27–33.

59. Ritter, J. E., Jr. 1978. "Engineering Design and Fatigue Failure of Brittle Materials", in *Fracture Mechanics of Ceramics, Vol. 4*. R. C. Bradt, D. P. H. Hasselmann and F. F. Lange, eds. NY: Plenum Press, p. 667.

60. Jakus, K., D. C. Coyne and J. E. Ritter. 1978. "Analysis of Fatigue Data for Lifetime Predictions for Ceramic Materials", *J. Material Science*, 13:2071.

61. Wiederhorn, S. M., E. R. Fuller, J. Mandel and A. G. Evans. 1976. "An Error Analysis of Failure Prediction Techniques Derived from Fracture Mechanics", *J. Am. Ceram. Soc.*, 59:403–411.

62. Evans, A. G. and S. M. Wiederhorn. 1974. "Proof Testing of Ceramic Materials—An Analytical Basis for Failure Prediction", *Int. J. Fracture*, 10:379.

63. Wilkins, B. J. S. and L. A. Simpson. 1974. "Errors in Estimating the Minimum Time-To-Failure in Glass", *J. Am. Ceram. Soc.*, 57(11):505.

64. Jacobs, D. F. and J. E. Ritter. 1976. "Uncertainty in Minimum Lifetime Predictions", *J. Am. Ceram. Soc.*, 59:481.

65. Weibull, W. 1939. "Statistical Theory of the Strength of Materials", *Ing. Vetensk. Akad, Handl.*, No. 151.

66. Ritter, J. E., N. Bandyopadhyay and K. Jakus. 1979. "Statistical Reproducibility of the Crack Propagation Parameter N in Dynamic Fatigue Tests", *J. Am. Ceram. Soc.*, 62:542.

67. Evans, A. G. and H. Johnson. "The Fracture Stress and Its Dependence on Slow Crack Growth", *J. Mater. Sci.*, 10:214.

68. Davidge, R. W., J. R. McLaren and G. Tappin. 1973. "Strength Probability Time (SPT) Relationships in Ceramics", *J. Material Science*, 8:1699–1705.

69. Wiederhorn, S. M. 1973. "Prevention of Failure in Glass by Proof-Testing", *J. Amer. Ceram. Soc.*, 56:227–229.

70. Ritter, J. E., Jr., P. B. Oates, E. R. Fuller, Jr. and S. M. Wiederhorn. 1980. "Proof Testing of Ceramics I—Experiment", *J. Material Science*, 15:2275.

71. Fuller, E. R., Jr., S. M. Wiederhorn, J. E. Ritter and P. B. Oates. 1980. "Proof Testing of Ceramics II—Theory", *J. Material Science*, 15:2282.

72. Xavier, C. and H. W. Hiibner. 1981. "Proof Testing of Alumina to Assure against Premature Failure", in *Science of Ceramics, Vol. 2*, Extended Abstracts, Stenungsund, p. 117.

73. Ritter, J. E. and S. A. Wulf. 1978. "Evaluation of Proof Testing to Assure against Delayed Failure", *Am. Ceramics Soc. Bull.*, 57:186.

74. Evans, A. G. and E. R. Fuller. 1975. "Proof-Testing: The Effects of Slow Crack Growth", *J. of Material Science and Engineering*, 19:69–77.

75. Pletka, J. and S. M. Wederhorn. 1982. "A Comparison of Failure Predictions by Strength and Fracture Mechanics Technique", *J. Material Science*, 17:1247–1268.

76. Weibull, W. A. 1951. "A Statistical Distribution Function of Wide Applicability", *J. Applied Mechanics*, 18:293.

77. Ritter, J. E., Jr., D. C. Greenspan, R. A. Palmer and L. L. Hench. 1979. "Use of Fracture Mechanics Theory in Lifetime Predictions for Alumina and Bioglass-Coated Alumina", *J. Biomed. Mater. Res.*, 13:251.

78. Richter, H., U. Seidelmann and U. Soltesz. 1980. "Slow Crack Growth and Failure Prediction for Alumina in Physiological Media: In Evaluation of Biomaterials", *Proc. 1st Eur. Conf. on Eval. Biomaterials*, Strassburg, 1977. G. D. Winter, J. L. Leray and K. de Groot, eds. NY: John Wiley & Sons, p. 227.

79. Billmeyer, F. W. 1971. *Textbook of Polymer Science, 2nd Ed.* NY: Wiley, p. 81.

80. Berry, G. C. and T. G. Fox. 1968. *Adv. Poly. Science*, 5:261.

81. Graessley, W. W. 1982. *Adv. Poly. Sci.*, 47:67.

82. deGennes, P. G. 1979. *Scaling Concepts in Polymer Physics*. Ithaca, NY: Cornell Univ. Press.

83. Tuminello, W. H. 1987. *Soc. of Plas. Eng. Antec*, p. 991.

84. Zeichner, G. R. and P. P. Patel. 1981. *Proc. 2nd Congress Chem. Eng.*, 6:333.

85. Tuminello, W. H., ibid.

86. Wunderlich, W. W. 1976. *Macromolecular Physics, Vol. 2*. NY: Academic Press.

87. Turi, E. A. 1981. *Thermal Characterization of Polymeric Materials*. NY: Academic Press.

88. Baxter, R. A. 1969. In *Thermal Analysis*. R. F. Schwenker and P. D. Garn, eds. NY: Academic Press, 1:65.

89. Wendlandt, W. W. 1965. *Thermal Methods of Analysis*, NY: Wiley Interscience.

90. Vallance, M. A., J. L. Castles and S. L. Cooper. 1984. *Polymer*, 25:1734.

91. Thamm, R. C. and W. H. Buck. 1978. *J. Poly. Sci., Polym. Chem. Ed.*, 16:539.

92. Lilaonitkul, A., J. C. West and S. L. Cooper. 1976. *J. Macromol. Sci., Phys. Ed.*, B12:563.

93. Matsuo, M., K. Geshi, A. Moriyama and C. Sawatari. 1982. *Macromolecules*, 15:193.

94. Jacques, C. H. M. 1977. In *Polymer Alloys*. D. K. Klempner and K. C. Frisc, eds. NY: Plenum Press, p. 287.

95. Hesketh, T. R., J. W. C. VanBogart and S. L. Cooper. 1980. *Polym. Eng. Sci.*, 20(1):190.

96. Leung, L. M. and J. T. Koberstein. 1985. *J. Polym. Sci., Polym. Phys. Ed.*, 23:1109.

97. Koberstein, J. T. and T. P. Russell. 1986. *Macromolecules*, 19:714.

98. Leung, L. M., J. T. Koberstein. 1986. *Macromolecules*, 19:706.

99. Struik, L. C. E. 1976. In *Annals New York Academy Science*. A. Goldstein and R. Simha, eds., 78:279.

100. Struik, L. C. E. 1978. *Physical Aging in Amorphous Polymers and Other Materials*. Amsterdam: Elsevier.

101. O'Reilly, J. M., J. J. Tribone and J. Greener. 1985. *Amer. Chem. Soc., Polym. Preprint*, 26(2):30.

102. Petrie, S. E. B. 1972. *J. Polym. Sci., Polym. Phys. Ed.*, 10:151.

103. Hodge, I. M. and A. R. Beren. 1982. *Macromolecules*, 15:762.

104. Hodge, I. M. and G. S. Huvard. 1983. *Macromolecules*, 16:371.

105. Beren, A. R. and I. M. Hodge. 1982. *Macromolecules*, 15:756.

106. Bair, H. E. and P. C. Warren. 1976. *Bull. Am. Phys. Soc.*, 24(3):288.

107. Bair, H. E., G. E. Johnson and B. Merriweather. 1978. *J. Appl. Phys.*, 49:4976.

108. Bair, H. E., G. E. Johnson and E. W. Anderson. 1980. *Polym. Prep., Am. Chem. Soc., Div. Polym. Chem.*, 2(2):21.

109. Howard, J. B. 1973. *Polym. Eng. Sci.*, 13:429.

110. Hedvig, P. 1977. *Dielectric Spectroscopy of Polymers*. NY: John Wiley & Sons.

111. McGrum, N. G., B. E. Reed and G. W. William. 1976. *Anealistic and Dielectric Effects in Polymeric Solids*. London: John Wiley & Sons.

112. Blythe, A. R. 1979. *Electrical Properties of Polymers*, NY: Cambridge.

113. Vallance, M. A., A. S. Young and S. L. Cooper. 1983. *Colloid and Polym. Sci.*, 541:261.

114. Wetton, R. E., W. J. MacKnight, J. R. Fried and F. E. Karasz. 1975. *Macromolecules*, 11:158.

115. Kurosaki, S. and T. Furumaya. 1960. *J. Polym. Sci.*, 43:137.

116. Ishida, Y. 1960. *Kolloid Z*, 168:29.

117. Coburn, J. C. "Dielectric Relaxation Process in PET", Ph.D. Dissertation, University of Utah, 1984.

118. Sandford, C. and L. Woo. 1988. *Radiation Physics and Chem.*, 31:671.

119. Sandford, C. and L. Woo. 1987. *Soc. of Plas. Eng.*, ANTEC, p. 1201.

120. Woo, L. and Wilson Cheung. 1988. *Soc. of Plas. Eng.*, ANTEC, p. 1352.

121. Bair, H. E., G. H. Bebbington and P. G. Kelleher. 1976. *Poly. Sci. Poly. Phy. Ed.*, 14:2113.

122. Woo, L. and W. Cheung. 1989. *Proc. North Am. Thermal Analysis Soc.*, 1:318.

7

Non-Destructive Testing of Virgin Mammary Prostheses: First Step in an Attempt to Characterize the Changes That Occur with These Implants *in Vivo*

DANIEL MARCEAU*
CATHERINE ROLLAND*
MICHAEL BRONSKILL**
ALAIN CARDOU*
ROYSTON PAYNTER*
ROBERT GUIDOIN*,1

ABSTRACT: Physical characterization of virgin gel-filled mammary prostheses has been achieved through a series of experiments involving only non-destructive test methods. The physical properties measured were density, luminous transmittance, coefficient of friction, compressive stiffness, dynamic response to a sine wave vibration and NMR relaxation times, T1 and T2. Although the collected data was intended to serve as a reference for quantification of the degradation phenomena observed in explanted mammary prostheses, they also proved useful for quality control purposes, suggesting that some of the tested products did not fully conform to the relevant ASTM standard specifications.

INTRODUCTION

During the last six years, we have received over 300 surgically excised prostheses and, as a first step in an attempt to characterize the changes that have occurred in these implants *in vivo* [1–12], we have used non-destructive test methods which preserve the overall integrity of the sample. It is worth noting that the currently applicable ASTM standards [13–16] do not incorporate this kind of testing. We developed an original protocol consisting of six experiments: measurement of the global density, measurement of the luminous transmittance, measurement of the coefficient of friction, measurement of the compressive stiffness, evaluation of the dynamic response to a sinusoidal vibration and measurement of nuclear magnetic reso-

nance (NMR) relaxation times. Since interpretation of the results necessitates comparison with a set of baseline data, the tests were first conducted on a series of virgin mammary prostheses. In this paper, the results pertain exclusively to virgin, silicone gel-filled mammary prostheses.

MATERIALS AND METHODS

Selection of Prostheses

The models of virgin prostheses selected for testing were chosen to cover the range of explanted devices already recovered through our retrieval programme. The final selection (23 specimens) included devices made by two important manufacturers: Dow Corning and Heyer Schulte. Table 1 lists the quantities and main characteristics of the selected models. An example of gel-filled mammary prosthesis is given in Figure 1.

It should be noted that two specimens were damaged during testing, thus explaining the progressive reduction in the number of tested prostheses as the experiments proceeded (Tables 1 through 8).

Experiments

Measurement of the Global Density

The global density (shell + silicone gel) of the mammary prostheses was determined using mass and volume measurements, in combination with the following equation:

$$\varrho = \frac{M_p}{V} \qquad (1)$$

where

ϱ = global density of the prosthesis (g/ml)
M_p = mass of the prosthesis (g)
V = volume of the prosthesis (ml)

1Correspondence: Dr. Robert Guidoin, Ph.D., Biomaterials Institute, Room Fl-304, St-François d'Assise Hospital, 10 de l'Espinay, Quebec City, QC G1L 3L5, Canada.

*Biomatériaux, Hôpital St-François d'Assise, Laboratoire de Chirurgie Expérimentale et Département de Génie Mécanique, Université Laval, Québec City, Canada
**Department of Medical Biophysics, University of Toronto and Ontario Cancer Institute, Toronto, Canada

Table 1. List of the tested mammary prostheses.

I.D. Code	Company	Type of Design	Nominal Volume (ml)	Number of Specimens N = 23
A	Dow Corning	Round, low-profile	150	2
B	Dow Corning	Round, low-profile	190	6
C	Dow Corning	Round, low-profile	305	1
D	Heyer Schulte	Oval	145	8
E	Heyer Schulte	Oval, low-profile	150	1
F	Heyer Schulte	Round	150	2
G	Heyer Schulte	Round	200	3

Table 2. Overall density of the prostheses.

I.D. Code	Mean Density (g/ml)	Standard Deviation (g/ml)	Number of Specimens N = 22
A	0.9760	0.0014	2
B	0.9772	0.0013	6
C	0.9730	—	1
D	0.9750	0.0018	7
E	0.9740	—	1
F	0.9735	0.0007	2
G	0.9746	0.0006	3

Table 3. Luminous transmittance of the prostheses.

I.D. Code	Mean Transmittance (%)	Standard Deviation (%)	Number of Specimens N = 22
A	88.5	0.9	2
B	86.3	1.0	6
C	91.7	—	1
D	90.3	0.9	7
E	88.6	—	1
F	90.4	0.2	2
G	90.6	0.8	3

Table 4. Coefficient of friction of the prostheses.

I.D. Code	Mean Coefficient of Friction (—)	Standard Deviation (—)	Number of Specimens N = 23
A	1.08	0.13	2
B	0.33	0.07	6
C	0.23	—	1
D	0.39	0.25	8
E	0.61	—	1
F	0.76	0.08	2
G	1.06	0.18	3

Table 5a. Compressive stiffness of the prostheses (loading).

I.D. Code	Mean Stiffness* (kN/m)	Standard Deviation (kN/m)	Number of Specimens N = 21
A	12.05	—	1
B	19.25	4.71	6
C	8.16	—	1
D	5.42	0.52	7
E	16.88	—	1
F	13.99	3.99	2
G	8.75	1.67	3

*Calculated at the 15 Newtons compressive force level.

Table 5b. Compressive stiffness of the prostheses (unloading).

I.D. Code	Mean Stiffness* (kN/m)	Standard Deviation (kN/m)	Number of Specimens N = 21
A	13.84	—	1
B	16.74	2.18	6
C	7.11	—	1
D	6.30	0.76	7
E	13.56	—	1
F	12.53	0.36	2
G	8.10	0.70	3

*Calculated at the 15 Newtons compressive force level.

Table 6. Natural frequency of the mass-prosthesis systems.

I.D. Code	Mean Natural Frequency (Hz)	Standard Deviation (Hz)	Number of Specimens N = 20
A	16.5	—	1
B	18.9	1.2	6
C	—	—	—*
D	11.0	0.5	7
E	17.2	—	1
F	15.7	0.5	2
G	12.7	1.0	3

*Too large for the test apparatus.

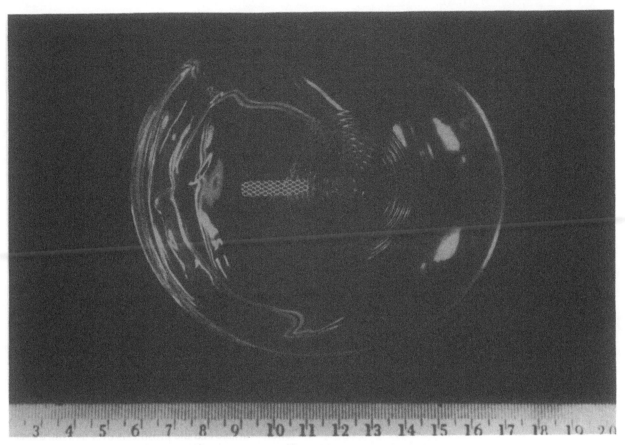

Figure 1. Example of a gel-filled mammary prosthesis.

The mass was measured using a digital balance (Mettler, PC 200) with a precision of ±0.01 gram. For the determination of volume, a specially designed apparatus was used that consisted of a 15.0 centimeter bore Plexiglas® reservoir (filled with distilled water) in which the prostheses were immersed by means of a 14.0 centimeter diameter aluminium piston. The reservoir was fitted with a V-notch nozzle that allowed precise control of the overflow so that, after zeroing with the piston only, the volume of water corresponding to the volume of the prosthesis could be collected in a beaker (Figure 2). The beaker was then weighed

on the digital balance, and conversion from mass to volume was made using the standard value for density of water (0.998 g/ml) under laboratory conditions (20°C and 101.33 kPa). Following careful calibration, the method proved to be precise to within 0.2 percent.

Measurement of the Luminous Transmittance

In this experiment, the prosthesis was used as the target and diffusion medium for a coherent beam of light (modified ASTM D 1003-61 Test Method) [17]. The luminous transmittance was calculated as follows:

$$T_t = \frac{I_{tb}}{I_{ib}} \times 100 \qquad (2)$$

Table 7. Damping coefficient of the mass-prosthesis systems.

I.D. Code	Mean Damping Coefficient (—)	Standard Deviation (—)	Number of Specimens $N = 20$
A	0.23	—	1
B	0.29	0.04	6
C	—	—	—*
D	0.15	0.02	7
E	0.22	—	1
F	0.21	0.01	2
G	0.15	0.01	3

*Too large for the test apparatus.

Table 8. NMR relaxation time measurements.

I.D. Code	T_1* (ms)	T_2** (ms)	Number of Specimens $N = 4$
A	359	138	1
B	356	124	1
C	352	120	1
G	348	100	1

*Estimated T_1 uncertainty ± 20 ms.
**Estimated T_2 uncertainty ± 10 ms.

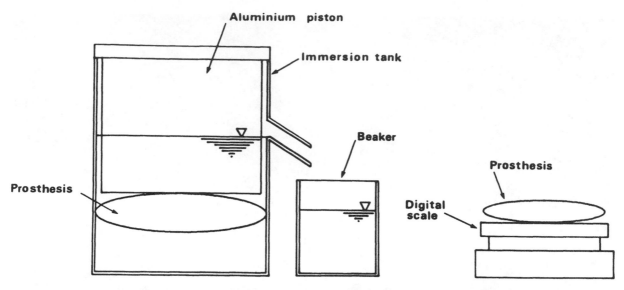

Figure 2. Density measurement kit.

where

T_t = total transmittance of the prosthesis (%)
I_{tb} = intensity of the transmitted beam of light (mW/cm²)
I_{ib} = intensity of the incident beam of light (mW/cm²)

The light source was a helium-neon laser (Hughes, Model 3225 HPC) that was selected because its polarized monochromatic radiation (λ = 632.8 nm) was known to have a low rate of diffusion. It was mounted on a horizontal rigid rest located on the left-hand side of the prosthesis to be tested (Figure 3). The prosthesis was clamped between the two thin Plexiglas® disks (0.65 centimeter thick and 1.50 centimeter apart) of a rotating support, the shaft of which laid a few centimeters below the laser beam level, so as to allow measurement of the transmittance at six different points on the specimen. These points were located at the vertices of a regular hexagon centered on the rotation axis and they were marked by small holes drilled into the disks. The incident beam of light was aimed to pass through the holes and the prosthesis, and then the transmitted light was collected in an integrating sphere (Labsphere, Model IAS 100WR) equipped with an appropriate detector (Labsphere, Model DA 100 R) and photometer–radiometer (Labsphere, Model 3000). A five percent "transmittance" filter was used in combination with the laser beam, in order to prevent saturation of the detector.

Measurement of the Coefficient of Friction

The kinetic coefficient of friction (modified ASTM D 1894-78 Test Method) [18] of the virgin mammary prostheses, sliding upon a reference surface made of Teflon®, was determined using a universal testing machine (Instron, Model 1130) and a specially designed set of receptacles, as shown in Figure 4. The prosthesis was nested between two Plexiglas® receptacles, the top one loaded to compress the prosthesis, and the one on the underside having three circular openings (20 millimeters in diameter in an equilateral triangle pattern) to allow direct contact between the Teflon® surface and the prosthesis over a defined area. The compressive load was kept constant at 1.0 kilogram and the total mass of the sliding system was measured using a digital balance. The underside receptacle was connected to the moving crosshead of the universal testing machine by means of a flexible stainless steel wire passing over a low-friction pulley, which converted the vertical movement of the crosshead into a horizontal one. The force required to keep the receptacles, load and prosthesis in a uniform rectilinear motion (200 millimeters/minute) was measured by the load cell (Instron, Model 2512-124) and the analog electrical output was transmitted to the integral X-Y recorder. The kinetic coefficient of friction was then calculated using the following equation:

$$\mu k = \frac{F_f}{M_t \cdot g} \tag{3}$$

where

μk = kinetic coefficient of friction (dimensionless)
F_f = mean friction force (N)
M_t = mass of the receptacles, load and prosthesis (kg)
g = gravitational acceleration (9.81 m/s²)

Measurement of the Compressive Stiffness

The Instron universal testing machine was also used for the determination of the compressive stiffness of

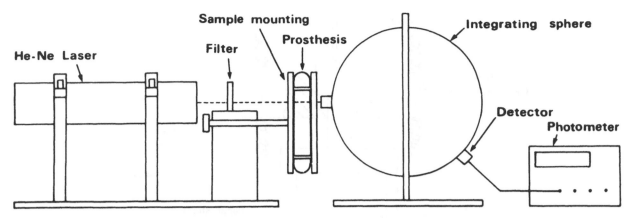

Figure 3. Luminous transmittance measurement system.

the prostheses. This time, the testing machine was fitted with an appropriate compression cage (Figure 5), made from a modified Hoffman/Turner mini-probe tester [19]. The prosthesis was placed between the two plates of the compression cage and, as they were brought together, the compressive force was recorded as a function of time (further converted into units of displacement by knowledge of the crosshead and paper chart speeds). The relative speed of the two compressing plates was kept to a minimum (50 millimeters/minute), in order to reduce the influence of the viscous effects in the material. The compressive

force was limited to a maximum value of 20 Newtons, known to be bearable by the prostheses [20], so as to allow measurement of the compressive stiffness during loading and unloading sequences. To prevent the prosthesis from sticking to the upper plate of the compression cage during the unloading cycles, a sheet of paper was interposed between the two. The compressive stiffness was calculated using the following equation:

$$K = \frac{\Delta F}{\Delta L} \qquad (4)$$

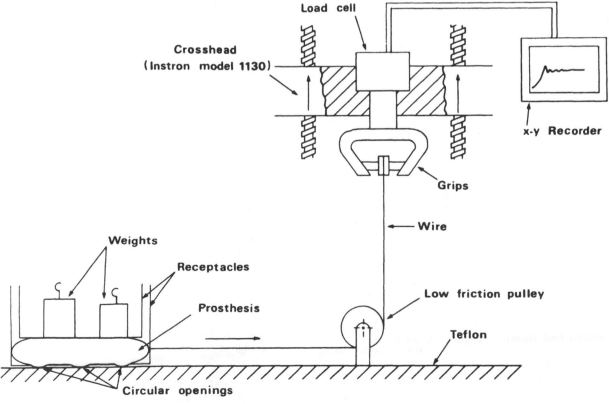

Figure 4. Friction measurement system.

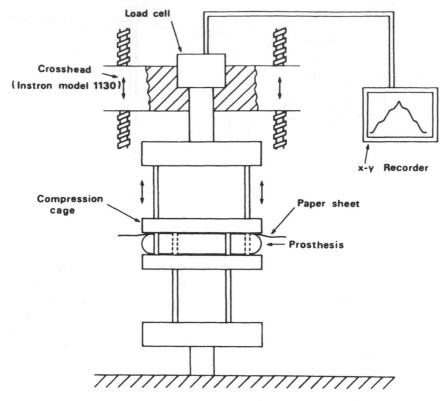

Figure 5. Stiffness measurement system.

where

K = compressive stiffness of the prosthesis (kN/m)
ΔF = change in compressive force (kN)
ΔL = displacement or change in thickness (m)

Evaluation of the Dynamic Response to a Sinusoidal Vibration

Evaluation of the dynamic response of the mammary prostheses to a sine wave excitation was realized through the use of a vibration exciter (MB Electronics, Model 2125) and a piezoelectric accelerometer (Brüel & Kjaer, Model 4339s). The exciter was used to impose a vertical sine wave displacement of constant amplitude to the bottom of a mass-prosthesis system (Figure 6), where the prosthesis played the role of a spring-dashpot combination placed between the mass and oscillating mounting.

For convenience, the prosthesis was nested between two Plexiglas® disks, the one on its underside being rigidly connected to the shaft of the exciter, and the one on its top carrying the load (total mass of the load and disk: 1.554 kilograms). A peripheral guiding system (not shown in Figure 6), composed of shafts and linear bearings, kept both disks parallel while allowing free relative vertical movement. The exciter was controlled through a function generator (Brüel & Kjaer, Model 3020) for waveform and frequency and through a power amplifier (MB Electronics, Model

PM25) for amplitude. The amplitude of the imposed and transmitted oscillations was evaluated by means of the piezoelectric accelerometer, connected to its own power amplifier (Brüel & Kjaer, Model 2805) and, through a DC-filter, to a spectrum analyzer (Schlumberger, Model 1510) and oscilloscope (Philips, Model PM3233).

The magnification factor was then calculated as:

$$B = \exp_{10} \left[(X - Y)/20 \right] \qquad (5)$$

where

B = magnification ratio (dimensionless)
X = amplitude of the transmitted oscillation (dB)
Y = amplitude of the imposed oscillation (dB)

and was plotted as a function of the frequency (range: 0–30 Hz).

Afterwards, the two fundamental viscoelastic models:

(1) mass supported by serial spring and dashpot (Maxwell)
(2) mass supported by parallel spring and dashpot (Voigt or Kelvin)

were simulated using the assistance of a microcomputer (hardware: Compaq Deskpro, 640 KBytes/software: Lotus 123), and their dynamic response was adjusted to the best fit with the experimental curves, in order to determine the equivalent values of the natural frequency and damping coefficient. The degree of fit was evaluated by summation of the squares of the errors between the corresponding experimental and theoretical values of the magnification ratios.

NMR Relaxation Time Measurement

Normally, measurement of NMR relaxation times requires placing a small quantity (<1 g) of the material to be measured in the narrow bore of the magnet of an NMR spectrometer. Remarkable progress has been made in recent years in the development of whole-body magnetic resonance imagers which produce detailed, cross-sectional images of the human body in any orientation. With a view to assessing the potential for *in vivo* monitoring of breast prostheses, it was decided to make preliminary baseline measurements of proton NMR relaxation times noninvasively using a magnetic resonance imager.

The imager used (Technicare Corp.) operated at 0.15 T with a corresponding proton frequency of 6.25 MHz. Individual prostheses were placed in the standard head coil and 0.7 centimeter thick single-slice images were obtained in the coronal plane, although the actual orientation of the prosthesis was arbitrary. T_1 relaxation time values were obtained using a special, interleaved pulse sequence (spin echo and inversion recovery) provided by the manufacturer, which produced an "observed" T_1 image based on a two-point fit to two images. T_2 relaxation times were calculated using a specially developed spin echo sequence using 8 echoes and non-selective 180° radio frequency pulses. As a quality control measure, all images were obtained with four calibration tubes in the field of view whose T_1 and T_2 values at 6.25 MHz were accurately known (Figure 7).

RESULTS

Density

The density of the mammary prostheses was found to be very well controlled by the manufacturers. In fact, all the data lay in the range from 0.973 g/ml to 0.979 g/ml (Table 2), which indicates that variations of less than 0.5% were detected among the different products. However, the specifications of the ASTM for breast implants [13] concern the volume rather than the density of the final products and, from this point of view, the tested prostheses were rarely compliant with the guidelines of the standard. Indeed, they were nearly all oversized, only four of them (from Dow Corning) being in full accordance with the specifications of the ASTM. Figure 8 illustrates the observed phenomenon.

Luminous Transmittance

Measurements of the luminous transmittance confirmed the relative optical homogeneity of the virgin gel-filled mammary prostheses (Table 3). Nevertheless, statistical analysis (bilateral Student t-test, $p < 0.01$) demonstrated that, although the differences detected between the Dow Corning and Heyer Schulte products were small, they were significant. Measured values of the luminous transmittance ranged from 84.9 to 91.7 percent.

Coefficient of Friction

Although the measurements of the coefficient of friction were carefully carried out, the experiments led to few conclusions. The overall values for the coefficient of friction lay between 0.07 and 1.17 (Table

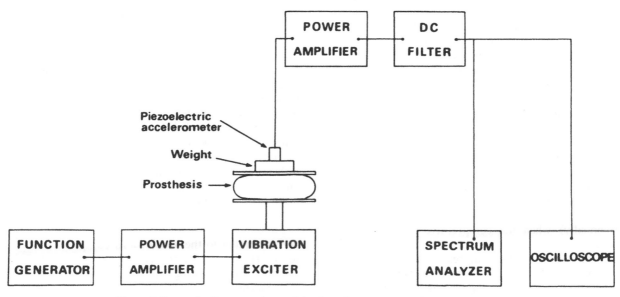

Figure 6. System for the measurement of the dynamic response to a sine wave excitation.

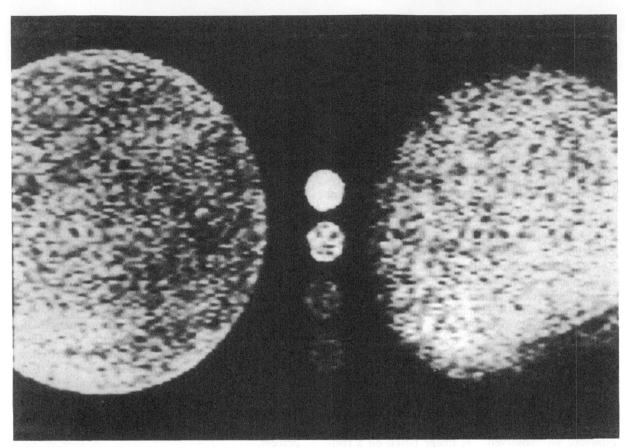

Figure 7. Cross-sectional magnetic resonance images of breast prostheses and four calibration tubes. The slice thickness was 0.7 cm and the image shown is the sixth echo of an eight-echo sequence. Late echo images have relatively poor signal-to-noise ratio.

4). A Chi-Square test ($p < 0.01$) failed to prove that the results of the measurements were normally distributed, for both the Dow Corning and the Heyer Schulte products. Futhermore, the test results were not always reproducible when obtained by different experimenters.

Figure 9 shows a typical recording of the friction force developed by the outer envelope of a prosthesis, as a function of time. Although small random variations were always present, a steady state condition was approached after some delay.

Compressive Stiffness

The curves of Figure 10 illustrate characteristic responses of the prostheses, during loading and unloading, in the compressive testing. There are three important points to note about these graphs. First, the maximum recorded force has no significance in itself. Transition from loading to unloading was initiated (manually) when the compressive force reached a value of 20 Newtons. However, as can be seen, the rate of change of the compressive force around the given threshold value was sometimes very high (e.g., prosthesis CPV15), making it physically impossible for the experimenter to reverse the process of loading

exactly when the compressive force reached its specified maximum level.

Secondly, one can note the presence of some "transition zones", where the slope of the recorded curves (i.e., the stiffness) changed abruptly from a positive to a negative value, or vice versa (e.g., at the 15 Newtons reference level). Although the exact nature of the physical changes that occurred within the prostheses at these precise moments is still unknown, sudden interruptions in their radial distensions were noticeable to the naked eye. As illustrated in Figure 10, the phenomenon was found to be of lesser importance during the unloading sequence.

Thirdly, the recorded curves of force-time are quite symmetric, except in the transition zones, indicating that only a minimum amount of energy was dissipated as heat during the total process. This proved that the crosshead's displacement speed was sufficiently low to minimize the influence of the viscous effects (if present) in the material.

Tables 5a and 5b show typical values of stiffness, corresponding to the 15 Newtons compressive force level. The results of the two series of calculations (loading and unloading) are similar but not identical. Considering the choice of the calculation site, near a transition zone, this could be expected. One may question the pertinency of selecting this compressive force reference level, but there were valid reasons that will be presented in the next section. Nonetheless, the data of Tables 5a and 5b demonstrate that the stiffness is related to the model of the prosthesis rather than to its volume or manufacturer. The models with a low profile design tend to be stiffer than the others (e.g., prostheses CPV09, CPV13, and CPV15 in Figure 10).

Dynamic Response to a Sinusoidal Vibration

The graphs of Figures 11 and 12 show the resonance curves (magnification ratio versus frequency) of some prostheses. We used the same selection as previously (cf., Figure 10), except that this time the prostheses were grouped by manufacturers, for ease of presentation. Those in Figure 11 are from Heyer Schulte, those in Figure 12 are from Dow Corning Ltd. In

these graphs the small triangles, squares and circles correspond to the values of the magnification ratio as calculated from Equation (5), and the continuous curves refer to the results of the numerical simulations performed using the Voigt (or Kelvin) viscoelastic model. The degree of fit can be appreciated by examination of the E values, corresponding to the summation of the squares of the errors.

As can be seen, the curves illustrated in Figures 11 and 12 form two families: a first, with high maximum magnification ratio ($\beta > 2.5$) and low resonance frequency ($\omega_r < 15$ Hz, the frequency that corresponds to the maximum of the magnification ratio); and a second, with low maximum magnification ratio ($\beta < 2.5$) and high resonance frequency ($\omega_r > 15$ Hz). These families correspond respectively to the normal and low-profile designs of prostheses, similar to the results of the stiffness measurements. Some of these

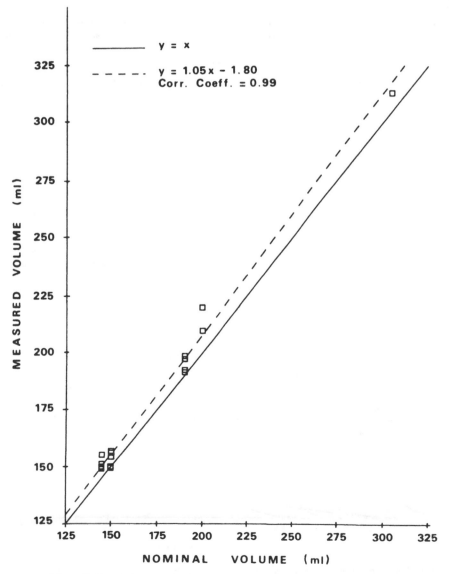

Figure 8. Correlation between the measured volumes and the nominal volumes.

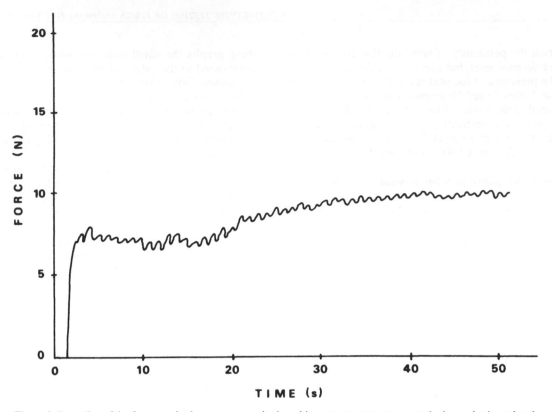

Figure 9. Recording of the force required to move a prosthesis and its support, at constant speed, along a horizontal path on a Teflon® surface.

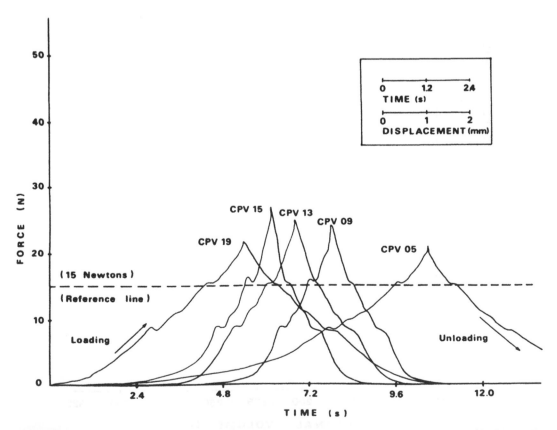

Figure 10. Recording of the force required to squeeze different mammary prostheses (CPV05—type D, CPV09—type E, CPV13—type A, CPV15—type B, CPV19—type G).

findings could be expected since the value of the resonance frequency is intimately related to that of the natural frequency ($\omega_r/\omega_n \cong 1.0$) which, in turn, is a function of the mass and stiffness of the oscillating system:

$$\omega_n = \frac{1}{2}\sqrt{\frac{K}{M_{osc}}} \qquad (6)$$

where

ω_n = natural frequency (Hz)
K = stiffness of the oscillating system (N/m)
M_{osc} = Mass of the oscillating system (kg)

We have compared the values of ω_n calculated from the numerical simulation of the Voigt viscoelastic model and from Equation (6), knowing the values of the stiffness, K, for the given experimental conditions. These conditions were that, at rest, an external force

of 15.25 Newtons (1.554 kg × 9.81 m/s² = 15.25 N) acted on the system, and was matched by an equal but opposite force developed by the prosthesis, due to its stiffness. This is why the values of the compressive stiffness of the prostheses were calculated in the previous section at the threshold of 15 Newtons.

Table 6 presents the grouped data for the natural frequencies of the mass-prosthesis systems as estimated from the numerical model. In Figure 13, these data are compared with those in Tables 5a and 5b. In this graph, the values of the natural frequency, as calculated from Equation (6), are plotted against those estimated from the numerical simulation. The dotted line represents the true relationship that was found to exist between the two series of data, and shows the two sets of figures to be closely related.

The other important aspect in comparing Figures 11 and 12 concerns the intensity of the magnification ratios. As predicted by the forced vibration theory, the intensity of the magnification ratios was found to be dependent on the damping characteristics of the mass-

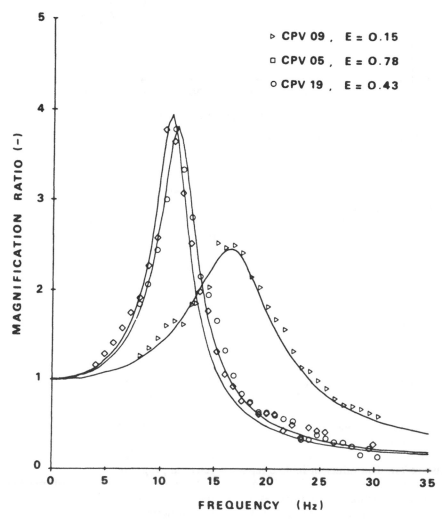

▷ **CPV 09 , E = 0.15**

▢ **CPV 05 , E = 0.78**

○ **CPV 19 , E = 0.43**

Figure 11. Resonance curves of some Heyer Schulte prostheses (CPV05−type D, CPV09−type E, CPV19−type G).

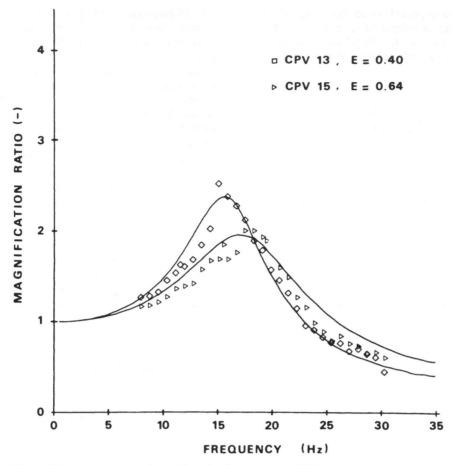

□ CPV 13 , E = 0.40

▷ CPV 15 , E = 0.64

Figure 12. Resonance curves of some Dow Corning prostheses (CPV13—type A, CPV15—type B).

prosthesis oscillating systems. These characteristics were quantified by means of a damping coefficient, estimated from the numerical simulations. Table 7 gives the mean calculated values of the damping coefficient for the different possible mass-prosthesis systems. As in the previous cases, the type of design—normal or low-profile—appears to be a better distinguishing factor than the form or manufacturer.

NMR Relaxation Times

The NMR relaxation times measured for four prostheses are shown in Table 8. Experimental uncertainties were estimated from the values obtained for the calibration tubes which were imaged simultaneously with the prostheses. These experimental uncertainties are fairly large (± 20 ms for T_1 and ± 10 ms for T_2) primarily due to the error associated with fitting exponential decays with 2 points (in the case of T_1) or 8 points (in the case of T_2). The values in Table 8 represent means measured over an area of 2 to 3 cm^3 in the 0.7 cm thick imaged sections of the prostheses. Within the experimental uncertainties, there are no significant differences in the measurement values of T_1 and T_2.

DISCUSSION

One may question the overall relevance of such experiments. This is the main problem of this investigation for which there is, in our opinion, no easy answer. Each test must be considered on a separate basis.

As far as the density measurements are concerned, they seem to be of little use. Indeed, the density of silicone is not very different from that of water and it is very unlikely that a global densitometric method, as we used, would detect infiltration of body fluids inside explanted prostheses. The method did prove to have the potential for evaluation of volumetric changes; however, the lack of consistency in the manufactured volume definitely compromises this possibility. The only remaining interest in the method lies in its use for the approximation of the nominal volume, in the case of the unidentified devices recovered through the retrieval programme.

The prospects for the use of transmittance measurements as an adequate test method for the determination of homogeneity or for the detection of chemical changes are more encouraging. Such a method will show its real potential only when the results of several destructive physico-chemical analyses are known. However, for now, the ease and rapidity of testing represent two major arguments in favor of this kind of experiment.

Concerning the coefficient of friction, the situation is quite confused. On one hand, it proved to be difficult to get accurate and reproducible data with our method. On the other hand, there is no proof that the observed variations in the values of the coefficient of friction did not reflect true changes in the surface properties of the prostheses. In fact, the sliding parts of the underside of the Plexiglas® receptacle certainly had some influence on the final measurements. Moreover, the parts of the tested prostheses that were in direct contact with the reference surface underwent a stick-slip sequence rather than a continuous sliding motion, as in the usual situation. The presence of silicone gel particles on the exposed areas of the prostheses may have contributed to their adhesion to the reference surface. However, although all the pros-

theses were carefully washed in distilled water before testing, nothing could really be done to improve the situation because of the sudation of the silicone gel through the external envelope, a fact admitted by the manufacturers [21].

One may also question the choice of Teflon® as the reference material over stainless steel, or even glass. Various possibilities were studied carefully and, after several preliminary tests, only two materials were found to be suitable (i.e., sufficiently non-adherent) to serve as a reference in the measurement of the coefficient of friction of the silicone implants: Teflon® and paper. Paper was rejected because of its low durability.

In view of these problems, it seems that the surface properties of the gel-filled mammary prostheses require further investigation, not only by measurement of the coefficient of friction, but also by other, perhaps destructive test methods.

Measurements of the compressive stiffness and

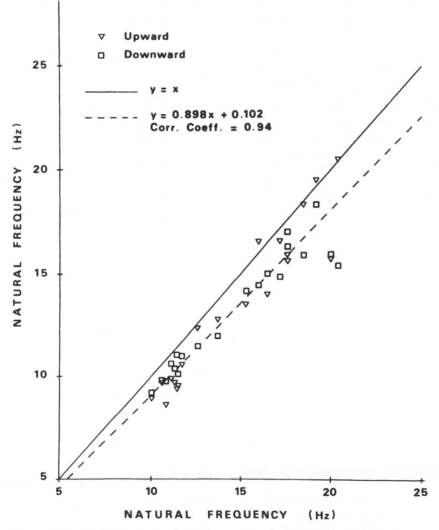

Figure 13. Correlation between the values of the natural frequencies calculated from Equation (6) (ordinate) and those estimated from the numerical simulation (abscissa).

evaluation of the dynamic response to a sine wave excitation proved that the prostheses could be adequately represented by a simple viscoelastic model. The peculiarity of the model resides in the fact that the characteristics of its elastic and viscous components are expected to vary as a function of the stress. This has already been proved in the case of stiffness, which is the characteristic of the elastic component in the material, by the non-linearity of the compressive force versus the time (and/or change in thickness) recordings; but it is still to be demonstrated with the damping coefficient, which is the characteristic of the viscous component in the material. In the case of compressive stiffness, the test is rapid (taking a few seconds) and easy to perform. In the second case (sinusoidal vibration), it is long and tedious. Indeed, for the complete determination of a stress-damping coefficient relationship, characteristic of a given prosthesis, one would need to produce a different resonance curve for each state of loading in order to get the corresponding value of the damping coefficient. Knowing that with the method of testing used here, a minimum of 90 minutes is required for the production of one of these curves, one can imagine the amount of work this characterization would require.

In its present, manually operated form, the evaluation of the dynamic response to a sine wave excitation cannot realistically be used to give a full determination of the stress-damping coefficient relationships. However, a full knowledge of the elastic and viscous characteristics of the mammary prostheses may well be a very useful tool for the identification of the chemical changes that seem to occur with them *in vivo*.

The NMR relaxation times are particularly intriguing. They represent considerable time ($\cong 30$ minutes positioning and imaging plus 30 minutes image-processing for each prosthesis) using a scarce and expensive resource. But magnetic resonance imaging is a non-invasive procedure and these measurements can be performed *in vivo*. Although relaxation time measurements from images are rather imprecise, further investigation is warranted to determine if changes in these relaxation times occur with time in implanted prostheses.

CONCLUSION

The previous discussion about the pertinency of the experiments performed on the virgin gel-filled mammary prostheses may seem rather negative to an outside observer. This is only partially true. Indeed, refinements appear possible in the less effective methods that may lead to better results. Moreover, a more selective use of some experiments (e.g., transmittance measurements in opacified explanted prostheses) is expected to be very useful in the identification, before destructive testing, of special features (e.g., mineral deposits) hidden to the naked eye. In the meantime, the reference data we have obtained

from these experiments will enable us to continue this investigation on the explanted mammary prostheses. It is also expected that some similar methods of testing could be developed for use with the other models of prostheses that were excluded from this study. Finally, we hope that the manufacturers may take an interest in the proposed test methods and use them as suggestions for the improvement of the work in their quality control departments.

LIST OF SYMBOLS

Variables (alphabetic order)

B = Magnification ratio (dimensionless)
F_f = Mean friction force (N)
ΔF = Change in compressive force (kN)
I_{ib} = Intensity of the incident beam of light (mW/cm²)
I_{tb} = Intensity of the transmitted beam of light (mW/cm²)
K = Compressive stiffness of the prosthesis (kN/m)
ΔL = Change in thickness (m)
M_{osc} = Mass of the oscillating system (kg)
M_p = Mass of the prosthesis (g)
M_t = Mass of the receptacles, load and prosthesis (kg)
T_t = Total transmittance of the prosthesis (%)
T_1 = NMR relaxation time (ms)
T_2 = NMR relaxation time (ms)
V = Volume of the prosthesis (ml)
X = Amplitude of the transmitted oscillation (dB)
Y = Amplitude of the imposed oscillation (dB)
λ = Wavelength (nm)
μ_k = Kinetic coefficient of friction (dimensionless)
ϱ = Global density of the prosthesis (g/ml)
ω = Frequency (Hz)
ω_n = Natural frequency (Hz)
ω_r = Resonance frequency (Hz)

Physical constant

g = Gravitational acceleration (9.81 m/s²)

ACKNOWLEDGEMENTS

This work has been supported in part by Health and Welfare Canada, Supplies and Services Canada and St-François d'Assise Hospital. We would like to thank Professors R. Lessard from the Department of Physics (Université Laval, Québec) and L. P. Boivin from the Department of Photometry and Radiometry (National Research Council, Ottawa) for their helpful suggestions and encouragement. We are indebted to Drs. P. Blais, G. Roy, C. Poirier, J. C. Forest and J. Couture for help and guidance. The technical assistance of Y. Gourdeau, K. Horth, C. Kingston, J.

Lacombe, G. Mongrain, D. Picard, M. Bosch, M. Wullschlegger and C. Stewart was greatly appreciated.

REFERENCES

1. Randal, J. May 15, 1983. "Bigger Breasts Are Not Necessarily Better. When Will the FDA Investigate Potential Perils of Silicone Implants?" *Washington Post.* 161:B1–B3.

2. Guérard, C. 1984. "La Chirurgie Esthétique: un bilan", *Madame au Foyer*, 19:88-98.

3. Rolland, C., R. Guidoin, D. Marceau, and R. Ledoux. 1989. "Non-destructive Investigations on 97 Surgically Excised Mammary Prostheses", *J. Biomed. Mat. Res. (Appl. Biomat.)*, 23(A3):285–298.

4. Vistnes, L. M. and G. A. Ksander. 1983. "Tissue Response to Soft Silicone Prostheses: Capsule Formation and Other Sequelae", L. R. Rubin, ed. in *Biomaterials in Reconstructive Surgery*. St. Louis: Mosby, pp. 516–528.

5. Gayou, R. M. 1979. "A Histological Comparison of Contracted and Non-Contracted Capsules Around Silicon Breast Implants", *Plast. Reconstr. Surg.*, 63:700–707.

6. Nicoletis, C. L. and B. Wlodarczyk. 1983. "Une Complication Rare des Protheses Mammaires. La Calcification de la Coque Rétractile Péri-Prothétique", *Ann. Chir. Plast. Esthet.*, 28:388–389.

7. Peters, W. J. and K. P. H. Pritzker. 1985. "Massive Heterotopic Ossification in Breast Implant Capsules", *Aesth. Plast. Surg.*, 9:43–45.

8. Capozzi, A., R. Du Bou, and V. R. Pennisi. 1978. "Distant Migration of Silicone Gel from a Ruptured Breast Implant", *Plast. Reconstr. Surg.*, 62:302–303.

9. Clegg, H. W., P. Bertagnoll, A. W. Hightower, and W. B. Baine. 1983. "Mammoplasty-Associated Mycobacterial Infection: A Survey of Plastic Surgeons", *Plast. Reconstr. Surg.*, 72:165–169.

10. Georgiade, N. G., D. Serafin, and W. Barwick. 1979. "Late Development of Hematoma Around a Breast Implant Necessitating Removal", *Plast. Reconstr. Surg.* 64:708–710.

11. Rubin, L. R. 1983. "Degradation of the Saline-Filled Silicone-Bag Breast Implant", in *Biomaterials in Reconstructive Surgery*. L. R. Rubin, ed. St. Louis: Mosby, pp. 260–272.

12. Schlenker, J. D., R. A. Bueno, G. Ricketson, and J. B. Lynch. 1978. "Loss of Silicone Implants After Subcutaneous Mastectomy and Reconstruction", *Plast. Reconstr. Surg.*, 62:853–861.

13. ASTM. 1981. "Standard Specification for Implantable Breast Prostheses", Designation F 703-81, American Society for Testing and Materials, Philadelphia, PA.

14. ASTM. 1978. "Standard Practice for Assessment of Compatibility of Nonporous Polymeric Materials for Surgical Implants with Regard to Effect of Materials on Tissue", Designation F 469-78, American Society for Testing and Materials, Philadelphia, PA.

15. ASTM. 1978. "Standard Classification for Silicone Elastomers Used in Medical Applications", Designation F 604-78, American Society for Testing and Materials, Philadelphia, PA.

16. ASTM. 1983. "Standard Test Methods for Rubber Properties in Tension", Designation D 412-83, American Society for Testing and Materials, Philadelphia, PA.

17. ASTM. 1983. "Standard Test Method for Haze and Luminous Transmittance of Transparent Plastics", Designation D 1003-61, American Society for Testing and Materials, Philadelphia, PA.

18. ASTM. 1983. "Standard Test Method for Static and Kinetic Coefficients of Friction of Plastic Film and Sheeting", Designation D 1894-78, American Society for Testing and Materials, Philadelphia, PA.

19. Hoffman, H. L. and R. J. Turner. 1975. "A New Method for Testing Burst Strength of Vascular Materials", Technical Report (Meadox Medicals), Oakland.

20. Peters, W. J. 1981. "The Mechanical Properties of Breast Prostheses", *Ann. Plast. Surg.*, 6:179–181.

21. Brody, G. S. 1977. "Fact and Fiction about Breast Implant Bleed", *Plast. Reconstr. Surg.*, 60:615–616.

Part 3

ADVANCED CONCEPTS

8

Microbial Adhesion to Biomaterials

ANTHONY G. GRISTINA, M.D.*,1
PAUL T. NAYLOR, M.D.*
QUENTIN N. MYRVIK, Ph.D.**
WILLIAM D. WAGNER, Ph.D.†

ABSTRACT: Man-made materials are increasingly being used as substitutes for damaged tissues in human hosts. At the current state of the art, however, biomaterials provide an adhesive substrata for bacteria and somehow diminish host defense and integration response, increasing the risk of infection. In addition, biomaterial-centered infections are resistant to antimicrobial treatment and often require that the device be removed before the infection can be eradicated. A greater understanding of the characteristics of and interactions between biomaterial surfaces, bacteria, tissue cells, and host defense mechanisms is required before long-term successful use of biomaterials can be achieved. In the future, advanced techniques such as ion implantation will be used to create biomaterial surfaces which will "direct" interactions with constituents of the surrounding biologic environment.

INTRODUCTION

Biomaterials are a billion dollar business. Successfully implanted biomaterials and devices decrease pain, prolong life, treat disease, and increase productivity. The world-wide use of prosthetic devices exceeds one million applications per year; the authors suggest 50,000 or more cases per year may become infected. Vascular devices such as aortofemoral grafts have an infection rate of 6% or more, and result in death or amputation in 30% of infections [1–4]. Orthopedic devices implanted deep in bone are less susceptible to infection. Total hip replacements have an infection rate of 0.1% to 1% [5–9], total knees a rate of 1% to 4% [10], and total elbows, a rate of 4% to 7% [11,12]. Central venous catheters have a 4% to 12% rate of bacteremia [13,14]. With prolonged use, 90% of patients with a total artificial heart experience biomaterial-centered infections, bacteremia and distant septic emboli, or death due to sepsis [15–17].

PATHOGENESIS

The pathogenesis of biomaterial-centered infections is based on the natural tendency of microorganisms to adhere to surfaces as a survival mechanism. Interestingly, both prokaryocytes and eukaryocytes adhere to and propagate upon surfaces or on some form of molecular scaffolding. The mechanisms used by cells to orient to surfaces may ultimately determine the fate of a biomaterial implant. Molecular and atomic interactions between biomaterials and tissue cells or bacteria are similar and include surface charge, van der Waals forces, hydrophobicity, and specific receptor–adhesion interactions.

HISTORY

The "foreign body effect" on infection is an accepted concept in medicine. However, the molecular mechanisms involved had not been investigated until recently. Elek and Conen first described the effect of foreign bodies in lowering the size of an infecting inocula in 1957 [18]. In 1963, it was suggested that bacteria used biomaterials as a scaffolding for growth and propagation [19]. Bayston and Penny cited slime produced by *Staphylococcus epidermidis* as a factor in virulence for plastic neurosurgical shunts in 1972

1Corresponding author.

* Section of Orthopedic Surgery, Wake Forest University Medical Center, 300 South Hawthorne Road, Winston-Salem, NC 27103

** Department of Microbiology and Immunology, Wake Forest University Medical Center, 300 South Hawthorne Road, Winston-Salem, NC 27103

† Department of Comparative Medicine, Wake Forest University Medical Center, 300 South Hawthorne Road, Winston-Salem, NC 27103

[20]. In 1975, Gibbons and van Houte described the adhesion of *Streptococcus mutans* to surfaces as a factor in the pathogenesis of dental caries [21]. In 1980, Ofek and Beachey cited bacterial adhesion to tissue cells as a fundamental mechanism of disease in man and animals [22]. In 1980 and 1981, Gristina et al. [23,24], Costerton and Irvin [25], Peters et al. [26], and Beachey [27] noted the association of adherent bacteria and biomaterial-centered infection.

FEATURES OF ADHERENT INFECTION AND MOLECULAR MECHANISMS

The characteristic features of implant-associated sepsis are: (1) a biomaterial or damaged tissue substratum; (2) adhesive bacterial colonization; (3) resistance to host defense mechanisms and antibiotic therapy; (4) specificity of phenomena (material, organism, location); (5) the presence of characteristic bacteria such as *S. epidermidis, S. aureus,* and *Pseudomonas aeruginosa;* (6) the transformation of nonpathogens or opportunistic pathogens into virulent organisms by the presence of a biomaterial substratum; (7) polymicrobial infection; and (8) persistence of the infection until the substratum is removed [28].

Bacteria may attach to surfaces using specific receptor–ligand or receptor–lectin–ligand interactions, or nonspecifically by charge-related, hydrophobic, and extracellular polysaccharide-based interactions. Colonization of surfaces in animal and plant hosts may also be symbiotic, such as the colonization of skin by *S. epidermidis* or of the gastrointestinal tract and oropharynx by nonvirulent organisms. An unusual feature of biomaterial-centered infections is the ability of normally commensal, autochthonous bacteria or opportunistic pathogens to become virulent and cause infection about the biomaterial, eventually spreading to adjacent tissue and distant sites. Adhesion to surfaces appears to cause phenotypic changes in bacteria which affect virulence. The presence of biomaterials may also disrupt normal macrophage oxidative response, motility, and phagocytosis. Tissue damage, an imbalance in host defenses, or an appropriate inoculum of a virulent pathogen may also allow colonization by pathogenic bacteria such as *S. aureus.*

The "Race for the Surface"

The fate of a biomaterial surface may be conceptualized as a "race for the surface" involving macromolecules, bacteria, and tissue cells. The presence of a biomaterial allows colonization by a small inocula of bacteria, disrupting potential colonization by tissue cells which orient and differentiate in relation to each other and specific macromolecules, not to relatively nonspecific, "inert" biomaterial surfaces.

Because of the nature of their surfaces and adsorption of organic materials, implanted biomaterials present a highly modified interface to potential colonizing cells. If tissue cells arrive first at a biomaterial surface and a secure bond can be established, bacteria will be confronted by a living, integrated cellular surface. If not traumatized or altered, an integrated tissue cell layer resists bacterial colonization through viable, intact cell membranes, and host defense mechanisms.

Bacteria are relatively ubiquitous in biologic environments and may colonize the biomaterial or compromised necrotic tissue at the implant site, resulting in infection and preventing tissue integration. Bacteria have developed methods for colonizing inanimate substrata and certain cell surfaces as a survival strategy. Therefore, bacteria have a high colonization potential for most substrata, while the colonization potential of more highly specialized tissue cells is low. Tissue cells are generally unable to dislodge adherent bacteria, and biomaterials are generally designed to be "inert", that is, they do not facilitate tissue integration. Thus, biomaterials currently being used represent the "eminent domain" of organic and inorganic moieties and bacteria, not tissue cells.

MOLECULAR MECHANISMS

The surfaces of implanted biomaterials are moderately perturbed or modified by chemical activities inherent to implantation procedures and occurring naturally in the biosystem. Although passivated and sterile before implantation, metallic and polymeric biomaterials become coated by surgical debris, blood, and cellular and matrix derivatives (Figure 1). In addition, a thin (10 to 200 Å) oxide layer forms almost immediately on metal alloys when they are exposed to the environment. This oxide layer represents the true interactive surface between metallic implants and constituents of the surrounding milieu [29].

The atomic structure, electronic state, oxidation layer, contamination level, and sequence of coating by glycoproteins on a biomaterial in a human host have not been defined, but can be assumed to be specific to the material, host environment, and the bacterium or tissue cell attempting adhesion or integration [13,30, 31]. Surface sites may also act as catalytic "hot spots" for molecular and cellular activities occurring at close ranges [30,32].

The surfaces of cells and most substrata are negatively charged. According to the theory of Derjaguin and Landau [33], and Verwey and Overbeek [34] (the DLVO theory), the energy of the interaction between two charged particles of like sign and magnitude is the sum of the repulsive electrostatic energy and the attractive energy of London-van der Waals forces [35]. Electromagnetic interactions between atoms and molecules with a similar fluctuation frequency produce an attractive force [35]. The repulsive energy decreases more rapidly with distance than the attractive energy [36,37]. Thus, one maximum and two minima of total potential energy are obtained over a range of separation distances [35]. Surface-to-surface cohesion is

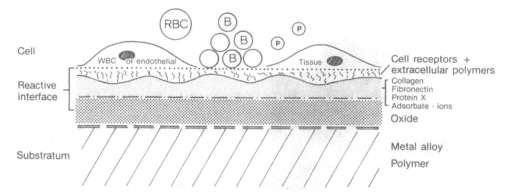

Figure 1. A biomaterial substratum interacts with available cells via a reactive interface, the passivated surface (metallic oxide or structured polymer surface layer), which is coated by an aggregated glycoprotein mosaic derived from the host environment. Bacterial extracellular polymers and receptors and outer membrane glycoproteins of cells in the biologic system then interact with this conditioning film. RBC = red blood cell; B = bacteria; P = platelets. Reprinted with permission from [28].

favored at the primary (less than 1 nm) and secondary (1 to 10 nm) minima of the bacteria. At distances between these minima the interacting forces cause repulsion. Adhesion at the primary minimum occurs only when the potential energy barrier between the diffuse electrical double layers of the contacting surfaces is overcome [35].

Although cell and surface charges are similar, isoelectric points on materials at the surface–liquid interface may vary with pH and tissue damage caused by surgery, trauma, and infection [38,39]. Corrosion of the biomaterial may also alter pH and charge [39].

Many bacteria and most surfaces have some degree of hydrophobicity [13,40]. Hydrophobic forces are exerted at distances as great as 15 nm, and at 8 to 10 nm are 10 to 100 times as great as van der Waals forces [41]. Hydrophobic interactions may attract particles to the primary attractive minimum, where short-range chemical interactions (ionic, hydrogen, and possibly covalent bonding) may occur with extracellular moieties. Hydrophobic receptor adhesion and chemical bonding are probably time-dependent, being initially reversible and secondarily more stable, but adhesion ultimately depends on system viability. Tissue cells interact with other cells or biomaterials via adhesive glycoproteins [42–44].

Bacteria may also interact specifically over distances greater than 20 nm using fimbriae or receptors [45]. Fimbriae may also react nonspecifically (by charged or hydrophobic interaction) with inorganic substratum elements [46]. Many pathogenic staphylococci have receptors for fibronectin, collagen and laminin [47–52] (Figures 2 and 3).

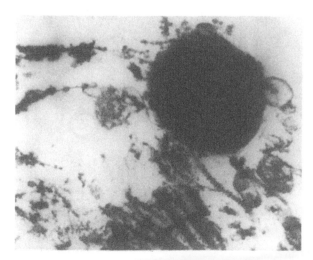

Figure 2. Transmission electron microscopy of rabbit articular cartilage illustrating direct bacteria-to-collagen fiber contact. Reprinted with permission from Voytek A. et al. "Staphylococcal adhesion to collagen in intra-articular sepsis". *Biomaterials*, 1988; 9:107–110.

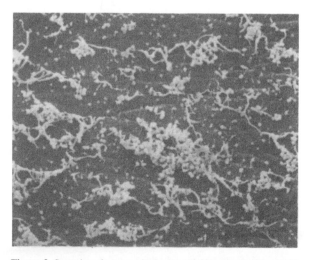

Figure 3. Scanning electron microscopy of articular cartilage at 24 h shows a more intense and regular pattern of distribution of cocci across the cartilage surface. Reprinted with permission from Voytek A. et al. "Staphylococcal adhesion to collagen in intra-articular sepsis". *Biomaterials*, 1988; 9:107–110.

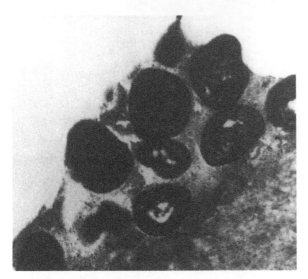

Figure 4. Ruthenium-red stained specimen of bacterial extracapsular polysaccharide enveloping organisms and cartilage. Extracapsular polysaccharide forms a continuum between organisms and cartilage substratum. Reprinted with permission from Voytek A. et al. "Staphylococcal adhesion to collagen in intra-articular sepsis". *Biomaterials*, 1988; 9:107–110.

polysaccharides which actively bind to biomaterial surfaces [54]. If environmental conditions such as temperature, nurtrients, antagonists and cation balance are favorable, bacterial propagation and infection occur.

Extracellular Polymers—The "Slime" and Biofilm

Shortly after attachment and adhesion (3 to 4 hours or less), if colony conditions are appropriate, bacteria produce extracellular polysaccharide polymers (Figures 4 and 5). This exopolysaccharide "slime" may be one of the pivotal factors in biomaterial-centered infections. The production of slime is strain-specific and nutrient-dependent.

Exopolysaccharides produced by coagulase-negative staphylococci are usually composed of neutral monosaccharides such as D-glucose, D-galactose, L-fucose, and L-rhamnose, and contain amino sugars and sialic acid [25,32,55–57]. Mannose has also been found in some strains of *S. epidermidis* [58]. Glycerol, hexosamine, phosphorus, glycine, alanine, and phenylalanine have also been identified as major components of slime [59]. Constituents of the exopolysaccharide vary within and between species.

Most studies of bacterial extracellular slime have been conducted before any size or charge fractionation of individual polymers occurs, and therefore the individual polymer constituents of the slime have not been determined. Extraction and characterization studies of the chemical composition of the extracapsular slime now being conducted in our laboratory have in-

Bacteria which produce slime may adhere to each other and to surfaces through polymer-to-surface interactions or in some cases, polymer-to-polymer interactions, consolidating adhesion and the formation of microcolonies [53]. Some species of *S. epidermidis* produce adhesion fractions in their extracapsular

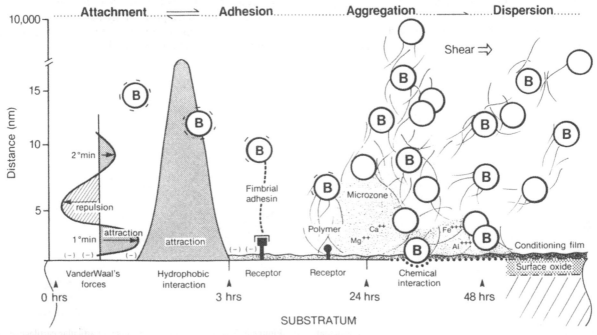

Figure 5. Molecular sequence in bacterial (B) attachment, adhesion, aggregation, and dispersion at substratum surface. A number of interactions may occur depending on the specificities of the bacteria or substratum system (graphics, nutrients, contaminants, macromolecules, species, and materials). Reprinted with permission from Gristina et al. "Biomaterial-centered infection: microbial adhesion versus tissue integration". *Science*, 1987; 237:1588–1595. Copyright 1987 by AAAS.

dicated that the total exopolysaccharide is rich in xylose (20%), galactose (16%), mannose (19%), and fucose (11%). The slime also contains glucosamine and galactosamine, and is largely electronegative [60]. Following dissociative extraction with chaeotropic agents and maintaining the native structure of the macromolecular components of the exopolysaccharide, general components have been isolated. By SDS polyacrylamide gel separation the characteristic Alcian blue positive exopolysaccharide product of bacterial colonies of *S. epidermidis* producing slime was found to consist primarily of material with a M_r of approximately 34 kDa. This material was eluted from DEAE-Sephacel with 0.3 M NaCl [61].

The production and function of polysaccharides varies depending on species, growth phase, and nutrient conditions. The integrity of the polysaccharide polymer is dependent on the availability of cations such as Ca^{2+} and Mg^{2+}. Controlled experiments defining the relationship of bacterial exopolysaccharides to substratum surface energy and to fluid medium qualities and constituents are needed [31,62].

The properties of bacterial polysaccharides have been summarized by Peters [63] (Table 1). The extracapsular polysaccharide serves not only as an adhesive mechanism but also appears to be related to virulence. The presence of slime has also been shown to confer resistance to host defense mechanisms [57,64–66]. The exopolysaccharide may act as an ion-exchanged resin which enhances nutrition, moderates susceptibility to phagocytosis, autogenicity and response to antibodies, and functions in surface adhesion, aggregation and polymicrobial interaction.

It has been proposed that the slime inhibits diffusion of antibiotics, but recent studies suggest that diffusion limitation is not a significant factor in bacterial resistance to antibiotics [67,68]. Studies have shown that significantly higher levels of antibiotics are required to kill surface-adherent bacteria than bacteria in suspension [63,69]. The mechanism of increased resistance to antibiotics appears to be based on phenotypic changes in bacteria which are induced by the surface environment.

Portions of the accumulated biofilm may eventually become detached from the microcolony secondary to hemodynamic forces or trauma. These inocula of pathogens represent a source of hematogenous septic emboli, distant seeding and secondary infection. The persistence of the biofilm appears to be a major factor in some chronic orthopedic infections [27,32,55,56, 70,71].

Glycoproteinaceous Conditioning Films

Upon implantation of biomaterials into host tissues, biomaterials are immediately exposed to ubiquitous serum and matrix glycoproteins such as fibronectin, albumin, fibrinogen, laminin, collagen and other proteins, and covalently bound, short chain oligosaccharides [31,62]. These protein and carbohydrate

Table 1. Biological properties of extracellular slime substance of S. epidermis.

1. Adhesin-like property
   * adhesion to mammalian cells (?)
   * attachment to polymer surfaces (?)
   * inter-cell adherence (cell-cluster-formation)

2. Interference with host defense mechanisms
   * inhibition of T-cell blastogenesis
   * inhibition of B-cell blastogenesis
   * inhibition of immunoglobulin production
   * enhancement of PMN adherence
   * inhibition of PMN chemotaxis
   * stimulation of PMN degranulation
   * inhibition of bacterial opsonization
   * inhibition of PMN chemiluminescence
   * inhibition of *S. epidermidis* uptake by PMN

3. Enhancement of *S. epidermidis* virulence in mice

4. Interference with the action of antistaphylococcal antibiotics

5. Heparin-like property

Reprinted with permission from [62]. Copyright 1988 by British Society for Antimicrobial Chemotherapy.

moieties rapidly coat the biomaterial surface via specific and nonspecific chemical interactions, changing the biological potential of the biomaterial surface, and providing receptor sties for bacterial or tissue adhesion [72].

Eukaryocytes adhere to fibronectin- and collagen-coated surfaces [73,74], and nerve cells have been shown to regenerate axons along laminin-coated surfaces [73]. Thus, conditioned surfaces are suitable for tissue integration.

Pathogenic bacteria also have receptors for conditioning film proteins, enhancing colonization of biomaterial surfaces. Several reports have demonstrated that *S. aureus, S. epidermidis,* and *E. coli* strains have specific receptors for fibronectin and collagen epitopes [47,75,76]. Studies of similiar strains of pathogenic and nonpathogenic bacteria have revealed that pathogenic bacteria display greater numbers of conditioning film protein receptors on their cell surfaces than do nonpathogenic bacteria [73].

In serum, fibronectin is a globular dimeric protein. When bound to surfaces or other matrix proteins, however, it assumes a more open form, exposing different binding domains. The physical state and quantity of bound proteins on a biomaterial surface dictates the interaction of these proteins with tissue and bacterial cells. Studies of fibronectin-coated biomaterials *in vitro* demonstrate that fibronectin bound at low concentrations enhances adherence by bacteria with fibronectin receptors, while a high concentration of bound fibronectin inhibits binding by the same bacteria [48,50,77]. Albumin may also decrease bacterial adhesion [52]. These results illustrate the differing roles conditioning surface molecules can play depending on protein concentrations and environmental conditions.

The initial surface free energy and the state of cleanliness of implanted materials has a dramatic influence on the adsorption of conditioning films and the subsequent adhesion of host tissue and bacterial cells [31,62]. Thus, surfaces may eventually be programmed to favor adhesion of tissue cells and resist invading bacteria.

The initial surface free energy and state of cleanliness of implanted materials dramatically affect the adsorption of conditioning films and the subsequent adhesion of host tissue and bacterial cells [31,62]. The low surface energy (22 dynes/cm²) of silicon- and stearate-covered surfaces does not favor adhesion. High surface energy, such as that of radio frequency glow discharge treated stainless steel, chrome-cobalt, and titanium, does favor bacterial adhesion.

Tissue Adhesion and Integration

Biomaterials and tissue transplants invariably stimulate host defense or immune mechanisms, regardless of their inertness or directed reactivity, or antigenicity. Integration may be defined as the functional assimilation of a transplanted tissue or tissue substitute by surrounding tissue without an intervening fibroinflammatory layer. Integration is achieved when tissue reaction to an implant approaches homeostasis; that is, a healthy, functional cell-to-biomaterial (100 to 200 Å) interaction.

Successful tissue integration of any biomaterial requires long-term physicochemical and biomechanical biocompatibility. Tissue cells such as endothelia, epithelia, and fibroblasts have receptors (integrins) for adhesive proteins which mediate integration [42–44]. Matrix proteins such as fibronectin, collagen, laminin, and fibrinogen are believed to provide an adhesive scaffolding for tissue cell receptors. Integration of skin, muscle, tendon, bone grafts, and organ transplants is possible to some extent, based on the presence of adhesive surfaces/proteins and the potential viability of the graft.

Autografts can be adaptively integrated, to a degree and after a period of time, depending on mediation by adhesive proteins and cell survival without an intervening inflammatory layer or "non-self"-stimulated response. Allografts are more difficult to integrate. The surfaces of allografts are immunogenic, inducing an inflammatory response before cellular integration occurs. Disruption of cell matrices and glycocalyx, cell necrosis, and the presence of an inflammatory layer may expose ligands for which bacteria have receptors, increasing susceptibility to bacterial colonization.

To some extent, titanium or titanium alloy implants currently in use approach integration with tissue [29, 78,79]. Polymers used in vascular devices are almost homeostatic. They resist clotting cascades and are reasonably coated by protein macromolecules, although true integration does not occur. In most sites, however, neither polymer nor metal surfaces achieve intimate, chemically bonded integration with tissue cells.

BIOMATERIAL SURFACES

The biocompatibility of a biomaterial is determined by its surface characteristics, which determine the elective adsorption of ions, glycoproteins, and extracapsular polysaccharides. These constituents in turn determine the adhesive or abhesive interaction with macromolecules, host cells, and bacteria.

Surface atomic and geometric configurations generally present active or unsatisfied binding sites (dangling bonds) and elemental segregations which are only indirectly related to the biomaterial's crystalline or amorphous bulk state [30,80–82]. The elemental composition of the atomic surface layers (0 to 10 Å) of a metal alloy (e.g., Ti6A14V) may be significantly different from its bulk phase composition because of segregation of specific elements at the surface [30]. Surface oxides which form on metallic implants may have more than one stoichiometry, and their integrity may be disrupted by grain boundaries and pinhole defects.

The atomic geometry and electron energy distribution of a clean metal or polymer surface affects the sequence, distribution, and content of initial adsorbates from the host environment (Figure 6). The surface geometry and energy states of nonmetallic crystalline or amorphous polymers are also subject to rearrangements based on their molecular composition or crystal structure and size. Even rigid polymers such as polymethylmethacrylate reorient their surface molecules because of relaxation mechanisms.

Metal surfaces are planar cuts through crystalline structures and generally have moderate-to-high surface energies (more than 40 dynes/cm) which are believed to be adhesive for tissue cells [31], and potentially capable of catalyzing chemical reactions [81, 83]. The geometric arrangement of metal atoms at the exposed surface plane, and thus the number of unsatisfied bonds, depends on surface cut orientation [81,83].

Surface diffusion plays an additional role in catalytic activity [81,83]. Molecules adsorbed to clean surfaces diffuse about freely as energy is acquired from thermal vibrations of the underlying lattice [83]. Therefore, molecular fragments interact more frequently than in free solution. Adsorption at specific sites may also lower the activation energy for specific chemical reactions, which may then proceed at a lower temperature [83]. Clean metallic surfaces, especially stainless steel and chrome-cobalt and titanium alloys, resist corrosion due to their elemental composition, crystalline homogeneity, and surface oxides [39]. Titanium and chrome-cobalt alloys appear to achieve closer and stronger binding with tissue cells than do polymers or bioglass [84,85].

Most *polymers* used in medicine are amorphous,

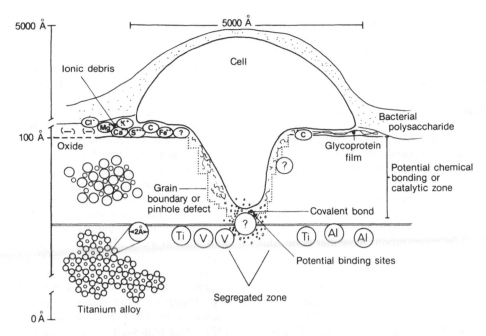

Figure 6. Schematic representation of the possible interaction between cells and a metal alloy at any atomic scale. A cell (bacterial or tissue cell) is shown at a defect or irregularity in Ti6A14V alloy oxide surface. Atomic geometry and electronic state direct the accumulation of ionic contaminants, resulting in catalytic processes. Ionic debris (area with ovals encircling dots), includes Cl^-, Mg^{2+}, K^+, Ca^{2+}, S^{3+}, C, Fe^{2+}, and unknown ions. Unsatisfied or dangling bonds are potential binding sites. Cell and surface perimeters are exaggerated because of the nonlinear scale. Reprinted with permission from Gristina et al. "Biomaterial-centered infection: microbial adhesion versus tissue integration". *Science*, 1987; 237:1588–1595. Copyright 1987 by AAAS.

although polytetrafluoroethylene, polyethylene, and polypropylene are partially crystalline [39]. Crystalline zones confer rigidity and amorphous zones confer toughness.

Solid polymers are nonequilibrium structures and adsorbates tend to satisfy their residual binding capacity, decreasing surface energy [86]. The resulting hierarchies are less complex than the high energy surfaces of metals or ceramics but are biologically relevant [87]. Increased rates of reaction may occur even on noncatalytic, two-dimensional planar surfaces because molecular contact is more likely in a planar or membrane system than in a three-dimensional one [88].

Although most high molecular weight medical polymers are believed to resist degradation by bacteria, some polymers contain low molecular weight plasticizers (polypropylene sebacate) which may be attacked by *P. aeruginosa* and *Serratia marcescens* [39]. The noncrystalline, porous structure of methylmethacrylate facilitates diffusion and molecular interaction.

Highly hydrophobic polymers are adhesive for many bacterial pathogens [13] (Figure 7). *S. epidermidis* has a higher rate of adhesion to polymers than does *S. aureus* [89]. Tissue cells adhere poorly to polymers such as methylmethacrylate and the interface is often inflammatory, especially after wear [29,90].

Most *ceramics and glass ceramics* used as dental

and orthopedic implants have crystalline structures. Bioactive glass ceramics are composed of crystals dispersed in an amorphous glass phase.

Bacteria probably do adhere to ceramics and glass ceramics, but the characteristics and clinical sig-

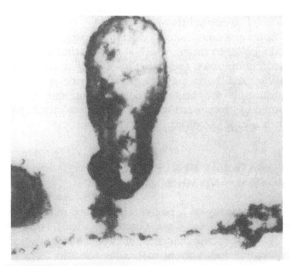

Figure 7. Transmission electron microscopy of extended-wear contact lens following colonization with *Pseudomonas*. Association of the bacterium with the lens surface is revealed through ruthenium red-stained macromolecules (original magnification, 85, 800×). Reprinted with permission from [58]. Copyright 1987, American Medical Association.

nificance of such infections require further study before any conclusions can be drawn. Studies of the comparable colonization of metals, polymers, and ceramics by *S. epidermidis* suggest that ceramics are less colonized than polymers [91].

Biological Surfaces

Fundamental mechanisms of adhesion also apply to biologic substrata. Individual cells or blood elements vary in their degree of surface receptivity for microorganisms.

Traumatized soft tissues are rich in nutrients, ligands, and adhesins, and may be colonized by bacteria with the appropriate receptors. Damaged tissues are unable to resist colonization. Avascular bone allografts have demonstrated a clinical infection rate of 5% to 14% [92].

Endothelial cells are surrounded by a well-developed glycocalyx. Disruption of this outer polysaccharide layer may expose fibronectin and receptor sites [93–95]. Bacterial adhesion to fibronectin and the presence of a biomaterial may help explain the colonization and infection of aortofemoral graft/vascular junctions by staphylococci and other bacteria [95,96]. Endothelial damage may also be a factor in site localization by trauma or by septic emboli in osteomyelitis.

Platelets also play a role in biomaterial infections. Gram-positive bacteria, *S. aureus, Str. pyogenes, Str. mutans,* and *Str. sanguis,* which are common causes of bacterial endocarditis, bind to fibronectin, fibrin, or platelets [47,48,51,97–99]. Trauma to natural heart valves, or conditioning of plastic valves by fibronectin, fibrin, and platelet vegetations may be an initial step in bacterial colonization. Bridging of platelets may allow bacteria to bind to damaged tissues [95, 99]; this is also a possible mechanism in trauma-induced osteomyelitis.

Bone is a composite of calcium phosphate crystals and a collagen matrix which is grossly similar to synthetic composites and partially crystalline polymers. Devitalized bone and allografts provide a passive substratum for bacterial colonization and a rich source of protein and mineral constituent metabolites for bacteria [32,70,75].

BIOMATERIAL DISRUPTION, BIOFILM, AND MICROZONES

The integrity of a biomaterial surface may be disrupted by trauma, wear, corrosion, toxins, viral effects, bacterial mechanisms, or chemical degradation. Structural and nutrient molecules released from the biomaterial bulk may be concentrated by colonizing bacteria.

Thus, adhesive, biofilm-enclosed and possibly polymicrobial colonies on the surface of a biomaterial may establish a microclimate within which optimal conditions are created and from which antagonistic environmental factors are excluded [100]. For example, iron may be sequestered within the microzone, preventing binding by host protein complexes (lactoferrin and transferrin) which would normally lower iron concentration levels below those required by pathogenic bacteria [101,102]. Excess iron may also be available to bacteria in a low pH or inflammatory environment as transferrin is saturated [102]. Iron may also accumulate in microcolonies due to localization of siderophores and acid metabolites. Iron has been linked to virulence for *S. aureus, S. epidermidis,* and *P. aeruginosa* and to adhesiveness and virulence of *E. coli* [103–106]. In excess quantities, iron may also inhibit macrophage function [101].

Corrosion of biomaterial surfaces releases metal ions such as Fe^{3+}, Mg^{2+}, Cr^{2+}, and Co^{3+}. Even with stable alloys such as stainless steel, corrosion (especially at grain boundaries) may occur due to wear or chemical interaction with biologic environments. Energy dispersive X-ray analysis of polymer surface has shown traces of iron, aluminum, and other substances [32]. Trace ions such as Mg^{2+} and Ca^{2+} may stabilize complex exopolysaccharides in gel form, enhancing cell-to-cell and cell-to-surface adhesion and increasing resistance to external antagonists [13,107]. Unstable polymers may be directly metabolized or may provide remnants of plasticizers, monomers, antioxidants, and stabilizers. Some synthetic polymers, such as polyester urethane and methylmethacrylate contain ester bonds which may be hydrolyzed by staphylococci [108].

HOST DEFENSE

Early concepts suggested that tissue damage caused by a foreign-body was responsible for increased susceptibility to infection [109–113]. Tissue damage was presumed to activate host defenses and stimulate the release of inflammatory mediators, including oxygen radicals and lysosomal enzymes. Bacteria served as additional inflammatory agents, amplifying tissue destruction. Activation of the complement system and the clotting cascade may have also contributed to the potentially destructive inflammatory response.

Conceptually, these ideas have merit when extensive tissue damage occurs and when the blood supply is disrupted. However, *S. epidermidis* is seldom a common etiologic agent of traumatic wound infections.

A singularly unique feature of *S. epidermidis* is its adhesion to polymer surfaces, the mechanisms of which are still unresolved [114–116]. Although some investigators have proposed that slime is not involved in primary binding, definitive data are not available to rule out this possibility. There is substantial evidence that slime-producing strains of *S. epidermidis* adhere to surfaces more readily than non-slime producing strains [23,117–120].

Extracellular slime may also inhibit host defense mechanisms. Slime from *S. epidermidis* has been reported to inhibit T-cell and B-cell blastogenesis, polymorphonuclear leukocyte (PMN) chemotaxis, opsonization, and chemiluminescence, and to enhance virulence of *S. epidermidis* in mice [63]. Johnson et al. showed that *S. epidermidis* grown on a plastic surface for 18 hours was less phagocytised by PMNs than was *S. epidermidis* grown on a plastic surface for 2 hours [120]. Because only the *S. epidermidis* grown for 18 hours was embedded in slime, this observation supports the suggestion that excess extracellular slime impairs PMN phagocytosis of embedded *S. epidermidis* [121].

Other researchers have suggested that slime protects embedded *S. epidermidis* from antibiotics, a common experience in the treatment of infections of polymers [122,123]. This observation is supported by the report that *S. epidermidis* is more resistant to various antibiotics when grown in a medium which favors slime production [69]. However, more recent studies suggest that limitation of diffusion is not the critical factor in resistance of biomaterial-adherent bacteria to antibiotics [67,68].

The interaction of professional phagocytes with a foreign body may somehow exhaust or preempt killing mechanisms. Klock and Bainton [124] observed that granulocytes exposed to nylon fibers retained their chemotactic response but had an impaired bactericidal response. Zimmerli et al. [125] reported that neutrophils inside Teflon cages placed in peritoneal cavities exhibited decreased phagocytic and bactericidal potential after one hour compared to neutrophils from peripheral blood. They also noted that superoxide production by neutrophils recovered from the Teflon cages was significantly reduced compared to neutrophils elicited from acute or chronic peritoneal exudates [126].

A similar pattern was noted when normal rabbit alveolar macrophages were exposed to polymethylmethacrylate spheres (~ 100 μm) for 3 or 18 hours and then challenged with phorbol myristate acetate (PMA) [61]. This possible mechanism of phagocyte impairment suggests that foreign body surfaces trigger a "slow burst" and "preempt" a second burst if the phagocyte subsequently encounters an infectious organism. It is almost certain that the killing capacity of such preempted phagocytes would be impaired.

While this "preemptive" theory could represent a general phenomenon in phagoctye-biomaterial interactions, host defenses may also be impaired by the protective nature of slime-enclosed microcolonies. However, because foreign bodies also enhance infections by non-slime-producing organisms (e.g., *S. aureus*), the presence of slime alone cannot fully explain the impairment of host defenses at the foreign body–tissue interface.

Antibiotics

Biomaterial-centered infections are generally resistant to antimicrobial treatment and cannot usually be eradicated until the biomaterial is removed. This resistance to antibiotic treatment, even after the infecting organism has been identified, is a perplexing problem.

Biofilm-enclosed bacteria are less susceptible and sensitive to antibiotics compared to the same organisms grown in suspension cultures. Data have revealed that when certain strains of *S. epidermidis* and *S. aureus* adhered to biomaterials, the minimum bactericidal concentration for various antibiotics increased from 2- to 250-fold, depending on the type of biomaterial and organism [69]. All organisms adhering to polymethylmethacrylate showed a greater resistance to antibiotics than the same organisms adherent to stainless steel [69]. It appears that a protective environment is created by the chemical composition of the biomaterial and the surrounding fluid, and the surface characteristics and metabolites of the adherent organisms.

PREVENTIVE TREATMENT AND FUTURE ADVANCES

Contemporary studies in microbiology, chemistry, and physics suggest the following investigative and therapeutic modalities.

Problems with biomaterial strength, design, and function have generally been solved. The remaining concern is to define the chemical and physical relationships of material surfaces at an atomic level and their interaction with organic and inorganic moieties. The characteristics of biomaterial surfaces and interfacial phenomena will be defined using advanced techniques such as scanning tunneling microscopy, Auger electron spectroscopy, and electron spectroscopy for chemical analysis.

Pathogens may be predicted for each type of surgery, material, and tissue system, so that correct preventive antibiotics can be chosen and the use of antibiotics which produce resistant strains of bacteria may be reduced.

Nonadherent bacteria are far more susceptible than adherent bacteria to antibiotics. Prophylactic antibiotics, delivered systemically or *in situ* in biomaterials, are effective because they act on bacteria in suspension populations (bacteremia) or before surface colonization can be consolidated and changes in host resistance occur. To a degree, the case for perioperative prophylactic antibiotics has already been proven—and is current practice in orthopedic and cardiovascular surgery.

Analogs may also be effective against biomaterial-centered infections. Peptides and oligosaccharides may be designed to saturate epitope or active receptor sites, thereby blocking or reversing bacterial adhesion and colony formation. Analogs and lectins preadsorbed to biomaterial surfaces may encourage adhesion of specific macromolecules or cells.

Precolonization or coating of biomaterial surfaces by healthy tissue cells or glycoproteins which do not provide receptors for bacteria before implantation

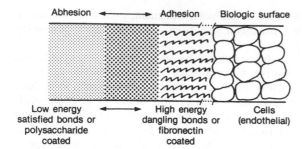

Figure 8. Biomaterial surface (left) is programmed by (1) surface energy state; (2) polysaccharide coating; or (3) glycoprotein coating for abhesion or adhesion. At site of junction with biologic surface (right), adhesion or integration by tissue cells (endothelial) is encouraged. Reprinted with permission from Gristina et al., "Infections from biomaterials and implants: a race for the surface". *Med. Prog. Technol.*, 1989. Copyright 1989 by Kluwer Academic Publishers.

may also protect against infection and accelerate bonding to adjacent tissue.

Modification of biomaterial surfaces may be the key to controlled biologic response (Figure 8). Surfaces will be created with idealized organic responses or programmed quantum states or energy levels. Adhesive or nonadhesive zones may be created to enhance biocompatibility and tissue integration or seeding. Ion implantation, chemical vapor deposition, and vacuum evaporation may be used to create surfaces which "direct" tissue or macromolecular integration, rather than allowing microbial colonization. Biomaterial surfaces of the future will be programmed, not for inertness, but for appropriate environmental reactivity.

REFERENCES

1. Lorentzen, J. E., O. M. Nielsen, H. Arendrup, H. H. Kimose, S. Bille, J. Andersen, C. H. Jensen, F. Jacobsen and O. C. Roder. 1985. *Surgery*, 98:81.
2. Hepp, W. and T. Schultze. 1986. *Thorac. Cardiovasc. Surg.*, 34:265.
3. Jensen, L. J. and H. H. Kimose. 1985. *Thorac. Cardiovasc. Surg.*, 33:389.
4. Sheth, N. K., T. R. Franson, H. D. Rose, F. L. A. Buckmire, J. A. Cooper, and P. G. Sohnle. 1983. *J. Clin. Microbiol.*, 18:1061.
5. Dougherty, S. H. and R. L. Simmons. 1982. *Curr. Probl. Surg.*, 19:269.
6. Eftekhar, N. S., and O. Nercessian. 1988. *Orthop. Clin. North Am.*, 19:557.
7. Eftekhar, N. S. 1987. *Clin. Orthop.*, 225:207.
8. Strathy, G. M. and R. H. Fitzgerald. 1988. *J. Bone Joint Surg.*, 70A:963.
9. Schutzer, S. F. and W. H. Harris. 1988. *J. Bone Joint Surg.*, 70A:724.
10. Jacobs, M. A., D. S. Hungerford, K. A. Krakow and D. W. Lennox. 1989. *Clin. Orthop.*, 238:159.
11. Ross, A. C., R. S. Sneath and J. T. Scales. 1987. *J. Bone Joint Surg.*, 69B:652.
12. Morrey, B. F. and R. S. Bryan 1987. *J. Bone Joint Surg.*, 69A:523.
13. Dankert, J., A. H. Hogt and J. Feijen. 1986. *CRC Crit. Rev. Biocompat.*, 2:219.
14. Maki, D. G. 1977. In: *Microbiological Hazards of Infusion Therapy*. I. Phillips, P. D. Meers and P. F. D'Arcy, eds. Lancaster, England: MTP Press, p. 99.
15. Gristina, A. G., J. J. Dobbins, B. Giammara, J. C. Lewis, and W. C. DeVries. 1988. *J.A.M.A.*, 259:870.
16. DeVries, W. 1988. *J.A.M.A.*, 259:849.
17. Didisheim, P., D. B. Olsen, D. J. Farrar, P. M. Portner, B. P. Griffith, D. G. Pennington, J. H. Joist, F. J. Schoen, A. G. Gristina and J. M. Anderson. 1989. *Trans. Am. Soc. Artif. Intern. Organs*, 35:54.
18. Elek, S. D. and P. E. Conen. 1957. *Br. J. Exp. Pathol*, 38:573.
19. Gristina, A. G. and G. D. Rovere. 1963. *J. Bone Joint Surg.*, 45A:1104.
20. Bayston, R. and S. R. Penny. 1972. *Devel. Med. Child Neurol.*, 14:25.
21. Gibbons, R. J. and J. V. van Houte. 1975. *Annu. Rev. Microbiol.*, 29:19.
22. Ofek, I. and E. H. Beachey. 1980. In *Bacterial Adherence: Receptors and Recognition, Series B*. E. H. Beachey, ed. London: Chapman and Hall, 6:3.
23. Gristina, A. G., J. W. Costerton, E. Leake and J. Kolkin. 1980. *Orthop. Trans.*, 4:405.
24. Gristina, A. G., J. W. Costerton, E. S. Leake, J. Kolkin and M. J. Wright. 1981. *Orthop. Trans.*, 5:332.
25. Costerton, J. W. and R. T. Irvin. 1981. *Annu. Rev. Microbiol.*, 35:299.
26. Peters, G., R. Locci and G. Pulverer. 1981. *Zentralbl. Bakteriol. Mikrobiol. Hyg. I Abt. Orig. B.*, 35:299.
27. Beachey, E. H. 1981. *J. Infect. Dis.*, 141:325.
28. Gristina, A. G., P. T. Naylor and Q. Myrvik. 1989. In *Molecular Mechanisms of Microbial Adhesion*. L. Switalski, M. Hook and E. H. Beachey, eds. New York: Springer Verlag, p. 177.
29. Albrektsson, T. 1985. *CRC Crit. Rev. Biocompat.*, 1:53.
30. Kasemo, B. and J. Lausmaa. 1986. *CRC Crit. Rev. Biocompat.*, 2:335.
31. Baier, R. E., A. E. Meyer, J. R. Natiella, R. R. Natiella and J. M. Carter. 1984. *J. Biomed. Mater. Res.*, 18:337.
32. Gristina, A. G., C. D. Hobgood and E. Barth. 1987. In *Pathogenesis and Clinical Significance of Coagulase-Negative Staphylococci*. G. Pulverer, P. G. Quie and G. Peters, eds. Stuttgart: Fischer Verlag, p. 143.
33. Derjaguin, B. V. and L. Landau. 1941. *Acta Physiochem. USSR*, 14:633.
34. Verwey, E. J. W. and J. T. G. Overbeek. 1948. *Theory of the Stability of Lyophobic Colloids*. Elsevier: London.
35. Watt, P. J. and M. E. Ward. 1980. In *Bacterial Adherence, Receptors and Recognition, Series B*. E. H. Beachey, ed. London: Chapman and Hall, 6:253.
36. Greig, R. G. and M. N. Jones. 1977. *Biosystems*, 9:43.
37. Curtis, A. S. G. 1973. In *Prog. Biophys. Mol. Biol.* J. A. V. Butler and D. Noble, eds., 27:317.

38. Lyklema, J. 1985. In *Surface and Interfacial Aspects of Biomedical Polymers*, J. Andrade, ed. *Surface Chemistry and Physics, Vol. 1*. New York: Plenum Press, p. 293.

39. Mears, D. C. 1979. *Materials and Orthopedic Surgery*, Baltimore, MD: Williams and Wilkins.

40. Jones, G. W. and R. E. Isaacson. 1984. *CRC Crit. Rev. Microbiol.*, 10:229.

41. Pashley, R. M., P. M. McGuiggan, B. W. Ninham and D. F. Evans. 1985. *Science*, 229:1088.

42. Gehlsen, K. R., L. Dillner, E. Engvall and E. Ruoslahti. 1988. *Science*, 241:1228.

43. Ruoslahti, E. and M. D. Pierschbacher. 1987. *Science*, 238:491.

44. Singer, I. I., S. Scott, D. W. Kawka, D. M. Kazazis, J. Gailit and E. Ruoslahti. 1988. *J. Cell Biol.*, 106:2171.

45. Christensen, G. D., W. A. Simpson, and E. H. Beachey. 1985. In *Bacterial Adhesion: Mechanisms and Physiologic Significance*. D. C. Savage and M. Fletcher, eds. New York: Plenum Press, p. 279.

46. Stenstrom, T.-A. and S. Kjelleberg. 1985. *Arch. Microbiol.*, 143:6.

47. Switalski, L. M., C. Ryden, K. Rubin, A. Ljungh, M. Hook and T. Wadstrom. 1983. *Infect. Immun.*, 42:628.

48. Hermann, M., P. E. Vaudaux, D. Pittet, R. Auckenthaler, P. D. Lew, F. Schumacher-Perdreau, G. Peters and F. A. Waldvogel. 1988. *J. Infect. Dis.*, 158:693.

49. Lopes, J. D., M. dos Reis and R. R. Brentani. 1985. *Science*, 229:275.

50. Vaudaux, P. E., F. A. Waldvogel, J. J. Morgenthaler and U. E. Nydegger. 1984. *Infect. Immun.*, 45:768.

51. Maxe, I., C. Ryden, T. Wadstrom and K. Rubin. 1986. *Infect. Immun.*, 56:695.

52. Deyme, M., A. Baszkin, J. E. Proust, E. Perez, G. Albrecht and M. M. Boissonnade. 1987. *J. Biomed. Mater. Res.*, 21:321.

53. Gibbons, R. J. and J. van Houte. 1980. In *Bacterial Adherence: Receptors and Recognition, Series B.* E. H. Beachey, ed. London: Chapman and Hall, 6:63.

54. Ludwicka, A., G. Uhlenbruck, G. Peters, P. N. Seng, E. D. Gray, J. Jeljaszewica and G. Pulverer. 1984. *Zentralbl. Bakteriol. Mikrobiol. Hyg. I, Abt.*, 258:256.

55. Gristina, A. G. and J. W. Costerton. 1984. *Orthop. Clin. North Am.*, 15:517.

56. Baltimore, R. S. and M. Mitchell. 1980. *J. Infect. Dis.*, 141:238.

57. Sutherland, I. W. 1978. In *Surface Carbohydrates of the Prokaryotic Cell.* I. W. Sutherland, ed. London: Academic Press, p. 27.

58. Slusher, M. M., Q. N. Myrvik, J. C. Lewis and A. G. Gristina. 1987. *Arch. Ophthalmol.*, 105:110.

59. Ichiman, I. and K. Yoshida. 1981. *J. Appl. Bacteriol.*, 51:229.

60. Gristina, A. G., E. Barth, L. X. Webb and Q. N. Myrvik. 1987. In *3rd ECCM Symposium: Foreign Body-Related Infections.* P. K. Peterson and A. Fleer, eds. Amsterdam: Excerpta Medica, p. 26.

61. Myrvik, Q. N., W. Wagner, E. Barth, P. Wood and A. G. Gristina. *J. Invest. Surg.* (in press).

62. Baier, R. E. 1982. *J. Biomech. Eng.*, 104:257.

63. Peters, G. 1988. *J. Antimicrob. Chemother.*, 21(Suppl. C):139.

64. Schwarzmann, S. and J. R. Boring, III. 1971. *Infect. Immun.*, 3:762.

65. Gwynn, M. N., L. T. Webb and G. N. Rolinson. 1981. *J. Infect. Dis.*, 144:263.

66. Nickel, J. C., J. B. Wright, I. Ruseska, T. J. Marrie, C. Whitfield and J. W. Costerton. 1985. *Eur. J. Clin. Microbiol.*, 4:213.

67. Nichols, W. W., S. M. Dorrington, M. P. E. Slack and H. L. Walmsley. 1988. *Antimicr. Agents Chemother.*, 32:518.

68. Nichols, W. W., J. J. Evans, M. P. E. Slack and H. L. Walmsley. *J. Gen. Microbiol.* (in press).

69. Naylor, P. T., R. Jennings, L. X. Webb and A. G. Gristina. 1988. *Orthop. Trans.*, 12:524.

70. Gristina, A. G., M. Oga, L. X. Webb and C. D. Hobgood. 1985. *Science*, 228:990.

71. Gristina, A. G. and J. W. Costerton. 1984. *Infect. Surg.*, 3:655.

72. Govan, J. R. W. 1975. *J. Med. Microbiol.*, 8:513.

73. Proctor, R. A. 1987. *Rev. Infect. Dis.*, 9(Suppl 4): S317.

74. Van Wachem, P. B., C. M. Vreriks, T. Beugeling, J. Feijen, A. Bantjes, J. P. Detmers and W. G. van Aken. 1987. *J. Biomed. Mater. Res.*, 21:701.

75. Vercellotti, G. M., J. B. McCarthy, P. Lindholm, P. K. Peterson, H. S. Jacob and L. T. Furcht. 1985. *Am. J. Pathol.*, 120:13.

76. Baier, R. E. 1983. *Ann. N. Y. Acad. Sci.*, 416:34.

77. Mohammad, S. F., N. S. Topham, G. L. Burns and D. B. Olsen. 1988. *Trans. Am. Soc. Artif. Intern. Organs*, 34:573.

78. Albrektsson, T. 1983. *J. Prosthet. Dent.*, 50:255.

79. Branemark, P. I., B. O. Hansson, R. Adell, R. Breine, J. Lindstrom, O. Hallen and A. Ohman. 1977. *Scand. J. Plast. Reconstr. Surg.*, 16:1.

80. Tromp, R. M., R. J. Hamers and J. E. Demuth. 1986. *Science*, 234:304.

81. Noonan, J. R. and H. L. Davis. 1986. *Science*, 234:310.

82. Engel, T. 1986. *Science*, 234:327.

83. Gomer, R. 1982. *Sci. Am.* 247(August):98.

84. Barth, E., H. Ronningen and L.F. Solheim. 1985. *Acta Orthop. Scand.*, 56:491.

85. Albrektsson, T., T. Arnebrandt, K. Larsson, T. Nylander and L. Sennergy. 1985. In *Transactions of the 5th European Conference on Biomaterials.* D. F. Williams, ed. Amsterdam: Elsevier, p. 151.

86. Andrade, J. D., D. E. Gregonis and L. M. Smith. 1985. In *Surface and Interfacial Aspects of Biomedical Polymers, Vol. 1, Surface Chemistry and Physics.* J. D. Andrade, ed. New York: Plenum Press, p. 15.

87. Andrade, J. D., L. M. Smith and D. E. Gregonis. 1985. *Surface and Interfacial Aspects of Biomedical Polymers, Vol. 1, Surface Chemistry and Physics.* J. D. Andrade, ed. New York: Plenum Press, p. 249.

88. Alberts, B., D. Bray, J. Lewis, M. Raff, K. Roberts and J. D. Watson. 1983. *Molecular Biology of the Cells.* New York: Garland Publishing, Inc.

89. Hsieh, Y.-L. and J. Merry. 1986. *J. Appl. Bacteriol.*, 60:535.

90. Kozinn, S. C., N. A. Johanson and P. G. Bullough. 1986. *J. Arthroplasty*, 1:249.

91. Oga, M., Y. Sugioka, C. D. Hobgood, A. G. Gristina and Q. N. Myrvik. 1988. *Biomaterials*, 9:285.

92. Burwell, R. G., G. E. Friedlaender and H. J. Mankin. 1985. *Clin. Orthop.*, 197:141.

93. Ryan, U. S. 1986. *Annu. Rev. Physiol.*, 48:263.

94. Birinyi, L. K., E. C. Douville, S. A. Lewis, H. S. Bjornson and R. F. Kempczinski. 1987. *J. Vasc. Surg.*, 5:193.

95. Hamill, R. J., J. M. Vann and R. A. Proctor. 1986. *Infect. Immun.*, 54:833.

96. Webb, L. W., R. T. Myers, A. R. Cordell, C. D. Hobgood, J. W. Costerton and A. G. Gristina. 1986. *J. Vasc. Surg.*, 4:16.

97. Christensen, G. D., W. A. Simpson and E. H. Beachey. 1985. In *Principles and Practice of Infectious Diseases, 2nd edition*. G. L. Mandell, R. G. Douglas, Jr., and J. E. Bennett, eds. New York: John Wiley and Sons, p. 6.

98. Baddour, L. M. 1988. *Rev. Infect. Dis.*, 10:1163.

99. Houdijk, W. P. M., P. G. de Groot, P. F. E. M. Nievelstein, K. S. Sakariassen and J. J. Sixma. 1986. *Arteriosclerosis*, 6:24.

100. Paerl, H. W. 1985. In *Bacterial Adhesion: Mechanisms and Physiologic Significance*. D. C. Savage and M. Fletcher, eds. New York: Plenum Press, p. 363.

101. Brown, M. R. W. and P. Williams. 1985. *Annu. Rev. Microbiol.*, 39:527.

102. Sriyoschati, S. and C. D. Cox. 1986. *Infect. Immun.*, 52:885.

103. Dho, M. and J. P. Lafont. 1984. *Avian Dis.*, 28:1016.

104. Bullen, J. J., H. J. Rogers and E. Griffiths. 1974. In *Microbial Iron Metabolism: A Comprehensive Treatise*. J. B. Beilands, ed. New York: Academic Press, p. 518.

105. Kochan I., J. T. Kvach and T. I. Wiles. 1977. *J. Infect. Dis.*, 135:623.

106. Weinberg, E. D. 1974. *Science*, 184:952.

107. Fletcher, M. 1985. *Bacterial Adhesion: Mechanisms and Physiologic Significance*. D. C. Savage and M. Fletcher, eds., New York: Plenum Press, p. 339.

108. Ludwicka, A., R. Locci, B. Jansen, G. Peters, and G. Pulverer. 1983. *Zentralbl. Bakteriol. Mikrobiol. Hyg. Abt. I Orig. B*, 177:527.

109. Dougherty, S. H. 1988. *Rev. Infect. Dis.*, 10:1102.

110. McGeehan, D., D. Hunt, A. Chaudhur and P. Rutter 1980. *Br. J. Surg.*, 67:636.

111. Alexander, J. W., J. Z. Kaplan and W. A. Alteneier. 1967. *Ann. Surg.*, 165:192.

112. Edlich, R. F., P. H. Panek, G. T. Rodeheaver, V. G. Turnbull, L. D. Kurtz and M. T. Edgerton. 1973. *Ann. Surg.*, 177:679.

113. Dougherty, S. H. and R. L. Simmons. 1982. *Curr. Probl. Surg.*, 19:221.

114. Hogt, A. H., J. Dankert, J. A. deVries and J. J. Feijen. 1983. *J. Gen. Microbiol.*, 129:2954.

115. Ludwicka, A., B. Jansen, T. Wadstrom, L. M. Switalski, G. Peters and G. Pulverer. 1985. In *Polymers as Biomaterials*. S. W. Shalaby, A. S. Hoffman, B. D. Ratner, and T. A. Horbett, eds. New York: Plenum Publishing Corp., p. 241.

116. Tojo, M., N. Yamashita, D. A. Goldmann and G. B. Pier. 1988. *J. Infect. Dis.*, 157:713.

117. Ishak, M. A., D. H. M. Groschel, G. L. Mandell and R. P. Wenzel. 1984. *J. Clin. Microbiol.*, 22:1025.

118. Christensen, G. D., J. T. Parisi, A. L. Bisno, W. A. Simpson and E. H. Beachey. 1983. *J. Clin. Microbiol.*, 18:258.

119. Davenport, D. S., R. M. Massanari, M. A. Pfaller, M. J. Bal, S. A. Streed and W. J. Hierholzer, Jr. 1986. *J. Infect. Dis.*, 153:352.

120. Christensen, G. D., W. A. Simpson, A. L. Bisno and E. H. Beachey. 1982. *Infect. Immun.*, 37:318.

121. Johnson, G. M., D. A. Lee, W. E. Regelmann, E. D. Gray, G. Peters and P. G. Quie. 1986. *Infect. Immun.*, 54:13.

122. Peters, G., R. Locci and G. Pulverer. 1982. *J. Infect. Dis.*, 146:479.

123. Sheth, N. K., T. R. Franson and P. G. Sohnle. 1985. *Lancet*, 2:1266.

124. Klock, J. C. and D. F. Bainton. 1976. *Blood*, 48:149.

125. Zimmerli, W., F. A. Waldvogel, P. Vaudaux and U. E. Nydegger. 1982. *J. Infect. Dis.*, 146:487.

126. Zimmerli, W., P. D. Lew and F. A. Waldvogel. 1984. *J. Clin. Invest.*, 73:1191.

9

The Healing Effects of Occlusive Wound Dressings

MARCEL F. JONKMAN, M.D., Ph.D.*

ABSTRACT: Since the discovery in 1962 that epithelialization is accelerated by wound occlusion with a moisture-retaining polyethylene film, occlusive therapy has made considerable advances. The first-generation occlusive dressings were of impermeable or of low-permeable plastic films without adhesive backing. The second-generation wound dressings, represented by medium-permeable polyurethane films and hydrocolloid dressings with an adhesive backing, were easy to handle, but had an insufficient vapor permeability that still led to wound fluid accumulation. In the third generation of wound dressings, the problems of wound fluid control was handled by using high water vapor permeable materials such as hydrogels and hydrophilized polyurethane films. In this paper, the mechanisms of accelerated epithelialization and improved dermal repair are discussed.

INTRODUCTION

Twenty-nine years ago, in a landmark article published in 1962, Winter showed that epithelialization can be accelerated if the wound is kept moist by using an occlusive polythene film [1]. It has been calculated from fresh partial-thickness wounds in Yorkshire pigs that epidermal cells migrate at a speed of about 0.5 mm per day over a moist wound surface, which is twice as fast as under a scab in dry wounds [2]. These observations were confirmed in experimental wounds on human volunteers [3]. A moist wound environment was also obtained when wounds were allowed to heal in a hot, humid, subtropical climate (Miami), rather than when they had to heal in a dry, cold, arctic climate (Fairbanks, Alaska) [4]. A moist wound environment thus enhances epithelialization.

Mechanisms of Action

The exact mechanism by which epithelialization is accelerated under occlusive wound dressings is still not exactly known. One plausible explanation is that keratinocytes migrate more easily over a moist wound surface than underneath a scab [5]. The reduction in speed of epidermal cell migration underneath scabs is explained by the 36- to 48-hour delay for scab formation until the watertable has reached a plane of equilibrium and by the divergence of energy needed by epidermal cells for collagenolytic [6,7] or phagocytic [8] activity to dissect themselves a way underneath the scab.

It is generally accepted that mitotic activity is not required for reaching epidermal continuity in linear incisions [9]. Interesting is that increased epidermal cell migration is accompanied by reduced mitotic activity of a yet unknown mechanism observation in stripped skin under occlusion [10]. Mitotic activity is prominently seen three days after wounding at a distance of 0.3 mm proximal from the migrating epidermal tongue [54]. The inhibition of cell mitosis is used when shielding psoriatic lesions with occlusive dressings [11,12].

Another explanation for accelerated epithelialization is that oxygen-permeable occlusive wound dressings increase the partial pressure of oxygen in the hypoxic wound environment under a scab [13]. However, in a recent paper Varghese found that an oxygen-permeable wound dressing (OpSite®) stimulates epithelialization at a rate similar to a non-oxygen-permeable wound dressing (Duoderm®), and that the wound environment remained in both conditions hypoxic [14]. They even proposed that actually a low partial oxygen pressure stimulates epithelialization, similar to fibroblast proliferation and angiogenesis, which is stressed by the group of Hunt [15].

Varghese also proposed that pH of the exudate might possibly play a role in wound healing, since he found a low pH under a hydrocolloid dressing to be

*Department of Dermatology, University Hospital, Oostersingel 59, 9713 EZ Groningen, The Netherlands

related to retarded microbial proliferation, especially to the reduction of *Pseudomonas aeruginosa* colonization, thus benefiting epidermal healing [14]. This effect was not related to P_{CO_2} level, since this did not differ in controls. In merchandising these propositions, a product such as Duoderm®/Granuflex® is said to produce an anaerobic, acidic environment. However, in a clinical trial on venous ulcers, the survival of *Pseudomonas aeruginosa*, a strict aerobe, under Duoderm®/Granuflex® makes this seem unlikely [16].

The fluid retained under occluded wounds is a source for bacterial proliferation. Although retained wound fluid is reported to be bactericidal by attracting neutrophils [17] and by activating complement C3 [18], there appears no doubt that microbial organisms accumulate more in occluded wounds than in air-exposed wounds [14,19]. Surprisingly, dermatitis or cellulitis seldom develop in or around occluded wounds, as has been reported in studies on split-skin donor sites covered with OpSite® [20] and venous leg ulcers covered with Duoderm®/Granuflex® [16]. Eaglestein even goes that far to propose that "bacteria and their metabolites could conceivably stimulate epidermal migration and healing" [21].

A less often heard proposition is that moistening of the wound by occlusion maintains an electrical potential between the wound and the surrounding skin thus stimulating epithelialization [22].

A very intriguing possibility for increased epithelialization is the increased concentration of local growth factors [21,23]. Buchan showed that the wound fluid collected under an occlusive film is similar in composition to human blood, which very likely contains an abundant amount of growth factors, although wound exudate contains more neutrophils, immunoglobulins and lysozyme, typical for the inflammatory response [24]. The Eaglestein group found that wound fluid, collected for 24 hours under a polyurethane occlusive dressing, had an inhibitory effect on outgrowth of epidermal explants, and concluded that increased epithelialization beneath occlusive dressings is not attributable to early wound fluid components [25]. However the same group also found that the stimulating effect of occlusion might be obtained by using an occlusive dressing for only a short period within 24 hours after wounding [26]. In contrast, the group of Hefton found that wound fluid, collected under an occlusive dressing, stimulated the proliferation of cultured epidermal cells [27]. This study emphasizes the stimulating role of growth factors likely present in wound fluid.

Possible candidates for local growth factors are interleukin-I, epidermal growth factor, transforming growth factor-α and -β, platelet-derived growth factor, and a yet unknown factor synthesized by keratinocytes themselves, as has been shown by Eisinger, who used supernatants of cultured epithelium to stimulate epithelialization in full-thickness wounds in pigs [28].

In addition to these mechanisms known in literature, we propose that epithelialization might even be more accelerated in the presence of a fibrin–fibronectin containing coagulum on the wound surface, which is used as a substratum for epidermal cell migration [29]. As we will show, such a fibrin–fibronectin coagulum is formed when using a high water vapor permeable wound dressing. A fibrin coagulum is not formed under truly occlusive conditions, such as when using medium-permeable wound dressings like OpSite®. Possibly, accumulation of watery exudate does not permit fibrin clotting into a three-dimensional network, or induces premature fibrinolysis. Although Buchan et al. have shown that the exudate under OpSite® contains twice as many leukocytes as do control blood samples [24], leukocytes are possibly not responsible for any increased fibrinolysis, since they produce little or no plasminogen activator and show only weak fibrinolytic activity, in contrast to endothelial cells [30].

Dermal Repair

The effect of occlusive dressings on dermal repair has recently received more attention. Winter has already found that dermal repair begins three days earlier in moist wounds than in dry wounds [2]. Linski found a decreased number of fibroblasts and a decreased breaking strength in incisions that had been dressed with an occlusive film [31]. However, Alvarez found [32], that wound occlusion increases collagen biosynthesis, and postulated that these seemingly contradictory findings might be explained by a delay of intermolecular cross-linking of the collagen fibrils under occlusive conditions. Recently, Dyson found [33], that the formation of granulation tissue was less extensive in full-thickness wounds covered with an occlusive dressing than in air-exposed controls. However, the moist wounds contained more capillaries directed to the wound surface, suggesting that angiogenesis was stimulated by the fluid exudate retained under the occlusive dressing. Furthermore, fibroblasts tended to exhibit a more parallel arrangement in the granulation tissue, typical of that of contractile myofibroblasts. This might explain the accelerated wound contraction observed under occlusive dressings, although final wound contraction was not altered compared with untreated controls. Leipzinger et al. also showed that occlusion does not effect ultimate wound contraction [34].

IDEAL REQUIREMENTS FOR A WOUND DRESSING

Numerous reviews have been concerned with the requirements needed for ideal wound dressing [35–41]. In our opinion, the following requirements are necessary. Ideally, a temporary wound dressing should:

(1) Have a high water vapor permeability or a high absorbance capacity to prevent fluid accumulation

(2) Adhere to the wound surface without damage to tissue at removal

(3) Not allow fibrovascular ingrowth with the underlying wound bed

(4) Form a bacterial barrier

(5) Be elastic also in dry state

(6) Reduce pain

(7) Be hemostatic

(8) Be cheap

(9) Be readily available

(10) Have a long shelf life and require minimal storage

(11) Be sterilizable

(12) Not be flammable

(13) Not be antigenic, allergenic, toxic, or carcinogenic

There is no material that wholly satisfies this list of requirements. Even human skin is not ideal, since its availability and shelf life are limited. It is obvious that the choice of dressing should be directed to the type of wound and the aim of the treatment, taking into consideration the balance of advantages and drawbacks of the chosen material.

However, *adherence* and *control of wound fluid* are the most important requirements.

Adherence

Tavis identified two distinct phases of adherence of wound dressings, a phase I and a phase II adherence [42]. We propose an extra *phase 0 adherence* preceding these phases. The sequence of adherence might thus be described as: an initial phase 0 adherence, in which the dressing "sucks" to the wound surface by capillary forces. Then, a *phase I adherence* within 5 hours, which is mediated by fibrin molecules present in the wound exudate and which correlates positively with the height of zeta potential of the dressing. The zeta potential might be increased by pre-coating the dressing with fibronectin [43].

Dressings with an open pore structure, such as autografts, allografts [44], sheets of collagen or calcium alginate [45], and synthetic artificial skins with an open porous bottom layer [46,47], will show a subsequent *phase II adherence* after 24 to 72 hours, characterized by fibrovascular ingrowth into the dressing. This fibrovascular ingrowth with the underlying dermis is undesirable in partial-thickness wounds, since the border with nonviable tissue will not be available as guidance for epidermal migration. Epidermal migration will then cease [48]. Moreover, tissue damage will result at removal, so that these dressings have to be changed daily to prevent tissue

incorporation, or should be left *in situ* until the wound has healed completely.

Control of Wound Fluid

Wound dressings might be classified as having a low (0–2 $g \cdot m^{-2} \cdot h^{-1} \cdot kPa^{-1}$), medium (2–15 $g \cdot m^{-2} \cdot h^{-1} \cdot kPa^{-1}$), or high (15–25 $g \cdot m^{-2} \cdot h^{-1} \cdot kPa^{-1}$) water vapor permeance (WVP). Erroneously they are often named "occlusive", "semi-occlusive", "semi-permeable", "vapor-permeable", or "high-vapor-permeable". Literally spoken, "occlusive" dressings are only those that trap the wound fluid by forming a watertight seal with the surrounding skin. Low vapor-permeable coverings might not at all be occlusive when the wound fluid leaks from under the dressing. Furthermore, the adjective "semi-permeable" literally means selectively permeable. For instance, the dressing might be permeable only for water but not for proteins or bacteria. Most polyurethane membranes are semi-permeable, but hydrophile gauzes are not. Thus the polyetherurethane wound dressing is at the same time occlusive (fibrin-mediated sealing to the wound margin), semipermeable (only for water vapor) and high-permeable.

The optimal water vapor permeability of a wound covering should be much higher than that of human skin. Although human skin grafts limit the wound's fluid production by reducing tissue edema, they lead to fluid retention if the graft is not expanded with meshed openings. "Semi-permeable" polyurethane films, such as OpSite®, which have a water vapor permeability four times that of human skin, still retain too much wound fluid [49].

Apparently, an ideal wound covering should be permeable to water vapor to such an extent that wound dehydration is prevented, but evaporation of superfluous wound fluid is allowed. We propose an optimum WVP at the lower limit of the range 20 to 25 $g \cdot m^{-2} \cdot h^{-1} \cdot kPa^{-1}$ [50]. A higher WVP than 25 $g \cdot m^{-2} \cdot h^{-1} \cdot kPa^{-1}$ might conceivably lead to wound desiccation. A free water surface has a WVP of about 27 $g \cdot m^{-2} \cdot h^{-1} \cdot kPa^{-1}$ (Figure 1).

Another solution to control excessive wound fluid is to create a dressing that absorbs superfluous exudate into the fabric. Representatives of this class are paraffin gauzes (Jelonet®, Optulle®, Xeroform®), collagen sheets (Tempocoll®, EZ-derm®, Mediskin®), nylon meshes (Biobrane®, Surfasoft® [51], nylon stockings [52]), and porous polyurethane foams (Lyofoam® [53]). However, these open dressings might allow fibrovascular ingrowth, or might become incorporated into the crust by coagulation of the absorbed fibrin in the fabric. Thus, changes of open dressings are necessary to prevent tissue ingrowth and a critical amount of fluid or viscous exudate is needed underneath to enable safe peeling-off from the wound without tissue damage. Opposite to this hypothesis, some encourage tissue ingrowth and crust incorporation to increase the drainage ability and adhesiveness of a temporary wound dressing [47]. However, the patient literally remains stuck to such a dressing, since removal of the dressing is only possible after healing is completed.

DESIGN DEVELOPMENT IN WOUND DRESSINGS

First Generation

After the recognition of speeded epithelialization with occlusive dressings by Winter in 1962, the first generation of experimental occlusive films were made of polyethylene, polypropylene, polyester or polyvinyl chloride [54]. These films were almost completely impermeable for water vapor, and for that reason are well known as wraps for food preservation. A transparent polyvinyl chloride film dressing (Stretch 'n' Seal®) is still recently recommended as temporary drape for burn wounds to prevent heat and water loss during waiting periods before operation and staff visits [55]. These fully occlusive films very soon result in accumulation of wound fluid. Typically, these first-generation films had no additional adhesive-backing.

Second Generation

Films

Industrial marketing was not encouraged until the mid 1970s, probably due to physicians' fears of wound infection when using occlusive wound dressings. The second generation of occlusive wound dressings soon appeared on the market [56], made from medical-grade polyurethane films such as OpSite®, Tegaderm®, Bioclusive®, MP 2080®, Uniflex®, Opraflex®, Ensure-It®, Thin Film Wound Dressing®, and Blister

Film®. Originally these products were designed for use as surgical-incision films [57], or as catheter and drain fixatives [58] and thus had an additional adhesive layer for fixation. However, it was not physicians but nurses who first advocated their use on leg ulcers [59] and pressure sores [60]. During the 1980s these products became more commonly accepted as being effective in speeding up healing of acute [20] and chronic wounds [61]. Nowadays, more than fourteen types of occlusive wound dressings are commercially available, most of which are made from polyurethanes [62].

However, many of these occlusive wound dressings overdo their task of keeping the wound moist. During the first days the wound superfluously produces exudate that accumulates into bullae under the dressing, and which may leak away [56], may need to be aspirated [20], may lead to tissue maceration [62], or may impair keratinization [63].

Since occlusive wound dressings do not adhere to a moist wound surface they need an additional adhesive backing for fixation to the surrounding intact dry skin. A major drawback of adhesive-backed dressings, whether as film dressing [56,32] or as hydrocolloid dressing [64], is that they adhere to the newly formed dry epidermis, which might be stripped away during dressing removal. Continuous pain might result from sticking and pulling of hairs from the surrounding normal skin under the dressing [65]. The adhesive backing also prohibits their use on erosions in bullous diseases, like epidermolysis bullosa, where the fragile epidermis is easily traumatized.

Hydrocolloids

In the early 1980s a new variant of occlusive dressings appeared on the market known as hydrocolloids, such as Duoderm®/Granuflex®, Comfeel®, Biofilm®, Dermiflex®, and Ulcer Dressing®. The surface of the

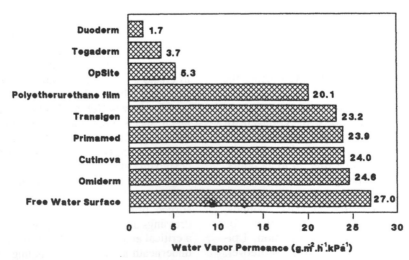

Figure 1. Water vapor permeance of some wound dressings and free water surface (from Erasmus and Jonkman, 1989 [50]).

dressing in contact with the wound is coated with an adhesive opaque hydrocolloid mass, which consists of polyisobutylene in which are dispersed granules containing gelatin, pectin and carboxymethylcellulose. When in contact with wound exudate, these granules absorb water, swell and eventually form a hydrophilic fluid gel. The hydrocolloid gel changes after some hours into a rather malodorous, yellow-brown fluid, which may leak aside. The hydrocolloid gel has no additional effect on epithelialization, since it accelerates proliferation of cultured epidermal cells to the same degree as the fluid exudate under occlusive film dressings [27].

Hydrocolloid dressings have an outer layer composed of a low-permeable plastic film. In Duoderm®/Granuflex® this outer layer is made from water-impermeable plastic film derived the first generation, and in Comfeel® it is identical to the medium-vapor-permeable OpSite®. Nevertheless, clinical successes have been claimed with hydrocolloid dressings in studies on burn wounds (no control group) [66], pressure sores (control Dakin's solution) [67], and venous ulcers (no statistical significance with paraffin gauze control) [16].

Biofilm® has, in contrast to the low-vapor-permeable hydrocolloids, an outer layer permeable to gases and water vapor composed of a hydrophobic polyester fabric, as shown *in vitro* by Thomas [68]. The open structure of Biofilm® would make this dressing penetrable for microorganisms, but it offers advantages over the other hydrocolloids in terms of its ability to cope with large volume of wound exudate, although no clinical data are available yet.

Third Generation

What actually is needed are wound dressings that keep the wound moist, prevent accumulation of wound fluid, and do not need an additional adhesive-backing. These dressings have in common a high water vapor permeability to evacuate superfluous fluid (Figure 1) [50]. Members of the third generation class are hydrogels, and hydrophilic polyurethane films like Omiderm®, Primamed®, Transigen®, and our experimental polyetherurethane film.

Hydrogels

Hydrogels are semitransparent (in contrast to opaque hydrocolloids) absorbent dressings containing 96% water reinforced with a network of polyester (Cutinova®) or polyethyleneoxide (Elasto-gel®, Spenco 2nd Skin®, Vigilon®). They are said to be non-adherent, but somtimes adhere very firmly to the wound.

The hydrogel layer is sandwiched between thin films for transport reasons. Both thin films should be removed before application to allow contact of the hydrogel with the wound surface and to enable a high water vapor permeability (Figure 1). A recent study by Jablonski and Tronnier [69] comparing a hydrogel (Cutinova®-plus) with a hydrocolloid (Duoderm®/Varihesive®) in addition to a polyurethane foam outer layer on chronic leg ulcers, demonstrated that the absorptive capacity and evaporative ability of the former enhances wound decontamination, granulation tissue formation, and subsequent wound closure. Non-adhering hydrogels are preferable in ulcers with surrounding dermatitis, which would otherwise worsen if adhesive dressings like OpSite®, or Duoderm® were used [23].

High Water Vapor Permeable Films

Omiderm® was the first non-porous polyurethane film on the market with a high water vapor permeability [70] (Figure 1). The hydrophilic property was obtained by grafting acrylamide on to a polyurethane film [71]. The high permeability for water vapor prevents wound desiccation as well as accumulation of wound fluid in partial-thickness wounds. The outer surface of the dressing tends to dry out, causing creasing and limited contraction, because the film is only elastic in the moist state, and becomes inelastic in the dry state [72]. Its use on full-thickness wounds (burned or excised) might result in wound fluid accumulation underneath, making frequent dressing changes necessary [72]. A new 1:1.5 meshed form is now available to allow passage of blood and exudate into an externally applied absorptive dressing [73].

Primamed® is a two-layer wound dressing of non-leaking polyurethane foam with a separate porous adhesive outer layer. Primamed® elongates but returns to its normal size after drying. This process might interfere with wound adhesion and thus might evoke fluid retention under the bubbling surface. Primamed® is delivered with an adhesive top layer which reduces its water vapor permeability about 50%.

Transigen® is a polyurethane film dressing with high water vapor permeability, but combines it with a sustained elasticity in dry state. It consists of a three-layer composite, composed of a non-adhering inner layer with pores for water penetration, an absorptive middle layer, and a hydrophilic polyurethane outer layer with high vapor permeability (Figure 1). The wound exudate collects between the inner and outer layers, where the wound fluid gelatinizes by selective evaporative water extraction. On theoretical grounds, this system will not profit from the growth-promoting characteristics of the gelatinous wound exudate because exudate components are not available for the growing epithelium, since they are collected between the inner and outer layer. Clinical reports of Transigen® are not available yet.

The experimental *polyetherurethane* film dressing designed by the author at the University of Groningen, in collaboration with the Department of Polymer Chemistry, is also a third-generation high water vapor permeable film [29]. The evaporative capacity allows condensation of the wound exudate into a gelatinous clot. This clot accelerates epithelialization more than a fluid exudate. The polyurethane film is unique, because it combines a high vapor permeability with high sustained elasticity, natural fibrin adherence, transparency, prevention of microbial penetration, prevention of tissue incorporation and easy all-time removal without breaking.

These exciting developments fine-tune the occlusive therapy of wounds regarding the control of fluid. The old Winternian concept of a moist wound environment has now been replaced by the concept that wound healing is most promoted in a gelatinous wound environment [29].

REFERENCES

1. Winter, G. D. 1962. *Nature (Lond)*, 193:293–294.
2. Winter, G. D. 1972. In *Epidermal Wound Healing*. H. I. Maibach and D. T. Rovee, eds. Chicago, IL: Year Book Medical Publishers, Inc., p. 71.
3. Hinman, C. D., H. Maibach and G. D. Winter. 1963. *Nature (Lond)*, 200:377.
4. Bothwell, J. W., D. T. Rovee, A. M. Downes, P. A. Flanagan, C. A. Kurowsky. 1972. In *Epidermal Wound Healing*. H. I. Maibach and D. T. Rovee, eds. Chicago, IL: Year Book Medical Publishers, Inc. p. 255.
5. Winter, G. D. and J. T. Scales. 1963. *Nature*, 197:91
6. Grillo, H. C. and J. Gross. 1967. *Dev. Biol.*, 15:300.
7. Gross, J. 1981. In *Cell Biology of the Extracellular Matrix*. Hay, ed. New York: Plenum Press, p. 217.
8. Ross, R. and G. Odland. 1968. *J. Cell. Biol.*, 39:152.
9. Rovee, D. T., C. A. Kurowsky, J. Labun, A. M. Downes. 1972. In *Epidermal Wound Healing*. H. I. Maibach and D. T. Rovee, eds. Chicago, IL: Year Book Medical Publishers, Inc. p. 159.
10. Fisher, L. B. and H. I. Maibach. 1972. *Br. J. Derm.*, 86:593.
11. Fryd, J. Almeyda, R. M. H. McMinn. 1970. *Br. J. Derm.*, 82:458.
12. Petzoldt, D. G., O. Braun-Falko and K. H. Wenig. 1970. *Arch. Klin. Exp. Dermatol.*, 238:160.
13. Silver, I. A. 1972. In *Epidermal Wound Healing*. H. I. Maibach and D. T. Rovee, eds. Chicago, IL: Year Book Medical Publishers, Inc., p. 673.
14. Varghese, M. C., A. K. Balin, D. M. Carter and D. Caldwell. 1986. *Arch. Dermatol.*, 122:52.
15. Knighton, D. R., I. A. Silver and T. K. Hunt. 1981. *Surgery*, 90:262.
16. Handfield-Jones, S. E., C. E. H. Grattan, R. A. Simpson and C. T. C. Kennedy. 1988. *Br. J. Dermatol.*, 118:425.
17. Buchan, I. A., J. K. Andrews, S. M. Lang, J. G. Boorman, J. V. H. Harvey Kemble and B. H. G. Lamberty. 1980. *Burns*, 7:326.
18. Holland, K. T., W. Davis, E. Ingham and G. Gowland. 1984. *J. Hosp. Inf.*, 5:323.
19. Mertz, P. M. and W. H. Eaglestein. 1984. *Arch. Surg.*, 119:287.
20. May, S. R. 1984. In *Burn Wound Coverings*. D. L. Wise, ed. Boca Raton: CRC Press, Inc., p. 53.
21. Eaglestein, W. H. 1984. *Clin. Dermatol.*, 2:107.
22. Jaffe, L. F. and J. W. Vanable. 1984. In *Clinics in Dermatology: Wound Healing*. W. H. Eaglestein, ed. Philadelphia, PA: JB Lippincott, p. 34.
23. Falanga, V. 1988. *Arch. Dermatol.*, 124:872.
24. Buchan, I. A., J. K. Andrews and S. M. Lang. 1981. *Burns,* 8:39.
25. Nemeth, A. J., P. Hebda, T. Fitzgerald and W. H. Eaglestein. 1986. *J. Invest. Dermatol.*, 86:497.
26. Eaglestein, W. H., S. C. Davis, A. L. Mehle and P. M. Mertz. 1988. *Arch. Dermatol.*, 124:392.
27. Madden, M. R., J. L. Finkelstein, E. Nolan, L. Stainano-Coico, C. L. Goodwin and J. H. Hefton. 1988. *J. Trauma*, 28:1091.
28. Eisinger, M., S. Sadan, I. A. Silver and R. B. Flick. 1988. *Proc. Natl. Acad. Sci. USA*, 85:1937.
29. Jonkman, M. F. 1989. *Epidermal Wound Healing Between Moist and Dry*. Thesis, University of Groningen, Groningen.
30. Astrup, T. 1968. *Biochem. Pharmacol. Suppl.*, 241.
31. Linsky, C. B., D. T. Rovee and T. Dow. 1981. In *The Surgical Wound*. P. Dineen and G. Hildick-Smith, eds. Philadelphia, PA: Lea & Febiger, p. 191.
32. Alvarez, O. M., P. M. Mertz and W. H. Eaglestein. 1983. *J. Surg. Res.*, 35:142.
33. Dyson, M., S. Young, L. Pendle, D. F. Webster and S. M. Lang. 1988. *J. Invest. Dermatol.*, 91:434–439.
34. Leipzinger, L. S., V. Glushko, B. DiBernardo, F. Shafaie, J. Noble, J. Nichols and O. Alvarez. 1985. *J. Am. Acad. Dermatol.*, 12:409–419.
35. Park, G. B. 1978. *Biomat. Med. Dev. Art. Org.*, 6:1.
36. Tavis, M. J., J. W. Thornton and R. H. Bartlett. 1978. *Surg. Clin. North. Am.*, 58:1223.
37. Pruitt, B. A., Jr. and N. S. Levine. 1984. *Arch. Surg.*, 119:312.
38. Alsbjörn, B. 1984. *Scand. J. Plast. Reconstr. Surg.*, 18:127.
39. Riel, S. de. 1984. In *Burn Wound Coverings, Vol. 1.* D. L. Wise, ed. Boca Raton: CRC Press, Inc., p. 1.
40. Quinn, K. J., J. M. Courtney, J. H. Evans, J. D. S. Gaylor and W. H. Read. 1985. *Biomaterials*, 6:369.
41. Queen, D., J. H. Evans, J. D. S. Gaylor, J. M. Courtney and W. H. Reid. 1987. *Burns*, 13:218.
42. Tavis, M. J., J. W. Thornton, J. H. Harney, E. A. Woodroof and R. H. Bartlett. 1976. *Ann. Surg.*, 184:594.
43. Morykwas, M., J. W. Thornton and R. H. Bartlett. 1987. *Plast. Reconstr. Surg.*, 79:732.
44. Demarchez, M., D. J. Hartmann and M. Prunieras. 1987. *Transplantation*, 43:896.
45. Barnett, S. E. and S. J. Varley. 1987. *Ann. R. Coll. Surg. Engl.*, 69:153–155.
46. Yannas, I. V. 1981. *The Surgical Wound*, P. Dineen, ed., Philadelphia, PA: Lea & Febiger, p. 171.
47. Lommen, E. 1988. *Artificial Skin*. Thesis, University of Groningen, Groningen.
48. Miller, T. A. 1974. *Plast. Reconstr. Surg.*, 53:316.

49. Lamke, L.-O., G. E. Nilsson and H. L. Reithner. 1977. *Burns*, 3:159.

50. Erasmus, M. E. and M. F. Jonkman. 1989. *Burns*, 15:371.

51. Kreis, R. W. and A. F. P. M. Vloemans. 1986. *Proceedings of the First Congress of the European Burns Association,* Groningen.

52. Levine, N. S., R. E. Salisbury, A. D. Mason and B. A. Bruitt. 1984. In *Burn Wound Coverings.* D. L. Wise, ed. Boca Raton: CRC Press, Inc., p. 79.

53. Davenport, P. J., P. L. Dhooghe and A. Yiacoumettis. 1977. *Burns*, 3:225.

54. Winter, G. D. 1971. In *Surgical Dressings and Wound Healing.* K. J. Harkiss, ed. Bradford: Bradford University Press, p. 46.

55. Wilson, G. and G. French. 1987. *Brit. Med. J.,* 294:556.

56. James, J. H. and A. C. H. Watson. 1975. *Brit. J. Plast. Surg.,* 28:107.

57. French, M. L. V., H. E. Eitzen and M. A. Ritter. 1976. *Ann. Surg.,* 184:46.

58. Smith & Nephew Ltd., Technical pamphlet. 1988.

59. Hammond, M. A. 1979. *Nursing Mirror,* 149:38.

60. Crisp, M. 1977. *Nursing Times,* 73:1202.

61. Alper, J. P., E. A. Welch and R. N. Maguire. 1984. *J. Am. Acad. Dermatol.,* 11:858.

62. Chvapil, M., T. A. Chvapil and J. A. Owen. 1987. *J. Trauma,* 27:278.

63. Fisher, L. B. and H. I. Maibach. 1972. *Br. J. Dermatol.,* 86:593.

64. Zitelli, J. A. 1984. *J. Dermatol. Surg. Oncol.,* 10:709.

65. Ehleben, C. M., S. R. May and J. M. Still. 1985. *Burns,* 12:122.

66. Hermans, M. H. E. and R. P. Hermans. 1986. *Burns,* 12:214.

67. Gorse, G. J., and R. L. Messner. 1987. *Arch. Dermatol.,* 123:766.

68. Thomas, S. 1987. *Report of the Welsh Centre for the Quality Control of Surgical Dressings.*

69. Jablonski, K., and H. Tronnier. 1988. *Aktuellen Dermatol.* (in press).

70. Golan, J., A. Eldad, B. Rudensky, Y. Tuchman, N. Sterenberg and N. Ben-Hur. 1985. *Burns,* 11:274.

71. Behar, D., M. Juszynski, N. Ben-Hur, J. Golan, A. Eldad, Y. Tuchman, N. Sterenberg and B. Rudensky. 1986. *J. Biomed. Mater. Res.,* 20:731.

72. Cristofoli, C., M. Lorenzini and S. Furdan. 1986. *Burns,* 12:587.

73. Eldad, A. and Y. Tuchman. 1987. Presented at the *Geneva International Congress of Burn Injuries, June 22–26.*

10

The Application of Synthetic Hydrogels for Cell Culture

SHOJI NAGAOKA, Ph.D.*,1
HIROSHI TANZAWA, Ph.D.*
JIRO SUZUKI, Ph.D.*

ABSTRACT: The adhesion and proliferation of mammalian fibroblasts (Flow 7000) on the surface of hydrophilic [copolymer of N-vinyl-2-pyrrolidone (NVP), methyl methacrylate (MMA)], and hydrophobic [polymethylmethacrylate (PMMA) stereocomplex] hydrogels with a wide range in water content, were studied morphologically and quantitatively.

It was demonstrated that cell proliferation by a static culture method on hydrogels decreased as the water content of the gels increased. However, it should be noted that the cell proliferation on PMMA hydrogels with a high water content is equivalent to that on glass petri dishes. The results obtained in the proliferation of cells on the surface of these hydrogels closely correspond to the state of cell adhesion.

When fresh medium or air was perfused from the side of the PMMA hydrogel membrane opposite to which the cells were proliferating (perfusion method), the cells continued to grow into a higher density than with the conventional static culture method. In the case of fresh medium perfusion, the degree of cell proliferation was dependent upon both the permeability of the membrane and the density of the membrane "scaffolding".

Virus multiplication in the cultured cells increased in proportion to the cell density, while the cell function was similar in both culture methods.

INTRODUCTION

In an *in vitro* culture of normal diploid cells, adhesion and spreading of cells on the substrate is needed for proliferation. As already reported by Rajaraman et al. [1], the morphology of a fibroblast cell during adhesion and growth on a substrate *in vitro* goes through four stages: attachment, growth of filopodia, cytoplasmic webbing, and flattening. These processes are affected by pericellular conditions. The development of a suitable substrate is one of the major steps needed to enhance *in vitro* cell cultures.

Many experimental results and mechanisms for cell adhesion and growth have been reported emphasizing the characteristics of the underlying substrates. It can be concluded that the extent of cellular adhesion is considerably affected by physical and chemical properties of the substrate surface.

While it is known that biocompatibility and permeability for hydrogels are excellent, few studies on the interaction between a hydrogel surface and a cell have been reported [2]. A series of hydrogel membranes with a wide range in water content can be made from various kinds of synthetic polymers, which have recently been developed at the author's laboratory for the purpose of utilizing them as biomedical materials. In the present study, the effects of the nature of the hydrogel substrate on the adhesion and growth of a normal diploid cell were examined by focusing on: (1) chemical composition, especially hydrophobic or hydrophilic; (2) water content; and (3) the effect of nutritional perfusion from the back side of the substrate.

MATERIALS AND METHODS

Synthetic Hydrogel Membranes

Synthetic hydrogel membranes used in this study were prepared and characterized as follows.

Hydrophilic Hydrogels

A cross-linked copolymer of N-vinylpyrrolidone and methylmethacrylate was selected as a nonionic hydrophilic polymeric material. A mixture of N-vinylpyrrolidone and methylmethacrylate, together

---

1Author to whom all correspondence should be addressed.

*Basic Research Laboratories, Toray Industries, Inc., 1111 Tebiro, Kamakura 248, Japan

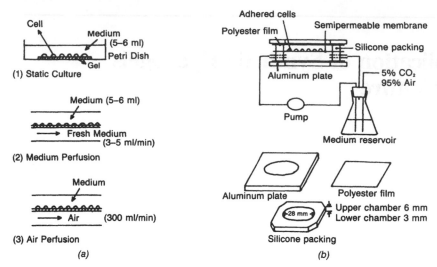

Figure 1. (a) Comparison of different culture methods, and (b) apparatus used for medium-perfusion culture.

with a $2,2^1$-azobis (2,4-dimethylvaleronitrile) initiator and a small amount of a cross-linking agent, was polymerized in the space between two glass plates. A polymer was obtained in the form of a thin sheet, swollen with water. The water content was regulated by changing the ratio of the comonomers. These hydrogel membranes had a water content of from 20 to 90%. The water content (%) of the membranes (W) was determined as follows:

$$W(\%) = \frac{\text{weight of wet membrane} - \text{weight of dried membrane}}{\text{weight of wet membrane}} \times 100$$

Hydrophobic Hydrogels

It is difficult to prepare a water-swollen membrane of a hydrophobic polymer such as polymethylmethacrylate in an ordinary process. However, we found a unique method for preparing polymethylmethacrylate (PMMA) membranes with high water content by utilizing the so-called stereocomplex formation between isotactic and syndiotactic PMMA. A dimethylsulfoxide (DMSO) solution of a mixture of isotactic and syndiotactic PMMA was found to exhibit a thermoreversible sol-gel transition due to stereocomplex formation. The solution was heated above its gelation temperature and was poured between two pre-heated glass plates. When the sandwiched solution was cooled, it changed to a gel which had enough strength to be held by hand. The gel was immersed into cold water containing ice, and a hydrogel membrane of PMMA was formed by replacing the DMSO in the gel by water. These membranes were transparent and uniform, although they contained a large amount of water.

Isotactic PMMA (isotacticity of more than 95%,

polymerized anionically in toluene using a Grignard reagent) and syndiotactic PMMA (syndiotacticity 55%, heterotacticity 32%, isotacticity 13%, polymerized by the conventional free-radical process) were used in this study. The stereoregularity of these polymers was determined from a triad NMR spectrum. The average viscosity molecular weight of these polymers was in the range of 1.30×10^5 to 1.45×10^6.

The ratio of the mixture of iso-polymer to syndio-polymer used was 1:5 by weight with the molecular weights of the polymers selected for suitable membrane formation. The water content of the membranes was adjusted by changing the polymer concentration of the DMSO solution in a range of 10 to 40%.

The water permeability of these membranes is very high compared to that of the commercially available cellulosic membrane. The molecular weight cut-off of these membranes was about 20,000. Details of these PMMA membrane properties have been reported elsewhere [3].

Cell Culture

A human neonatal foreskin diploid cell line (Flow 7000) was used in the form of a cell suspension. Eagle's MEM with 10% fetal calf serum was used as the medium for the cell suspension, which contained about 4×10^5 cells/ml.

Figure 1(a) shows the schematic representation of the cell culture methods. The static culture was achieved as follows: The cell suspension was poured over a sheet of hydrogel membrane placed in a petri dish, and was incubated at 37°C under air containing 5% CO_2. Two hours after inoculation (the attachment of the cells was accomplished about one hour after inoculation), the membrane was washed with phosphate-buffered saline and fixed with 2.5% glutaraldehyde normal saline solution.

The morphology of the cells adhering to the substrate was observed by phase-contrast microscopy and scanning electron microscopy. The fixation was done only to cultures terminated for photos.

After 48 hours of incubation at 37°C, cells proliferating on the surface of the membrane were observed with phase-contrast microscopy. The amount of cellular protein on the substrate was determined by Lowry's method after the proliferated cells were dissolved in 0.1N NaOH and the serum protein absorbed by the substrate was subtracted [4].

On the other hand, the perfusion culture with a membrane-type culture container shown in Figure 1(b) was perfused by air containing 5% CO_2 (300 ml/min), or by fresh medium (4ml/min) from the side opposite to which the cells grew. The thickness of the cell suspension above the membrane was 6mm.

RESULTS AND DISCUSSION

The Effect of the Water Content of Hydrogels on Cell Proliferation in a Static Cell Culture

In Figure 2, the amount of proliferated cells on the surface of the hydrophilic and hydrophobic hydrogels, 48 hours after inoculation, is plotted as a function of the water content of the hydrogels. In all the hydrogels, an increase of the water content caused a decrease in cell proliferation.

It is known that the "scaffolding" to which cells adhere is necessary for the proliferation of cultured cells. However, the mechanism by which the cells adhere to the "scaffolding" and proliferate remains unclear. One hypothesis on the cohesion between cells and substrate is as follows: Sugar proteins such as fibronectin in serum adhere to the substrate surface and change their higher order structures, then they create an integral connection with the receptor on the cellular surface [5]. An increase of the water content of the hydrogel results in a reduction of available polymer parenchyma, specifically the solid polymer part of the hydrogel, and also results in a decrease in the protein-substrate interaction. It should be noted that the cell proliferation on PMMA hydrogels with high water content is equivalent to that on a glass petri dish.

Figures 3(a,b) show phase contrast micrographs of proliferated cells. As shown in Figure 3(a), cells on the hydrophilic hydrogel (W = 45.7%) did not develop normal spindle-like structures. By contrast, cells on PMMA hydrogels with a similar water content (W = 51.5%) developed normal structures, as shown in Figure 3(b). Figures 4(a,b) are scanning electron micrographs of cells on the surface of the substrates 2 hours after inoculation. It is necessary for the substrate to have as much rigidity as possible to enable it to withstand stress caused by the deformity and extension of cells [6]. Compared to the amorphous hydrophilic substrate, PMMA stereocomplex

hydrogel has hydrophobic, rigid, micro-crystalline parts [3], where the proteins such as fibronectin are able to adhere easily through its high interfacial energy. Consequently, adhesion of the cell and alteration of the cell shape are promoted, leading to favorable conditions for active DNA synthesis and cellular proliferation.

Perfusion Culture by Using PMMA Hydrogel Membranes

The Effect of Perfusion on Cell Proliferation

The merit of culturing cells on a hydrogel membrane is that perfusion of a medium from the opposite side of the membrane makes it possible to supply oxygen and nutrients, and to eliminate metabolic wastes through the membrane. Therefore, we examined the effect of a perfusion on an *in vitro* cell culture by using a PMMA hydrogel membrane.

Figure 5 shows the amount of proliferated cells on the surface of a PMMA hydrogel membrane with a 73% water content and a 100 μm thickness in both static and perfusion cultures. For comparison, the results obtained with a glass petri dish and polystyrene petri dish are also shown. It is evident that perfusion from the backside of the membrane produces excellent results in cell proliferation. For example:

(1) The maximum amount of cells was several times higher than it was on the glass and polystyrene, with the cells proliferating in multiple layers on the surface of the gel.

(2) A maximum number of cells can be maintained for more than 2 weeks.

(3) The cells proliferate very quickly.

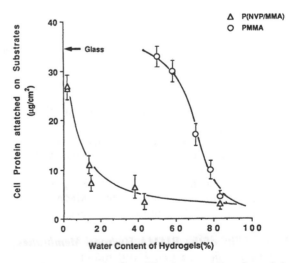

Figure 2. Amount of cell proliferation on the surface of the hydrophilic [P(MMA-co-NVP)] and hydrophobic (PMMA) hydrogel 48 hours after inoculation by static method as a function of their water contents. Mean ± SD (n = 5).

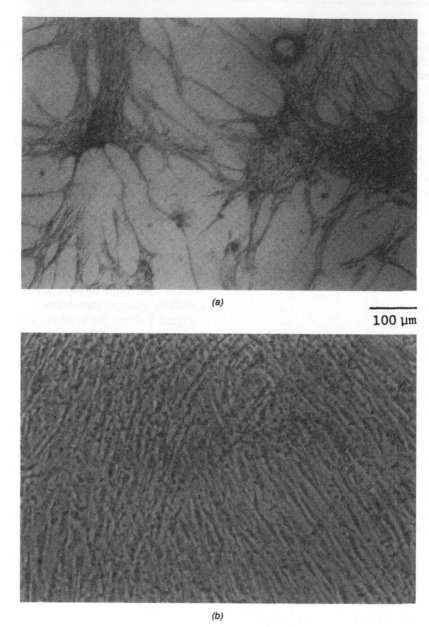

100 μm

Figure 3. Phase-contrast micrographs of Flow 7000 cells cultured by static method for 2 days on the surface of P(MMA-co-NVP) gel (water content = 45.7%) (a) and PMMA stereocomplex gel (water content = 51.5%) (b).

The molecular weight cut-off of the membrane is approximately 20,000. This indicates that constant maintenance by exchange of oxygen and soluble substances with middle and low molecular weight is effective in cell proliferation.

Figure 6 shows the phase contrast micrograph of the proliferated Flow 7000 cells on the PMMA hydrogel after perfusion of the culture for 14 days.

Permeability of the PMMA Hydrogel Membranes and Their Effect on Cell Proliferation in a Perfusion Culture

Substance exchange through the membrane is not only affected by the composition of the membranes, but also by other factors such as pressure, flow rate, and thickness of membrane. We investigated water content and membrane thickness, which have a major effect on the permeability of isotropic membranes like those made of PMMA hydrogel, in relation to cell proliferation.

MEMBRANE THICKNESS

Figure 7 shows the relationship between membrane thickness of a PMMA hydrogel (Iso/Syn = 1/5) with a constant water content of 65% and the amount of proliferated cells. The thinner membrane showed high permeability, which is advantageous for cell proliferation. Membrane-thickness dependency was seen in

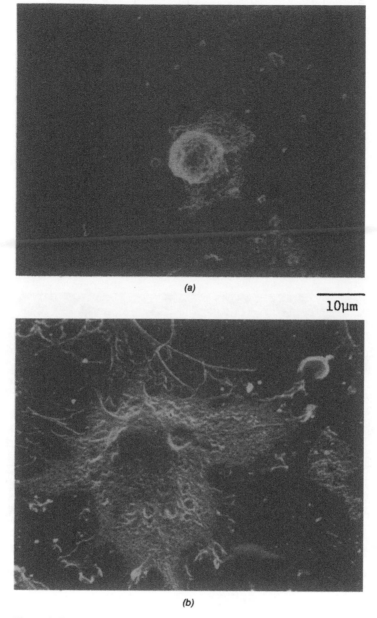

Figure 4. Scanning electron micrographs of a Flow 7000 cell cultured for 2 hours on the surface of P(MMA-co-NVP) gel (a) and PMMA stereocomplex gel (b). The water content of these hydrogels are given in Figure 3.

thicknesses ranging from 25 to 200 μm, indicating that the use of a thinner membrane allows more cell proliferation. Naturally, a similar membrane-thickness dependency was never seen in the static cultures.

When air containing 5% carbon dioxide was used as a perfusion substance, approximately twice the amount of cell proliferation, in comparison to the glass petri dishes, was observed. In this case, membrane-thickness dependency similar to that in the medium-perfusion cultures was not observed, although oxygen was supplemented to the cells through the membrane, and permeation rate of oxygen was related to membrane thickness. Flow 7000 cells which form a fibroblast can be successfully cultured through conventional cultivation and do not require so much

oxygen. Consequently, it is possible to supplement the necessary amount of oxygen even through thick membranes with low oxygen permeability.

WATER CONTENT

Figure 8 shows the amount of proliferated Flow 7000 cells on the surface of the PMMA hydrogels (membrane thickness; 100 ± 8 μm) in the perfusion culture as a function of water content of the membrane. The proliferation of the cells rose with an increase of the membrane water content of up to 80%, but began to decrease once the water content exceeded this value. This result may be attributable to the following reason—though increased water content of the

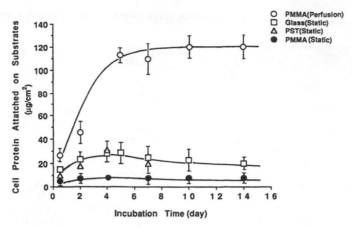

Figure 5. Growth of Flow 7000 cells on the surface of PMMA stereocomplex gel, glass, and polystyrene petri dish (Falcon®): ○, PMMA stereocomplex gel (medium perfusion); ●, PMMA stereocomplex gel (static); □, glass petri dish (static); △, polystyrene petri dish (static). The water content and the membrane thickness of PMMA stereocomplex gel used were 73% and 120 μm, respectively.

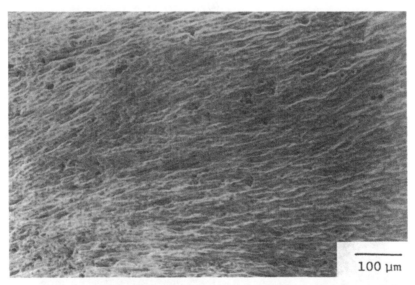

Figure 6. Phase-contrast micrograph of Flow 7000 cells cultured by medium perfusion method for 2 weeks on the surface of PMMA stereocomplex gel.

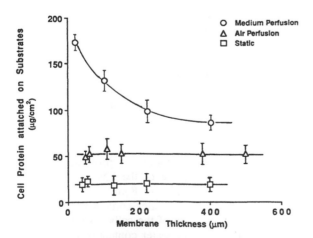

Figure 7. Relationship between membrane thickness in a PMMA hydrogel (Iso/Syn = 1/5) with a constant water content of 65 ± 2% and the amount of proliferated cells on it by static and perfusion method for 1 week.

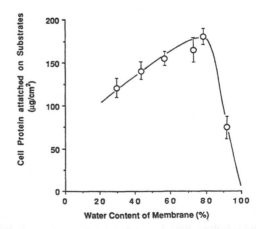

Figure 8. Amount of proliferated Flow 7000 cells on the surface of the PMMA hydrogels (membrane thickness = 100 ± 8 μm) in the perfusion culture as a function of water content of the membrane. Mean ± SD ($n = 5$).

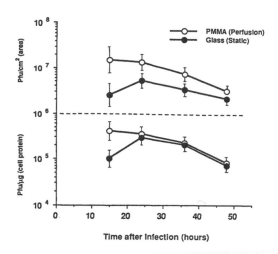

Figure 9. Comparison of Vesicular Stomatitis Virus reproduction in cells (in plaque forming unit, PfU) cultured for 5 days on the PMMA stereocomplex gel by medium perfusion method and on the glass petri dish by static method. The amount of cells on the surface of the PMMA stereocomplex gel is 3.7 times as much as that on glass.

substrate reduces the "scaffolding" necessary for cell adhesion and growth, it improves the permeability of the membrane.

The overall effect on the cell proliferation would be determined by the balance between these two opposing effects. When the water content is low, the permeability effect is dominant. But once the water content exceeds 80%, the nutritional perfusion effect is offset by a significant drop in "scaffolding" area. With the optimum water content (which is 80% in the case of PMMA hydrogel membrane), the amount of proliferated cells in the perfusion culture was about ten times higher than those of the static cultures.

Viability of Cells Proliferated on the Surface of a PMMA Hydrogel Membrane by Profusion Cultures

The method whereby viruses are inoculated into the cell culture, allowing secondary viruses to proliferate, is similar to the production process of various vaccines, and this method makes it possible to investigate the cell activity. Figure 9 shows the results of an experiment where Flow 7000 cells were infected with about 4 MOI (Multiplicity of Infection; the number of virus particles infected per cell) by using a Vesicular Stomatitis Virus. In this case, cells with higher activity produced more viruses [as indicated by plaque formation unit (PfU)].

In Figure 9, the abscissa represents the time after infection. The ordinate represents the degree of virus reproduction in the proliferated cells per unit area of

culture substrate for the upper curves and per unit cell protein (which means per amount of cells) for the lower curves. It was observed that the amount of reproduced virus per unit area of PMMA membrane (water content, 73%) was greater than that of the glass because the amount of cells proliferated on the PMMA membrane was 3.7 times higher than that of the glass. Development of such perfusion-culture devices using membranes with superior cell compatibility could greatly facilitate the production of biological products through cell-culture methods.

However, the amount of virus per amount of cells was the same for both substrates except immediately after infection, when occasionally the virus reproduction by the cells growing on the PMMA membrane was greater than that of the glass. This result suggests that the activity of the cells cultured on the PMMA membrane by the perfusion method is similar to that of the cells on glass.

CONCLUSIONS

Cell proliferation on hydrogels by the conventional static method decreased with an increase in the water content of the gels. The cell proliferation on the hydrophobic PMMA hydrogels was much greater than that on the hydrophilic copolymer of NVP and MMA hydrogels with a similar water content, and it is thought that the morphological change of the cells on the PMMA hydrogels correlates closely with their excellent proliferation.

Having produced a perfusion culture by utilizing the permeability of the PMMA hydrogel membranes with water contents up to 80%, cells continued to proliferate into much higher densities than those possible in the static culture method, though cell function was similar in both groups.

REFERENCES

1. Rajaraman, R. 1974. "The Morphology of a Fibroblast Adhered on Substrates", *Experimental Cell Res.*, 88:327.

2. Rosen, J. J. and Schway, M. B. 1979. "The Effect of Charged Substrate on the Cell Adhesion", *ACS Organic Coating and Plastic Chemistry*, 40:636.

3. Sakai, Y. and Tanzawa, H. 1979. "Poly(methyl methacrylate) Membranes", *J. Appl. Polymer Sci.*, 23:2089.

4. Lowry, O. H. 1951. "Protein Measurement with the Folin Phenol Reagent", *J. Biol. Chem.* 193:265.

5. Aoyama, H. and Takeichi, M. 1981. "Fibronectin", *Chemistry*, 36:95.

6. Maroudas, N. G. 1973. "Chemical and Mechanical Requirements for Fibroblast Adhesion", *Nature*, 244:353.

11

Chemically Modified Collagenous Amniotic Layer as a Wound Dressing Material

T. P. SASTRY*
K. PANDURANGA RAO*[,1]

ABSTRACT: The amniotic layer was carefully separated from human placenta and purified. 8 × 10 cm pieces of the amniotic layer were soaked in a solution of an antibacterial agent and subsequently cross-linked with glutaraldehyde. The amount of drug bound was estimated and found to be 40 microgrammes of sulfadiazine per 10 cm^{-2} and 120 microgrammes silver per 10 cm^2 indicating that silver was bound to the protein as well. The efficacy of the modified amniotic layer was tested by inflicting artificial cut wounds in the rabbits. The modified amniotic layers were inserted in the incision wounds, and the biopsies were taken at regular intervals for histopathological studies. The amniotic layers enhanced the healing; it appears that the sheets themselves transform into vascular spaces and do the healing to the surface in a remodelled fashion. Further, it was observed that there was no blood clot, exudate, or acute inflammatory reaction.

INTRODUCTION

Human collagenous amniotic membranes were used as early as 1910 by Davis [1] as a substitute for skin and by Sabella [2] in 1913 for the treatment of small skin defects. Chao et al.[3] were the first to use the dried and alcohol-preserved amniotic membrane for craniotomy wounds, to cover extensive dural defects and to prevent adhesions. Recently, attention has been drawn to the possible use of amnion as a biological dressing in the treatment of burns [4–7]. Allografts of skin from donors and cadavers were popularised by Brown et al. [8]. Bhatnagar et al. [9] suggested the use of xenografts from the intestines of cattle.

[1]Author to whom correspondence should be addressed.

*Polymer Division, Central Leather Research Institute, Adyar, Madras 600 020, India

The main drawback of using such membranes appears to be the difficulty of assuring adequate supplies and the difficulty of preserving them. Further, they could not be used for the management of infected wounds and burns. Dino et al. [4] studied the effects of human amniotic membranes in burns and suggested the organization of an amnion bank. 100% bacterial contamination occurred when the amnion in saline solution was kept at room temperature. Addition of 200,000 units of crystalline penicillin improved the viability to six weeks, especially if stored at 4°C. Rao et al. [10] used dry bovine and human amnion as a biological dressing. These authors claimed that the dried membranes obtained have a life span of at least 9 months. However, the dried amnion dressings will not adhere to the wound properly and the wound fluids will not be absorbed efficiently.

In the present investigation, we developed a novel technique for the preparation of collagenous amniotic wound and burn dressings, with the active drug covalently bonded to the membrane to ensure the controlled release of the drug. This alleviates the earlier difficulties of using dried amniotic membrane as well as the need for the maintenance of amniotic banks. Further, the amniotic wound dressing developed in present investigation can be used efficiently even in the infected wounds and burns.

MATERIALS AND METHODS

The placentas were collected aseptically from a nearby maternity hospital. The amnion layer was separated manually, then cleansed of blood in running water and thoroughly rinsed in isotonic solution.

Cross-Linking of Amniotic Membranes

Different concentrations of 25% glutaraldehyde, i.e., 0.04%, 0.08%, 0.1%, 0.2%, 0.3% were used along with 0.5% sodium chloride and 0.01% sodium

Table 1. Tensile strength and shrinkage temperature of amniotic membrane cross-linked with different concentrations of basic chromium sulfate.

Sl. No.	% Chrome Powder	Tensile Strength (kg/sq cm)	Elongation at Break (Percentage)	Temperature (°C)
1	0.04	26.10	80.00	120
2	0.08	46.30	65.70	120
3	0.10	117.70	48.95	121
4	0.20	58.15	63.90	121
5	0.30	53.00	45.50	121
6	0.40	43.50	46.50	121
7	Blank	38.25	99.36	64

acetate solutions to evaluate the optimum percentage of glutaraldehyde—that percentage which will impart maximum tensile strength to the amniotic layer. The pH was maintained at 7.4 and the amniotic layers were stirred in the solutions occasionally for three hours.

Similar studies were also done using the basic chromium sulfate as a cross-linking agent. Amniotic layers were treated in different concentrations of basic chromium sulfate solutions, i.e., 0.04%, 0.08%, 0.1%, 0.2%, 0.3% along with 0.5% sodium chloride. The pH was maintained at 3.2 and amniotic layers were stirred in solutions occasionally for three hours.

Later, the layers were removed from the solutions and rinsed in water thoroughly. Tensile strength and shrinkage temperature of the amniotic layers were then estimated. The results are given in Tables 1 and 2.

Coupling of Antibacterial Agent onto the Modified Amniotic Membrane

Optimum concentration of glutaraldehyde was used in all the subsequent experiments. The amniotic layers were cut into 10 × 8 cm pieces and placed in 0.1% sodium sulfadiazine solution for 3 hours. Later, the sulfadiazine solution was decanted and 0.08% glutaraldehyde solution was added to the amniotic layer. The layers were shaken for 3 hours. Thereafter, the layers were put in 0.1% silver nitrate solution for half an hour in the dark with intermittent thorough shaking. The layers were then washed with water and sterilized with ethylene dioxide. The layers were sealed in glass tubes containing isopropanol (98%).

Sterility Test of the Membranes

Sterility tests were done both aerobically and anaerobically using standard techniques [11]. No growth was seen in the respective media.

Estimation of Bound Silver Sulfadiazine

(1) Silver was estimated by atomic absorption spectrometric method.
(2) Estimation of sulfadiazine was done by AOAC (1980) method [12]. The amount of bound silver and sulfadiazine for 10 sq cm sheets of collagenous amniotic membrane are given in Table 3.

In vivo Experiments

Twelve rabbits were used for this experimental study. Hair was shaved (about 1 sq in area) on the right and left hind limb of each rabbit. A linear incision half an inch long and half an inch deep was made surgically under aseptic conditions on both hind limbs of the rabbit. In all the rabbits, the left side was taken as control and the right side was retained as test.

The control incisions were sutured with silk, after controlling the bleeding. In the experimental ones, a suitable piece of amniotic layer was cut and inserted horizontally in the wound. The skin was drawn up over the amniotic membrane and then sutured with silk. Biopsies from both control and test groups were taken periodically. The biopsy material consisted of pieces taken across the wound measuring less than 1/2

Table 2. Tensile strength and shrinkage temperature of amniotic membrane cross-linked with glutaraldehyde (25%).

Sl. No.	% of Glutaraldehyde Solution	Tensile Strength (kg/sq cm)	Elongation at Break (Percentage)	Shrinkage Temp. (°C)
1	0.04	30.65	42.30	82
2	0.08	83.50	55.50	83
3	0.10	67.25	42.05	83
4	0.20	44.50	63.45	82
5	0.30	27.25	126.45	82
6	Blank	38.25	99.36	64

Table 3. Amount* of bound silver and sulfadiazine in the amniotic membrane.

Amount of bound silver	: 120 microgrammes/10 sq cm
Amount of bound sulfadiazine :	40 microgrammes/10 sq cm

*The results are of an average of 6 different samples.

cm × 1/2 cm × 1/2 cm (length, depth and breadth). These were processed and embedded in paraffin, then the sections were stained with hematoxylin and eosin and, in some cases, Van Gieson stain.

RESULTS AND DISCUSSION

Histopathological Observations

The importance of tissue reactions to implant materials is becoming increasingly apparent as new materials and devices become available. It is essential to have an in-depth understanding of inflammatory and foreign-body reactions of implants before using them. Hence, a systematic wound-healing histopathological evaluation of the amniotic membrane was carried out in the present studies, using a rabbit model. Histologic examination of tissues across the wound revealed the following facts.

After 48 hours, the cavity of the control wound was filled with blood clot (Figure 1) and early inflammatory changes were visible in the margin.

In contrast, endothelialization and vascularization can be seen in the experimental wound by the third day [Figure 7(a,b)]. The endothelial cells are visible lining the vascularized sheets, which are seen as zigzag eosinophilic sheets.

After four days, it can be observed that there was down-growth of the epidermis (Figure 2) over the edge of the control wound. Blood clotting was also seen on the left side of the incision.

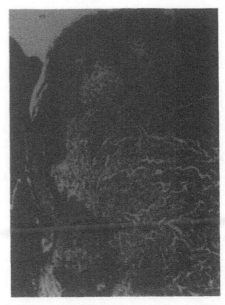

Figure 2. Wound over 4 days old. There is a downgrowth of the epidermis over the edge of the wound. The clot is seen along side on the left (135×).

After six days, the experimental wound was observed to have an intrinsic, horizontally oriented blood supply to the sheet (Figure 8).

After nine days, the epithelial union has occurred in the control wound, with a slight depression at the surface. The epithelium was defective at A and B (Figure 3).

No such defects were seen in the experimental wound. Horizontal vascularity was visible along the side of the amniotic layer. Here, the amniotic layer has acted as a scaffolding for the pattern (Figure 9).

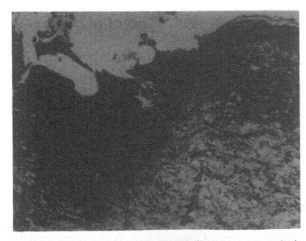

Figure 1. Photomicrograph of the wound after 48 hrs. The cavity is filled with blood clot. Early inflammatory changes are seen in the margin (135×).

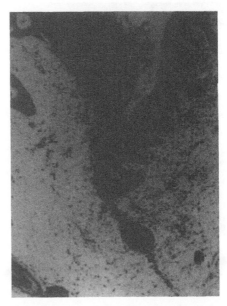

Figure 3. Histologic section of the wound after 9 days. The epithelial union has occurred with a slight depression over the surface. The epithelium is defective at A and B. C denotes the scab (135×).

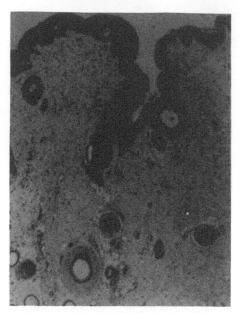

Figure 4. After 12 days, a depressed scar is observed and the defective epithelium is seen (A). The vertical orientation of the scar is observed with no remodelling (135 ×).

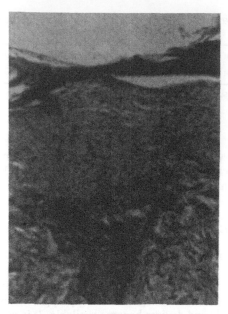

Figure 6. After 18 days, healing is complete and horizontal remodelling has occurred in the upper corium. Vertical fibroblastic disposition is seen in the lower corium (135 ×).

On the twelfth day, a depressed scar (Figure 4) and deficiency of epithelium was observed in the control wound. Vertical orientation of scarring was also seen, and no remodeling had taken place.

This contrasts with the horizontal orientation of the fibroblasts in the experimental wound [Figure 10(a)]. A slight depression of epidermis was observed. Figure 10(b) clearly illustrates the compact horizontally oriented collagen fibers and some amount of remodelling of the scar.

After fifteen days, healing in the control wound was nearly complete (Figure 5) but an epithelial depression at the point of injury was clearly visible.

In the experimental wound (Figure 11) the overhealed scar was observed and the incision track was absent. The collagen formation was dense and not fibrillar.

After eighteen days, healing in the control wound was complete, and horizontal remodelling could be seen in the upper corium (Figure 6).

In the experimental wound, complete horizontal orientation of fibroblasts was visible after eighteen days (Figure 12) and the epidermis was found to be intact. Even the slight depression of the epidermis over the scar, which was seen in the control wound, was not seen in the experimental wound.

Cross-Linking of Placental Collagen

The tensile properties of the artificial wound cover dressings are very important for the management of wounds and burns. Amniotic membrane by itself is very weak in its mechanical strength. Cross-linking methods are necessary to improve its mechanical properties. Human amniotic membrane was cross-linked using both glutaraldehyde and chrome to improve its tensile strength. Glutaraldehyde is widely used in protein chemistry as a cross-linking agent and it reacts primarily with the amino groups of proteins in biological systems. It has been used in the manufacture of medical devices, tissue bioprostheses, and as a sterilizing agent. Glutaraldehyde is also being used for improving the mechanical strength of collagen, which will be controlled by the degree and type of cross-

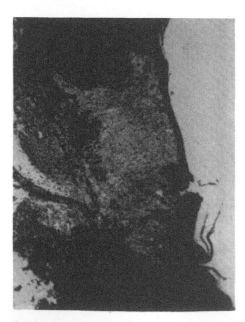

Figure 5. After 15 days, the healing is nearly complete. The scar has included an island of the epithelium. Below, the persistent vertically disposed vascularized granulation tissue is present (135 ×).

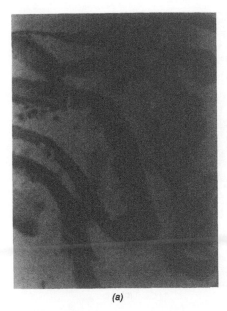

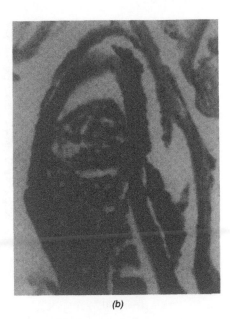

(a)

(b)

Figure 7. (a) Photomicrograph showing the amniotic layer placed after 3 days (135×). Note endothelialization and vascularization. (b) After 3 days (150×), the endothelial cells can be discerned lining the vascularized sheets which are seen as zigzag eosinophilic sheets.

links introduced. In the present study, we have introduced cross-links by reagents such as glutaraldehyde and basic chromium sulfate. The variations of tensile strength with the increase in the concentrations of glutaraldehyde and chromium sulfate are given in Tables 1 and 2. Collagen cross-linked with 0.1% basic chromium sulfate gave a highest tensile strength of 117.7 kg/sq cm. The tensile strength reduced from 117.7 to 43 kg/sq cm by further increase in the chromium sulfate concentration. The shrinkage temperature was

found to be 121°C, which agreed very well with standard results.

In the case of glutaraldehyde, 0.08% gave the best tensile strength of 83.5 kg/sq cm. The tensile strength decreased to 27.25 kg/sq cm by a further increase in the glutaraldehyde concentration to 0.3%. In both cases, the tensile strength shows a maximum and then falls off.

The results suggest that collagen is an elastic polymer that tends to be brittle when highly cross-

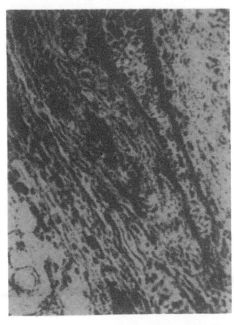

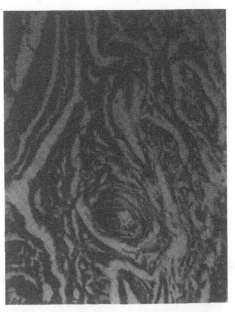

Figure 8. Horizontally oriented intrinsic blood supply to the sheet is seen (135×) after 6 days.

Figure 9. Note horizontal vascularity and arrangement of the collagen along side of the amniotic layer almost in its pattern (135×) after 9 days.

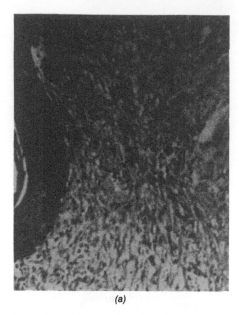 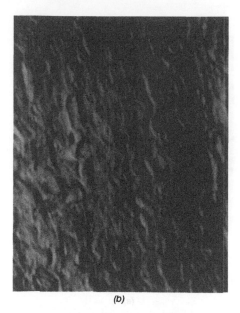

(a)   (b)

Figure 10. (a) After 12 days, there is a slight depression in the epidermis. Fibroblasts are oriented horizontally (135×). (b) After 12 days (150×), compact horizontally oriented collagen fibers and cells are seen. Some amount of remodelling of the structure of the scar is also seen.

linked. A glutaraldehyde-cross-linked amniotic layer showed a shrinkage temperature of 82–83°C. The optimum concentrations of chromium and glutaraldehyde were found to be 0.1 and 0.08% respectively, in regard to getting the highest tensile strength for the amnion layer. The optimum concentrations of cross-linking agents are reached when amplification of imperfections due to brittleness offsets any increase in strength gained by more cross-links. As the concentrations of cross-linking agents increase, the number of cross-linking sites per gram of collagen increase,

and the region of high cross-link density penetrates deeper into the fiber. In all our subsequent studies, we have used glutaraldehyde as a cross-linking agent at 0.08% concentration. It is well known that glutaraldehyde cross-linking exhibits a better blood compatibility. Glutaraldehyde introduces more cross-links, thereby yielding highly cross-linked collagen which is more resistant to bioattack than other cross-linking reagents. On the other hand, there is a controversy about toxicity of Cr^{3+}, but despite this glutaraldehyde is a promising cross-linking agent for biomaterials.

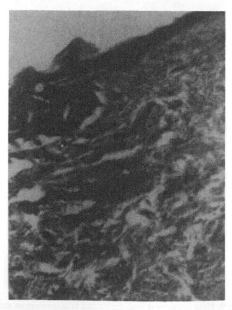

Figure 11. The over-healed scar after 15 days. The collagen is dense and the incision track is not seen (135×).

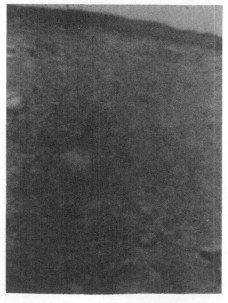

Figure 12. Horizontal orientation of the fibroblasts has occurred. Intact epidermis is seen after 18 days (135×).

Further, it was found that after cross-linking, amniotic membranes could be stored more than three years without any bacterial contamination.

In vivo Studies

The efficacy of the chemically modified human amnion has been established using rabbits as model animals. Incision wounds were treated as given in the experimental group. The following observations were made on the rabbit models which were treated by amniotic membranes, as compared to control. In the normal healing process, perpendicular remodelling of the wound incision is generally seen. Epidermal dipping is seen until the completion of the healing, and it is the blood clot which glues the cut surfaces. It takes a very long time for parallel remodelling to occur.

In test animals which were treated with amniotic membranes, it was observed that the amniotic layer acted as a scaffolding between the two cut surfaces, and that there was no dipping effect in one or both edges of the epidermis, depending on the contour of test surface of the animal. The graft gave some stability to the wound during the healing process. Being a very thin graft and the nutrients being diffusible, substances had a shorter distance to travel. In the healing process, the spaces were vascularized and contained blood. The interspaces induced the fibroblastic reaction. It looks as though the sheets themselves transformed into vascular spaces and did the healing in a remodelled fashion, parallel to the surface. There was no blood clot or exudate observed. No acute inflammatory reaction was seen. Therefore, it was inferred that the healing appears to be better after amniotic layer insertion.

The management of open or infected wounds still remains a difficult problem. The chemically modified amniotic membranes prepared by our method open up new potential avenues for commercial development. Keeping these avenues in view, this material was tried clinically for the healing of chronic ulcers in leprosy patients. It was found out that the modified amniotic membranes hastened the healing. Detailed clinical data will be reported elsewhere.

REFERENCES

1. Davis, J. S. 1910. "Skin Transplantation", with review of 50 Cases at John Hopkins Hospital JNH Report 15:307.
2. Sabella, N. 1913. "Use of the Fetal Membranes in Skin Grafting", *Med. Rec.*, NY 83:478.
3. Chao, Y. C., S. S. Humphry and W. A. Penfield. 1940. "A New Method of Preventing Adhesions: The Use of Amnioplasts in Craniotomy Wounds", *Br. Med. J.*, 1:517.
4. Dino, B. R., G. G. Eufemio and M. S. Devilla, "Human Amnion: The Establishment of an Amnion Bank and its Practical Applications in Surgery", *J. Phillip. Med. Ass.*, 42:357.
5. Robson, M. C., Krizec, T. J., N. Koss and J. L. Somberg. 1973. "Amniotic Membranes as a Temporary Wound Dressing", *Surg. Gynecol. Obstet.*, 136:904.
6. Colocho, G., W. P. Graham, A. E. Greene, D. W. Matheson and D. Lynch. 1974. "Human Amniotic Membrane as a Physiologic Wound Dressing", *Arch. Surg.*, 109:370.
7. Walker, A. B., D. R. Cooney and J. E. Allen. 1976. "Use of Fresh Amnion as a Burn Dressing", *J. Pediatric Surg.*, 12:391.
8. Brown, J. B., M. P. Fryer, P. Randall and M. Lu. 1953. "Postmortem Homografts as Biological Dressings for Extensive Burns and Denuded Areas", *Ann. Surg.*, 138:618.
9. Bhatnagar, S. K., R. Krishnan, T. C. Goel and Mahendrakumar. 1981. "Utility of Collagen Sheet as Skin Substitute", *J. Plast. Surg.*, 14:23.
10. Rao, T. V. and V. Chandrasekhram. 1981. "Use of Dry Human and Bovine Amnion as Biological Dressing", *Arch. Surg.*, 116:891.
11. 1980. *British Pharmacopoeia 2*, A186–A194.
12. 1980. *Official Methods of Analysis of the Association of Official Analytical Chemists, 13th Ed.* Washington, DC: AOAC, p. 631.

12

Composites of Collagen with Synthetic Polymers for Biomedical Applications

RITU BHATNAGAR*
ALOK R. RAY*,1

ABSTRACT The present review is concerned with the significance of and prospects for the use of biomaterials composed of a natural biopolymer, collagen, and synthetic polymers for biomedical applications. There is potential to produce hydrogels and composites tailor-made for specific clinical requirements. The necessity of obtaining a biocompatible material with reasonable tensile strength, tear strength, and resiliency is emphasized.

INTRODUCTION

Collagen is a potentially useful, naturally occurring biomaterial whose structure and modes of polymerization have been extensively studied [1,2]. A number of reviews on the chemistry and biology of collagen and the use of collagen as a biomaterial are available [3,4]. However, to date there is no review concerning the composites of synthetic polymers with collagen. This chapter reviews the research of the last ten years aimed at the preparation of implantable composite materials made from collagen with synthetic polymers.

Collagen is a major constituent of the connective tissue of skin, tendons, ligaments, cartilage, dentin and bone of all multicellular organisms. Collagen confers to the connective tissue many properties, of which the most important are its mechanical properties like strength and resiliency, the activation of coagulation of blood and a role in cellular growth [5,6]. These functions—along with two other characteristics, biocompatibility and biodegradability—have for many years led scientists to envisage biomaterials constituted principally of this protein.

Collagen is an excellent prosthetic substance in cases where regeneration of tissue is possible but inappropriate, and when the material is required to retain constant strength and shape within the body for a prolonged period [7]. Reconstituted collagen has been investigated for different applications including dialysis membrane, wound dressings and vitreous implants, and has been found to possess minimum antigenicity [8,9]. While native collagen fibres are known to possess high tensile strength, the chemical treatment necessary for isolation results in a non-fibrous gel with poor mechanical properties [10]. One major problem with the use of reconstituted collagen is the difficulty encountered in obtaining a film which can be handled easily without tearing. In such cases, synthetic polymers are more effective. The primary characteristics of a polymer to be used in biomedical applications are (a) it must have the chemical, physical and mechanical properties necessary to perform its function; (b) it must be reproducibly obtained as a pure material; (c) it must be able to be fabricated into the desired form without being degraded or adversely changed; (d) it must be sterilizable without a change in properties or form; and (e) it must exhibit no alteration of physical, chemical or mechanical properties when in contact with the biological environment [11].

A simple synthetic polymer is usually poor in tissue affinity, and is not easy to keep stationary at a given site. Such a material, if implanted at a site where force is applied at all times or which is in constant contact with the surroundings, is often dislocated. Thus, it is conceivable that bonding or mixing collagen with a synthetic polymer might produce a new material which combines the merits of both its components. These materials differ from synthetic polymers in their high tissue compatibility, and from collagen alone in that they do not undergo assimilation and absorption but hold a uniform shape and strength on implantation. The most common complication that arises with synthetic applications is the possibility of carcinogenesis in the later stages of implantation. The

1Author to whom correspondence should be sent.

*Centre for Biomedical Engineering, Indian Institute of Technology, and All India Institute of Medical Sciences, New Delhi 110016, India

Table 1. Types of collagen.

Type	Composition	Distribution
I	[α1 (I)]₂α2	Skin, tendon, bone, cornea
II	[α1 (II)]₃	Cartilage, vertebral disc, vitreous body
III	[α1 (III)]₃	Fetal skin, cardiovascular system
IV	[α1 (IV)]₃	Basement membrane

advantage of using a polymeric material that contains a natural constituent resembling tissue is that it is well-tolerated over long periods of time. Such bioactive polymeric materials are required for percutaneous devices, fixation of artificial organs, and some drug targetting as well.

COLLAGEN: STRUCTURE AND MECHANICAL PROPERTIES

The properties of this protein that make it suitable for fabrication into medical products are directly dependent on the characteristics of its amino acid composition, and the sequence which determines its three-dimensional structure and its interaction in the environment, among other mechanical properties.

The basic structure-unit of collagen is tropocollagen which consists of three strands, each about 1000 residues long. The chain composition depends on the type of collagen (Table 1).

There are hydrogen bonds between —NH groups of glycine residues on each strand and —CO— group on the other two strands. The triple-stranded helix is stabilized by cooperative interactions. Denatured collagen polypeptides assume a random coil configuration, and this material is gelatin.

Mature collagen, as found in nature, is insoluble because of inter- and intra-molecular covalent interactions that convert collagen into an infinite network of monomeric elements. The mechanical properties of

collagen are dependent on its chemical constitution, cross-links and helical structure.

The stress strain curve of a film of native collagen shows two distinct parts [12]. The first part corresponds to an elastic phase and the second to a viscoelastic phase. However, the denatured collagen film shows only a small elastic component, and the load and stretch values at break are only half those of native collagen. This shows that the native structure plays an important role in the mechanical properties of collagen. During the initial phase of a tensile test, the intra-molecular bonds give the protein pure elasticity. During the second phase, they break, the chains slide over each other, and necking appears. The remaining elasticity is due to the helical form of macromolecules.

CHEMICAL MODIFICATION OF COLLAGEN AND POLYMERS

The ability to solubilize collagen without destroying the basic rigid triple-helical structure is fundamental to the use of collagen as a biomaterial. The procedures for extraction, purification and characterization of collagen have been reviewed [13,14]. Introduction of cross-links into solubilized collagen, as well as restructuring and stabilizing the material, are also important aspects of the use of this polymer. Cross-links can be introduced by physical or chemical methods. Physical methods include simply drying, aging, heating or irradiating with UV or γ-rays. The most common chemical cross-linking agents are various aldehydes and chromic acid. The possible sites of reaction with collagen are primarily as follows: (a) amino groups, (b) guanidine groups, (c) hydroxyl groups [with formation of acetals, stable at neutral or alkaline pH $(R-OH + HCHO \rightarrow R-O-(CH_2OH)]$, (d) amide groups $(RCONH_2 + HCHO \rightleftharpoons RCONH-CH_2OH)$ and peptide linkage $(-CONH- + HCHO \rightleftharpoons -CON-CH_2OH)$.

Glutaraldehyde is the most common cross-linking

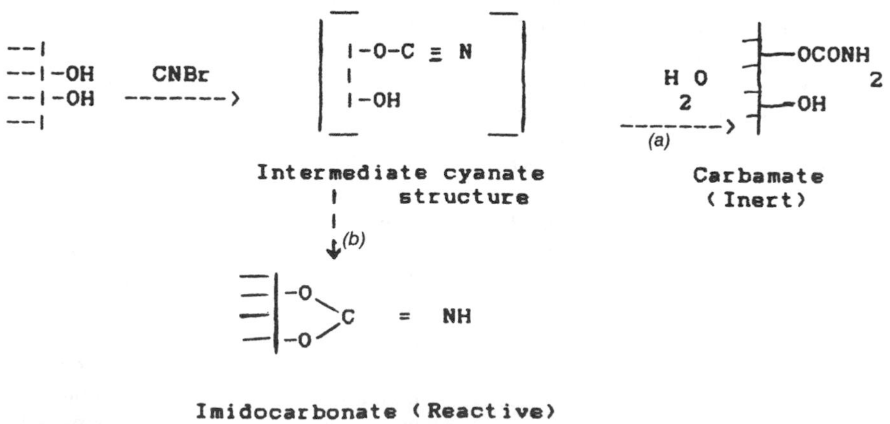

Figure 1. Chemical activation of polysaccharides by means of CNBr.

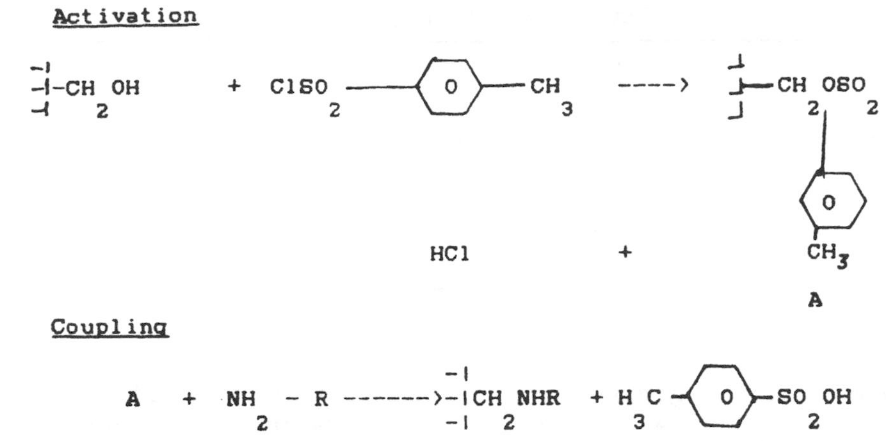

Activation

$$-\!\!\!|\!\!-CH_2OH \quad + \quad ClSO_2 \text{—} \bigcirc \text{—} CH_3 \quad ----> \quad \!\!\!|\!\!- CH_2OSO_2$$

$$\bigcirc$$
$$CH_3$$
$$A$$

$$HC1 \quad + $$

Coupling

$$A \quad + \quad NH_2 - R \quad ------>\!\!-|\!\!CH_2 NHR \quad + H_3C \text{—}\bigcirc\text{—} SO_2OH$$

Figure 2. Scheme for the coupling reaction by tosylation.

agent, although implants of collagenous material cross-linked with glutaraldehyde are prone to calcification, biodegradation, and low-grade immune reactions. Nimni et al. have tried to overcome these problems by enhancing cross-linking through (a) bridging of activated carboxyl groups with diamines and (b) using glutaraldehyde to cross-link the $-NH_2$ groups in collagen and the unreacted amines introduced by aliphatic diamines [15]. This cross-linking reduces tissue degradation and nearly eliminates humoral antibody reaction. Covalent bonding of diphosphonates, specifically 3-amino-1-hydroxypropane-1, 1-diphosphonic acid (3-APD), and chondroitin sulphate, to collagen reduces its potential for calcification.

Cellulose and polylvinylalcohol (PVA) possess hydroxyl groups, which provide a possibility for their surface modification. For immobilization of a bioactive molecule to such polyols, the cyanogen bromide (CNBr) activation method is widely utilized. Activation with other compounds such as p-toluene sulphonyl chloride, epichlorohydrin dialdehyde starch and diisocyanate has received less attention. Y. Tabata et al. [16] have shown that the CNBr activation method is able to couple covalently a large amount of collagen onto cellulose in a short-duration reaction time. The reaction scheme is given in Figure 1.

The cellulose film becomes weak and brittle after activation, but the PVA films do not. The reaction with CNBr deteriorates the cellulose substrate, presumably because of intermolecular cross-linking. The difference in the extent of cross-linking between cellulose and PVA films has been demonstrated by the changes in the degree of swelling and in the solubility characteristics of both the activated films. However, the extent of deterioration is not significant, so this activation method with CNBr may be employed if a high mechanical strength is not required for the substrate.

Denatured collagen can also be coupled by tosylation. The reaction scheme is shown in Figure 2.

The coupling reaction of proteins is much slower with tosylated film than with the CNBr activated film. In other words, the nucleophilic substitution of the tosyl groups by primary amino groups of protein is much slower than the reaction with imidocarbonates.

HYDROGELS

Chvapil et al. have prepared a material consisting of collagen sponge and glycol methacrylate with a density varying from a compact to a highly porous sponge-like material [17]. Mechanical properties, swelling capacity, trypsin digestion rate, structural stability, and the dynamics of tissue reactivity after subcutaneous and subperiostal implantation of this material, have been compared with collagen sponge and glycol methacrylate polymer alone. Collagen sponge with high porosity is quickly penetrated by connective tissue, which maintains the character of highly vascularized loose connective tissue. The combination of polymer gel with a collagen sponge increases the mechanical strength of the hydrophilic material. A typical porous sponge material had tensile strength almost three times greater than that of glycol methacrylate (gel-polymer) sponge alone.

Synthetic hydrogels that have properties similar to those of the tissue are made out of natural polymers such as collagen. Hydrogels have been prepared by the graft copolymerization of 2-hydroxyethyl methacrylate in combination with hydrophobic monomers, methylmethacrylate and glycidyl methacrylate onto soluble collagen using different cross-linking agents [18,19]. The procedure involves simultaneous graft copolymerization and cross-linking using methylene-bis-acrylamide, 1,4-butanediol dimethacrylate and hexamethylene urethane diacrylate as the cross-linking agent, and ceric ammonium nitrate as the initiator. The effect of various cross-linking agents on the water retention character of the hydrogels has been studied [20]. Hexamethylene urethane diacrylate cross-linked systems require a minimum amount of cross-linking agent to attain maximum water content in comparison to the other systems. No untoward rejection phenomena of these gels have been reported

Table 2. Mechanical properties.

Material	Young's Modulus (psi)	Tensile Strength (psi)	Strain %
Collagen fibre [27]	1.4×10^5	9–14×10^{13}	10
Silastic rubber	1.3	7–9×10^2	450
Silastic rubber/collagen	10	2.9–3.8×10^2	35
Urethane	22	$2.6 \times 2.9 \times 10^3$	600
Urethane/collagen	300	1.1×10^3	25

when implanted *in vivo* except the typical wound-healing process. These hydrogels are well tolerated and may be useful as vehicles for release of drugs and antibodies, and they have potential therapeutic applications.

Poly (2-hydroxyethyl methacrylate)–poly HEMA hydrogels are widely used, predominantly in ocular medicine (contact lenses) but also for various tissue implants. In spite of their biocompatibility, these gels, especially the macroporous ones, are prone to develop calcification. Cifkova et al. approached the problem through chemical or physical modification of polymers by collagen as a method of improving biocompatibility and consequently restricting the calcification processes [21]. Composite materials of poly HEMA and fibrillar collagen are prepared according to the method of Stol et al. [22]. The main principle of this method consists of mixing soluble poly HEMA and fibrillar collagen in a chosen weight ratio, followed by solvent evaporation, which gives a solid polymer. Calcification of the implanted material using radioactive tracer after three, six and twelve months of implantation, as well as histological examination of the implants and surrounding tissues, shows that the degree of calcification is directly proportional to the collagen content. Composites with 30% (w/w) or more collagen are biodegraded during long-term implantation, while those containing less than 20% (w/w) of fibrillar collagen are suitable for biomedical applications.

LAMINAR COPOLYMERS

Synthetic polymers may be coated with collagen to prepare laminar copolymers. Okamura, Hino, et al. [23], have devised a method to prepare such composites, which involves the following three steps.

(1) Active radicals are generated on the surface of the synthetic polymer by plasma discharge.
(2) Treated collagen of low antigenicity is coated into the polymer.
(3) Copolymerization is effected by γ-irradiation.

This method produces strong polymer bonding not only within the synthetic polymer and within the grafted collagen layer but also at the interface of the layers which cannot be readily separated. Shimizu et al. have prepared laminar copolymers from polyethylene (PE) film, polyvinylalcohol (PVA) film, silicon (Si) gum film, Teflon cloth, Polyflon® nonwoven cloth, silicon-coated Dacron mesh and collagen (Col) [24]. These copolymers require a strong peeling force of over 1000 g/cm to separate them. The collagen plastic copolymer film begins to adhere to the innate tissue one week after implantation. At two weeks, a thick layer of fibroblasts forms on the surface of the film. The grafted collagen film is identifiable by light microscopy. After three or four weeks, bridges of collagen fibrils 250–300 Å in diameter are formed between film surface and the living tissue, identifiable under electron microscope. With the course of time, collagen fibres thicken and the bonding of film and tissue continues to strengthen PE + Col exhibits strongest bonding, followed by PVA + Col and Sil + Col. However, all the copolymers maintain the capacity for extremely strong bonding for at least six weeks, and possess high tissue biocompatibility. Synthetic polymers like PE, PVA and Si films show no association with living tissue, even after four weeks of implantation. Collagen film adheres firmly to the innate tissue, and soon becomes unidentifiable by the naked eye. It is completely replaced by natural connective tissue after three weeks of implantation.

The mode of reaction of laminar composites with living tissue and the results of long term implantations have been studied by the same workers. The effects of ultraviolet radiation, glutaraldehyde treatment, and γ-radiation have been comparatively examined [25]. The composite bonds to the living tissue in such a manner that a portion of the collagen part is digested and absorbed, to be replaced by the invading connective tissue, and a part of collagen near the surface of the synthetic polymers escapes digestion to combine with the rabbit's own collagen fibre.

The mode of reaction of these composites is similar to real organisation and different from mere encapsulation. Composites radiated with 1–3 Mrads of γ-radiation prove desirable in both tissue affinity and duration of tissue bonding. The bonding force remains effective even 1.5 years later, while the composites radiated with 5 Mrad or more are poorer in these properties because of the destruction of collagen part. There is a large variation in the properties. Through use of ultraviolet radiation it is easy to control the degree of swelling of the collagen part. However, this method gives a lower bonding force than γ-radiation. The glutaraldehyde method allows the collagen to remain over a long time, but the composite has less tissue affinity than the other two methods.

Composites composed of collagen-coated urethane and Silastic rubber films are fabricated to give improved tear resistance, strength, and handling to the reconstituted films. Active centres are generated on the surface of Silastic rubber by glow discharge to enable collagen to bind to the polymer. The collagen glutaraldehyde solution binds to the urethane surface without glow discharge. The polymer/collagen composites show a decrease in tensile strength and elongation, and an increase in the Young's modulus relative to those of the original substrate films (Table 2).

Collagen and collagen composite implants adhere better to the muscle than to the substrate polymer films. Urethane has been rated with a response value of 1.5 versus 3.25 for the urethane/collagen composite, and Silastic® rubber rated a response value of 1.67 versus 3.12 for the Silastic® rubber/collagen. These ratings have been compared with a value of 3.3 for the collagen implant by the same coworkers [26]. It has also been suggested that these materials could be advantageous for uses such as percutaneous devices, where muscle ingrowth might prevent the implant from being expelled.

Collagen-synthetic polymer composite material, which possesses high tissue compatibility suitable for clinical use, is also applicable as a support for immobilization of enzymes. The enzymes trypsin and urokinase are bound to the collagen membrane layer, which has been activated by acyl azide formation of its carboxyl groups. The enzyme-bearing composite material shows excellent catalytic activity towards protein substrate, as well as a low molecular weight synthetic substrate [28]. The apparent affinity of immobilised urokinase for the substrate slightly decreases, but its intrinsic kinetic properties are not significantly affected. The *in vivo* fibrinolytic activity is maintained when this material is applied in rabbit blood vessels. The enzyme collagen-synthetic polymer composite materials can possibly find application in biomaterials and in artificial organs as functional biomaterials.

GENERAL CONCLUSIONS

The need for long-term implantable materials in medicine and surgery is increasing. Collagen and polymers alone do not suffice, but when a composite of the two is formed, the desirable properties of both are combined. Polymers add strength to the films for handling, while collagen improves the overall biocompatibility.

Collagen and polymers have been modified in a number of ways to link them chemically. Hydrogels

for use in ocular medicine have been synthesised and tested for their biocompatibility. Laminar copolymers offer the possibility of tailor-making biomaterials. Many synthetic polymers already in use for biomedical purposes with known physicochemical properties have been tried. Collagen and polymers are linked together through plasma discharge, UV treatment, γ-irradiation, and chemically by glutaraldehyde. Irradiation has two main effects on collagen—initiating random cross-links and breaking the tropocollagen molecule. Irradiation in air enhances the breakdown of collagen, whereas in a nitrogen atmosphere it delays degradation and increases cross-linking. It also inhibits fibre formation and antigenicity. Ultraviolet and gamma irradiation are useful methods of cross-linking collagen since no potentially toxic residues are introduced. The bonding force and the tissue affinity is effectively controlled by the radiation dosages. However, the chemical fixing agent, glutaraldehyde, is prone to calcification, and tissue affinity is also less than it is with other methods [22]. This area of preparation of composite materials from collagen with synthetic polymers has opened up new avenues for producing biomaterials tailor-made for specific uses.

REFERENCES

1. Stenzel, K. H., T. Miyata and A. L. Rubin. 1974. "Collagen as a Biomaterial", *Ann. Rev. Biophys. Bioeng.*, 3:231–253.

2. Pharriss, B. B. 1980. "Collagen as a Biomaterial", *JALCA*, 75:474–480.

3. Styrer, L. 1981. *Biochemistry.* San Francisco, CA: W. H. Freeman and Co., pp. 185–204.

4. "Collagen", in *Encyclopedia of Polymer Science and Engineering*. H. F. Mark, N. M. Bikales, C. G. Overberger and G. Menges, eds. Wiley Interscience publication, 3:699–727.

5. Huc, A. "Collagen Biomaterials—Characteristics and Applications", presented at the *80th Annual Meeting of the American Leather Chemists Association, Hot Springs, Virginia, June 25, 1984*.

6. Iverson, P. L., L. M. Partlow, L. G. Stensaas and F. Moatamad. 1981. "Characterization of a Variety of Standard Collagen Substrates: Ultrastructure, Uniformity and Capacity to Bind and Promote Growth of Neurons", *In Vitro*, 17:540–552.

7. Chvapil, M. 1980. "Reconstituted Collagen" in *Biology of Collagen.* A. Viidik and J. Vuust, eds. London, England: Academic Press, pp. 313–324.

8. Stenzel, K. H., J. F. Sullivan T. Miyata and A. L. Rubin. 1969. "Collagen Dialysis Membranes. Initial Clinical Evaluation", *Trans. Amer. Soc. Artif. Int. Organs*, 15:114–117.

9. Doillon, C. J., C. F. Whyne, S. Brandwein and F. H. Silver. 1986. "Collagen-Based Wound Dressings. Control of Pore Structure and Morphology", *J. Biomed. Mater. Res.*, 20:1219–1228.

10. Bruck, S. D. 1980. *Properties of Biomaterials in*

Physiological Environment. Florida: CRC Press, Inc., pp. 5–7.

11. Lyman, D. J. 1975. "Biomedical Polymers: An Introduction to Polymers" in *Medicine and Surgery* (Polymer Sci. and Tech. Series, Vol. 8). R. L. Kronenthal, Z. Oser and E. Martin, eds. New York: Plenum Press, pp. 29–32.

12. Huc, A. 1978. *Labo Pharma*, 275:307 in Ref. 5.

13. Miller, E. J. and R. K. Rhodes. 1982. In *Methods in Enzymology.* L. W. Cumniaghan and D. W. Frederikson, eds. New York, NY: Academic Press, Inc., 82:33–64.

14. Noda, H. 1955. "Physiochemical Studies on the Soluble Collagen of Rat Tail Tendon", *Biochima. et Biophysa. Acta*, 17:92–97.

15. Nimni, M. E., D. Cheung, B. Strates, M. Kodama and K. Sheikh. 1987. "Chemically Modified Collagen: A Natural Biomaterial for Tissue Replacement", *J. Biomed. Mater. Res.*, 21:741–771.

16. Tabata, Y., S. V. Lonikar, F. Horii and Y. Ikada. 1986. "Immobilization of Collagen onto Polymer Surfaces Having Hydroxyl Groups", *Biomaterials*, 7:234–238.

17. Chvapil, M., R. Holusa, K. Kliment and M. Stoll. 1969. "Some Chemical and Biological Characteristics of a New Collagen Polymer Compound Material", *J. Biomed. Mater. Res.*, 3:315–332.

18. Amudeswari, S., C. R. Reddy and K. T. Joseph. 1984. "Graft Copolymerization of 2-Hydroxyethylmethacrylate and Methyl Methacrylate onto Hide Powder", *Eur. Polym. J.*, 20:91–93.

19. Amudeswari, S., B. Nagarajan, C. R. Reddy and K. T. Joseph. 1986. "Short Term Biocompatibility Studies of Hydrogel Grafted Collagen Copolymers", *J. Biomed. Mater. Res.*, 20:1103–1109.

20. Amudeswari, S., C. R. Reddy and K. T. Joseph. 1986. "Hydrogels Based on Graft Copolymers of Collagen Synthesis", *J. Appl. Polym. Sc.*, 32:4939–4944.

21. Cifkova, I., M. Stol, R. Holusa and M. Adam. 1987. "Calcification of Poly(2-hydroxyethyl methacrylate) Collagen Composites Implanted in Rats", *Biomaterials*, 8:30–34.

22. Stol, M., M. Tolar and M. Adam. 1985. "Poly(2-hydroxylethyl methacrylate)—Collagen Composites which Promote Muscle Cell Differentiation *in vitro*", *Biomaterials*, 6:193–197.

23. Okamura, S. and T. Hino. U.S. Pat. 3, 868, 113 (1974) and U.S. Pat. 3, 955, 012 (1976).

24. Shimizu, Y., R. Abe, T. Teramatsu, S. Okamura and T. Hino. 1977. "Studies on Copolymers of Collagen and a Synthetic Polymer", First report, *Biomat., Med. Dev., Art. Org.*, 5:49–66.

25. Shimizu, Y., Y. Miyamoto, T. Teramatsu, S. Okamura and T. Hino. 1978. "Studies on Composites of Collagen and a Synthetic Polymer", Second report, *Biomat. Med. Dev., Art Org.*, 6:375–391.

26. Gilbert, D. L. and D. J. Lyman. 1987. "*In vitro* and *in vivo* Characterization of Synthetic Polymer/Biopolymer Composites", *J. Biomed. Mater. Res.*, 21:643–655.

27. Cooke, A., R. F. Oliver and M. Edward. 1983. "An *in vitro* Cytotoxicity Study of Aldehyde-Treated Pig Dermal Collagen", *Br. J. Exp. Path.*, 64:172.

28. Watanabe, S., Y. Shimizu, T. Teramatsu, T. Murachi and T. Hino. 1981. "The *in vitro* and *in vivo* Behaviour of Urokinase Immobilized onto Collagen Synthetic Polymer Composite Material", *J. Biomed. Mater. Res.*, 15:553–563.

13

Pressure-Sensitive Adhesives—
Effect of Rheological Properties

DON SATAS*

ABSTRACT: The use of pressure-sensitive adhesives in more recent medical applications is described. The performance of such adhesives in contact with human skin is difficult to relate to the standard tests carried out on pressure-sensitive adhesives because of the complexity of the adherend and the viscoelastic behavior of the adhesive. Dynamic measurement of the mechanical properties of the adhesive is very promising in the prediction of adhesive performance and is important in evaluating and compounding pressure-sensitive adhesives for medical and other applications. Test data of various medical adhesives is shown and compared to that of adhesives intended for other applications.

INTRODUCTION

Pressure-sensitive adhesives are used very widely for various hospital and first aid applications. Their uses vary greatly, from securing dressings and various medical devices to the skin, to restricting the movement of injured joints and muscles. Pressure-sensitive tapes and labels are also widely used in hospitals for packaging and other nonmedical applications. Overviews of medical tapes and other products can be found in several publications [1,2].

Although many of the medical uses of pressure-sensitive tapes are very old, new products and applications are still being developed, which indicates the versatility of these adhesives and assures their potential for future growth. Among more recent products are thin water-vapor-permeable films, pressure-sensitive adhesives for transdermal drug delivery, and electrically conductive adhesives for EKG and electrosurgery pads.

*Satas & Associates, 99 Shenandoah Road, Warwick, RI 02886

THIN FILM DRESSINGS

It has been recognized for a long time that thin, flexible tape backings and high moisture permeability are the main factors needed by adhesive tapes in order to minimize skin irritation. For this reason, thin polyurethane films have been utilized for hospital dressings and drapes [3]. Thin polyurethane film has a high moisture vapor transmission rate and is also highly flexible and conformable. When combined with a pressure-sensitive adhesive (based on acrylic or vinyl ether polymers) that has a sufficiently high moisture vapor transmission, it yields a product that does not cause skin maceration and that is transparent, allowing the inspection of the patient's skin without removal of the tape. These tapes have found applications such as surgical drapes and as tapes for holding intravenous needles in place.

In addition, these tapes are used for direct application over wounds, as opposed to utilizing an absorbent pad held down over the wound by pressure-sensitive adhesive. It is claimed that healing of the wound is accelerated under such conditions [4], although this wound-healing technique, employing occlusive dressings, is not universally accepted.

Dispensing of thin, sticky, and very flexible film dressings is difficult. Wrinkles can be formed easily unless the dressing is applied very carefully. Because of these difficulties many delivery methods have been proposed and have resulted in a host of patents [5,6,7].

TRANSDERMAL DRUG DELIVERY SYSTEMS

Transdermal drug delivery patches are best secured to the skin by pressure-sensitive adhesives. Usually the drug-containing patch is held to the skin by pressure-sensitive adhesive, in a construction analogous to the common wound dressing, where the absorbent pad is replaced by a drug-containing pad. The

185

adhesive requirements in such cases are no different from those of hospital tapes and dressings in general. Various drug delivery pad constructions have been reviewed by Cleary [8].

Transdermal delivery patches may be constructed utilizing pressure-sensitive adhesive as the reservoir for the drug as well as the medium for the transmission of the drug. In such cases, the adhesive is used for a dual purpose and the choice and design of the adhesive polymer becomes much more critical. Silicone adhesives are especially promising for such applications, because of their high drug-transmission rate [9] and their inertness. Pressure-sensitive adhesives which are more chemically reactive because of pending functional groups are more difficult to use with some drugs.

CONDUCTIVE ADHESIVES

Electrically conductive pressure-sensitive adhesives are used for EKG pads, for grounding systems in electrosurgical procedures, and for pain control devices. The conductive adhesive performs a double function: it secures the device to the skin, and also provides the path for the electrical current. Electrically conductive adhesives simplify the construction of such devices: it is not necessary to employ both conductive gel to transmit the electrical current and the adhesive to hold down the pad.

Electrical conductivity is usually achieved by employing hygroscopic materials, which absorb a large quantity of water containing dissolved salts.

ADHESIVE PROPERTIES

There are many requirements for pressure-sensitive adhesives which are to be used in medical applications. The adhesive should not cause skin irritation, chemical or allergenic. It should adhere firmly to the skin, and remain adhered under exposure to moisture such as perspiration or washing under a shower. The adhesive should also permit easy removal of the dressing or tape without causing excessive skin irritation.

There is no complete agreement in the industry as to what constitutes a good medical adhesive, because of the multitude of factors that affect the adhesive performance. The adhesive performance is determined by the rheological properties of the bulk adhesive and also by the surface properties and surface conditions of both adhesive and adherend. It is not simple, or sometimes even possible, to distinguish bulk from surface effects.

An interesting study on the effect of carboxylation of acrylic pressure sensitive adhesives is reported by Aubrey and Ginosatis [10]. In this study it was shown that bulk effects make the major contribution to the peel adhesion, although the interfacial effects, due to the presence of carboxylic groups, are also important.

Furthermore, these interfacial effects depend upon the peel rate. Such surface effects concern the energy expended to break the bonds established between the adhesive and the adherend.

There is an entirely different class of surface effects which pertain to the bond-formation process. The topography—rugosity—of the skin has an effect on the ease of bond establishment. The rougher the skin surface, the more difficult it is to establish a continuous bond between the adhesive and the skin. The ease with which such a bond is established depends upon the flow characteristics of the adhesive, i.e., its bulk properties. A poor adhesive-skin bond may also result because of the presence of oil or water on the skin surface. Such biological factors of skin adhesion have been discussed by Anasiewicz [11].

Interfacial conditions at the skin-adhesive boundary may also be affected after tape application. Adhesives may vary greatly in their resistance to moisture. Moisture from the perspiring skin or from the outside (i.e., washing or taking a shower) may enter at the adhesive-skin interface causing a loss of adhesion. The presence of surfactants at the adhesive surface will greatly accelerate moisture penetration. Some adhesives, especially polar acrylic polymers, can absorb a significant amount of moisture, which may lead to a significant loss of tack and adhesion. Komerska and Moffett [12] have suggested testing and adhesion to a collagen film, rather than to the standard stainless steel surface. It has been shown that aging at high humidity levels affects adhesion to collagen more than adhesion to a steel plate. Such methods could be helpful in predicting the adhesive's capability to retain a bond under moist conditions.

RHEOLOGICAL PROPERTIES

Rheological bulk properties of pressure-sensitive adhesives, however, are most important in determining the performance of adhesive to skin bond, once an adhesive of sufficient moisture resistance is chosen. Skin is a highly pliant substrate and as it flexes, the adhesive is subjected to stresses of varying magnitude and duration. Skin movements associated with an individual's activities are more readily transmitted in areas of "firm" skin than those of "flabby" skin [11]. It has been observed by many that a tape adheres better to the upper portion of the hand than to the palm, the latter clearly providing a much firmer skin surface, causing higher stresses in the adhesive. Thus, a soft adhesive which is capable of easy relaxation, causing a reduction of such induced stresses, is required for a good and lasting adhesion to skin.

Figure 1 shows the dependence of peel adhesion on peel rate for several acrylic adhesives, illustrating the behavior of various adhesive types [1]. A continuous line denotes the adhesive failure associated with a clean removal of the adhesive from the adherend (skin) surface. An interrupted line denotes cohesive

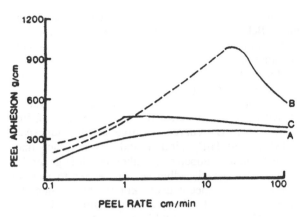

Figure 1. Dependence of peel adhesion on peel rate for some acrylic adhesives: (a) high cohesive strength industrial adhesive; (b) low cohesive strength adhesive; (c) medical tape adhesive.

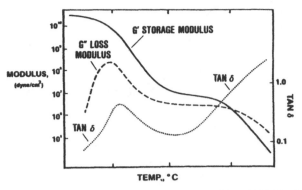

Figure 2. Viscoelastic properties of pressure-sensitive adhesives as a function of temperature (courtesy Hercules, Inc.).

failure, where an adhesive layer remains on the adherend after tape removal. Curve A shows the behavior of a typical fairly hard industrial adhesive which exhibits an adhesive failure at all peel rates. Curve B represents the peel behavior of a soft adhesive which fails cohesively at low and normal peel rates and exhibits adhesive failure only at higher peel rates. Such an adhesive will form a good and lasting bond to the skin, but it is not acceptable because it leaves adhesive residue which must later be removed. Adhesives of such performance characteristics are occasionally used for EKG pads to assure that they remain adhered during the testing. Curve C represents the peel behavior of a typical hospital tape adhesive. The adhesive is soft and fails cohesively at low peel rates. At higher peel rates, such as are used to remove the tape, the failure is adhesive and therefore clean. Flexing of skin is a relatively slow process falling within the region of cohesive failure. The adhesive must reach its ultimate elongation in order to fail cohesively. The skin displacement experienced in flexing is not even close to that required for cohesive failure. Thus, such an adhesive will not fail as a result of strains produced by skin flexing, unless its bond is weakened by some extraneous action.

Such considerations suggest that the rheological properties of hospital adhesives are extremely important and that their evaluation is an important criterion in the selection of adhesives for medical applications. Dynamic testing of the adhesive mechanical properties offers an evaluation of the adhesive performance unobtainable by the measurements of standard adhesive properties, such as tack, peel adhesion, and shear resistance.

Pressure-sensitive adhesives are viscoelastic materials, and both viscous and elastic properties determine their adhesive behavior. Furthermore, the extent of the viscous-elastic balance depends upon temperature and upon time, i.e., the rate of force application. The dynamic testing of rheological properties produces curves as shown in Figures 2 and 3. Figure 2

shows the mechanical properties of a pressure-sensitive adhesive as a function of temperature. G' —the curve of the storage modulus—represents the elastic component of the compound modulus, the energy which is recovered after force removal. Most rheometers measure the modulus in shear, but some might measure bending or tensile moduli. G'' —the curve of loss modulus—represents the viscous component, the energy which is lost and dissipated as heat. These two curves characterize the adhesive behavior. It has been shown that a polymer must have a G' below 10^7, preferably about 10^6 dyne/cm^2 at the temperature of application, in order to be pressure sensitive. Adhesives of a higher storage modulus do not exhibit sufficient flow [13].

The rheometer chart usually also shows the curve for tan δ (tan $\delta = G''/G'$). The tan δ curve (like the G'' curve) shows a maximum, which is close to the glass transition temperature of the adhesive.

Figure 3 shows G', G'', and viscosity (*) curves as a function of frequency of force application. While the temperature-time data is superimposable accord-

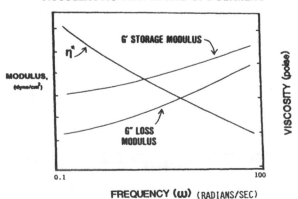

Figure 3. Viscoelastic properties of pressure-sensitive adhesives as a function of frequency (courtesy Hercules, Inc.).

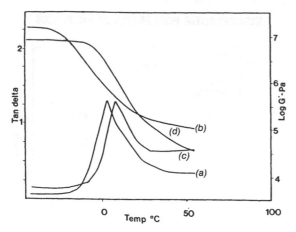

Figure 4. Tangent delta and storage modulus of medical adhesives as a function of temperature: (a) tangent delta of rubber/resin medical tape adhesive; (b) G' of rubber/resin medical tape adhesive; (c) tangent delta of acrylic finger bandage adhesive; (d) G' of acrylic finger bandage adhesive.

ing to the well-known WLF principle, frequency curves give the properties over a much narrower range and it is easier to observe small differences which might become hidden in the modulus-temperature curves.

Figure 4 shows the G' and tan δ values of two medical adhesives: one acrylic and the other natural rubber based [14]. Acrylic adhesives dominate medical applications, but natural rubber/resin blends are still used for some tapes. The value of G' is similar at room temperature for both adhesives, but the two curves diverge at both higher and lower temperatures. At higher temperatures, G' of the acrylic adhesive decreases faster than that of the natural rubber

adhesive, and the opposite is true at lower temperatures. Behavior at a higher temperature is related to that at a lower force application rate. The curves suggest that the acrylic adhesive will be softer and more conformable when flexed slowly, and harder when peeled at a higher peel rate. This property is much better represented in Figure 5 showing the G' values of several medical adhesives as a function of frequency [14]. G' curves of three acrylic adhesives tested exhibit fairly similar and lower values than those of natural rubber/resin adhesives. It is generally thought that acrylic adhesives are easier to remove and cause less mechanical skin irritation than the older-type natural rubber adhesives filled with zinc oxide. The latter type exhibits good adhesion to skin, but it also is more difficult to remove, and consequently may cause more mechanical irritation on removal.

Data like this are helpful in the selection and compounding of adhesives for hospital products. Rheological data of the adhesives considered are simply compared to the dynamic mechanical properties of a control adhesive obtained from a product known to perform well for a particular application. In addition, of course, attention must be paid to the effects of high humidity and other extraneous conditions.

Figure 6 compares G' of a medical adhesive to that of adhesives used for other applications [14]. Curve A represents the properties of a typical acrylic medical adhesive. Its storage modulus is substantially lower than that of industrial adhesives. Shown on the graph are: a hot melt adhesive for packaging tapes (curve B), a general purpose acrylic emulsion adhesive (curve D), and a rather firm acrylic solution adhesive (curve E). The exception is the G' of a soft removable

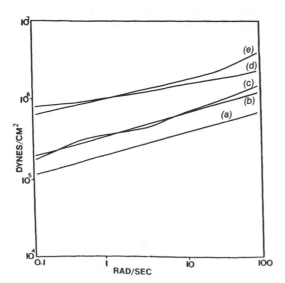

Figure 5. Storage moduli as a function of frequency of medical adhesives: (a) acrylic emulsion adhesive; (b) acrylic solution adhesive; (c) acrylic finger bandage adhesive; (d) rubber/resin medical tape adhesive; (e) rubber/resin medical adhesive.

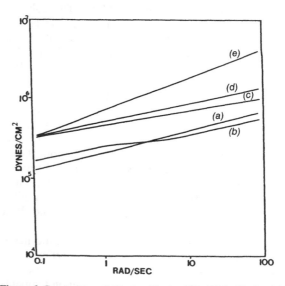

Figure 6. Comparison of G' of medical to industrial adhesives: (a) acrylic medical adhesive; (b) acrylic soft removable adhesive; (c) hot melt packaging adhesive; (d) acrylic emulsion adhesive for industrial tapes; (e) acrylic solution adhesive for industrial tapes.

adhesive (curve B). This adhesive has a low storage modulus and also a lower slope of the modulus/frequency curve. Low slope suggests that the adhesive does not show much change in peel adhesion with peel rate. G' at low frequencies is an indicator of the processes that take place over a longer time period (i.e., making of the bond). In the making of the bond process, the adhesive flows slowly to conform to the rugosity of the adherend (skin) surface. Tack measurements are supposed to indicate the adhesive behavior during bond making. The debonding process (peeling of the tape) takes place at higher shear rates and G' at the higher frequency range suggests the adhesive behavior when the bond is broken. Medical acrylic adhesives show a relatively low G' throughout the frequency range tested, indicating a low tack and a low peel force adhesive, which is the desirable combination for medical tapes.

Natural rubber/resin based adhesives in general exhibit a much higher level of G' (Figure 5), so it is no surprise that natural rubber based medical adhesives have a higher G' value than other adhesives. Obviously, simple inspection of G' curves is not sufficient to describe the behavior of the adhesive. Several authors have published their observations and suggested adhesive performance/mechanical property correlations based on more complex relationships [15,16,17].

It is believed that dynamic testing of the mechanical adhesive properties is going to be used much more often in the future, and that it will help to close the gap between the adhesive performance and the results of standard tests.

REFERENCES

1. Satas, D. and A. M. Satas. 1989. "Hospital and First Aid Products", in *Handbook of Pressure Sensitive Adhesive Technology, 2nd Ed.* D. Satas, ed. Van Nostrand: Reinhold.

2. 1972. *Professional Uses of Adhesive Tape, 3rd Ed.* Johnson & Johnson.

3. Hodgson, M. E. (assigned to T. J. Smith & Nephew, Ltd.) 1972. U. S. Patent 3,645,835.

4. Alper, J. C., et al. 1983. *Journal of the American Academy of Dermatology.* 8(39):347–353.

5. Grossman, F. and L. A. Sims. (assigned to American Hospital Supply Co.) 1983. U. S. Patent 4,372,303.

6. Johns, O. L. (assigned to Howmedica, Inc.) 1985. U. S. Patent 4,513,739.

7. Heinecke, S. B. (assigned to Minnesota Mining and Manufacturing Co.) 1986. U. S. Patent 4,598,004.

8. Cleary, G. W. 1984. "Transdermal Controlled Release Systems", in *Medical Applications of Controlled Release, Vol. 1.* R. S. Langer and D. L. Wise, eds. CRC Press, p. 203–251.

9. Baker, R. W., and H. K. Lonsdale. 1974. *Controlled Release of Biologically Active Agents.* T. C. Tanquary and R. E. Lacy, eds. Plenum Press, p. 15.

10. Aubrey, D. W. and S. Ginosatis. 1981. *J. Adhesion,* 12:189–198.

11. Anasiewicz, S. M. 1988. *TAPPI Journal,* 71(10):159–162.

12. Komerska, J. F. and N. Moffett. 1985. "Collagen Films as Test Surfaces for Skin-Contact Pressure Sensitive Adhesives", *Technical Seminar Proceedings, Pressure Sensitive Tape Council, Itasca, IL, May 8–10,* p. 108.

13. Dahlquist, C. A. 1989. In "Creep" *Handbook of Pressure Sensitive Adhesive Technology, 2nd Ed.* D. Satas, ed. Van Nostrand: Reinhold.

14. Satas, D. 1988. *Adhesives Age,* 31(9):28–32.

15. Chu, S. G. 1989. Viscoeleastic Properties. *Handbook of Pressure Sensitive Adhesive Technology, 2nd Ed.* D. Satas, ed. Van Nostrand: Reinhold.

16. Dale, W. C., J. K. Haynes, M. D. Paster and E. F. Alstede. 1987. "Measurement of Fundamental Mechanical Properties of Gelva Pressure Sensitive Adhesives and Their Relationships to Industrial Standard Testing", *Pressure Sensitive Tape Council Seminar Proceedings, Ilasca, IL, May 6–8,* p. 126.

17. Zosel, A. 1985. *Colloid and Polymer Sci.,* 263:541–553.

14

Foam Separation in Polyurethane-Covered Breast Prostheses

R. GUIDOIN*,1
C. ROLLAND*
P. E. ROY*
M. MAROIS*
P. BLAIS*

ABSTRACT: Pathological material was collected from 4 patients involved in post-surgical complications with polyurethane foam-coated mammary prostheses. This material included: prosthesis and capsule removed at prosthesis explantation for medical reasons (first and second patient), capsule removed following prosthesis implantation and prosthesis and capsule removed at prosthesis explantation (third patient), and lump excised two years after prosthesis explantation (fourth patient).

Evidence of deterioration processes and tissue interaction was evident as early as 12 days after the operation. In this short time, the polyurethane foam and the silicone-based adhesive that was used to bond it to the prosthesis surface became partly detached from the prosthesis core. Over longer time intervals, the tissue growth continued and a connective tissue layer was generated between the original foam cover and the surrounding fatty tissue. Then, larger solid entities dispersed in the tissue over a period of at least two years, suggesting that the half-life of prosthesis debris may be very long.

Our study emphasizes that it is of paramount importance to investigate mammary prostheses in three directions:

(1) A sound epidemiological study is needed to establish the in vivo durability of the prostheses, the success rate and the nature of major evolutive complications.
(2) A basic bench study is needed to characterize the prostheses and identify the degradation products, if any, and the kinetic of the reactions.
(3) An advisory board should be set up at the provincial or federal level to advise doctors and patients of the most appropriate forms of treatment in case of major complications.

INTRODUCTION

Polyurethane-covered mammary prostheses have been promoted since 1984 [1] as a major breakthrough in plastic and reconstructive surgery. It is claimed that the implants with their associated capsular tissue generally remain "soft" and therefore are less likely to require open or closed capsulotomy within five years after implantation [1,2]. However, serious complications have been reported. The difficulty in controlling infection, in the immediate post-operative period as well as later [3,4,5] and sometimes after attempts at removing the implants, is well documented [6,7,8]. Other complications such as allergic reactions to the polyurethane coating or its impurities have been described, and are common knowledge among users [2,9,10]. Painful prostheses have been reported by several authors [5,11,12] who noted immediate relief of pain upon removing the implants. Cases of lymphadenopathy [13], severe hematoma [1,10], unaesthetic wrinkling of the skin in patients with subcutaneous mastectomies [6,10,14] and easily ruptured prostheses [1,9] have also been described. Investigations by the U. S. Food and Drug Administration in 1988, alleged major deficiencies in production technology and manufacturing practices with respect to batches of products released prior to that date [15,16].

Histological studies on animal trials or with human explants confirm major foreign body reactions, capsular tissue anomalies and drastic physico-chemical changes in the prosthesis materials. The literature describes phenomena such as: "microfragmentation", "disintegration", "dissolution", "degradation", "phagocytosis" and "disappearing polyurethane covers" [7,9,11,18]. In spite of numerous implantations and adverse reactions, the polyurethane (PU) foam-

1Correspondence: Dr. Robert Guidoin, Ph.D., Biomaterials Institute, Room Fl-304, St-François d'Assise Hospital, 10 de l'Espinay, Quebec City, QC GlL 3L5, Canada.

*Faculty of Medicine, Laval University and Biomaterials Institute, St. François d'Assise Hospital, Quebec City, Canada

covered prostheses remain uncharacterized and their chemical composition has not been disclosed. The rate and mechanisms of biodeterioration are still unknown. The metabolites from the deteriorative process are also unknown, but the nature of the polyurethane is such that toxic and possibly animal tumorigenic entities are expected, specifically metabolites from toluene diamine isomers and urethane or urea-substituted benzenoids [17].

We hereby report systematic studies performed on specimens explanted from four patients.

MATERIAL AND METHODS

Implanted Material

Mëme® prostheses were manufactured between 1984 and 1987 by Natural-Y Surgical Specialties (Los Angeles, California) or by Cooper Surgical (Irvine, California). They were implanted and later explanted by several surgeons from different centres in Canada. The prostheses are now manufactured by Surgitek (Racine, Wisconsin) [2] and distributed in Canada by Réal Laperrière Inc. (Montréal, Québec). The products appear to be a close variant of the Natural-Y or Ashley [19,20] foam-covered prostheses which were sold in small numbers in the late sixties and seventies by various manufacturers (Markham Medical Specialties, Weck Surgical, Markham International Inc., 3T Inc., Aesthetech Inc., etc.).

These implants consist of a core that is similar to conventional gel-filled silicone breast prostheses of the "small, round, soft style" to which two 1–2 mm thick sheets (half shells) of open-pore polyurethane foam have been attached with a thick silicone adhesive and bonded together by a heat-sealing process around the circumference (Figures 1 and 2).

Clinical Material Collection

Material was collected from 4 patients involved in the post-surgical complications: 2 cases at prosthesis explantation for medical reasons, one case at early reoperation and at prosthesis explantation and one case involving an attempt to excise a lump two years after explantation of Mëme prostheses with associated capsular tissue. The samples were fixed and stored in 10% formalin solution until required for subsequent studies.

Macroscopic Observations

The capsular tissue and prostheses, as received, were investigated under binocular stereomicroscopes (Zeiss DV4C2, Oberkochen, Germany) at 1 to 15 times magnification and were photographed with a 35-mm camera (Contax 139 Quartz, Yashica, Mississauga, Ontario, Canada) mounted on a photomacrographic zoom system (Tessovar, Zeiss, Oberkochen, Germany) with 0.8 to 12.8 times magnification.

Light and Scanning Electron Microscopy

For histological studies and contrast enhancement of abiotic material, samples of capsular tissues were embedded in Epon 812 and stained with toluidine blue after conventional phosphate-buffered formalin fixation. Sudan IV and Mallory stains were also used for some specimens. Other pieces were fixed and stained with osmium tetroxide and sputter-coated with gold for observation with a scanning electron microscope (Jeol JSM 35CF, Soquelec, Montréal, Québec) in the secondary electron emission mode.

Microanalysis

An electron microprobe was used on selected specimens for element analysis and distribution studies (Princeton Gamma Tech, PGT System 4, multichannel energy dispersive spectrometer). Samples were coated with carbon to ensure conduction. Microanalysis was used principally to identify silicones and other non-biological inclusions.

CASE SUMMARIES

First Patient

This patient was a 34-year old woman who was given a bilateral augmentation mammaplasty using Mëme MP prostheses in June 1986. Twelve days later, the right breast prosthesis was removed following a severe intractable episode of infection associated with pathogenic staphylococcus. The prosthesis was recovered with most of its covering superficially intact.

Second Patient

This patient was 34 years old at time of implantation at the end of February 1986. In early May 1986, 2 months after implantation, a piece of non-contractile capsular tissue was excised from the right breast following exploratory surgery. Ten days later, she underwent additional procedures for drainage of a hematoma. Three other similar procedures were performed between May and July 1986. In July 1986, the right breast prosthesis and its capsular tissue were removed. Thus, from this patient, a prosthesis and two parts of one capsule, aged respectively 2 months and 4 months post-operatively, were recovered.

Third Patient

Little is known about this patient other than she was born in 1958. The prosthesis was received at the end of 1985. Since her medical records were not available, the date of implantation is unknown. Pathological observations on the capsule suggest that the device may have been *in situ* for about 4 to 6 months.

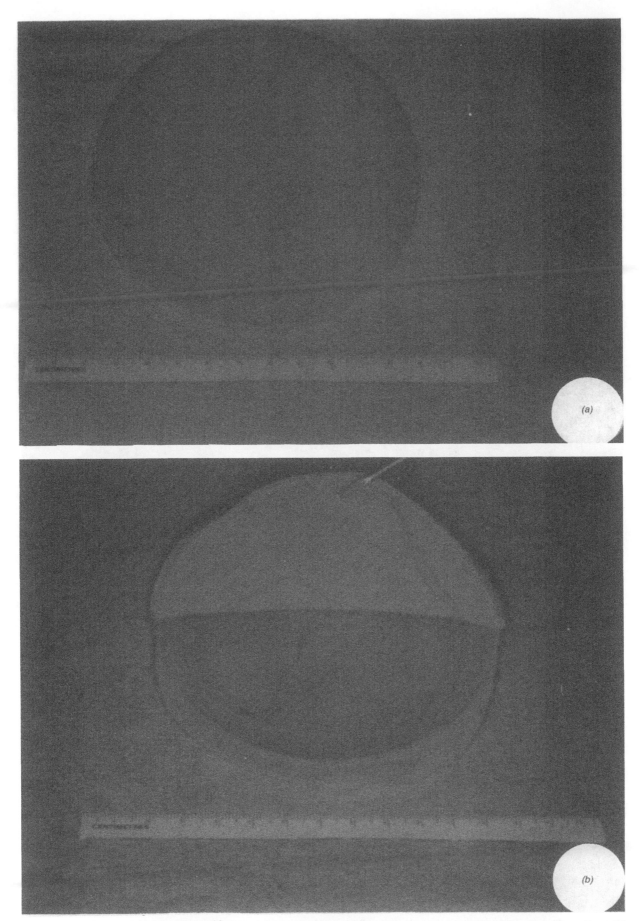

Figure 1. (a): Photograph of a new (intact) Mêeme prosthesis. (b): Same prosthesis, with the thin outer layer of polyurethane foam (about 1.5 mm thick), peeled back in order to reveal the adhesive-coated inner silicone core.

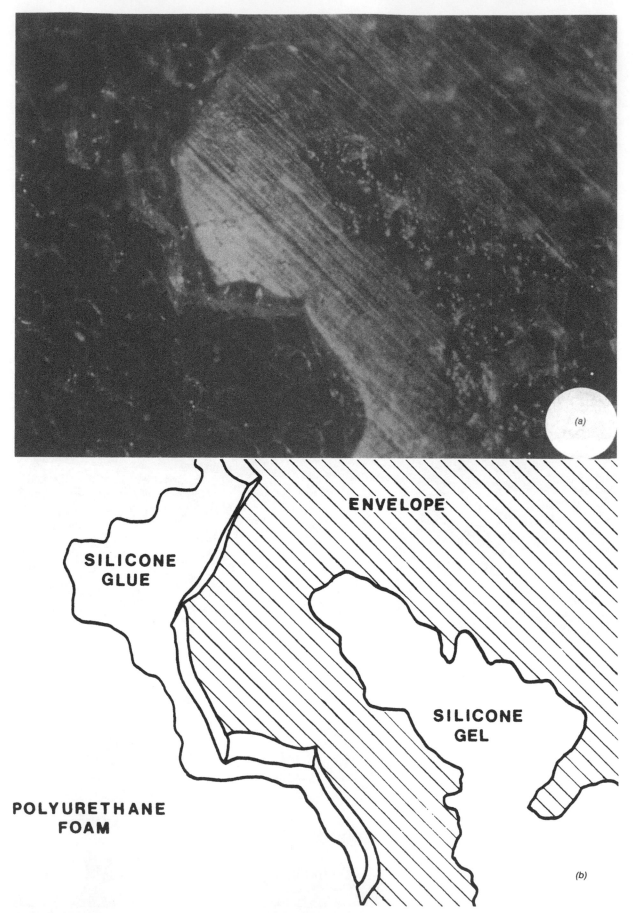

Figure 2. (a): Photograph of a virgin prosthesis showing wall section (from outer to inner): polyurethane foam, silicone glue, envelope and silicone gel (10 mm = 0.5 mm). (b): Diagram identifying different parts of the prosthesis as shown in 2(a).

Fourth Patient

This woman was a fibrocystic patient who underwent elective bilateral mastectomy with immediate reconstruction using Même prostheses in March 1985, when she was 37 years old. Infection appeared early on the right breast and the prosthesis was removed in April 1985. Similarly, the left implant was removed following an episode of infection and two Dow-Corning Silastic II prostheses were inserted in August 1985. In March 1986, two larger Dow Corning prostheses were inserted in order to correct some deformities. In the following 2 months, hematoma and infection were diagnosed in the right breast. On April 25th, 1986, a large area of skin was removed and Sofratulle® and regular dry dressings were applied on the open wound. One year later, new surgery was performed to reposition the breast and the nipple-areolar complex in the left breast. During this procedure, a 20/1000″ silicone sheet was inserted to separate the skin from the muscle in order to avoid the retraction of the skin towards the axilla. In April 1987, the silicone sheet was removed because of fluid build-up in the left breast. Another infection period immediately followed but was resolved in September 1987. In June 1988, a further reconstructive procedure was performed and in February 1989, curettage of fatty tissue and excision of non-malignant lumps were carried out in the right breast. The Silastic II right prosthesis was replaced. Samples consisting of two pieces of fibrofatty tissue, one taken from the infra-medial part of the right breast and another from the lateral part of the right breast, were removed. Fragments of sticky, opalescent white rubbery material, measuring from about 10 mm to less than 0.1 mm, were also recovered from the surgical site.

RESULTS

First Patient

The polyurethane foam cover still surrounds the prosthesis but does not adhere to the silicone shell. On closer macroscopic examination, the mottled silicone adhesive that is used to bond the polyurethane foam to the envelope is still visible on the internal side of the capsule. This shiny glue has now changed to a brown color. Although unaltered in some parts, in others it has become opaque. In a few large areas, this glue together with the embedded foam have disappeared to reveal the biological tissue which has developed inside the polyurethane foam pore structure (Figure 3).

Histologic observations at higher magnification show pores of the polyurethane foam invaded by red blood cells, inflammatory cells and macrophages. The fibrotic reaction is weak and appears concentrated on the outer (tissue side) of the foam. There is some non-adhering granulation tissue between the polyurethane particles. The innermost layers of foam (closest to the prosthesis) are invaded by dense non-staining gel-like foreign material without granulation tissue. These entities have vacuoles filled with another shiny foreign material. All tissues are impregnated by lipids which appear to have an affinity for the polyurethane foam. Sometimes, lipid pools are found within the macrophages.

Scanning microscope examination of the inner side of the capsule, which is in contact with the prosthesis, reveals the foam adhesive at different stages of degradation. The least degraded parts show large numbers of small dispersed vacuoles of about 20–100 μm. Polyurethane foam impressions, sometimes with residues of foam entrapped within the matrix, indicate that foam particles have broken and have been carried or dissolved away (Figure 4). In some places, the adhesive has crumbled and irregular erosion patterns have formed. In other areas, the material has become fissured or fragmented and parts of it have eroded deeply. Detached fragments, with polyurethane particles embedded in them or still attached to coherent foam masses, suggest that the silicone adhesive failed at the silicone–prosthesis shell interface before fragmentation of the foam took place (Figure 5).

Second Patient

The first sample of fibrous tissue collected after 2 months is about 2 mm thick. Remnants of the polyurethane foam network are still visible and are embedded in the tissue near the capsule–prosthesis interface. Early-stage granulation tissue is present nearest to the silicone shell interface. It shows an intense inflammatory reaction with giant cells, mastocytes and a non-staining foreign material presumed to be droplets of silicone oil. Within the middle layer of the capsule, granulation tissue is more mature; histiocytes and macrophages surround the polyurethane foam particles (Figure 6). The outermost part of the polyurethane layer is surrounded by a thin layer of new connective tissue without polyurethane foam. It acts as a boundary between the prosthesis and the adjacent fatty tissue.

The second capsule fragment corresponds to a post-implantation time of 4 months. The overall capsule wall is about 5 mm thick. Polyurethane zones are clearly visible on the side of the prosthesis shell. In some areas, the foam is not invaded by biological tissue. Histologic examination reveals a mature granulation tissue with pronounced macrophage activity. The polyurethane zones are surrounded by inflammatory cells, macrophages, red blood cells and some giant cells. The middle strata in the capsule contain intracellular vacuoles filled with the pervasive non-staining foreign material. Close to the fatty tissue, the outer layers form a thick zone of new granulation tissue. Less dense cellular collagen is oriented in bundles parallel to the surface of the prosthesis.

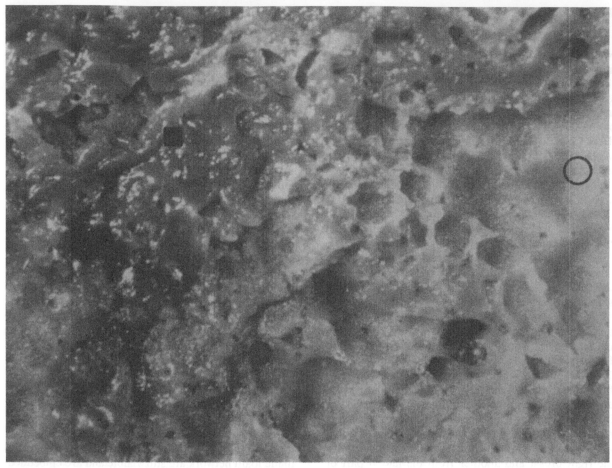

Figure 3. First patient. Part of the internal side of a capsule showing shiny brown glue which was nearly intact: ■, altered: ✪ and absent: ○ revealing the underlying biological tissue (40 mm = 1 mm).

Third Patient

The prosthesis, of very soft consistency, was ruptured at the time of arrival. There is free gel and some tissue associated with it. The tissue is about 2 mm thick and it engulfs the polyurethane foam. The cover is completely separated from the prosthesis and has a pronounced wrinkled appearance in several areas. Some folds in the foam are not invaded by tissue (Figure 7).

Stained sections show a regular, dense layer of collagenous tissue at the polyurethane–shell interface which was initially bound. The central polyurethane sections show multinucleated foreign body giant cells and mastocytes with many granulations. Small agglomerates of red blood cells are also present. Many vacuoles filled with a clear amorphous foreign material are present within tissue that has invaded the polyurethane layer. Collagenous foci are mixed with this granulation tissue and the relative volume of polyurethane to that of tissue appears elevated (Figure 8).

In one sample, a large piece of compacted abiotic material with the same stain uptake characteristics as that of polyurethane is found embedded in the granulation tissue. This piece is associated with translucent foreign material which is tentatively identified as silicone adhesive used to bond the polyurethane to the shell. The polyurethane part correlates with the peripherally fused external edge of the prosthesis.

By comparison with the other capsules and the maturation of granulation tissue, the duration of implantation of this prosthesis is estimated to be about 5 months. The polyurethane sections are invaded by different inflammatory and foreign body-type cells in association with a mature development of connective tissue. The thick collagenous tissue layer present close to the prosthesis is typical of later explantation.

Fourth Patient

The first sample consists mostly of fat cells. The second sample contains polyurethane debris embedded in adipose tissue. Under histologic examination, a large piece of compacted foam material is found. It is tentatively identified as remnants of the polyurethane cover from the heat-fused junction

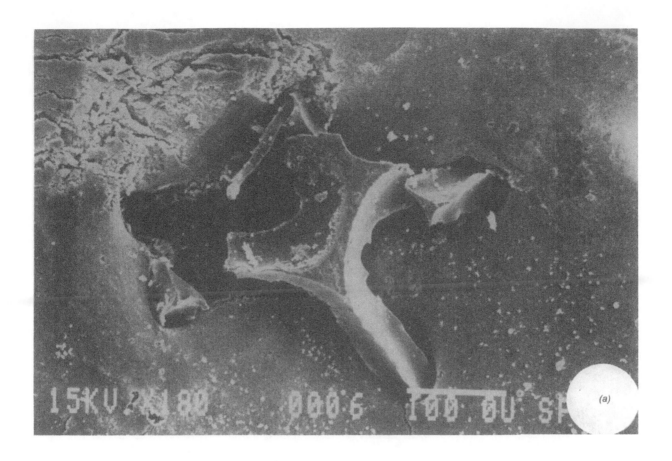

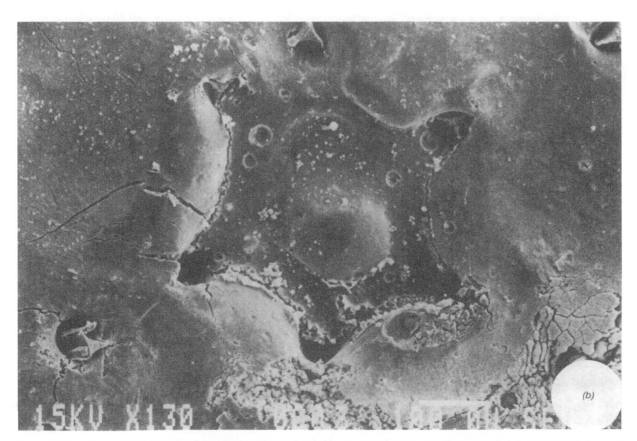

Figure 4. First patient. (a): Internal side of the capsular tissue showing broken polyurethane foam embedded in silicone glue. (b): Polyurethane foam impression, round vacuoles, severely fissured and crumbled adhesive.

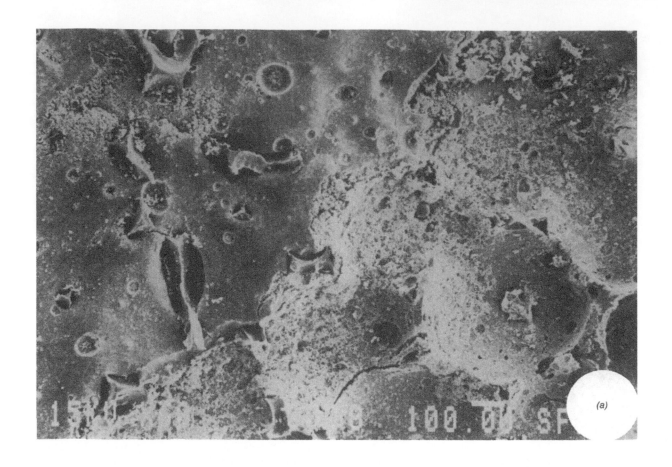

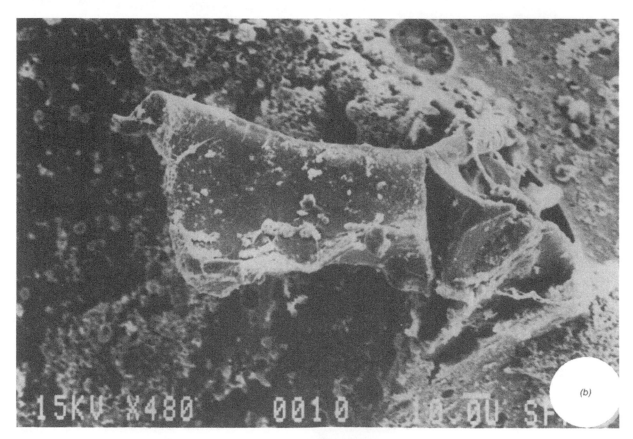

Figure 5. First patient. (a): Low-magnification view showing crumbled and vacuole-containing adhesive on the left and eroded glue on the right with severed polyurethane bridges. (b): Polyurethane fragment broken after erosion of the glue.

198

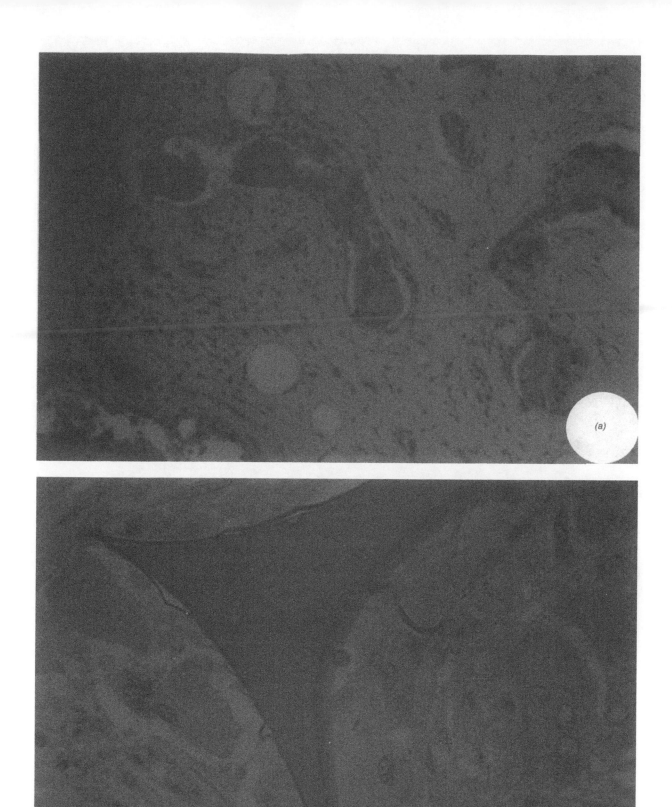

Figure 6. Second patient. (a): Early granulation tissue containing inflammatory cells distributed non-uniformly. The polyurethane areas are stained to an orange color by Sudan IV reagents. Multinucleated giant cells are proliferating peripherally. Foreign material containing oil vacuoles are present in tissue (Sudan IV stain, 240 mm = 1 mm). (b): The polyurethane areas appear uniformly blue with toluidine blue stain preparations. Many multinucleated giant cells are present around the foam particles (toluidine blue stain, 100 mm = 0.1 mm).

199

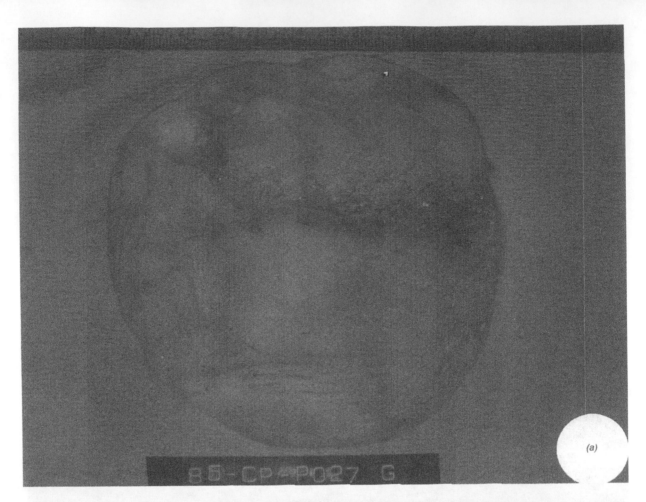

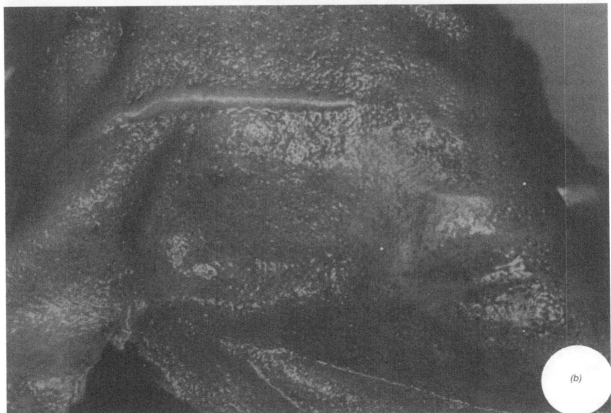

Figure 7. Third patient. (*a*): Explanted prosthesis from patient with the polyurethane cover completely removed from the envelope. The silicone shell is also ruptured and some of the gel is free. (b): Detached external capsule incorporating polyurethane foam.

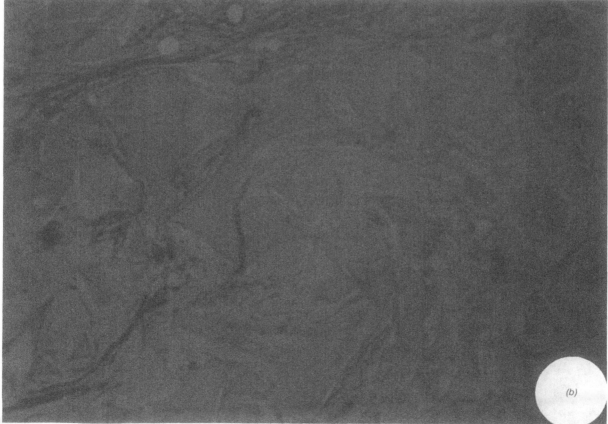

Figure 8. Third patient. (a): Section of polyurethane foam associated with fragments of foreign material believed to be remnants of the silicone glue. Red blood cells and mastocytes with granulation are observed within the granulation tissue. (b): Note large numbers of polyurethane pillars sections compared to the tissue surface. Collagenous foci and vacuoles are interspersed with granulation tissue.

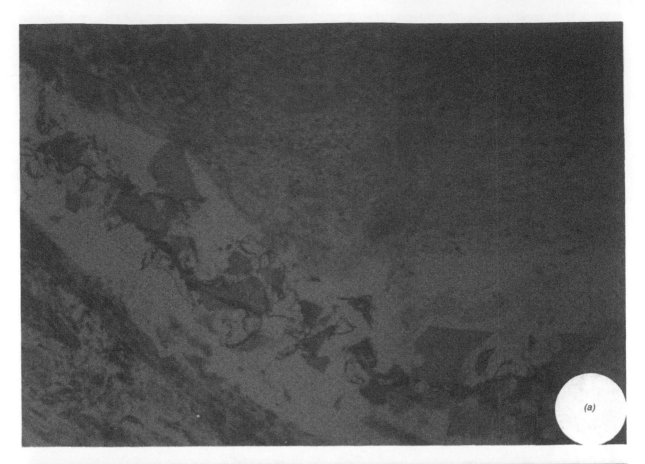

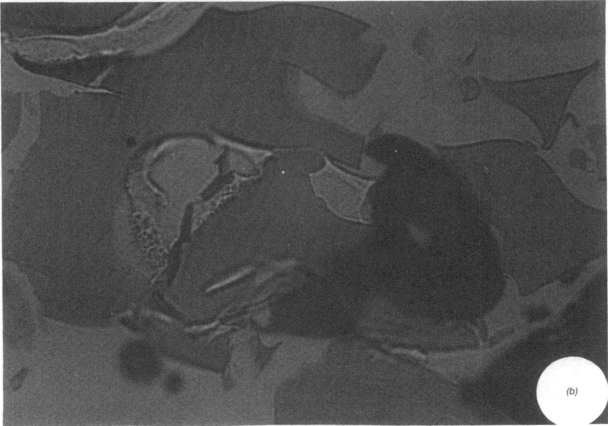

Figure 9. Fourth patient. (a): Large fragment of compacted polyurethane foam identified as the heat-fused junction of the two halves of the cover at the periphery of the prosthesis. A transparent foreign material identified as silicone glue is attached to the foam (250 mm = 1 mm). (b): Large piece of polyurethane engulfed by silicone adhesive, brownish lipids and parts of multinucleated giant cells (100 mm = 0.1 mm).

which is formed by the two halves of the cover as they meet at the periphery. The debris are similar to those found in the previous patient. Amid the tissue and polyurethane, a second foreign material was identified. It consists of particles irregular in shape and size. They appear to have been detached from the silicone adhesive which originally bonded the foam to the prosthesis (Figure 9). Scanning microscopy examination also reveals textile fibers of dressing as well as a piece of a foreign material (Figures 10 and 11). X-ray microanalysis of this material indicates that it contained silicon. This material may therefore have been a fragment of the adhesive.

A third sample taken during biopsy consists of a comparatively large thin fragment (1 cm) of rubbery foreign material which was subsequently identified as a silicone polymer by X-ray microanalysis. Its morphology correlates with the foam adhesive. It shows a smooth surface on one side and a mottled texture on the other (Figure 12).

DISCUSSION

These adventitiously collected prostheses and tissue samples provide significant insight on the behavior of currently sold polyurethane-coated prostheses. The observations confirm those of other workers who investigated reactions surrounding the earlier as well as the current versions of such coated implants [4,7,8, 11,12].

Evidence of deteriorative processes and tissue interaction are already evident 12 days after surgery:

- The polyurethane foam and the silicone adhesive that bonds it to the prosthesis surface become partly detached from the prosthesis core.
- The silicone glue appears to be attacked chemically and its properties are changed soon after implantation. Various stages of alteration of the adhesive are observed until its eventual break-up into very small fragments.
- The polyurethane embedded within the glue becomes progressively weaker and eventually breaks at the same time or just after the glue has mostly disappeared. This contributes to the early separation of the cover.
- Granulation tissue with inflammatory cells and macrophages already occupies foam spaces by the time the cover has detached.

Over longer time intervals, capsules show several possible tissue remodeling paths depending on the site.

- Close to the prosthesis (silicone) wall, there is granulation tissue containing macrophages and giant cells. This tissue develops more rapidly and profusely near the implant.

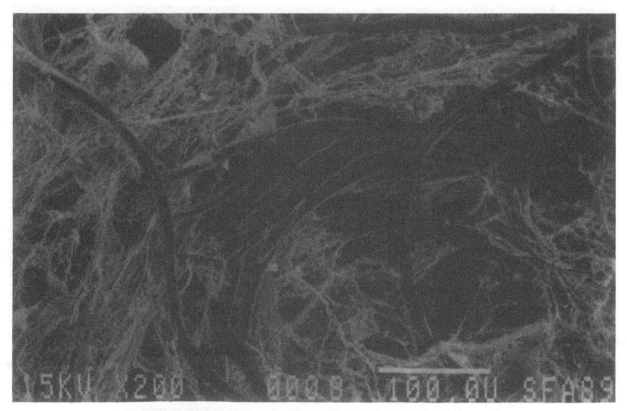

Figure 10. Fourth patient. Textile fibers of dressing observed on the surface of excised fat cells.

- Tissue growth continues outwardly from the polyurethane cover surface. It appears to proceed slowly and generate a connective tissue layer between the original foam cover and the surrounding fatty tissue in about 2–4 months.
- Collagenous tissue without polyurethane debris is also present in the space created by failure of the bond between the cover and the prosthesis inner shell. However, this was noted only in the older capsule. Overall, there appears to be patient- or prosthesis-related differences that could affect the evolution of the capsules.
- The silicone glue used to stick the foam to the prosthesis shell is present, but is altered after only 12 days. It is absent in capsules older than 2–4 months except for the very large pieces which would have taken much longer to break-up and disperse.
- Vacuoles filled with a clear and shiny foreign material similar to oil droplets are always present in the tissue from all four capsules. Their appearance and their behavior are typical of silicone oil products from the interior gel that diffuse through the envelope. Such oils have already been described in literature in connection with capsules surrounding the conventional (smooth wall) prostheses [21,22, 23]. A similar product is associated with parts of the tissue containing polyurethane fragments of the fourth patient, 2 years after removal of the foam-covered prostheses.
- The larger solid entities identified respectively as remnants of the heat-sealed polyurethane circumferential rim and foam adhesive suggest that the half-life of such prosthesis debris may be very long and may encapsulate separately to form palpable masses.

Because the widespread use of this implant on non-mastectomy patients is relatively recent, the value of anecdotal studies based on small numbers of explants is limited. It is therefore urgent to collect more pathological materials of this nature for systematic studies and to perform the appropriate chemical analyses on the degrading materials.

These preliminary observations do not answer all urgent questions. Rather, they invite further questions of equal if not greater importance. At present, the degradation of the polyurethane foam, the failure of the foam adhesive followed by its dispersion and degradation, the apparently variable nature of silicone-based products dispersed in capsules and the long and difficult resorption of this mass of debris should be addressed. When combined with the absence of knowledge regarding the nature and fate of degradation products and their metabolites, there is no basis to further enlarge the population of users. It

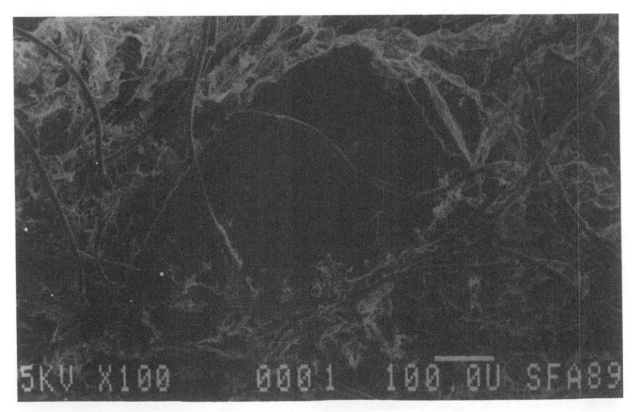

Figure 11. Fourth patient. Piece of silicone adhesive identified by X-ray microanalysis.

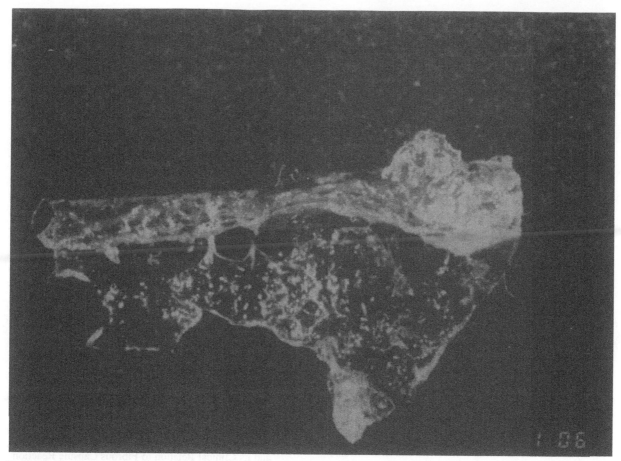

Figure 12. Fourth patient. Large, thin fragment of rubbery material identified as silicone foam adhesive by microanalysis (10 mm = 1 mm).

is essential to develop a data base that would quantify the risks associated with residual debris from the attempted removal of such prostheses. Further studies are needed to provide guidance in the clinical management of possible long-term problems arising from this product.

CONCLUSION

Prosthesis capsular tissues and fragments of breast tissue collected from patients who received polyurethane-coated prostheses show similar deterioration patterns and cellular activity which relate to the dwell time of the product *in vivo*. Outright separation of the foam coating from the silicone core appears to take place in as short a period as 2–3 weeks and loss of material is evident after 4–6 months. Biodeterioration does not take place uniformly. Complete surgical removal of polyurethane and silicone adhesive debris appears difficult if not impossible. Residual material can remain as histologically identifiable entities at least two years after repeated attempts at removing the prostheses and its spallation products. The erratic bonding and/or deteriorative characteristics of foam adhesives used with these prostheses add new dimen-

sions to the evaluation of their safety and the long-term health impact of these products on patients. Until appropriate biocompatibility and metabolic studies have been performed, it would seem prudent to minimize further clinical use of these products.

It has now become of paramount importance to investigate the performances of this controversial class of prostheses by:

(1) Initiating a sound epidemiological study to establish the *in vivo* durability of the prostheses, the success and failure rates and the nature of systemic and local complications
(2) Conducting a basic bench study to characterize the prosthesis and identify the degradation products, if any, and the kinetics of the reactions
(3) Establishing an advisory board which should be set up at the federal or provincial level to advise doctors and patients in regard to the management of complications

ACKNOWLEDGEMENTS

The technical assistance of S. Bourassa, K. Horth and R. Couture is appreciated. We are indebted to those people who gave us specimens and explanted prostheses. We extend our gratitude to Drs. T. How, G. Roy, J. C. Forest and C. Poirier for help and guidance.

REFERENCES

1. Herman, S. 1984. "The Même Implant", *Plast. Reconstr. Surg.*, 73:411–414.

2. Kerrigan, C. L. 1989. "Report on the Même Breast Implant", National Health and Welfare Canada.

3. Marion, R. B. 1984. "Polyurethane-Covered Breast Implant", *Plast. Reconstr. Surg.*, 74:728–729.

4. Umansky, C. 1985. "Infection with Polyurethane-Covered Implants", *Plast. Reconstr. Surg.*, 75:925.

5. Wilkinson, T. S. 1985. "Polyurethane-Coated Implants", *Plast. Reconstr. Surg.*, 75:925–926.

6. Capozzi, A. and V. R. Pennisi. 1981. "Clinical Experience with Polyurethane-Covered Gel Filled Mammary Prostheses", *Plast. Reconstr. Surg.*, 68:512–518.

7. Slade, C. L. and H. D. Peterson. 1982. "Disappearance of the Polyurethane Cover of the Ashley Natural-Y Prosthesis", *Plast. Reconstr. Surg.*, 70:379–382.

8. Okunski, W. J. and R. P. Chowdary. 1987. "Infected Meme Implants; Salvage Reconstruction with Latissimus Dorsi Myocutaneous Flaps and Silicone Implants", *Aesth. Plast. Surg.*, 11:49–51.

9. Eyssen, J. E., A. J. Von Weissowetz and G. D. Middleton. 1984. "Reconstruction of the Breast Using Polyurethane-Coated Prostheses", *Plast. Reconstr. Surg.*, 73:415–421.

10. Melmed, E. P. 1988. "Polyurethane Implants: a 6-year Review of 416 Patients", *Plast. Reconstr. Surg.*, 82:285–290.

11. Smahel, J. 1978. "Tissue Reactions to Breast Implant Coated with Polyurethane", *Plast. Reconstr. Surg.*, 61:80–85.

12. Jabaley, M. E. and S. K. Das. 1986. "Late Breast Pain Following Reconstruction with Polyurethane-Covered Implants", *Plast. Reconstr. Surg*, 78:390–395.

13. Truong, L. D., J. Cartwright, D. Goodman and D. Woznicki. 1988. "Silicone Lymphadenopathy Associated with Augmentation Mammaplasty", *Am. J. Surg. Pathol.*, 12:484–491.

14. Schatten, W. E. 1984. "Reconstruction of Breast following Mastectomy with Polyurethane-Coated Prostheses", *Ann. Plast. Surg.*, 12:147–156.

15. Anonymous. 1989. "Aesthetech Failed to Report Silicone Breast Prosthesis Failure", Medical Devices and Diagnostic Industry Reports, 15:W-6.

16. Gerstenberg, G. J. 1989. Regulatory Letter to R. Helbing, Surgitek Medical Engineering Corp., Racine, Wisconsin, USA, March 6.

17. Batich, C., J. Williams and R. King. 1989. "Toxic Hydrolysis Product from a Biodegradable Foam Implant", *J. Biomed. Mat. Res.; Applied Biomaterials*, 23, A3:311–319.

18. Brody, G. S. in Discussion. 1984. *Plast. Reconstr. Surg.*, 73:420–421.

19. Ashley, F. L. 1970. "A New Type of Breast Prosthesis: Preliminary Report", *Plast. Reconstr. Surg.*, 45:421–427.

20. Pangman, W. J. Compound Prosthesis. U. S. Patent No. 3,559,214, issued 1971.

21. Barker, D. E., M. I. Retsky and S. Schultz. 1978. "'Bleeding' of Silicone from Bag-Gel Breast Implants, and its Clinical Relation to Fibrous Capsule Reaction", *Plast. Reconstr. Surg.*, 61:836.

22. Wickham, G. and R. Rudolph. 1978. "Silicone Identification in Prosthesis-Associated Fibrous Capsules", *Science*, 199:437–439.

23. Mandel, M. A. and D. F. Gibbons. 1979. "The Presence of Silicone in Breast Capsules", *Aesth. Plast. Surg.*, 3:219–225.

15

Clinical Applications of Percutaneous Implants

MAGNUS JACOBSSON, M.D., Ph.D.*
ANDERS TJELLSTRÖM, M.D., Ph.D.*

ABSTRACT: Osseointegration is defined as a loaded implant surface in direct contact with living bone tissue at the light-microscopic level. In the following chapter the scientific background to osseointegration is reviewed and the clinical applications in otolaryngology derived from this concept. We routinely use commercially pure titanium implants for the Bone-Anchored Hearing Aid and for retention of Bone-Anchored Auricular and Orbital Prostheses. The integration of the implants into the bone tissue make possible the creation of reaction-free percutaneous passages. The clinical results of the Bone-Anchored Hearing Aid, Bone-Anchored Auricular and Orbital Prostheses and the percutaneous passages are also presented.

INTRODUCTION

The term osseointegration was coined by Bråne-mark et al. [1] in 1977 to describe a direct bone-to-implant interface observed in experimental and clinical investigations (Figure 1). Earlier, the development of a layer of intervening fibrous tissue between implant and bone tissue had been considered an inevitable result when a metal device was inserted into bone [2]. Albrektsson [3] published a clarification of the concept and defined osseointegration as a direct contact between a loaded implant surface and bone at the light-microscopic level. We maintain, in accordance with Albrektsson and Jacobsson [4], that at least 90% of the implant surface, at the level of cortical passage, be covered with bone for the term osseointegration to apply.

The first clinical application of this concept was in the field of dental implants. After many years of intensive experimental work, the method of direct anchor-

age of retention elements for intraoral reconstruction has progressed into a routine clinical procedure today [5]. Brånemark developed an oral implant for anchoring dentures in the edentulous jaw which, unlike dental implants anchored in fibrous tissue, gave excellent and lasting results. Although in the short term the results may be very convincing, long-term treatment results are very rare and the only reports that have been published in this respect deal with the Brånemark system. Adell [6,7] have followed up implants in the upper and lower jaw after intervals of 10, 15, and 20 years. The implant failures that these authors found occurred almost exclusively during the first 3 to 12 months after implantation. After this period very few implants were lost. The success rate after 10 years was better than 80% for implants in the upper jaw and better than 90% in the lower jaw. In a multicenter study of 11 international teams from North America, Europe and Australia, Albrektsson et al. [8] could show impressive long-term results for 1, 3 and 5 whole years from implant insertion. Fixture survival rate in the mandible for 5 years was 92.82% (195 implants), for 3 years 96.02% (1029 implants) and for one year 97.38% (2520 implants). The corresponding results for maxillary implants were for 5 years 100% (12 implants), for 3 years 89.02% (164 implants), and for 1 year 90.97% (631 implants).

Inspired by the promising results of Brånemark and associates, the method of direct-bone anchorage was attempted in the field of otolaryngology, at our clinic, starting in 1977. Some of our patients faced major obstacles to the leading of a normal life—obstacles which called for unconventional solutions. One patient category that had long endured in silence were those with maxillofacial disfigurement either congenital or after extensive tumour surgery. There simply had been no method available for safe retention of maxillofacial prostheses. The patients who were unable to use conventional air-conduction hearing aids due to chronically draining ears had to resort to sound vibrators attached either to glasses or to a steel

*ENT-Department, Sahlgren's Hospital, S-413 45 Gothenburg, Sweden

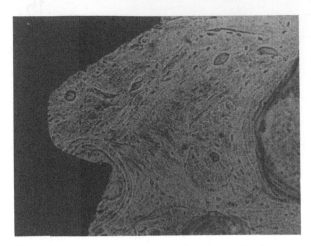

Figure 1. Osseointegration involves a direct bone-to-implant contact. On the left is seen the implant with a thread (black) and on the right is the mature bone tissue.

spring worn over the head. The use of osseointegrated fixtures to retain maxillofacial prostheses and bone-anchored hearing devices have, based on experimental and clinical experience, evolved into everyday clinical practice. Today over 280 patients operated on at our clinic wear bone-anchored hearing devices. Some 130 patients have been fitted with either orbital or auricular prostheses retained with the aid of osseointegrated fixtures.

The installation of the implants that we use is a two-step surgical procedure. The first step involves the insertion of the screw-shaped fixture, using a very controlled and minimally traumatic technique. After a healing period of 3–5 months, the second step is performed. This entails surgery for the actual skin penetration and the connection of an abutment to the fixture. This is also a procedure that has to be controlled by careful surgery. The key to success in constructing a reaction-free percutaneous passage, in our view, is to minimize the movements between soft tissue and implant surface. This is done by extensive subcutaneous tissue reduction at the second operation.

We believe that we are only at the beginning of a process that promises to develop into many new areas for the benefit of patients. One might ask: what is unique about osseointegration in otolaryngology? To put it succinctly, we believe the answer is: direct anchorage of an implant in living bone tissue and a reaction-free skin penetration with predictable long-term results. Below, we present the scientific background to our work as well as the experience and results we have attained in this special field of biology.

BONE TISSUE: ELEMENTARY CONSTITUENTS AND CELLULAR BASES

Bone is a connective tissue. The structure in and on which bone cells live is made up of three principal constituents. Collagen fibres make up nearly a third of

the dry weight of the bone matrix. Crystals, mainly in the form of mineral hydroxyapatite, form up two-thirds of the dry weight of bone matrix. The cement, which holds together the fibrils and the crystals consists of, among other substances, mucopolysaccharides, proteoglycans, lipids, carbonate, citrate, sodium, magnesium and fluoride [9].

The bone cells fall into more or less differentiated categories. The osteocyte is a well-differentiated, fixed-post mitotic cell incapable of further cell division [10] which is lodged within a lacuna in the mature bone tissue. The lacunae are arranged in a concentric pattern, the Haversian system, around a central vessel located in the Haversian canal. The osteocytes get their supply of nutrients and oxygen and dispose of waste products through a diffusion mechanism in interplay with these vessels. The cortical, Haversian bone is pierced, from its inner and outer surface, by the canals of Volkmann, through which the vascular supply to the Haversian canals is maintained [11]. The surfaces of the canals of Volkmann and the Haversian canals as well as the inner surface (endosteum) and the outer surface (periosteum) are lined with cells of osteogenetic capability [9]. These cells are chiefly the undifferentiated mesenchymal cells and the preosteoblasts and the osteoblasts [12]. The former cells are the precursors of the latter. The osteoblasts are actively engaged in the production and secretion of components of bone matrix [9]. When the cortical, Haversian bone is formed, the osteoblast becomes an osteocyte, trapped in its lacuna. The resorption of bone is mainly controlled by the osteoclasts. Their origin is disputed but two major theories have evolved, proposing that they are originated either from blood-bourne mononuclear precursors that unite to form multinucleated osteoclasts, or from local tissue precursors [12]. In reviews published in recent years, the blood-bourne origin of the osteoclast has been emphasised [13,14,15].

NORMAL BONE HEALING

The bone healing process is very complex and much remains to be investigated but, three main factors can be recognised: cytogenic impetus, osteogenetic cellular capability, and sufficient nutrition. These are elaborated below.

Cytogenic Impetus

The release of an osteogenetic inducer from the extracellular space (Bone Morphogenetic Protein) has been proposed by Urist et al. [16]. Piezoelectric signals are another factor considered to be of importance as a stimulus to bone repair [17,18,19]. Burwell [20] has introduced a theory proposing that dying cells in a fracture region could stimulate neighbouring cells to differentiate into bone-forming cells.

Osteogenetic Cellular Capability

Undifferentiated mesenchymal cells that are located along the blood vessels in the Haversian canals and the canals of Volkmann, as well as in the stroma of bone marrow are considered to be progenitors of the preosteoblasts which through mitosis evolve into osteoblasts [9,21]. The differentiation of new osteoblasts is a rapid process and it has been shown that already 24 hours after the fracturing of a rabbit costa there is a new layer of osteoblasts lining the original bone surface [22].

The osteoblasts surviving the fracture trauma are also an important source of osteogenetic capacity. The osteoblasts form an osteoid, which is the organic part of the bone matrix. An osteoblast in a 31-day old mouse can produce 0.17 mm³ matrix on average in a day [23]. By the action of alkaline phosphatase as a pyrophosphatase removing the pyrophosphate (a strong inhibitor of the calcification process), the osteoid becomes calcified and the callus is formed [9]. By a process known as creeping substitution [24] the callus becomes gradually lamellarised, i.e., organised in Haversian systems.

Sufficient Nutrition

A reduction in the metabolic rate of the bone cells close to the fracture may be one way to endure the reduced nutritional supply in the fracture area [25]. No bone regeneration is possible without access to functioning vessels. Rhinelander [26] estimated the vascular penetration rate in cancellous bone to be maximally 0.5 mm per day. Albrektsson [27] showed the vascular penetration rate to be 0.05 mm per day in cortical bone (creeping substitution).

FACTORS OF IMPORTANCE FOR THE ESTABLISHMENT OF OSSEOINTEGRATION

For osseointegration to occur it is of vital importance that certain factors be taken into consideration. Below are outlined some of these relevant considerations.

Material Biocompatibility

It is obvious that an implant must be free of toxic substances or that such substances must not be formed during the lifetime of the patient. The material should not cause allergy or have carcinogenic properties. The implant material should be accepted by the host organism's immune system and not be rejected. Silver and Howden [28] tested titanium biocompatibility in the rabbit ear chamber and found no cellular or vascular reaction. Titanium appeared to be tolerated as completely benign.

Implant Design—Macrostructure

The use of a threaded screw provides a form of interlocking with the bone tissue that allows full development of the strength of the bone for any direction of loading. The close apposition of the bone to the implant surface provides a similar transmission of load at the interface of the bone and implant, at the microscopic level.

Implant Surface—Microstructure

The tear-off strength (resistance to tensile force) will after complete osseointegration equal that of trabecular bone [30]. As a result of the manufacturing process, the Nobelpharma implants have a surface with microgrooves parallel to the threads. This is an aid to carrying stresses, provided the bone grows in close approximation to the surface roughness of the implant. If the bone tissue is not in close approximation to the implant, the roughness may be detrimental, because the peaks of roughness will then lead to stress concentrations and possible degradation of the bone tissue [31].

Status of the Implant Bed

Systemic diseases as well as the previous treatment of the organism, either systemically or locally to the implant bed, may greatly influence the fate of the implant. Rheumatoid arthritis has a negative influence on integration of implants, but diabetes mellitus has not been shown to have a decidedly negative influence on the fate of the implant. Severe osteoporosis is considered a relative contraindication [32]. Irradiation has a decidedly negative effect on bone healing as has been shown in several experimental studies [33–37].

Using divisible titanium implants, so-called Bone Growth Chambers, implanted in the proximal tibial metaphysis of rabbits, the healing pattern of bone tissue was studied both in normal and irradiated tissue. One implant was inserted in the irradiated leg and another in the control leg of each animal. The animals thus served as their own controls. It could be shown that single doses of 5 to 8 Gy Co⁶⁰ in rabbits lead to a reduction in bone formation of about 20%. At dose levels of 11, 15 and 25 Gy the reduction was about 65 to 75% [34]. A recovery in bone formation by a factor of almost 2.5, however, was seen after a recovery period of 12 months [36].

The information on the fate of clinically used implants in irradiated tissue is, unfortunately, scant. Jacobsson et al. [38] published a study of nine patients who had undergone external irradiation prior to the insertion of implants into the orbital or temporal regions. The absorbed dose to the implant region varied between 25 and 86 Gy normalised to 5 fractions of 2.0 Gy/wk, according to the cumulative radiation effect formula. The time interval between irradiation and implant insertion varied from 9 months to 37 years. Of the thirty-five implants installed, only five were lost because of lack of osseointegration. The follow-up time from implant insertion ranged from 15 to 44 months. Histological post-mortem specimens of clinically successful osseointegrated implants showed bone in direct apposition to the titanium oxide. There was no interposed soft tissue nor were there any signs of inflammatory reaction in the marrow space. Haversian systems were seen in the threads. Bone tissue was in direct contact with the implant on upper as well as on lower thread surfaces and all around the circumference of the implant. In contrast to this, the failed implants were surrounded by a coat of fibrous tissue.

Surgical Technique

In order to optimize the bone healing conditions, utmost care must be taken to avoid undue injury to the implant site during implant insertion. This means minimizing both bone cell death and damage to the microcirculation. It requires the use of sharp instruments, such as spiral drills and tap burrs, as well as a low drill speed and adequate cooling. Heat develops easily if adequate cooling is not used during surgery. Eriksson et al. [39] found that the use of a conventional drilling technique with rapidly rotating drills, despite a controlled cooling procedure, causes an average temperature elevation on the order of 89°C. This is worth remembering since retarded bone growth occurs after only 47°C for 1 minute [40]. On the other hand, if the surgical technique described for implants in this chapter is used, only minor and insignificant temperature elevations will occur [41]. In a study on the effect of the force used when inserting an implant in bone tissue Albrektsson et al. [42] could show that the removal torque of an implant after a healing period, was inversely proportional to the insertion torque used. In other words: a gentle surgical insertion technique will lead to better integration of the implant in the recipient bone bed.

Implant Movements and Overloading

It has been demonstrated that bone cell differentiation will become disturbed if the implant is exposed to movements relative to the bone tissue of the implant bed [43]. The screw-shape of the implant in part maximizes stabilization, but the risk of nonintegration is great if a load is put on an implant not yet properly integrated in the bone tissue [32].

IMPLANTS AND THE INTERFACE ZONE

The Interface

The interface zone between the implant and the bone tissue into which the implant is anchored is a very complex, dynamic, and continuously changing region. It is not to be regarded as a distinct boundary between implant and bone, but instead as a zone which is several hundred Ångströms thick and which contains a large variety of molecules and structures with crystalline and cellular elements [31].

Definition of "Interface Zone"

When the implant and tissue are brought into contact, a mutual interaction is initiated, i.e., the implant may induce changes in the biological system, which may in turn, via surface reactions, induce changes in the implant material. The interface zone is the region where such changes occur.

Properties of Solid Implant Materials

Before discussing in detail the implant made of commercially pure (c.p.) titanium and its surface characteristics, a brief review of properties of solid implants is in order. Solid implant materials are either polycrystalline, with crystallites made up of ordered arrangements of atoms, or amorphous, which means noncrystalline with a less-ordered atomic arrangement. Metals are often polycrystalline and composed of one kind of atom. Alloys are metallic mixtures. Metals and alloys have a high chemical reactivity. Ceramics are compounds between metals and other elements and usually polycrystalline. Glasses are amorphous. Carbon materials are amorphous, chemically inert and have favourable wear properties [44,45].

Processes at the Surface of Implant Materials

Most surfaces are heterogenous, due to imperfections. Mobility of atoms is higher along surfaces than in bulk metal, and many different reactions occur on the surfaces of implant materials. Segregation, which can occur during heat sterilization and autoclaving, means that bulk impurity of low concentration accumulates at the surface. Adsorption is either molecular, which means that the molecules stick to the surface in the original configuration, or dissociative, which means that the molecules at the surface become dissociated due to interaction with the surface. Adsorption is the primary reason for surface compositional changes. Desorption is the reverse process of adsorption. Absorption, finally, implies the dissolution of atoms on the surface into the bulk of the material [45].

Composition of Commercially Pure Titanium Implants

The bulk of the implants we use is commercially pure (c.p.) titanium. According to Avesta Jernverks AB, which is the source of the titanium, the composition is the following:

titanium	Ti	99.75%

iron	Fe	0.05%
oxygen	O	0.10%
nitrogen	N	0.03%
carbon	C	0.05%
hydrogen	H	0.012%

Structure of Commercially Pure Titanium Implants

The structure of this implant is polycrystalline, that is, it consists of randomly oriented crystallites whose sizes depend on the material processing [31]. During the manufacturing process and the cleaning procedure (ultrasonic cleaning, autoclaving) an oxide layer about 50 Å thick develops. The thickness of this layer is ten to twenty times larger than typical atomic dimensions. It is important to stress the fact that the oxide layer, which is the part of the implant which is in contact with the surrounding tissue, is thus in reality a ceramic material [31].

Oxides on Commerically Pure Titanium Implants

Titanium forms several oxides of different stoichiometry (TiO, Ti_2O_3, TiO_2) of which TiO_2 is the most common. Titanium is one of the most corrosion-resistant materials known, due to the high resistance of TiO_2 to chemical attack [44]. Titanium is virtually uncorrodable in near-neutral solutions, especially those containing the chloride ions which attack most metals and alloys [46]. This is one contributing factor to its high biocompatibility. For materials such as titanium oxide the electrostatic part of the energy needed to move a charged particle from the (highly conducting) aqueous medium into the oxide is inversely proportional to the dielectric constant, which is uniquely high for titanium dioxide. Similarly, denaturation effects are probably more likely on surfaces with low dielectricity constants, such as aluminium oxides, than on titanium dioxide [31].

Surface Spectroscopy of Commercially Pure Titanium Implants

Auger electron spectroscopic studies have shown that the oxide thickness on osseointegrated titanium implants increases continually during implantation. Also, calcium and phosphorus were found in the entire thickness of the oxides [47]. The chemical composition of titanium surfaces prepared according to the standard procedure used at Nobelpharma Company, is quite well known. Kasemo and Lausmaa [44] have compared this surface to the composition of bulk TiO_2 using surface-sensitive spectroscopic methods. It was found that the surface of the implant specimen is mainly TiO_2. Several chemical elements were present on the oxidised titanium surface that were absent on the reference TiO_2 sample such as carbon, nitrogen, chloride, sulphur and calcium.

Surface Analysis of Retrieved Commercially Pure Titanium Implants

An oxide layer 2000 Å thick was found on implants retrieved after 6 years in man, compared to unimplanted implants with 50 Å. In addition to this, varying amounts of Ca, P and S were found to be incorporated in the surface oxides of the retrieved implants [44].

Reactions between Commerically Pure Titanium Implants and Bone

When the implant and tissue are brought into contact, a process of interaction starts, i.e., the implant may induce changes in the biological system, which may in turn, via surface reactions, induce changes in the implant material. The interface zone is the region where such changes occur [45]. Several chemical processes can take place in the interface region. The increase in the thickness of the oxide layer over time is due to diffusion of oxygen from the bioliquid surrounding the implant into the oxide–metal interface or by diffusion of metal atoms/ions out to the oxide surface followed by oxidation or by hydroxide formation. Minerals such as calcium and phosphorus may also contribute to the growth of the oxide layer. The biomolecules initially adsorbed to the oxide layer may become desorbed and replaced by other biomolecules or may undergo such modifications as fragmentation [44]. The implant material chosen and its surface treatment are important in this last respect, as discussed in connection with surface energy and the dielectricity constant above.

These processes may be influenced by several factors. Important among those are the presence of impurities, an excess of metal atoms or oxygen vacancies, and sites where specific properties exist which influence the chemistry of the interface [31]. A spectrum of defect sites thus presents many possibilities for influencing chemical bond strength and the coordination between the implant surface and adjacent biomolecules. Upon insertion of an implant, the first reaction that will occur is diffusion of proteins and lipids to the implant surface. The proteins not irreversibly adsorbed can be exchanged for others. Structural and conformational changes are sure to occur in the adsorbed protein layer. After these initial reactions, which have a duration of up to a few minutes, diffusion into the implant surface may also take place [31]. Now, cells will start to interact with the surface and its protein layer. This will take place when the protein layer reaches a thickness of more than 1 nm [44]. Eventually, new bone may be formed.

In studies on implants in the abdominal wall of rats Thomsen [48] found that titanium implants induce a lower inflammatory response than do implants of polytetrafluoroethylene (PTFE) as determined by the number of polymorphonuclear granulocytes (PMN) and monocytes/macrophages in the extravascular space close to the implant. It is speculated that the outcome of the healing process is determined very early after implant insertion and that the interactions between inflammatory cells and the implant may play a decisive role in the development of tissue response. Thomsen states that it is possible that the adsorption pattern of the protein detected in the extravascular space determines the reactivity of the implant surface toward PMN and macrophages. Another possibility is that proteins become modified by interactions with the surface, which might lead to secondary events such as attraction, adherence, and activation of inflammatory cells.

Chemical Bonding Forces in the Interface Zone

Biomolecules may be bonded to the implant surface by several different forces, of which van der Waal's bonding is the weakest type. Bonds are also established between permanent electric dipoles. Hydrogen bonds are thought to be important in the interface, as are the strongest bonds, the covalent and ionic bonds [44].

Experimental Studies on the Interface Zone

Using an experimental method of TEM, Albrektsson et al. [49] were able to visualize the interface zone. A plastic plug implant technique was used, where a thin coat of titanium was vaporised on a plastic core implant. This implant with the covering titanium film was then sectioned for TEM. After an implantation period of six months and at more than 100,000 times magnification, the intact bone–metal interface could be studied. The collagen bundles of the bone tissue became gradually replaced by randomly arranged filaments at a distance of 0.1 to 0.5 μm from the titanium. These collagen filaments reached as close as 200 Å from the titanium surface. The last 200–300 Å to the implant surface were taken up by a partly calcified amorphous ground substance consisting of proteoglycans and glycoseaminoglycans.

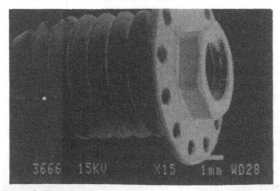

Figure 2. Scanning electron microscopic image of the fixture used for bone-anchored retention of hearing devices and prostheses in the auricular and orbital regions. The miniscule grooves on the threads can be seen.

These last 200–300 Å were thus devoid of collagen. There was no decalcified space found between titanium and tissue but the calcification was less pronounced in the last few hundred Å from the implant surface. The cellular processes that approached the implant surface were also separated from it by a layer of proteoglycans 200-300 Å thick. The proteoglycans are believed to act as a glue for adhesion between cell fibrils and other structures. The glycoseaminoglycans (mainly monosaccharides and chondroitinic sulphate) may play a role in forming hydrogen bonds to the implant surface [31]. The hydroxyl groups of the ground substance may act as important sites for the calcification process [50].

Surface Roughness

It has been demonstrated by several authors that rough implant surfaces bond better to bone tissue than do smooth surfaces [51,52]. Thomas and Cook [53] found that CP titanium cylinders implanted in the femora of dogs became directly bone-anchored if the surface was rough (sandblasted) whereas polished implants were surrounded by a coat of fibrous tissue. The forces that act between the implant and bone tissue can be divided into shear force and tensile force [30]. The shear force develops first through tissue ingrowth into the surface irregularities. During this early stage no tensile forces can be applied to the implant–bone interface, since this will lead to a separation. After a longer time complete osseointegration occurs, and only then can tensile forces be applied. The tear-off strength (resistance to tensile force) will, after complete osseointegration, equal that of trabecular bone. The roughness of the titanium surface is an aid to carrying stresses, provided that the bone grows in close approximation to the surface roughness of the implant (Figure 2).

Toxicity in Commerically Pure Titanium Implants

Titanium does leak from the implant, as evidenced by the occasional blackness of the tissue surrounding the implant. No adverse tissue effects have been demonstrated [31]. Proper ultrasonic cleaning will reduce this leakage and the subsequent blackening reaction [54]. Woodman and collaborators [55] studied metal concentration in the lung, liver, kidney, spleen and in muscle and lymph nodes adjacent to titanium-based fibre metal composite implants inserted as segmented bone replacements in the long bones of baboons. The authors followed the animals for up to 8 years. It was found that the titanium levels in the lung tissue increased up to 3 years after implantation but then reached a plateau without further increases. No evidence was found of any biochemical or hematologic toxicity. Persistent dietary intake of the metal results in some accumulation in the heart, lungs, spleen and kidneys, although no adverse effects have been observed following titanium ingestion [56].

Methods of Surface Preparation

The method used at our laboratory for cleaning the c.p. titanium implants involves ultrasonic cleansing in different solvents to remove oil, fingerprints, etc. This is followed by autoclaving at 130–140°C for 20 minutes. Several other techniques may come into use in the future, such as thermal spraying to produce porous and thick coatings, sputtering (deposition of the coating material in its atomic or molecular form), glow discharge with oxygen plasma to create a well-defined oxide layer, or ion implantation [45]. Baier and co-workers [57] recommend glow discharge with oxygen plasma for materials with high surface energy, followed by scrupulous care in specimen storage under contaminant-free liquids.

Clinical Evidence of Osseointegration

Several clinical methods have been attempted to demonstrate osseointegration, but unfortunately they can only provide a rough indication of true tissue response. It is important to note that clinical methods can be used only to indicate, not to verify, osseointegration, which is a concept defined at the light-microscopic level [4]. Performing a clinical mobility test, as proposed by several authors, and finding the implant mobile, is definite evidence of non-integration [1,6]. Unfortunately, the reverse is not true. In other words, the presence of clinical stability cannot be taken as evidence of osseointegration. Radiolucent zones around implants is a clear indication of non-integration, whereas the lack of such zones is not evidence of integration. The reason for this is that the optimal resolution capacity of radiography is in the range of 0.1 mm whereas the size of a soft tissue cell is in the range of 0.01 mm; thus a narrow zone of fibrous tissue may be undetectable by radiography. The clinical test of using a metal instrument to tap the implant and analyse the transmitted sound may, in theory, be used to indicate a proper osseointegration [4]. To our knowledge there is, however, no typical "sound diagram" defined for the osseointegrated implant, in contrast to the implant anchored in fibrous tissue.

Bone Apposition and Removal Torque of Commercially Pure Titanium Implants

We know from experimental studies in the rabbit [58] that full apposition of bone to the implant surface takes some time to develop. Johansson and partners [58] could show that 21 days after insertion of a threaded c.p. titanium implant in the rabbit tibia and femur the interface zone exhibited mostly soft tissue. Thirty days after insertion the morphological findings indicated a poor contact between implant and the bone, although more bone was observed in the threads compared to 21 days after insertion. At 90 and 180 days the amount of bone in the interface zone had increased but not until 360 days after implant insertion was there more than 90% overall contact between implant and bone at the cortical passage. In clinical practice, a 3–5 month healing period is recommended before an implant is fully loaded, in order to allow enough stability and bone-to-implant contact so that the implant is not lost [1].

We also know, from radiographic studies of clinical material [59] that an adequate load is important during the healing after this first period, as this will promote an increased corticalisation around the implant over longer periods of time. Johansson and co-workers [58] also measured the removal force for the titanium implants located in the femora and tibiae at varying time intervals after insertion. There was a sharp increase in the torque removal force during the first 90 days when an average of 61 Ncm for the femoral implants and 69 Ncm for the tibial ones was reached. The forces measured at one year were 85 Ncm for the femoral implants and 88 Ncm for the tibial implants. In a clinical study of 10 patients where c.p. titanium implants were removed 3 to 4 months after insertion the removal torque measured was an average of 42.7 Ncm with a range of 26 to 60 Ncm [60]. In a follow-up study to this [61], 24 patients with a total of 28 fixtures were studied and a positive correlation between the torque necessary for implant removal and the time of implantation was found. The correlation coefficient was 0.577. The removal torques varied from 20 to over 170 Ncm, with an average of 69.5 Ncm. The implants had been inserted between 3 months and 8 years earlier. A significant difference were found between the implants that had been inserted between 0 and 4 months compared to the implants that had been in place for between 4 months and 3 years, and those that had been in place for over 3 years. However, there was no significant difference in removal torque between implants that had been in place for from 4 months to 3 years and those that had been in place for over 3 years.

SKIN PENETRATION

Percutaneous implants are foreign objects penetrating surgically created skin defects. According to some authors [62,63] who conducted studies on polyethylene terephthalate velour percutaneous implants, failure occurs for several reasons, the main contributing ones being marsupialisation, permigation, avulsion, infection, and a combination of these. Marsupialisation occurs when the proliferating epidermal capsule surrounding the implant forms a sinus tract along the smooth surface of an implant. Permigation is the migration of connective tissue and epidermal cells into a porous implant surface. Avulsion pertains to the mechanical disruption of the interface between soft tissue and implant surface.

In one experiment, the collagen formed in the interstices of the porous implant was immature, and the turnover of collagen and glycoseaminoglycans was accelerated. The configurations and concentrations of collagen and glycoseaminoglycans were abnormal in a similar experiment [64]. The immaturity of the connective tissue in these instances appears to be related to the concentration of giant cells and polymorphonuclear granulocytes [65]. Yan and colleagues [66] using polyethylene terephthalate velour percutaneous implants, some of which were covered with c.p. titanium, found a greater collagen formation-rate around the c.p. titanium-covered velour. Lundgren [67] could demonstrate successful tissue ingrowth into monofilament polyester fabrics used as percutaneous implants. Infection was absent in a study of porous carbon percutaneous implants, although superficial surface colonization and infection did occur after deliberate application of pathogens [68]. Bacterial inhibition has been demonstrated with electrical stimulation of percutaneous silver implants [69].

In an experimental study, Gould and co-workers [70] concluded that the experimental evidence suggests that epithelial cells form a strong and possibly biomechanically resistant attachment to titanium *in vivo*. It is suggested that epithelial cells attach to titanium surfaces in the same way they attach to surfaces *in vivo*, i.e. by hemidesmosomes and basal lamina. Jansen et al. [71] studied attachment of guinea-pig epidermal cells to different substrates. Three main types of attachment were identified in the cell substratum interface: focal contacts, extracellular matrix contacts (ECM) and hemidesmosome-like contacts. This study failed to show any hemidesmosomes in the titanium epithelial interface. The nature of epithelial attachment to implant surfaces is thus a very complex issue where relatively little is known, but it seems clear that the adsorption and activation of certain plasma proteins play key roles in the subsequent cellular and molecular events that are critical to implant surfaces [72].

The term "contact guidance" refers to the possibility of influencing the growth-direction of epithelial cells in culture by preparing the substratum with grooves of microscopic dimensions. This process has been shown experimentally on titanium-covered silicon wafers and on epoxy stratum [73]. It is interesting to recognise that the c.p. titanium implants used for the attachment of osseointegrated hearing aids and auricular and orbital prostheses all have microgrooves at a 90 degree angle to the implant axis. The repair processes in a wound, such as those created at the insertion of a percutaneous implant, involve the migration of epithelial cells. The mechanism behind this is not clear, but it might be the result of the same haptotactic or chemotactic agent acting on all the cells individually; or the leading cells dragging the rest behind them; or the trailing cells leapfrogging over the leading cells; or some complex communication between individual cells [72].

Epithelial cells are packed closely together. The cells, having charged surfaces, tend to repel each other, and are held together by specialized contacts such as tight junctions (zonulae occludens), adhesive zones (zonulae adherens) and desmosomes (maculae adherens). The epithelial cells adhere to the underlying connective tissue with hemidesmosomes [74]. The underlying connective tissue determines the behaviour of the overlying epithelial cells. For example, a skin graft transplanted to the oral cavity remains a distinct area of skin due to the coding of the underlying connective tissue. Epithelial cells from a number of different sources behave in a similar and characteristic manner when their supporting connective tissue is altered in some way.

A fundamental characteristic of epithelium is to cover any exposed connective tissue surface. Ten Cate [74] suggests that past thinking about the reasons for implant success and failure has been erroneous because it rested on the principle of the ability or inability of epithelial cells to attach to implant surfaces and to provide a seal. Undifferentiated epithelial cells can attach with remarkable facility to a number of materials. Rather than focusing on these, Ten Cate suggests that we should focus on the underlying connective tissue. If the connective tissue is sound and void of inflammatory cells this will lead to a sound epithelium. If an implant is not stable, avulsion will occur, causing an inflammatory response in the connective tissue leading to epithelial migration and disturbance of the implant. Jansen and de Groot [75] using hydroxyapatite and titanium test implants found no adverse skin reactions around percutaneous stable tibial and cranial implants whereas similar implants placed in the dorsum of the test animals showed signs of epidermal migration downwards. These latter implants failed six weeks after insertion. It was concluded that the immobilization of the implant is important to achieve a good result.

In a review of naturally occurring skin penetrating devices Grosse-Siestrup and Affeld [76] discussed how nature has solved these problems. In the cow, the mobility of the skin close to the horn is decreased because the horn is firmly attached to the skull. Because of this the stress on the skin is transmitted by shear forces to the skull and not to the skin. The Babyrussa is a swine originating from the Celebes, Southeast Asia and it has a percutaneous tusk. The area of skin penetration consists of hairless epithelium. The authors state that the direct attachment of a skin-penetrating device to the bone underlying the skin is an effective and very simple solution to the problem of percutaneous penetration. There will be no forces applied to the skin if the percutaneous device is exposed to external forces. The osseointegrated skin-penetrating implants used at our clinic are good examples of this as is the LTI carbon percutaneous button used for signal transmission for artificial hearing. Grosse-Siestrup and Affeld [76] stress the importance of a two-stage surgical procedure to allow the subcutaneous healing to take place before the percutaneous part of the device is applied. Hall and partners [77] argue along the same lines in stating that some of the causes for failure are extrinsic forces (forces applied either to the skin or the implant by the external environment) and intrinsic forces (forces having to do with the body's growth and cell maturation).

In the system used by us, both the extrinsic and intrinsic forces are reduced by having the implant firmly attached to the underlying bone tissue, and the subcutaneous tissue reduction performed under the abutment connection procedure. This will minimize the movement between skin and the implant. Branemark and Albrektsson [78,79] in vital microscopic studies of human microcirculation, used titanium chambers inserted in a twin-pedicled skin tube on the inside of the upper left arm on a group of healthy volunteers. It was found that the integrity of the interface between skin and subcutaneous tissue and titanium was maintained. The chamber tissue reactions were evaluated by studying intravascular rheological phenomena. There were no long-standing inflammatory processes in the chamber tissue or in the regions of skin penetration.

In a case of skin infection around an osseointegrated implant for a hearing aid we took specimens from the soft tissue surrounding the implant and later removed the implant and surrounding bone tissue to study it histologically [80]. The implant had remained stable and no loss of osseointegration had occurred in spite of this long-standing infection. The soft tissues surrounding the implant at the skin level were heavily infiltrated with inflammatory cells. At 12 months after implant insertion, a leukocyte-rich exudate, consisting mainly of polymorphonuclear granulocytes (PMNGs) was seen close to the titanium surface at the skin–implant interface. The epidermis was partly eroded close to the abutment and the underlying connective tissue was replaced by monocytes/macrophages, lymphocytes and PMNGs. At 18 months granulation tissue replaced the connective tissue but the basally located collagenous tissue showed only minor signs of inflammation. Microscopic evaluation of the bone–implant interface showed no evidence of loss of contact between bone and implant. It was con-cluded that although the soft tissue overlying the bone tissue harbouring the osseointegrated implant is infected and granulation tissue is present, it is possible to maintain osseointegration.

In a study of patients who had been irradiated prior to the installation of implants, post mortem implants that were clinically osseointegrated, were studied histologically [38]. An intact epidermis as well as underlying connective tissue were in close apposition to the implant surface. The connective tissue was moderately vascularized and consisted of fibroblasts and scattered mononuclear cells. The connective tissue proper tended to become more dense deeper down into the soft tissue.

THE BONE-ANCHORED HEARING SYSTEM

Background

Since 1977, titanium implants for the attachment of bone-anchored hearing devices have been in use in Sweden. The system is today commercially available through Nobelpharma Inc., Sweden, under the name Nobelpharma Auditory System (NAS). To date we have installed 277 bone-anchored hearing devices at our clinic (Figure 3). Many patients have draining ears and poor hearing due to chronic otitis media, malformed ears, conductive or mixed hearing loss. Although surgical techniques to obtain disease-free and dry ears have led to better results over the last three decades, many patients still suffer from draining ears or have a conductive or mixed hearing loss that cannot, for different reasons, be improved surgically. Some patients require a hearing aid but are unable to use a conventional air-conduction instrument due to drainage, eczema of the ear canal, or allergic reaction to the plastic material of the insert. Such patients may be candidates for a conventional bone conduction hearing aid (BCHA). The most common indications for such a device are a chronically draining ear, an ear that starts to drain if the ear canal is occluded, a malformed ear, absent ear canals, and extensive conductive dysfunction which cannot be corrected surgically.

There are several disadvantages to the BCHA, such as discomfort, headache, skin irritation, and occasionally eczema due to the pressure that must be applied to the vibrator on the skull. The application of the bone vibrator with a steel spring over the head is often uncomfortable, awkward to apply and unstable. When pressure is supplied via "Hearing Eyeglasses", the function deteriorates with the flaccidity or bending of the frames. The quality of the transmitted sound is generally variable and of low fidelity. To avoid feedback the transducer and the electronic part have to be separated.

The Bone-Anchored Hearing System (NAS) provides a new type of direct bone-conduction hearing instrument for subjects with conductive or mixed

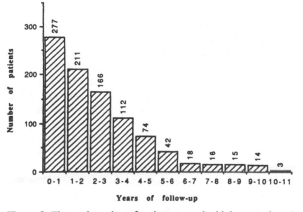

Figure 3. The total number of patients treated with bone-anchored hearing devices.

hearing loss. The sound processor (SP) or the bone-conductor is directly coupled to the temporal bone by means of a skin-penetrating bone-anchored implant and abutment. This makes it possible to aid patients who cannot be helped with a conventional device. In many ways the NAS has demonstrated superior performance characteristics over the BCHA. The advantages of the NAS are increased wearing comfort (it does not occlude the ear canal or exert any static pressure on the skull), improved speech intelligibility, especially in noisy surroundings, and the fact that the device fits into a single compact housing which is more cosmetically favourable and is easily concealed by most hairstyles [Figure 4(a,b)]. Also, due to high fidelity, less consumption of power, and lack of feedback, the patients' satisfaction has improved.

The audiometric indications for using a bone-anchored hearing device system are: (1) any patient who uses a conventional bone conduction hearing instrument; (2) any patient who uses an air-conduction hearing aid, with a chronically draining ear; or (3) any patient requiring amplification who cannot use a conventional air conduction hearing aid because of chronic middle ear disease or external ear disease.

The medical diagnoses for using a bone-anchored hearing device system are: (1) chronic otitis media op-

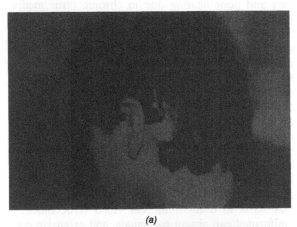

(a)

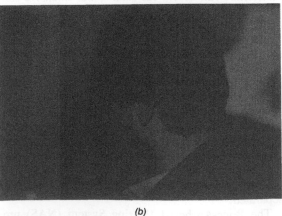

(b)

Figure 4. (a) The bone-anchored hearing device in place. (b) The hearing device is easily concealed by most hair styles.

erated or non-operated with conductive or mixed hearing loss; (2) conductive or mixed hearing loss with external ear disease; (3) radical mastoidectomy and meatoplasty with uncontrollable feedback when using an air-conduction aid; (4) chronic conductive loss in one ear and an uncurable sensorineural loss in the opposite ear; (5) congenital atresia when surgery is contraindicated; or (6) operated congenital atresia with hearing loss but draining ear if a mould is used.

The Bone-Anchored Hearing System

The titanium implant consists of a threaded cylindrical c.p. titanium screw with a perforated flange on top. Its dimensions are: diameter 3.75 mm, depth 3.0 or 4.0 mm. The skin-penetrating abutment is connected and fixed to the implanted screw with an internal screw. The inside of the abutment is fitted with a plastic insert, which is circumscribed by a silicon O-ring which holds the coupling in site and serves as a safety release if the sound processor is exposed to undue external forces. The vibrator piston of the sound processor fits into a slot of the plastic insert and is coupled by a 90-degree turning motion.

Surgical Procedure

The surgery is performed in two stages with an interval of 3–4 months. Local anesthesia is used in most cases, and the operation can be done as an out-patient procedure. The surgical field is prepared in the usual manner and the site of the hearing aid is marked out with surgical ink. A plastic dummy of the hearing aid is used in order to prevent the aid from touching the pinna, as this will produce acoustic feedback. The surgical field is then covered with plastic film in order to prevent contamination of the implant site in the bone. Even sterile fragments from the draping may jeopardize osseointegration and must therefore be avoided. The skin incision is made and a periostal flap is raised.

Drilling is started using a disposable cutting drill. The drillbits are used only once to ensure sharpness and thus less heat trauma. For the same reason the drill speed is kept fairly low—between 1500 and 3000 rpm. Drilling is never performed without ample cooling. The 2 mm guide burr is moved up and down, and the hole is enlarged slightly to allow the saline cooling fluid to reach the site and to keep the drillbits free of bone fragments [Figure 5(a)]. Widening the hole will also allow the surgeon to inspect the bottom of the hole to avoid penetrating the sigmoid sinus or the dura mater. The drill is fitted with a sleeve to keep it from penetrating too deeply. Initially drilling is performed with a sleeve to accommodate a 3 mm titanium screw/fixture. If, at this stage, there is still bone at the bottom, the sleeve is replaced with one for a 4 mm fixture. When the guide hole has been drilled and the depth has been established, the drill is changed to a spiral drill with a countersink. The same speed is used

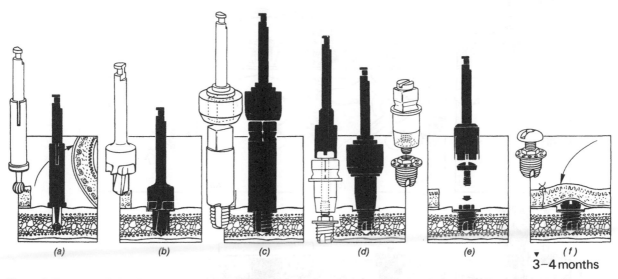

(a)   (b)   (c)   (d)   (e)   ▼ (f)

3-4 months

Figure 5. Fixture installation for the bone-anchored hearing device. (a) A 2 mm guide burr is moved up and down, and the hole is enlarged slightly. The drill is fitted with a sleeve to keep it from penetrating too deeply. The drill speed is kept fairly low—between 1500 and 3000 rpm. Drilling is never performed without ample cooling. (b) The drill is changed to a spiral drill with a countersink, used to obtain optimum contact with the flange of the fixture. This is of special importance if the bony surface is uneven or sharply angled. The direction of the implant is important. (c) The next step is to thread the hole which is done with a tap made of titanium in order to avoid contamination of the implant seat. The threading is also performed under adequate cooling with saline. The drill speed is now reduced to 8–15 rpm. Cooling is applied when the tap is unscrewed. (d) The screw-shaped titanium implant is mounted on a fixture mount without being touched by the gloved hand or anything but titanium instruments and then is introduced into the fixture seat at slow speed. The final tightening is performed manually with a ratchet wrench. For the sake of precision it is recommended that the previous steps be performed manually. (e) The internal threads of the fixture are protected by a cover screw. (f) The periostal flap is folded back and kept in place with a couple of Dexon® sutures. The skin incision is closed and an ordinary mastoid dressing is applied for one day, then removed after which only a small piece of plaster is needed.

and generous cooling applied. The hole will now be given its final width and direction [Figure 5(b)]. A countersink is used to obtain optimum contact with the flange of the fixture. This is of special importance if the bony surface is uneven or sharply angled. The direction of the implant is important because the shell of the hearing aid must not touch the skin, otherwise acoustic feedback will occur.

The next step is to thread the hole [Figure 5(c)]. This is done with a tap which is made of titanium in order to avoid contamination of the implant seat. The threading is also performed under adequate cooling with saline. The drill speed is now reduced to 8–15 rpm. Cooling is applied when the tap is unscrewed. The tap, which is never touched with anything but titanium-coated instruments and is kept in a titanium container, is constructed in such a way that the bone which is cut away during the threading is collected in the grooves on the sides of the tap and in its hollow lower part. The screw-shaped titanium implant is mounted on a fixture mount without being touched by the gloved hand or anything but titanium instruments and is then introduced into the fixture seat at slow speed [Figure 5(d)]. The final tightening is performed manually with a ratchet wrench. For the sake of precision it is recommended that the previous steps be performed manually. The internal threads of the fixture are protected by a cover screw [Figure 5(e)]. The periostal flap is folded back and kept in place with a couple of Dexon® sutures [Figure 5(f)]. The skin incision is closed and an ordinary mastoid dressing is ap-

plied for one day, then removed after which only a small piece of plaster is needed. The stitches are removed one week later. As this whole procedure aims at minimising tissue damage, cautery is not used. In fact, there is very seldom any need for cautery.

The second operation is performed 3–4 months later when osseointegration is expected to have taken place. Generally, this procedure is also performed under local anaesthesia. The surgical field is prepared in the usual manner. As it is seldom possible to palpate the implant through the skin, the surgical report should be consulted. Two conditions have to be fulfilled in order to establish a permanent reaction-free skin penetration. First, the skin most not move in relation to the implant. This means that the skin must be attached to the periosteum with a minimum of soft tissue in between. The second prerequisite is that there are no hair follicles adjacent to the skin-penetrating implant. This means that if the skin is hairbearing, a hairless-skin transplant has to be taken from a suitable place such as the post-auricular fold [Figure 6(a)]. After the incision has been made and the implant has been identified, the subcutaneous tissue is removed until the skin slopes nicely down towards the implant area [Figure 6(b)]. If the area is hairless the skin flap is thinned out as much as possible [Figure 6(c)]. The flange of the fixture is exposed and soft tissue and bony overgrowth is removed [Figure 6(d)]. The cover screw in the centre of the fixture is raised slightly to facilitate localising the fixture

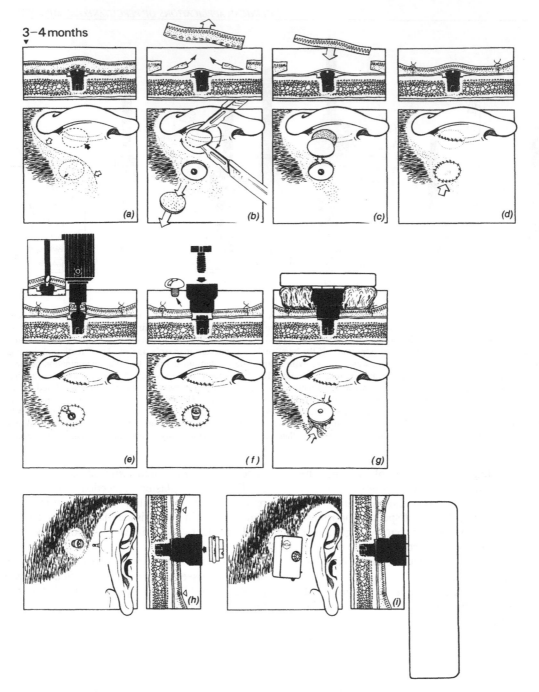

Figure 6. Second-stage operation for the bone-anchored hearing system. (a) The surgical field is prepared in the usual manner. Two conditions have to be fulfilled in order to establish a permanent reaction-free skin penetration. First, the skin must not move in relation to the implant. This means that the skin must be attached to the periosteum with a minimum of soft tissue in between. The second prerequisite is that there must be no hair follicles adjacent to the skin-penetrating implant. This means that if the skin is hairbearing, a hairless skin transplant has to be taken from a suitable place such as the post-auricular fold. (b) After the incision has been made and the implant has been identified, the subcutaneous tissue is removed until the skin slopes nicely down towards the implant area. If the area is hairless, the skin flap is thinned out as much as possible. Otherwise a hairless-skin transplant is obtained from the post-auricular fold. The flange of the fixture is exposed and soft tissue and bony overgrowth is removed. The cover screw in the centre of the fixture is raised slightly to facilitate localizing the fixture after the flap has been sutured into position, when the graft has been put in place. (c) The transplant is thinned to less than 1 mm thickness. (d) The skin transplant is sutured in place. (e) A hole is punched in the skin and the cover screw is removed. (f) The hearing aid coupling is secured to the fixture with an internal screw. (g) A plastic healing cap is snapped onto the coupling in order to keep the ointment-soaked gauze in place during the healing period. (h) Three to four weeks after the second stage operation, the patient can generally be fitted with the new hearing aid. A small plastic insert is placed inside the coupling and kept in place with the aid of an O-ring. (i) The hearing aid is then attached with its bayonet coupling. Using a master hearing aid the new BAHD is adjusted to fit the patient's hearing impairment.

after the flap has been sutured into position, when the graft has been put in place. A hole is punched in the skin and the cover screw is removed [Figure 6(e)].

The hearing aid coupling is secured to the fixture with an internal screw [Figure 6(f)]. A plastic healing cap is snapped onto the coupling in order to keep the ointment-soaked gauze in place during the healing period. This gauze dressing is about 10 mm wide and 50–70 cm long [Figure 6(g)]. It is changed after 5–6 days, at which time most of the stitches can often be removed. The site is left exposed for about 30 minutes to be aerated before a new piece of gauze is wound around the coupling. After a further 5–6 days the gauze is changed again. The compression, which serves as protection from post-op haematoma and swelling, should be used for about 2 weeks, after which time the coupling no longer needs any protection. The patient is asked to clean the area with soap and water and to apply a mild ointment like Terracortril with Polymyxin B® (Pfizer®) once or twice a week for the first few months.

Three to four weeks after the second-stage operation, the patient can generally be fitted with the new hearing aid. A small plastic insert is placed inside the coupling and kept in place with the aid of an O-ring [Figure 6(h)]. The hearing aid is then attached with its bayonet coupling [Figure 6(i)]. Using a master hearing aid the new NAS is adjusted to fit the patient's hearing impairment.

Follow-up of Patients Treated with the Bone-Anchored Hearing Device

A study [81] was conducted on 167 implanted ears, 166 of which had received The Bone Anchored Hearing System. No patient was lost to follow-up. Among the implanted ears, a range of conductive and mixed hearing handicaps were represented, including subjects with profound sensorineural hearing loss. Subjects of this study included those with conductive or mixed hearing loss due to chronic otitis media, ear malformations and otosclerosis. These patients were selected for a NAS as they could not benefit from conventional hearing aids.

After the second stage the subjects were studied at regular intervals (1 week, 2 weeks, 1 month, 3 months and thereafter every 6 months). At each of these outpatient visits, the skin around the implant was cleaned carefully and an evaluation of the skin status made. This evaluation system has been presented by Holgers and co-workers [82] and is graded from 0 to 4.

0 = No irritation. Epithelium debris removed if present.

1 = Slight redness, local treatment.

2 = Red and slightly moist tissue. No granuloma formation noted. Local treatment.

3 = Status as in 1 and 2, but with granulation tissue noted; local revision became necessary.

Table 1. Skin reactions around bone-anchored hearing devices.

Skin Reaction	Number of Patients	Percentage
0	130	77.8
1	23	13.8
2	3	1.8
3	10	6.0
4	1	0.6
Total	167	100.0

4 = Infection with removal of skin-penetrating implant.

The follow-up time varied from one month to nearly 10 years and comprised a total of 3284 months. Of the 167 implanted ears studied, the skin reactions were distributed as follows: skin reaction type 0: 103, skin reaction type 1: 23, skin reaction type 2: 3, skin reaction type 3: 10, skin reaction type 4: 1. In other words: of all 167 implants, 153 had skin reaction type 0 or 1, i.e., minimal skin reactions (Table 1). In all, 16 abutments were removed. One was removed due to a skin infection, five because of discomfort or psychological reasons, seven due to no improvement in hearing, two because of head trauma and finally one abutment was removed as the fixture had not become integrated (Table 2). Ten subjects were observed to have thick and movable skin around the abutment and underwent an extended subcutaneous tissue reduction to avoid future skin infections.

Audiological Results

A bone PTA threshold equal or better than 45 dB HL indicates that the NAS as a rule will give excellent hearing improvement with the present system. When the PTA bone thresholds are worse than 45 dB HL the hearing improvement depends on the actual cochlear reserve. In our material [81] about 50% of those with PTA bone thresholds between 46 and 65 dB HL considered themselves as improved. For most subjects in this group a more powerful model of the NAS, that has now been developed, may be beneficial.

The hearing as measured with sound field discrimi-

Table 2. Abutments removed from bone-anchored hearing devices.

Skin infection	1
Discomfort, psychological reasons	5
No hearing improvement	7
Head trauma	2
Fixture not integrated	1
Total	16

nation improved from an average of 14% unaided for the whole group to 81% with the NAS. A comparison with the subjects' old hearing aids showed an increase in speech discrimination from 50% to 66% at the same sound/noise ratio. Air-conduction hearing aids usually have a better sound reproduction than bone vibrators. This was, however, not very evident either in quiet or noisy surroundings in the patients studied by Lidén et al. [81]. According to the patients' subjective evaluation the advantages with the NAS were that it improved speech intelligibility, provided better sound quality, was easy to use, was cosmetically more attractive, and gave rise to less pressure on the head and less skin irritation.

Other Implanted Hearing Devices

The Xomed® Audiant Bone Conductor is another type of bone conductor. This type of hearing device consists of an internal device made of titanium-vanadium-aluminium into which has been mounted a rare earth permanent magnet encased in a polymer. It is surgically inserted into a precisely drilled and tapped hole in the temporal bone and is said to become osseointegrated within several weeks after surgery [83]. Electromagnetically coupled to this internal device is an external processor that transforms acoustic vibratory energy in the surrounding environment into an electromagnetic field that passes through the skin and into the magnet causing the latter, the skull and the cochlea, to vibrate. In our opinion, the loss of energy, as the vibrations pass through the thick soft tissue layer of the skull, must be substantial, as the limitation for bone-conduction thresholds is given as 25 dB or better for the three speech frequencies (500, 1000 and 2000 Hz) in the implanted ear by Gates et al. [83]. The corresponding recommendations for NAS is 45 dB at present. Another question that can be discussed is the choice of titanium-vanadium-aluminium for the implant. Several studies point to the lesser capacity for osseointegration with this type of material as compared to c.p. titanium [4] and to the potential toxicity of this same material as it contains aluminium which in a long-term study by Woodman et al. [55] on implants showed a continuous increase in blood level concentrations over many years. Aluminium also has been brought forward as a possible factor in the development of Alzheimer's disease.

Recommendations for the Use of the NAS

The only contraindication for providing a patient with a NAS is a pure sensorineural hearing loss with no ear canal problems. However, for an optimal result the following limitations should be taken into consideration when selecting patients for the NAS, even if they should not be considered as absolute contraindications.

(1) Mixed hearing loss with PTA bone-conduction thresholds (0.5–3.0 kHz) worse than 45 dB HL
(2) Speech discrimination score below 60% in quiet surroundings
(3) Emotional instability, delayed development and drug abuse
(4) Age less than 5 years

As mentioned above, a new superbass vibrator has now been developed and is commercially available, which will allow patients with mixed hearing loss and with PTA bone-conduction thresholds (0.5–3.0 Hz) of 45–60 dB HL to use the NAS.

Conclusions

• C.p. titanium implantation with a skin-penetrating abutment is a minor surgical procedure.
• The skin-penetrating abutment causes few adverse skin reactions, and most of these are easily corrected with subcutaneous tissue reductions.
• The subjects' own opinions about the NAS confirmed the positive results obtained with the audiological test results.
• The advantages of using NAS can be summarised as:
  (1) Better speech intelligibility
  (2) Better sound quality
  (3) Cosmetically more attractive
  (4) Ease of use
  (5) Less pressure on the head and less skin irritation
  (6) Diminished ear infections
  (7) Improvement of life quality

THE BONE-ANCHORED AURICULAR PROSTHESIS

Surgical methods for reconstructing the external ear have been previously published [84,85]. However, multiple procedures are often necessary, and although there are a number of skilled, specialist surgeons in the field, there is no simple method which ensures a predictable, cosmetically satisfactory result. This is especially true in cases where there is no cartilage or only very small remnants available. An auricular prosthesis may in many cases be a better solution. One problem is, however, how to retain the prosthesis. Methods such as skin pouches, glue, attachment to eyeglasses, etc. are used, but all have drawbacks and the patients often feel insecure with these types of retention. The use of tissue-integrated implants in the mastoid not only ensures safe retention but also gives the technician much greater leeway in choosing an appropriate material. The edges can be made thinner and will not become discoloured or brittle, as is often the case when glue is used. In short, a much better prosthesis can be made for the patient [Figure 7(a,b)].

Surgical Procedure—Auricular Prostheses

The surgery follows the same guidelines as the Bone-Anchored Hearing Aid. Two or three implants are placed in the mastoid. The positioning of the implants in relation to the external ear canal opening is important in order to obtain the optimum result. Based on our experience, the implants should be positioned 18–20 mm from the centre of the ear canal or, in atresia cases, the imagined ear canal opening. As

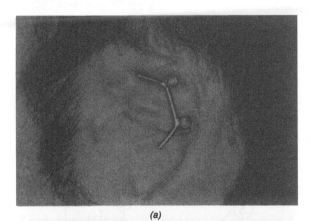

(a)

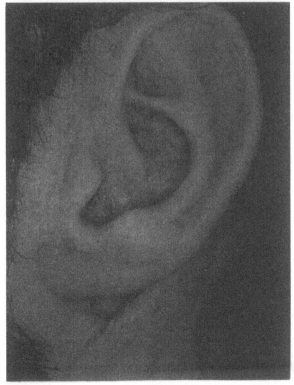

(b)

Figure 7. (a) The bar construction attached to the skin-penetrating abutments. (b) The auricular prosthesis in place.

will be shown in the follow-up section, the prognosis for osseointegration in the mastoid process is excellent, and today we prefer two implants to three or four. As illustrated in Figure 8.1 the position of the implants on the right side is one implant at 9 o'clock and one at 11 o'clock. The greater the distance is between the implants, the better. This will ensure easier cleaning of the skin. The first-stage surgical procedure is described in Figures 8.2–8.5.

At the second stage, performed 3–4 months after the first, the implants are identified and a careful subcutaneous tissue reduction is made (Figure 8.6). For best results, ear remnants are often removed at this stage in order to avoid having to hide skin buds and cartilage behind the prosthesis. The tragus is left untouched if it is of normal shape and position. If not, attempts can be made to create one, otherwise the tragus can be included in the silicone rubber prosthesis (Figure 8.7). The skin-penetrating cylinders—the abutments—are 4 mm high and are identical with those used intraorally. The screw for securing the cylinder to the fixture is however, somewhat shorter. Healing caps of intra-oral type are used to keep the skin down during the healing period and are changed according to the same schedule as for the NAS (Figure 8.8). If there is a hair in the penetration area we recommend that a hairless skin-graft be taken from the retro-auricular fold on the opposite side or from the inside of the upper arm. After 2 weeks the area is left open and after another 2–3 weeks healing has in most cases reached the stage where it is possible to start making the bar construction and the prosthesis.

The basic procedure for making the prosthesis and its retention device has been published by Tjellström and associates [86]. Over the last few years the technique has been refined and a new step-by-step description has been published by Jansson [87] (Figures 8.9–8.12). A master cast is made of the defect area using alginate as impression substance. Abutment replicas are included in this master cast. A bar construction is made to fit the abutments exactly. A wax ear is sculptured using the normal ear as a model. The wax ear is embedded in plaster and then flushed away, leaving a three-piece plaster mould. The silicone is mixed with curing agent, and colouring and flocking to simulate minor blood vessels are added. The mould is then filled with the silicone mixture and allowed to cure under the pressure and heat. One very critical detail is the preparation of the acrylic plate which will be embedded in the silicone. It is very important to have good bonding between the silicone and the acrylic plate where the retention elements for the bar are placed. After minor adjustments and some final extrinsic colouration, the prosthesis is delivered to the patient. The durability of the prosthesis is determined by several factors. In smokers there is a risk that after 1–3 years the prosthesis will become yellowish. Furthermore, oil, dirt and careless handling will shorten the service life of the prosthesis.

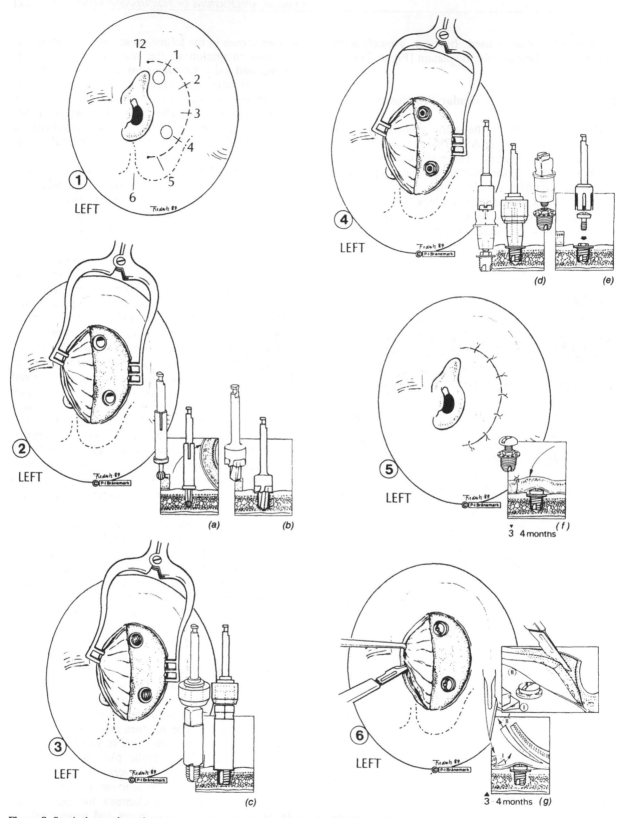

Figure 8. Surgical procedures for the bone-anchored auricular prosthesis. 8.1—The position of the implants on the left side is one implant at 1 o'clock and 4 o'clock. 8.2—(a) A 2 mm guide burr is moved up and down, and the hole is enlarged slightly. The drill speed is kept between 1500 and 3000 rpm and drilling is never performed without ample cooling. (b) A spiral drill with a countersink, used to obtain optimum contact with the flange of the fixture. 8.3—(c) The hole is threaded with a tap made of titanium in order to avoid contamination of the implant seat. 8.4—(d) The screw-shaped titanium is mounted on a fixture mount and introduced into the fixture seat at slow speed. (e) The internal threads of the fixture are protected by a cover screw. 8.5—(f) The periostal flap is folded back and kept in place with a couple of Dexon sutures. The skin incision is closed and an ordinary mastoid dressing is applied. 8.6—(g) After the incision has been made and the implant has been iden- tified, the subcutaneous tissue is removed until the skin slopes nicely down towards the implant area. If the area is hairless the skin flap is thinned out as much as possible. Otherwise a hairless skin transplant is obtained from the inside of the contralateral upper arm.

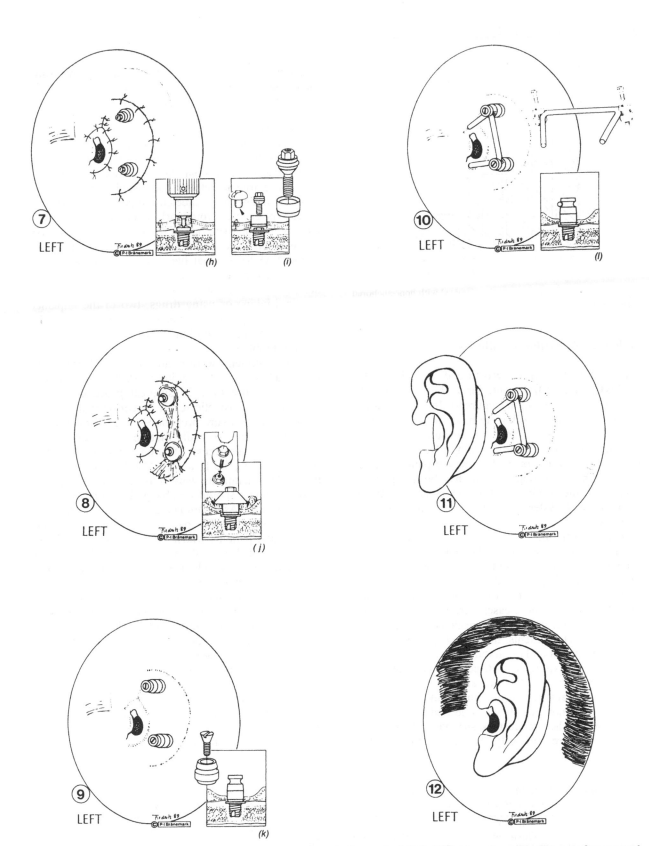

Figure 8 (continued). Surgical procedures for the bone-anchored auricular prosthesis. 8.7—For best results ear remnants are often removed at this stage in order to avoid having to hide skin buds and cartilage behind the prosthesis. The tragus is left untouched if it is of normal shape and position. If not, attempts can be made to create one, otherwise the tragus can be included in the silicone rubber prosthesis. (h) A hole is punched in the skin and the cover screw is removed. (i) The skin-penetrating cylinders—the abutments—are 4 mm high and are identical with those used intraorally. 8.8—(j) The screw for securing the cylinder to the fixture is, however, somewhat shorter. Healing caps of intra-oral type are used to keep the skin down during the healing period and are changed according to the same schedule as for the BAHD. 8.9—(k) After a healing period of 2–3 weeks, gold cylinders are mounted on the abutments. 8.10—(l) A bar construction is soldered onto the gold cylinders. 8.11—The auricular prosthesis, which is made of silicone rubber, is built on an acrylic plate into which clasps have been fitted. The clasps snap onto the bar construction. 8.12—The auricular prosthesis in place.

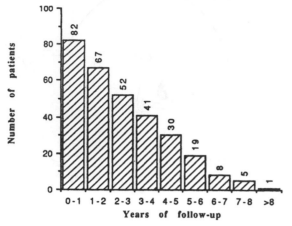

Figure 9. The total number of patients treated with bone-anchored auricular prostheses.

Follow-up Auricular Prostheses

In 1979 the first patient was treated according to this method in our department. Since then a further 81 have been operated upon (Figure 9). In Figure 9 all of the patients and the follow-up times are presented. In this group no one was lost to follow-up and the same principles are applied for recording adverse skin reactions as those used for the hearing-aid patients. Since every skin-penetrating implant has been registered separately, the number of observations is much larger than for the NAS despite the fact that there were fewer patients.

In Table 3 the number of observations in each skin reaction group is presented. The total number of fixtures placed in the mastoid for retention of auricular prostheses is 282, and 232 abutments were attached. Of these fixtures only two were found not to have integrated (Table 4). These cases were in the early phase of this study and abutments were attached despite lack of stability. The patients, however, experienced pain, so the abutments and the fixtures were removed. One other patient experienced discomfort and some tenderness when one of her implants was palpated. She had four implants for her prosthesis and was taken to surgery to remove the tender one and also an additional one at her request as she had difficulties in cleaning the area properly. This non-tender implant

was removed using an instrument made to measure the torque. The torque registered was 37 Ncm, which lies within the normal range. When an attempt was made to unscrew the tender fixture the meter broke at 136 Ncm and the fixture showed no sign of moving despite the considerable force applied.

Table 4 shows that four implants were removed due to skin infection. This patient in question was an alcoholic and a drug addict who had lost his ear in an accident. He deliberately infected the penetration area in order to be excused from work. In connection with removing the abutment one of the fixtures was removed for histology. The findings were identical with those of the NAS-fixture that had been removed and analysed. There were no signs of osteitis. After removal, healing was uneventful. Since the patient was no longer drinking or using drugs, two of the implants were again exposed and connected to abutments. He now takes proper care of the penetration zone and has no skin problems.

Three abutments were removed for psychiatric reasons in a boy with a congenital malformation who had undergone more than 30 surgical procedures. Not only must the cosmetic result be considered a catastrophe, but the many procedures and hospital visits have affected him so badly that he was unable to accept wearing a prosthesis. There were no adverse skin reactions during the 12 months that he wore his prosthesis. The abutments were removed but the fixtures were left intact should he change his mind when he becomes older. As mentioned earlier, it is of great importance to select the patients carefully. Immature persons and patients whose willingness to cooperate may be doubted, should only be treated after serious consideration. A psychiatric assessment may sometimes prove very useful.

A study of patients' opinions of auricular prosthesis has been made in collaboration with the University of Chicago, School of Dentistry [88]. The patients were asked to comment on several factors such as retention, color, and shape of the prosthesis, and its positioning. Of the forty-seven patients included in this study 40 considered their prosthesis as excellent, 6 as acceptable and one refused to answer. Forty-four patients used the prosthesis every day, the whole day, one only half the day and 2 only on occasion. The latter lived in a rural area without much contact with others.

Table 3. Skin reactions for the bone-anchored auricular prosthesis.

Skin Reaction	Number of Observations	Percentage
0	1,670	89.6
1	126	6.8
2	46	2.5
3	17	0.9
4	4	0.2
Total	1,863	100.0

Table 4. Reasons for removal of implants* for the bone-anchored auricular prostheses.

Reason	Number of Patients
Soft-tissue infection	4 (in 1 patient)
Discomfort	4 (in 3 patients)
Other	2 (in 2 patients)
Total	10

*A total of 232 abutments attached.

Those patients who had previously worn prostheses with other methods of retention were all satisfied and reported improved retention, easier positioning of the prosthesis, and better comfort.

TISSUE-INTEGRATED IMPLANTS IN CHILDREN

Initially only elderly patients were selected for the temporal bone implants, but the very favourable results and the need for the same type of prosthetic rehabilitation in younger patients convinced us to include children in this treatment program. As far as we know, there are only a small number of children who have been treated with intra-oral implants, the youngest being 8 years old at the time of implant insertion [89].

In a recent study [90], eighteen children with auricular malformations, such as atresia of the external auditory canal or Treacher-Collins syndrome, between ages of 7 and 17 years (mean age 10 years) operated upon before October 1987, were followed. A total of 40 standard titanium fixtures (Nobelpharma, Sweden) were inserted in the temporal bones of the patients. These fixtures were then used as bone anchorage for auricular epistheses (9 cases) and hearing aids (9 cases). Nine patients received one fixture each, two patients received two, four patients received three fixtures. Two of the patients had four fixtures installed each. In one case, the patient had three fixtures installed in the left temporal bone and four fixtures in the right. The surgical procedure is performed in two steps, as described above.

The patients have been followed with regular checkups for an average of four years and eight months (14 months–131 months) after fixture installation and four years and two months (10 months–125 months) after the abutment procedure. At each post-operative check-up the stability of the implant and skin reactions were recorded.

Results

Out of a total of forty implants studied in this material, one was lost due to non-integration into the bone tissue. This means a success rate of 97.5% for osseointegration for the period studied. The one implant that was lost supported a bone-anchored hearing aid. The implant failure occurred four months after the fixture insertion and one month after the abutment procedure. In two cases bone apposition was seen around the subcutaneous part of the abutment, causing an elevation of the skin around the implant, and leading to skin irritation. In one case this new bone formation was removed with a diamond burr under local anaesthesia and the adverse skin reaction disappeared. For the hearing aids there were a total of 102 observations of the skin reactions, 89 (87.25%) of which were classified as "grade 0"; 9 (8.92%) as "grade 1"; 2 (1.96%) as "grade 2" and 2 as "grade 3".

The corresponding results for the 330 observations on the prostheses were 258 (78.18%) "grade 0"; 52 (15.76%) "grade 1"; 15 (4.55%) "grade 2" and 5 (1.52%) "grade 3". For the whole material the skin reactions of grade 0 and 1 constituted 94.44% (Figure 10). Two patients were responsible for 14 (82.35%) of all grade 2 registrations, one of which (with 10 registrations of grade 2) had a difficult adolescent period, did not follow given instructions, and refused treatment.

Discussion

The fixture survival rate of 97.5% for osseointegrated implants in our material is as high as that for intra- or extra-oral implants in adults [6,7,8]. The small problems with adverse skin reactions is also well in line with studies on skin behavior around skin-penetrating implants in adults [82]. One practical problem in these young patients in the present study is, of course, the relatively thin cortical bone of the skull, as compared to adults. In addition, congenital deformities may complicate the anatomy further and the surgeon may encounter extremely thin bone tissue in some patients. On the other hand, these technical drawbacks are counterbalanced by the higher activity of fracture healing in children. According to Frost [91], the efficiency in producing bone of a newly generated osteoblast in a five year old is twice that of a newly generated osteoblast in a sixty year old person. Also, the absence of osteoporosis, which starts at the age of 35 [91], is another factor in favor of osseointegration in children. The two cases presented in this study in which bone apposition around the abutment had occurred are an indication of the very high bone formation capacity seen in children. In our experience, this has never been encountered in adult patients with skin-penetrating titanium implants.

Clinical indications of superior bone formation

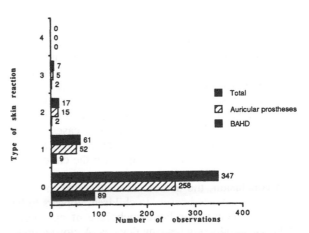

Figure 10. The skin reactions in children treated with skin penetrating implants for auricular prostheses and bone-anchored hearing devices.

capacity in children has been presented in case reports. Sluker [92] described a patient seven years old who had sustained a severe avulsion injury to the mandible. Spontaneous regeneration in the 6 cm gap was seen, with total healing. In another case report Nagase et al. [93] described spontaneous regeneration of the mandibular condyle following hemimandibulectomy by disarticulation and bone grafting in a 12 year old boy. Despite these indications of good bone healing capacity in children, it must be realised that the bone regeneration can vary substantially within the same tissue compartment, something evidenced by the asymmetrical healing of neurosurgical burr holes in the skull of a child [94]. The only other experience, to our knowledge, of bone-anchored implants in children has been presented by Scholz and d'Hoedt [95] who could show good healing capacity and implant acceptance in their patients.

One important factor in the context of any implants in children is the long-term aspect with respect to toxicity or carcinogenicity of the implant material. A Swedish child of 10 years of age today has a life expectancy of about 75 years. What will occur in the soft tissues and bone tissue in this long time period? No case of development of malignant tumours has been reported among the over 300,000 implants (extra- and intra-oral) that have been inserted up until now with the osseointegration technique, over a follow-up period of up to 20 years [89]. As suggested by Pedley et al. [96] a neoplastic change at the site of a solid implant develops in the cells of the fibrous capsule. The essence of osseointegration is the absence of a fibrous capsule around the implant, i.e., a direct contact between living bone and a loaded implant surface. The presence of a fibrous capsule is by our standards a failure. This may be one explanation to the absence of any neoplastic change in the 300,000 extra- and intra-oral implants.

The clinical experience both in the intra-oral and extra-oral application is that the majority of adverse soft tissue reactions occur in patients who for some reason do not cooperate and ignore given instructions [86]. This includes patients who have psychological problems, and patients with histories of alcohol and drug abuse. The difficulties with one of the children in this study could be fitted into the same group where problems could occur. This should be taken into consideration when the described technique is used in young patients. On the other hand, a malformed external ear or a hearing handicap that is difficult to correct with another technique could in some cases be the reason for a negative or aggressive attitude and a rehabilitation program could perhaps help the child overcome these problems.

In conclusion, the use of osseointegrated implants in carefully selected cases, in children, appears to be a reliable method for bone-anchorage of epistheses and bone-conduction hearing devices. A close follow-up and control of this patient category is especially important with respect to the long-term results.

THE BONE-ANCHORED ORBITAL PROSTHESIS

The same technique as the one described above has been used for retaining orbital prostheses [Figure 11(a,b)] although the prognosis for osseointegration in the bone rim of the orbit is not as good as in the mastoid. A total of 81 implants have been inserted, and 19 have been found not to be integrated. This gives a success rate of 76.5% [38,97]. The success rate for the implants that have been in place for more than 5 years is 75%. This is probably due to the fact that most of the implants that are lost, are lost in the early stages after the insertion, but it is also due to the fact that with improved clinical experience involving the osseointegration method, we have taken on more difficult cases than we would have attempted in the initial stages of clinical trials.

The incidence of infections around the implants has been 8.6% (7 cases). One fixture that was integrated was removed because it was positioned too close to another implant and gave rise to repeated skin irritation around the abutment. Several of these patients had undergone radiation treatment due to malignant disease, but even for the non-radiated cases the success rate is lower than for implants in the temporal bone region. The reasons for this are not clear. From the surgical point of view, there is a distinct difference between the hard cortical bone of the mastoid process and the chalky bone around the orbit, especially at the superior rim. Even in non-radiated patients we recommend an interval of at least 6 months between first- and second-stage surgery, and in radiated cases preferably 12 months. One patient (who had not received any radiation) lost all four implants within two weeks post-op due to a local infection. One year later, when the patient was taken into surgery again, the former implant sites had healed completely and only a slight impression in the bone was noted. This patient received four new implants which all integrated, and is now, two years after surgery, wearing his orbital prosthesis. Despite the somewhat less impressive primary results obtained with orbital implants, all the patients have enough implants left and are wearing their prostheses. The skin reactions are as favourable for these patients as for the NAS and auricular patients, with 93.2% skin reaction type 0.

CONCLUDING REMARKS

Today a vast number of different biomaterials are in use in clinical practice. This trend has increased enormously over the last decades. However, follow-up studies over longer time periods are scant. Although experimental models exist today where implant materials can be tested, clinical trials and careful follow-up over a sufficiently long period of time are also necessary before an implant material can be accepted for routine clinical practice. Commercially pure titanium appears to be very tissue-compatible, according to

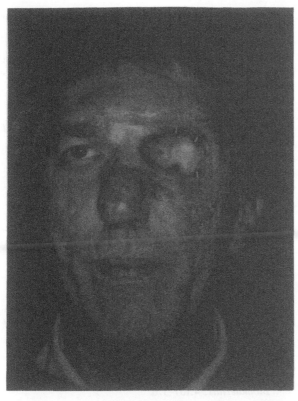

(a)

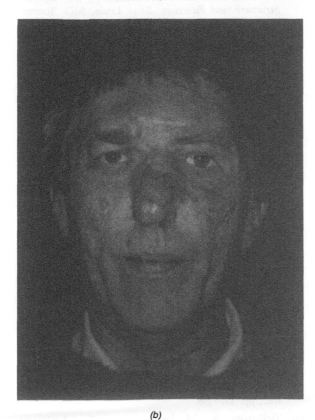

(b)

Figure 11. (a) Patient with an orbital defect following surgery. The skin penetrating abutments can be seen. (b) The same patient with the orbital prosthesis in place.

tests in animal models as well as in clinical use. The observation time for intra-oral use is more than 20 years, for extra-oral use more than 10 years.

Our conclusion is thus that the use of CP-titanium as implant material in combination with a surgical technique designed to minimize tissue trauma makes it possible to achieve osseointegration in the head and neck region. Furthermore, it is possible to establish and maintain a reaction-free skin penetration in the vast majority of patients, and no severe adverse reactions have been encountered.

REFERENCES

1. Brånemark, P. I., B. O. Hansson, R. Adell, U. Breine, J. Lindström, O. Hallén and A. Öhman. 1977. *Scand. J. Plast. Reconstr. Surg.*, 11 (suppl 16).

2. Southam, J. C. and P. Selwyn. 1971. *Br. J. Oral Surg.*, 8(3):211–221.

3. Albrektsson, T., P. I. Brånemark, H. A. Hansson and J. Lindström. 1981. *Acta Orthop. Scand.*, 52:155.

4. Albrektsson, T. and M. Jacobsson. 1987. *J. Prosth. Dent.*, 57:597–607.

5. Brånemark, P.I. 1985. "Introduction to Osseointegration", in *Tissue-Integrated Prostheses*. Brånemark, Zarb and Albrektsson, eds. Chicago, IL: Quintessence Publishing Co., Inc., pp. 11–76.

6. Adell, R., U. Lekholm, B. Rockler and P. I. Brånemark. 1981. *Int. J. Oral Surg.*, 10:387–397.

7. Adell, R. 1985. "Long-term Results", in *Tissue-Integrated Prostheses*. Brånemark, Zarb and Albrektsson, eds. Chicago, IL: Quintessence Publishing Co., Inc., pp. 175–186.

8. Albrektsson, T., B. Bergman, T. Folmer, P. Henry, K. Higuchi, I. Klineberg, W. R. Laney, U. Lekholm., V. Oikarinen, D. van Steenberghe, R. G. Triplett, P. Worthington and G. Zarb. 1988. *J. Prosthetic Dentistry*, 60:75–84.

9. Pritchard, J.′ J. 1972. "The Osteoblast", in *The Biochemistry and Physiology of Bone*. Bourne, ed. New York, NY, London, England: Academic Press, pp. 21–32.

10. Tonna, E. A. 1979. "Bone Tracers: Cell and Tissue Level Techniques", in *Skeletal Research: An Experimental Approach*. Simmons and Kunin, eds. NY, CA, England: Academic Press, pp. 487–496.

11. Copenhaver, W. M., R. P. Bunge and M. B. Bunge. 1971. In *Bailey's Textbook of Histology, 16th ed.* Baltimore, MD: Williams & Wilkins, pp. 136–154.

12. Owen, M. 1980. *Arthritis and Rheumatism*, 23:1073.

13. Hanaoka, H. 1979. *Clin. Orthop.*, 145:242–251.

14. Chambers, T. J. 1980. *Clin. Orthop.*, 151:283–292.

15. Bonucci, E. 1981. *Clin. Orthop.*, 158:252–261.

16. Urist, M. R., T. A. Dowell, P. H. Hay and B. S. Strates. 1988. *Clin. Orthop.*, 59:59–77.

17. Yasuda, I. 1953. *J. Kioto Med. Soc.*, 4:395–404. (Translated in *Clin. Orthop.*, 124:5–14, 1977).

18. Bassett, C. A. L. and R. O. Becker. 1962. *Science*, 137:1063–1081.

19. Colella, S. M., A. G. Miller, R. G. Stang, T. G. Stoebe

and D. M. Spengler. 1981. *J. Biomed. Mat. Res.*, 15:37–46.

20. Burwell, R. G. 1964. *J. Bone Jt. Surg.*, 46-B:110–129.

21. Young, R. W. 1963. *Clin. Orthop.*, 26:147–156.

22. Ham, A. W. and R. W. Harris. 1971. "Repair and Transplantation of Bone", in *The Biochemistry and Physiology of Bone III*. Bourne, ed. NY, England: Academic Press, pp. 338–356.

23. Baylink, D., J. Wergdal and C. Rich. 1970. *Clinical Research*, 18:183–192.

24. Axhausen, G. 1908. *Med. Klin.* (suppl), 2:23–58.

25. Albrektsson, T. 1979. "Healing of Bone Grafts". Thesis, University of Gothenburg, Sweden.

26. Rhinelander, F. W. 1974. *Clin. Orthop.*, 105:34–52.

27. Albrektsson, T. 1980. *Scand. J. Plast. Reconstr. Surg.*, 14:1–10.

28. Silver, I. A. and G. F. Howden. 1981. "The Use of the Rabbit Ear Chamber for Testing Biomaterials with Special References to Dental Materials", in *Fundamental Aspects of Biocompatibility II*. Williams, ed. Boca Raton, FL: CRC Press, pp. 259–266.

29. Skalak, R. 1985. "Aspects of Biomechanical Considerations", in *Tissue-Integrated Prostheses*. Brånemark, Zarb and Albrektsson, eds. Chicago, IL: Quintessence Publishing Co., Inc., pp. 117–128.

30. Steinemann, S. G., J. Eulenberger, P. A. Maeusli and A. Schroeder. 1986. *Adv. Biomater.*, 6:409–414.

31. Albrektsson, T., P. I. Brånemark, H. A. Hansson, B. Kasemo, K. Larsson, I. Lundström, D. H. McQueen and R. Skalak. 1983. *Ann. Biomed. Eng.*, 11:1–27.

32. Albrektsson, T. 1985. "Bone Tissue Response", in *Tissue-Integrated Prostheses*. Brånemark, Zarb and Albrektsson, eds. Chicago, IL: Quintessence Publishing Co., Inc., pp. 129–144.

33. Jacobsson, M. and T. Albrektsson. 1986. "Integration of Bone Implants in a Previously Irradiated Bone", in *Tissue Integration in Oral and Maxillo-Facial Reconstruction*. van Steenberghe, Albrektsson, Brånemark, Henry, Holt and Liden, eds. Amsterdam, The Netherlands: Excerpta Medica, pp. 110–116.

34. Jacobsson, M., A. Jönsson, T. Albrektsson and I. Turesson. 1985. *Int. J. Radiat. Oncol. Biol. Phys.*, 11:1963–1969.

35. Jacobsson, M., A. Jönsson, T. Albrektsson and I. Turesson. 1985. *Scand. J. Plast. Reconstr. Surg.*, 19:231–236.

36. Jacobsson, M., A. Jönsson, T. Albrektsson and I. Turesson. 1985. *Plast. Reconstr. Surg.*, 76:841–848.

37. Jacobsson, M., P. Kälebo, T. Albrektsson and I. Turesson. 1986. *Acta Radiol. Oncol.*, 25:57–62.

38. Jacobsson, M., A. Tjellström, T. Albrektsson, P. Thomsen and I. Turesson. 1988. *Ann. Otol. Rhinol. Laryngol.*, 97:337–340.

39. Eriksson, R. A., T. Albrektsson and B. Albrektsson. 1984. *Acta Orthop. Scand.*, 55:629–631.

40. Eriksson, A. R. and T. Albrektsson. 1985. *J. Oral Maxillofac. Surg.*, 42:701–711.

41. Eriksson, A. R. and R. J. Adell. 1986. *J. Oral Maxillofac. Surg.*, 44:4–7.

42. Jönsson, A. and T. Albrektsson. 1989. "Insertion and Removal Torque for Conical Titanium Implants" (in manuscript).

43. Albrektsson, T. 1983. *J. Prosth. Dent.*, 50:255–264.

44. Kasemo, B. and J. Lauksmaa. 1985. "Metal Selection and Surface Characteristics", in *Tissue-Integrated Prostheses*. Brånemark, Zarb and Albrektsson, ed. Chicago, IL: Quintessence Publishing Co., Inc., pp. 99–116.

45. Kasemo, B. and J. Lauksmaa. 1986. *CRC Critical Reviews in Biocompat.*, 2:335–380.

46. Williams, D. F. 1981. "Electrochemical Aspects of Corrosion in the Physiological Environment", in *Fundamental Aspects of Biocompatibility I*. Williams, ed. Boca Raton, FL: CRC Press, pp. 11–42.

47. McQueen, D., J. E. Sundgren, B. Ivarsson, I. Lundström, B. af Ekenstam, A. Svensson, P. I. Brånemark and T. Albrektsson. 1982. "Auger Electron Spectroscopic Studies of Titanium Implants", in *Adv. Biomat. Vol. 4, Clinical Applications of Biomaterials*. Lee, Allbrektsson and Brånemark, eds. New York, NY: John Wiley & Sons, pp. 179–185.

48. Thomsen, P. 1989. "Titanium and the Inflammatory Response", in *The Brånemark Osseointegrated Implant*. Albrektsson and Zarb, eds. Chicago, IL: Quintessence Publishing Co., Inc., pp. 25–35.

49. Albrektsson, T., P. I. Brånemark, H. A. Hansson, B. Ivarsson and U. Jönsson. 1982. *Advances in Biomaterials*, 4:167–176.

50. Ten Cate, A. R. 1980. *Oral Histology. Development, Structure and Function*. Saint Louis, MO, Toronto, Canada, London, England: C.V. Mosby Co.

51. Claes, L., P. Hutzschenreuter and O. Pohler. 1976. *Arch. Orthop. Unfallchir.*, 85:155–164.

52. Olmstead, M. L., O. Pohler, R. Schenk and R. B. Hohn. Progress Report. 1983. "Rough Titanium Screws: Biological Ingrowth Holding Power", Ohio State University, Dept. Vet.

53. Thomas, K. A. and S. D. Cook. 1985. *J. Biomed. Mater. Res.*, 19:875–894.

54. Albrektsson, T. 1985. *CRC Crit. Rev. Biocompat.*, 1:53–84.

55. Woodman, J. L., J. J. Jacobs, J. O. Galante and R. M. Urban. 1984. *J. Orthop. Res.*, 1:421–430.

56. Eneaux, C. P. 1955. *Can. Med. Assoc. J.*, 73:47–56.

57. Baier, R. E., J. R. Natiella, A. E. Meyer and J. M. Carter. 1986. "Importance of Implant Surface Preparation for Biomaterials with Different Intrinsic Properties", in *Tissue Integration in Oral and Maxillo-Facial Reconstruction*. van Steenberghe, Albrektsson, Brånemark, Henry, Holt and Liden, eds. Amsterdam, The Netherlands: Excerpta Medica, pp. 13–36.

58. Johansson, C., M. Jacobsson and T. Albrektsson. 1988. *Adv. Biomater.*, 8:87–92.

59. Strid, K. G. 1985. "Radiographic Results", in *Tissue-Integrated Prostheses*. Brånemark, Zarb and Albrektsson, ed. Chicago, IL: Quintessence Publishing Co., Inc., pp. 187–198.

60. Tjellström, A., M. Jacobsson and T. Albrektsson. 1988. *Int. J. Oral. Maxillofacial Implants*, 3:287–289.

61. Yamanaka, E., A. Tjellström, M. Jacobsson and T. Albrektsson. 1989. *Long-Term Observations on Re-*

moval Torque of Directly Bone-Anchored Implants. In manuscript.

62. von Recum, A. F. 1984. *J. Biomed. Mater. Res.*, 18:323-336.

63. von Recum, A. F., J. Yan, P. D. Schreuders and D. L. Powers. 1986. "Bone Healing Phenomena around Permanent Percutaneous Implants", in *Tissue Integration in Oral and Maxillo-Facial Reconstruction*. van Steenberghe, Albrektsson, Brånemark, Henry, Holt and Liden, eds. Amsterdam, The Netherlands: Excerpta Medica, pp. 159-169.

64. Schreuders, P. D., T. N. Salthouse and A. F. von Recum. 1988. *J. Biomed. Mater. Res.*, 22:121-135.

65. Gangjee, T., R. Colaizzo and A. F. von Recum. 1985. *Ann. Biomed. Eng.*, 13:451-467.

66. Yan, Y. J., F. W. Cooke, P. S. Vaskelis and A. F. von Recum. 1989. *J. Biomed. Mater. Res.*, 23:171-189.

67. Lundgren, D., J. P. Hakansson and P. Bodo. 1986. "Morphometric Analysis of Tissue Components Adjacent to Percutaneous Implants", in *Tissue Integration in Oral and Maxillo-Facial Reconstruction*. van Steenberghe, Albrektsson, Brånemark, Henry, Holt and Liden, eds. Amsterdam, The Netherlands: Excerpta Medica, pp. 173-180.

68. Krouskop, T. A., H. D. Brown, K. Gray, G. R. Shively, M. Romovacek, M. Spira and R. S. Runyan. 1988. *Biomaterials*, 9:398-404.

69. Spadaro, J. A., S. E. Chase and D. A. Webster. 1986. *J. Biomed. Mater. Res.*, 20:565-577.

70. Gould, T. R. L. 1986. "Clinical Implications of the Attachment of Oral Tissue to Permucosal Implants", in *Tissue Integration in Oral and Maxillo-Facial Reconstruction*. van Steenberghe, Albrektsson, Brånemark, Henry, Holt and Liden, eds. Amsterdam, The Netherlands: Excerpta Medica, pp. 253-270.

71. Jansen, J. A., J. R. de Wijn, Wolters-Lutgerhorst and P. J. van Mullem. 1986. "Adhesion of Guinea-Pig Epidermal Cells to Oral Implant Materials", in *Tissue Integration in Oral and Maxillo-Facial Reconstruction*. van Steenberghe, Albrektsson, Brånemark, Henry, Holt and Liden, eds. Amsterdam, The Netherlands: Excerpta Medica, pp. 271-277.

72. Carmichael, R. P., P. Apse, G. A. Zarb and C. A. G. McCulloch. 1989. "Role of the Soft Tissue", in *The Brånemark Osseointegrated Implant*. Albrektsson and Zarb, eds. Chicago, IL: Quintessence Publishing Co., Inc., pp. 39-78.

73. Cheroudi, B., T. R. Gould and D. M. Brunette. 1988. *J. Biomed. Mater. Res.*, 22:459-473.

74. Ten Cate, A. R. 1985. "The Gingival Junction", in *Tissue-Integrated Prostheses*. Brånemark, Zarb and Albrektsson, eds. Chicago, IL: Quintessence Publishing Co., Inc., pp. 145-154.

75. Jansen, J. A. and K. de Groot. 1988. *Biomaterials*, 9:268-272.

76. Grosse-Siestrup, C. and K. Affeld. 1984. *J. Biomed. Mater. Res.*, 18:357-382.

77. Hall, C. W., P. A. Cox and S. R. McFarland. 1984. *J. Biomed. Mater. Res.*, 18:383-393.

78. Brånemark, P. I. and T. Albrektsson. 1982. *Scand. J. Plast. Reconstr. Surg.*, 16:17-21.

79. Albrektsson, T., P. I. Brånemark and J. Lindström. 1982. "Transcutaneous Titanium Implants in Clinical Practice", in *Adv. Biomat. Vol. 4, Clinical Applications of Biomaterials*. Lee, Albrektsson and Brånemark, eds. New York, NY: John Wiley & Sons, pp. 157-166.

80. Jacobsson, M., A. Tjellström, P. Thomsen and T. Albrektsson. 1987. *Scand. J. Plast. Reconstr. Surg.*, 21:225-228.

81. Lidén, G., A. Ringdahl, A. Tjellström, M. Jacobsson, P. Carlsson and B. Hakansson. 1989. Submitted to *Ann. Otol. Rhinol. Laryngol.*

82. Holgers, K. M., A. Tjellström and L. M. Bjursten, et al. 1988. *Am. J. Otol.*, 9:56-59.

83. Gates, G. A., J. V. Hough, W. M. Gatti and W. H. Bardley. 1989. *Arch. Otolaryngol. Head & Neck Surg.*, 115:924-930.

84. Brent, B. 1977. *Plast. Reconstr. Surg.*, 59:475-484.

85. Brent, B. 1983. *Plast. Reconstr. Surg.*, 72:141-152.

86. Tjellström, A., E. Yontchev and J. Lindström, et al. 1985. *Otolaryngol. Head & Neck Surg.*, 93:366-372.

87. Jansson, K. and A. Tjellström. 1988. *How to Make an Auricular Prosthesis*. Göteborg Medical Service Video Library, videotape 19.

88. Fine, L., M. Jacobsson and A. Tjellström. 1989. "An Evaluation of Facial Prostheses Retained through Utilization of Osseointegrated Implants" (under preparation).

89. Brånemark. 1989. Personal communication.

90. Jacobsson, M., T. Albrektsson, and T. Tjellström. 1989. "Tissue-Integrated Implants in Children" (under preparation).

91. Frost, H. M. 1963. Bone Remodeling Dynamics. Springfield, IL: Charles C. Thomas Publ.

92. Sluker, S. J. 1985. *Max-Fac. Surg.*, 13:70-75.

93. Nagase, M., K. Ueda, I. Suzuki and T. Nakajima. 1985. *J. Oral Maxillofac. Surg.*, 43:218-227.

94. Sauer, N. J. and S. S. Dunlap. 1985. *Journal of Forensic Sciences, JFSCA*, 30:953-962.

95. Scholz, F. and B. d'Hoedt. 1983. *Dtsch. Zahnärztl. Z.*, 39:416-424.

96. Pedley, R. B., G. Mechim and D. F. Williams. 1981. "Tumour Induction by Implant Materials", in *Fundamental Aspects of Biocompatibility II*. Williams, ed. Boca Raton, FL: CRC Press, pp. 175-202.

97. Jacobsson, M. and A. Tjellström. 1988. "A 10-year Experience with Maxillo-Facial Bone-Anchored Implants", in *Otolaryngol. Head & Neck Surg.* (Special issue: Annual Meeting of the American Academy of Otolaryngology—Head and Neck Surgery), p. 170.

16

Development of a Bioadhesive Tablet

G. PONCHEL*
D. DUCHENE*.1

ABSTRACT: Bioadhesion is a technical innovation developed in order to improve the bioavailability and efficiency of various active ingredients. This method can be applied to solid or viscous dosage forms, but most of the studies concern tablets. Today, many bioadhesive polymers have been investigated, among which the most widely used is poly(acrylic acid). The formulation has to take into account the nature of the mucosa on which the tablet is to adhere and the type of activity required (local or systemic). It also has to consider the duration of release desired, and must therefore combine a matrix system with a bioadhesive polymer. The evaluation of such dosage forms is dual: bioadhesive potency (by tensile tests) and drug release (by dissolution and in vivo tests).

INTRODUCTION

In recent years, pharmaceutical research has shown an increasing interest in the development of controlled-release systems capable of improving the therapeutic efficiency of various active ingredients, with a concomitant decrease in secondary effects and a facilitation of use.

Bioadhesive forms have been proposed with the same objectives. In this field, bioadhesive tablets are new therapeutic forms, capable of adhesion on a mucosa for a sufficiently prolonged period of time. They are remarkable in that they not only allow the controlled release of an active ingredient, but, at the same time, they immobilize the pharmaceutical form on a mucosa at the best site for activity or resorption.

The knowledge of controlled-release techniques,

greatly developed during the past few years [1], has been swept along by the current development of controlled-release systems by the pharmaceutical industry. On the other hand, the study of bioadhesive forms is rather new in the pharmaceutical field. The combination of controlled-release concepts and bioadhesion constitutes a very promising therapeutic innovation.

Before explaining what bioadhesion is and what bioadhesive tablets are, it is interesting to recall that, some years ago, it was demonstrated that traditional dosage forms, whose composition included cellulosic polymers (such as hydroxypropyl-methylcellulose, ethylcellulose) or gelatin, had bioadhesive properties with respect to the oesophageal mucosa and the gastro-intestinal tract [2–7]. This adhesion, demonstrated for various pharmaceutical specialties [2,60], is generally undesirable because, due to its irregular appearance, it could result in variable bioavailability, detrimental for the patient. Furthermore, adhesion on the oesophageal mucosa of swine [3,6] or dogs [6] was proposed to explain the appearance of gastro-intestinal ulcerations observed with Oros systems containing indomethacin (Osmosin®).

If undesired and uncontrolled mucosa adhesion constitutes a limitation to the use of bioadhesive tablets for oral administration, the mastery of this phenomenon will lead to the development of very useful dosage forms. As a result, this led to the appearance on the market of polymers capable of "reliable" bioadhesion on certain mucosa. The use of bioadhesive tablets leads to improvement in local, topical and systemic activity.

THERAPEUTIC INTEREST OF BIOADHESIVE TABLETS

Bioadhesive tablets are designed to adhere to a specific mucosa. The various mucus-coated routes for drug administration include the ocular, nasal, buccal, respiratory, gastro-intestinal, rectal, urethral and

1Author to whom all correspondence should be addressed.

*Laboratoire de Pharmacie Galenique et Biopharmacie, URA 1218 CNRS, Faculte de pharmacie de Paris-Sud, 5 Rue Jean Baptiste Clement, 92296 Chatenay Malabry, France

vaginal routes. For obvious accessibility reasons, some mucosa are prohibited for tablets. However, many therapeutic applications can be (and have been) imagined for this kind of drug delivery system.

Prolongation of Residence Time

The prolongation of residence time for a drug dosage form is of major interest for drugs exhibiting low biological half-lives, such as nitroglycerin for the treatment of angina pectoris, or local anaesthetic drugs. The ability of bioadhesive tablets to prolong the period during which drug release is effective results from the immobilization of the dosage form on (or near) the absorbing mucosa.

Localization of a Drug Delivery System

Bioadhesive tablets can be immobilized on various mucosa. This localization has two main advantages: targetting the drug on locally-diseased mucosa, and immobilizing it at its "absorption window".

The targetting of drugs on locally-diseased mucosa is of special interest in the treatment of cervical or vaginal cancers, or of buccal diseases, such as aphthous stomatitis, and also for the reduction of pain by the local administration of morphine (for buccal cancers). Dental applications are equally possible: for local anaesthetic effects, or for the delivery of fluoride ions, for example. Two types of mucosa must be distinguished here: externally-accessible mucosa (buccal, vaginal or cervical), for which the patient is able to control adhesion, and gastro-intestinal mucosa for which adhesion has to be controlled by the polymeric device. At the present time, available polymeric devices are unable to adhere to a definite place on the gastro-intestinal tract [7–9]. Development of specific polymers capable of achieving high site specificity would be of great value in this area. However, for the moment, it is possible to use bioadhesive forms coated with polymers whose dissolution is pH-dependent.

Drugs are absorbed very differently from one mucosa to another. For example, iron, riboflavin and chlorothiazide are reported to have an "absorption window" in the gastro-intestinal tract. This means they are absorbed in a specific region of the digestive tract. For many well-known drugs, their absorption patterns are different through the various mucosa (buccal, nasal, rectal) [10–15]. Various studies have been reported for peptides [15–21], such as desmopressin, LHRH and insulin: they lead to the conclusion that absorption across these mucosa is better than across the gastro-intestinal mucosa. Furthermore, some of these mucosa avoid the enzymatic degradation of the drug, or hepatic first-passage effects, which are encountered with classical gastro-intestinal absorption. The immobilization of drugs on specific mucosa, or portions of mucosa, is of the highest interest.

Intimate Contact with an Absorbing Membrane

Due to the adhesion phenomenon, the bioadhesive tablet develops an intimate contact with the mucosa, which is an absorbing membrane. There is high drug concentration near the mucosa, and a high flux through the membrane is thus achieved.

As pointed out previously, many studies deal with the determination of absorbed quantities of drug through specific mucosa. However, many phenomena are involved at this stage. The mucus, which covers the mucosa, has a protective role stemming from its hydrophobicity. The mucus acts as a diffusion barrier for molecules and it is more generally directed against drug absorption.

Diffusion through the mucus layer depends mainly on the physicochemical characteristics of the active ingredient: its molecular weight, presence of electrically-charged groups, hydrophilicity or hydrophobicity, hydration radius, and the ability to form hydrogen bonds [22,23]. However, the very nature of the mucus also interferes in the diffusion process, due to glycoprotein concentration and type. Some modelizations of molecule absorption have been proposed for the gastro-intestinal tract [15,23] by considering the mucus as a macromolecular network. The physicochemical parameters of nasal drug absorption have also been studied [24]. It must be pointed out that the molecular weight of the drug seems to be the main parameter determining absorption. The upper molecular weight limit seems to be around 1000 daltons in order to obtain significant drug penetration into the gastro-intestinal mucosa [15]. Similar values are obtained for the nasal mucosa [21,25].

In order to enhance the penetration of drugs exhibiting high molecular weight, some studies are performed on enhancing agents concerned with different mucosa: gastro-intestinal [26] and nasal [27,28].

Finally, interactions between mucus and drugs have been studied for a number of products, such as tetracyclines [29–32] and other antibotics [22,23].

Therapeutic Applications of Bioadhesive Tablets

Table 1 reports some of the therapeutic applications of bioadhesive tablets, either already on the market, or under development.

BIOADHESION PHENOMENON

Bioadhesion Mechanism

Bioadhesive tablets are designed to adhere to mucosa. Bioadhesion is an interfacial phenomenon

Table 1. Active ingredients under development, undergoing clinical tests or already on the market, in the form of bioadhesive tablets.

Active Ingredient	Disease Concerned	Product under Development	Clinical Tests	Marketed	Ref.
Triamcinolone acetonide	Aphthous stomatitis	☐	☐	Aftach®	[34]
Dipotassium glycine lycine	Aphthous stomatitis	☐	☐	Pattel®	[35]
Lidocaine	Toothache	☐			[36,37]
Fluorides	Dental decay	☐			(dev.)
Morphine	Buccal analgesia	☐			(dev.)
Bleomycin	Cancers of the uterus by *Carcinoma colli*	☐*	☐		[38,39]
5-Fluorouracyl	Cancers of the uterus by *Carcinoma colli*	☐*	☐		[38]
Carboquone	Cancers of the uterus by *Carcinoma colli*	☐*	☐		[38]
Insulin	Insulin-dependent diabetes	☐			[34]
Metronidazole	Vaginal antifungal	☐			[40,41]
Nitroglycerin	Angina pectoris	☐	☐	Susadrin®	[42]
Prochlorperazine maleate	Dizziness, migraines and nausea	☐	☐	Buccastem®	

*Sticks prepared by compression.

which differs from conventional adhesion by the special properties and characteristics of the biological tissue.

For bioadhesion to occur, a succession of phenomena is required, whose relative importance depends on the nature of the bioadhesive polymer. First, an intimate contact must exist between the bioadhesive tablet and the mucosa. At this stage, several theories have been proposed to describe this mechanism of adhesion between two elements [1,43]: wetting theory, diffusion theory, mechanical interlocking theory, electronic transfer theory, and adsorption theory.

Depending on the nature of the polymer, one of these mechanisms may predominate over the others. In the case of poly(acrylic acid) polymers, it has been demonstrated that, after intimate contact has been established, it is possible to describe the phenomenon as a combination of polymer chain diffusion and mechanical interlocking into the mucus glycoprotein network, and establishment of secondary chemical and physical bonds (van der Waals forces between hydrophobic groups, and hydrogen bonds between hydrophilic groups) [1,43].

It appears that the mucus structure is as important as that of the polymer [22,44]. However, although slight differences in composition can exist between different types of mucosa [22,45], the glycoproteins, i.e., the basic component of the mucus, remain the same. Thus, bioadhesive polymers must possess molecular characteristics compatible with the glycoprotein structure. Polyanionic polymers, with high-charge density, such as poly(acrylic acid) polymers, are the best candidates for bioadhesive purposes [46].

Bioadhesive Polymer Evaluation

Based on the different theories concerning the bioadhesion mechanism, screenings of potentially bioadhesive polymers have been proposed in the literature. However, the final determination of their properties and classification must be based on experimental techniques of the measurement of bond strength. This knowledge is necessary for the formulator, and, although it is not the aim of this review, it is interesting to describe broadly some of the techniques reported in the literature.

Tests may be classified in three groups:

- mechanical measurements of the bioadhesive strength, including tear tests, either on artificial media [47–50] or on biological media (*ex vivo*) [4,5,40–42,51], and shear tests [46]
- stress relaxation measurements [52], or resistance to displacement tests [50,53]
- labelling tests (*in vivo* and *in vitro*) [54,55] by the use of radiolabelled or fluorescent probes

The principles of these tests are very different one from the other, and consequently they will give only comparative values rather than absolute strengths of adhesion.

For example, the mechanical tear tests, which are

the simplest to perform, will give varying results depending on the physical parameter measured. Park and Robinson [51] and other authors [43] measure only the maximum force necessary for the detachment of the bioadhesive polymer from a mucosa prepared *ex vivo*. Our research team recently developed a technique based on the determination of the work of adhesion of such a system, by measuring continuously force versus elongation during a tensile test [40, 41,56]. This parameter seems more accurate for the characterization of bioadhesive strength than the simple measurement of the maximum detachment force. Thus, under given experimental conditions, hydroxypropyl-methylcellulose and poly(acrylic acid) exhibit the same detachment force, but in the same time the second polymer requires three times more energy to be detached from the mucosa than the cellulosic polymer [57]. In this case, the simple measurement of the detachment force would not be sufficient to characterize the bioadhesive strength of these two polymers. Even when the same parameter is measured, some modifications during the experimental work leads to slight differences in the polymer classifications [43,44,47]. However, from this example, it is obvious that a polymer classification will be valid only for a given test, and must be considered as indicative. Table 2 gives an example of polymer classification, based on tear tests [44].

Bioadhesion tests are also used for the study of the influence of a number of physicochemical parameters. Two kinds of parameter have been studied, which can be classified in two groups: polymer-related factors and environmental factors. In the first case, inherent properties of the polymers can be studied in

connection with the interfacial phenomenon of bioadhesion. Acrylic acid-based polymers have been studied the most since they are the best candidates for bioadhesion. For these polymers, the following parameters have been investigated: cross-linking ratio [46,51,58], nature of the cross-linking agent [51,55], molecular weight, monomer nature [55], carboxylic group density [58], and polymer flexibility [58]. In the second case, parameters such as polymer hydration effect and swelling time [41], polymer electrical charge neutralization [35], effect of ionic species [46,51,57], pH of hydration medium [55,57], and presence of mucolytic agents [51] can be investigated using these methods.

Indeed, as a result of polymer evaluation studies, it appears that anionic polymers are better candidates for bioadhesion than neutral or cationic polymers. The nature of chemical groups borne by the polymer is important. Polymers containing hydroxyls and carboxyls are more mucoadhesive when adhesion to a soft mucosa is required, which is the case for all bioadhesive tablet applications.

We must emphasize that some of the mechanical tests used for the evaluation of the polymer bioadhesive properties will also be used for the measurement of the bioadhesive properties of the tablets.

Bioadhesive Polymers

Bioadhesive tablets are based on the use of a restricted number of polymers, although there are many kinds of bioadhesive polymer from synthetic and natural sources. They generally have two functions, since they ensure the adhesion and the controlled release of the drug. Table 3 shows the polymers used in commercialized bioadhesive tablets and products under development, with some of the commercial brand names of these products. From a practical standpoint, two groups of polymers are commonly used in tablet formulation: poly(acrylic acid) cross-linked polymers (cross-linking agents: divinylglycol for Polycarbophil®, and polyallylsaccharose for Carbopol® 934P) and hydrophilic cellulosic polymers.

DESIGN OF A NEW BIOADHESIVE TABLET

Many parameters related to the active ingredient, the polymeric system and the formulation have to be considered during the design of a bioadhesive tablet. First, the active ingredient must have pharmacokinetic properties compatible with this type of dosage form (examples of these problems were given above). Consideration of these data allows the choice of the mucosa onto which the bioadhesive tablet is to adhere.

The polymeric system has two functions in a bioadhesive drug delivery system: to immobilize the dosage form, and to ensure the controlled release of the active ingredient. However, a polymer exhibiting

Table 2. Relative bioadhesive performance of some test compounds (according to [44], with permission).

Substance	Muco-Adhesive Force[1]	Adhesive Performance[2]
Carmellose® (carboxy methylcellulose)	193	excellent
Carbomer 934 (carbopol®)	185	excellent
Polycarbophil®	—	excellent
Tragacanth	154	excellent
Sodium alginate	126	excellent
Hydroxyethyl-cellulose	—	excellent
Karaya gum	125	good
Gelatin	116	fair
Guar gum	—	fair
Pectin	100	poor
Povidone® [poly(vinylpyrrolidone)]	98	poor
Acacia	98	poor
Macrogol® (polyethylene glycol)	96	poor
Psyllium	—	poor

[1]Percentage of a standard tested *in vitro*.
[2]Assessed *in vivo*.

Table 3. Polymers encountered in some bioadhesive tablet formulations with some of their commercial denominations.

Polymer	Trade Name	Company	Reference
Poly(acrylic acid)	Carbopol® 934P Polycarbophil®	BFGoodrich Chemical Company	[34–38,] 40,41]
	Hiviswako® HVW 103	Wako Pure Chemical Industries Limited	
Natural polymers including modified hypromellose	Synchron®	Forest Laboratories	[42]
Hydroxypropyl- methylcellulose	Methocel®	Dow Chemical	[40,41]
Hydroxypropyl-cellulose	HPC	Nippon Soda Company	[35,38]
	Klucel®	Hercules	

good bioadhesive properties may have inadequate controlled-release capabilities. These two functions can therefore be consigned to two separate polymeric systems in the drug delivery system. Other considerations such as patient comfort must also be taken into account, since some mucosal cavities are rather small. Naturally, the activity level of the active ingredient in the organism will be of paramount importance for the localization of the drug in the polymeric device.

Figure 1 summarizes a few geometric possibilities which account for these different parameters. Two kinds of systems are presented here: monolithic systems and multicomponent systems.

In the first case, and for local action, simple matrix systems (Diagram 1) or compressed-rod systems (Diagram 2) are the simplest. Simple matrix systems have been developed for nitroglycerin delivery in the treatment of angina pectoris [42]. Compressed rods have been used by Nagai et al. for vaginal cancer treatment with various agents [17,38]. Diagram 3 shows a bioadhesive tablet coated with a gastro-resistant film. This system allows normal transit up to the intestine, where bioadhesion then comes into action.

The second case deals with multicomponent systems. When controlled release of the active ingredient cannot be achieved by the adhesive system itself, diagrams 4, 5, 6 and 7 show some possibilities. If drugs provoke irritation problems when in contact with a mucosa, or when they have to be released in a large mucosal area, it could be effective to place the controlled-release system on to the adhesive system of the drug delivery system. Diagram 4 in Figure 1 shows an example of such a bilayered system. On the contrary, if drug activity is to be very localized, the drug may be placed near the affected mucosa in the adhesive system and protection provided by an inert coating (Diagram 5). This is the case of the commercial product Aftach®, developed by Nagai et al. [17], for the treatment of aphthae. This bioadhesive tablet is a bilayered tablet with small dimensions (7 mm in diameter by 1.1 mm thick). The upper layer consists of lactose and has no adhesive properties, its role being to prevent the active ingredient (triamcinolone acetonide) from diffusing out of its activity site (aphtha), and to allow an easy placing of the bioadhesive tablet. The lower layer, which contains the active ingredient, is composed of hydroxypropyl-cellulose and poly (acrylic acid) (Carbopol® 934P), and constitutes the bioadhesive layer.

Diagrams 6 and 7 (Figure 1) show geometric arrangements that allow protection of drug controlled release from the environment. Nagai et al. [17,35,

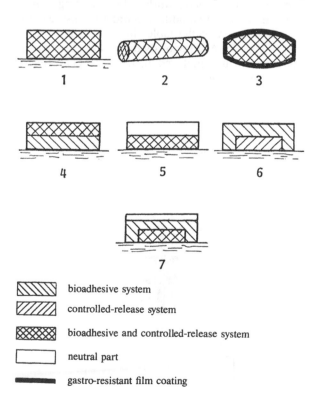

bioadhesive system

controlled-release system

bioadhesive and controlled-release system

neutral part

gastro-resistant film coating

Figure 1. A few possible geometric arrangements for bioadhesive tablets.

36,59] used features of diagram 6 for the drug delivery of insulin *per os*. In this case, the core is composed of a non-bioadhesive system (cocoa butter, glyceride bases and different penetration enhancers) containing insulin. It is then coated with a bioadhesive peripheral layer whose role is to stick to the buccal mucosa and also to protect the insulin from degradation and loss into the entire oral cavity. However, this system exhibited poor bioavailability capability.

Diagram 7 shows another possibility explored by Nagai for the delivery of lidocaine [37] for local anaesthetic purposes in toothache. In this case, the core contains the drug and is also bioadhesive. The first peripheral coating is also adhesive, but without drug, and is designed to stick slightly to human gums. Finally the system is top-coated by a non-adhesive layer that prevents the drug delivery system from sticking to the tongue or cheek mucosa.

Depending on the sophistication of the dosage form, the formulation of bioadhesive tablets will be more or less complicated. However, various manufacturing processes involved in their preparation are available, such as lyophilization for the preparation of raw materials, simple compression, double- or triple-layer compression, peripheral core coating by adapted compression techniques, and coating techniques.

EVALUATION OF BIOADHESIVE TABLETS

As bioadhesive tablets have two distinct functions, namely adhesion to tissue, and controlled-release properties, their evaluation must involve a characterization of these two properties.

Evaluation of Adhesive Properties

Bioadhesion of tablets will have to occur in the presence of many environmental factors, which have already been mentioned. It is therefore necessary, not only to have specific methods for the measurement of adhesion, but also to be able to evaluate the possible influence of these environmental factors.

Methods proposed in the literature characterize the adhesion of a tablet either to an inert support (*in vitro* methods) or to a biological support (*ex vivo* methods). *In vivo* methods, close to real conditions of dosage form utilization, require biological tissues similar to those on which the adhesion will really take place. They are more difficult to carry out than *in vitro* methods. To our knowledge, there are no *in vivo* methods for the study of the bioadhesion properties of tablets.

Ex vivo *Methods*

Nagai et al. [35] were probably the first to describe an apparatus with the purpose of measuring the adhesivity of bioadhesive tablets on oral mucosa. The apparatus (Figure 2) requires the use of a mouse peri-

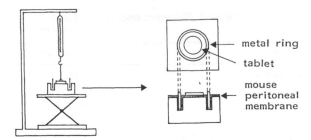

Figure 2. Apparatus used by Nagai et al. for the determination of adhesion on biological tissues [35] (with permission).

toneal membrane on which the dosage form is fixed for 10 minutes, and then wrenched away with a spring balance. The bioadhesive strength is evaluated as being the maximum detachment force which is recorded when the tablet is separated from the mucosa. For comparison purposes, this force can be related to the contact surface between the two systems.

Ponchel et al. [40,41] developed a system which measures the work of adhesion, and not just the maximum detachment force. This method uses a tensile apparatus Instron tester. The mucosa used is bovine sublingual or vaginal mucosa, which is stuck on to the holder connected to the lower clamp of the tester. A bioadhesive tablet is stuck on to the holder connected to the upper clamp of the tester. The system is then elongated at constant speed. The force necessary for detachment is continuously recorded, and enables the calculation of adhesion work. The operating conditions can be slightly modified in order to ensure complete immersion of the tablet in any desired media [57] (Figure 3). As previously discussed, these methods can also be employed in order to characterize polymer properties.

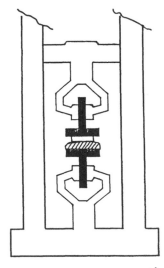

Figure 3. Apparatus used by Ponchel and Duchêne for the determination of adhesion on biological tissues.

In order to characterize the bioadhesive behaviour of tablets by the mean of viscoelasticity measurements, Peppas et al. [52] developed another method, based on the same apparatus. In this case, the system composed of the tablet adhering to the mucosa is subjected to a slight deformation: a force decay, due to viscoelastic modifications, is recorded and analyzed by using a Maxwell model.

It is necessary to mention two systems developed by Marvola [2,4,5,60] in order to measure the adhesion of a dosage form to the oesophagus (adhesion here being a disadvantage of classical formulations). These apparatuses (Figure 4) use segments of swine oesophagus maintained at 37°C in an oxygenated Tyrode solution. The solid dosage form under study is attached to a balance and inserted into the oesophagus. It is then progressively detached by increasing the charge on the opposite tray of the balance. Swisher et al. [6] used the same systems with dog and swine oesophagus. For the same purpose, Al-Dujaili et al. [3] developed a technique very similar to the technique of Nagai.

In vitro *Methods*

Recently, Forget et al. [61] developed an *in vitro* method for the measurement of the adhesion strength of tablets on artificial substrates (Figure 5). The technique uses sieves with varying mesh size as the artificial substrates. They are hydrated with a known quantity of liquid. The bioadhesive tablet, previously fixed to a metallic support, is then allowed to stick to the sieve surface for a given time. Afterwards, a tensile experiment is conducted, and the maximum detachment force is registered.

Factors Affecting Bioadhesion

The bioadhesive characteristics of a tablet are affected by two kinds of factor which are related to the tablet formulation and to the environmental conditions.

Influence of Formulation-Related Factors

To date, the influence of tablet formulation factors has not been widely investigated. However, it is quite clear that some of these are likely to have a certain influence on the bioadhesive properties of tablets. The type of lubricant is one of these factors. The presence of hydrophobic lubricants is capable of modifying the swelling capacity of tablets by modifying water penetration into the tablet structure. Consequently, hydrophobic lubricants can decrease the bioadhesive power of tablets, as has been demonstrated for magnesium stearate [42]. Studies of the incidence of porosity on tablet bioadhesion is also lacking at the present time, although this parameter may also modify tablet swelling behaviour.

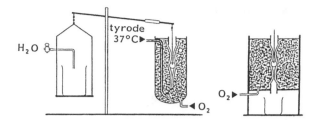

Figure 4. Apparatus used by Marvola et al. for the determination of adhesion on œsophaga [2] (with permission of the copyright owner, the American Pharmaceutical Association).

Influence of Environment-Related Factors

INFLUENCE OF HYDRATION CONDITIONS

The absorption of water by the tablet is necessary to induce the swelling of the bioadhesive polymer, which, in turn, is necessary for bioadhesion to occur.

Swelling, as mentioned earlier, allows the disentanglement of polymer chains and the development of interactions between the polymeric system and the glycoproteic network of the mucus. However, high swelling levels lead to a decrease in bioadhesion, since polymer chains will be rarefied at the tablet/mucosa interface. Such a phenomenon must not occur too early, in order to allow a sufficient action of the bioadhesive system. With polymers available at the present time, this phenomenon is a limitation for the use of bioadhesive tablets for gastro-intestinal drug delivery, since hydration conditions vary too much. Nevertheless, in other applications, complete swelling of the tablet allows easy detachment of the bioadhesive system after drug release.

Figure 6 shows that the bioadhesive strength decreases rapidly when small amounts of water are added at the surface of a tablet containing poly(acrylic acid). However, when a bioadhesive tablet is applied on a buccal mucosa, it is necessary to maintain it for a few minutes in order to allow the swelling of the bio-

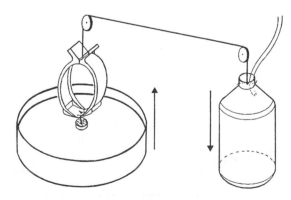

Figure 5. Apparatus used by Forget et al. for the determination of adhesion on artificial substrates [61] (with permission of *Editions de Santé*).

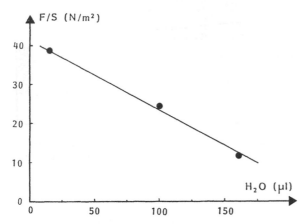

Figure 6. Effect of hydration on the bioadhesive strength of a poly(acrylic acid)-based tablet containing 50% w/w of metronidazole.

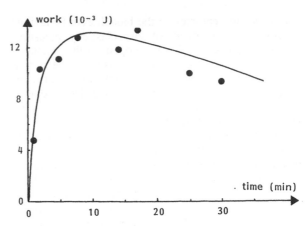

Figure 7. Effect of duration of applied strength on the bioadhesion of a hydroxypropyl-methylcellulose/poly(acrylic acid) system [41] (with permission of *J. Contr. Rel.*).

adhesive polymer and the development of its bioadhesivity. We have demonstrated [41], for a hydroxypropyl-methylcellulose/poly(acrylic acid) system, that an optimal swelling time is reached after 10 minutes under controlled hydration conditions (Figure 7).

INFLUENCE OF pH

The environment of a tablet placed in contact with a mucosa includes fluids which exhibit given pH and defined ionic contents [51,62,63]. Due to swelling, the absorption of liquid by the tablet can be significant so that the pH of the medium is able to modify the bioadhesivity of pH-sensitive polymers such as poly(acrylic acid) [1,51,55]. However, for high drug content tablets, we have shown that this parameter does not significantly affect bioadhesion [64].

INFLUENCE OF IONIC FORCE

Ionic force and ion nature can affect polymer conformity. Poly(acrylic acid) hydrogel properties are affected by the presence of divalent calcium ions [1], as shown in Table 4. However, it is not clear whether this is caused by a calcium/mucin interaction [46] or a calcium/poly(acrylic acid) interaction. Whatever the mechanism, we have shown that, even for highly drug-loaded tablets, ionic force has quite an influence on bioadhesive properties, detachment force and work of adhesion, depending on the nature of the mucosa.

INFLUENCE OF APPLIED STRENGTH

It is obvious that, to place a bioadhesive system, it is necessary to apply a defined force, necessary to ensure an intimate contact between the tablet surface and the mucosa. Robinson et al. [46,51] have shown that, for poly(acrylic acid)/divinylbenzene, poly(HEMA), or poly(acrylic acid) hydrogels, adhesion strength increases with applied force.

INFLUENCE OF MUCOSA TYPE

The nature of the mucosa on which the tablet is to be stuck may influence the strength of the bioadhesive bond which is created. Indeed, the quantity of mucus lining on this surface can vary widely depending on the type of mucosa. In fact, two mucus layers must be distinguished, one near the mucosa which is water-insoluble, and the luminal layer, which is water-soluble and may easily be washed away. Allen et al. [65] pointed out that the adherent mucus thickness in man is between about 50 and 450 μm, with an average value of 180 μm. However, somewhat lower values are proposed by some authors [59]. This layer is more or less adherent depending on the mucosa, and may be affected by many pathologic variables. However, for healthy mucosa, the mucin molecule arrangement, the "architecture" of the mucus, seems to be similar from one mucosa to another [66].

In Figure 8, microphotographs of bovine sublingual and vaginal mucosa, after preparation, show that the

Table 4. *Influence of the type of mucosa on the bioadhesion of tablets containing poly(acrylic acid), hydroxypropyl-methylcellulose and metronidazole (tests are carried out in the presence or absence of CaCl₂).*

CaCl₂		Sublingual Mucosa		Vaginal Mucosa	
g/l	Ionic Strength	F (N)	W (mJ)	F (N)	W (mJ)
0	0	1.9 ± 0.6	0.6 ± 0.3	2.8 ± 0.9	1.0 ± 0.5
100	2.77	1.5 ± 0.7	0.3 ± 0.2	2.9 ± 0.7	0.9 ± 0.0

vaginal mucosa has a large layer of mucus lining (coloured purple) on the epithelial cell basement (blue). On the other hand, the sublingual mucosa does not present any more mucus after preparation and coloration. Bioadhesion is affected by this parameter as reported in Table 4. Measurements of bioadhesivity were achieved by a tensile test [40,41] using a slightly modified technique which enables operation in aqueous media [56,64]. The parameters describing bioadhesion (maximum detachment force and work of adhesion) are significantly lower for the sublingual mucosa than for the vaginal one. This phenomenon remains the same when the aqueous medium contains divalent calcium ions.

Controlled-Release Behaviour and Clinical Aspects

Controlled-release behaviour is the other main property of bioadhesive tablets. Its evaluation is realized either *in vitro* (by the mean of classical dissolution experiments) or *in vivo*. These studies are often completed by clinical evaluation. Basically, it must be pointed out that parameters affecting controlled release of bioadhesive tablets are just the same as those affecting conventional hydrophilic matricial dosage forms: drug diffusion inside hydrogels, polymer/drug ratio, polymer swelling, chain relaxation, etc.

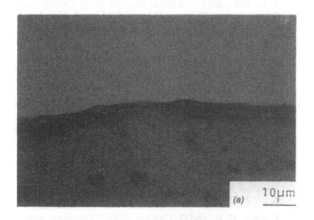

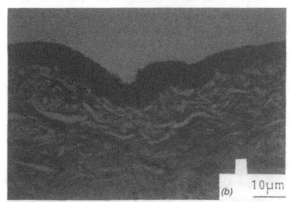

Figure 8. Microphotographs of bovine sublingual (a) and vaginal (b) mucosa.

Only three controlled-release systems have been used in bioadhesive tablets: a fatty-based system, and two polymeric systems: hydroxypropyl-cellulose/poly(acrylic acid) and hydroxypropyl-methylcellulose/poly(acrylic acid).

Fatty-Based System

In the case of the bioadhesive tablet containing insulin developed by Nagai's team [35], the controlled-release system is composed of a core of cocoa butter or glyceride (Witepsol® H15) added to sodium glycocholate and containing insulin. Unfortunately, blood sugar levels and plasma insulin levels in beagle dogs after administration remain very low, so that the bioavailability of insulin, compared with intramuscular administration, was 0.5%. However, in this case, it is quite clear that these low levels of absorbed insulin are not due to insufficient drug delivery, but rather are related to the properties of the drug itself.

Hyroxypropyl-Cellulose/Poly(acrylic acid) Systems

Evaluation of the controlled-release behaviour of hydroxypropyl-cellulose/poly(acrylic acid)-based systems follows the same scheme. In the case of the triamcinolone acetonide tablet designed by Nagai et al. [34,36] for aphthous stomatitis, this drug delivery system is more efficient than simple gels, since more of the drug remains for a longer period on the surface and in the tissue of the tongue of rats [17].

An interesting study of formulation parameters related to controlled-release properties has been carried out by Nagai's team for bioadhesive lidocaine tablets developed for local anaesthetic purposes [36,37]. Dissolution is slowed down when the drug/polymer ratio in the system decreases. *In vivo* investigations of the amount absorbed from human gums shows that 30% of the drug is absorbed after one hour of contact time, and that absorption lasts about 6 hours following the application of the bioadhesive tablet, in the case of the most efficient formulation. The anaesthetic effect expected lasts about 4 hours with this system.

Much longer release periods are obtained with these polymeric systems with carboquone [38] for vaginal application, since only 50% of the drug is released after 24 hours. With 5-fluorouracyl and bleomycin, 50 and 25% respectively of the drug is released after 2 hours. Moreover, it must be pointed out that release behaviour is unaffected by the geometry of the dosage form. Clinical application of these preparations to voluntary patients affected by *Carcinoma colli* leads to interesting results, such as the disappearance of side effects [17].

Other examples of controlled-release behaviour of bioadhesive tablets containing various drugs, such as indomethacin, tetracycline hydrochloride, isoproterenol hydrochloride, benzocaine, and dequalinium are given in a patent by Nagai [67].

Hydroxypropyl-Methylcellulose/Poly(acrylic acid) Systems

Our team has recently developed bioadhesive tablets containing metronidazole [40]. An analysis of metronidazole release as a function of time for a series of tablets with a wide range of compositions and poly(acrylic acid) contents leads to the conclusion that the drug release is highly non-Fickian. In this case, it seems plausible that the high drug loadings do not interfere with the chain relaxation process, so that drug diffusion into the hydrogel is not the only phenomenon. This result leads to the conclusion that the swelling behaviour of the system significantly affects the release pattern of metronidazole.

CONCLUSION

To our knowledge, the number of bioadhesive tablets on the world pharmaceutical market is lower than half a dozen. This must not be considered as a low quantity, the consequence of a poor value presented by this dosage form, but, on the contrary, as a proof of its advantages, involving very rapid commercial development of this pharmacotechnical innovation. In fact, the idea of using bioadhesion with the object of immobilizing a dosage form at its best level of resorption or activity is somewhat new, and the actual existence of pharmaceutical specialties, intended for local activity, such as Aftach® or Pattel®, or systemic activity, such as Susadrin® or Buccastem®, demonstrates, if anything, the interest of this kind of dosage form. Furthermore, bioadhesive tablets do not need special technology for their manufacture in the pharmaceutical industry.

We can be sure that, in a few years, there will be many bioadhesive forms on the market, not only with the purpose of improving the administration and efficiency of drugs by classical routes (oral, vaginal, rectal, ocular), but also to promote the administration of drugs by routes such as the nasal route, easier and more comfortable than the parenteral route.

REFERENCES

1. Park, K., S. L. Cooper and J. R. Robinson. 1987. "Bioadhesive Hydrogels", in *Hydrogels in Medicine and Pharmacy, Vol. III, Properties and Applications.* N. A. Peppas, ed. Boca Raton, FL: CRC Press.

2. Marvola, M., K. Vahervuo, A. Sothmann, E. Marttila and M. Rajaniemi. 1982. "Development of a Method for Study of the Tendency of Drug Products to Adhere to the Œsophagus", *J. Pharm. Sci.*, 71:975–977.

3. Al-Dujaili, H., A. T. Florence and E. G. Salole. 1986. "The Adhesiveness of Proprietary Tablets and Capsules to Porcine Œsophageal Tissue", *Int. J. Pharm.*, 34:75–79.

4. Marvola, M., M. Rajaniemi, E. Marttila, K. Vahervuo and A. Sothmann. 1983. "Effect of Dosage Form and Formulation Factors on the Adherence of Drugs to the Œsophagus", *J. Pharm Sci.*, 72:1034–1036.

5. Kannikoski, A., S. Mannermaa and M. Marvola. 1984. "The Effects of Some Tablet Film Coatings on the Adherence of Drug Products to the Isolated Porcine Œsophagus", *Acta Pharm. Fenn.*, 93:75–83.

6. Swisher, D. A., S. L. Sendelbeck and J. W. Fara. 1984. "Adherence of Various Oral Dosage Forms to the Œsophagus", *Int. J. Pharm.*, 22:219–228.

7. Fell, J. T., D. Harris, H. L. Sharma and D. C. Taylor. 1987. "The Use of Muco-Adhesive Polymers to Modify the Gastro-Intestinal Transit of Oral Pharmaceutical Formulations", *Polym. Prep.*, 28:145–146.

8. Harris, D., H. Sharma, A.-M. Smith, J. Fell and D. Taylor. 1987. "The Assessment of Muco-Adhesive Agents for Delaying Gastro-Intestinal Transit in Human Volunteers Using Gamma Scintigraphy", *Proc. Int. Symp. Control. Rel. Bioact. Mater.*, 14:12–13.

9. Davis, S. S. 1986. "Evaluation of the Gastro-Intestinal Transit of Pharmaceutical Dosage Forms Using the Technique of Gamma Scintigraphy", *STP Pharma.*, 2:1015–1022.

10. Daneshmend, T. K. 1986. "Systemic Absorption of Miconazole From the Vagina", *J. Antimicrobial Chemotherapy*, 18:507–511.

11. Hsu, C. C., J. Y. Park, N. F. H. Ho, W. I. Higuchi and J. L. Fox. 1983. "Topical Vaginal Drug Delivery, I. Effect of the Estrous Cycle on Vaginal Membrane Permeability and Diffusivity of Vidarabine in Mice", *J. Pharm. Sci.*, 72:674–680.

12. Hirai, S., T. Yashiki, T. Matsuzawa and H. Mima. 1981. "Absorption of Drugs from the Nasal Mucosa of Rat", *Int. J. Pharm.*, 7:317–325.

13. Fisher A. N., K. Brown, S. S. Davis, G. D. Parr and D. A. Smith. 1987. "The Effect of Molecular Size on the Nasal Absorption of Water-Soluble Compounds in the Albino Rat", *J. Pharm. Pharmacol.*, 39:357–362.

14. Su, K. S. E., K. M. Campanale and C. L. Gries. 1984. "Nasal Drug Delivery System of a Quaternary Ammonium Compound, Clofilium Tosylate", *J. Pharm. Sci.*, 73:1251–1254.

15. Cooper, E. R. and G. Casting. 1987. "Transport Across Epithelial Membranes", *J. Contr. Rel.*, 6:23–35.

16. Veillard, M. M., M. A. Longer, T. W. Martens and J. R. Robinson. 1987. "Preliminary Studies of Oral Mucosal Delivery of Peptide Drugs", *J. Contr. Rel.* 6:123–131.

17. Nagai, T. 1986. "Topical Mucosal Adhesive Dosage Forms", *Med. Res. Rev.*, 6:227–242.

18. Fjellestad-Paulsen, A., N. Tubiana-Rufi, A. Harris and P. Czernichow. 1987. "Central Diabetes Insipidus in Children, Anti-Diuretic Effect and Pharmacokinetics of Intranasal and Peroral 1-deamino-8-D-arginine Vasopressin", *Acta Endocrinological (Copenh)*, 115:307–312.

19. Morimoto, K., H. Akatsuchi, R. Aikawa, M. Morishita and K. Morisaka. 1984. "Enhanced Rectal Absorption of [Asu^{1,7}]-eel Calcitonin in Rats Using

Polyacrylic Acid Aqueous Gel Base", *J. Pharm. Sci.*, 73:1366–1368.

20. Harris, A. S., M. Ohlin, S. Lethagen and I. M. Nilsson. 1988. "Effects of Concentration and Volume on Nasal Bioavailability and Biological Response to Desmopressin", *J. Pharm. Sci.*, 77:337–339.

21. McMartin, C., L. E. F. Hutchinson, R. Hyde and G. F. Peters. 1987. "Analysis of Structural Requirements for the Absorption of Drugs and Macromolecules from the Nasal Cavity", *J. Pharm. Sci.*, 76:535–540.

22. Robert, C. et P. Buri. 1986. "Les mucus et son role dans l'absorption des médicaments", *Pharm. Acta Helv.*, 61:210–214.

23. Peppas, N. A., P. J. Hansen and P. A. Buri. 1984. "A Theory of Molecular Diffusion in the Intestinal Mucus", *Int. J. Pharm.*, 20:107–118.

24. Gibson, R. E. and L. S. Olanoff. 1987. "Physicochemical Determinant of Nasal Drug Absorption", *J. Contr. Rel.*, 6:361–366.

25. Y. W. Chien, ed. 1985. *Transnasal Systemic Medications*. Amsterdam: Elsevier.

26. Fix, J. A. 1987. "Absorption Enhancing Agents for the GI System", *J. Contr. Rel.*, 6:151–156.

27. Hersey, S. J. and R. T. Jackson. 1987. "Effect of Bile Salts on Nasal Permeability *in vitro*", *J. Pharm. Sci.*, 76:876–879.

28. Hirai, S., T. Yashiki and H. Mima. 1981. "Mechanisms for the Enhancement of the Nasal Absorption of Insulin by Surfactants", *Int. J. Pharm.*, 9:173–184.

29. Braybrooks, M. P., B. W. Barry and E. T. Abbs. 1975. "The Effect of Mucin on the Bioavailability of Tetracycline from the Gastro-Intestinal Tract, *In vivo, in vitro* Correlations", *J. Pharm. Pharmacol.*, 27:508–515.

30. Brown, D. T. and C. Marriott. 1979. "The Interactions of Some Tetracyclines with Purified Mucus Glycoproteins", *J. Pharm. Pharmacol.*, 31:87P.

31. Kearney, P. and C. Marriott. 1982. "The Effect of an Endogenous Mucus Layer on Tetracycline Absorption", *J. Pharm. Pharmacol.*, 34:71P.

32. Kellaway, I. W. and C. Marriott. 1975. "The Influence of Mucin on the Bioavailability of Tetracycline", *J. Pharm. Pharmacol.*, 27:281–283.

33. Aramaki, Y., J. Niibuchi, S. Tsuchiya and J. Hosoda. 1987. "Interaction of 3′,4′-Dideoxykanamycin B and Submaxillary Mucin", *Chem. Pharm. Bull.*, 35:320–325.

34. Nagai, T. and Y. Machida. 1985. "Advances in Drug Delivery, Mucosal Adhesive Dosage Forms", *Pharm. Int.*, 6:196–200.

35. Ishida, M., Y. Machida, N. Nambu and T. Nagai. 1981. "New Mucosal Dosage Form of Insulin", *Chem. Pharm. Bull.*, 29:810–816.

36. Nagai, T. and R. Konishi. 1987. "Buccal/Gingival Drug Delivery Systems", *J. Contr. Rel.*, 6:353–360.

37. Ishida, M., N. Nambu and T. Nagai. 1982. "Mucosal Dosage Form of Lidocaine for Toothache Using Hydroxypropyl-Cellulose and Carbopol", *Chem. Pharm. Bull.*, 30:980–984.

38. Machida, Y., H. Masuda, N. Fujiyama, M. Iwata and T. Nagai. 1980. "Preparation and Phase II Clinical Examination of Topical Dosage Forms for the Treatment of *Carcinoma colli* Containing Bleomycine, Carbo-

quone or 5-fluorouracyl with Hydroxypropyl-Cellulose", *Chem. Pharm. Bull.*, 28:1125–1130.

39. Machida, Y., H. Masuda, N. Fujiyama, S. Ito, M. Iwata and T. Nagai. 1979. "Preparation and Phase II Clinical Examination of Topical Dosage Forms for the Treatment of Carcinoma Colli Containing Bleomycin with Hydroxypropyl-Cellulose", *Chem. Pharm. Bull.*, 27:93–100.

40. Ponchel, G., F. Touchard, D. Wouessidjewe, D. Duchêne and N. A. Peppas. 1987. "Bioadhesive Analysis of Controlled-Release Systems, III. Bioadhesive and Release Behaviour of Metronidazole Containing Poly(acrylic acid)/hydroxypropyl-Methylcellulose System", *Int. J. Pharm.*, 38:65–70.

41. Ponchel, G., F. Touchard, D. Duchêne and N. A. Peppas. 1987. "Bioadhesive Analysis of Controlled-Release Systems, I. Fracture and Interpenetration Analysis in Poly(acrylic acid)-Containing Systems", *J. Contr. Rel.*, 5:129–141.

42. Schor, J. M., S. S. Davis, A. Nigalaye and S. Bolton. 1983. "Susadrin Transmucosal Tablets", *Drug Dev. Ind. Pharm.*, 9:1359–1377.

43. Robert, C., P. Buri and N. A. Peppas. 1988. "Experimental Method for Bioadhesive Testing of Various Polymers", *Acta Pharm. Technol.*, 34:95–98.

44. Longer, M. A. and J. R. Robinson. 1986. "Fundamental Aspects of Bioadhesion", *Pharm. Int.*, 7:114–117.

45. Mackenzie, I. C. and W. H. Binnie. 1983. "Recent Advances in Oral Mucosal Research", *J. Oral Pathol.*, 12:389–416.

46. Leung, S. H. S. and J. R. Robinson. 1988. "The Contribution of Anionic Polymer Structural Features to Muco-Adhesion", *J. Contr. Rel.*, 5:223–231.

47. Smart, J. D., I. W. Kellaway and H. E. C. Worthington. 1984. "An *in vitro* Investigation of Mucosa-Adhesive Materials for Use in Controlled Drug Delivery", *J. Pharm. Pharmacol.*, 36:295–299.

48. Gurny, R., J. M. Meyer and N. A. Peppas. 1984. "Bioadhesive Intra-Oral Release Systems, Design, Testing and Analysis", *Biomat.*, 5:336–340.

49. Ishida, M., N. Nambu and T. Nagai. 1983. "Ointment-Type Oral Mucosal Dosage Form of Carbopol Containing Prednisolone for Treatment of Aphtha", *Chem. Pharm. Bull.*, 31:1010–1014.

50. Ranga Rao, K. V. and P. Buri. 1987. "Design and *in vitro* Testing of Coated Microparticles for Bioadhesion", *Proc. 47th Int. Congress of Pharm Sci.*, p. 235.

51. Park, H. and J. R. Robinson. 1985. "Physicochemical Properties of Water-Insoluble Polymers Important to Mucin/Epithelial Adhesion", *J. Contr. Rel.*, 2:47–57.

52. Peppas, N. A., G. Ponchel and D. Duchêne. 1987. "Bioadhesive Analysis of Controlled-Release Systems, II. Time-Dependent Bioadhesive Stress in Poly(acrylic acid)-Containing Systems", *J. Contr. Rel.*, 5:143–149.

53. Peppas, N. A. and A. G. Mikos. 1986. "Experimental Methods for Determination of Bioadhesive Bond Strength of Polymers with Mucus", in *Interrelationships Between Gasto-Intestinal Physiology and Dosage Form Design.* J. R. Cardinal and E. G. Rippie, eds. Washington, DC: Academy of Pharmaceutical Sciences.

54. Park, K. and J. R. Robinson. 1984. "Bioadhesive

Polymers as Platforms for Oral Controlled Drug Delivery, Method to Study Bioadhesion", *Int. J. Pharm.*, 19:107–127.

55. Ch'ng, H. S., H. Park, P. Kelly and J. R. Robinson. 1985. "Bioadhesive Polymers as Platforms for Oral Controlled Drug Delivery, II. Synthesis and Evaluation of Some Swelling, Water-Insoluble Bioadhesive Polymers", *J. Pharm. Sci.*, 74:399–405.

56. Lejoyeux, F., G. Ponchel, D. Wouessidjewe, N. A. Peppas and D. Duchêne. 1988. "Assessment of a New Method for the Determination of Bioadhesion", *Proc. Int. Symp. Contr. Rel. Bioact. Mater.*, 15:348–349.

57. Lejoyeux, F., G. Ponchel, D. Wouessidjewe, N. A. Peppas and D. Duchêne. 1989. "Bioadhesive Tablets, Influence of the Testing Medium Composition on Bioadhesion", *Drug Dev. Ind. Pharm.*, 15:2037–2048.

58. Park, H. and J. R. Robinson. 1987. "Mechanisms of Muco-Adhesion of Poly(acrylic acid) Hydrogels", *Pharm. Res.*, 4:457–464.

59. Caramella, C., P. Colombo, A. Gazzaniga, G. Dondi and G. C. Santus. 1984. "Descrizione di Sistemi Terapeutici per Assorbimento Transmucosale", *Boll. Chim. Farm.*, 123:359–380.

60. Marvola, M. 1982. "Adherence of Drug Products to the Œsophagus", *Pharm. Int.*, 3:294–296.

61. Forget, P., P. Gazzeri, F. Moreau, M. Sabatier, C. Durandeau, J. P. Merlet et P. Aumonier. 1988. "Comprimés mucoadhésifs, Mesure de l'adhésivité *in vitro*", *STP Pharma.*, 4:176–181.

62. Duchêne, D., F. Touchard and N. A. Peppas. 1988. "Pharmaceutical and Medical Aspects of Bioadhesive Systems for Drug Administration", *Drug Dev. Ind. Pharm.*, 14:283–318.

63. Peppas, N. A. and P. A. Buri. 1985. "Surface, Interfacial and Molecular Aspects of Polymer Bioadhesion on Soft Tissues", *J. Contr. Rel.*, 2:257–275.

64. Lejoyeux, F., G. Ponchel, D. Wouessidjewe, N. A. Peppas and D. Duchêne. 1988. "Influence of the Composition of the Test Medium on the Adhesion of a Bioadhesive Tablet to a Biological Tissue", *Proc. Int. Symp. Contr. Rel. Bioact. Mater.*, 15:460–461.

65. Allen, A. and A. Leonard. 1985. "Mucus Structure", *Gastroenterol. Clin. Biol.*, 9:9–12.

66. Carstedt, I. and J. K. Sheehan. 1984. "Is the Macromolecular Architecture of Cervical, Respiratory and Gastric Mucins the Same?" *Biochem. Soc. Trans.*, 12:615–617.

67. Nagai, T., Y. Machida, Y. Suzuki, H. Ikura and Teijin Limited. 1979. UK Patent, GB 2 042 888 A, 27 February.

17

Synthetic Bioabsorbable Polymers

THOMAS H. BARROWS, Ph.D.*

ABSTRACT: Many types of surgically implantable devices that only function for a relatively short time *in vivo* can be made from polymers that are eliminated from the body by hydrolytic degradation and subsequent metabolism after serving their intended purpose. Although the first application for such bioabsorbable polymers was surgical suture, additional uses have been developed including clips, staples, pins, and mesh. Other applications of a more demanding nature such as fracture fixation implants and drug delivery devices are the subject of ongoing research. Copolymers and homopolymers of glycolide and lactide form an important class of bioabsorbable polymers as a result of their proven toxicological safety and commercial availability. Rates of strength loss and bioabsorption can be controlled by selecting an appropriate copolymer and processing the material under conditions that optimize the desired polymer morphology. Proprietary bioabsorbable polymer systems such as the "bioerodible" poly(ortho esters) appear well suited for zero-order drug delivery applications while stereocomplex blends of poly-L-lactide with poly-D-lactide offer superior mechanical properties needed for the fabrication of high-strength implants for orthopedic surgery.

INTRODUCTION

The use of polymers in surgically implantable devices has been successful due to the availability of a wide variety of commercial materials that could be adapted for medical applications. Dacron™, Lycra™, Teflon™, and Silastic™ are examples of familiar tradename polymers that are now clinically accepted biomaterials. As the need for more specifically defined polymer properties and *in vivo* performance characteristics increases, however, the possibility of utilizing known materials will diminish. Thus, polymers will need to be designed and synthesized to meet the requirements of future-generation devices. Implants which must "bioabsorb" clearly require special synthetic materials since most commercial polymers are required to be stable and those which are degradable, such as cellulose, are not usually degradable by enzymes present in human tissues.

Bioabsorbability can be defined as the ability of a tissue-compatible material to degrade at some time after implantation into nontoxic products which are eliminated from the body or metabolized therein. Although this term is preferred, it is often used interchangeably with the terms absorbable, resorbable, bioresorbable, and biodegradable. The term biodegradable refers to materials which experience accelerated degradation by the action of life forms present in the environment, for example bacteria and fungi. Bioabsorbable polymers also are biodegradable, but the converse may not be true. The terms resorbable and bioresorbable are derived from the word "resorption" which refers to loss of substance through physiological or pathological means. Absorbable and nonabsorbable are terms used by surgeons to differentiate between sutures that are bioabsorbable, such as catgut, and those that are not, such as silk.

The importance of bioabsorbability was noted by early surgeons such as Joseph Lister (1827–1912) who found that nonabsorbable suture material often served as a nidus for infection [1]. It is now known that the number of bacteria needed to establish infection can be reduced 10,000-fold by the presence of a silk suture. Even with the availability of modern antibiotics, infection associated with a surgical implant usually requires removal of the implant since the interface between tissue and foreign material creates a protected site for survival of bacteria [2]. Although bioabsorbable materials are still "foreign bodies" prior to absorption, the finite exposure time and typically mild inflammatory response to these synthetic

*Life Sciences Research Laboratory/3M, St. Paul, MN 55144

polymers is clearly advantageous. For example, a mesh made from bioabsorbable polyglycolic acid was found to be clinically superior to nonabsorbable polypropylene mesh in the repair of contaminated abdominal wall defects by significantly reducing the complication of chronic infection [3]. A possible explanation of this benefit results from *in vitro* studies which suggested that degradation products of polyglycolic acid possess antibacterial activity which could contribute to cleaning an infected wound [4].

A further advantage of bioabsorbable polymers over nondegradable materials relates to control over the rate at which mechanical properties deteriorate *in vivo*. Thus fracture fixation plates which gradually lose stiffness are postulated to provide a superior result compared to steel plates which ultimately weaken bone due to constant stress shielding [5]. The same concept of gradually transferring loads from the synthetic implant to natural tissue for the purpose of optimizing tissue regeneration and remodeling also applies to connective tissue [6] and vascular grafts [7–9]. In the case of pediatric surgery, bioabsorbable implants such as aortic patches that accommodate future growth and development are clearly beneficial [10].

Drug-releasing implants and injectable microspheres are prepared from bioabsorbable polymers both as a method of controlling the drug release rate and as a means of avoiding the accumulation of residual polymer with repeated dosing [11]. This approach is especially useful in the case of polypeptide drugs which cannot be effectively administered in traditional formulations [12]. Additional reasons for choosing bioabsorbable polymers over other materials range from the prevention of urinary tract stone formation to the benefit of radiotransparency during subsequent computerized tomographic scanning of the patient [13]. In general the trend in implantable devices appears to favor the use of bioabsorbable polymers for products which only serve a temporary function [14].

The following review will concentrate on polymers and copolymers of lactide and glycolide with brief mention of a few other polymers that appear promising based on preliminary experimental results. The reason for this emphasis is that lactide/glycolide polymers are now commercially available in grades that can be used directly in the manufacture of implantable devices (Appendix A). In addition, prospects for a relatively inexpensive FDA approval pro-

cess for new devices made from these polymers due to their proven safety makes them the materials of first choice for new product development programs. Thus, it is predictable that bioabsorbable devices will become more common in the near future, just as silicone rubber devices proliferated after that polymer was accepted as an implant material [15].

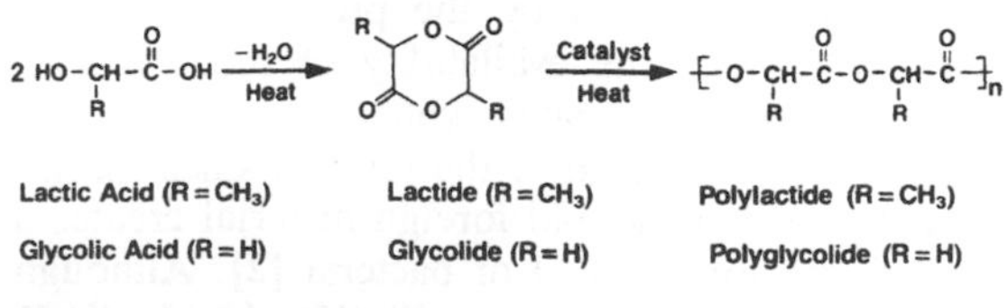

POLYLACTIDE

Synthesis

The synthesis of polylactic acid (PLA) and polyglycolic acid (PGA) was studied by Carothers in 1932 [16]. They are "new" materials only in the sense that previously observed hydrolytic susceptibility, originally regarded as an impediment to commercial utility, is now recognized as a desirable property for bioabsorbable polymers. Since lactic acid is a normal intermediate of carbohydrate metabolism in man, the use of this hydroxyacid as a monomer for polymer synthesis and its presence as a product of polymer hydrolysis are generally viewed as an ideal situation from the standpoint of toxicological safety [17,18]. The oligomers and polymers of lactic acid are not known to possess any pharmacologic action, presumably due to their insolubility. Oligomers with less than ten monomer units, however, have been claimed to possess plant growth stimulation activity [19].

Although lactic acid can be polymerized directly into polylactic acid, much higher molecular weight is achieved by first converting lactic acid into the cyclic diester known as lactide. Since lactide is the usual monomer used to synthesize PLA, the polymer is commonly known as polylactide. The ring-opening reaction, shown in Figure 1, is typically catalyzed with the use of stannous octoate [20,21].

Optical Isomerism

The optical isomerism of lactic acid has an important influence on monomer metabolism and polymer properties. This type of isomerism results from the fact that one of the carbon atoms (known as the asymmetric center) has four non-identical groups attached to it and thus is non-superimposible on its mirror image (the optical isomer). In order to make a correct structural assignment of each isomer it is helpful to visualize the tetrahedral asymmetric center with the smallest group (hydrogen) directly behind it. The remaining three groups are then given a priority based first on the atomic number of the atom bonded to the asymmetric carbon and secondly on the atomic number of the other atoms in the group. Thus the priority of the groups in lactic acid is $OH > CO_2H > CH_3$. These groups are viewed as spokes in a wheel which always turns in a direction such that the highest priority group changes places with the next highest priority group. Thus, as shown in Figure 2, if the

Lactic Acid ($R = CH_3$)   Lactide ($R = CH_3$)   Polylactide ($R = CH_3$)

Glycolic Acid ($R = H$)   Glycolide ($R = H$)   Polyglycolide ($R = H$)

Figure 1. Conversion of lactic (glycolic) acid into high molec. wt. polylactide (polyglycolide) requires preparation of high-purity lactide (glycolide) as an intermediate.

wheel turns to the right the configuration is R (from *rectus*, meaning right in Latin) and if it turns to the left the configuration is S (from *sinister*, meaning left in Latin). These configurations are also commonly known as D and L respectively.

The D and L lactic acids are physically and chemically identical in all regards except that each rotates a beam of polarized light to exactly the same degree as the other but in the opposite direction. The direction of rotation is designated by (+) or *d* for dextrorotation (to the right) and (−) or *l* for levorotation (to the left). Although the D and L configurations were originally based arbitrarily on optical rotation, configuration of the isomer should not be confused with its rotation since optical rotation values are determined experimentally and may be different or even reversed in different solvent systems.

Almost all the amino acids that occur naturally in proteins have the L configuration. Likewise, only L-lactic acid is produced in muscle tissue during vigorous exercise (anaerobic glycolysis). Excess lactic acid which accumulates in the blood is later recycled by conversion to glycogen in the liver. This metabolic pathway begins with the transformation of lactate to pyruvate by the enzyme lactate dehydrogenase which only accepts L-lactic acid [22]. Any D-lactic acid present in the bloodstream as a result of the hydrolysis of a poly-D-lactide implant would be excluded from this pathway and presumably excreted unchanged.

Pure L and D-lactic acid can be obtained by fermentation or culture techniques, whereas synthetic lactic acid is a racemic mixture, referred to as *dl*-lactic acid, which is an equal mixture of D- and L-lactic acid molecules. Since the optical rotations are equal and opposite, *dl*-lactic acid is optically inactive. As mentioned above, lactide is the cyclic dimer of lactic acid. It can now be seen that there are three different possible optical isomers of lactide: L-lactide, D-lactide, and *meso*-lactide (in which each lactide is made from one D and one L acid). The *dl*-lactide formed from *dl*-lactic acid is a mixture of all three isomers and has a melting point of 126°C whereas pure L-lactide (and therefore also D-lactide) has a melting point of 96°C [23].

Properties and Performance

Polylactide is typically available as either poly-L-lactide or poly-*dl*-lactide, although poly-D-lactide has recently become available from CCA Biochem (Appendix A). The differences between these two polymers result primarily from difference in crystallinity. Poly-L-lactide is a semicrystalline polymer whereas poly-*dl*-lactide is totally amorphous. Figure 3 shows a typical differential scanning calorimetry (DSC) trace for a sample of poly-L-lactide which was melted, then rapidly cooled into the glassy state. As the sample was slowly reheated, three different thermal transitions were observed: the glass transition (T_g), represented by an inflection in the baseline, the crystallization ex-

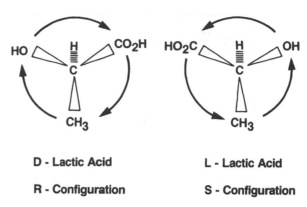

Figure 2. Optical (non-superimposible mirror image) isomers of lactic acid.

otherm (T_c) resulting from formation of crystalline structure, and the crystalline melting endotherm (T_m) resulting from the absorption of heat to melt the crystalline structure. The DSC trace for poly-*dl*-lactide had a similar T_g, but no T_c or T_m since no crystalline structure formation occurred and thus no crystalline melting was possible. Poly-*dl*-lactide is commonly used in drug delivery applications where it is desirable to have simultaneous loss of mass and strength. The absence of crystallites in poly-*dl*-lactide makes possible a monophasic matrix in which drugs can be well dispersed. It also results in improved solubility in common solvents, thus increasing the versatility of poly-*dl*-lactide in solvent-based processes for production of microspheres [24] and microcapsules [25].

Polymer crystallinity has enormous influence over physical properties and performance characteristics [26]. In the case of bioabsorbable polymers the degree of crystallinity also affects the bioabsorption process. Vert and Chabot polymerized mixtures of L-lactide and *dl*-lactide with increasing *dl*-lactide content and evaluated them as molded test bars [27]. The rates of tensile strength loss of the bars *in vivo* increased with increasing *dl*-lactide content in the polymer. After two months the strength of the poly-L-lactide sample was still 100% whereas the poly-*dl*-lactide had no strength, and the other polymers' final strengths depended on their degree of stereoregularity. Presumably moisture penetrated the amorphous

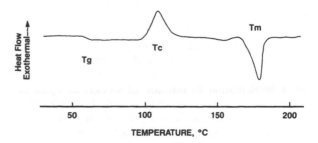

Figure 3. DSC thermogram obtained by the author on a sample of poly-L-lactide provided by Boehringer Ingelheim Co.

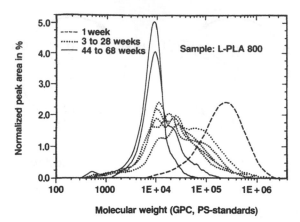

Figure 4. Molecular weight distributions of semicrystalline poly-L-lactide (500,000 molecular weight) at various times postimplantation. The multimodal distributions observed between 3 and 28 weeks and the single 10,000 molecular weight peak observed after 44 weeks were attributed to the accumulation of crystalline fragments having relatively greater hydrolytic stability than the amorphous phase. (Figure courtesy of Drs. Dieter Bendix and Günther Entenmann, Boehringer Ingelheim Co.)

phase with greater ease than the crystalline phase, and this led to rapid strength loss in samples with lower crystallinity. Alternatively, poly-*dl*-lactide may be more susceptible to hydrolysis than the amorphous regions of poly-L-lactide due to subtle differences in morphology as discussed below.

A detailed analysis of the changes in molecular weight distribution and crystallinity of high molecular weight poly-L-lactide during *in vitro* and *in vivo* degradation has been conducted by Bendix and Entenmann [28]. They found that both 500,000 and 800,000 molecular weight samples of poly-L-lactide with relatively narrow, symmetrical molecular weight distributions yielded broad, multimodal distributions of similar average molecular weight each, after only a few weeks *in vivo*. After 44 weeks the distribution resolved in both cases into a narrow, monomodal distribution at about 10,000 molecular weight, as shown for the 500,000 molecular weight sample in Figure 4. This was interpreted as the accumulation of highly crystalline fragments due to preferential degradation of amorphous regions. As shown in Figure 5, crystallinity decreased during the initial five weeks of implantation but was significantly higher at later time points. Percent crystallinity was determined from the DSC value for heat of fusion by assuming a value of 93 J/g for 100% crystalline polymer. To compare the degradation of crystalline and amorphous polymers *in vivo*, samples of totally amorphous poly-L-lactide were prepared by rapidly cooling molten polymer. The amorphous poly-L-lactide remained amorphous after implantation in rats for 12 weeks. Samples of both crystalline and amorphous poly-L-lactide with different initial molecular weights were reduced to the same average molecular weight after three weeks *in vivo* and degraded nearly simultaneously thereafter. Only the crystalline sample, however, gave a multi-

modal distribution. The similarity of degradation rates was an important finding because it demonstrated that amorphous poly-L-lactide does not necessarily degrade faster than semicrystalline poly-L-lactide, as would be predicted from the more rapid degradation of amorphous poly-*dl*-lactide. Identical results were obtained *in vitro* indicating that no special body fluid or enzymatic reaction was responsible for the observed degradation behavior.

Molded parts with high strength and stiffness are desired for internal fracture fixation device applications. Injection molding of semicrystalline polymers such as poly-L-lactide requires a rapid rate of crystallization to obtain a reasonable cycle time and small crystallite size. Since slow formation of large spherulitic crystallites often leads to a brittle material or one that becomes brittle with time, injection mold cavities are usually heated to the T_c where small crystallites can form to act as a reinforcement of the polymer matrix. Other than temperature control, however, injection molding provides very limited opportunity to control the development of preferred crystalline morphology. A review of the literature by Daniels has illustrated a wide range of reported properties for molded poly-L-lactide due to differences in the quality of the polymer used and the methods of fabrication [29]. Values for tensile strength ranged from 11.4 to 72 MPa.

Tunc has reported superior strength properties for injection-molded poly-L-lactide by stressing the molded parts to achieve orientation prior to crystallization [30]. This process, termed "orientrusion", produced samples with tensile strength of 300 MPa vs. 62 MPa before orientrusion. *In vitro* strength retention of this material was high after 12 weeks of incubation; whereas traditional "as polymerized" poly-L-lactide bone plate implants have been found to be very weak at this time postimplantation [31]. *In vivo* bioabsorption of 3.5 mm dia. orientruded intramedullary rods implanted in rabbits was about 65% complete after 2 years as measured by weight loss.

The exact time required for poly-L-lactide to bioabsorb has been found to depend on initial molecular weight, surface-to-volume ratio of the sample, and crystalline morphology. In addition, removal of low molecular weight material by extraction was found to reduce the rate of degradation [32]. Vert observed that fracture fixation plates of poly-L-lactide implanted in sheep started to exhibit histological features of degradation by three years only at their periphery [33]. No significant mass loss was noted after 4 years, although the plates had lost virtually all strength by that time. Molecular weight changes determined by gel permeation chromatography of these implants are shown in Table 1.

Fiber spinning allows a greater degree of control over polymer morphology since the filaments can be stretched during the crystallization process, which provides a dramatic improvement in tensile strength relative to unoriented filaments. Optimization of deformation rate and drawing temperature of poly-L-lactide has yielded fiber with tensile strength of 2.3 GPa [34]. Solution spinning gave fiber strength of 1.2 GPa [35]. In both cases the polymer chains were oriented by drawing which resulted in formation of crystal structure in alignment with the fiber axis. By contrast, poly-*dl*-lactide was found to be a poor fiber-forming material since molecular orientation obtained by drawing could not be preserved by subsequent crystallization due to its amorphous nature [23]. In any case, successful melt processing of polylactide requires that the polymer be substantially free of water, monomers, oligomers, and catalyst to minimize loss of molecular weight during extrusion [36].

The rate of strength loss *in vitro* and *in vivo* for poly-L-lactide fiber has been studied by Jamshidi, et al. [37]. Highly drawn and oriented fibers which were properly annealed retained 100% of their original strength (70 kg/mm²) five months after subcutaneous or intramuscular implantation in rabbits. At 10 months postimplantation the fibers still possessed 70% of their original strength. A high degree of strength retention was also observed for braided multifilaments of poly-L-lactide [38]. The rate of strength loss *in vivo* for these braided fibers in comparison to the commercial bioabsorbable sutures Vicryl™ and PDS™ (Appendix B) is shown in Figure 6.

A novel dry/wet spinning process for production of hollow, microporous fibers of poly-L-lactide has recently been described [39]. A mixture of poly-L-lactide (15%) and poly(vinylpyrrolidone) (5%) was spun from chloroform using a special die to produce the hollow fiber construction. The resultant filaments were then run through a coagulation bath which extracted the poly(vinylpyrrolidone) to form the porous structure. Drug-delivery implants were prepared from the hollow fibers by filling them with a suspension of the contraceptive hormone levonorgestrel in castor oil and sealing the ends with silicone rubber. Implantation of these devices in rats gave a virtually zero-order (2.4 micrograms per day) release of the drug for 180 days. Gamma-sterilization had an adverse effect on the hollow fiber properties and their release characteristics. Other investigators have demonstrated a linear relationship between irradiation dose and the reciprocal of the resultant molecular weight of poly-L-lactide [40]. The standard 2.5 Mrad sterilization dose caused a 50 to 60% drop in molecular weight al-

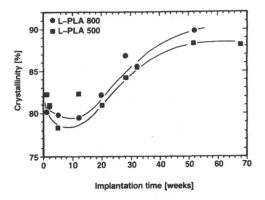

Figure 5. Crystallinity vs. time postimplantation for 800,000 molecular weight (L-PLA 800) and 500,000 molecular weight (L-PLA 500) samples of poly-L-lactide. (Figure courtesy of Drs. Dieter Bendix and Günther Entenmann, Boehringer Ingelheim Co.)

though this could be reduced to a 30% drop by conducting the irradiation in a high vacuum.

Composites and Blends

A promising approach to increasing strength and stiffness of polymers for use as fracture-fixation plates is the fabrication of fiber-reinforced composites [41]. There are several examples of the use of poly-L-lactide in this regard utilizing both bioabsorbable [42,43] and nonbioabsorbable [44] fiber reinforcements. Composite theory was used to design an optimum high-modulus carbon fiber laminae layup using polylactide as a thermoplastic binder and matrix [45]. This produced a partially bioabsorbable fracture-fixation plate with superior mechanical properties. It was predicted that the composite plate would gradually lose rigidity *in vivo* as the fracture healed due to bioabsorption of the polylactide. Unfortunately, water

Table 1. Molecular weight of poly-L-lactide bone plate residues postimplantation in sheep. *

Months *in vivo*	Molecular Weight
0–5	200,000
13	160,000
24	55,000
36	13,000
48	7,000

*Data tabulated from Reference [33].

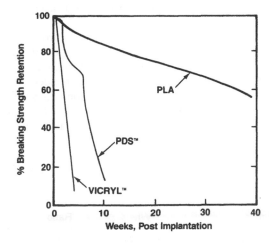

Figure 6. *In vivo* breaking strength retention of poly-L-lactide compared with commercial bioabsorbable sutures. (Reprinted with permission from Reference [38]. Copyright 1989, The American Chemical Society.)

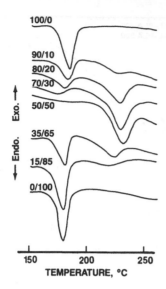

Figure 7. DSC thermograms of blend polymers from poly-L-lactide and poly-D-lactide. The ratios on the curves denote the blend ratios of poly-L-lactide to poly-D-lactide. (Reprinted with permission from Reference [47]. Copyright 1987, The American Chemical Society.)

absorption and subsequent delamination caused the plate to become flexible prematurely and it failed to provide adequate fracture fixation.

Polylactide has also been combined with minerals such as hydroxyapatite for use as a bone substitute [46]. As the polylactide in the polylactide-hydroxyapatite composite bioabsorbed, it was observed that new bone formed in direct contact with the remaining hydroxyapatite.

Mixtures of poly-L-lactide with a polyurethane have been used to fabricate compliant, microporous vascular grafts [9]. The concept behind this approach was to rely on the polyurethane elastomer component to provide compliance and the polylactide component to provide a temporary scaffold for attachment of host tissue, and ultimately to permit functional neoarterial wall regeneration.

A recent and intriguing approach to improving the physical properties of polylactide results from the discovery that poly-L-lactide forms a blend with poly-D-lactide. This discovery was made independently by Ikada et al. [47] and Murdock and Loomis [48]. The blending of poly-D-lactide with poly-L-lactide produced a stereocomplex having a crystalline phase

which melted about 45°C higher than the T_m of poly-L-lactide. As shown in Figure 7, the complex appeared upon addition of about 10% poly-D-lactide to poly-L-lactide. From the x-ray diffraction pattern of fibers of the 1:1 blend it was determined that the polymer chains involved in the stereocomplex formed a more compact helix than the individual poly-L- and poly-D-lactides. Consequently, the blend exhibited reduced solubility in organic solvents and substantially higher tensile strength, modulus, thermal stability, and hydrolytic stability [49]. High-strength fibers were prepared by mixing chloroform solutions of the individual polylactides, dry spinning the solutions, and drawing the resultant fibers in hot silicone oil at various temperatures and draw ratios [50]. Table 2 shows data on the highest-strength blend fiber in comparison to fibers obtained under similar conditions from the starting polylactides.

Additional experiments indicated the formation of stereocomplexes between copolymers of caprolactone containing L-lactate and D-lactate blocks [49]. In these examples, random copolymers of L-lactide blended with random copolymers of D-lactide also exhibited a 45°C higher melting crystalline phase. It was estimated that blocks of about 10 lactate units long were required to form a stereocomplex between copolymers made from lactides of opposite configuration.

POLYGLYCOLIDE

Synthesis

Glycolic acid (hydroxyacetic acid) like lactic acid is generally recognized as a safe substance in small doses due to its presence in edible plants such as sugar beets. Polyglycolic acid has been synthesized by heating glycolic acid, but this yielded low molecular weight polymer which was inadequate for achieving optimal properties. Thus conversion of glycolic acid to glycolide, purification of the glycolide, and ring-opening polymerization of the pure glycolide as shown in Figure 1 is the preferred synthetic approach [51].

Polyglycolide was first synthesized almost 100 years ago [52] and was known to be a potentially low-cost fiber-forming polymer since 1954 [53]. The "problem" of its hydrolytic instability was exploited in 1967

*Table 2. Fiber data on polylactides spun from chloroform solutions.**

Polymer	Molec. Wt.	Draw Ratio	Tensile Strength (kg/mm²)	Elastic Modulus (kg/mm²)	Tm (°C)	Heat of Fusion (cal./g)
Poly-L-lactide	400,000	8	68.4	725	184	36
Poly-D-lactide	360,000	8	65.9	703	182	35
1:1 Blend	—	25	220.5	2,889	245	54

*Data tabulated from Reference [50].

to yield the first commercially successful synthetic bioabsorbable suture [54]. As a result of the FDA approval process which treated synthetic bioabsorbable suture as a drug-like substance, the toxicological safety of polyglycolide is now well established [55].

Properties and Performance

Polyglycolide is a semicrystalline polymer (T_m 220°C) which is somewhat more difficult to process than poly-L-lactide due to its higher melting temperature and very limited solubility. It is freely soluble in hexafluoroisopropanol. Polyglycolide surgical suture produced by braiding melt-spun multifilaments has substantially replaced the use of catgut due to better tissue compatibility, reliable strength-retention characteristics, and predictable bioabsorption [56]. Pure polyglycolide multifilament suture retained about 20% of its initial strength after three weeks *in vivo* and was completely bioabsorbed by 4 months [57].

Chu has conducted numerous studies to elucidate details of the degradation process of polyglycolide fiber [58,59]. His proposed mechanism of degradation described hydrolysis occurring first in the amorphous phase, accounting for over half the loss in tensile strength and increasing the total crystallinity, followed by hydrolysis in the crystalline phase which resulted in a gradual decrease in the level of crystallinity. Furthermore, disorientation of crystals was postulated to make them more susceptible to hydrolytic attack than those well-oriented along the fiber axis. This conclusion is plausible for all semicrystalline bioabsorbable polymers since strength-retention and other properties have been found to vary widely under different conditions of thermal processing [29].

Poly(glycolide-co-trimethylene carbonate)

In spite of the success of braided polyglycolide suture, especially when coated with surfactant or low molecular weight bioabsorbable polymer compositions to improve handling, the high modulus of the polymer prevents its use as a monofilament suture. This problem was solved by copolymerization of glycolide with 30-40% trimethylene carbonate, a six-membered ring monomer shown in Figure 8. These two monomers were polymerized together such that the final product was a triblock copolymer with the central block in the molecule being about 85% poly(trimethylene carbonate) and the two terminal blocks being mostly polyglycolide [60]. This composition provided the best balance of fiber strength and flexibility as a monofilament and had superior *in vivo* strength-retention compared to pure polyglycolide suture. At 4 weeks postimplantation the copolymer (Maxon™) retained about 60% of original strength whereas polyglycolide (Dexon™) had virtually no strength left at that time. At 6 weeks Maxon™ retained about 30% of original strength and was completely bioabsorbed within 7 months [61]. Metabolism

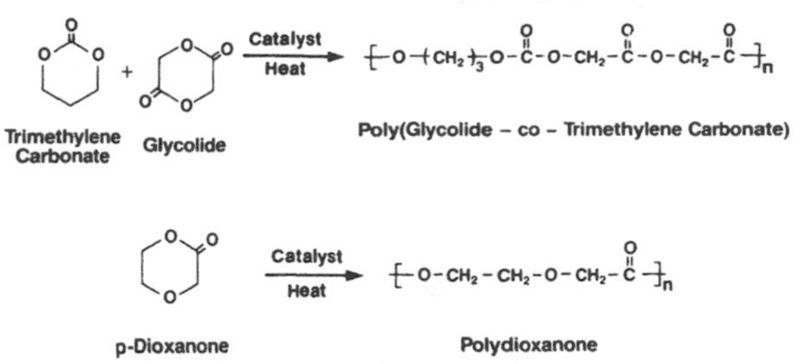

Figure 8. Monofilament bioabsorbable sutures are made from poly(glycolide-co-trimethylene carbonate) (Maxon™) and polydioxanone (PDS™).

experiments showed that most of the glycolate was excreted via urine whereas most of the carbonate was excreted via expired CO_2 and urine.

Molded Polyglycolide

Although polyglycolide is degraded by gamma irradiation and loses strength rapidly in the presence of moisture, these features have proven to be uniquely beneficial for fabrication of a "biofragmentable" device for intestinal surgery [62]. The purpose of this product was to provide a sutureless quick-connect device for constructing a secure inverting anastomosis of the large bowel with accurate serosa-to-serosa apposition. The device shown in Figure 9 was made of two identical segments molded from polyglycolide and 12.5% barium sulfate. Gamma irradiation facilitated both sterilization and accelerated disintegration at the appropriate time of 16 to 23 days. Thus the polymer "biofragmented" long before the bioabsorption process was complete and the resultant soft fragments were passed out in the stool. Clinical experience to date has shown the biofragmentable

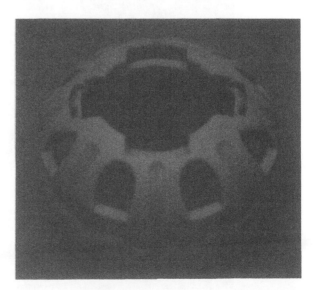

Figure 9. Biofragmentable bowel anastomosis ring molded from polyglycolide and barium sulfate. (Reprinted with permission from Reference [14]. Copyright 1986, Edward Arnold Publishers, Ltd.)

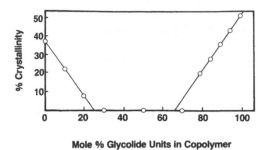

Figure 10. Percent crystallinities for L-lactide/glycolide copolymers as a function of composition determined by X-ray and DSC measurements. (Reprinted with permission from Reference [51]. Copyright 1979, Butterworth Scientific, Ltd.)

anastomosis ring (BAR) to be a safe alternative to sutures and staples for large bowel anastomosis [63].

Poly(glycolide-co-lactide)

Mixtures of lactide and glycolide were copolymerized together as an approach to controlling the rate of *in vivo* bioabsorption [64]. A more detailed study of the synthesis of these copolymers was reported by Gilding and Reed [51]. They found that the greater reactivity of glycolide in mixtures of lactide and glycolide led to glycolide being preferentially polymerized initially with incorporation of lactide into the polymer as glycolide was depleted from the mixture of monomers. Thus copolymers of glycolide and lactide tended to have broad composition ranges, not only within a given chain but also between chains

formed during the initial and final stages of the polymerization reaction.

Copolymerization of lactide and glycolide has provided a useful method of controlling the percent crystallinity of the resultant copolymer by simply varying the ratio of lactide to glycolide. Percent crystallinity, as determined from x-ray and DSC measurements, was found to be 52% for polyglycolide and 37% for poly-L-lactide. As shown in Figure 10, the copolymer compositions containing 25 to 70 mole percent of glycolide were amorphous. Use of *dl*-lactide instead of L-lactide extended the amorphous region from 0 to 70 mole percent glycolide since poly-*dl*-lactide is totally amorphous as mentioned previously. As was the case with the semicrystalline homopolymers of glycolide and L-lactide, semicrystalline copolymers were found to hydrolyze initially in the amorphous regions of the samples [65]. Thus the amorphous copolymers have been utilized for applications such as drug delivery where a single phase matrix is beneficial [66] and crystalline copolymer has been used in fabrication of fiber for use as surgical suture. The copolymer suture containing about 90% glycolide and 10% L-lactide, also known as polyglactin 910 or Vicryl™, retained strength slightly longer than pure polyglycolide suture and required only three months, about one month less, for complete bioabsorption *in vivo* [57].

A study of the amorphous copolymers of glycolide and L-lactide was conducted for the purpose of developing flexible injection-molded blood vessel ligating clips and interlocking staples for internal wound closure [67]. Samples of poly-L-lactide containing 25,

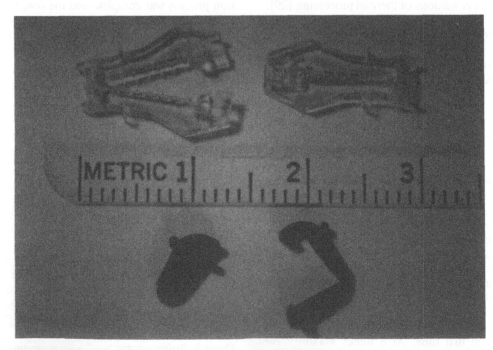

Figure 11. Bioabsorbable vessel ligating clips made of Lactomer™ (*above*) and PDS™ (*below*). (Reprinted with permission from Reference [14]. Copyright 1986, Edward Arnold Publishers, Ltd.)

30, and 35 percent glycolide implanted intramuscularly in rats were 23, 75 and 82 percent bioabsorbed after 12 weeks, respectively. Tensile strength retention after 3 weeks was 28, 32, and 8 percent, respectively. Thus the 30% glycolide copolymer (Lactomer™) was selected as the optimum composition for manufacture of clips and staples due to maximum strength-retention and a relatively rapid rate of bioabsorption. Tests performed on the actual strength of the locking mechanism of Lactomer™ clips *in vivo* revealed a 40 to 60% loss of strength after only one week [68]. This was still adequate, however, since only 96 hours of secure ligation were required for hemostasis.

Amorphous copolymers of lactide and glycolide have also been used clinically as implants to regenerate bony tissue in the cavity obtained after the curettage of mandibular cysts [69]. Pure poly-*dl*-lactide, however, appeared to give the best results with complete healing of the relatively small defect in 3 months. A 50:50 lactide:glycolide copolymer was used in combination with a partially purified bovine bone morphogenic protein as a delivery vehicle for this substance which resulted in the healing in monkeys of craniotomy defects that were too large to heal spontaneously [70]. Although ingrowth of new bone was observed, incomplete bioabsorption of the polymer at 4 months was considered to be a disadvantage.

POLYDIOXANONE

The synthesis of polydioxanone shown in Figure 8 is a ring-opening polymerization similar to the polymerization of glycolide except that the six-membered ring is a lactone monomer rather than a lactone dimer. The resultant semicrystalline polymer contains both ether and ester linkages and yields hydroxyethoxyacetic acid upon hydrolysis. Polydioxanone (PDS™) was used to develop the first commercially successful monofilament bioabsorbable suture [71]. These fibers retained 49 percent of original tensile strength after 6 weeks *in vivo*, 13 percent after 8 weeks, and were bioabsorbed in about 6 months with minimal tissue reaction. Preclinical studies gave no evidence of acute or chronic toxicological effects and radiolabeled polymer implants showed complete excretion of the degradation products with no accumulation in any tissues or organs. Fiber strength loss rates *in vitro* and *in vivo* were similar. The addition of enzymes *in vitro* did not substantially accelerate degradation of polydioxanone, but like polylactide and polyglycolide it was affected by gamma irradiation [72].

The prolonged strength retention of polydioxanone relative to other bioabsorbable sutures has been found to be an important advantage. Although the absolute strength of polydioxanone was lower than Vicryl™ or Maxon™ during the first 10 days *in vivo*, polydioxanone possessed greater strength beyond the initial 4

week period [73]. This has allowed surgeons to choose polydioxanone for procedures that traditionally indicated the use of nonabsorbable suture. In a randomized comparison of polydioxanone to polypropylene (nonabsorbable) for 284 abdominal wound closures, the use of polydioxanone resulted in significantly less dehiscence (0.7% vs. 6.4%), infection (8.6% vs. 15.4%), and wound pain (12% vs. 23%). After one year incisional herniation was the same (11%) in each group and thus unrelated to suture bioabsorbability [74].

Polydioxanone also was the first polymer to be used for bioabsorbable blood vessel ligating clips which replace the use of metallic hemostatic clips [75]. These clips, like the suture, are available in different sizes and are dyed with D & C Violet No. 2 dye for visability in the surgical field. Examples of polydioxanone (PDS™) and poly(L-lactide-co-glycolide) (Lactomer™) clips are shown in Figure 11. The Lactomer™ clips are now also available with violet dye. Note that the colorless Lactomer™ clips are perfectly clear since the amorphous copolymer is devoid of crystallites which might otherwise cause light scattering. Semicrystalline polydioxanone clips gave prolonged closure strength relative to Lactomer™ clips although both were deemed more than adequate for this application as mentioned previously [68].

POLYCAPROLACTONE

Polycaprolactone provides another example of a bioabsorbable polyester prepared by ring-opening polymerization of a lactone. In this case the lactone (ϵ-caprolactone) is a seven-membered ring in which a single ester moiety is linked together with five methylene units. Polycaprolactone is a hydrophobic, semicrystalline polymer (T_g $-60°C$, T_m $63°C$) which is degraded very slowly *in vivo* to yield ϵ-hydroxycaproic acid. Bioabsorption of polycaprolactone is initiated by nonenzymatic ester hydrolysis as occurs with the polymers discussed previously. The final stage of bioabsorption of polycaprolactone, however, was found to involve phagocytosis of polymer fragments by macrophages and giant cells, and degradation within these cells by lysosome-derived enzymes [76]. *In vitro* studies on polycaprolactone have established its sensitivity to microbial enzymes and, as expected, increased degradability of amorphous regions relative to the crystalline phase [77]. The permeability of polycaprolactone to various contraceptive steroids has made it an important candidate for the development of drug delivery implants [78].

An interesting feature of polycaprolactone is that copolymerization of lactide into the molecule provides a material that is much more flexible than either polylactide or polycaprolactone. An 80:20 copolymer of *dl*-lactide:caprolactone was used to produce flexible, suturable films that were successfully tested *in vivo* for the prevention of postoperative pleural and

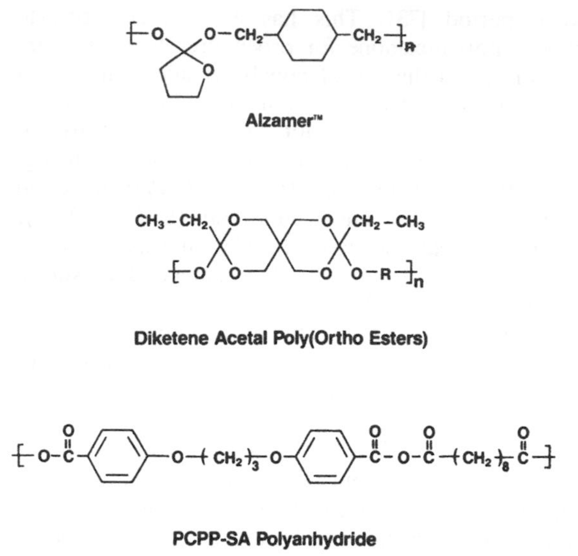

Alzamer™

Diketene Acetal Poly(Ortho Esters)

PCPP-SA Polyanhydride

Figure 12. Examples of bioerodible polymers used for controlled drug delivery.

pericardial adhesions [79]. These films maintained integrity for about one month postimplantation and were estimated by *in vitro* tests to bioabsorb in about five months. Histological examination of the copolymer films revealed no evidence of interference with the natural healing of adjacent tissues.

Caprolactone has also been copolymerized alternatively with glycolide [80] and trimethylene carbonate [81] to provide coatings for bioabsorbable sutures. Sutures treated with these coatings exhibited improved knot security and knot repositioning characteristics.

BIOERODIBLE POLYMERS

Although polymers and copolymers of lactide and glycolide are increasingly finding applications in the field of drug delivery research, the achievement of long-term zero-order release of water soluble drugs has presented a difficult challenge. Moisture uptake often results in drugs being leached out of the polymer

Diacid Chloride   **Amidediol**

PEA – x, y

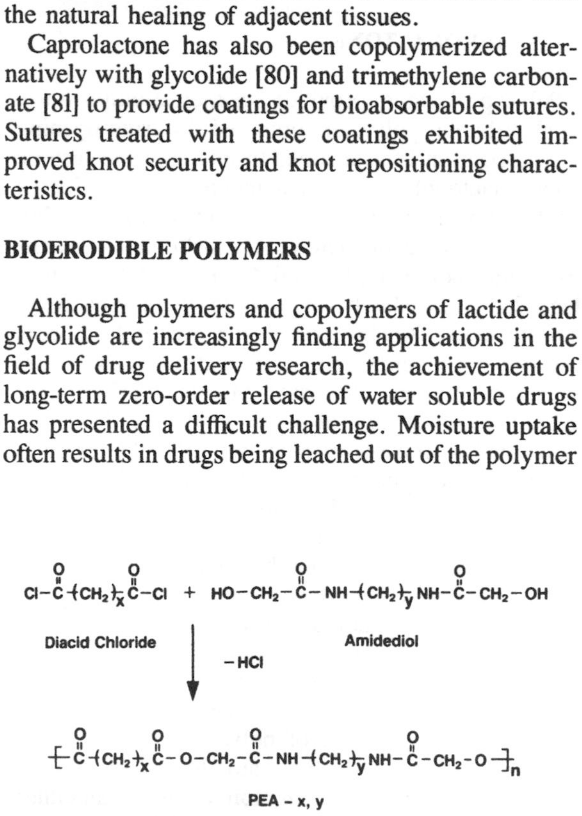

Figure 13. Poly(ester amide) formation from diacid chloride and amidediol. PEA-*x,y* refers to a poly(ester amide) where *x* is the number of methylene units in the diacid moiety and *y* is the number of methylene units in the diamine moiety.

matrix prior to the onset of bioabsorption. To overcome this problem and to create a bioabsorbable polymer matrix capable of zero-order release independent of the nature of the drug, the concept of "bioerodible" polymers was developed. In the ideal case a bioerodible polymer contains moisture-sensitive linkages but is so hydrophobic that moisture cannot penetrate its surface. Thus bioabsorption occurs by erosion of the surface and drug is released only as fresh surface is exposed due to the erosion process. Two types of polymers which approach this behavior are poly(ortho esters) and polyanhydrides.

One of the first poly(ortho esters) developed for drug delivery known as Alzamer™ is shown in Figure 12. *In vivo* degradation of this polymer yielded 1,4-cyclohexanedimethanol and 4-hydroxybutyric acid as hydrolysis products [82]. A more recent system developed by Heller involves reaction of polyols with the diketene acetal 3,9-*bis*(ethylidene-2,4,8,10-tetra-oxaspiro[5,5]undecane) to yield the poly(ortho ester) also shown in Figure 12 [83]. This system has an advantage in formulating dosage forms with heat or solvent sensitive drugs such as polypeptide hormones and growth factors since it is not necessary to melt, dissolve, or compress a preformed polymer. Instead a low molecular weight prepolymer is formed which is a viscous liquid at room temperature. The therapeutic agents can then be mixed into the prepolymer and the mixture cured at a temperature as low as 40°C to a solid material by the addition of a trifunctional polyol. For long-term controlled release it was necessary to add magnesium hydroxide to the poly(ortho ester) formulation. Since poly(ortho esters) are stable in base this protected the polymer from hydrolysis which otherwise would have resulted from a small amount of water that permeated the material in spite of its hydrophobicity. With this approach it was possible to achieve relatively constant blood plasma levels of levonorgestrel for one year in rabbits implanted with poly(ortho ester) rods containing 30% levonorgestrel and 7% magnesium hydroxide. The diketene acetal poly(ortho esters) also have recently been evaluated as possible matrix polymers for bioabsorbable polyphosphate glass reinforced fracture fixation plate materials [84].

An example of a bioerodible polyanhydride, shown in Figure 12, is a copolymer of poly[*bis*(p-carboxyphenoxy)propane] (PCPP) and poly(sebacic anhydride) (SA). Injection-molded samples of this polymer gave zero-order release rates of both the incorporated drug and the polymer hydrolysis products which in this case were the two dicarboxylic acids [85]. This polymer was found to have acceptable biocompatibility and the degradation products appeared to be nontoxic in preliminary tests [86].

POLY(ESTER AMIDES)

Several different types of polyesters containing amide linkages have been investigated as possible

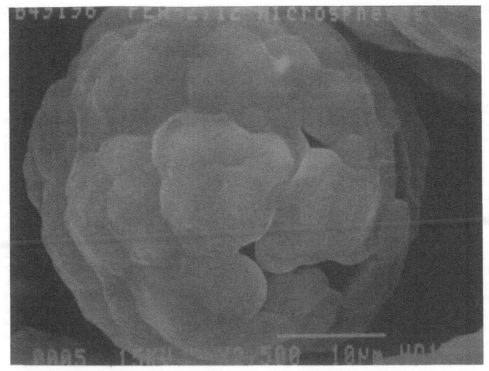

Figure 14. SEM of a single microsphere (38 microns dia.) of bioabsorbable poly(ester amide) showing spherulitic polymer crystal structure which formed during preparation of the microspheres by a solvent evaporation technique.

routes to achieving nylon-like properties in a bioabsorbable polymer [87]. A unique class of poly(ester amides) has been reported in which the amide linkages are preformed in a diol monomer synthesized from glycolic acid and various diamines [88]. This "amidediol" was then polyesterified with various diacid chlorides as shown in Figure 13. Fibers obtained by melt-spinning of PEA-2,6 and PEA-2,12 retained approximately 60% and 90% of initial tensile strength, respectively, after 4 weeks *in vivo*. Implantation of carbon-14 labeled filaments of these polymers revealed that PEA-2,6 was bioabsorbed in 9 months whereas PEA-2,12 was estimated to require about 3 years for complete bioabsorption. The disproportionately long bioabsorption time for PEA-2,12 was attributed to the water insolubility of the amidediol used in this polymer. Unlike water-soluble amidediols, the PEA-2,12 amidediol underwent extensive biotransformation and was excreted to a greater degree in feces rather than urine. Neither polymer, however, showed any appreciable accumulation of radioactivity in any tissues or organs during one year of implantation nor were any discernible toxic or adverse tissue reactions observed.

Both PEA-2,6 and PEA-2,12 are semicrystalline polymers with T_ms of about 165°C [89]. The spherulitic crystallites of PEA-2,12 can be seen clearly in Figure 14 which is a scanning electron micrograph (SEM) of polymer microspheres prepared by a solvent evaporation method [90]. This high magnification of a single sphere shows voids created by the loss

of amorphous material which has been transformed into higher density crystalline material. The surface of the sphere exhibits multifaceted bulges caused by the impacted growth of adjacent spherulites. Spherulitic crystal growth of this nature is typical of semicrystalline polymers in the absence of controlling factors such as nucleating agents or applied strain. As discussed previously, crystallite growth is generally avoided (by copolymerization) in drug delivery applications and exploited (by orientation) in fiber and other high-strength applications.

CONCLUSIONS

In the relatively short time that has elapsed since the first polyglycolide suture was introduced in 1970, high-quality lactide and glycolide homopolymers and copolymers have become commercially available to supply the growing need for bioabsorbable medical devices and drug delivery products. The choice of polyglycolide for use in the recently developed BAR device for colon surgery illustrates the value of a bioabsorbable polymer that is well-characterized and has a history of safe and efficacious clinical usage. Thus, patented new products can continue to be developed from this polymer while expiration of the original suture patent on polyglycolide has resulted in the development of generic bioabsorbable suture. Although drug delivery applications have been identified for lactide/glycolide polymers, especially in the form of injectable microspheres, general clinical use of these products must await the extensive testing that is required for any new drug formulation.

Advances in polylactide research have resulted in dramatic increases in the mechanical properties of this polymer due to optimization of "orientrusion" techniques and by formation of poly-L-lactide/poly-D-lactide blends. The spinning of polylactides into high-modulus stereocomplex fibers has created the opportunity for engineering a new generation of fiber-reinforced composites. These developments offer the possibility that fracture fixation of load-bearing bones may some day be treated with totally bioabsorbable implants that will permit better healing and not require surgical removal.

Research on new materials has yielded PDS™, Lactomer™, and Maxon™. These polymers have found applications beyond the suture in the form of clips, staples, pins, and mesh. Other proprietary bioabsorbable polymers are under development. Bioerodible poly(ortho esters) and polyanhydrides, for example, offer considerable promise in facilitating the administration of new polypeptide drugs and hormones created by genetic engineering technology. Thus bioabsorbable polymers clearly will continue to be utilized in the development of beneficial products in the future.

APPENDIX A—COMMERCIAL SOURCES OF LACTIDE AND GLYCOLIDE POLYMERS AND COPOLYMERS

1. Birmingham Polymers, Inc. (BPI)
   Avondale Commerce Park
   110 40th Street, No. 6, Bldg. 7
   Birmingham, Alabama 35222
   (205) 595-2231
2. Boehringer Ingelheim KG
   6507 Ingelhiem am Rhein
   Germany

   Sales in U.S.A.:
   Henley Chemicals, Inc.
   50 Chestnut Ridge Road
   Montvale, New Jersey 07645
   (201) 307-0422
3. CCA Biochem B.V.
   P.O. Box 21
   4200 AA Gorinchem
   Holland

   Sales in U.S.A.:
   Purac, Inc.
   1845 E. Rand Road, Suite 103
   Arlington Heights, IL 60004
   (312) 392-1540
4. DuPont Co., Inc.
   Chemicals & Pigments
   Customer Service Center
   Wilmington, DE 19898
   (302) 774-2290
   Toll Free 1-800-441-9442
5. Polysciences, Inc.
   400 Valley Road
   Warrington, PA 18976
   (215)343-6484

APPENDIX B—TRADEMARKS AND ACRONYMS FOR BIOABSORBABLE POLYMERS

1. Absolock™ — Polydioxanone vessel ligating clip. Ethicon, Inc.
2. Alzamer™ — Polyorthoester drug delivery matrix material (formerly Chronomer™). Alza, Inc.
3. BAR — Biofragmentable anastomosis ring.
4. Biodel™ — Poly[*bis*(p-carboxy-phenoxy propane anhydride)sebacic acid] drug delivery matrix. Nova Pharmaceutical, Inc.
5. Biofix™ — Polyglycolide pin for bone fragment fixation. Biofix-C™ is made from polydioxanone reinforced with polyglycolide fiber. Bioscience, Ltd., Tampere, Finland.
6. Capronor™ — Contraceptive steroid-releasing implant made of polycaprolactone. Research Triangle Institute, Inc.
7. Dexon™ — Braided polyglycolide surgical suture. American Cyanamid Co., Inc.
8. Drylac™ — Porous poly-L-lactide dressing for oral surgery. Osmed, Inc.
9. Ethipin™ — Polydioxanone pin for osteochondral fragment fixation. Ethicon, Inc.
10. Lactomer™ — Poly(L-lactide-co-30%-glycolide) vessel ligating clips and surgical staples. U.S. Surgical Corp., Inc.
11. Maxon™ — Poly(glycolide-co-trimethylene carbonate), also called polyglyconate, monofilament surgical suture. American Cyanamid Co., Inc.
12. Medisorb™ — Various copolymers and homopolymers of lactide and glycolide. DuPont Co., Inc.
13. Orthosorb™ — Orientruded poly-L-lactide for orthopedic surgery. Johnson & Johnson, Inc.
14. PCL — Polycaprolactone.
15. PDS™ — Polydioxanone monofilament surgical suture. Ethicon, Inc.
16. PEA — Poly(ester amide).
17. PGA — Polyglycolic acid, also called polyglycolide.
18. PLA — Polylactic acid, also called polylactide. PLLA stands for poly(L-lactic acid).
19. POE — Poly(ortho ester).
20. Resomer™ — Various copolymers and homopolymers of lactide and glycolide. Boehringer Ingelheim, KG, Germany.
21. Valtrac™ — BAR for intestinal surgery molded from polyglycolide and barium sulfate. American Cyanamid Co., Inc.
22. Vicryl™ — Poly(glycolide-co-10%-L-lactide), also called polyglactin 910, braided surgical suture. Ethicon, Inc.

REFERENCES

1. Fisher, R. B. 1977. *Joseph Lister*. New York: Stein and Day.
2. Rae, T. 1981. "Localized Tissue Infection and the Role

of Foreign Bodies", in *Fundamental Aspects of Biocompatibility*. D. F. Williams, ed. Boca Raton, FL: CRC Press, 2:139.

3. Dayton, M. T., B. A. Buchele, S. S. Shirazi and L. B. Hunt. 1986. "Use of an Absorbable Mesh to Repair Contaminated Abdominal-Wall Defects", *Arch. Surg.*, 121:954–960.

4. Edlich, R. F., P. H. Panek and G. T. Rodeheaver. 1973. "Physical and Chemical Configuration of Sutures in the Development of Surgical Infection", *Ann. Surg.*, 177:679–687.

5. Concoran, S. F., J. M. Koroluk, J. R. Parsons, H. Alexander and A. R. Weiss. 1980. "The Development of a Variable Stiffness, Absorbable Composite Bone Plate", in *Current Concepts of Internal Fixation of Fractures*. H. K. Uhthoff, ed. New York: Springer-Verlag, p. 136–145.

6. Rodkey, W. G., H. E. Cabaud, J. A. Feagin and P. C. Perlik. 1985. "A Partially Biodegradable Material Device for Repair and Reconstruction of Injured Tendons", *Am. J. Sports Med.*, 13:242–247.

7. Richardson, P. D., A. Parhizgar, H. F. Sasken, T. H. Chiu, P. Aebischer, L. A. Trudell and P. M. Galletti. 1986. "Tissue Characterization by Micromechanical Testing of Growths Around Bioresorbable Implants", in *Progress in Artificial Organs—1985*. Y. Nose, C. Kjellstrand and P. Ivanovich, eds. Cleveland: ISAO Press.

8. Greisler, H. P., D. U. Kim, J. B. Price and A. B. Voorhees. 1985. "Arterial Regenerative Activity after Prosthetic Implantation", *Arch. Surg.*, 120:315–323.

9. Leenslag, J. W., M. T. Kroes, A. J. Pennings and B. Van der Lei. 1988. "A Compliant, Biodegradable Vascular Graft: Basic Aspects of Its Construction and Biological Performance", *New Polymeric Mater.*, 1(2):111–126.

10. Bowald, S., C. Busch and I. Eriksson. 1979. "Arterial Regeneration Following Polyglactin 910 Suture Mesh Grafting", *Surgery*, 86:722–729.

11. Tice, T. R. and D. R. Cowsar. 1984. "Biodegradable Controlled-Release Parenteral Systems", *Pharm. Technol.*, (Nov.):26–35.

12. Hutchinson, F. G. and B. J. A. Furr. 1987. "Biodegradable Carriers for the Sustained Release of Polypeptides", *Trends Biotechnol.*, 5:102–106.

13. Wheeless, C. R. 1986. "Use of Absorbable Staples for Closure of Proximal End of Ileal Loops", *Obstet. Gynecol.*, 67:280–283.

14. Barrows, T. H. 1986. "Degradable Implant Materials: A Review of Synthetic Absorbable Polymers and Their Applications", *Clin. Mater.*, 1:233–257.

15. Devanathan, T. D. 1983. "Silicone Elastomers for Implantable Biomedical Devices", in *Biocompatible Polymers, Metals, and Composites*. M. Szycher, ed. Lancaster, PA: Technomic Publishing Co., Inc., pp. 769–779.

16. Carothers, W. H., G. L. Dorough and F. J. Van Natta. 1932. "Studies of Polymerization and Ring Formation. X. The Reversible Polymerization of Six-Membered Cyclic Esters", *J. Amer. Chem. Soc.*, 54:761–772.

17. Kulkarni, R. K., K. C. Pani, C. Neuman and F. Leonard. 1966. "Polylactic Acid for Surgical Implants", *Arch. Surg.*, 93:839–843.

18. "Polylactic Acid Surgical Dressing Material", U.S. Food & Drug Administration Premarket Approval Appl. No. P800012, Jan. 28, 1983.

19. Kinnersley, A. M., T. C. Scott, J. H. Yopp and G. H. Whitten. "Oligomeric Hydroxy Acids Regulating Plant Growth", PCT Intl. Appl. W08807815, April 6, 1987.

20. Aydin, O. and R. C. Schulz. 1982. "Poly-L-Lactide", *Macromolec Syn.*, 8:99–101.

21. Jamshidi, K., R. C. Eberhart, S. H. Hyon and Y. Ikada. 1987. "Characterization of Polylactide Synthesis", *Polym. Prepr.*, 28(1):236–237.

22. Mahler, H. R. and E. H. Cordes. 1966. *Biological Chemistry*, New York: Harper & Row, p. 430.

23. Kulkarni, R. K., E. G. Moore, A. F. Hegyeli and F. Leonard. 1971. "Biodegradable Poly(lactic acid) Polymers", *J. Biomed. Mater. Res.*, 5:169–181.

24. Bodmeier, R. and J. W. McGinity. 1987. "Poly(lactic acid) Microspheres Containing Quinidine Base and Quinidine Sulfate Prepared by the Solvent Evaporation Technique. I. Methods and Morphology", *J. Microencapsulation*, 4:279–288.

25. Leelarasamee, N., S. A. Howard, C. J. Malanga and J. K. H. Ma. 1988. "A Method for the Preparation of Polylactic Acid Microsapsules of Controlled Particle Size and Drug Loading", *J. Microencapsulation*, 5(2):147–157.

26. Van Krevelen, D. W. 1978. "Crystallinity of Polymers and the Means to Influence the Crystallization Process", *Chimia*, 32:279–294.

27. Vert, M. and F. Chabot. 1981. "Stereoregular Bioresorbable Polyesters for Orthopaedic Surgery", *Makromol. Chem.*, 5(suppl):30–41.

28. Bendix, D. and G. Entenmann. "Molecular Weight Distributions of Reimplanted Poly(L-lactides)", presented at *The World Congress on Implantology and Biomaterials, March 8–11, 1989, Paris, France*.

29. Daniels, A. U., M. K. O. Chang and K. P. Andriano. "Mechanical Properties of Biodegradable Polymers and Composites Proposed for Internal Fixation of Bone", *Appl. Biomater.*, (in press).

30. Tunc, D. C. and B. Jadhay. 1988. "Development of Absorbable, Ultra-High-Strength Polylactide", *Polym. Mater. Sci. Eng.*, 59:383–387.

31. Leenslag, J. W., A. J. Pennings, R. R. M. Bos, F. R. Rozema and G. Boering. 1987. "Resorbable Materials of Poly(L-lactide). VI. Plates and Screws for Internal Fracture Fixation", *Biomaterials*, 8:70–73.

32. Leenslag, J. W., A. J. Pennings, R. R. M. Bos, F. R. Rozema and G. Boering. 1987. "Resorbable Materials of Poly(L-lactide). VII. *In Vivo* and *In Vitro* Degradation", *Biomaterials*, 8:311–314.

33. Christel, P., F. Chabot and M. Vert. 1984. "*In Vivo* Fate of Bioresorbable Bone Plates in Long-Lasting Poly(L-lactic acid)", *Trans. Soc. Biomater.*, 7:279.

34. Postema, A. R. and A. J. Pennings. 1989. "Study on the Drawing Behavior of Poly(L-lactide) to Obtain High-Strength Fibers", *J. Appl. Polym. Sci.*, 37:2351–2369.

35. Gogolewski, S. and A. J. Pennings. 1983. "Resorbable Materials of Poly(L-lactide). II. Fibers Spun from Solution of Poly(L-lactide) in Good Solvents", *J. Appl. Polym. Sci.*, 28:1045–1061.

36. Jamshidi, K., S. H. Hyon and Y. Ikada. 1988. "Thermal Characterization of Polylactides", *Polymer*, 29:2229–2234.

37. Jamshidi, K., S. H. Hyon, T. Nakamura, Y. Ikada, Y. Shimizu and T. Teramatsu. 1986. "*In Vitro* and *In Vivo* Degradation of Poly-L-Lactide Fibers", in *Biological and Biochemical Performance of Biomaterials*. P. Christel, A. Meunier and A. J. C. Lee, eds. Amsterdam: Elsevier, p. 227–232.

38. Benicewicz, B. C., S. W. Shalaby, A. J. T. Clemov and Z. Oser. 1989. "*In Vitro* and *In Vivo* Degradation of Poly(L-lactide) Braided Multifilament Yarns", *Polym. Prepr.*, 30(1).

39. Schakenraad, J. M., J. A. Oosterbaan, P. Nieuwenhuis, I. Molenaar, J. Olijslager, W. Potman, M. J. D. Eenink and J. Feijen. 1988. "Biodegradable Hollow Fibres for the Controlled Release of Drugs", *Biomaterials*, 9:116–120.

40. Collett, J. H., L. Y. Lin and P. L. Gould. 1989. "Gamma-Irradiation of Biodegradable Polyesters in Controlled Physical Environments", *Polym. Prepr.*, 30(1):468–469.

41. McKenna, G. B. "The Development of Fiber Reinforced Polymer Composites for Orthopedic Applications", Ph.D. Thesis, University of Utah (Dec. 1976).

42. Kelley, B. S., R. L. Dunn and R. A. Casper. 1987. "Totally Resorbable High-Strength Composite Material", *Polym. Sci. Technol.*, 35(*Adv. Biomed. Polym.*):75–85.

43. Vert, M., H. Garreau, M. Audion, F. Chabot and P. Christel. 1985. "Totally Bioresorbable Composite System for Internal Fixation of Bone Fractures", *Trans. Soc. Biomater.*, 8:218.

44. Alexander, H., J. R. Parsons, A. B. Weiss and P. K. Bajpai. 1985. "Absorbable Composites as Orthopaedic Implants", *Trans. Soc. Biomater.*, 8:215.

45. Zimmerman, M., J. R. Parsons and H. Alexander. 1987. "The Design and Analysis of A Laminated Partially Degradable Composite Bone Plate for Fracture Fixation", *J. Biomed. Mater. Res.*, 21(A3):345–361.

46. Higashi, S., T. Yamamuro, T. Nakamura, Y. Ikada, S. H. Hyon and K. Jamshidi. 1986. "Polymer-Hydroxyapatite Composites for Biodegradable Bone Fillers", *Biomaterials*, 7:183–187.

47. Ikada, Y., K. Jamshidi, H. Tsuji and S. H. Hyon. 1987. "Stereocomplex Formation Between Enantiomeric Poly(lactides)", *Macromolecules*, 20(4):904–906.

48. Murdoch, J. R. and G. L. Loomis. 1988. "Polylactide Compositions", U.S. Patent 4,719,246.

49. Loomis, G. L., J. R. Murdock and K. Gardner. 1989. "New Materials from the Organization of Enantiomeric Polylactides", *Trans. Soc. Biomater.*, 12:73.

50. Ikada, Y. and S. Gen. 1988. "Polylactic Acid Fiber", European Patent Appl. 0288041.

51. Gilding, D. K. and A. M. Reed. 1979. "Biodegradable Polymers for Use in Surgery—Polyglycolic/Polylactic Acid Homo- and Copolymers: 1", *Polymer*, 20:1459–1464.

52. Bischoff, C. A. and P. Walden. 1893. "Glycolide and Its Homologs", *Ber.*, 26:262–265.

53. Lowe, C. E. 1954. "Preparation of High Molecular Weight Polyhydroxyacetic Ester", U.S. Patent 2,668,162.

54. Schmitt, E. E., and R. A. Polistina. 1967. "Surgical Sutures", U.S. Patent 3,297,033.

55. "Dexon™, Polyglycolic Acid Sutures", Summary of Basis of Approval, NDA 16-881, U.S. Food & Drug Administration, April 27, 1970.

56. Katz, A. R. and B. J. Turner. 1970. "Evaluation of Tensile and Absorption Properties of Polyglycolic Acid Sutures", *Surg. Gynecol. Obstet.*, 131:701–716.

57. Craig, P. H., J. A. Williams, K. W. Davis, A. D. Magoun, A. J. Levy, S. Bogdansky and J. P. Jones. 1975. "A Biologic Comparison of Polyglactin 910 and Polyglycolic Acid Synthetic Absorbable Sutures", *Surg. Gynecol. Obstet.*, 141:1–10.

58. Chu, C. C. 1985. "Degradation and Biocompatibility of Suture Materials", in *CRC Critical Reviews in Biocompatibility, vol. 1(3)*. D. F. Williams, ed. Boca Raton, FL: CRC Press, p. 261–321.

59. Chu, C. C. and A. Browning. 1988. "The Study of Thermal and Gross Morphologic Properties of Polyglycolic Acid Upon Annealing and Degradation Treatments", *J. Biomed. Mater. Res.*, 22:699–712.

60. Roby, M. S., D. J. Casey and R. D. Cody. 1985. "Absorbable Sutures Based on Glycolide/Trimethylene Carbonate Copolymers", *Trans. Soc. Biomater.*, 8:216.

61. Katz, A. R., D. P. Mukherjee, A. L. Kaganov and S. Gordon. 1985. "A New Synthetic Monofilament Absorbable Suture Made from Polytrimethylene Carbonate", *Surg. Gynecol. Obstet.*, 161:213–222.

62. Ritter, T. A., A. L. Kaganov and J. P. Budris. 1985. "Modification of Polyglycolic Acid Structural Elements to Achieve Variable *In Vivo* Physical Properties", U.S. Patent 4,496,446.

63. Cahill, C. J., M. Betzler, J. A. Gruwez, J. Jeekel, J. C. Patel and B. Zederfeldt. 1989. "Sutureless Large Bowel Anastomosis: European Experience with the Biofragmentable Anastomosis Ring", *Br. J. Surg.*, 76:344–347.

64. Cutright, D. E., B. Perez, J. D. Beasley, W. J. Larson and W. R. Posey. 1974. "Degradation Rates of Polymers and Copolymers of Polylactic and Polyglycolic Acids", *Oral Surg.*, 37:142–152.

65. Fredericks, R. J., A. J. Melveger and L. J. Dolegiewitz. 1984. "Morphological and Structural Changes in a Copolymer of Glycolide and Lactide Occurring as a Result of Hydrolysis", *J. Poly. Sci.*, 22(*Poly. Phys. Ed.*):57–66.

66. Kitchell, J. P., D. L. Wise. 1985. "Poly(lactic/glycolic acid) Biodegradable Drug-Polymer Matrix Systems", *Methods. Enzymol.*, 112:436–448.

67. Kaplan, D. S. and R. R. Muth. 1985. "Polymers for Injection Molding of Absorbable Surgical Devices", U.S. Patent 4,523,591.

68. Hay, D. L., J. A. von Fraunhofer, N. Chegin and B. J. Masterson. 1988. "Locking Mechanism Strength of Absorbable Ligating Devices", *J. Biomed. Mater. Res.*, 22:179–190.

69. Chanavaz, M., F. Chabot, M. Donazzan and M. Vert. 1986. "Further Clinical Applications of Bioresorbable PLA 37.5 GA 25 and PLA 50 Polymers for Limited Bone Augmentation and Bone Replacement", *Adv. Biomater.*, 6(*Biol. Biomech. Perf. Biomater.*): 233–238.

70. Ferguson, D., W. L. Davis, M. R. Urist, W. C. Hurt and E. P. Allen. 1987. "Bovine Bone Morphogenetic Protein (bBMP) Fraction-Induced Repair of Craniotomy Defects in the Rhesus Monkey (*Macaca Speciosa*)", *Clin. Orthop. Rel. Res.*, 219:251–258.

71. Ray, J. A., N. Doddi, D. Regula, J. A. Williams and A. Melvegar. 1981. "Polydioxanone (PDS); A Novel Monofilament Synthetic Absorbable Suture", *Surg. Gynecol. Obstet.*, 153:497–507.

72. Williams, D. F., C. C. Chu and J. Dwyer. 1984. "Effects of Enzymes and Gamma Irradiation on the Tensile Strength and Morphology of Poly(p-dioxanone) Fibers", *J. Appl. Poly. Sci.*, 29:1865–1877.

73. Sanz, L. E., J. A. Patterson, R. Kamath, G. Willett, S. W. Ahmed and A. B. Butterfield. 1988. "Comparison of Maxon Suture with Vicryl, Chromic Catgut, and PDS Sutures in Fascial Closure in Rats", *Obstet. Gynecol.*, 71(3):418–422.

74. Cameron, A. E., C. J. Parker, E. S. Field, R. C. Gray and A. P. Wyatt. 1987. "A Randomized Comparison of Polydioxanone (PDS) and Polypropylene (Prolene) for Abdominal Wound Closure", *Ann. R. Coll. Surg. Engl.*, 69(3):113–115.

75. Schaefer, C. J., P. M. Colombani and G. W. Geelhoed. 1982. "Absorbable Ligating Clips", *Surg. Gynecol. Obstet.*, 154:513–516.

76. Woodward, S. C., P. S. Brewer, F. Moatamed, A. Schindler and C. G. Pitt. 1985. "The Intracellular Degradation of Poly(ε-caprolactone)", *J. Biomed. Mater. Res.*, 19:437–444.

77. Jarrett, P., C. Benedict, J. P. Bell, J. A. Cameron and S. J. Huang. 1983. "Mechanism of the Biodegradation of Polycaprolactone", *Polym. Prepr.*, 24(1):32–33.

78. Pitt, C. G., M. M. Gratzl, G. L. Kimmel, J. Surles and A. Schindler. 1981. "Aliphatic Polyesters II. The Degradation of Poly(DL-lactide), Poly(ε-caprolactone), and their Copolymers *In Vivo*", *Biomaterials*, 2:215–220.

79. Nakamura, T., S. Hitome, T. Shimamoto, S. H. Hyon, Y. Ikada, S. Watanabe and Y. Shimizu. 1987. "Surgical Application of Biodegradable Films Prepared from Lactide-ε-Caprolactone Copolymers", *Adv. Biomater.*, 7:759–764.

80. Jarrett, P. K., D. J. Casey and L. T. Lehmann. 1988. "Caprolactone Block Copolymers as Coatings for Surgical Articles", U.S. Patent 4,788,979.

81. Jarrett, P. K., D. J. Casey and L. T. Lehmann. 1988. "Bioabsorbable Caprolactone Copolymer Coating for a Surgical Article", U.S. Patent 4,791,929.

82. Sendelbeck, S. L. and C. L. Girdin. 1985. "Disposition of a Carbon-14 Labeled Bioerodible Polyorthoester and Its Hydrolysis Products, 4-Hydroxybutyrate and Cis, Trans-1,4-Bis(hydroxymethyl)Cyclohexane, in Rats", *Drug Metab. Dispos.*, 13:291–295.

83. Heller, J. 1988. "Synthesis and Use of Poly(ortho esters) for the Controlled Delivery of Therapeutic Agents", *J. Bioact. Biocompat. Polym.*, 3:97–105.

84. Andriano, K. P., A. U. Daniels, W. P. Smutz, R. W. B. Wyatt and J. Heller. 1989. "Initial Histological and Mechanical Comparison of Several Biodegradable Fiber Reinforced Polymers", *Trans. Soc. Biomater.*, 12:76.

85. Leong, K. W., B. C. Brott and R. Langer. 1985. "Bioerodible Polyanhydrides as Drug-Carrier Matrices. I. Characterization, Degradation, and Release Characteristics", *J. Biomed. Mater. Res.*, 19:941–955.

86. Leong, K. W., P. D. Amore, M. Marletta and R. Langer. 1986. "Bioerodible Polyanhydrides as Drug-Carrier Matrices. II. Biocompatibility and Chemical Reactivity", *J. Biomed. Mater. Res.*, 20:51–64.

87. Barrows, T. H. "Bioabsorbable Poly(ester amides)", in *Biodegradable Polymers*. S. J. Huang, ed. Munich: Hanser (in press).

88. Barrows, T. H., G. J. Quarfoth, P. E. Blegen and R. L. McQuinn. 1988. "Comparison of Bioabsorbable Poly(ester-amide) Monomers and Polymers *In Vivo* Using Radiolabeled Homologs", *Proc. Polym. Mater. Sci. Eng.*, 59:376–379.

89. Barrows, T. H., J. D. Johnson, S. J. Gibson and D. M. Grussing. 1986. "The Design and Synthesis of Bioabsorbable Poly(ester-amides)", in *Polymers in Medicine II*. E. Chiellini, P. Giusti, C. Migliaresi and L. Nicolais, eds. New York: Plenum, p. 85–90.

90. Barrows, T. H. unpublished data.

18

Bioadhesion and Factors Affecting the Bioadhesion of Microparticles[1]

K. V. RANGA RAO*
P. BURI*

ABSTRACT: In order to understand the mode of adhesion of polymers to mucus or soft tissues and to help the formulator in designing suitable bioadhesive dosage forms, the essential features of the structure of mucus, the mechanism of mucoadhesion, and the various techniques reported in the literature to screen the polymers for bioadhesion are reviewed briefly. The potential of bioadhesive microparticles to increase the bioavailability of nasally or orally administered drugs is obvious from the literature.

Several factors which may influence the bioadhesion of polymer-coated microparticles were studied in detail and the results are presented. Increase in the nominal viscosity of the polymer in the coat increased the adhesion of the particles to the intestine but not to the stomach. This shows that polymer chain length is important for bioadhesion. Strong adhesion of hydroxypropylmethyl-cellulose (HPMC)-coated particles to the intestine, when the amount of mucus was minimal, indicates that HPMC has a strong affinity for epithelial cells. Increase in the thickness of the HPMC coat increased the adhesion, but this did not occur with polycarbophil (PC). Synergistic increase in the viscosity due to the presence of both HPMC and sodium carboxymethylcellulose (Na CMC) in the coat did not increase the adhesion. PC and Na CMC-coated particles adhered less well to the duodenum than to the jejunum. All the particles adhered less well to the distal end of small intestine than to the jejunum. The contact time and moisture content are important for the celluloses, but not for PC. Viscosity and the structure of the mucus are important for the mucoadhesion. The results revealed

that polymers of high molecular weight and/or polymers having ionizable groups can adhere strongly to the mucus of the gastro-intestinal tract.

BACKGROUND

Definition

Bioadhesion may be defined as the adhesion between two biological materials (e.g., bacterial adhesion to intestinal epithelium or adhesion of mucus to epithelial cell surfaces) or the adhesion of a biological material to an artificial substrate or vice-versa (e.g., bacterial adhesion to glassware or adhesion of α-cyanoacrylate esters, commonly called "super glues", to teeth or bones). Polymers adhering to biological tissues have been used for many years in surgery, dentistry and orthopaedics. For a pharmaceutical technologist, bioadhesion may be defined as the adhesion, by interfacial forces, of a dosage form containing a synthetic or natural polymer to soft tissues like the mucous layer or epithelial cell layer in the presence of water for extended periods of time. The main objectives of bioadhesive dosage forms are: (1) to increase the bioavailability of a drug due to longer contact times at the site of absorption, (2) to deliver the drug specifically at the site of absorption, and (3) to minimize the frequency of administration, leading to better patient compliance. The subject is gaining popularity in recent years and the topic has been reviewed by a few authors [1–8].

Under normal circumstances, the bioadhesive dosage form is expected to adhere to the mucus or epithelial cell surfaces and release the drug. Hence, to understand the phenomenon of adhesion between the polymer and the mucus, one must know about the structure of the mucus and the mechanism of its adhesion to polymers.

[1]Presented partly at the 15th International Symposium on Controlled Release of Bioactive Materials held at Basel, Switzerland in Aug. 1988.

*School of Pharmacy, University of Geneva, 30 quai Ernest Ansermet, CH-1211 Geneva 4, Switzerland

STRUCTURE OF THE MUCUS

Mucus is a highly viscous and translucent gel secreted by the goblet cells of the epithelium. Its thickness is heterogeneous and composition varies with the source (nasal, gastric, intestinal, bronchial, vaginal, etc.), sex, and state of health. For example, gastric mucus consists of ~95% water, 1% electrolytes, 0.5–1% each of proteins, lipids and glycoproteins [9,10]. The proportions of electrolytes and glycoproteins are slightly higher in nasal mucus [11,12]. The glycoprotein fraction of mucus is mainly responsible for its gel-like structure and consists of 20% protein and 80% sugar with an average molecular weight of 2×10^6 [13]. About 25–40% of human bronchial mucus glycoproteins were found to be lipids [14]. The chemical composition and the physicochemical properties of various submaxillary gland glycoproteins were reviewed [15].

Mucous glycoproteins consist of a protein core with long-chain branched oligosaccharide side chains covalently attached, predominantly by *O*-glycosidic linkages via the serine and the threonine amino acid components. About one carbohydrate side chain is attached to every four amino acids present in the peptide backbone of the glycoprotein [16]. The number of sugar residues in each side chain varies from two to twenty, with an average value of eight. Each carbohydrate side chain terminates with a sialic acid group having a pKa of ~2.6 [17] or with a L-fucose. Thus the typical mucous glycoprotein can be considered as an anionic polyelectrolyte at pH greater than 2.6. Some of the molecular parameters of the mucin glycoprotein of various animals and man have been reviewed [1]. The conformation of the glycoprotein depends on the number and sequence of amino acids and sugars present in it. The polymer chains are entangled within and between each other by disulphide and secondary bonds like electrostatic and hydrophobic interactions, and are responsible for the gel-like structure of the mucus. The mucous layer along with the water present around it protects the underlying mucosa from mechanical damage and also acts as a selective permeability barrier. The structure of the mucus and its role in the absorption of drugs has been reviewed [18].

MECHANISM OF BIOADHESION

For the adhesion of a polymer to soft tissue or mucus, an intimate contact first has to be established between them. This is possible only when the spreading coefficient of the adhesive on the adherend (i.e., tissue or mucus) is positive. When the bioadhesive polymer spreads on the adherend, a strong interaction may be produced by:

(1) Physical or mechanical bonds
(2) Chemical bonds

Physical or Mechanical Mechanism of Bioadhesion

When a bioadhesive polymer is in contact with the mucus, the polymer chains get hydrated and due to the concentration gradient, they penetrate into the glycoprotein network of the mucus. Once diffused, they are able to match their adhesive sites with those on the substrate to form an adhesive bond. Since this occurs in the presence of water, it is often called wet adhesion. The rate of penetration depends on the diffusion coefficient of the polymer in the mucus ($\sim 10^{-10}$ to $10^{-16} \mathrm{cm^2 \cdot s^{-1}}$ [19,20]) and also on the affinity between them. The amount of water present at the interface and the time for which the adhesive and the adherend are in contact with each other also influence the strength of the adhesive bond formed between them. Therefore, polymers having a flexible and more mobile polymer backbone and lighter side chains can diffuse into the cross-linked and complex mucus at a faster rate than those of the cross-linked polymer. It has been reported that the adhesive forces increase as the molecular weight increases until a plateau value is reached [21].

Chemical Mechanism of Bioadhesion

Polymers that have very reactive functional groups and can form covalent bonds with the proteins of the biological tissues can adhere permanently. This type of linkage is not practical, since the compatibility of the majority of the polymers with tissues has not been well studied. However, polymers having a high affinity for the mucus (i.e., having nearly the same solubility parameters) and possessing polar groups such as hydroxyl, carboxyl or other ionic groups can also interact with the mucus through hydrogen bonding or van der Waals attractions [22]. The bioadhesive and the adherend should be in close contact with each other for this interaction to occur (e.g. London dispersion forces act when the adherend and the adhesive are at a distance of ~4 Å). Although these interactions are weak, a strong adhesion can occur when numerous such contacts exist between them. In an attempt to understand the optimum structural features needed for bioadhesion, copolymers of acrylic and methacrylic acids with variations in charge density and hydrophobicity were prepared. When their adhesion to rabbit stomach tissue was studied, it was observed that the charge density is more important [23]. The expanded nature of the polymeric network was found to be closely related to the adhesion of anionic loosely cross-linked polymers to mucus [24].

METHODS TO STUDY BIOADHESION

Before designing any bioadhesive dosage form, it is necessary to select a polymer which can adhere well to the mucus by screening several candidate polymers.

Several methods reported in the pharmaceutical literature to test the bioadhesive property of polymers have been reviewed [6,8]. These methods may be classified as (1) *in vitro/in situ* techniques and (2) *in vivo* techniques.

In vitro/in situ Techniques

Tests to evaluate the adhesive strength of adhesives/glues/mucilages were reported in the literature nearly three decades ago [25,26]. These methods were later adapted by the researchers to test the adhesion between bioadhesive polymers and soft tissues. In all these techniques, the force required to detach the polymer from the tissue or mucus was measured, i.e., the adhesive bond between the polymer and the mucus or tissue is destroyed by shear/peeling/tensile forces. In the majority of techniques, the polymer sample is placed on one [27–29] or between two soft tissue layers [30] in an appropriate buffer or saline solution. The tissues used were either the mucosal surfaces of the rabbit stomach [30], or mucous membranes of the oesophagus of various animals [31–34], or mouse peritoneal membrane [35], or bovine sublingual membrane [29], etc. Alternately, a glass plate is coated with the polymer and allowed to interact with mucus by dipping the glass plate in mucin solution [21]. Park and Robinson classified bioadhesive polymers in a different way [36]. The principle of their technique is as follows.

The lipid bilayer of the cell membrane of cultured human conjunctival cells was labelled by adding a lipid-soluble fluorescent probe, pyrene. When a polymer to be tested (which can adsorb to cell membrane) is added to this, the fluorescence exhibited by the cell membrane decreases proportionally with the polymer adsorption. This means that the greater the fall in the fluorescence, the greater is the adsorption of polymer to the cell membrane. According to this technique, anionic polymers are good binders and carboxylated anions are better than sulphated polyanions. Bridges et al. [37] studied the adhesion of several N-(2-hydroxypropyl)methacrylamide (HPMA) copolymers containing pendent sugar residues or quaternary ammonium groups to rat intestine *in vitro* and reported that cationic derivatives of the polymer adhered very strongly to all regions of the intestine. They also reported [38] a delay of 5 hours in the transit time when a polycationic HPMA copolymer was administered into the stomachs of rats by intubation. This was attributed to the strong electrostatic affinity between the cationic polymer and the anionic mucus.

Although all these indirect methods give quantitative results, they are not close to the real *in vivo* situation prevailing when a microparticle is in contact with the mucus. Hence, we developed a simple, quantitative and realistic *in situ* technique [39] to screen both the soluble and insoluble polymers and the polymer-coated microparticles for bioadhesion. In this method [39], the rat jejunum or stomach was cut and spread on a polyethylene support with the help of pins. Uncoated or coated particles were then placed uniformly as a monolayer on the mucosa of the stomach or the intestine. The tissue was then placed in a desiccator maintained at >80% relative humidity and room temperature for 20 min to allow the polymer to hydrate and to interact with the glycoprotein, and also to prevent the drying of the mucus.

After 20 min, the mucosas of the stomach and the intestine were washed for 5 min with 0.1N HCl and Sörensen phosphate buffer (pH 6.0), respectively at room temperature at a rate of 22 ml/min using a peristaltic pump. After 5 min, the percent of the beads washed away was determined by weighing the residue collected. The quantity of the polymer dissolved during washing being very small compared to the weight of the glass beads, it was considered negligible. The retention of polycarbophil or Carbopol-934 coated poly(hydroxyethylmethacrylate) microspheres in the intestine was studied. It was observed that only the polycarbophil-coated microspheres showed bioadhesion, for about 2 hours. Interestingly, tensiometric methods revealed that both the polymers have the same mucoadhesive strength [40].

The duration of adhesion of the polymer or polymer-containing dosage form to mucus is normally studied by monitoring the clearance of radio-labelled polymers from the organ. Ch'ng et al. [30] introduced surgically a capsule containing chromium[51]-labelled polymers into the stomachs of anaesthetised rats, and later allowed the animals to recover by exposing them to fresh air. Periodically the animals were sacrificed, the intestine was cut into 20 equal parts and the radioactivity was measured. They reported that nearly 50% of the polycarbophil remained in the stomach even 10 hours after administering the capsule. Longer et al. [41] mixed chlorothiazide-containing albumin beads with polycarbophil granules (both 0.5 mm diameter) and introduced surgically a capsule containing them into the stomachs of rats as mentioned earlier. Plasma drug levels in the rats showed a longer duration of action and greater bioavailability for the bioadhesive dosage form than for either albumin beads or drug powder alone. Khosla and Davis [42] administered a capsule having a mixture of Amberlite IRA 410 resin beads (0.5 to 1 mm diameter) and polycarbophil to fasted volunteers and found that the polycarbophil did not retard the gastric emptying of pellets for more than 1 hour. Harris et al. [43] also conducted a similar study and reported that neither polycarbophil nor Carbopol-934 increased the gastric and intestinal transit times significantly. Technetium-99m-labelled microspheres of albumin, starch, and DEAE-dextran (40 to 60 μm) were administered intranasally to humans and their clearance was followed for 3 hours by gamma-scintigraphy. The half-life of clearance for the starch microspheres was found to be 240 min as compared to 15 min for the powder and liquid control formulations [44]. This was attributed to the adhesion of the swollen starch microspheres to the nasal mucosa. When starch microspheres (48 μm) were loaded with gentamicin and an absorption enhancer, lysolecithin, the availability of nasally administered gentamicin in sheep was increased to about 50% of the intravenous dose as compared to less than 1% for the simple gentamicin solution [45]. Blood level-time profiles of several gentamicin formulations when administered intranasally and intravenously are shown in Figure 1.

FACTORS INFLUENCING THE ADHESION OF MICROPARTICLES

Gamma-scintigraphic studies revealed that the gastric transit time of pellets and single-unit dosage forms can be prolonged considerably by administering them with food. Intestinal transit time was found to be unaffected by the dosage size and density [46,47]. O'Reilly et al. [48] reported that the mean gastric emptying time of Amberlite IRA 410 pellets (0.7 to 1.3 mm diameter) in healthy volunteers was about 3 to 4 hours when administered before, during, or with the meal. However, particle size is very critical if the formulation is to be administered into the nose or trachea or eye. Bioadhesive microparticles of various sizes (ranging from 40 μm to 500 μm) were administered orally [41] and nasally [44]. Adhesion of microparticles to the mucus was achieved by (1) simply mixing the drug-containing particles with the bioadhesive polymer [41], or (2) coating the particles with the bioadhesive polymer [49], or (3) using particles of water-swellable and bioadhesive polymer [45]. Using our simple *in situ* technique [39] various factors influencing the bioadhesion of microparticles

were studied, namely: (a) nominal viscosity of the polymer, (b) the amount of the polymer content in the coat, (c) the mixture of anionic and nonionic celluloses in the coat, (d) the nature of the tissue, (e) the contact time between the particles and the mucus, (f) the moisture content on the mucosa, and (g) the viscosity of the mucus. The mean (n = 6) results obtained are given in this chapter in Figures 3 to 8. Standard deviations are shown as open heads on the histograms.

Materials

Hydrophilic polymers, viz., hydroxypropylmethylcellulose (HPMC) 4000, 15,000 and 100,000 cP and methylcellulose(MC) 4000 cP, sold as Methocel K4M, K15M, K100M and A4M Premium, respectively, by Colorcon Ltd., Orpington, U.K. were used. MC 25 and 1500 cP, sold as Methocel MC 25 and 1500 cP, respectively, were obtained from Fluka AG, Buchs, Switzerland. Polycarbophil (PC), sodium carboxymethylcellulose (Na CMC) and pectin (PT), marketed as Carbopol EX-55 (BFGoodrich, Cleveland, Ohio, U.S.A.), Blanose 7H4F (Aqualon, Delaware, U.S.A.) and Pectin purum (Fluka AG), respectively, were also used to coat the microparticles. N-acetyl-L-cysteine (AC) was also obtained from Fluka. To avoid the influence of the core on the bioadhesive property of the polymer coat (particularly while evaluating the mucoadhesion of the polymers and while studying the various factors affecting the bioadhesion), glass beads of 0.45 to 0.5 mm diameter (ABS, Geneva, Switzerland) and crystals of acetyl salicylic acid, >630 μm (Siegfried, Zofingen, Switzerland) were chosen as model particles and model drug, respectively.

Methods

The glass beads or aspirin crystals were first coated with the polymers using the miniature air-suspension apparatus designed by us for this purpose [50]. After coating, the coated particles were tested for bioadhesion. Representative photographs showing the adhesion of aspirin crystals coated with different polymers to the stomach and intestine are shown in Figure 2. In order to check the influence of the thickness of the mucous layer for bioadhesion, the mucus present on the intestine was gently scraped off before placing the microparticles.

Influence of the Nominal Viscosity of the Polymer

Glass beads were coated with 4% w/w of MC and HPMC of different nominal viscosities and tested for bioadhesion. The results are given in Figure 3. Increase in the nominal viscosity of MC and HPMC did not increase the degree of adhesion of the coated microparticles to the stomach, whereas adhesion to the intestine did increase with the viscosity. It was evi-

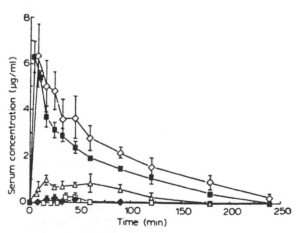

Figure 1. Intranasal and intravenous administration of gentamicin to sheep (mean ± S.E.M.). (□) intranasal gentamicin solution (5 mg/kg) (n = 2); (◆) intranasal gentamicin solution (5 mg/kg) containing 2 mg/ml lysophosphatidylcholine (0.026 mg/kg) (n = 3); (△) intranasal gentamicin (5 mg/kg) in combination with starch microspheres (n = 3); (◇) intranasal gentamicin (5 mg/kg) in combination with starch microspheres and lysophosphatidylcholine (0.2 mg/kg) (n = 3) and (■) intravenous gentamicin solution (2 mg/kg) (n = 3).

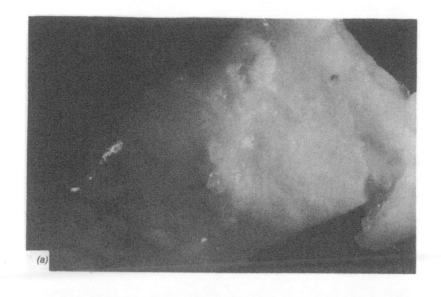

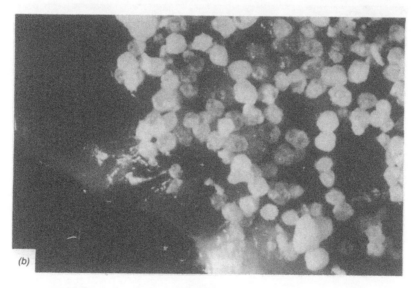

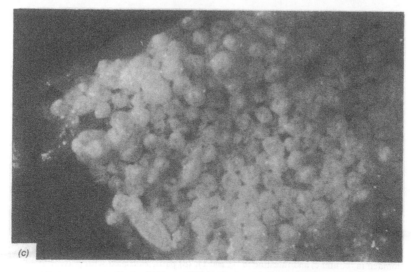

Figure 2. Adhesion of acetylsalicylic acid crystals on the mucosa of the rat stomach (a, b, and c) and intestine (d, e, and f) (p. 263): (a) uncoated particles; (b) particles coated with polycarbophil; (c) particles coated with sodium carboxymethylcellulose 4000 cP.

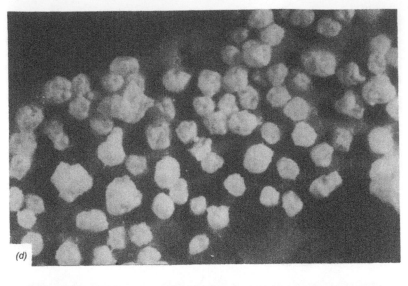

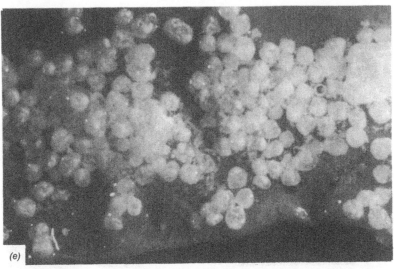

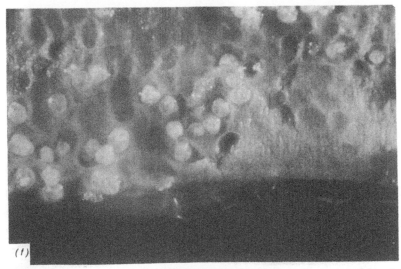

Figure 2 (continued). Adhesion of acetylsalicylic acid crystals on the mucosa of the rat stomach (a, b, and c) and intestine (d, e, and f): (d) particles coated with polycarbophil; (e) particles coated with hydroxypropylmethylcellulose 4000 cP; (f) particles coated with methylcellulose 1500 cP.

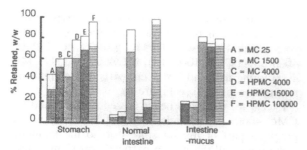

Figure 3. Adhesion of drug particles to stomach, normal intestine, and intestine with minimum amount of mucus, when coated with polymers of different nominal viscosities. A, B and C correspond to methylcellulose 25, 1500 and 4000 cP, respectively. D, E and F correspond to hydroxypropylmethylcellulose 4000, 15,000 and 100,000 cP, respectively.

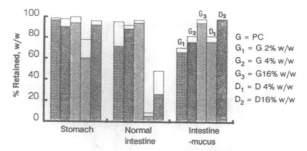

Figure 4. Adhesion of drug particles to stomach, normal intestine, and intestine with minimum amount of mucus, when different amounts of polymer were present in the coat. G_1, G_2, and G_3 correspond to drug particles coated with 2%, 4%, and 16% w/w of polycarbophil. D_1 and D_2 correspond to drug particles coated with 4% and 16% w/w of hydroxypropylmethylcellulose 4000 cP.

dent from the data obtained with the two nonionic cellulose ethers that when the viscosity of the polymer was above a certain value, the polymer adheres strongly to the intestinal mucus. Thus, when the viscosities of the MC and HPMC were 4000 and 100,000, respectively, their chain lengths might have been sufficient to penetrate deep into the glycoprotein network. Significant adhesion of HPMC to the intestine with minimum mucus (most of the mucus was removed gently before placing the particles) indicates that the epithelial cells have strong affinity for the HPMC.

Influence of the Amount of the Polymer in the Coat

For this purpose, glass beads were coated with different amounts of polycarbophil (2%, 4%, and 16% w/w) and HPMC 4000 (4% and 16% w/w). The findings are shown in Figure 4.

Increase in the amount of HPMC 4000 in the coat (i.e., thickness of the coat) increased the degree of adhesion of the particles to the stomach, natural intestine, and intestine with minimum mucus (Figure 4). This may be because more polymer chains become relaxed when exposed to a humid atmosphere, and hence more chains penetrate into the mucus. Owing to the presence of the carboxyl groups in PC, its adhesion to mucus was reported to be stronger [3] and hence even when the polymer content was minimal in the coat, its adhesion was very strong. But for cellulose ethers like HPMC and MC, 2% w/w of the polymer in the coat was insufficient to adhere to the mucus, indicating that some minimum thickness of their coat is needed for strong adhesion. To confirm the influence of the thick coat, particles of PC, Na CMC, HPMC 4000 and 100,000, MC 1500 and pectin were prepared by dry compression and placed (50 mg) on the intestine. All these particles formed a gel-like layer and adhered strongly to the intestine, and hence no difference was seen between them.

Influence of the Mixture of the Anionic and Nonionic Polymers in the Coat

It is well established that a synergistic increase in the viscosity occurs when an anionic polymer (like Na CMC) and a nonionic polymer (like HPMC) are mixed, owing to the stronger hydrogen bonding between the carboxyl groups of Na CMC and the hydroxyl groups of the HPMC [51]. Hence, to check its influence on bioadhesion, the glass beads were coated (4% w/w) with a mixture of HPMC 4000 and Na CMC 4000 (1:1) and MC 1500 and Na CMC 4000 (1:1). These particles were tested and an increase in adhesion was seen only with those of HPMC and Na CMC and that too on normal intestine alone (see Figure 5).

This suggests that the synergistic increase in the viscosity need not increase bioadhesion and that the individual polymer chain length or its molecular weight is more important.

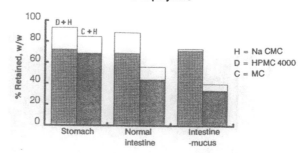

Figure 5. Adhesion of drug particles to stomach, normal intestine, and intestine with minimum amount of mucus, when coated with a mixture (1:1) of anionic and nonionic cellulose ethers. D + H correspond to the mixture of sodium carboxymethylcellulose 4000 cP and hydroxypropylmethylcellulose 4000 cP; C + H correspond to the mixture of sodium carboxymethylcellulose 4000 cP and methylcellulose 4000 cP.

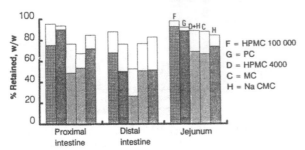

Figure 6. Adhesion of polymer-coated drug particles to proximal intestine, distal intestine and jejunum. Drug crystals were coated with: (F) hydroxypropylmethylcellulose 100,000 cP; (G) polycarbophil; D + H correspond to the mixture (1:1) of sodium carboxymethylcellulose 4000 cP and hydroxypropylmethylcellulose 4000 cP; (c) methylcellulose 1500 cP and (H) sodium carboxymethylcellulose 4000 cP.

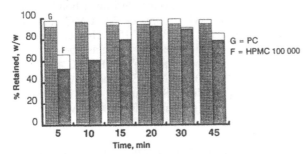

Figure 7. Adhesion of polymer-coated drug particles to jejunum when they were kept in contact with each other for various periods of time. (G) polycarbophil and (F) hydroxypropylmethylcellulose 4000 cP.

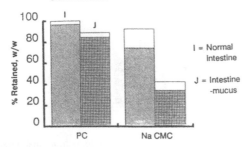

Figure 8. Adhesion of polycarbophil (PC) and sodium carboxymethylcellulose 4000 cP (Na CMC) coated drug particles to (I) normal intestine and (J) intestine with minimum mucus.

Influence of the Nature of the Tissue

Since the composition of the mucus varies in different regions of the GI tract, adhesion of particles coated with 4% w/w of HPMC 100,000, PC, HPMC 4000 + Na CMC 4000 (1:1), MC 4000, and Na CMC 4000 to the first and last 5 cm parts of the small intestine was tested (see Figure 6).

Except for the glass beads coated with PC and Na CMC 4000, the particles adhered less well to the proximal part of the intestine than to the jejunum. Adhesion of all the coated particles was significantly less at the distal end of the small intestine compared with the jejunum.

Influence of the Contact Time Between the Particles and the Mucus

In order to know the optimum contact time needed for the formation of the strong adhesive bond between the coated particles and the tissue, particles coated with PC (16% w/w) and HPMC 100,000 (4% w/w) were placed on the jejunum and kept in the desiccator for 5 to 45 min. Later, the tissue was washed with the buffer as described earlier (see Figure 7).

It was observed that the adhesion of PC-coated beads was same from 5 to 45 min and for those coated with HPMC 100,000, the adhesion reached a maximum at 20 min and later decreased, perhaps due to the dissolution of the polymer coat. This shows that contact time is critical for soluble polymers like HPMC.

Influence of the Moisture Content on the Tissue

In order to know whether the content of water present on the tissue influences bioadhesion, the moisture present on the tissue was blotted gently with a fine tissue paper before placing the microparticles. Particles coated (4% w/w) with Na CMC 4000 and PC were used for this study. Results are shown in Figure 8.

Removal of the moisture from the intestinal mucosa (using a fine filter paper) decreased the adhesion of Na CMC 4000-coated particles to the intestine from 74% to 35%. PC-coated particles adhered strongly even when the moisture was minimum. This study suggests that the moisture content is important for soluble polymers like celluloses and not so important for insoluble polymers like polycarbophil. Since the moisture needed for the relaxation of the polymer chains is different for different polymers, the fall in the adhesion of Na CMC-coated particles may be attributed to the incomplete relaxation of the polymer chains of Na CMC.

Influence of the Viscosity of the Mucus

The mucolytic activity of N-acetyl-L-cysteine (AC) was reported to be maximum at pH 9 and when kept in contact with the mucus for 1 hour [52]. Rat intestinal mucosa was found to be unaffected when the concentration of AC was 4% w/v [53]. Therefore, to study this factor, 0.05 and 0.01 ml of 4% w/v of a freshly prepared solution of AC (pH adjusted to 9 with sodium hydroxide solution) were added to the mucosa of the jejunum and kept aside at room temperature before placing the PC-coated (4% w/w) glass beads. Later the study was completed in the usual manner. The adhesion was unaffected by 0.05 ml of AC. However, in the presence of 0.1 ml of AC, only 26.37 ± 6.08% of the particles adhered as compared to 88.8 ± 3.3% in the absence of AC. This indicates that the structure and the viscosity of the mucus are important for bioadhesion.

CONCLUSIONS

Research in the area of bioadhesive drug delivery systems has become very popular in recent years. Bioadhesive microparticles are preferred to macromatrices since the former cause minimum irritation to the mucosa and can be administered through different routes for both topical and systemic applications. A better understanding of (1) the strucutre of the mucus, (2) the mechanism of interaction between the polymer and the mucus, and (3) various technological factors which may influence the adhesion of the dosage form to the mucus, will enable the researchers to prepare biocompatible, stable and bioadhesive polymers, and ultimately clinically useful bioadhesive drug delivery systems. From our specific study, the following conclusions can be drawn.

Increase in the nominal viscosity and thickness of the HPMC coat increased the adhesion. Coating the particles with a mixture of anionic and nonionic polymers had no beneficial effect. Particles adhered better to the jejunum than to the proximal or distal end of the intestine. Contact time and moisture content were important for soluble polymers like celluloses but not for insoluble polymers like polycarbophil. The structure and viscosity of the mucus are important for adhesion.

ACKNOWLEDGEMENT

We are grateful to Dr M. Ali F. Hussein, Geneva, for reading the manuscript. Permission to publish Figure 1 from *Int. J. Pharm.*, 46(1988):261–265 was granted by Professor P. F. D'Arcy, Editor-in-Chief, *Int. J. Pharm.* and Professor L. Illum, University of Nottingham. We are thankful to both of them.

REFERENCES

1. Park, K., H. S. Ch'ng and J. R. Robinson. 1984. "Alternative Approaches to Oral Controlled Drug Delivery: Bioadhesives and *in situ* Systems", in *Recent Advances in Drug Delivery*. J. M. Anderson and S. W. Kim, eds. New York, NY: Plenum, pp. 163–183.
2. Nagal, T. and Y. Machida. 1985. *Pharm. Int.*, 6:196.
3. Peppas, N. A. and P. Buri. 1985. *J. Controlled Release*, 2:257.
4. Longer, M. and J. R. Robinson. 1986. *Pharm. Int.*, 7:114.
5. Mikos, A. G. and N. A. Peppas. 1986. *S.T.P. Pharma.*, 2:705.
6. Duchene, D., F. Touchard and N. A. Peppas. 1988. *Drug Dev. Ind. Pharm.*, 14:283.
7. Duchene, D., G. Ponchel, D. Wouessidjewe, F. Lejoyeux and N. A. Peppas. 1988. *S.T.P. Pharma.*, 4:688.
8. Park, K., S. L. Cooper and J. R. Robinson. 1988. "Bioadhesive Hydrogels", in *Hydrogels in Medicine and Pharmacy, Vol. III, Properties and Applications*. N. A. Peppas, ed. Boca Raton, FL: CRC, pp. 151–175.
9. Spiro, R. G. 1970. *Ann. Rev. Biochem.*, 39:599.
10. Labat-Robert, J. and C. Decaeus. 1979. *Path. Biol.*, 24:241.
11. Pfaltz, C. R., ed. 1979. *La Muqueuse Nasale, ses Problemes, Forum Medici.*, Nyon, Switzerland: Zyma S. A., No. 11.
12. Melon, J. 1968. *Acta Oto-Rhino-Laryngol. Belg.*, 22:1.
13. Scawen, M. and A. Allen. 1977. *Biochem. J.*, 163:363.
14. Slater, H. S., G. Lamblin, A. Le Treut, C. Galabert, N. Houdret, P. Degand and P. Roussel. 1984. *Eur. J. Biochem.*, 142:209.
15. Gottschalka, A. and A. S. Bhargava. 1972. "Submaxillary Gland Glycoproteins", in *Glycoproteins: Their Composition, Structure and Function*. A. Gottschalka, 2nd ed. Amsterdam: Elsevier, pp. 810–829.
16. Horowitz, M. I. 1977. "Gastrointestinal Glycoproteins", in *The Glycoconjugates*. M. I. Horowitz and W. Pigman, eds. Vol. I. New York: Academic Press, pp. 189–213.
17. Johnson, P. M. and K. D. Rainsford. 1972. *Biochim. Biophys. Acta*, 286:72.
18. Robert, C. and P. Buri. 1986. *Pharm. Acta Helv.*, 61:210.
19. Gilmore, P. T., R. Falabella and R. L. Laurence. 1980. *Macromolecules*, 13:880.
20. Tirrel, M. 1984. *Rubb. Chem. Technol.*, 57:523.
21. Smart, J. D., I. W. Kellaway and H. E. C. Worthington. 1984. *J. Pharm. Pharmacol.*, 36:295.
22. Chen, J. L. and G. N. Cyr. 1970. "Compositions Producing Adhesions through Hydration", in *Adhesion in Biological Systems*. R. S. Manly, ed. New York, NY: Academic Press, pp. 163–181.
23. Park, H. and J. R. Robinson. 1985. *J. Controlled Release*, 2:47.
24. Leung, S. S. and J. R. Robinson. 1988. *J. Controlled Release*, 5:223.
25. de Bruyne, N. A. 1951. *Adhesion and Adhesives*, New York: Elsevier.
26. de Bruyne, N. A. 1957. *Nature*, 180:262.
27. Wang, P. Y. and D. H. Forrester. 1974. *Trans. Am. Soc. Artif. Int. Organs*, 20:504.
28. Reich, S., M. Levy, A. Meshorer, M. Blumental, R. Yalon, J. W. Sheets and E. P. Goldberg. 1984. *J. Biomed. Mater. Res.*, 18:737.

29. Ponchel, G., F. Touchard, D. Duchene and N. A. Peppas. 1987. *J. Controlled Release*, 5:129.

30. Ch'ng, H. S., H. Park, P. Kelly and J. R. Robinson. 1985. *J. Pharm. Sci.*, 74:399.

31. Marvola, M., K. Vahervuo, A. Sothmann, E. Marttila and M. Rajaniemi. 1982. *J. Pharm. Sci.*, 71:975.

32. Marvola, M., M. Rajaniemi, E. Marttila, K. Vahervuo and A. Sothmann. 1983. *J. Pharm. Sci.*, 72:1034.

33. Al-Dujaili, H., A. T. Florence and E. G. Salole. 1986. *Int. J. Pharm.*, 34:75.

34. Robert, C., P. Buri and N. A. Peppas. 1988. *Acta Pharm. Technol.*, 34:95.

35. Ishida, M., Y. Machida, N. Nambu and T. Nagai. 1981. *Chem. Pharm. Bull.*, 29:810.

36. Park, K. and J. R. Robinson. 1984. *Int. J. Pharm.*, 19:107.

37. Bridges, J. F., J. F. Woodley, R. Duncan and J. Kopecek. 1988. *Int. J. Pharm.*, 44:213.

38. Bridges, J. F., J. F. Woodley, R. Duncan, P. Kopeckova and J. Kopecek. 1987. *Proc. Int. Symp. Controlled Release Mater.*, 14:14.

39. Ranga Rao, K. V. and P. Buri. September 1987. *Proc. 47th Int. Cong. Pharm. Sci. F.I.P.*, Amsterdam, Abstract No. 281.

40. Lehr, C.-M., J. A. Bouwstra, F. G. J. Poelma, J. J. Tukker and H. E. Junginer. 1988. *Proc. 3rd Int. Conf. Drug Absorption September*, p. 66.

41. Longer, M. A., H. S. Ch'ng and J. R. Robinson. 1985. *J. Pharm. Sci.*, 74:406.

42. Khosla, R. and S. S. Davis. 1987. *J. Pharm. Pharmacol.*, 39:47.

43. Harris, D., H. Sharma, A. Smith, J. Fell and D. Taylor. 1987. *Proc. Int. Symp. Controlled Release Mater.*, 14:12.

44. Illum, L., H. Jorgensen, H. Bisgaard, O. Krogsgaard and N. Rossing. 1987. *Int. J. Pharm.*, 39:189.

45. Illum, L., N. Farraj, H. Critchley and S. S. Davis. 1988. *Int. J. Pharm.*, 46:261.

46. Davis, S. S. 1985. *J. Controlled Release*, 2:27.

47. Wilson, C. G. and N. Washington. 1988. *Drug Dev. Ind. Pharm.*, 14:211.

48. O'Reilly, S., C. G. Wilson and J. G. Hardy. 1987. *Int. J. Pharm.*, 34:213.

49. Ranga Rao, K. V. and P. Buri. 1988. *Proc. Int. Symp. Controlled Release Mater.*, 15:103.

50. Ranga Rao, K. V. and P. Buri. 1989. *Acta Pharm. Technol.*, 35:256.

51. Walker, C. V. and J I. Wells. 1982. *Int. J. Pharm.*, 11:309.

52. Sheffner, A. L. 1963. *Ann. N. Y. Acad. Sci.*, 106:298.

53. Schiller, M., J. L. Grosfeld and T. S. Morse. 1971. *Am. J. Surg.*, 122:22.

Part 4

BLOOD COMPATIBILITY AND VASCULAR PROSTHESES

19

Nonthrombogenic Graft Copolymers

HAJIME MIYAMA*

ABSTRACT: Use of graft copolymers as nonthrombogenic material is very practical, because it is not difficult to modify a conventional polymer in such a way that the trunk of the graft copolymer provides mechanical support and the side chains provide nonthrombogenicity. Various kinds of nonthrombogenic polymers are introduced briefly, and the synthesis and application of heparinized graft copolymers and hydrophilic graft copolymers having poly(ethylene oxide) side chains are described. Particularly, for the latter polymer, correlation between platelet adhesion and plasma protein adsorption is discussed.

INTRODUCTION

In order to develop medical application of plastics for artificial internal organs, many nonthrombogenic polymers have been synthesized. The synthesis has been carried out by changing the composition and microstructure of the polymer surface or by binding an antithrombogenic reagent such as heparin to the polymer. However, most of the polymers do not have both excellent nonthrombogenicity and satisfactory mechanical strength. Therefore, it is more practical to modify conventional polymers such as poly(vinyl chloride) or polyacrylonitrile because various polymers of desired mechanical and physical properties are available. In particular, the use of graft copolymers is very effective because it is not difficult to design graft copolymer in such a way that the trunk of the graft copolymer provides the mechanical support and side chains provide nonthrombogenicity. The author will introduce heparinized graft copolymers and graft copolymers having poly(ethylene oxide)

(PEO) side chains as examples of nonthrombogenic graft copolymers.

NONTHROMBOGENIC POLYMERS

To design nonthrombogenic polymers, there are many approaches, as follows:

(1) When a cloth of synthetic fibres such as poly(ethylene telephthalate) is brought in contact with blood, a thrombus layer is formed initially on the surface of the cloth. Then adhesion and growth of endothelium occurs on the thrombus layer, which leads to the formation of neointima or pseudointima. This gives excellent nonthrombogenicity to the cloth [1].

(2) Pharmaceutical reagents such as urokinase or heparin are immobilized to the polymer [2]. The former reagent decomposes fibrin to dissolve the thrombus. The latter prevents activation of coagulation factors and platelets to give thrombogenicity to the polymer.

(3) Platelet adhesion and morphologic change of the adhered platelets are suppressed by microphase-separated structures of polymers such as 2-hydroxymethyl methacrylate/styrene block copolymer [3].

(4) Grafting of hydrophilic groups to bulk polymer [4] or polymer surface [5] prevents platelet adhesion, to give nonthrombogenicity to the polymer.

Recently Noishiki et al. [6] combined the first and second approaches and developed a small-caliber vascular graft by a cross-linking method incorporating slow heparin release collagen and natural tissue compliance. All of these approaches may be applied to the synthesis of nonthrombogenic graft polymers. In this report, the second and fourth ap-

*Consultant, Doctor of Science, Kataseyama 3-14-10, Fujisawa 251, Japan

proaches will be introduced by referring mainly to studies on the graft polymers.

HEPARINIZED GRAFT COPOLYMERS

Immobilization of Heparin

As described above, one of the approaches to developing nonthrombogenic polymers is to incorporate pharmacologically active agents within polymers. This approach, especially involving immobilization of heparin and prostaglandin, was well reviewed by Kim et al. [2] The most widely studied pharmaceutical agents are heparin, prostaglandin and urokinase. Sometimes combinations of these agents have been studied [2,7]. In order to immobilize the agent within the polymer, many methods have been reported such as physical adsorption, blending or dispersion, ionic bonding, and covalent bonding. In the former three methods, the polymer releases the agent which prevents blood coagulation in blood flow. In the covalent bonding method, the agent is fixed within the polymer or on the polymer surface, and is not released from the polymer.

A study of the heparin-releasing material was initiated by Got et al. [8] who bound heparin ionically to a cationic surfactant adsorbed onto the graphite surface. Leininger et al. [9] modified the method and synthesized a polymer having quaternary amine groups which bind heparin ionically. Both of the materials release heparin by an ion exchange mechanism with anions of blood flow, but are not tough enough to be used practically. Thereafter, Miyama et al. [10] photochemically synthesized poly(vinyl chloride) graft copolymer having quaternary amine groups which were heparinized. Tanzawa et al. [11] evaluated the heparinized polymers and developed them into an antithrombogenic catheter which is now in practical use. A similar method was used to obtain heparinized polyacrylonitrile graft copolymer [12]. Also, polyurethane has been well studied as a matrix for heparin-releasing polymer. The interaction of platelets with plasma proteins adsorbed to the surface of heparinized polyurethane was reviewed by Ito [13]. Ito et al. [14] synthesized polyetherurethaneurea having tertiary amino groups, then quaternized and heparinized the polymer. They found from *in vivo* tests that either platelet adhesion and activation or thrombus formation decreased by quaternization and further by heparinization of polyurethaneureas, which agreed with an *in vitro* blood clotting test [15].

Long-term application of the heparin-releasing polymer for medical use is not expected. Covalently bound heparin is considered to meet the long-term nonthrombogenicity standards. Many studies on covalently immobilized heparin polymers have been published [2]. Various polymers such as silicone, polyvinyl alcohol, methyl methacrylate copolymers, agarose, styrene–butadiene–styrene elastomer, colla-

gen, cellulose and polyurethane were used as matrices [2,16]. In particular, blood compatibility of the heparinized polyurethanes having alkyl [17] or poly (ethylene oxide) [18,19] spacer arms was evaluated fully and in detail.

Among the above described heparinized polymers, there were not many heparinized graft polymers. However, heparinized graft polymer is very important from academic and practical viewpoints because the trunk of the graft polymer takes the part of mechanical support, while the side chains take the part of blood compatibility and other functions, as described below. Therefore, as typical examples, heparinized poly(vinyl chloride), polyacrylonitrile and polyurethane graft copolymers will be explained in detail.

Heparinized Poly(vinyl chloride) Graft Copolymers

Miyama et al. [10] carbamated poly(vinyl chloride) by the following reaction.

$$- CH-CH_2 - \; + \; NaSCSN(C_2H_5)_2 \; \rightarrow \; - CH-CH_2 - \; + \; NaCl$$
$$| \qquad\qquad\qquad\qquad\qquad\qquad\qquad\qquad |$$
$$Cl \qquad\qquad\qquad\qquad\qquad\qquad\qquad SCSN(C_2H_5)_2$$

To the modified polymer, methoxypoly(ethyleneglycol) methacrylate (SM),

$$CH_3$$
$$|$$
$$CH_2 = C - C - (OCH_2 CH_2)_n - OCH_3$$
$$||$$
$$O$$

and N,N-dimethylaminoethyl methacrylate (DAEM),

$$CH_3$$
$$|$$
$$CH_2 = C - C - O - (CH_2)_2 - N(CH_3)_2$$
$$||$$
$$O$$

were simultaneously photografted. Dimethylamino groups of the graft polymer were quaternized to give positive charges. To the positive charges of the polymer, antithrombogenic heparin molecules which have negative charges were ionically bound. Here the trunk of the graft copolymer takes the part of mechanical support, the hydrophilic group (SM) the part of biocompatibility, and the heparinized group the part of nonthrombogenicity, respectively. In order to avoid contamination by plasticizer, commercial graft copolymer of vinyl chloride, ethylene and vinyl acetate (Graftmer R_3) was used instead of poly(vinyl chloride) with plasticizer. The kinetics of photochemical synthesis of the graft polymer was studied in detail [20].

Tanzawa et al. [11,21] evaluated the heparinized copolymer. Catheters made of the heparinized polymer (about 30 cm in length, 0.3 cm O.D., and 100–200 μm in wall thickness) were inserted through the right femoral vein into the inferior vena cava of a dog under intravenous pentobarbital sodium anesthesia. The right femoral vein was ligated at the site of insertion of the catheter. Prior to the implantation into the inferior vena cava, the catheter was filled with sterilized Ringer's solution, and its distal end was closed with a Teflon plug, so that the blood did not enter the lumen of the catheter. After two weeks, the dogs were sacrificed by acute exsanguination from the aorta and examined at autopsy for the thrombus formation around the catheters.

The *in vivo* results are shown in Table 1 together with the chemical composition of the heparinized polymers. Neither the polymers of low water content nor those of high water content showed good *in vivo* results. Those of medium water content (Group 2) gave the best result. On the other hand, release of heparin from the polymer surface was measured by circulating canine ACD plasma through the catheters. The ACD plasma used was stored frozen at $-74\,°C$ in siliconized glass bottles and thawed quickly in 5 min by heating in a warm bath at $38\,°C$. Twenty ml of ACD plasma were circulated through a catheter for 16 to 17 hr at flow rates of 50 ml/min. Heparin content was measured at intervals of 60 min, utilizing a one ml sampling. After each sampling, 1 ml of fresh plasma was added to keep the total amount of the circulating plasma volume constant.

The results showed that the heparin release rate for Group 1 is low and that for Group 3 is high, and that the critical elution rate to give *in vivo* thromboresistance is around 4×10^{-8} g/cm²/min. Further, it was confirmed that the elution rate kept constant for Group 2 but decreased rapidly for Group 3. Thus, it

was concluded that ionically bounded heparin is released from the polymer surface into blood and that the release rate depends upon heparin content and water content. The heparin release mechanism was considered to be controlled by two steps: (1) the dissociation of the ionic complex between heparin and the cationic sites of the polymer, and (2) the diffusion of dissociated heparin through the polymer matrix. The first step is mainly determined by the number of heparin molecules bound to the cationic sites. The latter step largely depends upon the water content of the polymer, which differs considerably for each polymer group as shown in Table 1. It was found from the study that the heparinized polymer having a heparin content of about 15% and water content of about 30% has the best nonthrombogenicity.

Mori et al. [22] studied the effect of released heparin on the process of thrombus formation, and proposed that the continuous existence of a certain amount of free heparin near the polymer surface prevents the release of some thrombus-inducing substances from adherent platelets. They also proposed that the heparinized polymer having a sufficient water and heparin content provides sufficient concentration of free heparin in the interface between the polymer and blood by balancing the loss of heparin from the polymer surface into the bloodstream with the heparin diffusion from the inside of the polymer. Also, Basmadjian and Sefton [23] proved that the above described value of the critical heparin elution rate is valid, by using mathematical models to predict surface concentrations that result from the release of heparin into flowing blood and stagnant or well-mixed plasma.

The best heparinized polymer showed nonthrombogenicity for more than 3 months in the *in vivo* test and excellent results for up to 3 weeks of implantation in clinical tests [22]. The catheter made of the heparinized polymer is commercialized under the name of "Anthron" by Toray Industries, Inc. Here, the catheter is prepared by coating inner and outer surface of a polyurethane tube with the heparinized polymer to

Table 1. Composition, properties and blood compatibility of heparinized poly(vinyl chloride) graft copolymers (from p. 250 of Reference [21]).

	Sample No.	Graft (%)	SM (%)	DAEM (%)	Ad. Hep.	W (%)	N ● (meq./g)	SNP (m Volt)	Smoothness	*In vivo* Results
	103	15	0	15	15	27	0.84	−33	○	×
1	102	22	0	22	15	28	0.88	−32	○	×
	113	17	2	15	12	27	0.76	−32	○	×
	107	22	5	17	13	(48)	0.83	−28	○	△
2	110	30	12	18	13	37	0.76	−25	○	○
	23	32	16	16	7	49	0.80	−19	○	○
3	109	42	23	19	12	76	0.77	−13	○	△
	111	55	20	35	16	80	1.04	−21	×	×

SM: methoxypolyethyleneglycol methacrylate, W: water content/dry polymer, DAEM: 2-dimethylaminoethyl methacrylate, SMP: standard membrane potential, Ad. Hep.: heparin content/dry polymer, Smoothness: surface condition.

Table 2. Properties of quaternized and heparinized polyacrylonitrile graft copolymer (from p. 899 of Reference [12]).

Sample Number	Quaternized Polymer		Heparinized Polymer		
	Water Content	N+ Content	Water Content	Heparin Content	Release Rate* of Heparin
	wt%	mmol·g⁻¹	wt%	g·g⁻¹	µg·cm⁻²·min⁻¹
1	22	0.18	21	0.036	—
2	34	0.27	33	0.098	1.3
3	39	0.61	33	0.202	—
4	46	0.30	44	0.116	5.7
5	49	0.53	43	0.187	14.7

*Initial release rate of heparin.

give flexibility to the catheter. The tube is also used as a bypass tube for surgery of pancreas cancer, etc.

Miyama et al. [12] used polyacrylonitrile instead of poly(vinyl chloride) in the synthesis of heparinized graft copolymer. At first, acrylonitrile (AN) was photopolymerized by using carbon tetrabromide as an initiator in dimethylsulfoxide (DMSO) solution. The obtained polymer (PANBr) contained 10–20 bromine atoms per polymer molecule and was photosensitive. To PANBr, SM and DAEM were photografted in DMSO. Tertiary amino groups of the DAEM part of the polymer were quaternized and then heparinized. Preliminary tests [24] showed the following results: (1) water content of the quaternized polymer increased proportionally to ethylene oxide (EO) content, (2) the amount of platelet adhering to the heparinized polymer decreased with an increase of EO content according to an *in vitro* test, (3) the higher the water content of the heparinized polymer, the higher was the release rate of heparin. Here, kinetics of photochemical synthesis was studied in detail [25].

In Table 2, properties of the quaternized and heparinized copolymers used for *in vivo* tests are shown [12]. An *in vivo* test was carried out by Noishiki's method [26] as follows. A pliable and soft suture of about 10 cm in length was coated with the test polymer. For the experiment, a dog under general anesthesia was used. An 18 gauge needle was inserted into a peripheral vein and the polymer-coated suture was then inserted through the needle into the lumen of the vessel. After the needle was withdrawn, the end of the suture was fixed near the area of the vessel puncture. After a given period of time, the animal was sacrificed by acute exsanguination under general anesthesia and heparin administration. The vein in which the suture was inserted was opened and observation was carried out macroscopically and by means of light microscopy.

The results of the *in vivo* test are shown in Figure 1. For nonheparinized cationic polymer (NH3PAN) which corresponds to Sample No. 4 in Table 2, red thrombus formation incorporating red blood corpuscles and fibrins was observed. However, no thrombus formation was observed for any of the heparinized

polymers as shown in the pictures. Also, no fibrin precipitation was noted by light microscopic observation. Stress–strain curves, tensile strength, and elongation of the heparinized polyacrylonitrile copolymer and the heparinized poly(vinyl chloride) copolymer (HRSD) showed that the heparinized polyacrylonitrile copolymers are tougher than HRSD. Therefore, the former seems to be very promising for medical applications.

Heparinized Polyurethane Graft Copolymers

Polyurethanes have excellent mechanical properties and *in vivo* durability and are widely used as biomedical polymers. Although both ionic and covalent heparinization of polyurethanes have been tried as described above, only the latter study will be introduced here.

Han et al. [18] modified surfaces of commercial polyurethanes by grafting PEO and heparinization as follows. Polyurethane (PU) sheet (Pellethane 2363-80A; Upjohn Co.) was extracted with methanol and immersed in toluene. Following this, octoate and hexamethylene diisocyanate (HMDI) were added. The reacted sheet was washed in toluene and then anhydrous ether to yield PU-HMDI. The PU-HMDI sheet was reacted with PEO in benzene with stannous octate to produce PU-PEO. Direct immobilization of heparin onto PU-HMDI was carried out by reacting the PU-HMDI sheet with formamide or water solution containing heparin and PU-HMDI-Hep(FA) or PU-HMDI-Hep(H₂O) was obtained. Immobilization of heparin onto PU-PEO via glutaraldehyde (GA) linkage to prepare PU-PEO-GA-Hep was performed by a modification of Peppas' method [27]. Finally, the PU-PEO sheet was treated with HMDI as in the preparation of PU-HMDI, and reacted with heparin as in the direct immobilization of heparin onto PU-HMDI. Thus PU-PEO-HMDI-Hep was obtained. The reaction scheme and surface chemical structure of each modified PU were confirmed by attenuated total reflection infrared and electron spectroscopy for chemical analysis, respectively. In order to estimate the surface heparin concentration, the toluidine blue

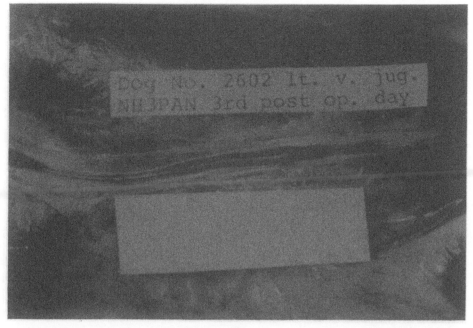

(a)

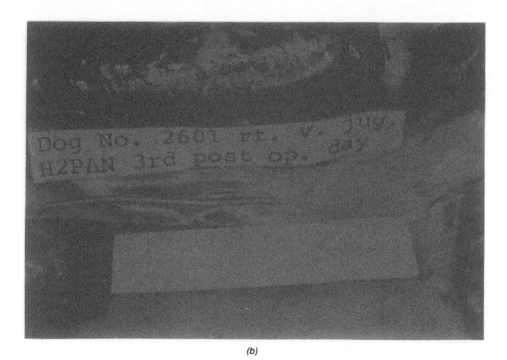

(b)

Figure 1. Open views of peripheral vein in which a suture coated with the polymer was inserted. (a) non-heparinized cationic polymer of Sample No. 4, (b), (c) and (d) heparinized polymers, Sample No. 2, 4 and 3, respectively (from p. 901 of Reference [12]).

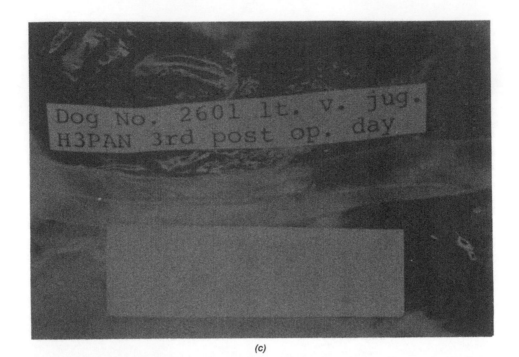

(c)

(d)

Figure 1 (continued). Open views of peripheral vein in which a suture coated with the polymer was inserted. (a) non-heparinized cationic polymer of Sample No. 4, (b), (c) and (d) heparinized polymers, Sample No. 2, 4 and 3, respectively (from p. 901 of Reference [12]).

dye depletion method [28] was used. The hydrophilicity of the surface was evaluated by Wilhelmy plate method [29].

The concentrations of immobilized heparin on modified PU sheets varied insignificantly from 1.45 to 1.48 $\mu g/cm^2$ but showed a slight decrease with increasing chain length of the PEO spacer for PU-PEO-GA-Hep and PU-PEO-HMDI-Hep. The PU control surface showed values of advancing and receding contact angles of a typical hydrophobic surface. Heparinized surfaces PU-PEO-GA-Hep and PU-PEO-HMDI-Hep showed a complete wetting behaviour on receding. This was considered to be due to the synergistic effect of the hydrophilic PEO grafting and the ionic $-SO_3H$ groups of heparin. Data on the nonheparinized sheets will be discussed later.

Moreover, Han et al. [19] evaluated the blood compatibility of the modified PU sheets. They found from *in vitro* and *ex vivo* tests that the heparinized PU-PEO surfaces displayed enhanced blood compatibility due to the synergistic effects of PEO and heparin. Among their results, those of the activated partial thromboplastin time (APTT) test, the prothrombin time (PT) test and the heparin bioactivity test will be introduced. The former two tests were carried out by the Fibrometer method [30] and the one-stage prothrombin time method [31], respectively. The last one performed as follows [32].

Heparin usually forms heparin-antithrombin III (ATIII)-thrombin (T) complex with ATIII in plasma. Therefore, by making heparin complexes with excess amounts of thrombin and determining the amount of thrombin consumed with Chromozym TH(Tos-Gly-Pro-Arg-pNA, Boehringer Mannheim), bioactivity of heparin can be measured indirectly. Here, thrombin acts as a catalyst in the splitting of paranitroaniline (pNA) from Chromozym TH. The pNA release rate is determined by measuring the absorbance at 405 nm. The quantity of heparin in the plasma was analyzed by utilizing the Heparin Low Dose Kit (Boehringer Mannheim). Here, APTT, PT and chromogenic tests relate to the bioactivity of intrinsic blood coagulation factors, that of extrinsic blood coagulation factors and the thrombin neutralization activity of immobilized heparin, respectively. Results of the APTT tests showed a prolongation of clotting times for the heparinized PU sheets compared with those for PU control or PU-PEO sheets, but those of PT tests did not show any significant increases in the prolongation of clotting times. Therefore, this indicates that the immobilized heparin influences the intrinsic blood coagulation factors rather than the extrinsic ones. Results of the chromogenic tests showed that the concentration of active heparin is around 10–27% irrespective of the chain length of PEO or the concentration of immobilized heparin. These values were much lower than expected in spite of the high mobility of PEO spacers. The authors suggested that this was probably due to the damage of immobilized heparin molecules during the reaction process.

HYDROPHILIC GRAFT COPOLYMERS

Blood Compatibility of Hydrophilic Polymers

In the early 1960s it was believed that hydrophobic surfaces were blood-compatible. Lyman et al. [33] proposed that the more hydrophobic the surface (the higher the surface free energy) the less thrombogenic it would be. However, this proposition was disproved later when many exceptional cases were found. Thereafter, the blood compatibility of hydrophilic polymers or hydrogels attracted the attention of many researchers. Here, a hydrogel is a kind of polymer–water complex containing a large amount of water. Its biological performance depends on its hydrophilicity, chemical composition, types and number of cross-links, presence of functional groups, quasi-organized water structure, porosity and the interaction between the components of the environment and the gel [34]. Relating to the blood compatibility of materials, Andrade et al. proposed [35,36] the minimal interfacial free energy hypothesis, stating that as the interfacial free energy approaches zero, the driving force for plasma protein adsorption decreases. They considered that hydrogels are blood compatible because of low interaction between the surface and plasma proteins or cells. On the other hand, Ratner et al. [37] proposed the hydrophilic–hydrophobic ratio hypothesis, stating that suitable proteins will be adsorbed and remain adherent if the polar and apolar surface characters are properly balanced.

Coleman et al. [38] tested the two typical hypotheses by using methacrylate polymers and copolymers, and found that neither hypothesis could explain their data on the platelet adhesion and coagulation time. Ikada et al. [5] claimed that hydrophilic chains extended from the graft polymer are highly resistant to thrombus formation. Although none of the hypotheses can explain completely the interaction between the surface and blood components, many trials to synthesize nonthrombogenic hydrophilic polymers or hydrogels have been carried out. Here again, graft polymers are very favorable because trunk polymers and side chains provide mechanical support and hydrophilicity, respectively. Various trunk polymers such as poly(vinyl chloride) [4], polyethylene [5], polyurethane [18,19], polyacrylonitrile [39,40], silicone [41], and fluoro polymer [42] were used as trunk polymers. Here, various hydrophilic polymers such as acrylates and acrylamides were used as side chains. Among the hydrophilic polymers used as side chains, PEO is very attractive because of its high protein-resistant property. Characteristics and application of PEO to blood-compatible polymers were well described by Lee et al. [43] They considered that PEO was an effective polymer for protein-resistant surfaces because of its low interfacial free energy with water, unique solution properties and molecular conformation in aqueous solution, hydrophilicity, high surface mobility and steric stabilization effects. More detailed discussion was given by them. Also, a great deal of interesting data on graft polymers having PEO side chains was collected, and will be introduced below.

Graft Polymers Having PEO Side Chains

Poly(vinyl chloride) Graft Polymers Having PEO Side Chains

Mori, Nagaoka, et al. [4,44] synthesized poly(vinyl chloride) graft copolymers with long PEO side chains and evaluated their blood compatibility. The synthesis was carried out photochemically according to the method of Miyama et al. [10]. Methoxypoly(ethylene-glycol)methacrylate (abbreviated as MnG) with PEO chains of various lengths (n) ($n = 4, 9, 15, 23, 50, 100$ as side chains) was photografted to dithiocarbamated poly(vinyl chloride). The *in vitro* test of the graft copolymer (PVC-g-MnG) was carried out as follows. The blood was withdrawn from the rabbit carotid and placed in a siliconized glass tube containing trisodium citrate aqueous solution. Platelet-rich plasma (PRP) and platelet-poor plasma (PPP) were prepared by conventional methods. The platelet counts (about $2 \times 10^5/\mu l$) in PRP were adjusted by diluting the PRP with the PPP. The membranes of the graft polymers were soaked in PRP at 37°C for 3 hrs. The membranes were then fixed with glutaraldehyde saline solution. The amount of platelet adhered to the membranes was measured by an amino acid analyzer.

Since the water content of the PVC-g-MnG increased linearly with the content of the EO grafted onto the PVC, the PVC containing water ranging from 40–45% was used for the *in vitro* test. Results are shown in Figure 2 [44]. Here, PMMA-co-MnG is random-type hydrogels prepared from copolymers of methyl methacrylate and methoxypoly(ethyleneglycol)monomethacrylates. The amount of adhered platelets (relative value to glass = 1.0) decreases with an increase in the PEO chain length (n) and to almost negligible value at $n = 100$. The graft-type hydrogels show weaker platelet adhesion. The *in vivo* test showed a similar dependence of blood elements ad-

sorption on the PEO chain length for the PVC-g-MnG. They also measured oxygen permeation of the graft- and random-type hydrogels [44]. The oxygen permeability of both hydrogels increased with an increase in PEO chain length where the graft-type hydrogels showed higher values. In the previous report [45], Nagaoka et al. observed a decrease of NMR ^{13}C line width of PEO chain with an increase in water content and PEO chain length for random-type copolymer. They claimed that long PEO chain enhances motion of PEO chains (corresponding to narrowing of ^{13}C line width) and that this effect coupled with the volume-restriction effect causes the decrease of platelet adhesion. The same discussion was applied for the graft-type polymer. Further, oxygen permeation data for the graft-type copolymer indicated existence of higher-order structure in the graft-type hydrogels. This was supported by the microphase-separated structure of the graft-type hydrogels, which was not observed for the random-type hydrogels. As a conclusion, they suggested that the volume-restriction effect resulting from the formation of long-chain PEO on the surface effectively suppresses the adsorption of blood elements and prevents the denaturation of blood elements.

Mori et al. [46,47] studied interactions between PVC-g-MnG hydrogels and circulating platelets by implanting tubes fabricated from the graft polymer between the jugular vein and the carotid artery of rabbits. The adherence of platelets to the tubes significantly decreased with an increase in PEO chain length (n), and the PVC-g-MnG tubes with long-chain PEO effectively suppressed decreases in platelet counts and in clot retraction ability, and also the enhancement of platelet adhesiveness during the arteriovenous shunt. From these findings, they proposed that a long PEO chain with high flexibility and hydrophilicity contributes to the enhancement of volume restriction and osmotic repulsion effects which prevent the adherence of platelets and also minimize denaturation of the circulating platelets.

A transmission electron micrograph of the cross section of the PVC-g-M100G implanted in the peripheral veins of a dog for 14 days, which was photographed by Dr. Y. Noishiki, is shown in Figure 3. A double layer of plasma proteins is clearly observed in the interface between the polymer surface and the blood. Mori et al. [4,46] considered that the long-chain PEO protracting from the surface into the blood in some way constructed the double layer, because the distance of 40 Å between the inner and outer layers was close to the average end-to-end distance of the PEO chain and the double layer was not recognized in the PVC-g-MnG with short-chain PEO. From these findings, it was concluded that the double layer plays a role as buffer to minimize denaturation of blood elements, and that the buffer action of the double layer is caused by the superior flexibility, hydrophilicity and biocompatibility of the long-chain PEO.

Recently, Nagaoka et al. [48] proposed that the mo-

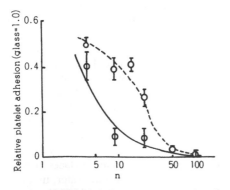

Figure 2. Effect of PEO chain length (n) on platelet adhesion to polymer surface. ⊕: PVC-g-MnG, ○: PMMA-co-MnG (from p. 177 of Reference [44]).

Figure 3. Transmission electron micrograph of a cross section of PVC-g-M100G implanted in the peripheral vein of a dog (photographed by Dr. Y. Noishiki). A mark under the picture shows 1000A.

tion of the PEO side chains with water molecules bound to the PEO units causes microscopic water flow, which prevents the local stagnation of blood components and the adhesion of platelets. On the other hand, Tanzawa [49] proposed that a definite structure of water molecules on the hydrogel surface prevents the platelet adhesion.

Polyacrylonitrile and Polyurethane Graft Polymers Having PEO Side Chains

Miyama et al. [39,40] synthesized polyacrylonitrile graft copolymers containing PEO and dimethylamine side chains and evaluated their blood compatibility. The synthesis was carried out photochemically as described above [12]. To the brominated polyacrylonitrile, methoxypoly(ethyleneglycol)monomethacrylate MnG and dimethylaminoethylmethacrylate DAEM were photografted at various feeding ratios in dimethyl sulfoxide. Interfacial free energy γsw between the graft copolymer film and water was calculated according to the equation of Andrade et al. [50] from the contact angle between an air bubble and the film, and the contact angle between an octane bubble and the film. Values for the contact angles were obtained in water kept at 25°C by using a contact angle goniometer. The half-width of the 1H-NMR signal at about 3.5 ppm was used as a measure of the mobility of the PEO side chain. The spectra were measured by using a model JNM-GX 207 JEOL NMR spec-

trometer with 10 mg of each of the polymers dissolved in 0.6 ml of DMSO-d$_6$. Platelet adhesion was measured according to the *in vitro* test described above [4,10].

From preliminary results [39], it was found that the water content increased almost proportionally to the weight % of EO content in the graft polymer. Also, interfacial free energy increased with an increase in the degree of grafting of PEO, and therefore with an increase in the water content. The line-width of the 1H-NMR spectra was narrower for the longer PEO chain, which indicated that the mobility of the PEO chain increased with an increase in the PEO chain length. The number of platelets adherent to the graft polymer PAN-g-M23G was smaller than that of the PAN-g-M4G. However, the adhesion increased for PAN-g-M100G. These results contradict those for PVC-g-MnG. The relationships between platelet adhesion and water content for both graft polymers are compared in Figure 4 [51]. The platelet adhesion to the PAN-g-MnG is much smaller than that to the PVC-g-MnG. The researchers did not explain the difference in the adhesion behaviour between the two graft polymers and suggested that one of the factors affecting the difference is a small amount of DAEM which was added to prevent gelation during the photografting process.

In order to clarify the effect of DAEM, polyacrylonitrile graft copolymers containing various amounts of PEO and dimethylamine (DA) side chains were synthesized to examine their physical, mechanical and nonthrombogenic properties [40]. The results are shown in Table 3. Here, M23G is used as PEO component and an *in vivo* test was performed by Noishiki's method. In Figures 5 and 6, the relationship between water content and EO content, and between the 1H-NMR line width and water content, are shown, respectively. For the graft copolymers with a low DAEM content (<1%), a linear relationship was observed as

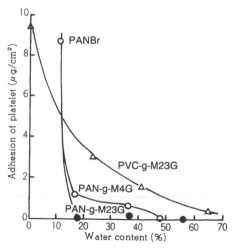

Figure 4. Relation between adhesion of platelet and water content for PVC-g-MnG and PAN-g-MnG (from p. 902 of Reference [51]).

Table 3. Composition, water content, γsw, and amount of platelets of polyacrylonitrile graft copolymers. (from p. 224 of Reference [40]).

Sample No.	Composition (wt%)			Water Content (%)	γsw (erg/cm²)	Adhered Platelets (μg/cm²)	*In vivo*** Test
	Trunk Polymer	M23G	DAEM				
D-1	74.35	25.65	0.01	23	0.5	0.00	○
D-2	66.97	32.90	0.13	30	0.8	0.00	○
D-2′	70.89	28.78	0.38	29	0.7	—	○
D-3	66.19	33.15	0.66	36	1.0	0.00	○
D-4*	50.17	45.72	4.11	53	1.3	0.14	×
D-5*	57.01	30.71	12.28	51	2.6	0.59	×
D-6*	69.10	17.50	13.40	29	3.6	—	×
D-7*	64.33	23.40	12.27	35	2.3	—	×
D-8*	59.65	28.55	11.80	45	2.7	—	×
D-9	42.88	56.65	0.47	61	0.5	0.00	○
D-10 (PAN-Br)	—	—	—	12	4.1	28.90	×

*These samples are classified as those of high DAEM content.
**○, no thrombus formation; × thrombus formation.

reported previously [39]. However, for the graft polymers with a high DAEM content (>1%), the data deviated from the linear relationship. The water content of the latter graft copolymers was higher than that of the former when the EO side chains were the same. Values of γsw, in Table 3 are high for the graft copolymers with high DAEM content, even for those with higher water content. Andrade et al. [50] reported that γsw of poly(hydroxymethyl methacrylate) and related polymers decreased with an increase in hydrophilicity of the polymer. However, for the present graft copolymers, an increase in the DAEM component increased γsw, that is, it reduced the wettability of the polymer surface. This deviation may be due to the tertiary amine groups of DAEM. As reported by Nagaoka et al. [44,45], the half-width of the NMR signal originated from PEO is a measure of the mobil-

ity of the PEO side chain, that is, the narrower the half-width the higher the mobility of the PEO side chain. However, the data for the graft copolymers with high DAEM content deviated from the normal curve and showed a wider half-width than those polymers with low DAEM content. This result suggests that an increase in DAEM content reduces the mobility of the PEO side chains. Based on the *in vitro* data in Table 3, it appears that the graft copolymers

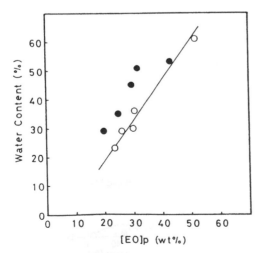

Figure 5. Relation between the water content and EO content of the graft copolymers. ○: low DAEM content, ●: high DAEM content (from p. 227 of Reference [40]).

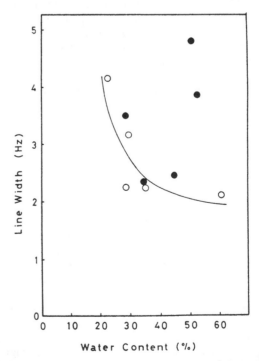

Figure 6. Relation between half-width of ¹H-NMR signal for PEO side chain and water content of graft copolymers. ○: low DAEM content, ●: high DAEM content (from p. 227 of Reference [40]).

with >1% DAEM content had an appreciable amount of platelet adhesion even when the water content was high. On the other hand, the copolymers with <1% DAEM content had no platelet adhesion even when the water content was not high. According to the *in vivo* test, after insertion for 24 h the trunk polymer (D-10) showed thrombus formation incorporating red blood corpuscles and fibrins, but the graft copolymers did not show any thrombus formation. After insertion for 7 days, red thrombus formation was observed for the graft copolymers with >1% DAEM content, but no thrombus formation for those with low DAEM content. They explained the results as follows. The DAEM parts of the graft copolymer are localized on the polymer surface which increases γsw, prevents the motion of the PEO chains and the microscopic water flow on the surface, and promotes the stagnation of the blood components.

For the synthesis of the above-described graft polymer PAN-g-MnG, the photografting method was used because PAN was very inert to conventional methods of thermal grafting. However, from the viewpoint of the simplicity of the synthetic process, it is desirable to develop a method of thermal grafting. Miyama et al. [52] developed a new method of thermal grafting via thioamide formation, where ammonium peroxydisulfate was used as an initiator. Preparation of thioamide polyacrylonitrile (TPAN) and the grafting were performed as follows. Into a three-necked flask, definite quantities of PAN and diemethylformamide (DMF) were introduced and stirred for 30 min during Ar bubbling. Into the solution, H_2 gas was bubbled. The solution was poured into methyl alcohol to precipitate TPAN. The polymer was washed with methyl alcohol, precipitated in DMF, washed with methyl alcohol and dried in vacuum. Definite quantities of TPAN, DMSO, M23G and ammonium peroxydisulfate were mixed and reacted. After adding hydroquinone monomethylether to stop the polymerization, the solution was concentrated in vacuum to one half of the original volume. The solution was poured into an aqueous solution of methyl alcohol to precipitate the graft copolymer. The copolymer was reprecipitated in DMSO, then washed and dried in vacuum. The grafting was confirmed by IR absorption and NMR spectrum. The kinetics and mechanism of graft polymerization were studied in detail to find the optimum conditions for the synthesis. Water content of the graft copolymer increased with an increase in the grafted M23G, and the interfacial free energy between the polymer and water decreased with an increase in grafting. The behaviour was very similar to that of the graft polymer obtained by the photografting method. Since the graft copolymer obtained by the present method had almost the same chemical structure and physical properties as that obtained by the photochemical method, it is expected that the graft copolymer has excellent nonthrombogenic properties. As a result of *in vivo* tests according to the Noishiki's method, the graft copoly-

mers showed no thrombus formation after an insertion for 7 days, while the trunk polymer showed appreciable thrombus formation. The graft copolymer also showed excellent mechanical strength.

Han et al. [18] synthesized the PEO grafted polyurethanes as described earlier. Wilhelmy plate contact angle data showed that the receding contact angle of the PU-PEO decreased, the advancing contact angle increased, and the contact angle hysteresis $\Delta\theta$ increased with increasing PEO chain length. Han et al. tried to explain the results by the reorientation or relaxation effect of the polymer chain on the surface [53]. That is, the hydrophobic groups of polymers orient toward the surface in air, minimizing surface free energy. When an initially dried PU-PEO surface comes into contact with water, the reorientation time of PEO chain molecules increases with higher molecular weight, resulting in a higher advancing contact angle and a higher $\Delta\theta$. Also, the swelling of the PU-PEO increased with the increasing molecular weight of the grafted PEO, which caused high mobility of the polymer chains.

The results agreed well with the NMR study of Nagaoka et al. [44,45]. The platelet adhesion to the PU-PEO surfaces was very insignificant compared to the PU control, and it decreased with increases in the molecular weight of PEO [19].

PROTEIN ADSORPTION ON HYDROPHILIC GRAFT POLYMER SURFACE

Protein Adsorption and Blood Compatibility

When a foreign surface is in contact with blood, the surface becomes covered with plasma protein layers, which leads to interactions with blood cells and finally to thrombus formation. Blood–polymer surface events are illustrated in the literature [54]. Thus, the adsorbed protein layer plays an important role in the blood compatibility of the foreign surface. However, not much is known about the adsorption of proteins on the material surface. The adsorption behaviour seems to depend on the chemical structure and characteristics of the material surface. Therefore, it is very important to clarify details of the dependence.

The adsorbed protein layer is considered to be a monomolecular layer of Langmuir type. Hanson et al. [55] showed that relations between the amount of albumin, γ-globulin and fibrinogen adsorbed on surface of Cuprophane or poly(vinyl chloride) are expressed by an adsorption isotherm of Langmuir type, respectively. The dependency of the equilibrium adsorption on the surface characteristics of various polymers was studied by many researchers. Lyman et al. [56] examined the amount of albumin adsorbed onto the surface of polyetherurethaneurea from aqueous albumin solution and compared the result with platelet adhesion to the same polymer surface. Thus it was found that the amount of adsorbed albumin shows a maximum and the platelet adhesion a minimum for the polymer having an optimum polyether length. Hoffman et al. [57] examined the *in vivo* nonthrombogenicity of silicon grafted with 2-hydroxyethyl methacrylate (HEMA) and ethylmethacrylate (EMA) and adsorption of fibrinogen on its surface, where composition of HEMA and EMA was varied. It was found that the surface which adsorbs more fibrinogen is more thrombogeneic.

The results described above suggest that the albumin-adsorbed surface suppresses the platelet adhesion but the fibrinogen-adsorbed surface increases the platelet adhesion. Kim et al. [58] proposed that fibrinogen or γ-globulin forms a complex with the platelets but that albumin does not. This may be because the former proteins have saccharide chains but the latter has no chains, which make a complex with the glycoprotein of the platelets. Akaike et al. [59] showed from study on conformation change of albumin adsorbed onto the surface of polyioncomplex that the platelet adhesion is not suppressed by the quantity of the adsorbed albumin, but by the conformation change of the adsorbed albumin. Okano et al. [60] studied competition adsorption of albumin and γ-globulin on the surface of HEMA-styrene block copolymer and found that albumin is adsorbed preferentially on the hydrophilic domain of the surface, while γ-globulin is adsorbed on the hydrophobic domain. Ikada et al. [5] proposed that the low protein adsorbability and the good blood compatibility of hydrophilic grafted surface can be attributed to the diffuse surface structure of the grafted chains.

Since blood contains many kinds of proteins, interaction between foreign surfaces and plasma proteins cannot be discussed by a simple equilibrium adsorption. Vroman et al. [61] found that when a foreign surface is exposed to undiluted plasma, a relatively limited adsorption of albumin, γ-globulin and fibrinogen occurs compared with the adsorption of the same proteins from less concentrated solution. Further, Vroman's group [62] found a phenomenon designated as the "Vroman effect", involving the fact that proteins replace one another at the surface in an ordered sequence. In these phenomena, fibrinogen initially adsorbed from plasma onto a hydrophilic surface, such as glass, decreased with time, an effect which was due to the displacement of fibrinogen by high molecular weight kininogen (HMWK). The phenomena were confirmed in detail by Brash et al. [54]. Also, the adsorption kinetics of protein mixtures used to explain the Vroman effect were studied by Cuypers et al. [63]. From these studies, it is considered that intrinsic coagulation factors are activated by HMWK displaced with fibrinogen adsorbed on a surface. On the other hand, hydrophobic surface adsorbs fibrinogen strongly, which prevents the Vroman effect, but the surface also adsorbs platelets strongly. Therefore, the nonthrombogenicity of a polymer surface is not discussed from the viewpoint of a balance of hydrophilicity and hydrophobicity alone. At any rate, not much

data have been reported on plasma protein adsorption on hydrophilic polymer surfaces. Some data concerning protein adsorption on the surfaces of graft polymers having PEO side chains will be introduced below.

Protein Adsorption on Graft Polymers Having PEO Side Chains

Nagaoka et al. [44] examined *in vivo* adsorption of rat plasma proteins on surfaces of PVCg-M9G and PMMA-co-M9G and found that the protein adsorption increased with increasing water content, which was higher for the graft polymers than for the random polymers. The behaviour was similar to that for platelet adhesion. No further discussion about the results was reported.

As described above, Miyama et al. [40] found from an *in vivo* test that graft copolymers having EO and DA side chains showed excellent nonthrombogenicity at a low DAEM content and that the nonthrombogenicity decreased with an increase in DA content. To clarify the mechanism of the phenomenon, they examined the relation between adhesion of platelets and adsorption of plasma proteins on the polymer surfaces [64]. Synthesis and evaluation of the physical properties of the polymers were the same as described above [12,40]. Here, methoxypoly(ethylene-glycol)methacrylate M23G was used.

The platelet adsorption was measured by a "column method" which was developed by Kataoka et al. [65]. The polymer was coated on glass beads (48–60 mesh, Toshiba Ballotini Co.). Then 1 g of precoated beads were closely packed in a poly vinyl chloride tube. Blood was withdrawn by cardiopuncture from a Wistar male rat into 0.25% sodium citrate aqueous solution. PRP was separated by centrifugal operation for 20 min at 900 rpm. From the PRP, platelets were precipitated by centrifugal operation for 15 min at 2000 rpm. The platelets were suspended in Hanks' balanced salt solution (HBSS), to which N-2-hydroxyl-N′-2-sulfoethylpiperazine (HEPES) was added to keep the pH at 7.3. The platelet concentration in this solution was approximately 1×10^7 cells/ml. When rat serum albumin (RSA) or rat γ-globulin (RγG) was added to the solution, a 0.1% solution of each in HBSS was added, keeping the same cell count and pH. The platelet suspension from a disposable syringe was passed through the column with the use of a Precidol Model 5003 infusion pump for 3.5 min at a flow rate of 0.4 ml/min. The number of platelets in the solution before and after the elution was determined by a Coulter counter. Retention of the platelets was calculated according to the following equation:

$$(1 - [P]/[P]_0) \times 100$$

where $[P]_0$ and $[P]$ were concentrations of the platelets before and after the elution. The rentention value was an average of four runs.

Table 4. Composition and water content of polyacrylonitrile graft copolymers (from p. 58 of Reference [64]).

Sample No.	Composition (wt%)			Water Content (wt%)
	Trunk Polymer	M23G	DAEM	
1	70.6	29.4	0.0	32
2	61.9	36.7	1.4	34
3	64.0	29.8	6.3	29
4	62.4	30.0	7.6	31
5	66.3	25.2	8.5	29
6	66.4	21.8	11.9	24
7	56.3	24.1	19.6	33

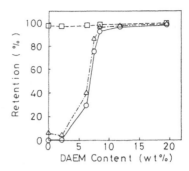

Figure 7. Effect of RSA on the relation between platelet retention and DAEM content. □: no RSA is present either in solution or on polymer surface, △: no RSA is present in solution but is present on surface, ○: RSA is present both in solution and on surface (from p. 59 of Reference [64]).

A measurement of the adsorbed protein was carried out as follows. About 2 g of glass beads (150–200 mesh) precoated with the polymer were immersed in 10 ml HBSS-HEPES, containing 0.2 mg RSA or Rγ G and incubated at pH 7.3 for 6 h at 30°C. The concentrations of the proteins were measured before and after incubation by adding Coomassie Brilliant Blue G-250 to the solution and measuring absorption at 595 nm. The amount of the proteins adsorbed was calculated from the difference in the protein concentration before and after the incubation.

Composition and water content of the graft copolymers are shown in Table 4, where the average molecular weight of the PANBr used for the photografting was in the range of 7.3×10^5 to 8.1×10^5. Figure 7 shows the relation between the platelet retention and the DAEM content of the polymer. When RSA was absent both in the platelet suspension and on the coated polymer, the retention was almost 100% irrespective of the DAEM content. When RSA was present on the polymer surface or both in the solution and on the polymer surface, the retention was almost zero for the polymers with a low DAEM content and increased with an increase in DAEM content for polymers with a DAEM content higher than 1.4 wt%. When Rγ G was present, a similar tendency was observed. On the other hand, the adsorption of albumin on the polymer surface reached a maximum when DAEM content was 1.4%, which coincided with the start of the increase in platelet retention, and decreased gradually thereafter as shown in Figure 8. Similar behaviour was observed in γ-globulin adsorption. From these results, the following important conclusions were obtained:

(1) The presence of plasma proteins is required to prevent platelet adhesion on the surfaces of polymers having PEO chains.

(2) The proteins adsorbed on the polymer surface are responsible for the prevention of platelet adhesion.

Recently Miyama et al. [66] synthesized PAN-g-MnG having different numbers of EO unit ($n = 4, 9, 23$ and 110) and tried to find a dependence of both

platelet adhesion and protein adsorption on the PEO chain length. Experimental details were similar to those in the previous report [64]. The degree of the protein adsorption on the polymer surface was on the order of RPF > Rγ G > RSA. Reduction of platelet retention for the protein-coated polymer was also on the same order as that of the protein adsorption. A typical example is shown in Figure 9. The results support the conclusion of the previous report [64] that the protein adsorbed on the polymer surface prevents the platelet adhesion. Both the protein adsorption and the platelet adhesion failed to show a dependence on the PEO chain length. The addition of Ca^{2+} hardly increased the platelet adhesion. Since the presence of both Ca^{2+} and fibrinogen activates platelets, it is expected that the addition of Ca^{2+} increases markedly the platelet adhesion. The obtained effect was too small to conclude that the adherent platelets were activated. This indicates that both the protein adsorption and the platelet adhesion proceed via the same mechanism, perhaps via physicochemical adsorption.

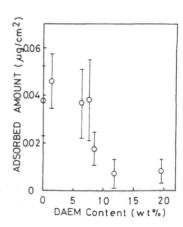

Figure 8. Relation between the amount of RSA adsorbed on a unit area of polymer surface and the DAEM content of polymer (from p. 60 of Reference [64]).

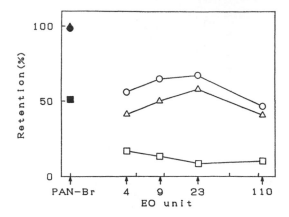

Figure 9. Relation between platelet retention and the number of EO units. ○,●: uncoated, △,▲: RSA-coated, □,■: RPF-coated (full marks correspond to trunk polymer PANBr) [66].

These results are inconsistent with the conclusion of Nagaoka et al. [48] that the motion of the PEO side chains prevents the local stagnation of blood components and the adhesion of platelets, and that the effect is more marked for the polymer having longer PEO side chains. Rather, the results are consistent with the findings of Mori et al. [4] who concluded that the adsorbed proteins penetrate into the PEO layer to form a microheterogeneous PEO/protein layer as shown in Figure 3 and that this proteinaceous layer prevents the adhesion of the platelets. Since contact time between the polymer and the platelet was limited, from several minutes to 30 minutes in the column method, the results of Miyama et al. may be limited to the initial reversible or physicochemical adsorption of platelets. The competitive adsorption and desorption of plasma proteins, as well as the activation and deformation of the adsorbed proteins, must be studied to confirm the dependence of platelet adhesion on the PEO length.

In order to obtain further information on recent development of biocompatible polymers, consult the excellent book of Professor K. Kataoka et al. [67] which was very useful in writing this review. Also, the author wishes to express his thanks to Professor K. Kataoka, Doctors H. Tanzawa and Y. Noishiki for their helpful advice.

REFERENCES

1. Noishiki, Y. 1976. *J. Biomed. Mater. Res.*, 10:759–767.
2. Kim, S. W., C. D. Ebert, J. Y. Lin and J. C. McRea. 1983. *Trans. ASAIO J.*, 6:76–87.
3. Okano, T., S. Miyahara, I. Shinohara, T. Akaike, Y. Sakurai, K. Kataoka and T. Tsuruta. 1981. *J. Biomed. Mater. Res.*, 15:393–402.
4. Mori, Y., S. Nagaoka, H. Takiuchi, T. Kikuchi, N. Noguchi, H. Tanzawa and Y. Noishiki. 1982. *Trans. ASAIO*, 28:459–463.
5. Ikada, Y., H. Iwata, F. Horii, T. Matsunaga, M. Taniguchi, M. Suzuki, W. Taki, S. Yamagata and Y. Yonesawa. 1981. *J. Biomed. Mater. Res.*, 15:697–718.
6. Noishiki, Y., T. Miyata and K. Kodaira. 1986. *Trans. ASAIO*, 32:114–119.
7. Ebert, C. D., J. C. McRea and S. W. Kim. 1969. In *Controlled of Bioactive Materials*. J. Baker, ed. New York: Academic Press, p. 107.
8. Gott, V. L., J. D. Whiffen, D. E. Koepke, R. L. Daggett, W. C. Boake and W. P. Young. 1964. *Trans. ASAIO*, 10:213–217.
9. Leininger, R. I., C. W. Cooper, R. D. Falb, and C. A. Grode. 1966. *Science*, 152:1625–1626.
10. Miyama, H., N. Harumiya, Y. Mori and H. Tanzawa. 1977. *J. Biomed. Mater. Res.*, 11:251–265.
11. Tanzawa, H., Y. Mori, N. Harumiya, H. Miyama, M. Hori and N. Oshima. 1973. *Trans. ASAIO*, 14:188–194.
12. Miyama, H., N. Fujii, A. Kuwano, S. Nagaoka, Y. Mori and Y. Noishiki. 1986. *J. Biomed. Mater. Res.*, 20:895–901.
13. Ito, Y. 1987. *J. Biomater. Res.*, 2:235–265.
14. Ito, Y., M. Sisido and Y. Imanishi. 1986. *J. Biomed. Mater. Res.*, 20:1139–1156.
15. Ito, Y., M. Sisido and Y. Imanishi. 1989. *J. Biomed. Mater. Res.*, 23:191–206.
16. Raghunath, K., G. Biswas, K. P. Rao, K. T. Toseph and M. Chvapiul. 1983. *J. Biomed. Mater. Res.*, 17:613–621.
17. Ebert, C. D., S. W. Kim. 1982. *Thrombosis Research*, 26:43–57; Heyman, P. W., C. S. Cho, J. C. McRea, D. B. Olson and S. W. Kim. 1985. *J. Biomed. Mater. Res.*, 19:419–436.
18. Han, D. K., K. D. Park, K-D Ahn, S. Y. Jeorg and H. A. Kim. 1989. *J. Biomed. Mater. Res.*, 23:87–104.
19. Han, D. K., S. Y. Jeory and Y. H. Kim. 1989. *J. Biomed. Mater. Res.: Applied Biomaterials*, 23:211–228.
20. Miyama, H., N. Fujii, Y. Shimazaki and K. Ikeda. 1983. *Polymer Photochem.*, 3:445–461.
21. Mori, Y., H. Tanzawa, H. Harumiya, H. Miyama, Y. Idezuki, N. Oshima and M. Hori. 1978. *Jpn. Artif. Organs*, 2:247–252.
22. Mori, Y., S. Nagaoka, Y. Masubuchi, M. Itoga, H. Tanzawa, H. Watanabe and Y. Idezuki. 1978. *Trans. ASAIO*, 24:736–744.
23. Basmadjian, D. and M. V. Sefton. 1983. *J. Biomed. Mater. Res.*, 17:509–518.
24. Miyama, H., N. Fujii, T. Nakamura, S. Nagaoka and Y. Mori. 1983. *Kobunshi Ronbunshu*, 40:691–696.
25. Miyama, H., N. Fujii, K. Ikeda and A. Kuwano. 1985. *Polymer Photochem.*, 6:247–257.
26. Noishiki, Y. 1982. *Jpn. J. Artif. Organs*, 11:794–797.
27. Peppas, N. A. and E. W. Merrill. 1977. *J. Biomed. Mater. Res.*, 11:423–434.
28. Smith, D. K. and A. K. Mallia. 1980. *Anal. Biochem.*, 109:466–473.
29. Smith, L., C. Doyle, D. E. Gregais and J. D. Andrade. 1982. *J. Appl. Polym. Sci.*, 26:1269–1276.
30. Mason, R. G., R. W. Shermer and N. F. Rodman. 1972. *Am. J. Pathol.*, 69:271–284.
31. 1972. *Laboratory Medicine Hematology, 4th Ed.* J. B. Miale, ed. St. Louis: C. V. Mosby Co., pp. 1267–1295.

32. 1984. *Medical Hematology, 1st Ed.* R. Hall and R. G. Malia, eds. London: Butterworth, pp. 629–632.

33. Lyman, D. J., W. M. Muir and J. J. Lee. 1965. *Trans. ASAIO*, 11:301–306.

34. Bruck, S. D. 1973. *J. Biomed. Mater. Res.*, 7:387–404.

35. Andrade, J. D. 1973. *Med. Instrm.*, 7:110–121.

36. Andrade, J. D., H. B. Lee, M. S. Johns, S. W. Kim and J. B. Hibbs, Jr. 1973. *Trans. ASAIO*, 19:1–7.

37. Ratner, B. D., A. S. Hoffman, S. R. Hanson, L. A. Harker and J. D. Wiffen. 1979. *J. Polym. Sym.*, 66:363–375.

38. Colman, D. L., D. E. Gregonis and J. D. Andrade. 1982. *J. Biomed. Mater. Res.*, 16:381–398.

39. Miyama, H., A. Kuwano, N. Fujii, S. Nagaoka, Y. Mori and Y. Noishiki. 1985. *Kobunshi Ronbunshu*, 42:623–628.

40. Miyama, H., N. Fujii, N. Hokari and H. Toi. 1987. *J. Bioactive and Biocompatible Polym.*, 2:223–231.

41. Inoue, H. and S. Kohama. 1984. *J. Appl. Polym. Sci.*, 29:877–889.

42. Otsuhata, K., M. T. Razzak, Y. Tabata, F. Ohashi and A. Takeuchi. 1985. *Nihon Kagaku Zasshi*, 10:1935–1944.

43. Lee, J. H., J. Kopeck and D. J. Andrade. 1989. *J. Biomed. Mater. Res.*, 23:351–368.

44. Nagaoka, S., H. Takiuchi, K. Yokota, Y. Mori, H. Tanzawa and T. Kikuchi. 1982. *Kobunshi Ronbunshu*, 39:173–178.

45. Nagaoka, S., A. Takeichi, K. Yokota, Y. Mori, H. Tanzawa and T. Kikuchi. 1982. *Kobunshi Ronbunshu*, 39:165–171.

46. Mori, Y., S. Nagaoka, H. Takiuchi, R. Terada, S. Nishiumi, H. Tanzawa, A. Kuwano and H. Miyama. 1984. *Progress in Artif. Organs–1983*, 2:852–830.

47. Mori, Y., S. Nagaoka, H. Takiuchi, R. Terada, S. Nishiumi, H. Tanzawa, A. Kuwano and H. Miyama. 1984. *Jpn. J. Artif. Organs*, 13:1143–1146.

48. Nagaoka, S., Y. Mori, H. Tanzawa, Y. Kikuchi, F. Inagaki, Y. Yokota and Y. Noishiki. 1987. *ASAIO J.*, 10:76–78.

49. Tanzawa, H. 1987. *Jpn. J. Artif. Organs*, 15:16–18.

50. Andrade, J. D., R. N. King, D. E. Gregonis and D. L. Colman. 1982. *J. Polym. Sci.*, 66:313–336.

51. Miyama, H. and Y. Noishiki. 1985. *Byoutai Seiri*, 4:898–903.

52. Miyama, H., H. Shimada, N. Fujii and Y. Nosaka. 1988. *J. Appl. Polym Sci.*, 35:115–125.

53. Holly, F. J. and M. F. Refojo. 1975. *J. Biomed. Mater. Res.*, 9:315–326.

54. Brash, J. L. 1987. *Ann. N.Y. Acad. Sci.*, 516:206–221.

55. Hanson, Y. K., K. Chuang, E. F. King and R. Mason. 1978. *J. Lab. Clin. Med.*, 92:483–496.

56. Lyman, D. J., L. O. Metalf, D. Albo, K. F. Richards and J. Lamb. 1974. *Trans. ASAIO*, 20:474–479.

57. Hoffman, A. S., T. A. Horbett and B. D. Ratner. 1977. *Ann. N.Y. Acad. Sci.*, 283:372–382.

58. Kim, S. W., E. S. Lee and R. G. Lee. 1974. *Trans. ASAIO*, 20:449–455.

59. Akaike, T., Y. Sakurai, K. Koswuge, Y. Senba, K. Kuwana, S. Miyata, K. Kataoka and T. Tsuruta. 1979. *Kobunshi Robunshu*, 36:217–222.

60. Okanao, T., K. Kataoka, K. Abe, Y. Sakurai, M. Sunada and I. Shinohara. 1984. *Progress in Artif. Organs–1983*, 2:863–866.

61. Vroman, L., A. Adams, M. Klings, G. Fischer, P. C. Munoz and R. P. Solensky. 1977. *Ann. N.Y. Acad. Sci.*, 28:65–76.

62. Vroman, L., A. Adams, G. C. Fischer and P. C. Munoz. 1980. *Blood*, 55:156–159.

63. Cuypers, P. A., G. M. Williams, G. M. Willems, H. C. Hemker and W. Th. Thermens. 1987. *Ann. N. Y. Acad. Sci.*, 516:244–252.

64. Miyama, H., K. Ikegami, Y. Nosaka, K. Kataoka, N. Yui and Y. Sakurai. 1988. *Artificial Heart 2: Proc. 2nd Int. Symp. Artif. Heart and Assist. Device*. Tokyo: Springer Verlag, pp. 57–61.

65. Kataoka, K., M. Maeda, T. Nishimura, Y. Nitadori and T. Tsuruta. 1980. *J. Biomed. Mater. Res.*, 14:817–823.

66. Miyama, H., O. Miyahara, Y. Nosaka, K. Kataoka, N. Yui and Y. Sakurai (submitted to *J. Biomater. Sci.*).

67. Kataoka, K., M. Okano, N. Yui and Y. Sakurai. 1988. *Seitai Tekigousei Polymer (Biocompatible Polymers)*. Tokyo: Kyouritsu Shuppan.

20

Expanded PTFE Prostheses as Substitutes in the Abdominal Aorta of Dogs: A Comparative Study of Eleven Different Grafts

JAMAL CHARARA, Ph.D.*
ROBERT GUIDOIN, Ph.D.*,1
TIAN JIAN RAO, M.D.**
MICHEL MAROIS, M.D.*
JUAN BORZONE, M.D.†
YVES MAROIS, M.Sc.*
CAMILLE GOSSELIN, M.D.*
NATHAN SHEINER, M.D.†

ABSTRACT: Eleven models of expanded PTFE arterial prostheses were implanted as infrarenal aortic substitutes in dogs to determine how the modifications in the structure of the grafts influence the healing characteristics. The eleven types included homogenous, reinforced, ringed and reinforced, helix-supported, double-helix-supported, graphite-lined, helix-supported graphite-lined and double-layered designs. They were implanted for predetermined periods ranging from 4 hours to 6 months, to demonstrate different sequences of healing. Scanning electron microscopy showed that, in all graft structures, the endothelialization of the luminal surface of the grafts never extended more than a few millimeters from the anastomoses. Light microscopy demonstrated that the double-layered model experienced the fastest and most extensive fibrous tissue incorporation compared to the other models that showed less fibrous tissue infiltration. The helix external support model showed considerably reduced penetration of blood elements and, thus, fibrous tissue proliferation: the structure of the wall is compressed, resulting in a structure that is less porous and less likely to heal. These results are reported as part of our ongoing program to characterize the arterial substitutes.

1Correspondence: Dr. Robert Guidoin, Ph.D., Biomaterials Institute, Room Fl-304, St-François d'Assise Hospital, 10 de l'Espinay, Quebec City, QC GIL 3L5, Canada.

*Biomaterials Unit, St. François d'Assise Hospital and Laboratory of Experimental Surgery, Laval University, Quebec City, Canada

**Visiting professor from the Laboratory of Cardiovascular Surgery, Shanghai Chest Hospital, Shanghai, People's Republic of China

†Lady Davis Research Institute and Jewish General Hospital, and McGill University, Montreal, Canada

INTRODUCTION

Peripheral vascular surgery procedures frequently require the implantation of alternative blood conduits for the restoration of the distal blood flow. In the absence of suitable autogenous vein grafts, chemically processed biological grafts and synthetic materials have been used as vascular prostheses [1–3]. The expanded polytetrafluoroethylene (PTFE) grafts are now the most widely used for such purposes [4]. Since they were first used with reservation as a venous substitute by Soyer in 1972 [5], PTFE grafts have undergone multiple clinical trials as arterial blood conduits. Indeed, they have been used for hemodialysis [6], extra-anatomical bypass [7–9], femoro-popliteal and distal replacement [10–16]. Several authors have reported less than acceptable results, while most surgeons have achieved good to excellent patency rates. It appears therefore that there is still room for improvement. The different models rely mostly on design modifications by the manufacturers in quest of the best blood conduit [17–21].

Ideally, a vascular graft should achieve excellent patency rates, have good handling characteristics, be non-immunogenic, present good healing characteristics, be durable, and not deteriorate over long-term implantation. Thus, they must have acceptable mechanical properties, be impervious at implantation to prevent blood oozing from the interstices, and possess an appropriate porosity to allow extensive healing. Much information concerning these properties of PTFE grafts was accrued from several clinical and experimental studies, on which the development of new PTFE structures was based. In order to improve the mechanical and thromboresistance properties of the most widely accepted models, major structural changes were introduced by the manufacturers [17,18] and several new models were developed. We hereby report the evaluation of eleven of these models.

While the clinical performance of these expanded

PTFE grafts has been reported extensively, the comparison of the healing characteristics of the different types of grafts has still not been investigated systematically. The present study was carried out to examine eleven types of expanded PTFE grafts, particularly the healing characteristics and the benefits of the carbon impregnation, the external helix support, the reinforcing layer and the concentric rings. In parallel, new methods for testing the *in vitro* properties of these grafts are in progress in this laboratory, but they cannot assess the complete system in its real biological environment. Despite differences in the blood properties between dogs and humans, dogs are still widely used because of the accumulated experience. Each model of PTFE grafts was implanted as an infrarenal aortic substitute for a series of prescheduled periods ranging from 4 hours to 6 months. The healing characteristics of these prostheses were investigated after the animals' sacrifice using light microscopy and scanning electron microscopy.

MATERIALS AND METHODS

Selection of Prostheses

The expanded PTFE vascular graft originates from pure PTFE resin which is preformed and then extruded into thin wall tubes under high pressure. After extrusion, the tubes are made microporous by a novel mechanical stretching process which produces a highly porous material. The material is then sintered, i.e., heated and fused above its melting temperature, to acquire its permanent stability. The expanded PTFE is made of solid nodes of PTFE interconnected by numerous thin microfibrils of PTFE. The fibrils are oriented with the longitudinal axis of the graft while the nodes are perpendicular to this graft axis.

Eleven types of commercially available PTFE grafts of various configurations were selected and are described in Table 1. They originate from 5 different manufacturers:

(1) Grafts manufactured by Impra Inc., Tempe Arizona, U.S.A. Five different models were investigated, namely:

- Impra Regular: an expanded PTFE tube whose wall is homogenous and 0.64 mm thick[2] (Figures 1 and 2)
- Impra Thin Wall: a homogenous tube with 0.45 mm of wall thickness whose microstructure is equivalent to that of the previous one
- Impra Graphite Lined: a homogenous wall with abundant particles of carbon incorporated on and into the inner surface which

is exposed to the bloodstream. Those particles penetrate up to a third of the thickness of the wall.

- Impra Flex graft: a homogenous tube with 0.64 mm of wall thickness. It is supported by an external helical coil (5 mm distance between rings) (Figures 3 and 4).
- Impra Flex graft Graphite Lined: an Impra Spirograft with particles of carbon incorporated in the wall and on the flow surface

All Impra models have a double blue guideline running parallel to the main axis.

(2) Grafts manufactured by W. L. Gore and Associates, Flagstaff, Arizona, USA. Three different models were investigated, namely:

- Reinforced Gore-tex®: an expanded PTFE tube whose nodules are at a 30 microns distance. This conduit is externally reinforced by a thin layer of expanded PTFE of low porosity. The wall thickness is 0.64 mm (Figures 5 and 6).
- Gore-tex® Thin Wall: the same structure as the Reinforced Gore-tex® with the wall thickness reduced to 0.39 mm
- Ringed Gore-tex®: a Reinforced Gore-tex® tube of regular thickness which is externally supported by concentric (3 mm apart each other) individual rings (Figures 7 and 8)

(3) Graft manufactured by Sumitomo of Japan, and distributed by Johnson and Johnson, Anaheim, California, U.S.A.

- Vitagraft®: has two distinct layers. Inside, the structure is equivalent to the one of the Impra with nodules perpendicular to the blood flow, about ⅓ of total wall thickness, and interrelated by microfibrils. Outside, the nodules are bunched into large ridges, i.e., 0.5 mm in width, with grooves up to 1 mm (Figures 9 and 10). This ridge structure comprises about ⅔ of the wall thickness. This graft has been discontinued.

(4) Graft manufactured by Bard Implants: a homogenous PTFE tube supported externally by a double helix of polypropylene. Wall thickness was 0.62 mm and internodal distance was 20–30 μm. This graft has been discontinued.

(5) Graft manufactured by the Shanghai Institute of Plastic Research. This Chinese PTFE is an homogenous PTFE tube whose structure is similar to the Impra Regular.

Surgical Protocol

The operations were performed in dogs according to the protocol previously established in this laboratory [22]. All animals were anesthetized with intravenous sodium pentobarbital (30 mg/kg), and were

---

[2]Wall thickness was measured with a micrometer Model CS-49-055 (Custom Scientific Instrument Inc., Whippany, New Jersey, U.S.A).

Table 1. Structural characteristics of the different grafts implanted.

Graft	Manufacturer	External Wrapping	External Support	Carbon Treated
Impra Regular	Impra Inc., Tempe, Arizona, U.S.A.	No	No	No
Impra Thin Wall	Impra Inc., Tempe, Arizona, U.S.A.	No	No	No
Impra Graphite Lined	Impra Inc., Tempe, Arizona, U.S.A.	No	No	Yes
Impra Flex graft	Impra Inc., Tempe, Arizona, U.S.A.	No	Spiral support	No
Impra Flex graft Graphite Lined	Impra Inc., Tempe, Arizona, U.S.A.	No	Spiral support	Yes
Reinforced Gore-tex®	W. L. Gore & Associates, Flagstaff, Arizona, U.S.A.	Yes	No	No
Gore-tex® Thin Wall	W. L. Gore & Associates, Flagstaff, Arizona, U.S.A.	Yes	No	No
Ringed Gore-tex®	W. L. Gore & Associates, Flagstaff, Arizona, U.S.A.	Yes	Individual concentric rings	No
Vitagraft	Sumikomo Electric Ind. Ltd., Osaka, Japan	No*	No	No
Bard PTFE	Bard Implants, Billerica, Massachusetts, U.S.A.	No	Double helix support	No
Chinese PTFE	Shanghai Institute of Textile Research, Shanghai, P.R. China	No	No	No

*Vitagraft has two distinct layers—a thin inner layer plus a thicker outer layer with a structure "en nid d'abeilles".

given halothane upon request. The animals were intubated and were maintained mechanically ventilated using a Bird Mark 14 respirator.

A segment of the infrarenal abdominal aorta was excised and replaced with a 6 cm segment of vascular prosthesis 6 mm in diameter, according to Table 2. All animals received a dose of 0.5 mg/kg of heparin 5 minutes prior to arterial clamping. End-to-end anastomosis was performed with continuous suturing by means of 5-0 polypropylene suture (Prolene, Ethicon,

Table 2. Implantation versus patency for short (4, 24 and 48 hours), medium (1, 2 and 4 weeks) and long-term (3 and 6 months) implantation.

Graft	Short Term	Patency Rate (%)	Medium Term	Patency Rate (%)	Long Term	Patency Rate (%)	General Patency Rate (%)
Impra Thin Wall	3/3	100	3/3	100	2/2	100	100
Impra Regular	3/3	100	3/3	100	2/2	100	100
Impra Graphite Lined	4/4	100	4/4	100	2/2	100	100
Impra Flex graft	6/6	100	5/5	100	2/2	100	100
Impra Flex graft Graphite Lined	6/6	100	5/4	80	10/8	80	85.7
Reinforced Gore-tex®	4/4	100	4/4	100	2/2	100	100
Gore-tex® Thin Wall	3/3	100	3/3	100	2/1	50	87.5
Ringed Gore-tex®	6/4	66.6	6/6	100	4/4	100	87.5
Vitagraft	3/3	100	3/2	66.6	2/2	100	87.5
Bard PTFE	3/2	66.6	3/3	100	2/2	100	87.5
Chinese PTFE	2/2	100	3/2	66.6	2/1	50	71.4

Patency rate of all Gore-tex® models: 91.17%.
Patency rate of all Impra models: 95%.

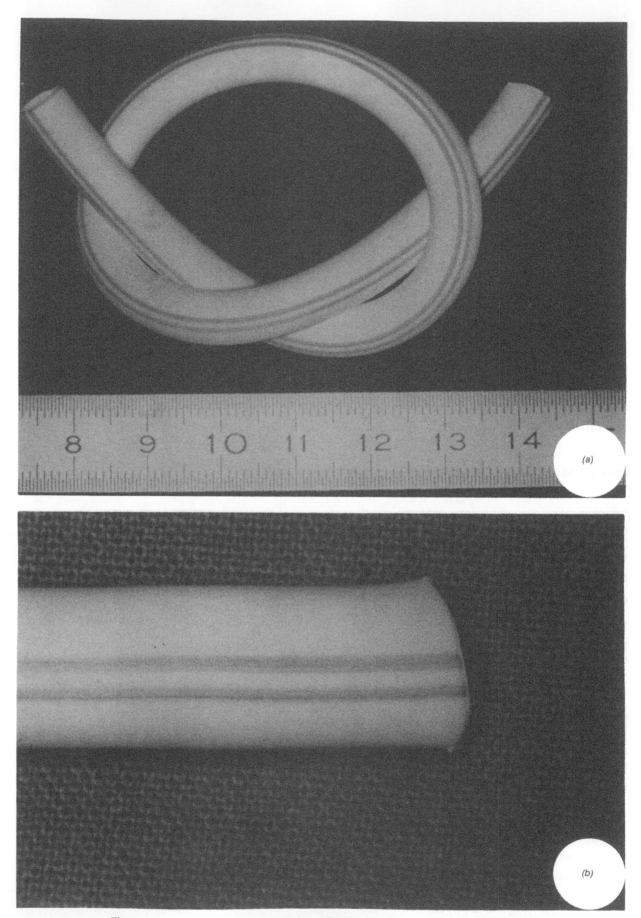

Figure 1. Photographs showing the virgin Impra Regular: (a) general view; (b) magnifying view.

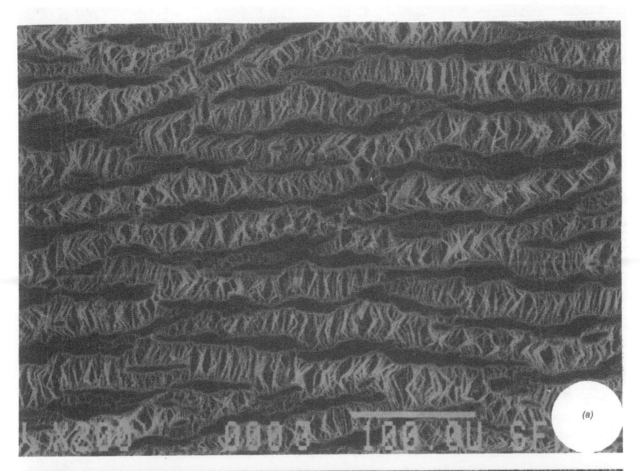

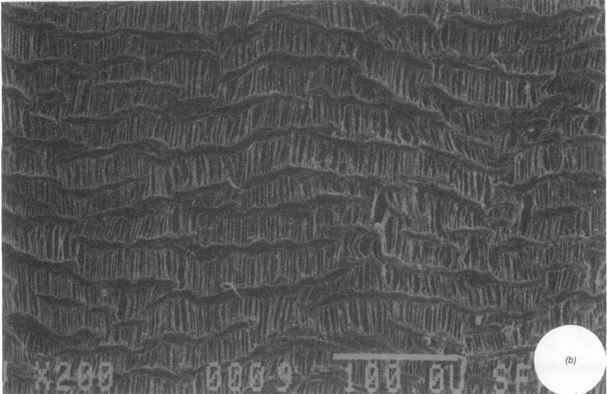

Figure 2. Scanning electron photomicrographs of the virgin Impra Regular showing the similarity between the inside [(a) ×200] and outside [(b) ×200] wall structures.

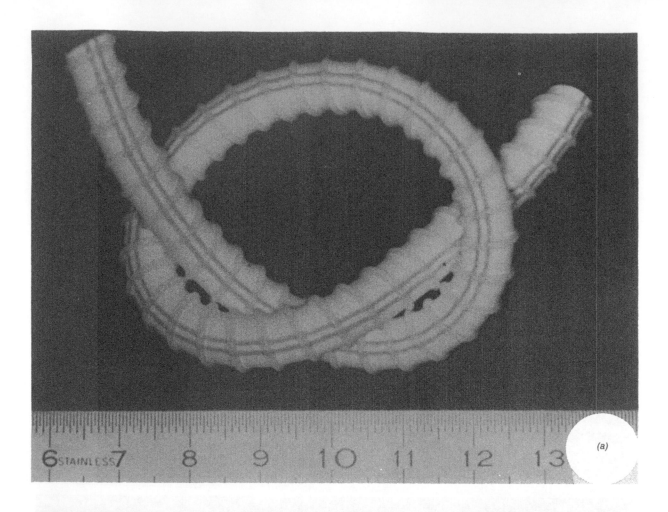

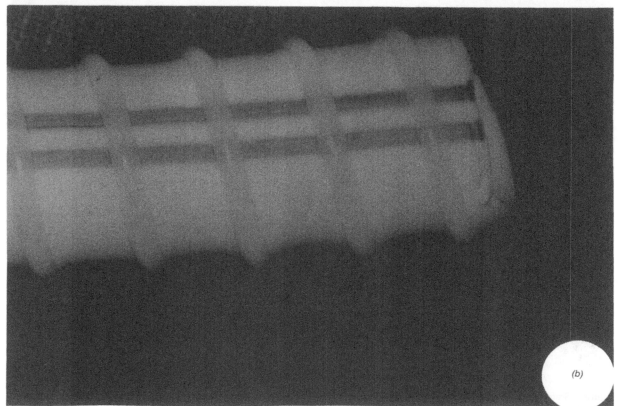

Figure 3. Photographs of the virgin Impra Flex graft: (a) general view; (b) magnifying view showing the external spiral support.

292

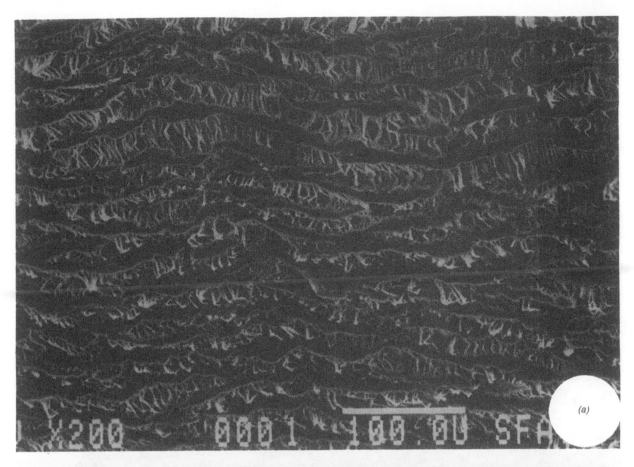

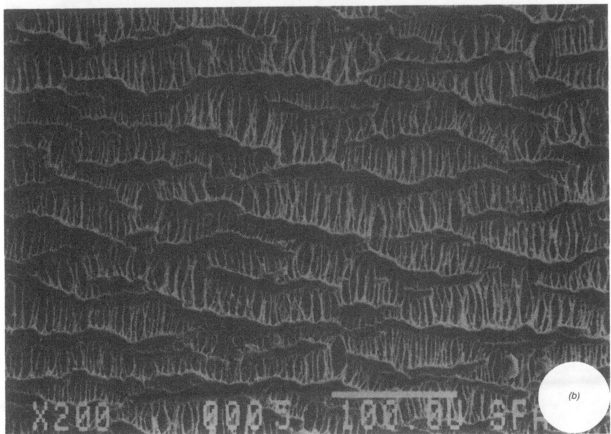

Figure 4. Scanning electron photomicrographs of the virgin Impra Flex graft: [(a) ×200] interior; [(b) ×200] exterior.

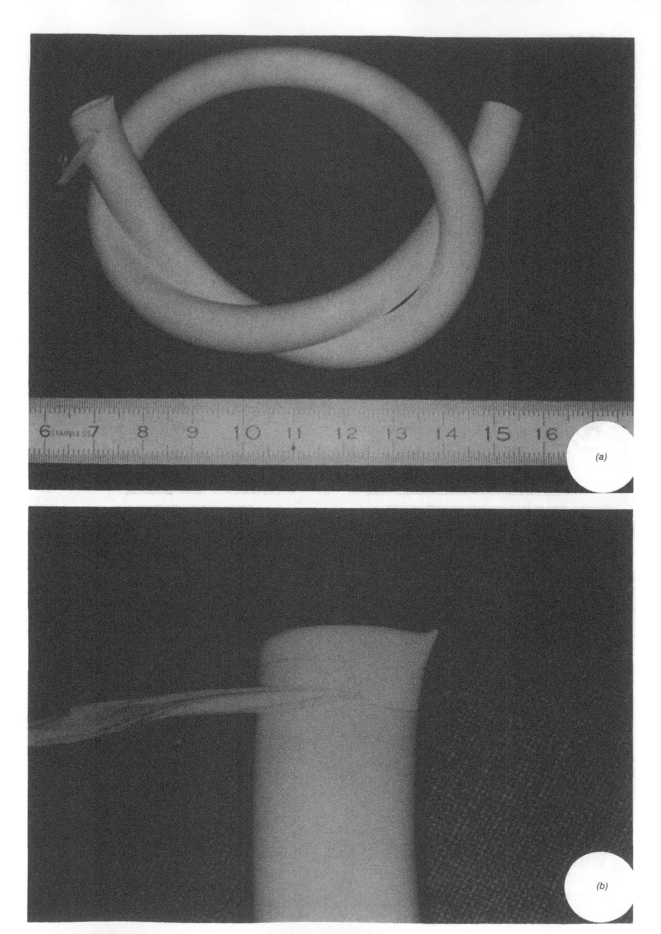

Figure 5. Photographs of the virgin Reinforced Gore-tex® graft: (a) general view; (b) magnifying view showing the external wrap of the graft.

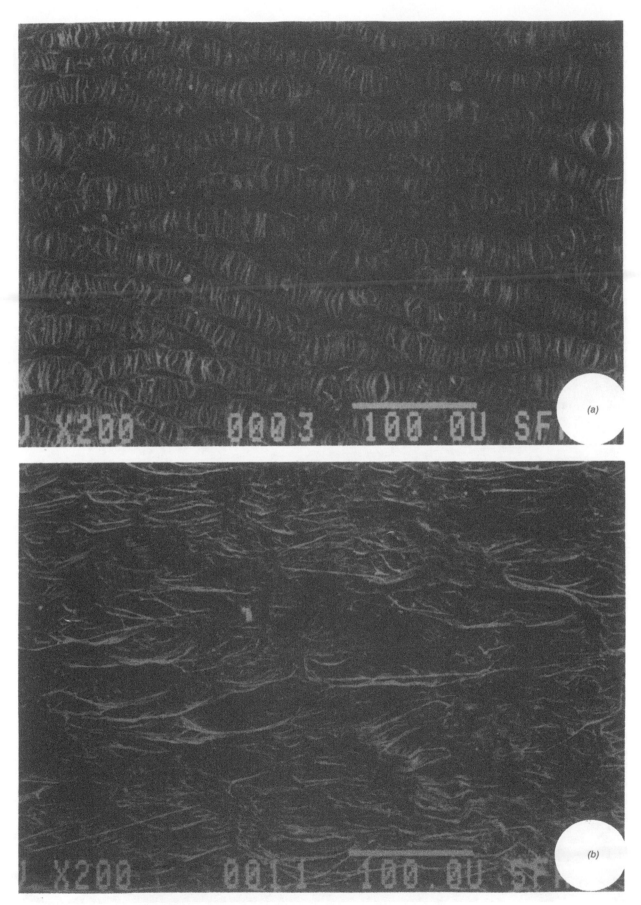

Figure 6. Scanning electron photomicrographs of the virgin Reinforced Gore-tex® graft comparing the structures of the inner wall and the outer wrap: (a) interior; (b) exterior.

295

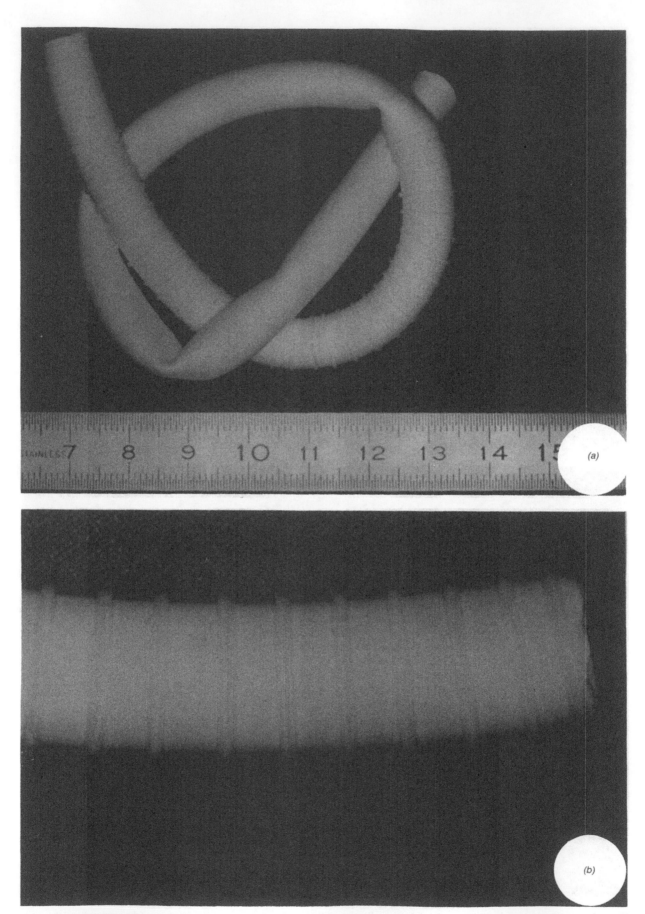

Figure 7. Photographs of the virgin Ringed Gore-tex® graft: (a) general view; (b) magnifying view showing the individual and concentric supporting rings.

296

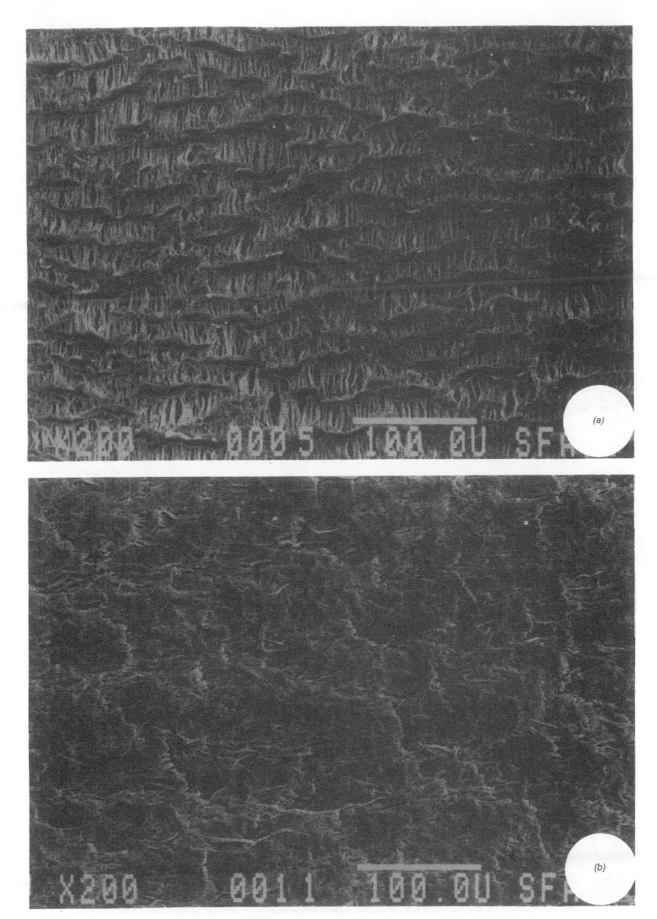

Figure 8. Scanning electron photomicrographs of the virgin Ringed Gore-tex® graft: (a) inside; (b) outside.

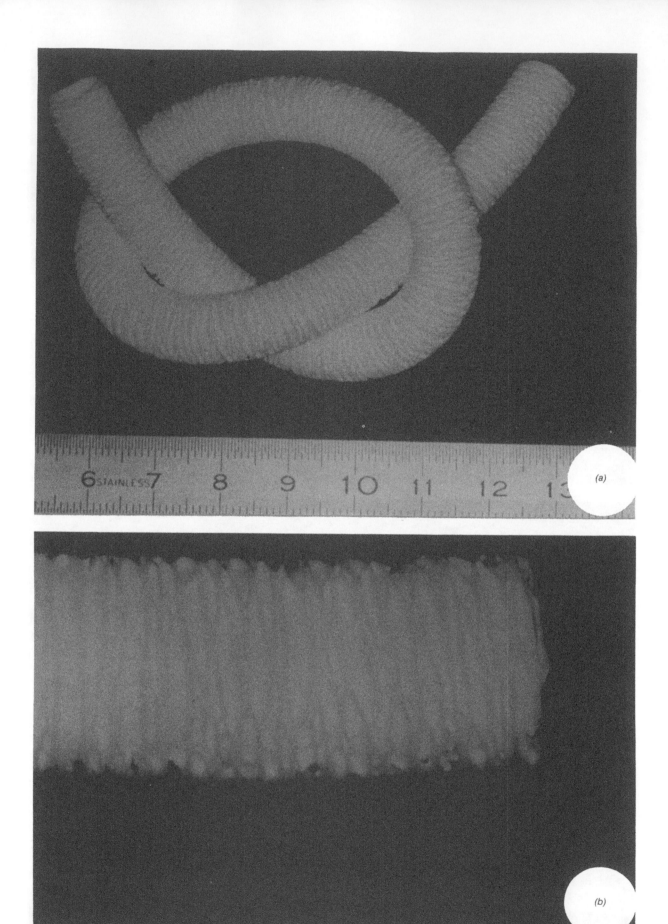

Figure 9. Photographs showing the virgin Vitagraft: (a) general view; (b) magnifying view.

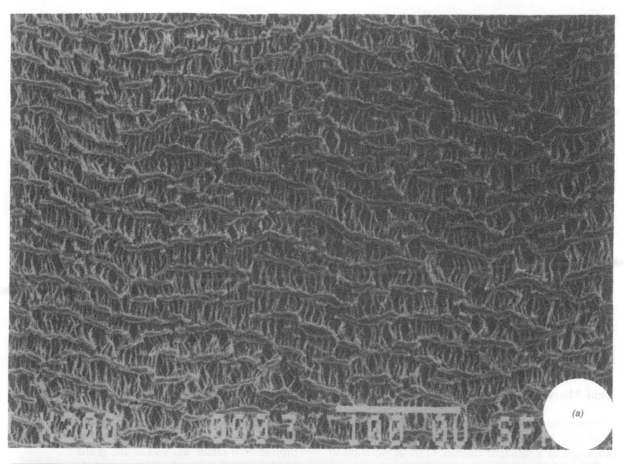

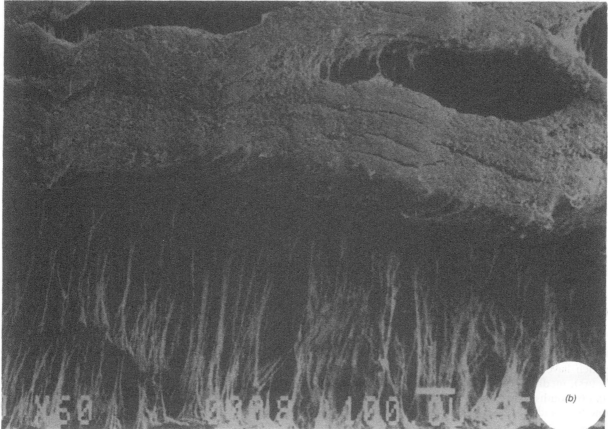

Figure 10. Scanning electron photomicrographs showing the inside [(a) ×200] and outside [(b) ×60] of the virgin Vitagraft.

Peterborough, Ont.). The abdomen was closed in layers using 2-0 polypropylene suture. The animals were injected antibiotics daily for 5 days.

Specimen Collection

The animals were sacrificed as scheduled at intervals of 4 hours, 1 day, 2 days, 1 week, 2 weeks, 1 month, 3 months and 6 months after implantation. The entire graft including both anastomotic segments was surgically excised, opened longitudinally, rinsed with heparinized saline and fixed in a buffer solution of 2% glutaraldehyde.

Macroscopic Examination

The grafts were first examined for gross morphology and photographed by a specially designed system (Tessovar®, Zeiss, Oberkochen, Germany) for magnifications of 0.4 to 12.8. Representative samples of various segments were selected for light microscopy and scanning electron microscopy (SEM).

Light Microscopy

Representative samples of grafts were immersed in 10 to 20% buffered formaldehyde, and subsequently processed in a standard manner [23]: dehydration in graded mixtures of ethanol, cleaning in toluene, and impregnation in paraffin. Then, the segment was sectioned with a microtome to a thickness of 4 μm. The sections were then stained with hematoxylin-eosin and Weighert preparation for elastic tissue, Masson's trichrome stain for collagen, Dahl's stain for calcification and Gram's stain for the assessment of bacteremic colonization.

Scanning Electron Microscopy

Samples were post-fixed in 1% carbodihydrazide and 1% osmium tetroxide, rinsed in distilled water, and dehydrated in graded solutions of ethanol, then transferred in absolute acetone. After critical point drying using liquid CO_2 as the transfer medium, the samples were coated with gold under vacuum and were examined in SEM at a 15 to 25 KV accelerating voltage.

RESULTS

Implantations performed in 117 dogs were uneventful. Table 2 summarizes the patency rates of the grafts which have been grouped for short- (4, 24 and 48 hours), medium- (1, 2 and 4 weeks) and long-term (3 and 6 months) durations of implantation. At 4 hours, one Bard and one Ringed Gore-tex® graft were thrombosed. After 24 hours, all the grafts were patent. Within 48 hours, one Ringed Gore-tex® had acquired an occlusive thrombus. By 1 week, one Vitagraft was

occluded. One Chinese graft showed an occlusive thrombus after 2 weeks. One out of 3 Impra Flex graft Graphite Lined was occluded after 1 month, and 2 out of 8 after 3 months. At 6 months, one Gore-tex® Thin Wall and one Chinese graft were occluded.

This table indicates also that 31 of 34 (91.17%) Gore-tex® grafts [Thin Wall (87.5%) and Ringed Gore-tex® (87.5%), Reinforced Gore-tex® (100%)] and 57 of 60 (95%) Impra grafts [Impra Thin Wall, Impra Regular, Impra Graphite Lined and Impra Flex graft (100%), Impra Flex graft Graphite Lined (85.7%)] were patent. Bard and Vitagraft showed an 87.5% patency rate, but the Chinese graft showed only a 71.4% patency rate.

Macroscopic Observations

All models experienced a similar macroscopic healing sequence over the 6 months of implantation (Figure 11), i.e., antithrombogenicity and/or thrombotic accumulation, fibrinolytic reaction of the host, anchorage of a thrombotic matrix along the suture lines, pannus reorganization with endothelial-like cells on the flow surface. Mild variations appeared to be related either to the differences in manufacturing or in the thrombohematologic differences in properties between dogs, and were mostly related to the fibrous proliferation inside the wall of the grafts.

After 4 hours of implantation, most of the grafts acquired large and irregular amounts of red surface thrombi but some remained free of thrombotic deposits. With the onset of fibrinolytic activity within 24 to 72 hours after implantation, the mass of thrombi almost disappeared. Then, a new phase of deposition of blood species began, including wall penetration with some particularities in the case of supported grafts. The inner surface of the Impra Flex graft, beneath the helix support, was clearly clean of any blood deposit or cell penetration [Figure 11(a)]. At 2 weeks, the surfaces of the grafts were entirely covered by a thin layer of fibrin enmeshing some blood deposits with some mural thrombi [Figure 11(b)]. A thrombotic matrix was anchored along the suture lines. Within 1 to 6 months, the grafts were covered with a thick external fibrous tissue. The pannus and the inner surfaces were smooth and glistening, with localized flattened red thrombi [Figures 11(c) and 11(d)].

Pathological Investigations

Although the amount and the content of the thrombotic matrix deposits did vary in the short-term group of animals due to variations in the thrombohematological characteristics of the hosts, there were few differences in the evolution of the healing. After 4 hours, the graft luminal surfaces were irregular with an intense red appearance, due to the accumulation of a thick thrombus consisting of a mass of leukocytes, platelets and red blood cells that were immersed in a disorganized fibrin network (Figure 12).

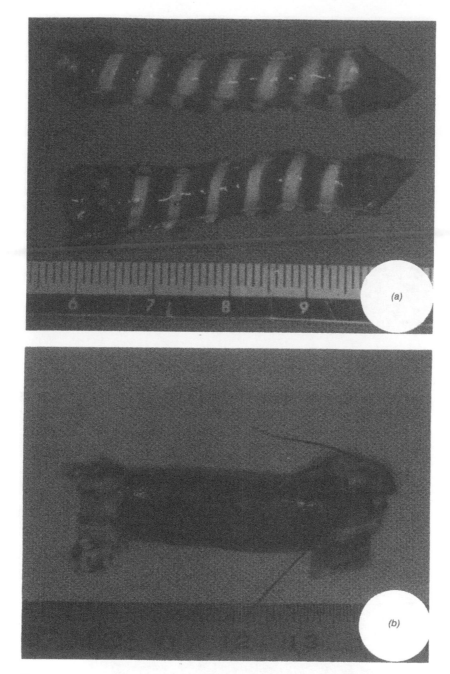

Figure 11. Macroscopic views of various explanted PTFE grafts. (a) Impra Flex graft after 24 hours of implantation, showing reduced accumulation of thrombi due to fibrinolytic activity developed by the host. The influence of the external helix support is evident: the microporous structure is compressed and no blood species can penetrate the area underneath. (b) Impra Regular after 2 weeks of implantation, showing the presence of fibrin deposits and some mural thrombi.

After 24 hours, a large amount of the thrombotic matrix disappeared since the fibrinolytic activity of the animals had caused partial lysis. For the Reinforced Gore-tex® graft, several thrombi developed within the initial layer of fibrin-erythrocytes along the luminal surface. During this time period, the wall facing the outer ring of the Impra Flex graft Graphite Lined was compressed (Figure 13). Furthermore, the ring and the reinforcing wrap of the Ringed Gore-tex® graft were detached from the graft wall (Figure 14).

After 48 hours, the flow surfaces of the prostheses consisted primarily of exposed microfibrils to which platelets and leukocytes were attached, as in the Chinese graft illustrated in Figure 15. Moreover, cellular

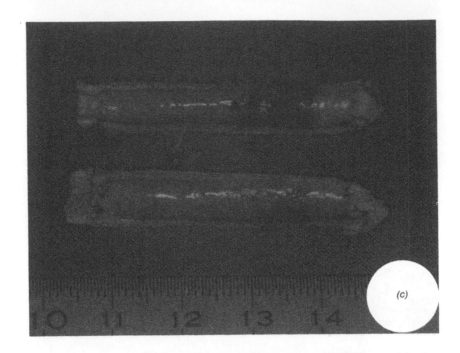

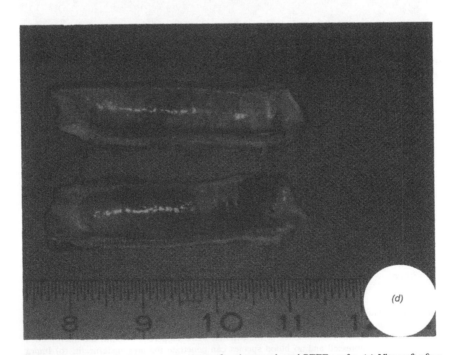

Figure 11 (continued). Macroscopic views of various explanted PTFE grafts. (c) Vitagraft after 3 months, showing that the entire surface was smooth and glistening with localized red thrombi. (d) Bard PTFE after 6 months, showing a well-encapsulated graft both internally and externally.

infiltration into the Impra Flex graft Graphite Lined was delayed by the carbon particles (Figure 16).

After 1 week, a few endothelial-like cells were observed over the Impra Thin Wall graft and Vitagraft; the latter was occluded. The patches of endothelialization were extending from the proximal suture lines. Most of the luminal surfaces of the grafts remained visible and exposed to the bloodstream. Thrombotic deposits accumulated along the suture lines as illustrated in Figure 17 (Impra Thin Wall).

Within 2 weeks, the flow surfaces were covered by a thin fibrin network in which few blood elements

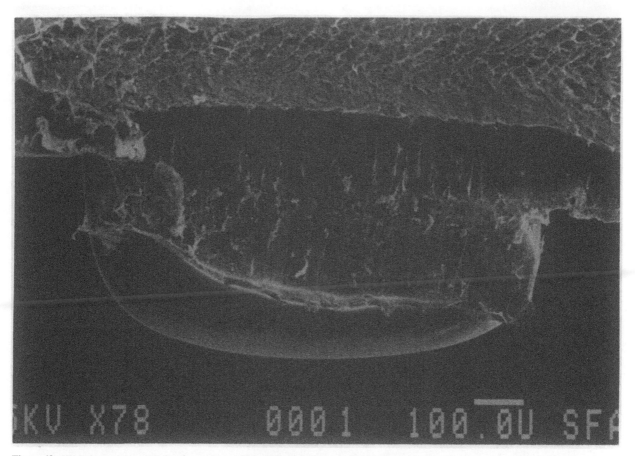

Figure 12. SEM photomicrograph showing an Impra Thin Wall graft, 4 hours after implantation. Clotting was very cellular with platelets, red blood cells and leukocytes trapped in an open fibrin network (×1000).

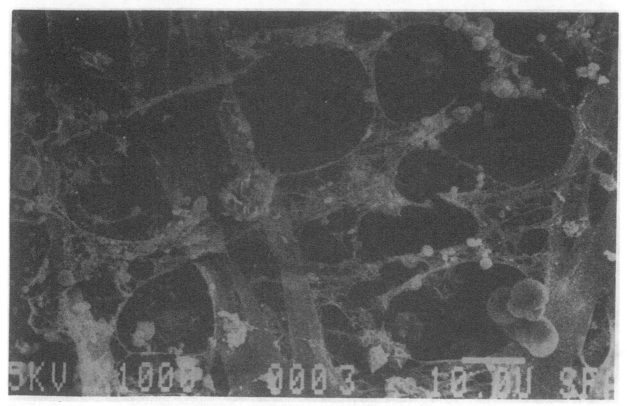

Figure 13. SEM photomicrograph of an Impra Flex graft Graphite Lined. After 24 hours, the inner surface was irregular with a thick and detached coagulated matrix. The wall was completely compressed in the region under the external support (×60).

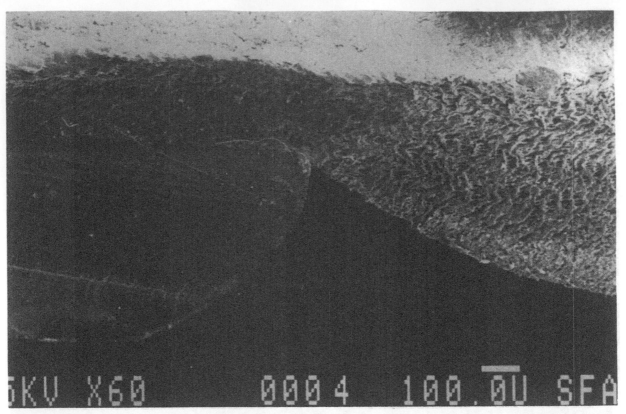

Figure 14. SEM photomicrograph showing a Ringed Gore-tex® graft implanted for 4 hours. The outer reinforcing wrapping of the graft attached to the supporting ring was slightly unstuck (This external ring has caused a partial compression of the graft wall) (×78).

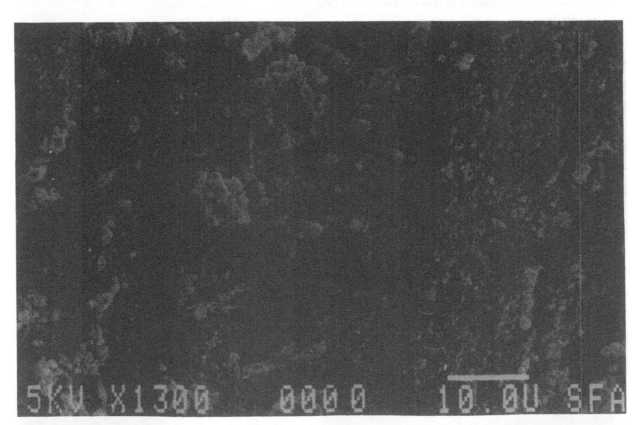

Figure 15. SEM photomicrograph of a Chinese graft after 48 hours of implantation. The thrombotic matrix had almost disappeared due to the fibrinolytic mechanism of the host. There are, however, few fibrin deposits, platelets and red cells trapped inside the graft structure, which showed some minor damages (×1300).

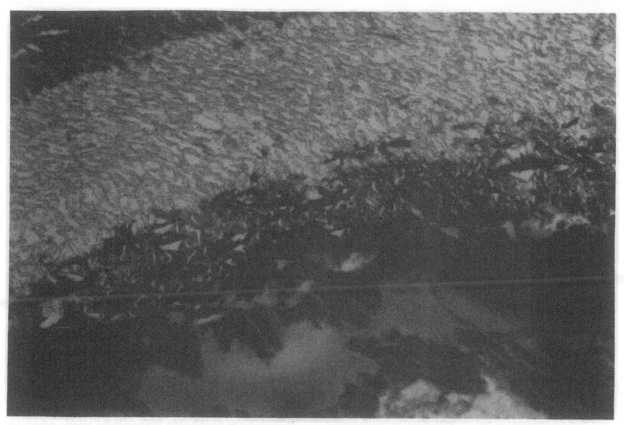

Figure 16. Light microscope photomicrograph of a section through the Impra Flex graft Graphite Lined after 48 hours of implantation, showing a thin thrombus extending over the inner surface. Graft wall was filled with cellular infiltration that was controlled by the carbon deposits (×100).

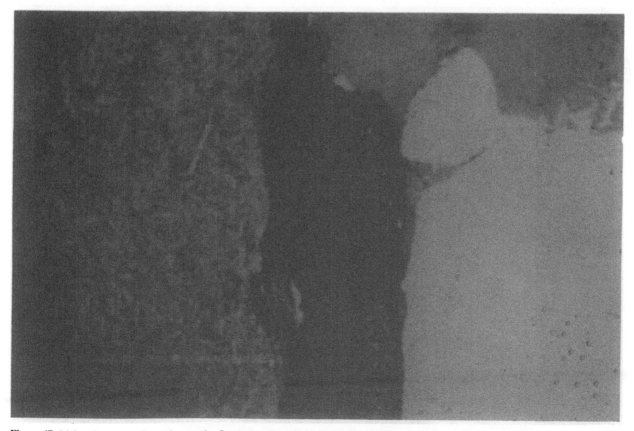

Figure 17. Light microscope photomicrograph of a section through the Impra Thin Wall graft after 1 week of implantation, showing that the graft wall is filled with blood elements. The luminal surface is covered by a variably thick thrombus (×400).

were immersed. At this time, endothelialization had started in all grafts. Sporadic islands of endothelial-like cells were located only near the anastomoses. Vasa-vasorum were observed near the suture line in the Ringed Gore-tex® graft.

After 1 month there were more areas of healing, as indicated by the presence of pannus ingrowth over the luminal surfaces from the adjacent native vessels. The cells formed a continuous carpet, bridging the anastomotic sites and much of the protruding sutures.

By 3 months, the whole graft lumens had a glistening appearance, and the fibrin was compact. Thrombus-coated areas were rarely seen after this length of implantation, and cells were increasingly extended over the inner surface from the suture lines (Figure 18). However, the central region of the grafts remained poorly healed, except in one Gore-tex® Thin Wall graft in which a collagen layer was observed (Figure 19). The wall structure of Vitagraft was filled with granulous tissue which might have caused some wall damage (Figure 20). In addition, dilation appeared on the structures of the Chinese graft.

At 6 months, no major differences in the surfaces were seen when compared with those at 3 months. Regions of cellular development were limited to the vicinity of the anastomoses and did not invade the central part of the graft (Figure 21).

DISCUSSION

More than fifteen years have elapsed since the introduction of expanded PTFE as a blood conduit. This material is one of the most chemically inert polymers known, and the PTFE graft engenders very little tissue or blood reaction. The material is believed to undergo little or no biological or chemical deterioration. However, the earlier models of expanded PTFE grafts did have some incidence of aneurysmal dilatation because they had insufficient radial strength to resist the pulsatile pressure of arterial blood flow [24–27]. This problem was addressed in two ways, depending on the manufacturers: W. L. Gore introduced the concept of external wrapping with a thin and much less porous film of expanded PTFE to increase the radial strength, whereas Impra increased the radial strength of the grafts by increasing the wall thickness. Since then, it appears that grafts have suffered less frequently from late structural lesions [28–30], but one must be cautious about predicting very long term stability for those improved products. Indeed, Formichi [31] has reported that a few reinforced Gore-tex® prostheses retrieved after several months of implantation in humans experienced some deteriorations where the external wrapping had been removed or damaged at implantation. In the present study, only

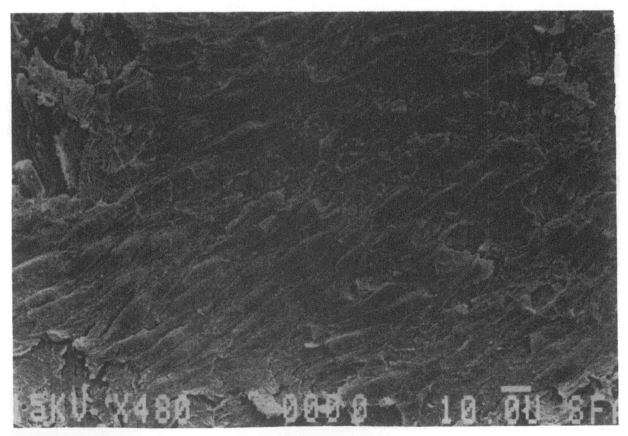

Figure 18. SEM photomicrograph of the Chinese graft after 1 month of implantation. A pannus coated with endothelial-like cells is visible along the anastomoses (×480).

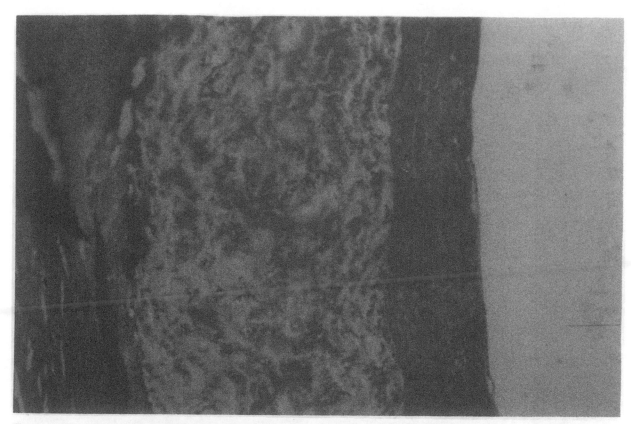

Figure 19. Light microscope photomicrograph of a section through the Gore-tex® Thin Wall graft after 3 months of implantation showing a thrombus layer covering the inner surface with abundant collagen (× 100).

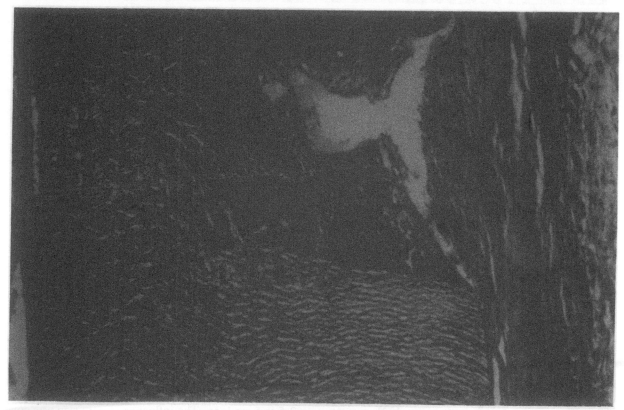

Figure 20. Light microscope photomicrograph of a section through Vitagraft after 3 months of implantation, showing a variably thin layer extended over the inner surface. In this figure, both inner and outer layers of the wall graft structure are distinguishable. Infiltration of the wall by granulous tissue might cause some damage (× 100).

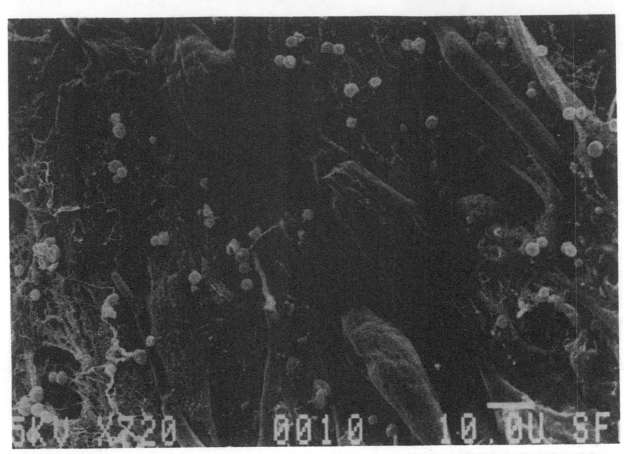

Figure 21. SEM photomicrograph showing the healing of the Impra Flex graft Graphite Lined after 6 months of implantation. Healing had advanced and endothelial-like cells were oriented with the direction of the blood flow (× 720).

one Ringed Reinforced Gore-tex® graft showed a poor adhesion of this external wrapping after 24 hours of implantation. However, no aneurysmal dilatation was observed in spite of some microscopic radial distension of the Chinese graft implanted for 3 months.

It is believed that the external wrapping of the Reinforced Gore-tex® models controls tissue ingrowth, and thus interferes with fibroblastic infiltrations into the graft mid wall. When reporting the pathological investigations about explanted Gore-tex® and Impra grafts used as blood access devices in hemodialyzed patients, Mohring concluded that the two models behaved in different ways [32]. The uniform structure of the Impra allowed rapid penetration of connective tissue, resulting in an organized cellular neointimal lining on the luminal surface. In the Gore-tex® grafts, the penetration of fibrous tissue into the graft wall was less pronounced, and these grafts generally exhibited a cell-free flow surface.

The hypothesis that a cellular invasion of the wall of the prosthesis by fibrous tissue is an essential step in the healing process and the long-term patency of arterial grafts, and an important criterion in selecting which commercial PTFE graft to use [33], was recently questioned by Camilleri [34]. He observed that the walls of 26 patent grafts remained essentially free

from fibrous tissue penetration after implantation times from 1 to 60 months.

Also, in this study, the Reinforced Gore-tex® grafts have experienced less rapid and less extensive tissue penetration than other grafts tested. The Thin-Walled Gore-tex® showed cellular ingrowth as early as 24 hours, while the other models (Reinforced and Ringed Reinforced Gore-tex®) showed it after 2 weeks. Thus, our results do not confirm that the Impra and Gore-tex® grafts behaved very differently for up to six months of implantation. They were seen to have similar degrees of cellular penetration and similar patency rates (Gore-tex® 91.77% to Impra 95%).

The cellular invasion of the wall may be controlled by the porosity of the structure. The ideal pore size for matching healing and patency in arterial grafts remains controversial. Campbell [35] obtained an 88% patency with grafts that had a pore size less than 22 μm, compared with only 53% patency in those with pore size greater than 34 μm. Florian [36] reported excellent results using PTFE with 100 μm pore size. This discrepancy was attributed by Hanel [18] to the short grafts used in the latter study, which were only 2.5 to 5 cm long. The influence of pore size was confirmed to some extent by the present study, in the case of the Vitagraft (with the ridged outer surface). The penetration of the wall by fibrous tissue was more pronounced and more intense than it was in the other models, and a relatively earlier surface cell development was observed. The Vitagraft has two distinct layers, as previously discussed—a thin layer with typical internodal spacing and slightly less axial orientation of the fibers, plus a thicker outer layer that is macroporous with more than 20 times the internodal spacing of the Gore-tex® or the Impra models [21].

Our study reflects not only the effects of structure and pore size on tissue ingrowth and patency, but also the effects of the PTFE external spiral supports. These supports were added to prevent kinking of the graft when crossing an area of flexion, such as the knee joints. Because the PTFE grafts are quite soft, Clark, in the discussion of Soyer's paper [5], pointed out that the kinking leads to decreased blood flow and then thrombosis. This point of view, however, was challenged by Kempczinsky [20], who found no pressure gradient and no decrease of blood flow, when PTFE grafts kinked crossing the bent knee joint.

Our observations demonstrated the effect of the outer supporting ring on cell penetration. The ring compressed the graft wall, reducing pore size in this area and consequently controlling to a large degree the cellular infiltration into the wall. The only exception was the double-helix-supported Bard PTFE. These results are not fully conclusive yet, and continued evaluation of its effects *in vitro* is recommended.

Another objective of this study was to investigate the suitability of the Impra models, in which graphite was incorporated into the wall structure. Graphite placed in the blood stream is thought to reduce thrombosis. Such a thromboresistance is attributed to its electronegativity [19]. Cellular blood elements, as well as fibrinogen and platelets, are known to be negatively charged at normal pH. Therefore, natural intima which is relatively negative plays a significant role in natural antithrombogenesis. Another theory suggests that, because of the ability of carbon to absorb whatever it comes into contact with, its exposure to blood causes immediate protein deposition. Thus, blood compatibility depends on carbon's ability to maintain a layer of anti-thrombogenic proteins at the carbon–blood interface without causing alterations in the protein molecules that initiate thrombosis [37].

Thus, whether the prevention of thrombosis may be dependent upon the electrical properties of carbon or upon its ability to absorb proteins is not certain. Our experience with the carbon layer has not been conclusive and consequently, in our opinion, the use and the role of graphite treatment should be reevaluated.

While endothelialization of the flow surface is an important factor in maintaining long-term patency of vascular grafts, the pattern of healing is still unknown [38]. Previous studies of endothelial healing in grafts have suggested that endothelium can arise from sources in the adjacent artery or capillaries derived from surrounding granulation tissue [39–42]. However, in our studies the endothelialization of all the grafts was still incomplete. The grafts follow the same healing sequence, requiring an initial layer of fibrin, leading to fibroblasts and collagen proliferation prior to the deposition of endothelial-like cells over the flow surface. By using short segments in dogs, the endothelial-like cells mostly cover the entire luminal surface, but this is not the usual clinical experience in humans. The use of longer grafts leads to incomplete healing, with the central region only covered with an acellular collagen layer [23]. Hence, the length of cellular proliferation from the anastomoses could serve as an indicator of the extent of healing. It is still too early to recommend cell-seeding of expanded PTFE grafts implanted in humans. The experiments carried out in animals are fascinating but the animals are healthy and the patients frequently present associated diseases.

CONCLUSION

The multiplicity of the differently constructed models of expanded PTFE arterial grafts appears to be confusing, and it is mandatory to separate each for ease of identification. Following surgery, we did not observe any significant differences in patency rates. Our observations can be summarized as follows:

- The fibrous tissue penetration from the outside to the inside wall of wrapped PTFE is slowed by the addition of an external wrapping, provided this wrapping adheres well and is not damaged.
- A better cell infiltration into the wall and cellular lining is achieved in those grafts with a homogenous structure.
- The addition of an external support results in compression of the wall structure where it is applied; such alterations may modify the physical properties of the grafts as well as the healing characteristics.
- The treatment with carbon has limited influence, if any, on the healing characteristics.

Our *in vivo* observations in animals are informative but must be compared with clinical results. Observations such as those of Camilleri, who observed that cellular invasion is not necessary for high patency [34], are of paramount importance.

ACKNOWLEDGEMENTS

The technical assistance of Jacques Bastien, Suzanne Bourassa, Karen Horth, Denise Lafrenière-Gagnon, Denis Martel, Louisette Martin, Nicole Massicotte and Gilles Mongrain is greatly appreciated. The authors are indebted to Drs. John Awad, Jean Couture, Gérard Roy, Jean-Claude Forest, Claude Poirier, Pierre-Albert Levaillant and Olivier Goëau-Brissonnière for help and guidance. This work has been supported by the Medical Research Council of Canada (Grant MT-7879) and the Quebec Heart Foundation. The grafts were kindly provided by W. L. Gore and Associates, Impra Inc., C. R. Bard, Johnson and Johnson and the Shanghai Institute of Plastic, the sutures by Ethicon, the antibiotics by Schering and the heparin by Allen and Hanburys.

REFERENCES

1. Weisel, R. D., K. W. Johnston, R. J. Baird, A. D. Frezner, T. K. Oates and I. H. Lipton. 1981. "Comparison of Conduits for Leg Revascularization", *Surgery*, 89:8–15.

2. O'Donnell, T. F., Jr., S. P. Farber, D. M. Richmond, R. A. Deterling and A. D. Callow. 1982. "Above-Knee PTFE Femoropopliteal Bypass Graft: Is It a Reasonable Alternative to the Below Knee Reversed Autologous Vein Graft?" *Surgery*, 94:26–31.

3. Julian, T. B., J. Loubeau and R. J. Stremple. 1982. "Polytetrafluoroethylene or Saphenous Vein as a Femoropopliteal Bypass Graft?" *J. Surg. Res.*, 32:1–6.

4. Quinones-Baldrich, W. J., V. Martin-Paredero, J. D. Baker, R. W. Busultil, H. I. Machleder and W. S. Moore. 1984. "Polytetrafluoroethylene Grafts as the First Choice Arterial Substitute in Femoropopliteal Revascularization", *Arch. Surg.*, 119:1238–1243.

5. Soyer, T., M. Lempinen, P. Cooper, L. Norton and B. Eiseman. 1972. "A New Venous Prosthesis", *Surgery*, 72:864–872.

6. Palder, S. B., R. L. Kikman, A. D. Whittemore, R. M. Hakin, J. M. Lazarus and N. L. Tilney. 1985. "Vascular Access for Hemodialysis. Patency Rate and Results of Revision", *Ann. Surg.*, 202:235–239.

7. Campbell, C. D., D. H. Brooks, R. D. Siewers, R. L. Peel and H. T. Banson. 1979. "Extra-anatomic Bypass with Expanded PTFE", *Surg. Gyn. Obstet.*, 148:525–530.

8. Fletcher, J. P., J. M. Little and J. Loewenthal. 1980. "Initial Experience with PTFE Extraanatomic Bypass", *Am. J. Surg*, 139:696–699.

9. Courbier, R., J. M. Jausseran and P. Bergeron. 1982. "Axillo-femoral Bypass Material of Choices", In *Extraanatomic and Secondary Arterial Reconstruction*. R. M. Greenhagh, ed. Pitman Press, pp. 122–130.

10. Campbell, C. D., D. H. Brooke, N. W. Webster, D. L. Diamond, R. L. Peel and H. T. Bahnson. 1979. "Expanded Microporous Polytetrafluoroethylene as a Vascular Substitute: A Two Year Follow-up", *Surgery*, 85:177–183.

11. Simone, S. T., Jr., B. Dubner, A. R. Safi, P. Delguerria, M. A. Shah, L. Zagoun and F. A. Reichel. 1981. "Comparative Review of Early and Intermediate Patency Rates of PTFE and Autologous Saphenous Vein Grafts for Lower Extremity Ischemia", *Surgery*, 90:991–999.

12. Yeager, R. A., R. W. Hobson, II, T. G. Lynch, Z. Jamil, B. G. Lee, K. Jain and R. Keys. 1982. "Analysis of Factors Influencing Patency of Polytetrafluoroethylene Prostheses for Limb Salvage", *J. Surg. Res.*, 32:1–6.

13. Geiger, G., J. Hoevels, L. Storz and H. P. Bayer. 1984. "Vascular Grafts in Below-Knee Femoro-Popliteal Bypass. A Comparative Study", *J. Cardiovasc. Surg.*, 25:523–529.

14. Bennion, R. S., R. A. Williams, B. E. Stabile, M. A. Fox, M. L. Owens and S. E. Wilson. 1985. "Patency of Autologous Saphenous Vein Versus Polytetrafluoroethylene Grafts in Femoro-Popliteal Bypass for Advanced Ischemia of the Extremity", *Surg. Gyn. Obstet.*, 160: 239–242.

15. Ascer, E., F. J. Veith, S. K. Gupta, G. Krasowski, R. M. Samson, L. A. Scher, S. A. White-Flores and S. Sprayregen. 1985. "Six-Year Experience with Expanded Polytetrafluoroethylene Arterial Grafts for Limb Salvage", *J. Cardiovasc. Surg.*, 26:468–472.

16. Gupta, S. K., E. Ascer and F. Veith. 1987. "Expanded Polytetrafluoroethylene Arterial Grafts: An Eight-Year Experience", in *Modern Vascular Grafts*. P. N. Sawyer, ed. NY: McGraw Hill Book Company, pp. 181–189.

17. Heydorn, W. H., J. W. Geasling, W. Y. Moores, L. O. Lollini and A. C. Gomez. 1979. "Changes in the Manufacture of Expanded Microporous Polytetrafluoroethylene: Effects on Patency and Histological Behavior When Used to Replace the Superior Vein Cava", *Ann. Thor. Surg.*, 27:173–177.

18. Hanel, K. C., C. McCabe, W. M. Abbott, J. Fallon and J. Megerman. 1982. "Current PTFE Grafts. A Biomechanical Scanning Electron and Light Microscopic Evaluation", *Ann. Surg.*, 195:456–462.

19. Goldfarb, D., J. A. Houk, J. L. Moore and D. L. Gain. 1977. "Graphite-Expanded Polytetrafluoroethylene: An Improved Small Artery Prosthesis", *Trans. Amer. Soc. Artif. Intern. Organs*, 23:268–274.

20. Kempczinsky, R. F. 1979. "Physical Characteristics of Implanted Polytetrafluoroethylene Grafts." *Arch. Surg.*, 114:917–919.

21. McClurken, M. E., J. M. McHaney and W. M. Colone. 1986. "Physical Properties and Test Methods for Expanded Polytetrafluoroethylene (PTFE) Grafts", in *Vascular Graft Update: Safety and Performance*. ASTM STP 898, H. E. Kambic, A. Kantrowitz and P. Sung, eds. American Society for Testing and Materials, Philadelphia, pp. 82–94.

22. Guidoin R., P. A. Levaillant, M. Marois, C. Gosselin, L. Martin, C. Rouleau, P. Garneau, H. P. Noël and P. Blais. 1980. "Les Prothèses en Polyéthylènetétéphlate (Dacron®) Comme Substituts Artériels. Evaluation des Greffes Commerciales Comme Substituts de L'aorte Abdominale de Chien", *J. Mal. Vasc.*, 5:3–12.

23. Goëau-Brissonnière O., R. Guidoin, M. Marois, B. Boyce, J. C. Pechère, P. Blais, H. P. Noël and C. Gosselin. 1981. "Thoraco-Abdominal Bypass as a Method for Evaluating Vascular Grafts in the Dog", *Biomat. Med. Devices Artif. Organs*, 9:195–212.

24. Campbell, C. D., D. H. Brooks, M. W. Webster, R. P. Bondi, J. C. Lloyd, M. F. Hybes and H. T. Bahnson. 1976. "Aneurysm Formation in Expanded Polytetrafluoroethylene Prostheses", *Surgery*, 79:491–493.

25. Roberts, A. K. and N. Johnson. 1978. "Aneurysm Formation in an Expanded Microporous Polytetrafluoroethylene Graft", *Arch. Surg.*, 113:211–213.

26. Courbier, R., J. M. Jausseran, M. Reggi and G. Chiche. "Les prothèses artérielles en polytétrafluo-

roéthylène. Premiers résultats cliniques", *J. Mal. Vasc.*, 4:151–155.

27. Mohr, L. L. and L. L. Smith. 1980. "Polytetra-fluoroethylene Graft Aneurysm. A Report of Five Aneurysms", *Arch. Surg.*, 115:1457–1470.

28. Graham, L. M. and J. J. Bergan. 1982. "Expanded PTFE Vascular Grafts. Clinical and Experimental Observations", in *Biologic and Synthetic Vascular Prostheses*. J. C. Stanley et al., eds. NY: Grune and Stratton, pp. 563–586.

29. Bergan, J. J., J. P. Harris, N. D. Rudo and S. T. Yao. 1982. "Update of PTFE Grafts", in *Current Critical Problems in Vascular Surgery*. F. J. Veith, ed. NY: Appleton-Century Crofts, pp. 105–122.

30. Vaughan, G. D., K. L. Mattox, D. V. Feliciano, A. G. Beall, Jr. and M. E. DeBakey. 1979. "Surgical Experiences with Expanded PTFE as a Replacement Graft for Traumatized Vessels", *J. Trauma*, 19:403–408.

31. Formichi, M., R. Guidoin, J. M. Jausseran, J. Awad, W. Johnston, M. King, R. Courbier, M. Marois, C. Rouleau, M. Batt, J. F. Girard and C. Gosselin. 1988. "Expanded PTFE Prosthesis as Arterial Substitutes in Man: Late Pathological Findings in 73 Excised Grafts", *Ann. Vasc. Surg.*, 2:14–26.

32. Mohring, K., H. W. Asbach and H. W. Bersh, et al. 1978. "Clinical Implications of Pathomorphological Findings in Vascular Prostheses", in *Dialysis Transplantation Nephrology*. R. Hawkins, ed. Great Britain: The Pitman Press, pp. 582–583.

33. Ansel, A. L. and J. M. Johnson. 1982. "Prevention and Management of Polytetrafluoroethylene Grafts. Complications in Peripheral Vascular Reconstructions", *Am. J. Surg.*, 144:228–230.

34. Camilleri, J. P., V. N. Phat, P. Bruneval, V. Tricottet, A. Balaton, J. N. Fissinger and J. M. Cormier. 1985. "Surface Healing and Histologic Maturation of Patent Polytetrafluoroethylene Grafts Implanted in Patients for up to 60 Months", *Arch. Pathol. Lab. Med.*, 109:833–837.

35. Campbell, C. D., D. Goldfarb and R. Roc. 1975. "A Small Arterial Substitute, Expanded Microporous Polytetrafluoroethylene: Patency Versus Porosity", *Ann. Surg.*, 182:138–143.

36. Florian, A., L. H. Cohn, G. J. Dammin and J. J. Collins, Jr. 1976. "Small Vessel Replacement with Gore-tex (Expanded Polytetrafluoroethylene)", *Arch. Surg.*, 111:267–279.

37. Sharp, W. V. 1983. "Present Status of Carbon Grafts", in *Vascular Grafting, Clinical Applications and Techniques*. C. B. Wright, ed. Boston: John Wright PSG Inc., pp. 326–330.

38. Kuwano, H. M. Hashizume, Y. Yang, A. M. Kholloussy and T. Matsumoto. 1986. "Patterns of Pannus Growth of the Expanded Polytetrafluoroethylene Vascular Graft with Special Attention to the Intimal Hyperplasia Formation", *Am. Surg.*, 52:663–666.

39. Clowes, A. W., A. M. Gown, S. R. Hanson and M. A. Reidy. 1985. "Mechanisms of Arterial Graft Failures. I. Role of Cellular Proliferation in Early Healing of PTFE Prostheses", *Am. J. Pathol.*, 118:43–45.

40. Clowes, A. W., T. R. Kirkman and M. M. Clowes. 1986. "Mechanisms of Arterial Graft Failures. II. Chronic Endothelial and Smooth Muscle Cell Proliferation on Healing Polytetrafluoroethylene Prostheses", *J. Vasc. Surg.*, 3:877–886.

41. Clowes, A. W., T. R. Kirkman and M. A. Reidy, 1986. "Mechanisms of Arterial Graft Healing. Rapid Transmural Capillary Ingrowth Provides a Source of Intimal Endothelium and Smooth Muscle in Porous PTFE Prostheses", *Am. J. Pathol.*, 123:220–230.

42. Clowes, A. W., R. K. Zacharias and T. R. Kirkman. 1987. "Early Endothelial Coverage of Synthetic Arterial Grafts: Porosity Revisited", *Am. J. Surg.*, 153:501–504.

21

Interrelation of Protein Adsorption and Blood Compatibility of Biomaterials

V. I. SEVASTIANOV, Ph.D., Dr. Sci.*

ABSTRACT: A review of recent research on the interrelation of protein adsorption and blood compatibility is presented. The mechanism of surface passivation, determined by the physicochemical properties of the biomaterials, is considered. Also analyzed is the influence of the composition and structure of the adsorbed protein layer on short- and long-term processes such as blood and tissue cell reaction, thrombosis, thromboembolization, infections and inflammatory response, and calcification. Up-to-date approaches to the development of blood-compatible biomaterials are analyzed, based on the regulation of their adsorptional characteristics.

INTRODUCTION

The blood compatibility of biomaterials is a complex problem. On one hand, protein adsorption is known to be the first stage of blood/surface interaction. In the majority of studies on the mechanism of the blood compatibility of biomaterials, attempts have been made to establish relationships between the physicochemical properties of the surface and its adsorptional characteristics [1–12]. On the other hand, it is evident that the blood compatibility of medical devices depends on many parameters, as is shown in Figure 1. Therefore, the positive role of certain adsorptional parameters in a biomaterial's blood compatibility, proven in model experiments *in vitro*, *in vivo* and *ex vivo*, does not mean for sure that the medical device will also be blood-compatible.

In addition the correlation between thrombus formation on subendothelium and the mechanism of blood/foreign surface interaction should be sought with great care. Table 1 lists a number of the factors

that have been described as important in the research on thrombus formation on subendothelium [13]. Interestingly, fibrinogen (FG), which is thought from *in vitro* studies to be necessary for platelet activation, appears not to be involved significantly in thrombus formation, as is indicated by normal values of thrombus dimensions on subendothelium in afibrinogenemia [14]. This conclusion may be related to the ability of the von Willebrand factor (VWF) to substitute for FG in binding to the platelet membrane [15–17].

No biomaterial is known not to adsorb protein to a certain extent. Therefore, it remains necessary to obtain optimal, in terms of blood compatibility, parameters of the protein adsorption/desorption processes. Figure 2 represents the main events that take place during the interaction of a biomaterial with blood, and establishes the role of protein adsorption.

Taking into account current knowledge of the process of protein adsorption on the solid/liquid interface and the blood compatibility of biomaterials [1–12,18], the interrelation between these mechanisms will be considered separately for short-term contact and long-term contact with blood. The parameters of the adsorbed protein layer that most probably influence the blood compatibility of biomaterials are presented in Table 2. The contribution of these parameters to the biomaterials' blood compatibility will be analyzed in this chapter.

PROTEIN ADSORPTION AND THE SHORT-TERM BLOOD COMPATIBILITY OF BIOMATERIALS

Let us discuss the role of the main parameters of protein adsorption (Table 2) on short-term blood compatibility, namely thrombosis and embolization, in terms of the reactions of the blood cells, the activation of the blood coagulation system, and the activation of the complement system.

*U.S.S.R. Research Center of Blood Compatible Biomaterials, Institute of Transplantology and Artificial Organs, Moscow, 123436, U.S.S.R.

Table 1. Influence of various components on thrombus formation [13].

	Degree of Influence
Plasma Components	
Platelet count	+ + + +
Hematocrit	+ + + +
Ca++ ion	+ + + +
PGI₂ (PGE₁)	+ + + +
Heparin	+
Aspirin	+ +
Von Willebrand factor	+ + +
Fibrinogen	±
Procoagulant factors	+ + + +
Vessel Wall Components	
Collagen	+ + + +
Von Willebrand factor	?
Other adhesive proteins (fibrinogen, fibronectin)	?
Tissue factor	?
Platelet Related Components	
GPIb	?
GPIIb-IIIa	+ + + +
Dense granules	+ + +
α-Granules	?

Composition of the Adsorbed Protein Layer

Studies of serum albumin (SA), fibrinogen (FG) and γ-globulin (γ-Gl) adsorption on the surface of a number of hydrophobic polymers by IR–ATR method revealed initially that the quantity of adsorbed protein is independent of surface properties and is determined only by the nature of the protein [19]. Later it was shown [20] that the surface properties play a considerable role in protein adsorption from plasma and solutions. Most researchers consider that blood compatibility might be determined by the composition of the

Table 2. The parameters of adsorbed protein layer probably influencing blood compatibility of biomaterials.

1. The character of the formation of the irreversibly adsorbed protein layer.
   - rate of the passivation
   - composition
   - thickness (monolayer, multilayer)
   - structure (surface distribution and conformation)

2. The ratio of irreversibly and reversibly adsorbed protein layers.

3. The character of the desorption processes.
   - exchange and displacement
   - conformation of desorbed proteins

adsorbed protein layer [21–28]. After studies on the positive influence of relative albumin concentration in the adsorbed protein layer (surface albuminization degree) on hemocompatibility [25,26], numerous reports appeared supporting this supposition *in vitro* and *in vivo* [11,27].

Due to the positive effect of adsorbed albumin on the blood compatibility of the polymer, the degree of surface albuminization is widely used as a criterion of blood compatibility [28]. This has led to a new development in processing of blood-compatible polymers possessing high affinity to SA [29–32].

The main argument in favor of the influence of protein layer composition on surface hemocompatibility is the fact that the albumin coating provides for decreased platelet adhesion, whereas, when the surface is precoated with FG and γ-Gl, platelet adhesion is increased. The notion that the degree of albuminization should be used as a criterion for surface hemocompatibility quickly became popular due to the attractive biochemical hypothesis of Lee and Kim [19,33] explaining the positive effect of surface passivation with albumin by the absence of saccharide residues in albumin molecules. Later there appeared other suppositions about antithrombogenic properties of surfaces coated with albumin [34] stressing the following: (1) competitive adsorption of SA, limiting the availability of binding sites on the polymer for FG, which promotes platelet adhesion and aggregation; (2) participation of SA in spontaneous isomerization of PGH₂ to PGD₂, a potent platelet functional inhibitor; and (3) binding of albumin with products of arachidonate metabolism at the blood/polymer interface, preventing platelet recruitment.

However, analysis of experimental data on the relationship between the composition of the adsorbed layer and the surface hemocompatibility reveals a number of contradictions.

This can be shown on the basis of recent works, which concern the proofs of thrombogenicity of FG and antithrombogenicity of SA. The results of some studies questioned "antithrombogenic" and "thrombogenic" role of albumin and fibrinogen, respectively, in the blood compatibility of surface. Anderson et al. showed [35] that an albumin coating improved the short-term blood compatibility of Dacron® by all the methods employed in this study. Moreover, an albumin coating not only inhibited platelet adhesion, but also significantly decreased the high levels of platelet release. This group also investigated the effect of preclotting on the reactivity (count, platelet factor 3 (PF-3), PF-4, β-thromboglobulin, aggregatibility) of a vascular graft prosthesis of a crimped Dacron bionit, using an *in vitro* perfusion system [36]. Platelet activation by Dacron was initially rapid and then leveled off, whereas the platelet activation with preclotted Dacron began more slowly, but reached much greater levels after three hours of *in vitro* perfusion. Contradicting this, Saski et al. [37] reported that platelet activation occurred after 15 weeks of implan-

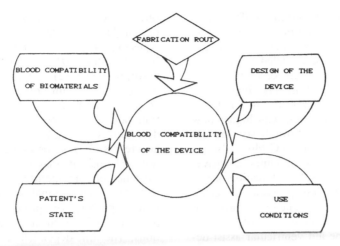

Figure 1. Important factors influencing blood compatibility of medical devices.

tation, and that no obvious differences were observed in the behavior of vascular grafts treated *in vivo* with one of the following methods: fibrin precoating, autoclaving after soaking in albumin, and conventional whole-blood preclotting.

Blood compatibility of the cross-linked polyether/polysiloxane networks was evaluated using an *in vitro* platelet retention test and ^{125}I-fibrinogen adsorption experiments from human plasma and buffered saline [38,39]. Networks which adsorbed the largest amounts of fibrinogen were found to have the greatest reactivity with platelets. Data from this test, however, suggests that the amount of surface-bound FG is not the sole mediator of platelet/surface interactions. The authors explain the obtained effect by the conformational changes of FG produced by adsorption.

The thrombogenic role of fibrinogen and other adhesive proteins (von Willebrand factor, fibronectin) was established in the studies of platelet adhesion on uncoated and coated polyethylene [40]. It was observed that platelet adhesion is promoted by these adsorbed proteins. Von Willebrand factor is the most active protein according to the amount of cells, while platelet spreading is the most extensive on fibronectin-coated surfaces. This work [40] revealed that adsorption of IgG results in platelet aggregation at the surface, and platelet adhesion is inhibited by adsorbed albumin.

Horbett et al. [41] briefly reported that platelet adhesion did not correlate with fibrinogen adsorption to glass. These results may suggest that other plasma proteins besides fibrinogen have an important influence on platelet adhesion.

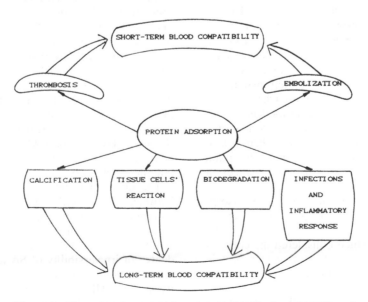

Figure 2. The role of protein adsorption in the blood compatibility of biomaterials.

As to the amounts adsorbed, opinions differ. A plateau of the surface concentration depends on protein and polymer type and is on the order of 0.2 to 2.0 μg/cm^2. Such quantities can be modeled as monomolecular layers [67–42]. For a number of polymers, proof of the multilayer adsorption was obtained [11, 43–45]. Based on the discovered transfer form, monolayer-to-multilayer adsorption with higher flow rate, the concept of "protein" thrombosis was advanced, in particular for adsorbed FG [46]. Also, as with the hemocompatibility of the albumin monolayer in the early stages of the logical continuation of implantation, a "multilayer protein passivation mechanism" for long-term antithrombogeneity was proposed [45]. Detailed analyses of the segmented polyurethane surfaces of diaphragm-type left ventricular assist devices (LVAD) implanted for a term varying from 1 week to 1 month in goats, showed that thrombus could be formed occasionally even after long-term implantation, even when the passivation was considered to be completed. Subsequently, stable multilayers were formed with loosely bound intact proteins at the blood/surface interface to help prevent thrombus formation.

Therefore, the process of passivation of the surface of irreversibly adsorbed protein, as opposed to the influence of the composition of the adsorbed layer on the surface's hemocompatibility, should be primarily considered. The positive role of irreversibly adsorbed protein layers in the hemocompatibility of hydrophobic surface has been independently revealed by several authors [47–51]. It may be explained by the possible result of emboli generation because of a weak affinity for plasma proteins with surfaces.

The Kinetics of the Formation of the Irreversibly Adsorbed Protein Layer

At present it is known that the Langmuir model cannot adequately describe protein adsorption. The majority of the models for protein adsorption proposed up to now are based on an assumption of the existence of several states for adsorbed protein molecules on the surface. These states of adsorbed protein may be interpreted from different physical approaches.

For example, there are a number of models considering the adsorbed states as stages of conformational alterations of adsorbed proteins [7,8,10]. There is also a lot of reliable data proving that protein adsorption may result in significant conformational changes of protein molecules [1–12].

Another way of giving a meaning to a set of adsorptional states consists of introducing the heterogeneity for the protein/surface interaction. In particular it was the theoretical model which considered the effect of surface heterogeneity on the formation of a protein layer irreversibly adsorbed onto a hydrophobic surface [11,51].

The main assumptions of the model of initial stages of kinetics of formation on an irreversibly adsorbed protein layer are as follows (Figure 3): (1) adsorbed protein has two states "P" and "D" according to the types of adsorptional centers: "the centers of irreversible adsorption" (P) and the "centers of irreversible desorption" (D); (2) decrease in adsorbed protein "D" is linked only with conversion into denatured state "D", followed by desorption; and (3) protein adsorption can occur in both state "P" and state "D", but desorption proceeds only from state "D". Formation of an irreversibly adsorbed protein layer with concentration [P] (μg/cm^2) may be formally explained by the existence of corresponding "surface centers" (P) and (D) (or conformational states of protein) with their ratio depending on protein type, physicochemical properties of the surface, and experimental conditions. The time-dependent character of this ratio determines the form of a kinetic curve.

The analytical solution of the model is:

$$[P] = C_1 [1 - \exp(-k_1 t)]$$
$$+ C_2 [1 - \exp(-k_4 t)] + (k_3 - k_6)t \qquad (1)$$

where k_1 and k_4 are effective rate constants of adsorption and desorption (sec^{-1}), respectively, in transitional regions ($0 < t \ll k_1^{-1}$; k_3 and k_6 are effective rates of adsorption and desorption (μg/cm^2/sec), respectively, in the diffusion region ($t \gg k_1^{-1}$). This equation describes six types of kinetic curves observed experimentally (Figure 4).

The obtained kinetic parameters of SA and FG adsorption from plasma, namely k_1, k_4, k_3 and k_6 depend on the type and chemical composition of the surface. The ratios of k_1/k_4 and k_3/k_6 characterize the degree of irreversibility of protein adsorption on the surface in the transitional and diffusion areas, respectively. The parameter $\beta_i = k_1 k_3 / k_4 k_6$ (i = SA, FG) stands for the common degree of irreversibility of protein adsorption equal to the ratio of the constants-of-adsorption rates to the constants-of-desorption rates in transitional and diffusion areas. This reflects the role of the formation of an irreversibly adsorbed layer (or the degree of affinity of surface) for a given protein.

While the degree of irreversibility of SA adsorption increases (Table 3), the value of the relative index of platelet adhesion (RIPA) decreases for all studied polymers (Spirmen correlation coefficient between β_{SA} and RIPA = -0.91 where $p < 0.005$). It should be noted that in the upper part of the Table 3 there are polymers with good antithrombogenic properties.

The obtained values of the correlation coefficient between β_{SA} and RIPA supported the positive role of albuminization in the blood compatibility of polymers. In addition, it allowed the following generalization to be made: the higher the value of β_{SA} and the degree of irreversibility of SA adsorption, the higher the probability of a given polymer's blood compatibility *in vivo*. All the existing polymers can be distributed into the following groups according to their affinity to SA and FG: (1) $\beta_{SA} < 1$, $\beta_{FG} < 1$; (2)

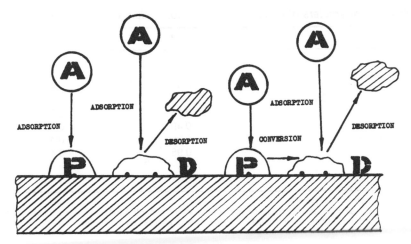

Figure 3. General outline of the physical processes occurring in irreversible adsorption of protein. *A*, circulating protein; *P*, irreversible adsorption centers or conformational state of adsorbed protein in the form "*P*"; and *D*, irreversible adsorption centers or conformational state of adsorbed protein in the form "*D*".

$\beta_{SA} > 1$, $\beta_{FG} < 1$; (3) $\beta_{SA} > 1$, $\beta_{FG} > 1$; and (4) $\beta_{SA} < 1$, $\beta_{FG} > 1$ (Table 4). The SA preadsorption is much better revealed in group 2 than in polymers of the first group, which have a low affinity of SA and FG adsorption. In addition, increasing the bulk activation of the coagulation and complement systems due to the desorption of the conformationally altered protein components, it also brings about energetic heterogeneity of the blood-contacting surface because of the low probability of the formation of the continuous protein layer at small values of β_{SA} and β_{FG}. The latter largely promotes both the growing number of adherent platelets and their morphological changes, followed by the release of platelet coagulation factors.

Table 4 demonstrates that although Pellethane®, which belongs to the third group, has a high affinity to FG, it reveals low adhesivity to platelets (Table 3). It was assumed that polymers with a high value of FG would tend to form fibrin rapidly with low probability of thrombus formation, thus displaying high blood compatibility.

The hypothesis of the positive role of high adsorption and low desorption rates of FG ($\beta_{FG} > 1$) in surface hemocompatibility of hydrophobic biomaterials is confirmed by the time-dependent character of FG adhesivity to platelets [34,41,52]. Thus, it was found *in vivo* that the transitional complex emerging during polymerization of FG into fibrin (induced by the Hageman factor activation) is highly attractive to platelets [54]. After the formation of fibrin film the quantity of adherent platelets decreases [34,41,52,53]. Also it was demonstrated *in vivo* that platelets do not adhere to "converted" (having lost its antigenicity FG [55], i.e., the shorter the time for transition of native FG into its "converted" form, the lower the probability of platelet adhesion. So, since during the formation of the first adsorptional monolayer, blood proteins are subjected to the most considerable conformational changes, high values of β_{FG} provoke quick passivation

of the surface with "converted" proteins, resulting in rapidly forming fibrin film. *In vivo* this is followed by rapidly forming fibrin film, which accelerates, for example, the formation of neointima on the surface of a vascular graft [37,56–58]. This conclusion has been supported by the results of Horbett et al. [53]. Using the model of a deposition baboon ^{125}I-FG from plasma *in vitro* or from blood *in vivo*, they found that

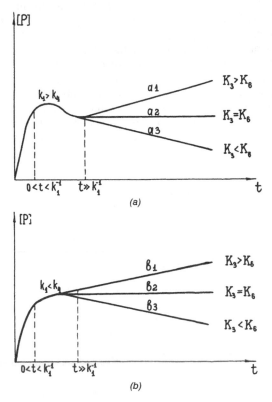

Figure 4. General form of the theoretical curves (a) $k_1 > k_4$; $C_1 > 0$; $C_2 < 0$—curves a_1, a_2, a_3; (b) $k_1 < k_4$; $C_1 > 0$; $C_2 > 0$—curves b_1, b_2, b_3.

Table 3. Parameters of irreversible protein adsorption and platelet adhesion.

Polymer	β_{SA}[a]	β_{FG}[a]	RIPA[b]
Biomer® (Ethicon, Inc.)	5.50	0.70	0.50
Pellethane® (UpJohn)	3.43	1.60	0.70
PTFE	0.97	0.28	1.0
Silicon rubber MSK-1 on the base of PDMS (medical grade)	2.25	0.39	1.0
PU-11p (MDI, PIBA, BD)	0.40	0.48	1.3
Vitur (PU) (MDI, PTMG, ED)	0.35	0.43	1.8
Low-density polyethylene	0.95	0.44	2.0
Silicon rubber on the base of PDMS	0.01	0.40	3.5

[a]t = 37°C, static, ^{191}I-SA, ^{125}I-FG, from human plasma.
[b]t = 37°C, static, in chamber without air, ^{51}Cr-rabbit platelets, time of incubation—60 min. RIPA (relative index of platelet adhesion) = the ratio of the number of platelets adhering to the surface of the sample tested to the number of platelets on the surface of the standard (glass slides).

most polymers with high initial *in vitro* FG adsorption, followed by a decrease, had low FG deposition behavior *in vivo* and were also minimally destructive of platelets.

Hence, the positive effect of albuminization and fibrinization on the surface's hemocompatibility will be conditioned by its physicochemical properties, which eventually define the degree of irreversibility of adsorption. In this context, it becomes clear why the attempts to increase antithrombogenicity of biomaterial surface by preadsorption of SA or passivation with fibrin film have failed. Preadsorption of SA will be most effective for the polymers of group 2 ($\beta_{SA} > 1$, $\beta_{FG} < 1$), while the passivation fibrin film fits for the polymers of group 4 ($\beta_{SA} < 1$, $\beta_{FG} > 1$). For the biomaterial of group 3 ($\beta_{SA} > 1$, $\beta_{FG} > 1$) all ways mentioned of increasing hemocompatibility will do. At the same time, for polymers of the first group ($\beta_{SA} < 1$, $\beta_{FG} < 1$), physical preadsorption of proteins will not significantly increase antithrombogenicity. Here only physical or chemical modification of the surface, inducting necessary changes in its adsorptional properties to SA and FG, will be sufficient.

Table 4. Four adsorptional types of surfaces and their blood compatibility.

Intervals of the Values of			
NN	SA	FG	Example
1	$\beta_{SA} < 1$	$\beta_{FG} < 1$	Industrial polyether (ester) urethanes and silicon rubber (low blood compatibility)
2	$\beta_{SA} > 1$	$\beta_{FG} < 1$	Biomer® (high blood compatibility)
3	$\beta_{SA} > 1$	$\beta_{FG} > 1$	Pellethane® , Avcothane® (Cardiothane) (high blood compatibility)
4	$\beta_{SA} < 1$	$\beta_{FG} > 1$	Surfaces with covalent immobilized heparin (high blood compatibility)

The Mechanism of Improvement of Biomaterials' Blood Compatibility

Recently, a theoretical model [59,60] has been developed to explain the reversible and irreversible protein adsorption in kinetic regime by assuming continuous energetical heterogeneity (CEH) for protein/surface interaction (Figure 5). The mathematical approach is based on the approximation of the "controlling band", which is accurate for wide monotonous distributions of the energetical characteristics of protein/surface interaction. Different ways of correlating energy of activation E_{ad} and heat of adsorption Q for the adsorptional centers are introduced. There is a negative correlation between E_{ad} and Q (Figure 6) and a positive correlation between E_{ad} and Q with the existence of surface diffusion of the protein (Figure 7). Lateral diffusion leads to redistribution of adsorbed molecules from the centers of irreversible adsorption. The suggested model of protein adsorption allows us to explain the experimental data on HSA adsorption involving PDMS and Quartz (Qu) surfaces, but not involving conformational changes or protein/protein interactions.

Linear approximation of the kinetic curves and isotherms in the semilogarithmic form for HSA adsorption from solution onto Qu corresponds (according to CEH) to the negative correlation between E_{ad} and Q and the rectangular distribution of the energy characteristics of protein/surface interaction [56,60] (Figure 6). HSA adsorption on PDMS under the same experimental conditions proceeds at a constant rate, which is characteristic of protein/surface systems with a positive E_{ad}–Q correlation. Firstly, protein occupies the centers of adsorption with minimal energy of activation E_{ad}. These centers also have the minimal value of Q. Due to lateral diffusion, adsorbed molecules are redistributed to the centers with higher heat of adsorption Q (Figure 7). And the following protein will adsorb on the same centers "1". In other words, the occupation of the surface centers proceeds through the "gate", through the centers with low E_{ad}.

It is hard to determine what variant of "energetical

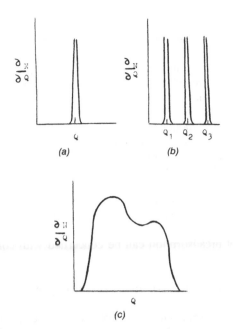

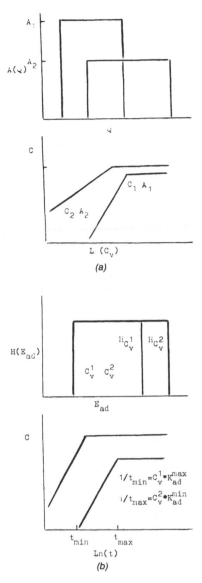

Figure 5. The progress of the hypotheses of energetical heterogeneity: (a) the Langmuir surface; (b) the set of centers with different heats of adsorption; (c) the continuous distribution of the energetical density of adsorptional centers $\partial N/\partial Q$ in the heat of adsorption Q.

heterogeneity" of protein/surface interaction will be preferential in terms of blood compatibility. One can only suppose that in the case of negative correlation between E_{ad} and Q for the surface/protein system, the protein in the first monolayer will be tightly bound with the surface and the effects of "exchange" and "replacement" will be negligible ("static" passivating layer). In the case of positive correlation between E_{ad} and Q, even for a hydrophobic material, we have the probability of partial exchange of proteins in the adsorbed state ("dynamic" passivating layer), which proceeds through the centers with low values of E_{ad} and Q, i.e., through the "gate".

Sevastianov et al. [61] analyzed the kinetics of SA adsorption onto bare and albuminized quartz (Qu), and the distribution of the density of adsorptional centers by energy E_{act} of adsorption for coated and uncoated Qu surfaces on the basis of the CEH theory.

The general view of kinetic curves of adsorption is represented in Figure 8. Not only was a significant decrease in the total amount of adsorbed protein observed, but so was a change in the character of adsorption for the passivated surface in comparison with the uncoated surface. Indeed, the kinetics of HSA–FITC adsorption onto uncoated silica can be well approximated by a straight line in $F \sim \ln(t)$ coordinates (Figure 9), but that for coated Qu surface yields a straight line in $\ln(F) \sim \ln(t)$ coordinates (Figure 10). This supports the model of adsorption onto albuminized surfaces described by the Freundlich equation. Consequently with passivation the transition from rectangular to exponential distribution of adsorptional centers is realized.

Figure 6. Isotherms (a) and the kinetic curves (b) for adsorption onto surface with rectangular distribution $A(Q)$ and $H(E_{ad})$ in the assumption (for kinetics) of negative correlation between the energy of activation E_{ad} and heat of adsorption Q. C_v—bulk protein concentration; K_{ad}—rate constant of adsorption.

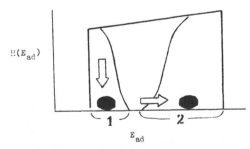

Figure 7. The scheme of protein adsorption onto energetically heterogeneous surfaces with positive correlation between E_{ad} and Q. When the surface/protein interaction can be characterized by continuous distribution $H(E_{ad})$, the real situation can be reduced to the case of two centers: "1"—reversible adsorption; "2"—irreversible adsorption.

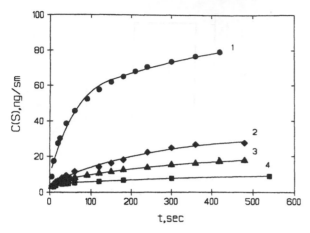

Figure 8. Kinetics of the HSA adsorption from PBS (pH = 7.35) onto uncoated (1) and coated quartz surfaces. C_v = 0.1 mg/ml, T°K = 297 ± 1; γ = 2000 sec^{-1}; the total time of preadsorption (t_p) equals to the sum of the time of adsorption (t_{ad}) and the time of desorption (t_{des}) of unlabelled HSA (2), t_p = 2 min; (3), t_p = 7 min; (4), t_p = 30 min.

From the analysis of the experimental data the authors inferred that:

- Albuminization of Qu surfaces results in a striking decrease in the total amount of adsorptional centers proportional to the duration of preadsorption.
- Passivation changes the character of the energetical distribution of adsorptional centers based on their E_{act} from rectangular to exponential.
- Passivation causes a growth in the fraction of adsorptional centers with high E_{act}. Conse-

quently, the passivated surface becomes more energetically homogeneous than the original one.

- With the increase in the duration of passivation procedure, the energetical distribution becomes more uniform.

Thus, the model of CEH allows us to explain the positive effect of passivation as a blocking of high-energy centers that may activate thrombosis.

Nevertheless some of the experimental data cannot be explained within the scope of this theory. For example, transformation of energetical distribution, decrease in the density of all adsorptional centers, and the dependence of the surface properties on the total time of preadsorption can be concerned with conformational changes of adsorbed proteins.

Structure of a Passivated Protein Layer

The experimental results obtained to date reveal the secondary role played by the composition and the amount of irreversibly adsorbed protein in determining the surface's blood compatibility, as compared with the structure of this initial layer of proteins. Mori et al. [62] investigated by FTIR the amount of adsorbed bovine serum albumin (BSA), bovine γ-globulin (BγG) and bovine plasma fibrinogen (BPF) on the polymer films of the A-B-type block copolymers, consisting of polystyrene (PST) or poly (methylmethacrylate) (PMMA) and poly(γ-benzil L-glutamate) {P[Glu(oBzL)]}, and the degree of denaturation of adsorbed proteins from a single solution in static conditions. A positive correlation was found *in vitro* between thrombus formation and the degree of denaturation of all adsorbed proteins only.

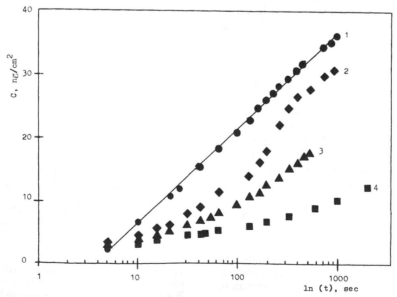

Figure 9. Kinetics of the HSA adsorption onto uncoated and coated quartz surfaces in semilogarithmic coordinates. Symbols are as in Figure 8. The experimental data are multiplied by 0.4.

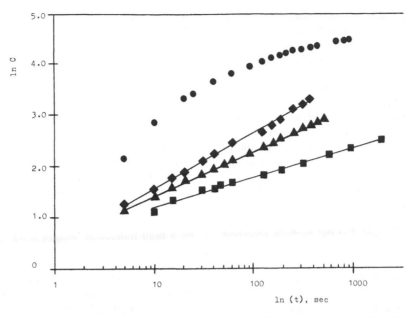

Figure 10. Kinetics of the HSA adsorption onto uncoated and coated quartz surfaces in bilogarithmic coordinates. Symbols are as in Figure 8.

Platelet adhesion from washed ^{51}Cr-platelet suspension to polymer films coated with one of the proteins showed that the activation of adhered platelets was suppressed when the degree of denaturation of coated proteins was lower. In the same experiments using platelet-rich plasma, neither the number of platelets adhered, nor the degree of activation of the platelets was correlated with the composition of the polymer films.

Therefore, these experimental and theoretical results clearly showed that with the lower extent of denaturation of adsorbed proteins, the adhered platelets are less activated, thus leading to a slower rate of thrombus formation.

The works of Cooper and coworkers [63–65] can be presented to illustrate the necessity of careful interpretation of the experimental data on the role of the composition of adsorbed layer in the blood compatibility of the surface. Analyzing the results of these and other works, let us consider in detail the influence of such characteristics of an irreversibly adsorbed protein layer as its surface distribution and conformation on the blood compatibility of biomaterials.

The heterogeneity of protein formation on surfaces of fluoropolymers and polyethylene was demonstrated by different authors [66–72]. In particular, a positive correlation was found between a surface's tendency to form a thick uniform adsorbed layer and its hemocompatibility. It was also found that the organization of protein films depends both on the protein nature and on the polymer's physicochemical properties [69]. FG and especially SA molecules are more extensive and closely packed on LTI carbon surfaces than on Fluorofilm Teflon® [67]. But the organization of the protein layers on LTI carbon is also different, with

FG not exhibiting the reticulated network to the same degree, and SA exhibiting less of the sparse microaggregation which had been previously observed for the Teflon® material. Thus LTI carbon surfaces may bind albumin and FG adsorbates more tenaciously than Teflon® and other hydrophobic surfaces possibly by virtue of interactions with high-energy, surface-functional oxygen groups and, particularly for FG, by interactions with surface pores. The results are consistent with the concept of an immobilized, dense protein film, which may be unreactive with blood.

On poly(tetrafluoroethylene), poly(vinylidene fluoride), and poly(vinyl fluoride), hemoglobin and fibronectin were localized into islands, i.e., bare areas of polymer exist, and the degree of coverage of the polymer surface increased with increasing polymer critical surface tension. The fibronectin was found to cover a larger fraction of each polymer surface than hemoglobin [68].

In addition, the degree of coverage of the polymer surface depends on protein affinity for the surface. Protein affinity was found to increase with increasing biomaterial surface-water free energy in the order PEU < PVC < PE < SR [43]. In general, the binding strength of the proteins for these surfaces increases in the order IgG < α_2M < Tfr < SA < FG.

The results of a kinetic investigation [44] indicate that time-dependent changes in the conformation of the adsorbed protein molecules and of the polymer surface occur on the solid surface toward a higher affinity of the molecules for the solid state. According to the experimental results [44] it is suggested (as in Reference [43]) that higher adsorption should occur on a surface with a larger interfacial free energy.

At first, in the studies of acute surface-induced

thrombosis in the canine *ex vivo* model, Park et al. [63] came to the conclusion that the thrombogeneity of a surface (PVC, PE, SR) was related to the composition of the initial protein layer. Specifically, the composition of this layer determines the extent of platelet activation and the adhesive strength between platelets and the polymer surface.

Later, both Park [65] and other authors [66–73] obtained evidence of the importance not only of the composition of the adsorbed layer, but of its microstructure (or microheterogeneity) for determining blood compatibility.

On glass surfaces it was observed [65] that fibrinogen always formed multimeric aggregates even at surface concentration much lower than a monolayer coverage. It has been assumed that the surface-adsorbed FG undergo conformational changes to a biochemically more active form which has a high affinity for platelet receptors [74]. Authors [75] proposed, as an alternative to the conformation hypothesis, the multiple-binding hypothesis. This hypothesis suggests that the surface-adsorbed FG may present continuous, multiple binding sites which substantially increase the interaction with platelet receptors.

But it was found that the adsorbed FG has a different structure at hydrophobic and hydrophilic quartz surfaces [76]. At a hydrophobic surface the FG molecules appeared as a 46 nm nodose rod consisting of 6–7 nodes with a diameter of 4 nm. At a hydrophobic surface the molecule appeared as a binodular or trinodular rod with a node diameter of 5–9 nm, connected with a thin filament to form a 40 nm rod.

Evidently that different structure (different distribution) of proteins is closely connected with the conformational changes of proteins both in the adsorbed and desorbed states.

Kang et al. [82] showed that the antithrombogenicity of A–B block copolymers of four different compositions depends upon the extent of platelet adhesion and the activation on the material, which is dependent in turn on the conformation of plasma proteins adsorbed on the material. The number of adhered platelets and the rate of serotonin release increased when plasma proteins underwent conformational change. In some cases an increase in the quantity of adherent platelets by one order can be related to the contact of blood with air, resulting in denaturation of the protein molecules [83] or to the presence of gas nuclei deposited in the surface's microroughness [84].

In light of the above-mentioned thesis concerning the positive role of surface passivation with protein (degree of irreversibility of SA and FG adsorption) in the hemocompatibility of biomaterials, the following working theory as to the relationship between protein molecular structure and the mechanism of the polymer/blood interaction may be advanced [11]: the part played by conformational changes of protein molecules during the adsorption/desorption process is both positive (surface passivation with irreversible adsorbed protein layer) and negative (the initiation of

blood/enzyme systems, in particular bulk activation of the coagulation and complement systems because of the desorption of the surface-activated protein components). It is noteworthy that the positive role of the surface passivation depends on its rate, especially for hydrophobic biomaterials. For hydrophobic materials, the positive effect of the high degree of irreversibility of SA adsorption on the hemocompatibility of the surface may be specified in terms of rapid passivation by SA and simultaneous decrease in the probability of adsorption of other proteins, in particular FG. This results in a considerable reduction in the activation factors of coagulation induced by the surface. For example, it was generally shown that a part of FG on the surface of the biomaterial is rather quickly replaced by a high molecular weight kininogen necessary for activating XIII factor [85]. This speculation does not belittle the importance of the reaction of platelets with glycoproteins (FG and γ-globulin), catalyzed by glycosyl transferase of the cell membrane, which explains the reduced adhesiveness of platelets to adsorbed SA [19].

Speaking about the passivation of the biomaterial's surface with protein, one should definitely distinguish the cases of hydrophilic and hydrophobic surfaces. In general, protein molecules are assumed to change conformation to a larger extent on a hydrophobic surface than on a hydrophilic one. Note that the terms "polar" and "nonpolar" (or "apolar") are more fundamental [77] than "hydrophilic" and "hydrophobic", but the latter are more commonly used. The repulsive force normally acting between native protein molecules is probably decreased for conformationally changed molecules adsorbed onto a hydrophobic surface. This means that one can expect closer packing of protein molecules on a hydrophobic surface [78,89]. That is, hydrophilic surfaces differ from hydrophobic ones in providing only insignificant conformational changes in proteins during the formation of the passivating layer [79–81]. The loosely bound protein monolayer is formed on the hydrophilic surface, whereas the multilayer with the first tightly bound protein layer is formed on the hydrophobic surface. For the true hydrophilic surface we have the dynamic passivating layer (the effects of exchange and replacement), and for the hydrophobic one the protein adsorbed in the first layer does not practically interact with protein in other layers. The partial exchange in this case, as was mentioned above, can take place for the system of biomaterial/protein with a positive correlation between E_{ad} and Q [59,60].

Reliable reports have appeared [47–49,91,93] showing that the good hemocompatibility of certain hydrophobic materials was not related to the "repulsion" of protein molecules, as for a hydrophilic surface, but on the contrary, to the ability of the surface to form a homogeneous protein film tightly bound with the surface.

The hypothesis of the minimal quantity of adsorbed protein, explaining in particular the high hemocompatibility of such materials different in surface energy properties—polymers like LTI carbon and polyethyleneoxide—is true for very hydrophilic surfaces. Analysis of the composition and organization of the protein layer adsorbed on the surface of LTI carbon and polyethyleneoxide, supports the possibility that the biomaterial's hemocompatibility correlates to its ability to form a dense, loosely immobilized protein layer [70,94,95].

For example [94], a newly developed hydrophilic having long polyethyleneoxide chains showed excellent antithrombogenicity when evaluated by the insertion of the polymer-coated suture into the peripheral vein. In macroscopic observation, there was no thrombus on the polymer inserted into the vein. However, by SEM analysis, platelet and white blood cells were noticed sporadically on the polymer. By means of TEM of the cross section of the polymer implanted for 2 to 72 days, an adsorbed film of plasma protein was observed on the polymer surface.

The slower the formation of multilayer (the transition from irreversible adsorption to reversible) on the surface of hydrophobic material (low degree of irreversible adsorption, β_i), the greater is the amount of "denatured" protein desorbing into the bulk.

Practically all the authors of the cited studies have attempted to establish the correlation between a surface's hemocompatibility and the conformational changes of only the adsorbed protein molecules. With very few exceptions [27,86], the possibility of the negative influence of desorbed molecules on the blood, accountable for bulk activation of various enzyme/blood systems, has not been considered.

The activation of the complement system induced by the surface of a biomaterial may serve as a proof of the desorption of denatured protein molecules.

The protein nature of the complement components and the interaction of the surface with blood causes processes, necessarily inducing structural alterations in the macromolecules and possibly resulting in the step-by-step activation of the complement system.

In fact, the initiation of the cascade mechanism of complement activation is accompanied by conformational changes in the complement components playing a central role in the classical (C1) and alternative (C3) pathways of complement activation [87,88]. Using the methods of enzyme-linked immunosorbent assay and ellipsometry [89] it was found that C3 adsorbed onto hydrophobic silicon had a conformation exposing antigenic epitopes which are only accessible in C3 denatured by sodium dodecyl sulfate or C3 that has been biologically activated.

There are reasons for the influence of the degree of complement activation by a biomaterial's surface on its hemocompatibility [54,90]: (1) the activated complement mediates the chemotaxis and promotes adhesion of leukocytes to the surface. The alternative pathway results in the release of chemotactic factors C3a and C5a, which promote the adhesion of polymorphonuclear leukocytes to the surface. The leukocytes increase the quantity of adherent platelets and the probability of thrombus formation, (2) activated complement promotes the formation of leukocyte-platelet embolies.

Recently, a kinetic model of complement activation by a foreign surface, which provided for obtaining the expression for the rate constant of complement activation induced by a foreign surface (k_{ind}) [86], was proposed and experimentally confirmed.

Table 5 contains the values of $\bar{k}_{ind}$ for a number of polymer materials. One can conclude that the relative constant $\bar{k}_{ind}$ is dependent on the surface type. For polymers presented in Table 5, $\bar{k}_{ind}$ varies from 0.070 ± 0.002 for Pellethane® to 2.13 ± 0.05 for polydimethylsiloxane. Table 5 also contains the results of the evaluation of the hemocompatibility for the polymers in vitro as determined by platelet adhesion (RIPA) and the degree of irreversible adsorption of SA (β_{SA}). The Spirmen correlation coefficients (β) were calculated for pairs of RIPA and β_{SA}, $\bar{k}_{ind}$ and RIPA, $\bar{k}_{ind}$ and β_{SA}. They are equal to −0.96 ($p < 0.001$), 0.71 ($p < 0.025$), and −0.88 ($p < 0.001$), respec-

Table 5. Quantitative characteristics of biomaterial hemocompatible properties.

Materials	$\bar{k}_{ind}$[a] (± SD)	RIPA[b] (± SD)	β_{SA}[c]
Pellethane (UpJohn)	0.070 ± 0.002	0.7 ± 0.1	3.43
Biomer (Ethicon, Inc.)	0.25 ± 0.01	0.5 ± 0.1	5.50
Low-density polyethylene	0.65 ± 0.02	2.0 ± 0.4	0.95
LDPE (primary reference material Abiomed)	0.97 ± 0.02	1.7 ± 0.3	1.6
Cuprophane (Enca)	1.00 ± 0.02	0.8 ± 0.1	1.49
Vlacefan (cellulose hydrate)	1.20 ± 0.03	1.8 ± 0.2	0.44
Diacell (cellulose hydrate)	1.60 ± 0.03	2.2 ± 0.3	0.54
Silurem (PU–PDMS copolymer)	1.38 ± 0.03	0.6 ± 0.1	2.03
Vitur (PU)	1.96 ± 0.03	1.8 ± 0.3	0.35
Polydimethylsiloxane (primary reference material, NHLBI–DBT)	2.13 ± 0.05	2.3 ± 0.4	0.30

[a]$\bar{k}_{ind} = \bar{k}^i_{ind}/\bar{k}^{st}_{ind}$; the standard surface is Cuprophane, $n = 3$.
[b]$t = 37\,°C$, static, in chamber without air, 51-Cr-rabbit platelets, time of incubation—60 min; RIPA (relative index of platelet adhesion) = the ratio of the number of platelets adhered to the surface of the sample tested to the number of platelets on the surface of the standard (glass).
[c]$t = 37\,°C$, static, 131-I-SA from human plasma, $n = 5$.

tively. The obtained values of correlation coefficients between the criteria of blood compatibility (RIPA β_{SA}) and relative rate constant ($\bar{k}_{ind}$) support the assumption of the close relationship between the character of the formation of irreversibly adsorbed protein layers and platelet adhesion and the degree of complement activation.

There may be two principal pathways for the complement activation by the polymer surface. The complement is activated either directly by the polymer surface or by the preadsorbed protein layer. In both cases, the degree of complement activation ($\bar{k}_{ind}$) should be dependent on the adsorptional properties of the surface. Furthermore, this is the only way that the nature of the polymer can influence the degree of conformational change in the complement components, so the initiation of the cascade mechanism in the volume solution is for desorption of the adsorbed complement components. Thus, the ease of desorption may be a controlling factor in the activation of the complement systems by polymers.

From this point of view, the registered value of $\bar{k}_{ind}$ reflects the complement consumption by adsorption/desorption processes at the blood/polymer interface, and the negative correlation between the degree of irreversible adsorption of SA and $\bar{k}_{ind}$ is quite explainable. According to the radioisotopic method used, the value of β_i (i = SA, FG) characterizes only the formation of irreversible protein layers. The greater the tendency of the polymer surface to irreversible adsorption (i.e., the higher the degree of surface passivation with protein), the lower the desorption rate of the conformational altered molecules in the volume solution, and therefore the higher the bulk complement activation. Certainly the adsorptional properties of the surface depend not only on its physicochemical characteristics but also on the nature of the adsorbed protein. Thus, one can expect a strong correlation between the degree of irreversible adsorption of the two main plasma proteins SA and FG and the conformational changes and desorption of the complement components. Nevertheless, unlike the value of β_i, the value of $\bar{k}_{ind}$ characterizes the degree of structural alterations in both irreversible and reversible layers. The lower the relative rate constant of the induced complement activation, the lower the denaturative action of the surface on the protein macromolecules.

The results obtained make it possible to suggest that the reaction of a complement system in a given patient will be essentially dependent on the type of polymers in the extracorporeal and implanted devices. Moreover, the effect of one and the same polymer will depend of the individual reactivity of a patient's complement system. The rate constant for the spontaneous complement activation (k_{sp}) is proposed as the criterion for the individual reactivity of the complement system.

So, in the formation of the first protein layer, tightly bound with the surface, there is a high probability of conformational changes [45,96,97] that have a lot to do with physicochemical surface properties. Therefore the desorption of protein molecules during this period can have a negative effect on the blood. The only situation in which the inference for increasing hemocompatibility of materials with decreased quantity of adsorbed molecules is valid is that of reversible adsorption [98,99].

In other words, the more rapidly the first dense adsorbed protein layer with homogeneous distribution is formed, the higher the probability that the surface is hemocompatible. Fulfillment of this condition makes hemocompatibility certain, but only for short-term use. All available methods of protein pretreatment (passive exposure, protein cross-linking, and covalent linkage of albumin to the polymer) possess limitations in long-term use due to biological degradation and spontaneous denaturation with time. Methods which have been developed to selectively enhance the affinity of polyetherurethanes, cellulose derivatives, nylon, and polyester surfaces for albumin by covalently binding C_{16-18} aliphatic chains, graphically prove the necessity of combining irreversible and reversible adsorption components for substantially improved blood compatibility of polymers in long-term use [29–32]. This technique provides for rapidly forming dense and homogeneous protein layers on the polymer surface, while allowing the *in vivo* replacement of denatured and desorbed albumin by endogenous native albumin onto a surface having high affinity for this protein.

PROTEIN ADSORPTION AND LONG-TERM BLOOD COMPATIBILITY OF BIOMATERIALS

Infections and Inflammatory Response

Infections and inflammatory responses are major complications of long-term implantation of cardiovascular devices (ventricular assist device (VAD) and total artificial heart (TAH) [100,101]), especially beyond 30 days of implantation. Existing experimental and clinical studies on blood compatibility of artificial organs connected with the above-mentioned processes consider mainly cellular/biomaterial interactions. For example, concerning the role of proteins in biomaterial-induced inflammatory response, the mediators of cell response appearing as a result of biomaterial-induced complement activation (C3a,b,d; C4b; C5a) [101–103], macrophage activation and release on implant surfaces (Interleukin 1) [104] are studied. Only Kossovsky et al. [105,106] made an attempt to relate the conformational changes of protein in an adsorbed state (in terms of immunogenicity) and inflammatory reaction. The model system consisting of syngeneic guinea pigs, silicone oil and pooled serum, has yielded data supporting the supposition that silicon–protein complexes may be immunogenic. The reactions are consistent with both an acute type I

IgE-mediated hypersensitivity response as well as with a type IV cell-mediated delayed hypersensitivity reaction.

With regard to the identity of the immunogenic agent, the two favored hypotheses based on current protein antigen theory [107] are as follows.

The first involves the exposure of a determinant on a denatured protein irreversibly adsorbed on silicone, thus making the silicon–protein complex antigenic. The second proposes the exposure of a determinant on a catalytically denatured and desorbed protein.

The nature of the relation between infection and the blood compatibility of biomaterials in terms of thrombus formation and thromboembolization and implantable cardiovascular devices is poorly understood [100]. This is largely true for the relationship of inflammatory response to the processes of protein adsorption in presence of biomaterial surface. However it is obvious that, for example, selective adherence of certain bacteria to surfaces will be determined by the structure and composition of irreversibly adsorbed protein layer, particularly the degree of specific adsorption of such proteins as fibrinogen, fibronectin, vibronectin, factor XII, and high-molecular weight kininogen. The factors and mechanisms thought to be involved in bacterial interactions with biomaterial surfaces have been reviewed by A. G. Gristina [108]. For instance, initial events in blood/material interactions can lead to the formation of platelet–fibrin thrombi. Early platelet–fibrin thrombi, less than 48 hours in age, are more susceptible to bacterial incorporation than the healing fibrin layer [109,110].

Thus, the conformational changes of proteins both in adsorbed and desorbed states, such as for the events of short-term blood compatibility of biomaterials, play a certain role in biomaterial-induced infections and inflammatory response.

Tissue Cells' Reactions

The ability of a blood surface (especially vascular grafts) to activate tissue repair mechanism and to be assimilated within the natural tissue is an important characteristic of biomaterials intended for long-term implantation [111]. In general, protein adsorption to the surfaces plays a key role in irreversible endothelialization. The ability of a biomaterial to adsorb certain proteins from blood can dictate whether it is capable of supporting cell attachment, spreading and growth (Figure 11) [112]. The presence of specific cell attachment sites on certain protein molecules for cell membrane receptors is also well known [113].

It was found that the attachment, spreading and proliferation of different types of tissue cells onto various surfaces depend on the composition of the adsorbed serum proteins [114–116], the conformation of adsorbed proteins [117] and protein adsorption/desorption and exchange processes on biomaterials [118].

Unfortunately, current experimental results present a set of contradictions in this area. Moreover, there exist contradictory opinions about the relationship between the stages of endothelialization. On one hand, it has been reported that better attachment and wider spreading of cells stimulate the cell growth [119–121]. On the other hand, it has been demonstrated that they suppress it [112,123].

Because of this, the main aim of this part of the chapter is to present briefly the experimental data, most of which concern fibronectin (FN) and human endothelial cells (HEC).

Plasma fibronectin (PFN) is known to promote cell adhesion [124]. However, in various experiments the amount of surface-bound PFN did not directly correlate with its activity of promoting fibronectin spreading [117], adhesion of baby hamster kidney cells [125] and HEC adhesion and growth [116,126,127]. These differences in cell behavior on the surfaces of biomaterials might be explained by the different molecular orientations (different conformational states) of adsorbed PFN [117,126].

Lindblad et al. [128] have reported that PFN-coated surfaces, which should have enhanced HEC adhesion, demonstrated a 6.0% cell attachment, which is lower than the 11.6% observed with a blood coating alone. This supports the hypothesis that endogenous (cellular) fibronectin (cFN) may be more important for HEC adhesion, spreading and proliferation than the

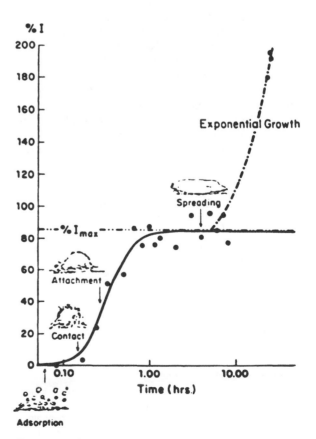

Figure 11. Different stages of cell–biomaterial interaction (from Reference [112]).

adsorbed PFN [116,128]. Two other proteins produced by endothelial cells, von Willebrand factor and thrombospondin, may also be involved in adhesion and/or spreading of the cells [129,130]. Besides, upon biomaterial-induced activation, macrophages can synthesize a regulatory protein Interleukin 1 (IL1) [104]. By stimulating fibroblast activity [131], IL1 induces the proliferation of endothelial and smooth muscle cells [132,133].

Significant changes in mouse 3T3 cell spreading and PFN adsorption were observed when either serum concentration or polymer type was varied [113]. The spreading of 3T3 cells in serum was found to be well correlated with the degree of fibrinogen adsorption to the surfaces, but attachment was not correlated with fibronectin adsorption. It was suggested that the amount of adsorbed proteins having binding sites with cells is a critical factor controlling cell interactions with biomaterials [113,134]. The presence of specific cell attachment sites on certain biological molecules, and their interaction with cell membrane receptors, is well known [135]. For example, apart from PFN the adsorption of other serum proteins, such as vibronectin [114], may influence cell adhesion. The role of the composition of the adsorbed protein layer, which depends on the surface properties of the biomaterial (especially surface wettability and surface charge), in the reactions of tissue cells is shown also by several authors [116,120,135,136]. But van Wachem et al. [116] did not find the difference between adhesion and proliferation of HEC onto uncoated and serum-precoated biomaterials (except tissue-culture polystyrene (TCPS), and Schakenraad et al. [120] reported that the absolute values for the spread and growth of human fibroblasts for different surfaces (including TCPS) are higher in the presence of serum than in the absence of serum. This contradiction can be explained by different behavior of HEC and human fibroblast in their interactions with the surfaces of biomaterials. It

should be taken into account when attempting to generalize the experimental data received from different cell cultures.

Calcification of Biomaterials

One of the limiting factors in the long-term use of implanted polymer systems and devices is calcification, which causes the loss of implant functional properties [137]. The process of the calcification of polymer surfaces induces various physicochemical and biochemical reactions, including cellular degradation of surrounding tissues [138,139]. The rate and intensity of calcification depend on many factors: external, internal and humoral [138–141]. The levels of calcium, phosphorus, specific proteins, lipids and phosphatase activity are all humoral factors that influence calcification. These parameters play a significant role in the deposition of calcium complexes onto the surfaces of materials with subsequent transition of soluble calcium salts to insoluble ones [140–143].

Among the possible factors initiating calcification [144] there are events classified as short-term effects, longer-term effects and long-term effects (Table 6). It should be noted that the development of the initial stages of calcification begins immediately upon the contact of the biomaterials with blood. For example, there exists a metastable equilibrium of protein-bound (mainly albumin-bound), ligand-bound and ionized calcium fractions in normals serum [145]. This equilibrium can be shifted by systemic dysfunction or by local changes (i.e., pH, conformational alterations of protein, release or deposition of calcium in dead adherent cells, etc.) in the presence of the biomaterial surface.

Pedersen [146] showed that there was no saturation in binding of SA with calcium at the physiological levels of SA and Ca^{++}. Only 10% of the total number of binding sites (n) in the molecule of SA were occupied with calcium. Authors present different data on the number of binding sites for Ca in the molecule of SA varying from 5–8 [147] or 12 to 19 and more [146,148]. Therefore it can be proposed that the increase in the number of binding sites and decrease of association constant K_α during the incubation of silicone rubber, based on PDMS with serum in the conditions of hypercalcemia ($[Ca^{++}] > 1.6$ mM/L) [149,150], are caused by the conformational changes of macromolecules induced by adsorption-desorption events proceeding at the polymer/blood interface. Moreover, it was observed that the interaction of polymer samples with serum beyond 20 hours provoked the change of the mechanism of protein–calcium binding from noncooperative to cooperative.

Actually it was shown [151,152] that the key role in the binding capacity of an SA molecule is played by its ability to exist in different conformational states. The conformational changes of the SA molecule can be local, affecting only a certain binding site, or they can result in more profound structural transformations of

---

Table 6. Possible events initiating the process of biomaterial calcification [144].

1. *Short-Term Effects (Hour or Less)*

    (a) ion interaction, imbalance and complexation
    (b) protein and lipid adsorption
    (c) cell collisions and changes (cell adhesion and aggregation)

2. *Longer-Term Effects (Hours to Days)*

    (a) changes in protein and lipid adsorption
    (b) continued cell adhesion, aggregation and destruction

3. *Long-Term Effects (Days to Months)*

    (a) deposition of different substances including calcium, phosphorus, phospholipids, etc.
    (b) transition from soluble forms of calcium phosphate into insoluble ones under participation of special enzymes

the globule [153,154]. The influence of the polymer in the conformational changes of bovine serum albumin (BSA), labelled with a fluorescent probe 8-anilino-1-naphthalene sulfonic acid (ANS) [156], was studied in the solution with physiological and pathological levels of calcium [155]. Unfortunately, the conformational changes of a protein molecule were evaluated only according to the change of association constant for SA with ANS, because of the inaccuracy of graphical determination of a number of binding sites. No change of association constant was detected in the presence of the samples of low-density polyethylene (LDPE) and polyurethane (PU) based on MDS, PDMS and BD both at physiological and pathological levels of calcium ($[Ca^{++}]$ = 5mM/L) in contrast to the protein incubated without polymer. However, the incubation of BSA solution with SR caused a decrease in the association constant of SA with ANS from (2.9 ± 0.3) 10^{-4} L/M^{-1} to (2.3 ± 0.2) 10^{-4} L/M^{-1} (Figure 12). This different behavior of three hydrophobic materials can be explained by the different characteristics of the passivating protein layers which formed, specifically involving the degree of irreversibility of SA adsorption β_{SA} which was equal to 0.95, 0.35, and 0.01 for LDPE, PU, and SR respectively (Table 3). The decrease in the value of β_{SA} testifies to an increase in the amount of protein desorbed in the denatured state [11]. This caused the registered effects, establishing the influence of SR surface on the complexation of SA with calcium or ANS under conditions of the experiment chosen.

Among the determining factors in the initial stages of the biomaterials' calcification are the blood lipid fractions, in particular the fractions of fatty acids (FA). It was shown that an increase in the concentration of longchain fatty acids promotes the formation of tightly bound complexes of protein (albumin)–fatty acid–calcium (Pr–FA–Ca) [157]. It was reported [158] also that the increase in HSA ability to bind Ca was caused by the conformational changes of protein in the complex of HSA–FA and that the adsorption of macrocomplexes containing Ca on the biomaterial's surface, especially in the presence of microdefects, can provoke the formation of a calcification nucleus [159].

It could be supposed [20] that in presence of plasma proteins FA is removed from the polymer surface to form and interface localized negative charge suspension. This suspension can lead to a high concentration of Ca^{++} in the local region of biomaterial's surface. In general the redistribution of ions on biomaterial/blood interfaces due to different adsorption/desorption processes can result in a local increase in the concentration of not only Ca but also of phosphates, phospholipids, lipids, specific proteins and enzymes, which can initiate or promote calcification.

Therefore it was a matter of particular interest to study the influence of FA's concentration on its complex-formation with Ca ions and proteins [159,160], and also on the adsorption of such com-

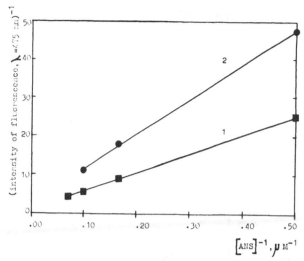

Figure 12. Titration curves of Tris-solution of bovine serum albumin (BSA) with ANS probe: 1—incubation of BSA without silicon rubber K_α = (2.9 ± 0.3) 10^{-4} *L/M*; 2—incubation of BSA with silicon rubber (4 cm^2/ml) K_α = 2.3 ± 0.2 10^{-4} *L/M*. Experimental conditions: 2.5 mg/ml of BSA solution in Tris, pH = 7.4; time of incubation 20 hours; $[Ca^{++}]$ = 5 mM/L; T = 310°K.

plexes on the surface. Table 7 shows that with the increase in FA's concentration in serum the number of binding sites (n), the association constant K_α, and the association constant for the first binding sites ($K_\alpha n$) all increase. Moreover, the addition of about 10 mM/L of FA results in the transition to another mechanism of protein–calcium binding, from noncooperative to cooperative (the Hill's coefficient more than 1.0). The presence of polymer (SA) samples has no influence on the complex-formation. This can be explained by the weak influence of polymer surface on the balance of calcium fractions in serum, in contrast with the effect of FA.

On the contrary, the quantity of adsorbed albumin and the deposition of calcium increased, and the value of ionized calcium decreased, when FA was added in concentrations of more than 3 mM/L (Figure 13). Thus, the obtained results demonstrate that the formed complexes have adsorbed on the polymer surface under the excess of FA.

For evaluation of the contribution of molecular and cell factors to the calcification of biomaterials, an *in vivo* model of subcutaneous implantation of diffusion

Table 7. Effect of palmitate potassium (FA) on the process of the formation of calcium complexes. *

(ΔFA) mM/L	n	k	nk	n_H
0	6.2	560	3,481	0.95
1	5.0	830	4,186	0.84
3	4.1	1,240	5,091	0.90
7	4.0	4,460	17,686	0.90
10	3.6	37,160	134,958	1.29

*The time of incubation is 5 hours, T°K = 310°.

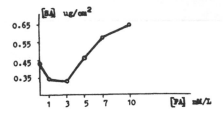

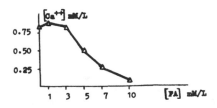

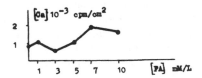

Figure 13. Dependence of: adsorbed ^{131}I-HSA on the silicon rubber, the level of ionized calcium in serum, [45]Ca deposition on the silicon rubber, on the concentration of palmitate potassium (FA).

chambers from polyethyleneterephthalate filters (0.56 mkm) in rabbits was used [161]. The presence of calcium on the bovine pericardium surfaces in the cage system (Table 8) indicates the possibility of biomaterials' calcification without direct contact with cells. At the same time the activation and aggregation of cells involves the processes of trans-, endo- and exocytosis, secreting lysosomal enzymes, specific proteins, phospholipids [162,163] which take an active part in calcification. For example, the cell adherent to the chamber's surface spreads and the formed pseudopods penetrate into the pores, releasing the products of activation into the chamber (Figure 14). The direct interaction of cells with implanted samples (without chamber) promotes and accelerates the process of calcification. Calcium deposition is clearly observed on the bovine pericardium surfaces. Figure 15 shows representative scanning electron micrographs of bovine pericardium before implantation, after 40 days' subcutaneous implantation in the diffusion chamber, and after 40 days' implantation without the diffusion chamber.

Corresponding X-ray energy dispersion analysis (EDAX) confirms the high levels of calcium in the subcutaneous implants, as compared to the implants from the diffusion chambers and the bovine pericardium before the implantation.

The calcium contents of the samples show the importance of humoral factors, in particular the calcium levels and the presence of vitamin D for the initiation of biomaterial calcification (Table 8). It is well known that vitamin D promotes synthesis of calcium-binding protein, intensifying the adsorption of calcium in the intestine. In addition, vitamin D takes part in the

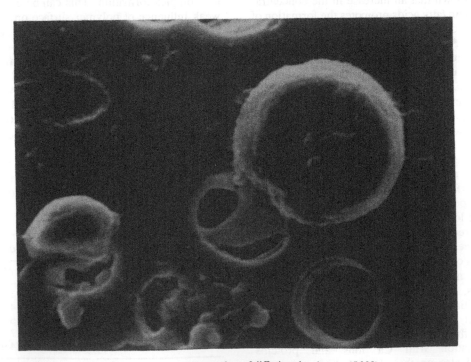

Figure 14. The cell on the surface of diffusion chamber (× 15,000).

Table 8. The content of calcium in the pericardium samples depending on conditions and period of implantation.

The Group of Animals and the Conditions of Implantation	The Period of Implantation		
	20	40	60
	The Content of Ca (μg/mg dry wt)		
1. Group (control) without chamber into chamber	30.0 ± 12.0 2.3 ± 0.7	56.4 ± 14.0 22.7 ± 5.4	107.5 ± 20.5 31.5 ± 6.5
2. Group (CaCl₂) without chamber into chamber	13.8 ± 4.2 3.5 ± 0.7	— —	215.0 ± 22.6 68.6 ± 8.9
3. Group (vit. D) without chamber into chamber	70.4 ± 10.2 44.3 ± 4.5	210.4 ± 27.3 168.2 ± 21.4	212.0 ± 16.0 197.0 ± 21.7

Unimplanted samples—2.5 ± 0.7 μg/mg dry wt.

redistribution of lipids (cholesterol, etc.), thereby presumably facilitating the flux of ions and macromolecules into and out of cells [164].

Also, the examination of a silicon rubber surface by SEM with EDAX showed the presence of calcium-containing depositions on the polymer surface implanted both into and without diffusion chamber. These depositions represent a localized slightly elevated area with irregular but recognizable margins (Figure 16).

Figure 17 represents the distribution of calcium, phosphorus, and the ratio of calcium to phosphorus for one of the common depositions. It should be noted that the distribution and appearance of depositions were the same for the samples (with and without chambers). Thus, these experiments support the hypothesis that the processes of formation and adsorption of the calcium–protein–lipid complexes can induce biomaterial calcification without direct contact with cells.

Combining the *in vivo* and *in vitro* experimental data, we suggested the hypothetical scheme of biomaterial calcification (Figure 18). According to this scheme there may be two pathways of the development of calcification. The first way is the most common one, with the degradation of cells being the primary step of biomaterial-associated calcification [138,143]. The second way is the development of biomaterial calcification without direct contact of the surface with cells. Both in the first and second cases, the initial stages represent the molecular processes at the biomaterial/blood interface (Figure 18).

Thus, the proposed mechanism of biomaterial-associated calcification takes into account the molecular and cellular interaction of biomaterials with blood. It is assumed that initial stages of calcification are the

Table 9. The principles and methods of prevention of biomaterial calcification.

1. Possible ways to protect biomaterials from destructive effects of medium	1. (a) Coating with dense regular structure (pyrocarbon, etc.) (b) Polymer coating of bioprosthetic valve (dextran, etc.)
2. The inhibition of calcium complexation	2. (a) Cuspal diphosphonate preloading (b) Methods of medical therapy (warfarin, etc.)
3. The inhibition of adsorption of calcium complexes on polymer surface	3. Immobilization of physiologically active agents
4. The prevention of conversion of soluble calcium phosphates salts into insoluble forms	4. The application of diphosphonate compounds
5. The extraction of phospholipids from prosthetic surface	5. The use of pretreatment with detergent compounds
6. The alteration of the biomaterial structure	6. (a) Regulation of surface distribution in microphase separated systems (b) Increase of cross-linking of collagen or cardiac valve bioprosthesis
7. The decrease of cracking load on prosthetic area undergoing the most destructive changes	7. Modification of valve design and fabrication

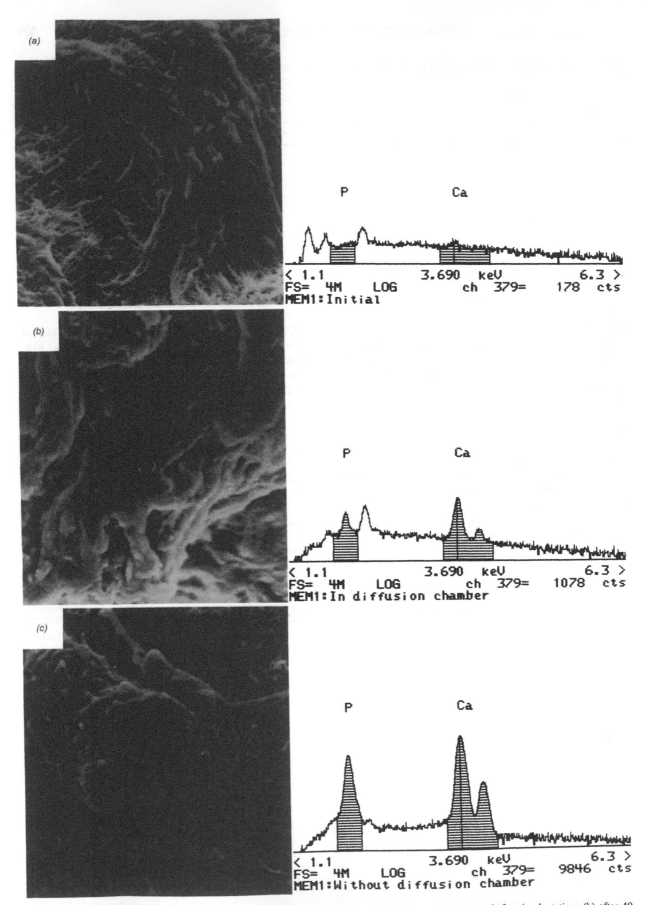

Figure 15. The results of SEM (× 10,000) and EDAX of bovine pericardium treated by glutaraldehyde: (a) before implantation, (b) after 40 days of implantation in diffusion chamber, (c) after 40 days of implantation without diffusion chamber.

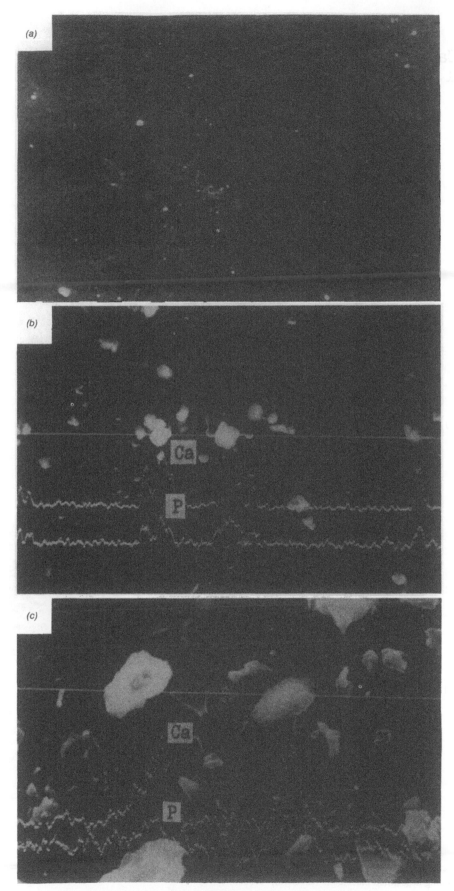

Figure 16. The results of SEM (×1000) and EDAX of silicone rubber: (a) before implantation, (b) after 60 days of implantation in diffusion chamber, (c) after 60 days of implantation without diffusion chamber.

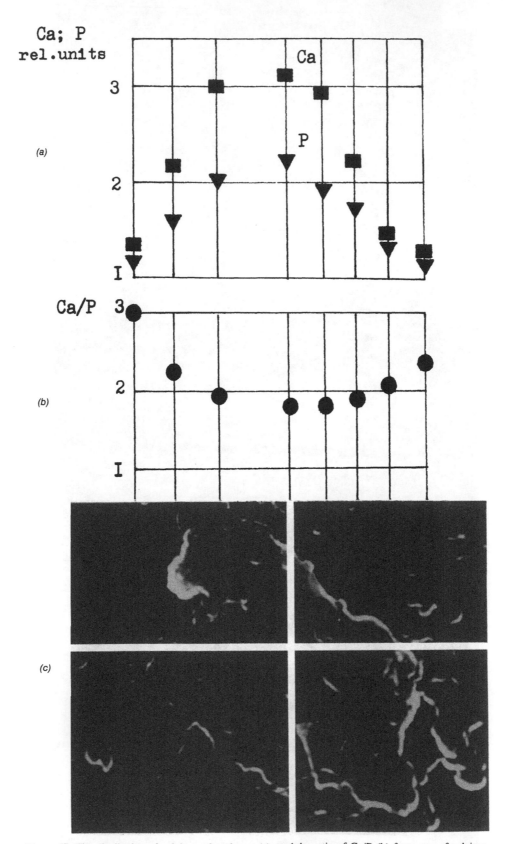

Figure 17. The distribution of calcium, phosphorus (a), and the ratio of Ca/P (b) from one of calcium-containing depositions on silicone rubber (c), (×5000).

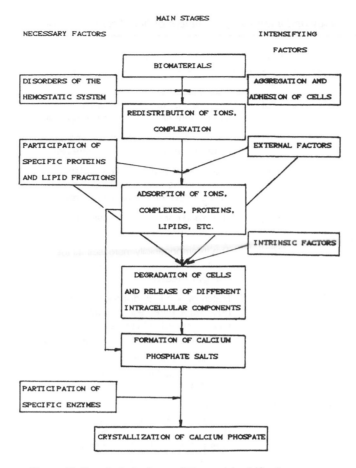

Figure 18. Hypothetical scheme of biomaterial calcification.

following: The surface induces the conformational changes of proteins both in adsorbed and desorbed states. This causes a change in the balance of calcium fractions in blood, promoting formation of calcium complexes with proteins or with lipids and proteins. The deposition of these complexes on the surface is the potential nucleus of calcification. The surface distribution of these depositions depends on the physicochemical and physicomechanical characteristics of a polymer's surface. These should be taken into account when working out methods of preventing biomaterial calcification (Table 9).

As follows from the paragraphs above, adjusting first of all the conformational changes of proteins induced by adsorption-desorption processes at the surface/blood interface, and such promoting factors as composition and surface distribution of the adsorbed protein layer, one can increase the hemocompatibility of biomaterials for short-term contact with blood as well as for long-term implantation.

PROTEIN ADSORPTION AND PHYSICOCHEMICAL PROPERTIES OF BIOMATERIALS

As we have already noted, the blood compatibility of medical devices depends not only on physico-chemical properties of biomaterials but on a number of other factors also (Figure 1). However, in many cases we have only one method of increasing the blood compatibility of the device: changing the physicochemical properties of the biomaterials listed in Table 10 [6].

"Polar" Biomaterials and "Apolar" Biomaterials

It should be noted that almost all the physico-chemical properties of biomaterials (Table 10) affect the energetical parameters of the surface. That is why the majority of hypotheses considering the mech-

Table 10. Important physicochemical properties of blood-compatible biomaterials [6].

- surface composition (polar/apolar, acid/base, H-bonding, ionic charges, immobilized biomolecules)
- surface molecular motions (polymer chain ends, loops and their flexibility)
- surface topography (roughness, porosity, imperfections, gas microbubbles)
- domains (distribution and sizes)
- tendency to biodegradation, erosion or corrosion
- surface crystalline/amorphous structure

Table 11. Surface energy and interfacial parameters of blood-compatible biomaterials (hypothesis).

Author	Year	Ref.	Conclusion	Energy Criteria of Blood Compatibility
1	2	3	4	5
Zisman, W. A.	1964	[165]	The material with minimal critical surface tension will be blood-compatible.	$\gamma_c \rightarrow 0$ (10–15 dyne/cm)
Lyman, D. J.	1965	[167]	The blood compatibility of a biomaterial increases as surface energy increases.	
Baier, R. E.	1970	[166]	The material with the critical surface tension in the range of 20–30 dyne/cm will have low thrombogenic potential.	$\gamma_c = 20\text{–}30$ dyne/cm
Andrade, J. D.	1973	[168]	The blood-compatible biomaterial must have the minimal interfacial free energy.	$\gamma_{SL} \rightarrow 0$ (1–3 dyne/cm)
Nyilas, E.	1975	[169]	The thrombogenicity increases as the polar contribution to the surface free energy increases.	$\gamma_S^d/\gamma_S \gg \gamma_S^p/\gamma_S$
Kaelble, D. H.	1977	[48]	Materials with high dispersion and low polar surface free energies will be more blood-compatible than those with low dispersion and high surface free energy.	$\gamma_S^d/\gamma_S^p \gg 1$
Ratner, B. D.	1979	[170]	The balance of polar and apolar sites on a surface may be important for its blood compatibility	$\gamma_S^d/\gamma_S^p \cong 1$
Ruckenstein, E.	1984	[91]	Surface with the minimal interfacial free energy will be blood-compatible if the dispersions and the polar surface free energies for the biomaterial and blood are equal respectively.	$\gamma_{SL} \cong 1\text{–}3$ (dyne/cm) $\gamma_S^p \cong \gamma_L^p$ $\gamma_S^d \cong \gamma_L^d$

anisms of polymer interaction with blood, especially with proteins, primarily analyze the influence of the surface's energy characteristics on its hemocompatibility.

Therefore, in the research on hemocompatible materials, attempts are made mostly to establish relationships between the energetical properties of the material and its adsorptional and blood-compatible characteristics [48,91,165–170].

Table 11 includes the various hypotheses and theories that had been put forward during the past 25 years. The supporters of "hydrophobic" criteria of blood compatibility (W. A. Zisman, R. E. Baier, E. Nyilas and D. H. Kaelble) consider biomaterial hemocompatibility to be connected with the affinity of the surface for a strong homogeneous protein film, i.e., with the effect of irreversible "passivation". The "hydrophilic" theory of blood compatibility (D. J. Lyman, J. D. Andrade and E. Ruckenstein) stresses the minimization of protein adsorption during the biomaterial's interaction with blood, i.e., ideally the blood-compatible biomaterial should not adsorb protein. In the hypothesis of an optimum polar/apolar ratio, an attempt is made to find a trade-off between the supporters of "hydrophilic" and those of "hydrophobic" hypotheses of biomaterial blood compatibility.

But the more detailed analysis of the works that served as a basis for the suggested hypotheses (Table 11) shows that these two opposite approaches (hydrophobization or hydrophilization of surfaces) to the creation of hemocompatible biomaterials are actually based on the same concept. Specifically, all the speculations of the authors can be represented by the following scheme of "one root" (Figure 19).

For an "apolar" hydrophobic surface, the greater the degree of irreversible protein adsorption in the first monolayer (or the less the time of the formation of the first tightly adsorbed layer of protein) [11] and the faster the transition to "multilayered proteinaceous passivation" [45], the higher is the probability of the biomaterial's blood compatibility. If these two conditions of blood compatibility for a hydrophobic surface are satisfied, a loosely bound layer of "intact" proteins is formed at the blood/surface interface. In such a regime of multilayer adsorption, the negative influence of conformational changes of protein during the formation of the first monolayer on the activation of enzyme systems and blood cells will be negligible.

For a "polar" surface (Figure 19) with interfacial energy on the order of 1–3 dyne/cm the blood compatibility is provided by the formation of a mechanically stable but loosely bound monolayer of "intact" proteins at the solid/blood interface (the regime of monolayer adsorption) [171].

That is, the main difference in the mechanism of blood compatibility for a "polar" and an "apolar" surface, according to the suggested scheme (Figure 19), consists in the regimes of the formation of the loosely bound layer of "intact" proteins at the blood/surface interface (monolayer and multilayer regimes).

For both cases the predominance of albumin in the adsorbed layer is not an obligatory but a promoting factor in the surface's blood compatibility. However, SA will play a great positive role in the case of multilayer adsorption on the hydrophobic surface followed by the considerable conformational changes of proteins in the first adsorptional layers [45,172]. The preferential adsorption of SA decreases both the amount of platelet-adhesive proteins [63] and the degree of conformational changes [63,173].

From the "Concept of Correspondence" to the "Concept of Complementarity"

One should be very careful with terms "hydrophilic" and "hydrophobic" surfaces used by different authors. For example, it was reported that protein adsorption, platelet adhesion, serotonin and β-thromboglobulin release from adhered platelets were suppressed on very hydrophobic and very hydrophilic surfaces of polypeptide derivative [174] and of other several biomaterials [174,175]. However, the water contact angle for "very hydrophobic" surface was about 40°

and that for "very hydrophilic" surface was about 60°–70°, i.e., these materials have both hydrophilic and hydrophobic properties. Moreover, numerous experimental studies [172,176-180] show that the blood compatibility of hydrophilic and hydrophobic homopolymers is lower than that of block copolymers with hydrophilic and hydrophobic phases.

For instance [82], A–B block copolymers having water contact angles form 60° to 85° do not induce either conformational changes in adsorbed plasma proteins, increases in the number of adhered platelets, or changes in the rate of serotonin release.

One of the first explanations for the high hemocompatibility of microphase systems involves the high affinity of hydrophilic areas to serum albumin and of hydrophobic areas to fibrinogen and γ-globulin [180]. Accordingly, the regularity of the protein adsorptional layer lowers the probability of redistribution of membrane proteins in adherent platelets, and decreases their morphological alterations. Another hypothesis [62] explains the blood compatibility of some block copolymers by the fact that the surfaces of block copolymers with certain compositions suppress the denaturation of adsorbed proteins and the activation of adhered platelets.

The intima of a blood vessel is a typical heterogeneous system with alternating hydrophilic and hydrophobic regions. Blood and biomaterials also represent multicomponent systems, and all protein molecules contain polar and apolar regions several Å in size [6]. For this reason, describing a microheterogeneous

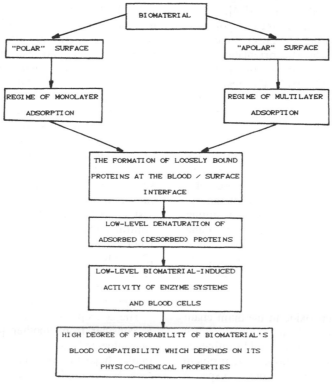

Figure 19. "One root" of two main energetical approaches to blood compatibility of biomaterials.

system with such macroparameters as the average of the energetical characteristics is incorrect. When developing blood-compatible biomaterials (especially multiphase ones) we must take into account more than just the equality of the values of the polar and dispersive components of the surface free energy of the biomaterial and the blood, respectively (the so-called "concept of correspondence") [91,181]. It is reasonable to try to correlate protein adsorption on the biomaterial surface with the distribution of dispersive and polar components, as well as with the averaged values of these components for the surface free energy of a biomaterial and that of the outermost protein layer. In other words, for a high biomaterial blood compatibility, the "complementarity" between hydrophilic and hydrophobic regions of the surface between the regions of loosely bound macromolecules should be satisfied. These ideas represent the further extension of the "concept of correspondence" developed by Lyman [167], Andrade [168] and Ruckenstein et al. [91] sequentially. The same conclusion [182] was made after the analysis of antithrombogenicity of polyetherurethaneurea having tertiary amino groups and its heparinized derivative.

When developing blood-compatible biomaterials in terms of the mutual correspondence of the distribution of dispersive and polar components during contact with blood [49,183], those factors that can influence the dynamic of the composition of the adsorbed protein layer should be taken into account. It should be noted that the time of establishing the equilibrium of the components of the surface free energy varies from 10 days to 1 month, depending on the dynamics of biomaterial/blood interface [184].

It was observed that different degrees of polymer chain flexibility followed by the formation of a corresponding subsurface characteristic orientation, can influence the blood-compatibility of the polymer when immersed in blood [185,186]. The rearrangement of the surface structure of the biomaterials brings about a decrease in the solid/blood interfacial free energy, due to a decrease in the dispersion component of the surface free energy. At the same time, the surface polar component increases [184]. This conclusion is valid not only for flexible polymers with sufficient segment mobility but also for more relatively rigid materials, such as polymethyl methacrylate [91]. Thus, the surface autoregulation, resulting in a decrease in the amount of adsorbed protein and the degree of its conformational changes, takes place in accordance with the concept of complementarity to corresponding blood energetical characteristics.

The ability of this surface to "adjust" to its microenvironment is exhibited most strikingly by the biomaterials based on polyethyleneoxide in the main chain [177,187,188] or in the side chain [188,189]. Since different chain mobilities may considerably influence the energy characteristics of the surface, the problem of the microstructure of the surface acquires a special significance. Indeed, the results of *in vitro* studies

[190] indicate that the initial adsorption of the plasma proteins and blood cells onto the surface of the block copolymer and, ultimately, its thrombogenicity are mediated, in part, by a combination of morphological order and surface mobility. The microstructure of crystalline and amorphous phases also plays a great part in the heterogeneity of the block copolymer's surface and finally in the character of the distribution of polar and dispersion components of the surface free energy in the outermost layer of biomaterials [11,12, 191–199].

Summarizing the data obtained independently by several groups, one can propose that the increase in blood compatibility of flexible biomaterials with the crystalline/amorphous type of microdomain structure may be achieved by

- forming a homogeneous mixed phase in the polymer (or, in other words, of a mixed phase of high microheterogeneity related to the higher degree of hard and soft chain association and to the dimension of crystalline and amorphous phases not exceeding 10 nm
- balancing the crystalline and amorphous phase distributions in a biomaterial
- lowering the content of hard segments and increasing the content of the soft ones in the mixed phase by the absence of full-phase segregation
- creating a supermolecular structure of a globular type with higher content of the soft block in the mixed phase of the surface biomaterial layer

The best biomaterials, which allow the values of the distribution of polar and dispersion components of surface free energy to vary are multiphase materials with hydrophilic and hydrophobic microdomains, or graft copolymers having hydrophilic–hydrophobic chains [12,177,179,188,193] with certain surface mobility [200].

The limiting case of such an approach is the development of multiblock copolymers with a certain flexibility of chains, possessing amphiphilic surfaces on the molecular level. The combination of these properties promotes the rapid transition of the biomaterial's surface into equilibrium (concerning energetical parameters) with the microenvironment of physiological systems and primarily with blood proteins. The most fruitful studies in this direction are carried out in the laboratories of S. W. Kim [177,188,200], J. Feijen [201], Okano [176,180,193] and Ito [12], with positive results, proving the efficiency of the approach to the development of blood-compatible biomaterials based on the "concept of complementarity".

The concept of complementarity makes it possible to consider from another point of view the role of physiologically active compounds [200,202] (in particular, heparin) covalently immobilized onto the surface. For example, one can propose that the increase in the blood-compatible properties of the surface is conditioned not only by the anticoagulant effect of immobilized heparin, but by the "enrichment" of the surface with various hydrophilic and hydrophobic groups, i.e., the extension of the set of values of polar and dispersion components. The presence of hydrophilic spacers increases on one hand the effect of surface "autoregulation" according to the "concept of complementarity" and on the other hand its hydrophilicity, that is, the average of the polar component of the biomaterial's surface energy. The latter is important because for all block copolymers for contact with blood used at present, even the "concept of correspondence" for polar components of surface and blood is not satisfied. Really, the polar component of blood is approximately equal to 50.8 dyne/cm, whereas for polyetherurethanes this value is about 10 dyne/cm [49,92].

CONCLUSION

The complicated relationship of adsorptional and blood-compatible properties of biomaterials is determined by the structure and composition of the passivating protein layer and also by the mechanism of its formation. These parameters depend primarily on the energetical properties of the biomaterial/blood interface. In terms of the "concept of complementarity", considered in the last part, an ideal blood-compatible material should possess amphiphilic surfaces having not only the averages of polar ($\gamma^p \rightarrow$ 50.8 dyne/cm) and dispersion ($\gamma^d \rightarrow$ 21.8 dyne/cm) components of the surface energy close to those of blood, but also the character of their distribution should be similar to that of blood (proteins). Also, a hydrophilic material will form the homogeneous protein monolayer loosely bound to the surface and with minimal conformational changes.

The designing of a surface so microheterogeneous on the molecular level, considering surface and protein structure mobility, is a very complicated problem [203], which is unlikely to be solved in the near future.

A more realistic approach is to synthesize multiblock copolymers with various hydrophobic and hydrophilic groups (preferably the latter) grafted onto a space with random surface distribution. Macromolecular chain mobility with a wide set of functional groups can lead to the fulfillment of the "conditions of complementarity" in the process of mutual reconstruction of the structures of the surface and the protein at the blood/material interface.

Another approach is realized in the regime of the hydrophobic-hydrophilic balance of the surface. In this case the blood compatibility of biomaterials is determined by the rate of transition from the formation of a homogeneous protein layer tightly bound to the surface to multilayer adsorption. An example of such an approach is the synthesis of multiblock copolymers with hydrophilic and hydrophobic blocks in the main chain.

Such high-performance amphiphilic materials with sufficient reliability allow the initial stages of the blood/surface interaction to proceed favorably. These initial stages will play the primary role in determining short-term blood compatibility, and if successful will promote the formation of the pseudointima developed by endothelial cells without biomaterial-associated calcification.

REFERENCES

1. Vroman, L. and E. Leonard, eds. 1977. *Behavior of Blood and Its Components at Interfaces, Ann. N.Y. Acad. Sci.* New York: N.Y. Acad. Sci., Vol. 283.

2. Williams, D. F. and R. D. Bagnell. 1981. "Adsorption of Proteins on Polymers and Its Role in the Response of Soft Tissue", in *Fundamental Aspects of Biocompatibility, Vol. 2.* D. F. Williams, ed. Boca Raton, FL: CRC Press.

3. Cooper, S. I. and N. A. Peppas, eds. 1982. *Biomaterials: Interfacial Phenomena and Applications, Adv. Chem. Ser.* Washington, D.C.: ACS, Vol. 199.

4. 1983. *Biocompatible Polymers, Metals, and Composites.* M. Szycher, ed. Lancaster, PA: Technomic Publishing Co., Inc.

5. 1984. *Polymers as Biomaterials.* S. W. Shalaby, A. S. Hoffman, B. D. Ratner and T. A Horbett, eds. New York: Plenum Press.

6. Andrade, J. D., ed. 1985. *Surface and Interfacial Aspects of Biomedical Polymers, Vol. 2, Protein Adsorption.* New York: Plenum Press.

7. Ivarsson, B. and I. Lundström. 1986. *Critical Rev. in Biocompatibility*, 2:1–96.

8. Feast, W. J. and H. S. Munro. 1987. *Polymer Surfaces and Interfaces.* John Wiley & Sons Ltd.

9. Brash, J. L. and T. A. Horbett, eds. 1987. *Proteins at Interfaces. Physicochemical and Biochemical Studies.* Washington, D.C.: Amer. Chem. Soc., Vol. 343.

10. Leonard, E. F., V. T. Turitto and L. Vroman, eds. 1987. *Blood in Contact with Natural and Artificial Surfaces, Ann. N.Y. Acad. Sci.* New York: N.Y. Acad. Sci., Vol. 516.

11. Sevastianov, V. I. 1988. *CRC Crit. Rev. Biocompat.*, 4:109–154.

12. Ito, Y. and Y. Imanishi. 1989. *CRC Crit. Rev. Biocompat.*, 5:45–104.

13. Turitto, V. T., H. J. Weiss, H. R. Baumgartner, L. Badimon and V. Fuster. 1987. In *Blood in Contact with Natural and Artificial Surfaces, Ann. N.Y. Acad. Sci.* E. F. Leonard, V. T. Turitto and L. Vroman, eds. New York: N.Y. Acad. Sci., 516:453–463.

14. Turitto, V. T., H. J. Weiss and H. R. Baumgartner. 1984. *J. Clin. Invest.*, 74:1730–1741.

15. Ruggery, Z. M., L. De Marco, L. Gatti, R. Bader and R. R. Montgomery. 1983. *J. Clin. Invest.*, 72:1.

16. Gralnick, H. R., S. B. Williams and B. S. Coller. 1984. *Blood*, 64:797.

17. Plow, E. F., A. Srouji, D. Meyer, G. Marguerie and M. H. Ginsberg. 1984. *J. Biol. Chem.*, 259:5388.

18. Andrade, J. D., ed. 1985. *Surface and Interfacial*

Aspects of Biomedical Polymers, Surface Chemistry and Physics. New York: Plenum Press, Vol. 1.

19. Lee, R. G. and S. W. Kim. 1974. *J. Biomed. Mater. Res.*, 8:393–398.

20. Kim, S. W., S. Wisniewski, E. S. Lee and M. L. Winn. 1977. *J. Biomed. Mater. Res. Symp.*, 8:23–31.

21. Ihlenfeld, J. V. and S. L. Cooper. 1979. *J. Biomed. Mater. Res.*, 13:583–591.

22. Lee, R. G., C. Adamson and S. W. Kim. 1974. *Throm. Res.*, 4:485.

23. Chittur, K. K., D. J. Fink, Leninger and T. B. Hutson. 1986. *J. Colloid. Interface Sci.*, 110:419–435.

24. Lelah, M. D., T. G. Grasel, J. A. Pirerce and S. L. Cooper. 1986. *J. Biomed. Mater. Res.*, 20:433–468.

25. Lyman, D. J., L. C. Metcalf, D. Ir. Acbo, K. F. Richards and J. Lamb. 1974. *Trans. Am. Soc. Artif. Intern. Organs*, 20:474–478.

26. Kim, S. W., A. G. Lee, H. Oster, D. Lentz, L. Coleman, J. D. Andrade and D. Olsen. 1974. *Trans. Am. Soc. Artif. Intern. Organs*, 20:449–453.

27. Brash, J. L. 1983. In *Biocompatible Polymers, Metals and Composites.* M. Szycher, ed., Lancaster, PA: Technomic Publishing Co., Inc., pp. 35–52.

28. Brash, J. L. and S. Unijal. 1979. *J. Polym. Sci.*, C66:377–389.

29. Eberhart, R. C., N. S. Munro, J. A. Frautchi, M. Lubin, F. G. Clubb, C. W. Miller and V. I. Sevastianov. 1987. In *Blood in Contact with Natural and Artificial Surfaces, Ann. N.Y. Acad. Sci.* E. F. Leonard, V. T. Turitto and L. Vroman, eds. New York: N.Y. Acad. Sci., 516:78–95.

30. Grasel, T. G., J. A. Pierce and S. L. Cooper. 1987. *J. Biomed. Mater. Res.*, 21:815–842.

31. Munro, M. S., R. C. Eberhart, N. G. Maki, B. E. Brink and W. J. Fry. 1983. *ASAIO J.*, 6:65–75.

32. Pitt, W. G., T. G. Grasel and S. L. Cooper. 1988. *Biomaterials*, 9:36–46.

33. Lee, E. S. and S. W. Kim. 1979. *Trans. Am. Soc. Artif. Intern. Organs*, 25:124–131.

34. Addonizio, V. P. and R. W. Colman. 1982. *Biomater. Med Devices Artif. Organs*, 3:9–15.

35. Kottke-Marchant, K., J. M. Anderson, Y. Umemura and R. E. Marchant. 1989. *Biomaterials*, 10:147–155.

36. Kottke-Marchant, K., J. M. Anderson and A. Rabinovitch. 1986. *Biomaterials*, 7:441–448.

37. Saski, T., T. Matuzaki and N. Yamomoto. 1985. *Jinkozoki*, 14:1000.

38. Pekala, R. W., M. Rudoltz, E. R. Lang, E. W. Merrill, J. Lindon, L. Kuchner, G. McManama and E. W. Salzman. 1986. *Biomaterials*, 7:372–378.

39. Pekala, R. W., E. W. Merrill, J. Lindon, L. Kushner and E. W. Salzman. 1986. *Biomaterials*, 7:379–385.

40. Poot, A., T. Bengeling, J. P. Casenave, A. Bantjes and W. G. van Aken. 1988. *Biomaterials*, 9:126–132.

41. Horbett, T. A. and K. Mack. 1986. *Trans. Soc. Biomater.*, 9:46.

42. Lensen, H. G., W. Breemhanr, C. A. Smolders and J. Fejen. 1986. *J. Chromatogr.*, 376:191.

43. Young, B. R., W. G. Pitt and C. L. Cooper. 1988. *J. Colloid. Interface Sci.*, 124:28–43.

44. Lee, S. H. and E. Ruckenstein. 1988. *J. Colloid. Interface Sci.*, 125:365–379.

45. Vroman, L. 1974. *Science*, 184:585–586.

46. Mastuda, T., H. Tanaka, K. Hayashi, E. Taenaka, S. Takaichi, M. Umezu, T. Nakamura, T. Tanaka, S. Takatani and T. Akutsu. 1984. *Trans. Am Soc. Artif. Intern. Organs*, 30:353–358.

47. Williams, D. F. and R. D. Bagnall. 1981. In *Fundamental Aspects of Biocompatibility.* D. F. Williams, ed. Boca Raton, FL: CRC Press, 2:113–127.

48. Kaelble, D. H. and J. Moacanin. 1977. *Polymer*, 18:475–482.

49. Ruckenstein, E. and S. V. Gourisankar. 1986. *J. Colloid. Interface Sci.*, 109:557–566.

50. Sevastianov, V. I., E. A. Tseytlina, A. V. Volkov and V. I. Sumakov. 1984. *Trans. Am. Soc. Artif. Intern. Organs*, 30:137–141.

51. Sevastianov, V. I., A. V. Volkov, O. N. Rodin, L. I Valuev and N. A. Plate. 1981. *Doklad. Acad. Nauk. SSSR*, 260:383–386.

52. Pitt, W. G., K. Park and S. L. Cooper. 1986. *J. Colloid Interface Sci.*, 111:343–362.

53. Horbett, T., C. M. Cheng, B. D. Ratner, A. S. Hoffman and S. R. Hanson. 1986. *J. Biomed. Mater. Res.*, 20:739–772.

54. Szycher, M. 1983. In *Biocompatible Polymers, Metals, and Composites.* M. Szycher, ed. Lancaster, PA: Technomic Publishing, Co., Inc., pp. 1–34.

55. Vroman, I. 1983. In *Biocompatible Polymers, Metals, and Composites.* M. Szycher, ed. Lancaster, PA: Technomic Publishing Co., Inc., pp. 81–88.

56. Moore, W. S., J. M. Malone and K. Keown. 1980. *Arch. Surg.*, 115:1379–1383.

57. Izumi, Y. 1984. *Jpn. Assoc. Thorac. Surg.*, 32:1205–1209.

58. Szycher, M., C. Fransblan and B. Faris. 1981. *J. Biomed. Mater. Res.*, 15:247–253.

59. Sevastianov, V. I. and A. N. Asanov. 1988. *Trans. of the 3rd World Biomaterials Congress*, 11:91.

60. Kulik, E. A. and V. I. Sevastianov. *J. Colloid Interface Sci.* (in press).

61. Kalinin, I. D. and V. I. Sevastianov. *J. Colloid Interface Sci.* (in press).

62. Mori, A., Y. Ito, M. Sisido and Y. Imanishi. 1986. *Biomaterials*, 7:386–392.

63. Park, K., D. F. Mosher and S. L. Cooper. 1986. *J. Biomed. Mater. Res.*, 20:589–612.

64. Murthy, K. D., S. R. Simmons, R. M. Albrecht and S. L. Cooper. 1988. *J. Colloid Interface Sci.*, 125:176–189.

65. Park, K., S. J. Gerndt and H. Park. 1988. *J. Colloid Interface Sci.*, 125:702–711.

66. Iordanskii, A. L., B. P. Ulanov, L. A. Zimina and G. E. Zaikov. 1979. *Dokl. Akad. Nauk. SSSR*, 249:480–483.

67. Eberhart, R. C., M. E. Lynch, F.N. Bilge, J. F. Wissinger, M. S. Munro, S. R. Ellsworth and A. J. Quattrone. 1982. In *Biomaterials: Interfacial Phenomena and Application, Adv. Chem. Ser.* S. L. Cooper and N. A. Peppas, eds. Washington, D.C.: ACS, 199:293–316.

68. Paynter, R. W., B. D. Ratner, T. A. Horbett and H. R. Thomas. 1984. *J. Colloid Interface Sci.*, 101:233–242.

69. Rudee, M. L. and T. M. Price. 1985. *J. Biomed. Mater. Res.*, 19:57–68.

70. Ricitelli, S. D., F. H. Bilge and R. C. Eberhart. 1984. *Trans. Am. Soc. Artif. Intern. Organs*, 30:420–423.

71. Eberhart, R. C., M. S. Munro, J. R. Frautchi and V. I. Sevastianov. 1987. In *Protein at Interfaces. Physico-Chemical and Biochemical Studies.* Washington, D.C.: ACS, 343:378–400.

72. Eberhart, R. C., L. Prokop, J. Wissinger and M. Wilkov. 1977. *Trans. Amer. Soc. Artif. Intern. Organs*, 23:134–139.

73. Sheehan, S. J., S. M. Rajah and R. C. Kester. 1989. *Biomaterials*, 10:75–79.

74. Tomikawa, M., O. Iwamoto, S. Olsson, S. Soderman and B. Blombäck. 1980. *Thromb. Res.*, 19:869–879.

75. Mosher, D. F. 1981. In *Interaction of the Blood with Natural and Artificial Surfaces.* E. W. Salzman, ed. New York: Dekker, p. 85.

76. Nygren, H. and M. Stenberk. 1988. *J. Biomed. Mater. Res.*, 22:1–11.

77. Hoffman, A. S. 1986. *J. Biomed. Mater. Res.*, 20:IX–XI.

78. Absolom, D. R., W. Zing and A. W. Neumann. 1987. *J. Biomed. Mater. Res.*, 21:161–171.

79. Lee, J. H., J. Kopecek and J. D. Andrade. 1989. *J. Biomed. Mater. Res.*, 23:351–368.

80. Absolom, D. R., Z. Policova, T. Bruck, C. Thomson, W. Zingg and A. W. Neumann. 1987. *J. Colloid Interface Sci.*, 117:550–564.

81. Sandwick, R. K. and K. J. Schray. 1988. *J. Colloid Interface Sci.*, 121:1–12.

82. Kang, I.-K., Y. Ito, M. Sisido and Y. Imanishi. 1988. *Biomaterials*, 9:138–144.

83. Olsen, D. A. 1973. "Biophysical Interactions of Blood Proteins with Polymeric and Artifical Surfaces", in *Progress and Membrane Science*, J. F. Danielli, ed. New York: Pergamon Press, 6:331–364.

84. Ward, C. A., B. Ruegsegger, D. Standa, W. Zingg and M. A. Herbett. 1977. *Am. J. Physiol.*, 233:100–105.

85. Brash, J. L., C. F. Scott, P. Ten Hove and R. W. Coleman. 1985. *Trans. Soc. Biomater.*, 8:105.

86. Sevastianov, V. I. and E. A. Tseytlina. 1984. *J. Biomed. Mater. Res.*, 18:969–978.

87. Bauer, J. and G. Vater. 1981. *Biochim. Biophys. Acta*, 670:129–133.

88. Isenman, D. E. and N. R. Cooper. 1981. *Mol. Immunol.*, 18:331–339.

89. Elwing, H., B. Nilsson, K.-E. Svensson, A. Askendahl, U. R. Nilsson and I. Lundström. 1988. *J. Colloid Interface Sci.*, 125:139–145.

90. Fukumura, H., K. Hayashi, S. Yoskikawa, M. Miya, N. Yamamoto and I. Yamashita. 1987. *Biomaterials*, 8:74–76.

91. Ruckenstein, E. and S. V. Gourisankar. 1984. *J. Colloid Interface Sci.*, 101:436–451.

92. Sharma, C. P. 1981. *Biomaterials*, 2:57–59.

93. Baszkin, A. and D. J. Lyman. 1980. *J. Biomed. Mater. Res.*, 14:393–403.

94. Noishiki, Y. 1985. "*In Vivo* Evaluation of Biocompatibility", *Jinkozoki*, 14:713–718.

95. Howbold, A. D. 1983. "Blood/Carbon Interactions", *ASAIO J.*, 6:88–99.

96. Morrissey, B. W. 1977. In *Behavior of Blood and Its Components at Interfaces, Ann. N.Y. Acad. Sci.* L. Vroman and E. F. Leonard, eds. New York: N.Y. Acad. Sci., 283:50–64.

97. Sanado, T., Y. Ito, N. Sisido and Y. Imanishi. 1986. *J. Biomed. Mater. Res.*, 20:1179–1195.

98. Coleman, D. L., D. E. Gregonis and J. D. Andrade. 1982. *J. Biomed. Mater. Res.*, 16:381–192.

99. Hoffman, A. S., B. D. Ratner, T. A. Horbett, L. O. Reynolds, C. S. Cho, L. A. Harker and S. R. Hanson. 1984. in *Progr. Artif. Organs—1983.* Cleveland: ISAIO Press, 2:819–824.

100. Didisheim, P., D. B. Olsen, D. J. Farrar, P. M. Portner, B. P. Griffith, D. G. Pennington, J. H. Joist, F. J. Schoen, A. G. Gristina and J. M. Anderson. 1989. *ASAIO Trans.*, 35:54–70.

101. Anderson, J. M. 1988. *ASAIO J.*, 11:101–107.

102. Kottke-Marchant, K., J. M. Anderson, K. M. Miller, R. E. Marchant and H. Lazarus. 1987. *J. Biomed. Mater. Res.*, 21:379–397.

103. Marchant, R. E. and J. M. Anderson. 1986. *J. Biomed. Mater. Res.*, 20:37–50.

104. Miller, K. M. and J. M. Anderson. 1988. *J. Biomed. Mater. Res.*, 22:713–731.

105. Kossovsky, N., J. P. Heggers and M. C. Robson. 1987. *J. Biomed. Mater. Res.*, 21:1125–1133.

106. Kossovsky, N., J. P. Heggers, R. W. Porsons and M. C. Robson. 1983. *Plas. Reconstr. Surg.*, 71:795–802.

107. Cooper, S. L., P. R. Young and M. D. Ledah. 1981. In *Interactions of the Blood with Natural and Artificial Surfaces.* E. Salzman., ed. New York: Dekker, pp. 1–35.

108. Gristina, A. G. 1987. *Science*, 237:1588–1595.

109. Freedman, L. R. and J. Valone, Jr. 1979. *Prog. Cardiovasc. Dis.*, 22:169–180.

110. Durack, D. T., P. B. Beeson and R. G. Petersdorf. 1973. *Br. J. Exp. Pathol.*, 54:142–151.

111. Anderson, J. M. 1986. *Proc. of the 23rd Japanese Soc. for Artif. Organs, Tokyo*, pp. 1705–1712.

112. Vogler, E. A. and R. W. Bussia. 1987. *J. Biomed. Mater. Res.*, 21:1197–1211.

113. Horbett, T. A. and M. B. Schwey. 1988. *J. Biomed. Mater. Res.*, 22:763–793.

114. Knox, P. and S. Griffiths. 1980. *J. Cell. Sci.*, 46:97–112.

115. Grinnell, F., D. G. Hays and D. Minter. 1977. *Exp. Cell. Res.*, 110:175–190.

116. van Wachen, P. B., C. M. Vreriks, T. Beugeling, J. Feijen, A. Bantjes, J. P. Detners and W. G. van Aken. 1987. *J. Biomed. Mater. Res.*, 21:701–718.

117. Grinnell, F. 1983. In *Biocompatible Polymers Metals, and Composites.* M. Szycher, ed. Lancaster, PA: Technomic Publishing Co., Inc., pp. 673–699.

118. Feijen, J., T. Beugeling, A. Bantjes and C. Th. Smit Sibinga. 1979. "Biomaterials and Interfacial Phenomena", *Adv. Cardiovasc. Physics*, 3:100.

119. van Wachen, P. B., T. Beugeling, J. Feigen, A. Bantjes, J. P. Detners and W. J. van Aken. 1985. *Biomaterials*, 6:403–407.

120. Schakenraad, J. M., H. J. Busscher, C. R. H.

Wildevuur and J. Arends. 1986. *J. Biomed. Mater. Res.*, 20:783–784.

121. Horbett, T. A., M. B. Schway and B. D. Ratner. 1985. *J. Colloid Interface Sci.*, 104:28–39.

122. Imai, Y., A. Watanabe and Masuhara. 1983. *J. Biomed. Mater. Res.*, 17:905–912.

123. Rajaraman, R., D. E. Rounds, S. P. S. Yen and A. Rembanm. 1974. *Exp. Cell. Res.*, 88:327–339.

124. Grinnell, F. 1978. *Int. Rev. Cytol.*, 53:65.

125. Grinnell, F. 1987. In *Blood in Contact with Natural and Artificial Surfaces, Ann. N.Y. Acad. Sci.* E. F. Leonard, V. T. Turitto and L. Vroman, eds. New York: N.Y. Acad. Sci., 516:280–290.

126. McAuslan, B. R. and G. Johnson. 1987. *J. Biomed. Mater. Res.*, 21:921–935.

127. van Wachen, P. B., A. H. Hogt, T. Beugeling, J. Feijen, A. Bantjes, J. P. Detners and W. G. van Aken. 1987. *Biomaterials*, 8:323–328.

128. Lindblad, B., S. W. Wright, R. L. Sell, W. E. Burkel, L. M. Graham and J. C. Stanley. 1987. *J. Biomed. Mater. Res.*, 21:1013–1022.

129. Reinders, J. H., Ph. de Groot, J. Dawes, N. R. Hunter, H. A. A. van Heugten, J. Zandbergen, M. D. Gonsalves and J. A. van Moorik. 1985. *Biochim. Biophys. Acta.*, 844:306–313.

130. Mosher, D. F., M. J. Doyle and E. A. Jaffe. 1982. *J. Biol. Chem.*, 93:343.

131. Schmidt, J. A., S. B. Mizel, D. Cohen and E. Green. 1982. *J. Immunol.*, 128:2177.

132. Dinarello, C. A. 1984. *Interleukin 1, Ref. Infect. Dis.*, 6:51.

133. Martin, B. M., M. A. Gimbrone, Jr., E. R. Unanue and R. S. Cotran. 1981. In *Plasma and Cellular Modulatory Proteins.* D. H. Bing and R. A. Rosenbaum, eds. Boston: Center for Blood Research, Inc., pp. 83–94.

134. Kang, I.-K., Y. Ito, M. Sisido and Y. Imanishi. 1989. *J. Biomed. Mater. Res.*, 23:233–239.

135. McAuslan, B. R., G. Johnson, G. N. Hannan, W. D. Norris and T. Exner. 1988. *J. Biomed. Mater. Res.*, 22:963–976.

136. Ito, Y., Y. Imanishi and M. Sisido. 1987. *Biomaterials*, 8: 464–472.

137. Schoen, F. J., G. P. Clagett, J. D. Hill, D. E. Chenoweth, J. M. Anderson and R. C. Eberhart. 1987. *Trans. Am. Soc. Artif. Intern. Organs*, 33:824–833.

138. Levy, R. J., F. J. Schoen and G. Golomb. 1986. *CRC Crit. Ref. Biocompat.*, 2:147–187.

139. Schoen, F. J., H. Harasaki, K. M. Kim, H. C. Anderson and F. J. Levy. 1988. *J. Biomed. Mater. Res.; Appl. Biomater.*, 22A1:11–36.

140. Bruek, S. D. 1982. *Med. Progr. Technol.*, 9:1–16.

141. Coleman, D. L., D. Lim, T. Kessler and J. D. Andrade. 1981. *Trans. Am. Soc. Artif. Intern. Organs*, 27:97–103.

142. Boskey, A. L. and A. S. Posner. 1973. *J. Phys. Chem.*, 77:2313–2317.

143. Nose, Y., H. Harasaki and J. Murray. 1981. *Trans. Am. Soc. Artif. Intern. Organs*, 27:714–720.

144. Salzman, E., ed. 1981. *Interactions of the Blood with Natural and Artificial Surfaces.* New York: Dekker.

145. Siggaaro-Anderson, O., J. Thode and J. J. Wandrup. 1980. *YF CC-EPPH Workshop.* Kopenhagen, pp. 163–190.

146. Pedersen, K. O. 1971. *Scand. Clin. Lab. Invest.*, 28:459–469.

147. Carr, C. W. 1953. *Arch. Biochem. Biophys.*, 43:147–156.

148. Anderson, M. F. 1977. *Clin. Chem.*, 23:2122–2126.

149. Rosanovz, I. B., A. V. Gorshkov and V. I. Sevastianov. 1988. *Med. Technika*, 5:15–19.

150. Rosanova, I. B., V. I. Sevastianov and S. W. Kim. *J. Biomed. Mater. Res.* (in press).

151. Johanson, K. O., O. B. Wetlanfer, R. G. Reed and Th. Tr. Peters. 1981. *J. Biol. Chem.*, 256:445–450.

152. Wetlaufer, O. B. 1981. *Advanc. Protein Chem.*, 34:76–83.

153. Besarab, A., A. Deguzman and J. W. Swanson. 1981. *J. Clin. Path.*, 34:1361–1367.

154. Aguanno, J. J. and J. H. Ladenson. 1982. *J. Biol. Che.*, 257:8745.

155. Sevastianov, V. I. and I. B. Rosanova. (unpublished data).

156. Conti, F., R. Fiorovanti, F. Malebra and E. Wanke. 1974. *Biophys. Structure and Mech.*, 1:27.

157. Wortsman, J. and R. Traykoff. 1980. *Amer. J. Physiol.*, 238:E104-E107.

158. Sorkina, D. A. 1988. *Vopros. Med. Chemi.*, 2:8–16.

159. Sevastianov, V. I. and I. B. Rosanova. 1988. *Trans. of 3rd World Biomaterials Congress*, 11:462.

160. Sevastianov, V. I. and I. B. Rosanova. 1989. *Artif. Organs*, 13:364.

161. Rosanova, I. B., B. P. Mishenko, V. P. Zaitsev, S. L. Vasin and V. I. Sevastianov. *J. Biomed. Mater. Res.* (in press).

162. Marchant, R. E., J. M. Anderson, A. Hiltner, E. J. Castillo, J. Gleit and B. D. Ratner. 1986. *J. Biomed. Mater. Res.*, 20:799–815.

163. Spilizewski, K. L., R. E. Marchant, J. M. Anderson and A. Hiltner. 1987. *Biomaterials*, 8:12–17.

164. Boskey, A. L. 1986. In *Cell Mediated Calcification and Matrix Vesicles.* Ali Yousuf, ed. Elsevier Sci., Publ., B.V., pp. 175–179.

165. Zisman, W. A. 1964. In "Contact Angle, Wettability, and Adhesion", F. M. Fowkes, ed. *Adv. Chem. Ser.*, 43:1.

166. Baier, R. E. 1970. In *Adhesion in Biological Systems.* R. S. Manly, ed. New York: Acad. Press.

167. Lyman, D. J., W. M. Muir and I. J. Lee. 1965. *Trans. Amer. Soc. Artif. Intern. Organs*, 11:301–317.

168. Andrade, J. D. 1973. *Med. Instrum.*, 7:110–120.

169. Nyilas, E., W. A. Morton, D. M. Lederman, T. H. Chin and R. D. Cumming. 1975. *Trans. Am. Soc. Artif. Intern. Organs*, 21:55–69.

170. Ratner, B. D., A. S. Hoffman, S. R. Hanson, L. A. Harker and J. D. Whiffen. 1979. *J. Polym. Sci. Polym. Symp.*, 60:363–375.

171. Lee, S. H. and E. Ruckenstein. 1987. *J. Colloid Interface Sci.*, 117:172–178.

172. Lelah, M. D. and S. L. Cooper. 1986. *Polyurethanes in Medicine.* Boca Raton: CRC Press.

173. Ito, Y., M. Sisido and Y. Imanishi. 1986. *J. Biomed. Mater. Res.*, 20:1139–1155.

174. Kang, I.-K., Y. Ito, M. Sisido and Y. Imanishi. 1988. *J. Biomed. Mater. Res.*, 22:595–611.

175. Ikado, Y., M. Suzuki and Y. Tamada. 1984. In *Polymers as Biomaterials*. S. W. Shalaby, A. S. Hoffman, B. D. Ratner and T. A. Horbett, eds. New York: Plenum Press, pp. 135–147.

176. Okano, T., T. Aoyagi, K. Kataoka, K. Abe, Y. Sakuai, M. Shimada and I. Shinohara. 1986. *J. Biomed. Mater. Res.*, 20:919–927.

177. Grainger, D., T. Okano and S. W. Kim. 1987. In *Adv. Biomed. Polym.*, C. G. Gebelain, ed. Plenum Publ. Corp., pp. 229–247.

178. Nojiri, C., T. Okano, D. Grainger, K. D. Park, S. Nakahama, K. Suzuki and S. W. Kim. 1987. *Trans. Am. Soc. Artif. Intern. Organs*, 33:596–600.

179. 1985. *Design of Multiphase Biomedical Materials*. Tsuruta, T., ed. Tokyo.

180. Okano, T., S. Nishiyama, I. Shinohara, T. Akaike, Y. Sakurai, K. Kataoka and T. Tsurata. 1981. *J. Biomed. Mater. Res.*, 15:303.

181. Barbucci, R., A. Baszkin, M. Benvenuti, M. Costa and P. Ferruti. 1987. *J. Biomed. Mater. Res.*, 21:443–457.

182. Ito, Y., M. Sisido and Y. Imanishi. 1989. *J. Biomed. Mater. Res.*, 23:191–206.

183. Andrade, J. D. and W.-Y. Chen. 1986. *Surf. and Interface Analysis*, 8:253–256.

184. Ruckenstein, E. and S. H. Lee. 1987. *J. Colloid Interface Sci.*, 120:153–161.

185. Reichert, W. N., F. E. Filisko and S. A. Barenberg. 1982. In *Biomaterials: Interfacial Phenomena and Applications, Adv. Chem. Ser.* S. L. Cooper and N. A. Peppas, eds. Washington, D.C.: ACS, 199: 177–194.

186. Andrade, J. D. and V. Hlady. 1986. *Adv. Polym. Sci.*, 79:1–63.

187. Merrill, E. W. and E. W. Salzman. 1983. *ASAIO J.*, 6:60–64.

188. Grainger, D. W., S. W. Kim and J. Feijen. 1988. *J. Biomed. Mater. Res.*, 22:231–239.

189. Mori, Y. and S. Nagaoka. 1982. *Trans. Am. Soc. Artif. Intern. Organs*, 28:459–463.

190. Barenberg, S. A., J. M. Anderson and K. A. Mauritz. 1981. *J. Biomed. Mater. Res.*, 15:231–245.

191. Sevastianov, V. I. and O. V. Laksina. 1986. *J. Colloid Interface Sci.*, 112:279–289.

192. Sevastianov, V. I., R. C. Eberhart and S. W. Kim. 1988. *ASAIO J.*, 11:10–18.

193. Yui, N., K. Sanui, N. Ogata, K. Kataoka, T. Okano and Y. Sakurai. 1986. *J. Biomed. Mater. Res.*, 20:929–943.

194. Grasel, T. G., W. G. Pitt, K. D. Murthy, T. G. McCoy and S. L. Cooper. 1987. *Biomaterials*, 8:329–340.

195. Yui, N., K. Kataoka, Y. Sakurai, T. Aoki, K. Sanui and N. Ogato. 1988. *Biomaterials*, 9:225–229.

196. Boota, J. G. F., L. van der Does and A. Bantjes. 1986. *Biomaterials*, 7:393–399.

197. Maruyama, A., T. Tsurita, K. Kataoka and Y. Sakurai. 1988. *Biomaterials*, 9:471–481.

198. .Goodman, S. L., T. G. Grasel, S. L. Cooper and R. M. Albrecht. 1989. *J. Biomed. Mater. Res.*, 23:105–123.

199. Mineura, N., S. Aiba, Y. Fujiwara and N. Koshizaki. 1989. *J. Biomed. Mater. Res.*, 23:267–279.

200. Park, K. D., T. Okano, C. Nojiri and S. W. Kim. 1988. *J. Biomed. Mater. Res.*, 22:977–992.

201. van Damme, H. S. and J. Feijen. *J. Colloid Interface Sci.* (in press).

202. Kim, S. W. and J. Feijen. 1985. *CRC Crit. Rev. Biocompatibility*, 1:229–260.

203. Horsley, D., J. Herron, V. Haldy and J. D. Andrade. 1987. In *Proteins at Interfaces: Physico-Chemical and Biochemical Studies, Symposium Ser.* J. L. Brash and T. A. Horbett, eds. Washington, D.C: ACS, 343:290–305.

Modified PHEMA Hydrogels

PATRICIA A. DAVIS*
SAMUEL J. HUANG*
LUIGI NICOLAIS**
LUIGI AMBROSIO†

ABSTRACT: PHEMA hydrogel is modified using two techniques aimed at keeping such property as high water content in the swollen state. The first method is copolymerization with maleic acid or maleic anhydride. The copolymer containing maleic acid displays properties similar to those of PHEMA, but the copolymer with maleic anhydride hydrolyzes faster than PHEMA. The second modification technique employed is incorporation of linear poly(caprolactone) into PHEMA. Significant improvement in strength and toughness resulted without chemical grafting between the components or considerable reduction in water absorption capacity.

INTRODUCTION

The term *hydrogel* refers to a broad class of polymeric materials which swell extensively, but do not dissolve in water. They include many natural materials of both plant and animal origin. Because of the similarity between synthetic and natural hydrogels, these gels have been used in a wide variety of biomedical applications, and the number is growing. Presently, these applications include suture coatings, contact lenses and artificial organs. Such a wide range of uses requires easy manipulation of physical properties—attainable by changing monomers and/or polymerization conditions. Since biocompatibility apparently depends on water content, characterization of the amount of imbibed water in the swollen gel is essential.

The conceptualization and initial development of synthetic polymeric hydrogels especially intended for biomedical applications was accomplished by Wichterle and Lim [1] who described the potential use of cross-linked poly(2-hydroxyethyl methacrylate), (PHEMA) gels as biomaterials in a 1960 article. Since then a tremendous interest in hydrogels for a variety of biomedical applications followed.

Hydrogels are polymeric networks held together by either cross-links or weak cohesive forces such as hydrogen or ionic bonds. These networks imbibe large quantities of water (or organic liquids) without dissolution. Swelling ability in different solvents depends on the type of cross-links; thus, a hydrogel may swell in one solvent but not in another. Covalently cross-linked hydrogel systems are insoluble in any solvent that does not break the cross-links. Evidently, there are various types of hydrogels. Swelling behavior depends on chemical structure, cross-link density, and on the presence of ionic groups.

Usually hydrogels retain a significant fraction of water. The water content is defined as:

$$\frac{\text{swollen mass} - \text{dry mass}}{\text{dry mass}} \times 100\% \qquad (1)$$

There are several factors, favorable and inhibitive, which influence the degree of hydrogel swelling. Some of the favorable influences on swelling are osmotic potential, strong interactions with water, high free volume, high chain flexibility and low cross-link density. A few of the inhibitive factors affecting swelling are weak interactions with water, low free volume, low chain flexibility, and high cross-link density. Thus, strong positive interactions between chemical groups on the polymer chain and water, such as hydrogen bonding, increase the driving force for swelling.

As water enters the polymer, the chains extend and exert a resistive force because swelling places the chains into less entropically desired configurations.

*Institute of Materials Science, University of Connecticut U-136, Storrs, CT 06268

**Department of Materials Production and Engineering, University of Naples, Piazzale Tecchio, Naples, 80125 Italy

†Institute of Composite Materials Technology, C. N. R., University of Naples, Piazzale Tecchio, Naples, 80125 Italy

When this resistive force balances the osmotic force driving water into the polymer, the equilibrium degree of swelling is reached.

Because a high cross-link density of the network or a stiffer polymer backbone intensifies the resistive force to chain extension, a more highly cross-linked system or a polymer with a stiffer backbone will swell less. Finally, if the free volume in the polymer is too low, water may be unable to penetrate the polymer matrix to initiate the swelling process. All the factors influencing hydrogel swelling are controllable by the choice of monomer and polymerization conditions.

Many different polymeric structures can be classified as hydrogels. Table 1 [2] lists monomers used in hydrogel syntheses, while Table 2 [2] lists the polymers that can be converted into hydrogels. In Table 1, the types of monomers listed are divided into four categories; namely, neutral, acidic or anionic, basic or cationic, and cross-linker. Most of the monomers are hydrophilic and have strong positive interactions with water. Thus, the resulting hydrogels displaying high degrees of swelling.

One way of reducing the extent of swelling in water is by copolymerization of the hydrophilic and hydrophobic monomers. Sometimes hydrogels are created by conversion of already existing polymers. Table 2 lists examples of such polymers. Note that PHEMA results from the polymerization of the neutral monomer, listed in Table 1 as hydroxymethyl methacrylate. This polymer is usually referred to a poly(2-hydroxyethyl methacrylate) or PHEMA, and is the system of choice for our research.

Polymers fabricated from the structures listed in Tables 1 and 2 are insoluble in aqueous media after they have been made into hydrogels. The polymer chains are interconnected by covalent bonds. It is obvious from the quantity of listed monomers and convertible polymers that many different hydrogels with widely varying properties are possible.

Hydrogels are fabricated into useful forms using a variety of techniques, where the specific approach depends on the polymer type. Figure 1 [3] displays schematically some of these fabrication methods. Cast films [Figure 1(a)] are frequently used as coatings for

Table 1. Monomers used in hydrogels preparation [2].

Table 2. Converted polymers used as hydrogels [2].

$$\{CH_2-CH\}\ \longrightarrow\ \{CH_2-CH\}$$
$$\underset{C=O}{\overset{O}{|}} \qquad OH$$
$$CH_3$$

$$\{CH_2-CH=CH-CH_2\}\ \longrightarrow\ \{CH_2-CH-CH-CH_2\}$$
$$OH\quad OH$$

(+) (+) (+) (+) / (−) (−) (−) ⟶ Polyelectrolyte Complex

$$\{CH_2-CH\}\ \longrightarrow\ \{CH_2-CH\}\{CH_2-CH\}\{CH_2-CH\}$$
$$CN \qquad CN \quad \underset{NH_2}{\overset{C=O}{|}} \quad CO_2H$$

$$CH_2=C\overset{CH_3}{\underset{CO_2C_2H_4OH}{<}}\ +\ \{CH_2-CH\}\,(N=O)\ \longrightarrow\ \text{Mixture of 2 Polymers}$$

$$OCN-R-NCO\ +\ HO\{CH_2-CH_2-O\}_x H\ \longrightarrow\ \left[\overset{O}{\overset{\|}{C}}-HNR-NH-\overset{O}{\overset{\|}{C}}O\{CH_2-CH_2-O\}_x\right]$$

Natural $\left\{HN-CH-\overset{O}{\overset{\|}{C}}\right\}_x \underset{R_y}{}\ \longrightarrow\ $ Reconstituted $\left\{HN-CH-\overset{O}{\overset{\|}{C}}\right\}_w \underset{R_z}{}$

other materials usually requiring noncovalent forces to prevent dissolution of the polymer in an aqueous media. Such films are either hydrophobically or covalently bonded to the material of interest. An example of the use of this type of coating is the work of Tollar et al. [4]. Indeed, as early as 1969, Tollar and his colleagues used PHEMA hydrogel as a coating for surgical sutures with excellent results. Also, they successfully loaded the gel coating with antibiotics to facilitate wound healing.

Figure 1(b) shows the preparation of the molded cross-linked hydrogel network. Such a network is formed by injecting a mixture of monomer, cross-linking agent and initiator into a mold. Sometimes a solvent is also added to the mixture as diluent to yield a more porous gel. Hydrogels prepared in this manner have been used in such applications as plastic surgery for breast augmentation [5], as artificial membranes in corneal surgery [6], in otolaryngology for covering ear drum perforations and nasal pyramids [7], and as prosthesis for the ureter [8].

Surface grafting [Figure 1(c)] of hydrogels to other polymers is a fabricating technique in which the hydrophilic polymer is made water-insoluble by bonding it to an insoluble substrate. Only the substrate needs to be in a specific shape, because the graft follows the contours of the substrate polymer. Ratner and Hoffman [9] discuss in detail techniques for preparing grafted hydrogels.

Interpenetrating polymer networks can be prepared by forming cross-linked hydrogel systems within other polymer networks [Figure 1(d)] where both are topologically independent but inseparable. Such systems are used to mechanically strengthen hydrogels. We used a modification of this technique to prepare strengthened versions of PHEMA hydrogel [10].

Synthesis and fabrication of hydrogels are intimately related. The fabrication technique usually dictates the polymerization conditions. For example, IPN preparation requires synthesis of the gel within another network while surface grafting requires the presence of a substrate during polymerization. The

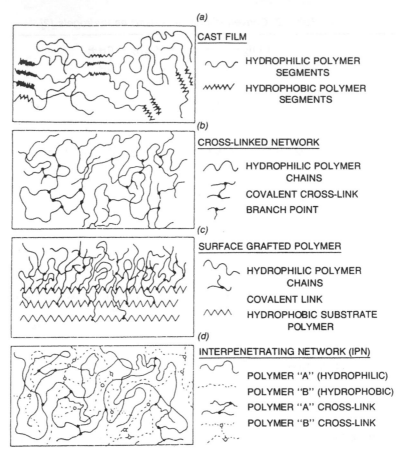

Figure 1. Fabrication of hydrogels [3].

porosity of hydrogel systems depends on synthesis conditions, and affects their mechanical and physical properties. If the monomer is polymerized in the presence of a solvent good for both itself and the polymer formed, an optically clear gel results. This type of hydrogel is called "homogenous" or "microporous". The porosity of these systems is related to the void space between individual polymer chains.

If the monomer is polymerized in a solvent good for itself, but poor for the polymer, simultaneous polymerization-cross-linking-precipitation (microsyneresis) results in a macroporous gel. This type of gel appears white or translucent. The macroporous or "heterogenous" hydrogels have true void spaces in their structures which can allow cellular ingrowth when they are used as implant material.

The possibility of tissue ingrowth into the hydrogel matrix makes these materials very attractive for biomedical use. This and other attributes such as permeability to small molecules, (i.e., metabolites); soft consistency; and low interfacial tension between the gel and aqueous solutions are the intriguing biocompatible-dependent properties which have generated such interest in hydrogels as potential biomaterials. Moreover, ease of purification, adjustable mechanical properties, and equilibrium water content, along with sterilizability by heat, chemical,

or radiation means without significant damage to the hydrogel renders this class of materials ideal for biomedical use.

High permeability to small molecules allows for the extraction of unreacted molecules, initiator decomposition products, and extraneous materials to produce a highly purified network. High purity is a necessity for biomaterials, because otherwise impurities can leach from the implant and produce adverse effects on the surrounding tissues. Moreover, these impurities can travel to distant parts of the body and damage vital organs. Also, low molecular weight metabolites can diffuse through the hydrogel to body tissue where they are needed as nutrient.

The soft consistency of hydrogels minimizes mechanical frictional irritation to surrounding tissue. The low interfacial tension between the hydrogel surface and aqueous solution should reduce the tendency of proteins in body fluids to adsorb to the gel and to unfold upon adsorption [9]. Thus, protein activity would not be adversely affected by the presence of the hydrogel in the body.

Table 3 [9] is a brief list of some of the biomedical applications of synthetic hydrogels. This table lists three categories of hydrogels in biomedical use. They are coatings, "homogenous" materials, and devices. The wide range of biomedical applications for hydrogels can be attributed to both their satisfactory performance upon *in vivo* implantation in either blood contacting or tissue contacting situations and their ability to be fabricated into a large number of morphologies.

The ease with which the physical forms of hydrogels can be altered allows for adjustment of physical properties to match specific applications. However, particular hydrogel composition that may be suitable for one biomedical application may have to be significantly modified for a different application. The hydrogel system must be matched to the intended biomedical use. Fortunately, hydrogels are flexible in this respect.

Matching hydrogels to specific biomedical uses requires a means of characterizing the gels. Although the presence of imbibed water within the gel is not a guarantee of excellent biocompatibility, it is believed to be intrinsically related. Unfortunately, the hydrogel interface with water presents a unique and complex situation. It is suggested that water may be quasiorganized within hydrogels [11].

Many types of hydrogels exist. And the literature is full of works involving them. Since PHEMA is the hydrogel of choice for our work and it is the most widely used, the following discussion is limited to PHEMA hydrogel.

Preparation of PHEMA hydrogels was first described by Wichterle and Lim [1] in 1960. Although the linear polymer was first prepared as early as 1936 by DuPont scientists, they did not polymerize the monomer in the presence of a cross-linking agent in an aqueous media as Wichterle and Lim did in 1960 [9]. Since 1960, PHEMA has become the most widely used and studied synthetic hydrogel.

Refojo and Yasuda [12] described the synthesis of PHEMA by several methods in detail. These methods are bulk polymerization of the polymer, followed by bulk cross-linking with a cross-linking agent; the introduction of cross-links into the polymer in solution; and the simultaneous polymerization and cross-linking of monomer-cross-linking agent mixtures.

The last method proved to be the most advantageous because the formation of the hydrogel can be quickly achieved at low temperatures by using redox initiator systems. Also, gels of any shape are readily obtained since the starting materials are all liquid.

Bulk polymerization of 2-hydroxyethyl methacrylate (HEMA) with a free radical initiator proceeds in a fashion similar to the bulk polymerization of methyl methacrylate (MMA). The resulting polymer resembles poly(methyl methacrylate), (PMMA), but is harder and brittler. Immersion of the cross-linked polymer into water results in gradual swelling, to the point where the polymer becomes soft.

In contrast, the homopolymer produced from polymerization of purified HEMA without cross-linking agent is soluble in a water-ethanol mixture when polymerized to low percent conversions. At low percent conversion, cross-linking through chain transfer is avoided. However, the polymer is insoluble at high percent conversion. The authors [12] suggested that cross-links are introduced in the high percent conversion polymer by both an undetermined amount of residual difunctional monomer [ethylene glycol dimethacrylate, (EDMA)], and by chain transfer within the polymer. The water content of this particular bulk-polymerized PHEMA gel was found to be 37.5% after the polymer was allowed to swell in water at room temperature for about one year.

The PHEMA hydrogel literature is vast. This polymer, its composites, copolymers and blends have been and are being studied and in innumerable laboratories in the world and on many levels.

Since the 1960s, the structural and chemical properties of PHEMA have been researched with zeal. Some of these properties are: molecular weight between cross-links [13,14]; the coefficient of the diffusion of water [15–17] and other solutes [18–21] into the gels; the equilibrium percent swelling of the gel in water [2,6,12] and other solvents [17,23,24], and the effect of cross-linking agent [14], diluent type [25], and the presence of solutes [17] on swelling; polymerization conditions [26]. Other properties are polymer–sol-

Table 3. A brief list of the biomedical applications of synthetic hydrogels [9].

Coatings	"Homogeneous" Materials	Devices
Sutures	Electrophoresis gels	Enzyme therapeutic systems
Catheters	Contact lenses	Artificial organs
IUDs	Artificial corneas	Drug delivery systems
Blood detoxicants	Vitreous humor replacements	
Sensors (electrodes)	Estrous-inducers	
Vascular grafts	Breast or other soft tissue substitutes	
Electrophoresis cells	Burn dressings	
Cell culture substrates	Bone ingrowth sponges	
	Dentures	
	Ear drum plugs	
	Synthetic cartilages	
	Hemodialysis membranes	
	Particulate carriers of tumor antibodies	

vent interaction parameters [14,24]; water organization within the gel [27,28]; the types of materials that leach out of PHEMA after preparation, in conjunction with the time frame for purification of the gel [29], along with the irritation effects of these compounds on the biological tissue [30,31]. These are just some of the chemical and physical characteristics of PHEMA-type hydrogels analyzed during the past thirty years.

There is substantial disagreement in the literature among the different groups who measure the chemical and structural properties of hydrogels of PHEMA and its copolymers and blends. One example is the determination of the molecular weight between cross-links, Mc, of cross-linked PHEMA hydrogels from volume fractions measurements using the modification of the Flory-Rehner equation by Peppas et al. [14]. They arrived at Mc values ranging from 800–3700 Daltons and refuted the values of 8,660–67,180 reported by Migliaresi et al. [13].

The results of Migliaresi et al. [13] were obtained from rubber elasticity theory and shear stress measurements. An important factor to note is the vastly different PHEMA preparation methods used by the two groups. The samples prepared by Peppas et al. [14] were simultaneously polymerized and cross-linked in the presence of 40 weight-percent water at 60°C for 12 hours with 0.5 weight-percent benzoyl peroxide, (BPO), initiator. On the other hand, sample preparation by Migliaresi et al. [13] involved simultaneous polymerization and cross-linking in the presence of either diacetin, poly(N-vinyl pyrrolidone) (PNVP), or glycerol at 90°C for 1 hour with 0.1 weight-percent azobisisobutyronitrile, (AIBN), or BPO initiator. With such a great difference in polymerization techniques, little chemical basis for comparing results from these two works can be found. One immediately realizes that using five times the amount of initiator and carrying out the reaction to high conversion, where chain transfer will occur to promote even more cross-linking, might easily result in a tighter network.

Along these same lines, one finds coefficients of the diffusion of water into these gels varying by as much as two orders of magnitude [13,16,17,32]. Also, there are disagreements as to whether this diffusion process is Fickian [13,16,17,33].

The determination of the thermal, mechanical, and viscoelastic properties of PHEMA-type hydrogels appears to be less controversial than the investigations of chemical properties. Early mechanical property studies involved application of the kinetic theory of rubber elasticity [34,35] to understand the deformation behavior of PHEMA and the effects of swelling solvent [36,37] and diluent [38]. Loss and compliance moduli were measured by Janacek and Ferry [39]. They determined the dynamic mechanical properties of PHEMA using the torsion pendulum [40].

In addition, the effects of side group chain length and chemical make-up on the glass transition temperature (T_g) of the hydrogel were investigated by Ilavsky et al. [41,42]. How the presence of low molecular weight substances affected the T_g of these gels was studied by Janacek [43]. A recent work by Roorda et al. [28] used DTA to thermally study swollen PHEMA hydrogels. In this work, they refuted the existence of different thermodynamic phases of water in hydrogels explained by Bruck [11] and Jhon and Andrade [27].

The incorporation of particulates such as SiO_2 [44] and glass beads [45,46] and their effects on the viscoelastic properties of PHEMA gels were investigated. A major motivation for these works was the attempt to improve the mechanical properties of the swollen hydrogel. The authors had some success in this regard. Janacek [47] provides an excellent review of the thermo-mechanical behavior of PHEMA and other hydrogels.

A more recent emphasis is noted in the research of PHEMA-type hydrogels in the area of biomedical characterization of the biological processes that ensue immediately and on a long-term basis following implantation. Early works, such as that of Barvic et al. [48] investigated, on a systemic level, the effects of functional groups incorporated into the skeleton of PHEMA on the biological tolerance of the organism.

Also, the effect of gel porosity on the healing-in of the implant was researched by Sprincl et al. [49,50] on both a short-term [49] and long-term basis [50]. They found that higher-porosity gels had narrower encapsulation with newly formed capillaries penetrating into the implant after 30–90 days. However, after 360 days, the low-porosity gels were completely healed-in, while the high-porosity gels remained encapsulated as described for the 30–90 days results.

To add more to these implant results, Imai's and Masuhara's recent work [51] on the long term tolerance of PHEMA concluded with the finding that PHEMA is tumorigenic only in rats but not in hamsters and guinea pigs. The authors suggest a correlation between thick avascular capsule formation and tumor development at the tumor site. Thin fibrous capsule formation was observed in the hamsters and guinea pigs without subsequent tumorigenesis.

Cifkova's study [31] of the irritation effects of the materials that leach out of PHEMA found no irritation to biological tissue because the substances did not accumulate in the tissue in concentrations great enough to cause irritation. In addition, early [52] and recent [53] orthopedic implantations of PHEMA and a PHEMA/PMMA blend into bone to stimulate bone healing were performed. The results indicated that bone formation indeed occurred [52] and polymer resorption took place after adhesion of macrophages onto the polymer [53].

Current research in this area of biological studies of PHEMA-type hydrogels after implantation concentrates more on surface studies of implants in order to fathom the events that affect biocompatibility on the microscopic level. One example is the work of Brynda et al. [54] studying protein sorption onto PHEMA measured by fluorescence labels. They found sorption, then desorption of the proteins which they attributed to protein–polymer bond instability. The motivation for this study is the assumption that protein adsorption on the implant surface is an important step in implant rejection.

A prevalent school of thought noted in the literature concerning protein adsorption to implant surface is that hydrophilic–hydrophobic microdomains influence the adsorption of proteins onto the materials surface; and thus, platelet adhesion is affected. One early work [55] following this line of thought used PHEMA/polystyrene (PS) block copolymers. Protein adsorption onto the polymer was indeed reduced and this was attributed to the hydrophilic–hydrophobic microdomains on the polymer surface. More work in this area, this time by Okano et al. [56,57] on PHEMA/PS and PHEMA/poly(dimethyl siloxane) (PDMS) block copolymers, led to the same results. They concluded that the presence of these microdomains—structured in alternate lamellae, led to selective protein adsorption. This, in turn, prevented platelet activation.

Studies of cell adhesion onto PHEMA/PS and PHEMA/poly(ethyl methacrylate) (PEMA) [58] reported excellent cell adhesion with the suggestion that the equilibrium water content of the gels is an important factor for cell adhesion. When adsorption of blood elements onto PHEMA/PNVP copolymeric hydrogel-coated silicone was investigated [59], the authors found reversible adsorption onto the hydrophilic surface with less denaturation of the adsorbed proteins.

A work on the adsorption of trypsin onto PHEMA/ PS copolymeric microspheres and its enzymatic activity [60] found less trypsin adsorption onto the more hydrophilic surfaces. This adsorbed trypsin displayed better enzymatic activity than that adsorbed to a more hydrophobic surface. A study on coagulase negative staphylococci adhesion to PHEMA/PEMA copolymers [61] reported a decrease in adhesion rate as the percentage HEMA in the copolymer increased. At the human level, Bowers and Tighe [62–64] found that unsaturated lipids adhered to the surface of PHEMA contact lenses. This reduced the compatibility of the gel and created patient intolerance.

Human serum complement activation by PHEMA, PMMA and silicone was studied by Gobel et al. [65]. PHEMA displayed lower C3a and C4a uptake than PMMA and silicone. Payne and Horbett [66] also studied complement activation, but on PHEMA/ PEMA copolymers. They found significant complement activation caused by copolymers with 60 percent or more PHEMA. The authors concluded that PHEMA is an activator of the human complement system in heparinized plasma. More recently, Horbett and Schway [67] correlated fibronectin adsorption onto PHEMA/PEMA copolymers with the spreading of mouse 3T3 cells. According to them, PHEMA ex-

hibited absolutely no fibronectin uptake. These results are in direct contrast to those of Payne and Horbett [66].

Rat lymphocyte adsorption onto PHEMA/poly-(amine) (PA) graft copolymers was quantitatively studied by Maruyama et al. [68]. Fewer lymphocytes adsorbed to the copolymers with original shape retention than to the homopolymers. The conclusion, here, was that the heterogeneity of the graft copolymer surface suppressed cellular activation. Also, rat peritoneal macrophage adhesion to PHEMA/PEMA copolymers was investigated [69]. The rate of adhesion decreased as the copolymer hydrophilicity increased. The amount of hydrophilicity is proportional to the quantity of PHEMA in the copolymer. Along these same lines, Poly(ethylene) (PE)/PHEMA blends generated less thrombus formation than PE, according to Brynda et al. [70].

Some biomedical surface studies were performed on etched PHEMA-type hydrogels. McAuslan and Johnson [71] researched adhesion and growth of vascular bovine aortal endothelial cells onto etched PHEMA. Increased adhesion and growth was found with the creation of more surface-COOH groups. Instead, Smetana [72] found improved intraocular biocompatibility of etched PHEMA/PMMA copolymer gel in rabbits.

Since the 1960s, PHEMA-type hydrogels have continued to be applied clinically in humans for various uses. The studies of Kliment [5] in plastic surgery and Majkus [7] in otolaryngology cited earlier were performed on human subjects. Currently, Bowers and Tighe [62–64] are investigating the mechanisms by which commercially available hydrogel long-term-wear contact lenses are rendered incompatible during use. Horak et al. [73–75] are using spherical PHEMA particles to suppress pulmonary hemorrhage and hemoptysis in their patients. They inject these spheres into the arteries at the site of hemorrhage and quick blood coagulation ensues because of thrombus formation on the particles' surfaces. Subsequent X-ray tracking of the particles later made radiopaque by incorporation of iodine, indicated that the spheres do not resorb [75].

Animal subjects, primarily the dog [8,52] and rabbit [76–78], have been continuously used for screening prostheses fabricated from PHEMA-type hydrogels. For example, Michnevic and Kliment [76] used hydron reinforced with polyester netting to anchor sutures in the resection of liver in rabbits. Recently, Yoshida et al. [77] studied the slow release of testosterone from radiation-polymerized PHEMA testicular prosthesis. The prosthesis was implanted subcutaneously in the back of castrated rabbits. They found non-constant release of the drug because fibrous tissue adhered to the surface of the implant and depressed drug release.

Ronca et al. [78] replaced the Achilles tendon of the rabbit with a PHEMA/poly(ethylene terephthalate) (PET) fiber artificial tendon. This prosthesis was pre-

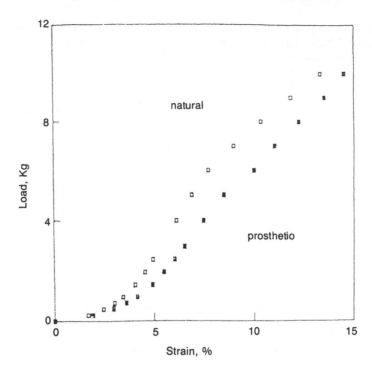

Figure 2. Stress–strain curves of muscle-tendon complex prepared by Ronca et al.; natural tendon (left) and prosthesis (right).

pared in a manner which mimics, in a simplified manner, the structural heirarchy of natural tendon. The PET fibers were crimped, then embedded into the PHEMA matrix. From their *in vivo* studies, the authors found no toxic cellular or tissue reaction. Instead, ingrowth of collagen along the fiber axis occurred. In addition, mechanical testing of the implanted and natural tendon–muscle complexes after forty-five days disclosed similar stress–strain curves (see Figure 2).

As is evident from above, PHEMA hydrogels are widely used as biomaterials. Their softness and high water content in the water-swollen state impart the quality of natural tissue [3]. High water permeability allows for ease of purification before implantation. Likewise, diffusion of biofluids and nutrients through the prosthesis after implantation is permitted. These two factors are important for biocompatible materials. Unfortunately, PHEMA hydrogel possesses low mechanical strength and tear resistance. This limits its biomedical applications to low-strength uses such as contact lenses and suture coatings.

We have been examining different ways of improving the mechanical properties of PHEMA while maintaining those desirable biocompatible attributes. Copolymerization of HEMA with maleic acid (MAC) and maleic anhydride (MAH) and incorporation of biocompatible and biodegradable PCL [79] and PCL oligomeric diols into PHEMA hydrogel are the techniques attempted in order to improve the mechanical properties of the swollen networks.

At the same time, some degree of softness, high equilibrium water content, and high permeability is maintained. In short, the positive attributes which makes PHEMA hydrogel exceedingly biocompatible are to be preserved. Furthermore, some of these modified PHEMA hydrogels such as the blends with PCL will allow natural tissue ingrowth since PCL degrades to leave voids in the network. In this way, the implant can be anchored in the body, as may be desired in certain applications. Also, in the case of PHEMA/PCL blends, combining hydrophilic and hydrophobic components could have enormous potential for blood-contacting biomedical applications, as is mentioned previously in the discussion of surface analysis of PHEMA hydrogels and blends.

Our modified PHEMA hydrogel networks are evaluated in terms of their thermal, mechanical, and swelling properties, morphology, hydrolysis behavior, and *in vitro* degradation. The results are discussed in the following pages.

MODIFIED POLY(2-HYDROXYETHYL METHACRYLATE) HYDROGELS

Since PHEMA hydrogel has poor mechanical strength, we explored several ways of improving the strength of this hydrogel without sacrificing the properties which impart good biocompatibility. Polymer blends and random copolymers were investigated. The blends were composed of cross-linked PHEMA and linear poly(caprolactone), (PCL). The random copolymers were of HEMA monomer polymerized with maleic anhydride and maleic acid.

This first section describes the syntheses and analyses of PHEMA copolymers—with maleic acid and maleic anhydride along with PHEMA/PCL blends incorporating different molecular-weight linear PCL. Water absorption, hydrolysis in different buffers, and degradation behavior, along with dynamic and static mechanical properties of these water swollen systems were compared to those of PHEMA.

The PHEMA/PCL blends were prepared as follows. PCL (MW ~ 35,000 or 2000) was dissolved in HEMA monomer at 60°C. After allowing the solution to cool, 0.5 weight-percent EDMA and 0.1 weight-percent AIBN were added. The percent initiator and cross-linking agent were calculated with respect to HEMA. For the copolymers, 10 weight-percent MAC or MAH was dissolved in HEMA monomer at room temperature prior to the addition of cross-linking agent and initiator.

Mixed solutions were poured into molds fabricated from silicone gasket, sandwiched by two pieces of Mylar-lined glass plates. Molds were heated at 90°C for one hour. After cooling, each hydrogel film was placed in distilled water for purification through the leaching-out of unreacted reagents. The PHEMA/PCL blend samples were white opaque gels, while all the other hydrogels were clear and transparent. Table 4 lists the samples prepared from these materials and the weight-percentages of their components.

Analysis techniques include water absorption, static and dynamic mechanical analysis, differential scanning calorimetry, hydrolysis, *in vitro* degradation and scanning electron microscopy. Water absorption of the hydrogels was followed by a recording of changes in the sample mass during exposure to distilled water using Equation (1). These water absorption data were also used to determine the equilibrium amount of water absorbed by each hydrogel and the average diffusion coefficient of a waterfront into the networks.

Static mechanical analysis consisted of testing dogbone samples (ASTM D638-86) of the swollen modified PHEMA networks, in tension on an Instron Universal Tester, Model 1122 at room temperature. A strain rate of 0.1/min was used. Tensile stress was related to the initial cross-sectional area of the sample. Differential scanning calorimetry of these hydrogel samples was carried out on a DuPont DSC 1000 Thermal Analysis Unit at a heating rate of 10°C/min.

Dynamic mechanical analysis of rectangular-shaped samples of both water swollen and dry hydrogels were tested in the bending mode on a Polymer Laboratory DMTA Model Mk11 dynamic mechanical analyzer. DMA experimental parameters used were strain value of 4X and frequency of 1 Hz. The samples were heated at a rate of 5°C/min.

In addition to the water-swollen and dry hydrogels tested on this DMA, autoclaved, water-swollen hydrogel samples were tested immediately after autoclaving. This batch of tests was performed to ascertain if the steam-autoclaving dramatically affected the mechanical properties of the hydrogels in their swollen states. Since steam-autoclaving subjects the hydrogels to conditions (temperature greater than 100°C in steam) favorable for hydrolysis of the esters linkages that make up the cross-links, this is a valid concern. Moreover, some hydrogels were tested twice on the DMA to verify reproducibility of the results obtained.

Hydrolysis of the hydrogels involved placing dry disc-shaped samples of the hydrogels in pH buffers 4.0, 7.4, and 10.4 in a water bath held at 37°C. Again, sample mass change with respect to the dry mass was the method used to monitor the effects of the buffers on the samples. Scanning electron microscopy of these samples followed.

In vitro degradation proceded as follows. Three water-swollen disc-shaped samples of each of the hydrogels were steam-autoclaved and then exposed to pond sludge containing active microorganisms. The sludge was raked from the bottom of Duck Pond on the University of Connecticut's campus. This sludge has been assayed and contains such microorganisms as *Cryptococcus laurentii*—a user of PCL carbon as a food source [79]. The intact sludge was used with the hope that it might have contained other microor-

Table 4. A list of modified hydrogel samples and their compositions.

Hydrogel	Description
PHEMA	Cross-linked poly(2-hydroxyethyl methacrylate) 0.5 wt% EDMA (cross-linking agent, ethylene dimethacrylate) 0.1 wt% AIBN (initiator, 2,2′-azobisisobutyronitrile)
PHEMA/PCL 90/10 blend	0.5 wt% EDMA; 0.1 wt% AIBN {wrt HEMA} 10 wt% Poly(caprolactone) {MW ~ 35,000}
PHEMA/PCL-2000-Diol 75/25 blend	0.5 wt% EDMA; 0.1 wt% AIBN {wrt HEMA} 25 wt% PCL-Diol {MW ~ 2,000}
PHEMA-MAC 90-10 copolymer	0.5 wt% EDMA; 0.1 wt% AIBN 10 wt% Maleic acid
PHEMA-MAH 90-10 copolymer	0.5 wt% EDMA; 0.1 wt% AIBN 10 wt% Maleic anhydride

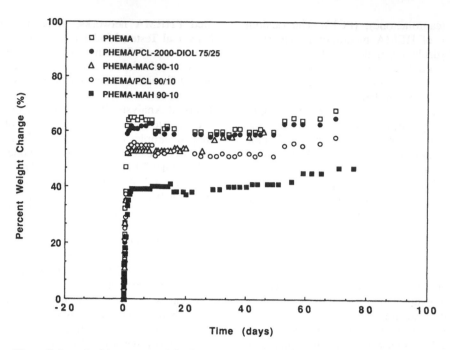

Figure 3. A graph of the percent weight change of the modified PHEMA hydrogel during water absorption. The percent weight changes are calculated with respect to the dry weights of the hydrogels. The legend in the figure identifies the samples.

ganisms yet unknown to us which could successfully use PHEMA as a food source.

Control flasks containing the same pond sludge were steam-autoclaved for twenty minutes to sterilize the sludge and kill all living microorganisms prior to introducing the control samples into the flasks. Both the control flasks and sample flasks were stirred continuously on a mechanical stirrer table at room temperature throughout the duration of the experiment. The control flasks were not disturbed until the end of the experiment, to prevent spurious contamination through handling. As mentioned for the above experimental methods, sample weights were continuously recorded during the experiment. Solution pH and temperatures were not recorded.

After removal of the samples from the flasks, each sample was dried in a vacuum oven at 25°C for 48 hours. These dried samples were then viewed under the scanning electron microscope for changes in structure. Both the controls and the samples were analyzed under the SEM.

Water absorption is one of the first parameters used for comparing hydrogels. The ability to absorb large quantities of water imparts the softness, porosity, and ease of purification characteristics that are much desired for biomedical application. Figure 3 is a plot of the percent weight gained by the modified PHEMA hydrogels while exposed to distilled water at room temperature for approximately seventy-five days. The percent weight changes were calculated with respect to the dry weights of the hydrogel samples.

Several general attributes are noticeable in all the curves in Figure 3. Each sample gained its equilib-

rium weight within the first twenty-four hours of the experiment. In some cases, there was an apparent overshoot in weight change. However, this overshoot is within the error (4 weight-percent) associated with this experimental method even though each weighing of the samples was performed after removal of surface water. This percent error was arrived at by repeating the experiment and comparing results.

The most important aspect about these water absorption curves was the relative positions of the curves to each other, because the percent weight gain was interpreted as the amount of water absorbed by the hydrogel network. The PHEMA-MAH copolymeric sample curve displayed considerably lower equilibrium percent water absorbed—only 40 weight-percent water. Thus, it was obviously different from the other samples in water absorption behavior.

Pure PHEMA absorbed the greatest amount of water, followed by the PHEMA/PCL blend containing low molecular weight PCL. PHEMA-MAC 90-10, and PHEMA/PCL 90/10 networks absorbed slightly less water than PHEMA. These results indicated that the approaches to modifying PHEMA hydrogel by copolymerization with MAC and blending with PCL do not adversely affect the ability of the networks to absorb large amounts of water.

In order to better understand the water absorption behavior of these hydrogels, we determined the coefficient of diffusion of water front into each network during swelling. The water-absorption data from the first twenty-four hours were replotted as shown in Figure 4.

The following is an explanation of the Y-axis of the

Table 5. A list of the equilibrium water absorption and coefficients of diffusion values obtained for the modified PHEMA hydrogels.

Hydrogel	Percent Equilibrium Water Absorption (%)	Coefficient of Diffusion D, (cm² sec⁻¹)
PHEMA	64	1.4×10^{-7}
PHEMA/PCL-2000 75/25	62	7.2×10^{-6}
PHEMA-MAC 90-10	59	9.9×10^{-6}
PHEMA/PCL 90/10	55	1.2×10^{-7}
PHEMA-MAH 90-10	41	4.0×10^{-6}

graph in Figure 4. The sample mass, M_t, is defined as the mass of the sample at time, t, minus its dry weight; or

$$M_t = M - M_i \qquad (2)$$

where

M = the sample mass at time, t, including water absorbed and dry mass

M_i = the mass of the dry sample

M_t = the mass of the water absorbed at time, t. The equilibrium mass of sample is defined as M_∞.

This value is the point beyond which the mass of the sample no longer changes. In our case the equilibrium mass was taken at approximately the thirty-day point in the water absorption experiments.

The following equation [80] was used to calculate the diffusion coefficients using the equation of the lines described above and depicted in Figure 4.

$$D = 0.049/(t/L^2)_{1/2} \qquad (3)$$

where

D = diffusion coefficient in cm²/sec

$(t/L^2)_{1/2}$ = the value of t/L^2 for which M_t/M_∞ is equal to 1/2

t = time in seconds

L = sample thickness in centimeters

Equation (3) is used to determine the diffusion coefficient into a sheet from the initial gradient of the sorption curve. This equation holds as long as this gradient is linear up to $M_t/M_\infty = 1/2$.

The equation of the line obtained from plotting M_t/M_∞ against $(t/L^2)^{1/2}$ was used to calculate the value of (t/L^2) for which M_t/M_∞ is equal to 0.5. The number obtained was then used in Equation (3) to calculate D in cm²/sec. In brief, the slopes of the lines in Figure 4 reflects the relative values of the coefficients of diffusion of the samples, in that a steeper line represents a higher D value.

The PHEMA network displayed the highest value for the coefficients of diffusion of a water front into the networks (see Table 5 for quantitative values of the equilibrium amount of water absorbed by the networks and coefficients of diffusion). The value of 1.4×10^{-7} cm²/sec recorded for PHEMA was close to that of 1.6×10^{-7} cm²/sec reported by Migliaresi et al. [15]. This particular reference was chosen because of the similarity in hydrogel preparation.

The PHEMA/PCL 90/10 blend displayed a surprisingly high coefficient of diffusion compared to the other modified PHEMA hydrogels. On the other hand, the PHEMA-MAH copolymer displayed the lowest coefficient of diffusion of water, indicating that it is considerably more hydrophobic or has less free volume than the other networks. In this aspect, the coefficient of diffusion results for the PHEMA-MAH copolymeric networks parallel those of the equilibrium percent water absorption.

The most surprising observation from these coefficient of diffusion results is that the PHEMA/ PCL-2000-Diol 75/25 blend displayed a coefficient of diffusion value of almost one-half that of the PHEMA network. But, to the contrary, both networks absorbed practically the same equilibrium amount of water (see Figure 4). A direct correlation between the coefficient of diffusion of a water front into these networks and the equilibrium amount of water absorbed is not evident in this case (see Table 5). However, in general, the coefficient of diffusion of water results apparently displayed the differences between these modified PHEMA hydrogels more clearly than the equilibrium percent water absorption results.

The primary motive for preparing these modified PHEMA hydrogels was to improve the mechanical properties of PHEMA hydrogel in the water-swollen state. Therefore, static mechanical analysis of the water-swollen networks was performed on an Instron in order to compare stiffness, ultimate stress and ultimate strain differences. Table 6 lists the ultimate static mechanical properties of these hydrogels.

Table 6. Ultimate static mechanical properties of modified hydrogels.

Hydrogel	Average σ_b (KPa)	Average ϵ_b (%)	Average E (KPa)
PHEMA/PCL 90/10	670	63	2000
PHEMA-MAC 90-10	300	80	570
PHEMA	340	50	780
PHEMA/PCL-2000 75/25	300	83	750
PHEMA-MAH 90-10	200	36	860

Table 7. An explanation of the assignment of the peaks in the DMA thermograms to the structural segments of the hydrogel systems. Figure 5 is a diagram of the PHEMA chain segments.

Segment Type in Motion	Transition Temperatures (°C)	
	Dry Hydrogels	Swollen Hydrogels
Polymer backbone (T_g) (α-peak)	110–120	−4–4
Cross-links (β-peak)	79–98	−24−−34
Pendant side groups (γ-peak)	−78−−74	−99−−84
PCL melt	55–56	55–60
Unassociated water		68–95
Associated water		93–120

From the list in Table 6, one notes that the PHEMA/PCL 90/10 blend exhibited the highest breaking stress and Young's modulus. In contrast, the pure PHEMA-MAC 90-10 copolymeric hydrogel registered the lowest Young's modulus value. However, the lowest ultimate stress was displayed by the PHEMA-MAH 90-10 copolymer. Again, the PHEMA/PCL 90/10 blend exhibited excellent extension with the PHEMA-MAH copolymer showing the lowest percent strain.

The PHEMA/PCL 90/10 blend containing high molecular weight PCL was clearly the most mechanically superior of the hydrogel systems in the swollen states. Although the interaction of this network with water in terms of equilibrium percent water absorbed is noticeably less than that of PHEMA, its coefficient-of-diffusion results and exceptional mechanical properties indicate that this blend retains the hydrogel attributes discussed above. Thus, dynamic mechanical experiments were carried out to better clarify this issue.

Two primary motivations underlay the DMA analysis. First, differential scanning calorimetry analysis of these networks proved to be too insensitive to yield any information about their glass transition temperatures. Secondly, a better understanding of the thermomechanical and dynamic mechanical behavior of these systems is essential for deciding which is the correct network for a particular biomedical application.

The results of dynamic mechanical experiments performed on these modified hydrogels (see Table 7) indicate a significant difference in peak positions between the tan δ spectra of dry and swollen hydrogels. The major, or α peak that was found in the range of 110–121 °C is shifted to the range of −4–4 °C when the samples are water-swollen. The α transition is assigned to that of the glass transition temperature, T_g. This considerable change in the peak position is attributed to the presence of water in the swollen hydrogels. Water plasticizes the hydrogels, but freezes below 0 °C. Thus, the plasticizing effect is not seen until solid water melts in the range of −4–4 °C. In contrast, plasticization of the more hydrophobic PCL component in the blended hydrogels is not evident. These samples display the tan δ peaks associated with

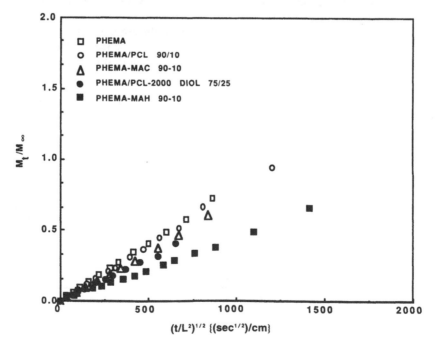

Figure 4. Plots of M_t/M_∞ vs. $(t/L^2)^{1/2}$ used to determine the coefficient of diffusion of the water front into the modified PHEMA hydrogel samples. The legend in the graph explains the lines.

PCL melt in the expected temperature range of 55–60°C.

Other peak shifts are apparent when comparing the DMA tan δ results of the dry and swollen networks. The shoulders of the swollen samples' T_g peaks, or β peaks are transposed to the range of −34−−24°C. Also, small, low temperature γ peaks are displaced from the range of −94−−78°C for the dry hydrogels to the range of −99−−90°C in the plots of the water-swollen networks.

Additional peaks, intermediate in size, are evident in the ranges of 68–94°C and 93–120°C. These new peaks are assigned as followed. The lower temperature peaks in the range of 68–94°C are considered to be tan δ peaks involved with the boiling of unassociated water. Those peaks found in the range of 93–120°C are considered to be generated from the boiling of associated water.

The terminology of associated and unassociated water is explained in terms of the bonding of the water molecules with polar portions of the hydrogel. Associated water is regarded as the water consisting of molecules that are hydrogen-bonded to the polar molecules of the hydrogel. The 2-hydroxyethyl side chain on PHEMA is an example of a polar moiety that can hydrogen bond with water molecules. By contrast, unassociated water is composed of those molecules that do not interact with PHEMA. The term "bulk water" is often used to describe this portion of the water in the swollen hydrogel [27]. Table 7 explains the assignments of the tan peaks discussed above and Figure 5 diagrams these PHEMA chain segments described above.

A recent work by Roorda et al. [28] in which water in PHEMA hydrogel was thermally analyzed using differential thermal analysis (DTA) and adiabatic calorimetry (AC), refuted this concept of different thermodynamic classes of water in hydrogels. They maintained that the condensation of evaporated water on the inside of the sample pans is responsible for the erroneous results and interpretations of dual water phases reported by many researchers. Unfortunately, these effects do not exist in the DMA tests performed on the samples. Moreover, two distinguishable peaks are reproducibly produced in the tan δ spectra of these hydrogel networks.

In addition to characterizing the thermo-mechanical behaviors of these gels, the DMA was used to com-

pare the hydrogels after they were subjected to autoclaving. Table 8 lists the major tan δ peak positions and E' at 37°C of the autoclaved and non-autoclaved swollen hydrogels. The gels displayed minor changes in their DMA response in terms of tan δ peak positions. However, while the PHEMA/PCL 90/10 blend showed a sharp drop in E' at 37°C after autoclaving, the other blend, PHEMA/PCL-2000-Diol 75/25 underwent a great deal of embrittlement. Cleavage of the cross-links is believed to be responsible for some of these changes in DMA response.

We have discussed water absorption and diffusion, as well as the thermo-mechanical and dynamic mechanical behaviors of these hydrogel systems. The remainder of this section addresses the results obtained from exposure of these networks to different buffers at 37°C and exposure to active pond sludge, to determine hydrolysis and in vitro degradation responses, respectively.

The hydrogel samples were exposed to pH buffers 4, 7.4, and 10.4, then dried at 25°C for 100 hours. Then they were rinsed in 1 μM HCl solution and redried under vacuum for 211 hours. Rinsing with dilute HCl was done to replace the buffer acid groups that may have conjugated with the bases produced by chain scission at the ester linkages. Hydrogen ions from HCl should exchange for these acid groups.

Almost none of the gels experienced weight loss beyond the percent error of 4% for this experimental method. Only the PHEMA-MAH 90-10 sample exposed to pH 10.4 buffer experienced significant weight loss. An 11% weight loss is recorded for this sample after exposure to HCl. Apparently the MAH rings in the backbone of this copolymer open in high-pH buffer, making it capable of accepting cations. The HCl rinsing step provided H⁺ ions that exchange for the buffer cations.

Figures 6–8 are photomicrographs of some of the hydrolysis samples. In Figure 6, one sees a photo of the surface of the PHEMA-MAH 90-10 sample exposed to pH 10.4. Tiny, deep holes are visible on this sample surface. Figure 7 is a photo of the PHEMA hydrolysis sample exposed to pH 4.0. This type of unetched surface is seen for all the PHEMA samples as well as the PHEMA-MAH 90-10 samples exposed to the other buffer solutions. Basically, it is concluded that these samples did not undergo significant hydrolysis.

Table 8. DMA tan δ peaks and E' at 37°C of the autoclaved and unautoclaved swollen modified PHEMA hydrogels.

Autoclaved & (Non-Autoclaved) Swollen Hydrogel	α-peak (°C)	β-peak (°C)	E' at 37°C (KPa)
PHEMA	0 (−2)	−27 (−32)	750 (631)
PHEMA-MAC 90-10	0 (−1)	−25 (−25)	750 (724)
PHEMA-MAH 90-10	−2 (−4)	−28 (−34)	944 (955)
PHEMA/PCL 90/10	4 (1)		1060 (1440)
PHEMA/PCL-2000 75/25	6 (4)		1780 (1350)

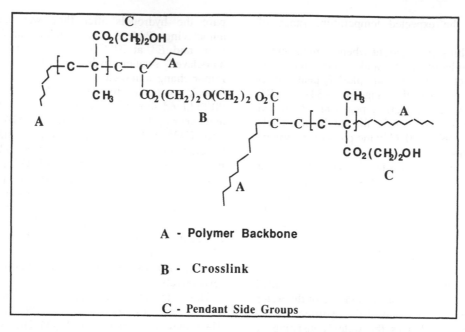

Figure 5. A schematic diagram of PHEMA polymer chain to assist in explaining the assignment of the peaks in the DMA thermograms to the structural segments of the hydrogel network.

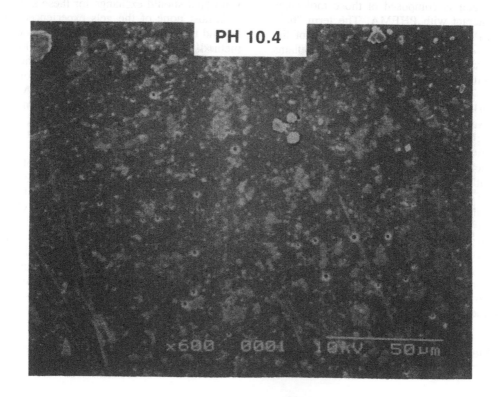

Figure 6. SEM photomicrograph of PHEMA-MAH 90-10 hydrolysis samples (pH buffer 10.4).

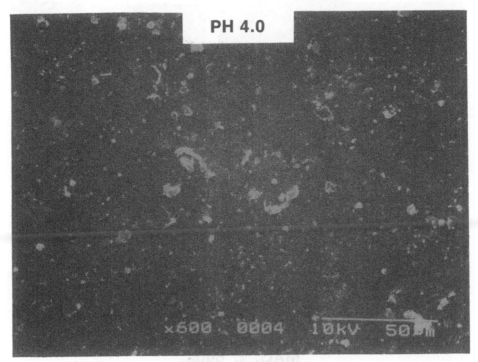

MAG. = 600X

Figure 7. SEM photomicrograph of PHEMA hydrolysis samples (pH buffer 4.0).

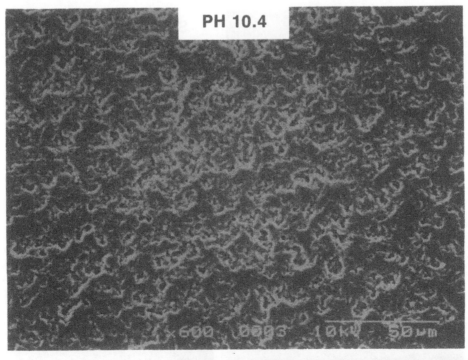

MAG. = 600X

Figure 8. SEM photomicrograph of PHEMA/PCL-2000 Diol 75/25 hydrolysis samples (pH buffer 10.4).

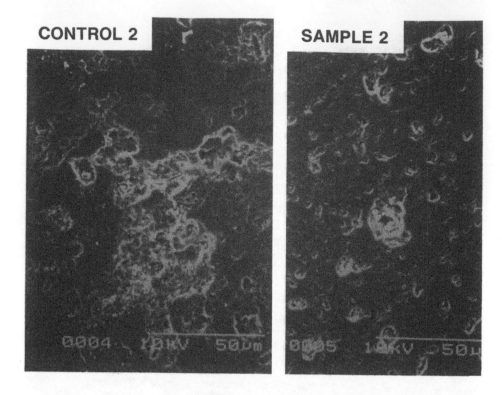

CONTROL 2

SAMPLE 2

MAG. = 600X

Figure 9. SEM twin photomicrograph of a PHEMA-MAH 90-10 degradation sample (on right) and its control (on left).

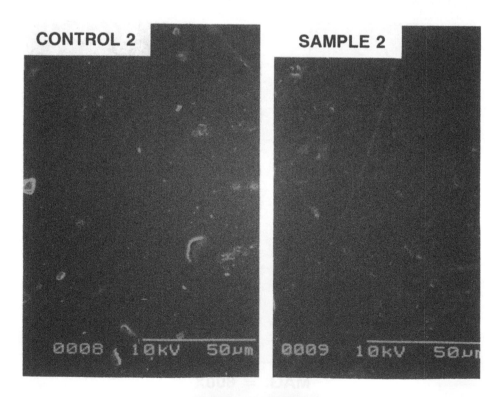

CONTROL 2

SAMPLE 2

MAG. = 600X

Figure 10. SEM twin photomicrograph of a PHEMA degradation sample (on right) and its respective control (on left).

The PHEMA/PCL-2000-Diol 75/25 hydrolysis sample shown in Figure 8 was exposed to pH 10.4 buffer. Significant surface irregularity, accompanied by voids, is evident. Although this type of surface irregularity is typical of incompatible polymer blends, the presence of voids is not. Also, these voids are considerably more larger than those seen in Figure 6.

A similar situation is seen in the photomicrographs of the degradation samples and controls. In fact, Figure 9 is a twin SEM photomicrograph of one of the PHEMA-MAH 90-10 samples and its corresponding control. On the left, one sees a picture of the sample at a magnification of $600 \times$ with the picture of the control on the right. Holes are evident in both photos, but a greater quantity is seen in the picture of the degradation sample. Also, these holes are deeper than the ones in the picture of the control. The samples of this particular hydrogel became more and more difficult to handle towards the end of the experiment because of their fragility.

In contrast, Figure 10 is a photomicrograph similar to that in Figure 9, but for a PHEMA degradation sample and control. Voids on the scale of those seen in Figure 9 are not present. It can be concluded that degradation of PHEMA hydrogel by pond sludge microorganisms did not occur.

Another set of photomicrographs are presented in Figure 11. This set is of a PHEMA/PCL-2000-Diol 75/25 hydrogel degradation sample and control. A similar situation to that seen in the PHEMA-MAH hydrogel degradation sample and control is noted, but the topographies of the eroded sample and control surfaces are different. The voids are of a much smaller size and are more numerous. Also, on the left in the photo of the sample, two surface layers of the sample are evident. A great deal of the top layer has not yet been completely eroded. This type of erosion is typical of enzymatic degradation. In contrast, the uniform surface erosion seen in the photo of the control is typical of non-specific hydrolysis.

These results for PHEMA/PCL-2000-Diol 75/25 are expected since the active pond sludge contains *Cryptococcus laurentii*—a known user of PCL carbon as a food source [79] by means of hydrolysis. Moreover, *Cryptococcus laurentii* is capable of utilizing the lower molecular weight PCL faster than the higher molecular weight PCL. Recall that the difference in molecular weights between the two PCLs is considerable. The PCL-diol has a molecular weight of 2000 while the high molecular weight PCL has a molecular weight of 35,000 [81]. The sample blend containing lower molecular weight PCL is degraded at a slightly faster weight.

The photomicrographs of the other hydrogels are as follows. The photomicrograph of PHEMA/PCL 90/10 is similar to that of PHEMA/PCL-2000-Diol 75/25. That of PHEMA-MAC 90-10 is like the photomicrograph of PHEMA. From the SEM pictures, two types of behaviors are noted. Either both the sample and control surfaces are smooth, or both are pitted. This observation can be explained by simultaneous hydrolysis and enzymatic degradation. The networks more susceptible to hydrolysis are easier to degrade and a correlation can be drawn between the results reported in Figures 6–8 and Figures 9–11.

First, in comparing the PHEMA-MAH 90-10 hydrolysis (Figure 6) and degradation (Figure 9) photomicrographs, one notes a similarity in the types of voids present. This is also true for the PHEMA/PCL-2000-Diol 75/25 hydrolysis (Figure 7) and degradation samples (Figure 11). In contrast, both sets of photos of PHEMA hydrogel samples are unpitted and assumed to be more resistant to hydrolysis as well as degradation.

Because of the interesting properties of the PHEMA/PCL blends, we looked more in-depth into this type of modification of PHEMA hydrogel. The following section describes our work on blends containing PHEMA and high molecular weight PCL.

POLY(2-HYDROXYETHYL METHACRYLATE)/ POLY(CAPROLACTONE) BLENDS

The results of the work on the modified PHEMA hydrogels indicated that blending linear high molecular weight PCL into PHEMA represents an elegant way of improving the strength of the swollen PHEMA hydrogel without sacrificing the excellent properties of PHEMA. Some of these properties are high water content, softness, and ease of purification after processing to remove low molecular weight impurities. Such impurities can elicit strong tissue reaction that may hinder favorable tissue–implant interaction. With this in mind, a series of PHEMA/PCL blends were prepared covering the concentration range of 0–25 weight-percent PCL (MW ~ 35,000) in cross-linked PHEMA.

Hydrogels of the PHEMA/PCL blends are compared to that of pure PHEMA with the following analysis methods: water absorption, differential scanning calorimetry (DSC); static mechanical analysis, scanning electron microscopy (SEM), peformed concurrently with extraction of the linear component with ethyl acetate; and dynamic mechanical analysis, (DMA).

PCL (MW ~ 35,000) was dissolved in HEMA monomer at 60°C. After allowing the solution to cool, 0.5 weight-percent EDMA and 0.1 weight-percent AIBN were added. The percent initiator and cross-linking agent were calculated with respect to HEMA. Hydrogel preparation is described in the previous section. Table 9 lists the blends prepared from these materials and their specifications.

Pure PHEMA hydrogel is a transparent material in both the swollen and dry states; however, the networks containing PCL are opaque. Figure 12 depicts this contrast. On the right is a sample of pure hydrogel. A sample of PHEMA/PCL 90/10 (90 wt% PHEMA and 10 wt% PCL) is on the left. The inability of the

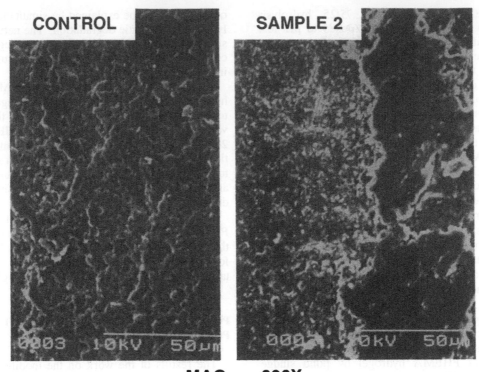

MAG. = 600X

Figure 11. SEM twin photomicrograph of a PHEMA/PCL-2000 Diol 75/25 degradation sample (on right) and its control (on left).

latter to transmit light suggests that its components are phase-separated. Swollen networks are soft and rubbery, but the dry networks prove to be harder and brittler.

Figure 13 shows the results of the water absorption experiments. The equilibrium percent water absorbed and the normalized equilibrium percent water absorbed are featured in the plot. The normalized values are ratios of the equilibrium percent water absorbed to the weight fraction PHEMA in each network. Both

curves fall off with increasing weight percent PCL. The plot shows that the blends retain less water in the swollen state than PHEMA hydrogel itself, at least for PCL concentrations higher than 10 weight-percent.

Figure 14 contains DSC thermograms of the networks along with those of cross-linked pure PHEMA and linear PCL. The thermogram of pure PHEMA is at the top of the figure with that of pure PCL at the bottom. Most of the blends lack the second order transition observed in the pure component's thermo-

Table 9. A list of PHEMA/PCL blends and their descriptions.

Hydrogel	Description
PHEMA	Cross-linked poly(2-hydroxyethyl methacrylate) 0.5 wt% EDMA (cross-linking agent, ethylene dimethacrylate) 0.1 wt% AIBN (initiator, 2,2′-azobisisobutyronitrile)
PHEMA/PCL 95/5 blend	0.5 wt% EDMA; 0.1 wt% AIBN {wrt HEMA} 5 wt% Poly(caprolactone) {MW ~ 35,000}
PHEMA/PCL 90/10 blend	0.5 wt% EDMA; 0.1 wt% AIBN {wrt HEMA} 10 wt% Poly(caprolactone) {MW ~ 35,000}
PHEMA/PCL 85/15 blend	0.5 wt% EDMA; 0.1 wt% AIBN {wrt HEMA} 15 wt% Poly(caprolactone) {MW ~ 35,000}
PHEMA/PCL 80/20 blend	0.5 wt% EDMA; 0.1 wt% AIBN {wrt HEMA} 20 wt% Poly(caprolactone) {MW ~ 35,000}
PHEMA/PCL 75/25 blend	0.5 wt% EDMA; 0.1 wt% AIBN {wrt HEMA} 25 wt% Poly(caprolactone) {MW ~ 35,000}

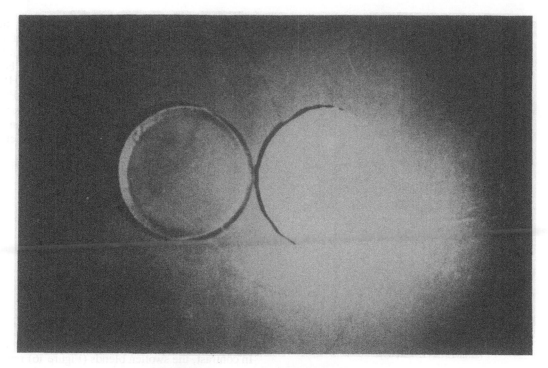

PHEMA   **PHEMA/PCL 90/10**

Figure 12. A photograph of pure PHEMA on the left and PHEMA/PCL 90/10 blend on the right. Pure PHEMA is transparent but the blend is opaque, a result of phase separation of the components.

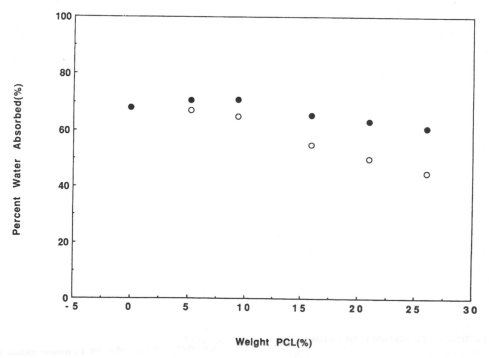

Figure 13. Equilibrium and normalized equilibrium percent water absorbed by the networks. (●) are data of the equilibrium percent water absorbed and (○) are the normalized values. The normalized equilibrium percent water absorbed values are calculated by dividing the equilibrium percent water absorbed by the weight percent PHEMA of the network.

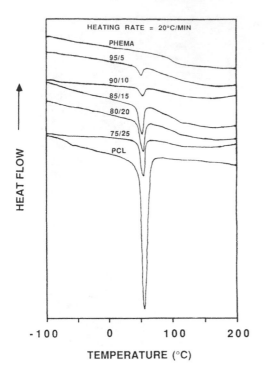

Figure 14. DSC thermograms of blends and components. Heating rate was 20°C/min. (Sample mass = 10.0 ± 0.5 mg; second heating recorded under nitrogen atmosphere.)

grams. However, there are some indications of second order transitions in a few of the thermograms. For example, the thermogram of PHEMA/PCL 90/10 displays such a transition at about −70°C. This transition appears to be the expected glass transition of PCL reported at −62°C. Also, the PHEMA/PCL 80/20 thermogram shows another second order transition near 110°C, which reflects the glass transition of PHEMA. Absence of second order transitions could mean that the sensitivity of the DSC may be taxed with regards to these transitions.

PCL melt peaks (~57°C) are apparent in all but the pure PHEMA thermogram. The size of the peak increases steadily with the percentage of PCL without significantly shifting position. PCL melt peak size reflects the percent PCL in these blends.

A look at the average breaking stress of the dry networks reveals a decrease as more PCL inclusions are added (Figure 15). The term "inclusions" is used for reasons evident in the SEM morphology study discussed below. This general trend in Figure 15 agrees with the theories and data presented by Danusso and Tieghi [81]. They show that the mechanical stress to fracture decreases with increasing filler content in rigid matrix particulate composites. Dry cross-linked PHEMA behaves as a rigid matrix and PCL appears as particulates in these networks.

The authors evaluated models and data from several sources covering cases of adhesion and non-adhesion between the matrix and its inclusions. In summary, non-adhesion composites exhibit a steady decrease in

breaking stress with increase volume-percent inclusions, as is evident in Figure 15. In the case of adhesion, first a decrease is noted followed by a minimum and an increase [81]. In contrast, PCL spheres behave as points of stress concentration in the brittle PHEMA matrix. The ultimate stress falls off as more PCL is added to the system. Comparing these results to the predictions of the Nicolais-Narkis equation [82] reveals a more acute loss of strength than predicted by theory.

The Nicolais-Narkis equation is:

$$\frac{\sigma_c}{\sigma_P} = (1 - 1.21\ V_f^{2/3}) \qquad (4)$$

where

σ_c is the strength of the composite
σ_P is the strength of the particulates
V_f is the filler content

The line in Figure 15 is a plot of the Equation (4) for the case of PCL particulates in a dry PHEMA matrix.

In contrast, the swollen blends (Figure 16) reveal an increase in fracture stress with increase in volume-percent PCL. This increase in strength suggests that interfacial adhesion exists between PCL inclusions and the swollen PHEMA network. Otherwise, the breaking stress would decrease with more PCL as shown in Figure 15. Allen et al. [83–86] and Hourston and his colleagues [87,88] found that tensile strength increases with the amount of the linear phase in their blends. In addition, Janáček [47] reported a four-fold increase in the tensile strength of swollen PHEMA reinforced with 0.194 volume-fraction SiO_2. Physical interaction between the components is a likely factor in such systems and has not been ruled out in these PHEMA/PCL networks. With this in mind, covalent chemical bonding between PCL and PHEMA was investigated.

Chemical grafting between the components was considered as a possible reason for the increase in strength noted in the swollen state. A PHEMA/PCL 90/10 blend network was extracted with ethyl acetate in a Soxhlet extractor to test this hypothesis. The extracted sample lost 8 percent of its weight and contained spherical voids when viewed under the SEM. Also, a color change accompanied extraction. The sample changed from an opaque off-white color to pristine white. This latter white color results from the presence of micropores within the sample.

Figure 17 shows SEM photomicrographs of unextracted and extracted networks. Note the micropores in the bottom photograph of the extracted network. They represent sites once occupied by ethyl acetate soluble PCL. Thus, the PCL phase exists mostly as inclusions in the cross-linked PHEMA matrix. Covalent bonding between PCL and PHEMA is apparently not a factor. The increase in ultimate tensile strength seen in the swollen networks occurs without chemical grafting between PCL and PHEMA.

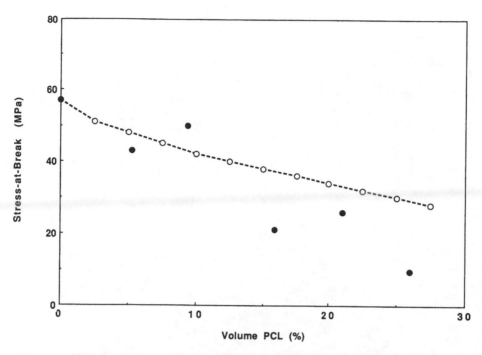

Figure 15. Average stress-at-break of dry networks. Note the decrease in fracture stress as volume PCL increases. (●) are data points for the fracture stress of the dry PHEMA/PCL networks. The line with -○- represents a plot of the Nicolais-Narkis equation, which predicts the strength of our particulate reinforced composites with brittle matrix. The decrease for these blends is greater than predicted by theory.

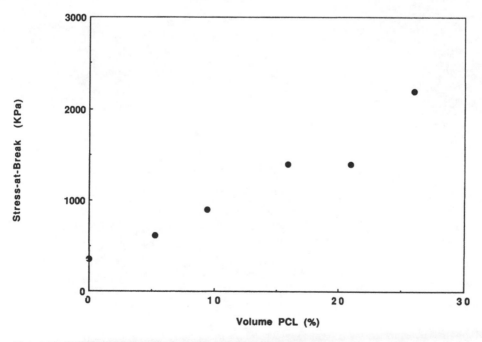

Figure 16. Average stress-at-break of swollen networks. Note the increase in fracture stress with volume PCL in comparison to Figure 15.

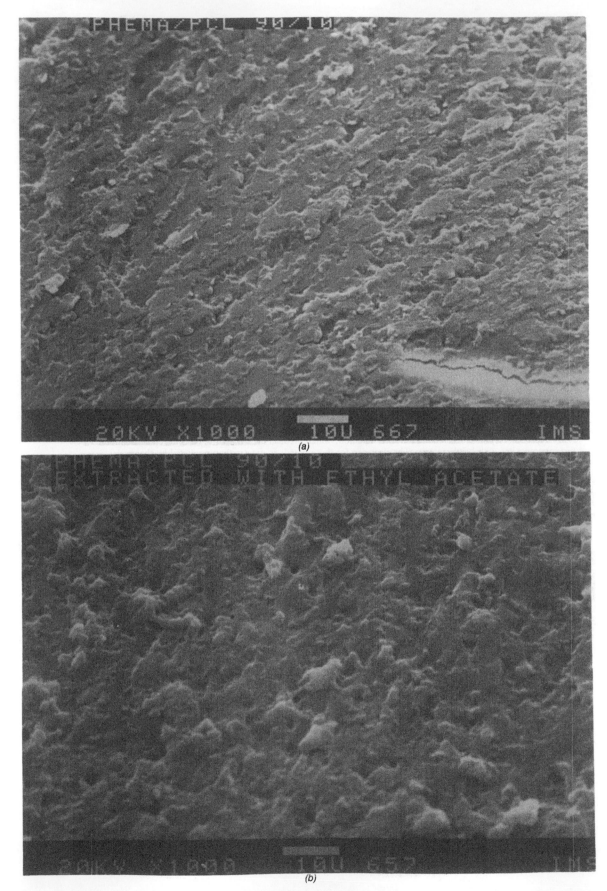

Figure 17. SEM photomicrographs of a PHEMA/PCL 90/10 blend. The top photograph is of an unextracted sample, while the bottom picture is of a sample extracted with ethyl acetate. Note the voids in the bottom photomicrograph that are not in the top one. These voids represent sites occupied by PCL before extraction.

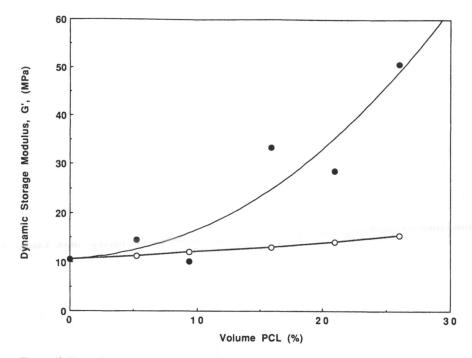

Figure 18. Dynamic storage modulus of swollen networks at 36°C (●) -○- forms a line representing a plot of the Mooney equation which predicts the increase in shear modulus for our particulate reinforced composites with rubbery matrix. The increase seen for the blends is considerably more than predicted by theory.

DMA storage modulus results revealed an increase in G' with percent PCL for the swollen networks. No change in G' of the dry networks was expected. Figure 18 is a plot of the storage moduli of the swollen networks recorded at 37°C. A greater increase is noted when the data are compared to predictions of the shear modulus from the Mooney equation [89].

The Mooney equation is:

$$\ln G/G_1 = k_E\nu_2/(1 - \nu_2/\nu_m) \qquad (5)$$

where

G and G_1 are the shear moduli of the filled and unfilled polymer, respectively

ν_m is the maximum packing faction ($=0.74$ for hexagonal close packing and 0.524 for simple cubic packing, etc.)

k_E is the Einstein coefficient ($=2.5$ for dispersed spheres)

The dashed line in Figure 18 is a plot of Equation (5) for our networks in the swollen state.

Nicolais et al. [45] studied the ultimate tensile properties of swollen PHEMA hydrogel filled with glass beads. They found an initial decrease in tensile modulus with increasing filler content followed by an increase at higher filler concentrations. In an earlier work, Ilavsky et al. [44] studied SiO_2-filled PHEMA hydrogel. They observed an increase in the elastic modulus which they attributed to restriction of PHEMA chain mobility because of physical interac-

tions between SiO_2 and the hydrogel. In our case, the size of the PCL inclusions are between 2–10 μm in diameter (see voids in bottom picture of Figure 17). This filler size may be comparable to that of the SiO_2 inclusions. Surface interactions between PHEMA and PCL may play a role because of the large PCL surface area, and could lead to chain mobility restriction. This, in turn, can result in the large increase noted in the fracture stress of the swollen networks.

CONCLUSION

PHEMA hydrogel is modified using two techniques aimed at maintaining high water absorption capability. The first method involves copolymerization with small amounts of maleic acid (MAC) and maleic anhydride (MAH). Secondly, blends of cross-linked PHEMA and linear poly(caprolactone) (PCL) of different molecular weights are prepared. Although it has poorer water absorption capability, the copolymeric hydrogel containing MAH showed faster degradation and hydrolysis compared to PHEMA. Blends of linear PCL in cross-linked water swollen PHEMA displayed unusual improvement in ultimate tensile strength without chemical grafting between the components. The opposite trend is noted for the dry networks tested under similar conditions. Equilibrium swelling analysis indicates that the PHEMA component retains its high water content characteristic in the presence of PCL. Since end-use of these biomaterials will be in the water-swollen state, these results are encouraging. Thus, important mechanical properties are improved without loss of necessary biocompatible aspects.

ACKNOWLEDGEMENTS

Support for our research by U. S. Army Contract DAAG29-85-K-0222 is gratefully acknowledged. P. Davis also thanks the National Research Council's Ford Foundation Predoctoral Fellowships for Minorities Program for financial support. A research grant from Aeritalia made possible the work performed at the University of Naples by the primary author. We gratefully thank Professor Silvana Saiello for her help in taking the SEM photomicrographs.

REFERENCES

1. Wichterle, O. and D. Lim. 1960. *Nature*, 185:117.
2. Ratner, B. 1981. *Biocompatibility of Clinical Implant Materials*. D. Williams, ed. Boca Raton, FL: CRC Press, Ch. 7.
3. Hoffman, A. S. 1975. *Polymers in Medicine and Surgery*. R. Kronenthal, et al., eds. New York: Plenum Press, Vol. 8.
4. Tollar, M. et al. 1969. *J. Biomed. Mater. Res.*, 3:305.
5. Kliment, K. et al. 1968. *J. Biomed. Mater. Res.* 2:237.
6. Refojo, M. 1969. *J. Biomed. Mater. Res.*, 3:333.
7. Majkus, V. et. al. 1969. *J. Biomed. Mater. Res.*, 3:443.
8. Kocvara, S. et. al. 1967. *J. Biomed. Mater. Res.*, 1:325.
9. Ratner, B. and A. Hoffman. 1976. *Hydrogels for Medical and Related Applications*. J. Andrade, ed. Washington, DC:ACS, Ch. 1.
10. Davis, P. et al. 1988. *J. Bio. Comp. Polym.*, 3:205.
11. Bruck, S. 1973. *J. Biomed. Mater. Res.*, 7:387.
12. Refojo, M., H. Yasuda. 1965. *J. Appl. Polym. Sci.*, 9:2425.
13. Migliaresi, C. et al. 1981. *J. Biomed. Mater. Res.*, 15:307.
14. Peppas, N. et al. 1985. *J. Biomed. Mater. Res.*, 19:397.
15. Refojo, M. 1965. *J. Appl. Polym. Sci.*, 9:3417.
16. Migliaresi, C. et al. 1984. *Polymer*, 25:686.
17. Moynihan, H. et al. 1986. *Polym. Eng. Sci.*, 26:1180.
18. Refojo, M. 1967. *J. Appl. Polym. Sci.*, A1, 9:3417.
19. Ratner, B. and I. Miller. 1973. *J. Biomed. Mater. Res.*, 7:353.
20. Spacik, P. and M. Kubin. 1973. *J. Biomed. Mater. Res.*, 7:201.
21. Drobnik, J. et al. 1974. *J. Biomed. Mater. Res.*, 8:45.
22. Korsmeyer, R. et al. 1986. *J. Polym. Sci., Polym. Phys. Ed.*, 24:409.
23. Dusek, K. 1969. *Collec. Czech. Chem. Commun.*, 34:3309.
24. Bahar, I. et al. 1987. *Macromolecules*, 20:1353.
25. Carfagna, C. et al. 1983. *Polymers in Medicine I*, E. Chielini and P. Giusti, eds. New York: Plenum Press., pp. 311.
26. Kumakura, M. et al. 1983. *Eur. Polym. J.*, 19:621.
27. Jhon, M. and J. Andrade. 1973. *J. Biomed. Mater. Res.*, 7:509.
28. Roorda, W. et al. 1988. *Biomaterials*, 9:494.
29. Brynda, E. et al. 1985. *J. Biomed. Mater. Res.*, 19:1169.
30. Stol, M. et al. 1988. *Biomaterials*, 9:273.
31. Cifkova, I. et al. 1988. *Biomaterials*, 9:372.
32. Horak, D. et al. 1986. *Biomaterials*, 7:467.
33. Barr-Howell, B. and N. Peppas. 1987. *Eur. Polym. J.*, 23:591.
34. Janacek, J. and J. Hasa. 1966. *Collec. Czech. Chem. Commun.*, 31:2186.
35. Hasa, J., J. Janacek. 1967. *J. Polym. Sci., Part C.*, 16:317.
36. Hasa, J., M. Ilavsky. 1969. *Collec. Czech. Chem. Commun.*, 34:2189.
37. Ilavsky, M., J. Hasa. 1969. *Collec. Czech. Chem. Commun.*, 34:2199.
38. Janacek, J. and J. Ferry. 1970. *Rheologica Acta*, 9:208.
39. Janacek, J. and J. Ferry. 1969. *Macromolecules*, 2:370.
40. Janacek, J. and J. Ferry. 1969. *Macromolecules*, 2:379.
41. Ilavsky, M. et al. 1967. *J. Appl. Polym. Sci., Part C*, 16:329.
42. Ilavsky, M. et al. 1968. *Collec. Czech. Chem. Commun.*, 33:3197.
43. Janacek, J. and J. Kolarik. 1967. *J. Appl. Polym. Sci., Part C*, 16:279.
44. Ilavsky, M. et al. 1972. *Intern J. Polym. Mater.*, 1:187.
45. Nicolais, L. et al. 1975. *Polym. Eng. Sci.*, 15:35.
46. Acierno, D. et al. 1975. *J. Polym. Sci., Polym. Phys. Ed.*, 13:703.
47. Janacek, J., 1973. *J. Macromol. Sci. Rev. Macromol. Chem.*, C9(1):1.
48. Barvic, M. et al. 1971. *J. Biomed. Mater. Res.*, 5:225.
49. Sprincl, L. et al. 1971. *J. Biomed. Mater. Res.*, 4:447.
50. Sprincl, L. et al. 1973. *J. Biomed. Mater. Res.*, 7:123.
51. Imai, Y., E. Masuhara. 1982. *J. Biomed. Mater. Res.*, 16:609.
52. Rubin, R. and J. Marshall. 1975. *J. Biomed. Mater. Res.*, 9:375.
53. Korbelar, P. et al. 1988. *J. Biomed. Mater. Res.*, 22:751.
54. Brynda, E. et al. 1978. *J. Biomed. Mater. Res.*, 12:15.
55. Shimada, M. et al. 1983. *Eur. Polym. J.*, 19:929.
56. Okano, T. et al. 1986. *J. Biomed. Mater. Res.*, 20:919.
57. Okano, T. et al. 1986. *J. Biomed. Mater. Res.*, 20:1035.
58. Lyndon, M. 1986. *Br. Polym. J.*, 18:22.
59. Seifert, L. and R. Greer. 1985. *J. Biomed. Mater. Res.*, 19:1043.
60. Kamei, S., et al. 1986. *Colloid Polym. Sci.*, 264:743.
61. Hogt, A. et al. 1986. *J. Biomed. Mater. Res.*, 20:533.
62. Bowers, R. and B. Tighe. 1987. *Biomaterials*, 8:83.
63. Bowers, R. and B. Tighe. 1987. *Biomaterials*, 8:172.
64. Bowers, R. and B. Tighe. 1987. *Biomaterials*, 8:89.
65. Gobel, R. et al. 1987. *Biomaterials*, 8:285.
66. Payne, M. and T. Horbett. 1987. *J. Biomed. Mater. Res.*, 21:843.

67. Horbett, T. and M. Schway. 1988. *J. Biomed. Mater. Res.*, 22:763.

68. Maruyama, A. et al. 1988. *Biomaterials*, 9:471.

69. Lentz, A. et al. 1985. *J. Biomed. Mater. Res.*, 19:1101.

70. Brynda, E. et al. 1987. *Biomaterials*, 8:57.

71. McAuslan, B. and G. Johnson. 1987. *J. Biomed. Mater. Res.*, 21:921.

72. Smetana, Jr., K. et al. 1987. *J. Biomed. Mater. Res.*, 21:1247.

73. Horak, D. et al. 1986. *Biomaterials*, 7:188.

74. Horak, D. et al. 1986. *Biomaterials*, 7:467.

75. Horak, D. et al. 1988. *Biomaterials*, 9:367.

76. Michnevic, I., K. Kliment. 1971. *J. Biomed. Mater. Res.*, 5:17.

77. Yoshida, M. et al. 1987. *Biomaterials*, 8:124.

78. Ronca, D. et al. 1987. *Min. Ort. Traum.*, 38:807.

79. Jarrett, P. et al. 1984. *Polymers as Biomaterials*. S. W. Shalaby et al., eds. New York: Plenum Press, p. 181.

80. Crank, J. 1975. *The Mathematics of Diffusion, 2nd Ed.* Oxford: Clarendon Press.

81. Danusso, F. and G. Tieghi. 1986. *Polymer*, 27:1385.

82. Nicolais, L. and M. Narkis. 1971. *Polym. Eng. Sci.*, 11:194.

83. Allen, G. et al. 1973. *Polymer*, 14:597.

84. Allen, G. et al. 1973. *Polymer*, 14:604.

85. Allen, G. et al. 1974. *Polymer*, 15:19.

86. Allen, G. et al. 1974. *Polymer*, 15:28.

87. Hourston, D. J. and Y. Zia. 1984. *J. Appl. Polym. Sci.*, 29:2951.

88. Hourston, D. J. and Y. Zia. 1984. *J. Appl. Polym. Sci.*, 29:2963.

89. Sheldon, R. 1982. *Composite Polymeric Materials*. New York: Applied Science Publ.

23

Cellular Immune-Reactivity to Synthetic Materials Used in Vascular Prostheses: *In vivo* Studies in Rats

YVES MAROIS*
YAHYE MERHI*,1
RAYNALD ROY*
MICHEL MAROIS*
CHARLES J. DOILLON*
ROBERT GUIDOIN*,2

ABSTRACT: The immunogenicity and biocompatibility of biomaterials used as blood vessel conduits were assessed by the quantification of blood T lymphocyte subsets (T helper and T suppressor cells), using a cytofluorometric technique and by light microscope observation. One cm² disc of grafts made from woven polyester (Dacron®), expanded polytetrafluoroethylene (ePTFE), and woven polyester whose luminal surface was coated with a tetrafluoroethylene plasma, were implanted in the peritoneal cavities of rats. Animals were sacrificed at 1, 2 and 6 weeks post-implantation. At 1 week, the percentage of T helper cells and T suppressor cells in the woven polyester and ePTFE groups were significantly lower than in the control group (wounded rats). Moreover, the ratio T helper/T suppressor cells at 1 week was found to be higher in the woven polyester ($p = 0.04$) and in the ePTFE group ($p = 0.03$) when compared to the ratio of the control group. At 2 and 6 weeks, no difference in the percentage of T cell subsets was observed for all groups. Pathological examination showed a severe inflammatory reaction to woven polyester grafts and plasma TFE polyester grafts, while a moderate reaction to ePTFE grafts was observed.

INTRODUCTION

The implantation of any biomaterial triggers a cascade of events at the interface and in the vicinity of the implant, events which determine the biocompatibility fate of the graft. The primary response involved is an acute inflammatory reaction at the implantation site. White blood cells migrate to and are then activated at the implantation site. This invasion is controlled by various chemotactic factors [1]. The macrophage is mainly involved in the inflammatory response by interacting with the implant and by releasing secretory products which leads to the formation of a fibrous capsule. Furthermore, the appearance of foreign body giant cells (cellular differentiation of monocytes/macrophages) corresponds to a parameter of chronic inflammation [2].

The immunological response to vascular grafts has not been extensively investigated, and there is a need to further understand the cellular reactivity to different biomaterials and to determine their degree of biocompatibility. Most studies have relied on morphologic observations of the inflammatory reaction to biomaterials [3,4] or using a hollow implant system [5,6,15]. A secondary T cellular immune reactivity towards Dacron® and PTFE [8], and Interleukin 1 (IL-1) production *in vitro* by monocytes towards biomedical polymers [9] were also demonstrated. Recently, we have investigated the cellular immune mobilization after the intraperitoneal implantation of albumin-coated vascular grafts in mice [10].

In order to better assess the biocompatibility of the synthetic materials used in vascular grafts and the mobilization of the immune system towards implants, T cell subpopulations (T helper and T suppressor cells) were quantified by cytofluorometry after three different biomaterials used in the construction of vascular prostheses were implanted in the peritoneal cavities of rats.

MATERIALS AND METHODS

Graft Selection

Three types of materials used in vascular prostheses were investigated: the Reinforced Gore-tex® (W. L.

1Current Address: Laboratoire de Pathologie Expérimentale, Institut de Cardiologie de Montréal, Montréal, Canada.

2Correspondence: Dr. Robert Guidoin, Ph.D., Biomaterials Institute, Room Fl-304, St-François d'Assise Hospital, 10 de l'Espinay, Quebec City, QC GlL 3L5, Canada.

*Faculté de Médecine, Université Laval, Institut des Biomatériaux, Hôpital St-François d'Assise et Unité de Recherche Inflammation, Immunologie et Rhumatologie, Centre Hospitalier de l'Université Laval, Québec City, Canada

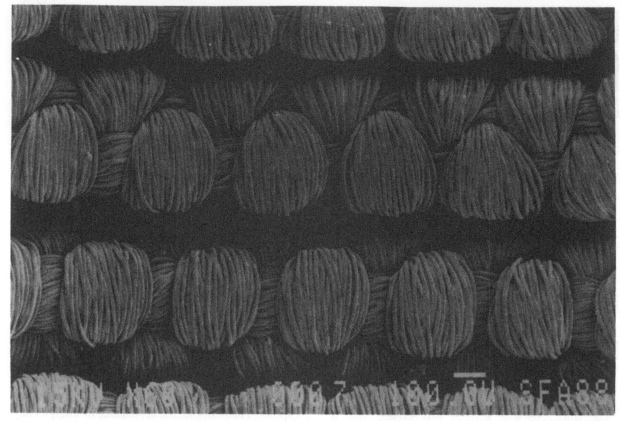

Figure 1. Woven DeBakey (Dacron®) prosthesis: in a 1/1 plain weave structure made of texturized yarns, each one incorporating 108 filaments. The inside and outside present the same morphology (×60).

Gore and Associates, Flagstaff, AZ, U.S.A.), an expanded polytetrafluoroethylene (ePTFE); the Woven DeBakey (Bard Cardiosurgery Division, C. R. Bard Inc, Billerica, MA, U.S.A.), a woven polyester; and the Atrium Plasma TFE (Atrium Medical Corp., Hollis, NH, U.S.A.), a woven polyester whose luminal surface is treated with a tetrafluoroethylene plasma.

- The Woven DeBakey (Figure 1) and the Atrium Plasma TFE (Figure 2) were both woven polyesters. However, the filaments were thinner in the case of the Atrium (Table 1). In addition, the Woven DeBakey was crimped while the Atrium Plasma TFE was not, but it was supported by an external helically-wound polypropylene monofilament. The luminal surface of the Atrium Plasma TFE was coated with a plasma of tetrafluoroethylene which modifies the surface properties. Thus, the body fluids and tissues were more likely to be in direct contact with fluoroethylene than the polyester.
- The Gore-tex® graft (Figure 3) was an expanded tetrafluoroethylene in which the nodes were at a 30 micron distance and were interconnected with microfibrils. The fibrils were oriented along the longitudinal axis of the

graft, while the nodes were perpendicular to the graft axis. The graft was externally reinforced by a thin layer of expanded PTFE of low porosity. The wall thickness was 0.64 mm. The prosthesis was manufactured from pure PTFE resin which was preformed and then extruded into thin wall tubes under high pressure. After extrusion, the tubes were modified into a highly microporous structure by a novel mechanical stretching process. The material was then sintered (i.e., heated and fused above its melting temperature) in order to obtain a permanent and stable structure.

Animal Experimentation

Male Sprague Dawley rats, weighing 175–200 g (Charles River Inc., St. Constant, Quebec, Canada) were divided into 4 groups: 1 control group and 3 experimental groups. Four rats were evaluated in each group at three different follow-up periods. For the experimental groups, the different grafts were cut into small 1 cm² discs, sterilized by gamma radiation (2,5 Mrad). Each disc was inserted into the peritoneal cavity of each rat by means of a trocar 12.5 cm long and 0.4 cm diameter in a sterile environment. In the control group, the rats were submitted to a surgical

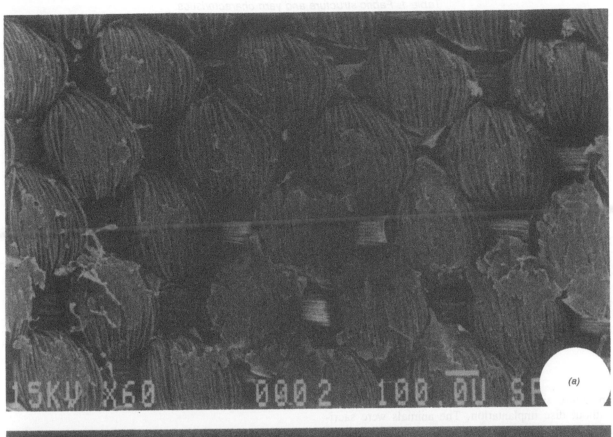

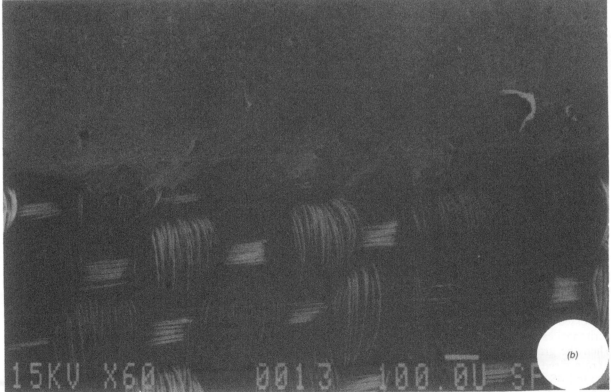

Figure 2. Atrium Plasma TFE prosthesis: in a 1/1 plain weave and noncrimped. The flow surface is coated with a plasma TFE [(a): ×60] and the external side is supported by a helically wound polypropylene monofilament (arrow) [(b): ×60].

Table 1. Fabric structure and yarn characteristics.

	Atrium Plasma TFE	Woven DeBakey
Manufacturer	Atrium Medical Corporation	Bard Cardiosurgery
Type	Woven	Woven
Fabric construction	1/1 plain weave	1/1 plain weave
Thickness (mm)	0.30*	0.25
Porosity %	58.4	64
Mass per unit area (g/m²)	172*	165
Woven fabric count (ends/cm, picks/cm)	46/43	56/34
Type of multifilament yarn (warp/weft)	texturized/flat	texturized
Nominal linear density (dtex)	180/112	180
Approximative filament count	216/96	108
Filaments diameter (microns)	9.0 ± 0.7/ 10.6 ± 0.3	12.5

*Without support

procedure similar to the one described above, but without disc implantation. The animals were sacrificed at 1, 2 and 6 weeks post-implantation.

Indirect Immunofluorescence

Heparinized blood was collected at 1,2 and 6 weeks post-implantation and leukocytes were obtained by centrifugation on a Ficoll-Hypaque gradient. Suspensions of lymphocytes (1×10^6 cells/ml) were incubated with a murine anti-rat monoclonal antibody T helper specificity (Cedarlane, Hornby, Ontario, Canada) and anti-T suppressor specificity (Ingram & Bell, Don Mill, Ontario, Canada) for 30 min at 4°C. After washing, the binding of monoclonal antibodies was detected with a fluoresceinated goat anti-mouse antibody (Coulter, Miami, FL, U.S.A.). After several washes, cells were quantified with an EPICS C flow cytometer at 488 nm (Coulter Electronics Inc., Miami, FL, U.S.A.).

Pathological Evaluation

At the time of sacrifice, all grafts were retrieved and processed for pathological investigations. Briefly, the peritoneal cavity of the rat was opened longitudinally. Then the graft and the tissue surrounding the graft were excised and fixed by a 2% glutaraldehyde solution in PBS. Five micron sections in paraffin were cut and stained with Hematoxylin-Eosin and Masson's Trichrome. The inflammatory reaction, the presence of foreign body giant cells and the fibrotic tissue were blind-graded.

Statistical Analysis

The results of cytofluorometry were expressed as mean percentage (S.D.) and the experimental groups were compared to the control group by a one-way analysis of variance (Anova test). In the control group and the experimental groups, each result was the mean of four rats. A probability level of more than 0.05 was considered statistically insignificant.

RESULTS

Cytofluorometric Study

Blood total T cell population was similar for all groups. At 1 week post-implantation, the percentages of T helper cells of either the woven polyester (Dacron®) group [59.5 (1.0); $p = 0.028$] or ePTFE group [60.0 (1.0); $p = 0.034$] were significantly lower than that found in the control group. The percentages of T suppressor cells of either the ePTFE group [26.7 (2.5); $p = 0.004$], woven polyester (Dacron®) group [24.5 (4.2); $p = 0.003$] or Atrium Plasma TFE [31.5 (2.4); $p = 0.04$] were statistically lower than in the control group. At 2 and 6 weeks, the percentages of T helper and T suppressor cells of the three experimental groups were not significantly different from the control group (Table 2).

At 1 week, the ratio of T helper to T suppressor cells in either the ePTFE group [2.2 (0.3); $p = 0.044$] or the woven polyester (Dacron®) group [2.5 (0.4); $p = 0.031$] were significantly higher than the ratio in

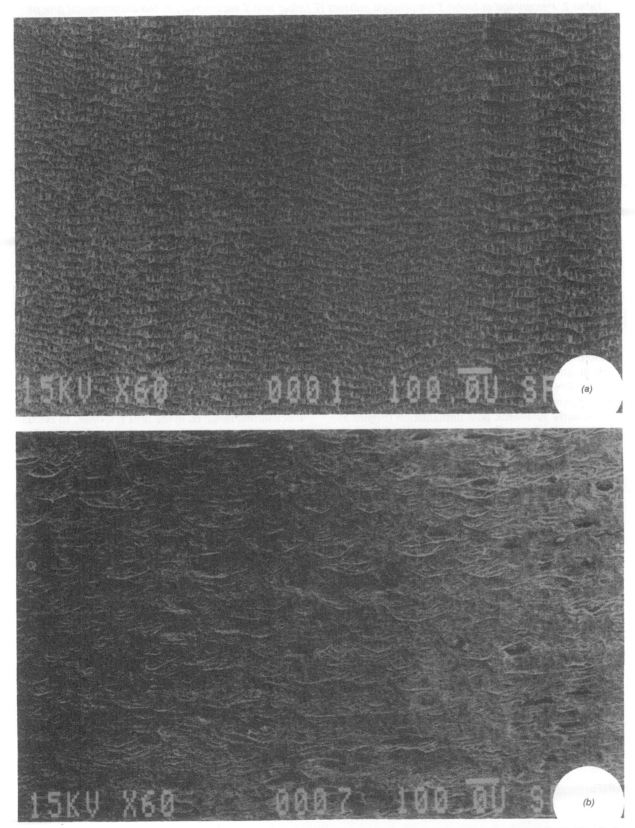

Figure 3. Gore-tex prosthesis: internal surface. It is composed of Teflon nodules at a 30 micron distance and interconnected with microfibrils [(a): ×60]. It is externally reinforced by a thin layer of expanded PTFE of low porosity [(b): ×60].

Table 2. Percentage of blood T lymphocyte subsets (T helper and T suppressor) in the experimental groups determined by cytoimmunofluorescence at 1, 2 and 6 weeks post-implantation.

Experimental Groups	1 Week		2 Weeks		6 Weeks	
	T Help.	T Supp.	T Help.	T Supp.	T Help.	T Supp.
Control	67.0 (5.1)	35.8 (2.2)	63.3 (9.1)	33.7 (22.0)	55.0 (11.8)	23.0 (6.3)
ePTFE	60.0 (1.0) ($p = 0.034$)	26.7 (2.5) ($p = 0.004$)	53.5 (9.7)	31.0 (2.9)	49.0 (1.8)	27.8 (4.2)
Woven polyester (Dacron®)	59.5 (1.0) ($p = 0.028$)	24.5 (4.2) ($p = 0.003$)	60.3 (3.8)	28.0 (5.9)	45.8 (6.6)	20.0 (4.3)
Atrium Plasma TFE	62.8 (8.5)	31.5 (2.4) ($p = 0.04$)	63.5 (4.7)	22.5 (5.1)	45.0 (6.2)	19.7 (5.5)

All results mean (SD) of 4 animals.

the control group [1.9 (0.1)]. At 2 and 6 weeks post-implantation, the ratios found for the three experimental groups were similar to the ratio in the control group (Figure 4).

Pathological Investigations

Table 3 summarizes the pathological reaction of each prosthesis implanted for 1,2 and 6 weeks. The woven polyester (Dacron®) group was identified as the group promoting the most severe inflammatory reaction as early as 1 week post-implantation (Figure 5). Foreign body giant cells were observed and the presence of collagen increased gradually. In the Atrium Plasma TFE group, the inflammatory reaction was close to the one observed in the Dacron group. In the ePTFE group, a slight inflammatory reaction was detected in the first two weeks of implantation. At 6 weeks, the reaction revealed the presence of numerous foreign body giant cells surrounding the ePTFE graft (Figure 6).

DISCUSSION

Inflammatory and immunological reactions are complex mechanisms, where lymphocytes and monocytes/ macrophages are extensively involved in secreting mediators such as macrophage inhibitor factor (MIF), macrophage activating factor (MAF) and IL-1. These reactions are probably observed in contact with biomaterials.

Immunological studies of vascular grafts are mandatory in order to assess the biocompatibility and the mechanisms involved in the host response. In evaluating the biocompatibility, a majority of studies have relied on morphologic observations in describing inflammatory reaction at the implant interface [3–5]. A hollow implant system of different constructions permits investigation of the cell behaviour towards biomaterials [6,7,14,15]. Cavallini et al. [8] observed a cellular-immune reaction in patients receiving Dacron and PTFE vascular prostheses. In addition, Miller and Anderson [9] reported the synthesis of IL-1 by hu-

Table 3. Tissue reaction to different materials observed in the experimental groups at 1, 2 and 6 weeks post-implantation.

Experimental Groups	Duration of Implantation	Acute Inflammatory Reaction	Foreign Body Giant Cells	Collagen
Woven polyester (Dacron®)	1 week	+ + +	+ +	+
	2 weeks	+ +	+ + +	+ +
	6 weeks	+ +	+ + +	+ + +
Atrium Plasma TFE	1 week	+ + +	+	+
	2 weeks	+ +	+ +	+ +
	6 weeks	+	+ + +	+ +
ePTFE	1 week	+ +	+ +	+
	2 weeks	+ +	+ + +	+
	6 weeks	+	+ + +	+ +

−: Absent.
+: Discrete.
+ +: Moderate.
+ + +: Severe.

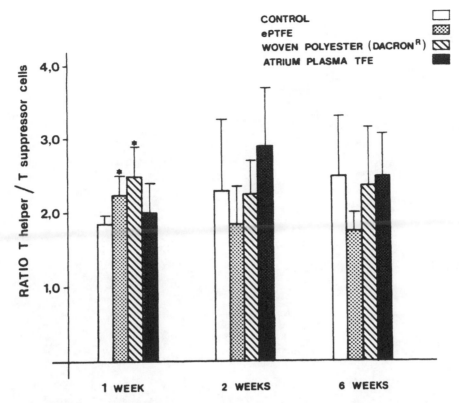

Figure 4. Ratio of blood T helper/T suppressor cells from animals where either a woven polyester (Dacron®), ePTFE or Atrium Plasma TFE grafts have been implanted at 1, 2 and 6 weeks post-implantation. At 1 week, Dacron® and ePTFE groups are statistically (*) different from the control group. Control group corresponds to animals operated on but without implanted grafts.

man monocytes/macrophages in contact with vascular materials. Recently, we have proposed to quantify T cell subsets as a valuable index of biocompatibility for albumin-coated vascular prostheses [10].

In the present investigation, the implantation of synthetic biomaterials used in vascular prostheses results in a decrease in T helper and T suppressor cells at 1 week. The decrease in T helper and T suppressor cells may be compensated for by an increase in T cytotoxic or killer cells towards the biomaterials, because the total blood T cells is similar for all the experimental groups. On the other hand, the mobilization of T cell subsets to either the immune organs or towards the implants can be suggested. T cell subpopulations in each experimental group returned to the control values at 2 and 6 weeks. However, the foreign materials are not so extensively infiltrated by lymphocytes as grafts. This may correspond to the isolation of the implant by a fibrotic capsule.

The ratio of T helper to T suppressor cells of the woven polyester and ePTFE was higher than the control group 1 week after implantation. The high ratio T helper/T suppressor cells observed in this study cannot by itself account for a possible rejection process because extensive lymphocyte infiltration was not observed in histology as in the case of allografts [21,22].

Polyester (Dacron®) is acknowledged as an *inert* biomaterial [16]. However, such a statement should be revised because observations of intense inflammatory reactions are not uncommon [3,17,18]. This study suggests a cellular immunological reaction induced by this biomaterial. Dacron and PTFE seem to modulate T cell subpopulations shortly after implantation (1 week) as shown by the high ratio of T helper/T suppressor cells observed. In patients, Cavallini et al. [8] have shown specific reactivation of T cells and mononuclear cells when exposed to Dacron and/or PTFE antigens. They concluded that a stronger cellular immune response occurs towards Dacron than ePTFE vascular substitutes. The study of the IL-1 production by human monocytes in reaction to biomaterials has shown a high reactivity for Dacron and an intermediate one for PTFE [9]. However, the question of the immunological reaction induced by expanded PTFE vascular graft is not clear. Some investigators have demonstrated a normal foreign body reaction composed of macrophages and foreign body giant cells at the periadventitial interface of the graft [15,19] as we have observed. On the other hand, others claim that ePTFE grafts elicit no foreign body reaction [3]. The comparison between the tissue reaction to polyester graft Dacron® and that to Atrium suggests that the coating of TFE plasma reduced the inflamma-

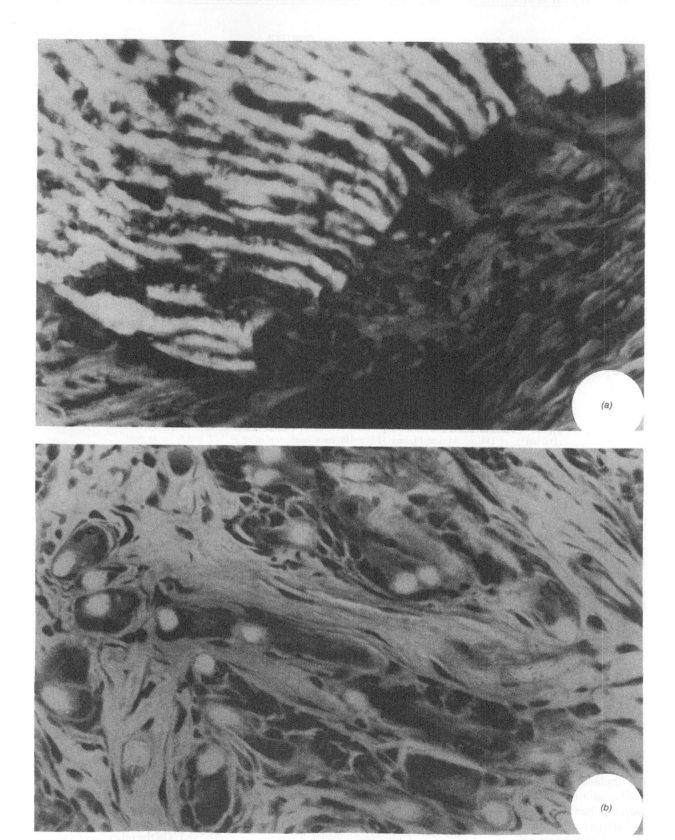

Figure 5. Woven polyester (Dacron®) implants at 1 week [(a): ×400] and 6 weeks [(b): ×400]. The inflammation is intense at 1 week with foreign body giant cells surrounding the polyester fibers. At 6 weeks, the foreign body reaction (giant cells) is severe and still present within a collagenous fibrous tissue.

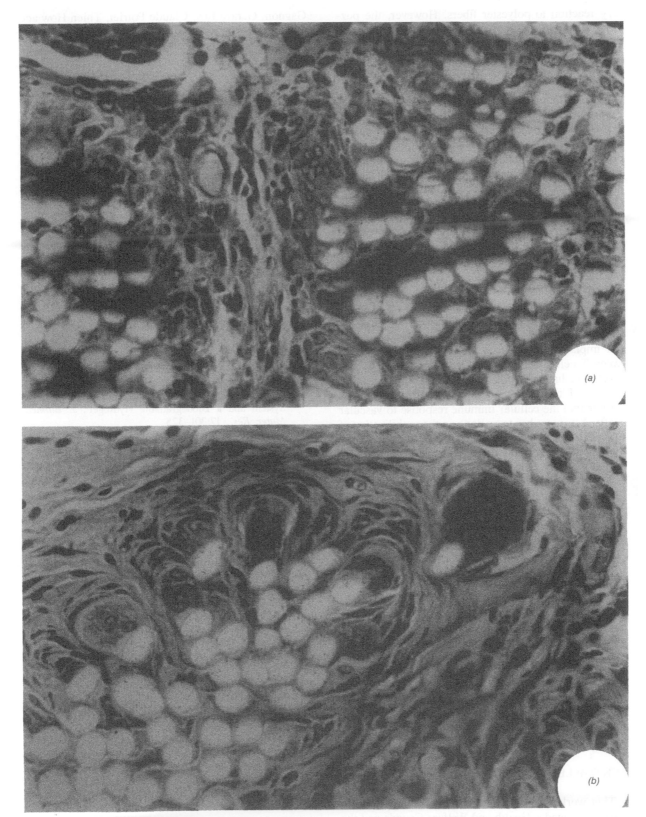

Figure 6. Tissue reaction after implantation of ePTFE [(a): ×400] and Atrium plasma TFE [(b): ×400] grafts in the peritoneal cavity of rats for 6 weeks. Numerous foreign body giant cells are present around the materials. In (a), inflammatory reaction is observed while in (b) a fibrous tissue is formed around the materials.

tory reaction to polyester fibers. However, the puzzling results of the *in vivo* implantations in dogs and analysis of surgically excised grafts in patients may suggest that other factors or cellular reactions are involved. The question therefore remains unanswered [23,24].

Cellular immune reactivity should be considered as a parameter of biocompatibility and could partially explain the graft failures observed with these synthetic materials when used as small-diameter vascular prosthesis. The inflammatory cells surrounding the site of implantation promote the production of coagulation factors which can affect the fate of these grafts. Other secretory factors released by activated cells can directly influence the formation of a stenotic fibrous capsule. An intense inflammatory reaction at the anastomoses could lead to neointimal fibrous hyperplasia [20]. However, in medium- and large-diameter vascular conduits, tissue reaction could be minimized by high blood flow.

It is becoming increasingly clear, as a result of recent immunological research on biomaterials, that the acute inflammatory reaction following foreign material implantation involves intimate relationships between T cell subpopulations, inflammatory cells and several mediators of inflammation. The quantification of blood T cell subpopulations has helped us to look further into the cellular immune response to vascular grafts. Yet, more has to be done on the mobilization of immune cells and the secretory products released by these cells at the implant site. Indeed, blood samples may not totally reflect the local reaction to biomaterials. The role of lymphokines and monokines released by inflammatory cells as a marker of biocompatibility should be further investigated in order to better understand the immunogenic potential of vascular grafts.

CONCLUSION

Cytofluorometric quantification of T cell subpopulations in rats implanted with three different biomaterials used in the construction of vascular grafts has shown some variations in the cellular behaviour of T cell subpopulations. According to previous histopathological studies, the degree of immunogenicity of various graft materials, in decreasing order, was as follows: woven polyester Dacron®, Atrium Plasma TFE and ePTFE.

ACKNOWLEDGEMENTS

This work was supported in part by Supplies and Services Canada, Health and Welfare Canada and the Medical Research Council of Canada. The skillful technical assistance of Simone Lille, Roger De la Durantaye, Karen Horth and Suzanne Bourassa is greatly appreciated. We are indebted to Drs. Denis Gagnon, Gérard Roy, Claude Poirier, Thien How and Paul-Emile Roy for help and guidance.

REFERENCES

1. Ziats, N. P., K. M. Miller and J. M. Anderson. 1988. "*In vitro* and *in vivo* Interactions of Cells with Biomaterials", *Biomaterials*, 9:5–13.
2. Mariano, M. and W. G. Spector. 1974. "The Formation and Properties of Macrophage Polykaryons (Inflammatory Giant Cells)", *J. Pathol.*, 113:1–9.
3. Burkel, W. E. and R. H. Kahn. 1982. "Biocompatibility of Prosthetic Grafts", in *Biologic and Synthetic Vascular Prostheses*. James C. Stanley, ed. New York: Grune & Stratton, pp. 221–247.
4. Woodward, S. C. and T. N. Salthouse. 1986. "The Tissue Response to Implants and Its Evaluation by Light Microscopy", in *Handbook of Biomaterials Evaluation: Scientific, Technical and Clinical Testing of Implant Materials*. A. F. von Recum, ed. New York: Macmillan Publ. Co., pp. 367–378.
5. Salthouse, T. N. 1984. "Some Aspects of Macrophage Behaviour at the Implant Interface", *J. Biomed. Mat. Res.*, 18:395–401.
6. Marchant, R. E., A. Hiltner, C. Hamlin, A. Rabinovitch, R. Slobokin and J. M. Anderson. 1983. "*In vivo* Biocompatibility Studies. 1. The Cage Implant System and a Biodegradable Hydrogel", *J. Biomed. Mater. Res.*, 17:301–325.
7. Marchant, R. E., J. M. Anderson, E. Castillo and A. Hiltner. 1986. "The Effects of an Enhanced Inflammatory Reaction on the Surface Properties of Cast Biomer", *J. Biomed. Mat. Res.*, 20:153–168.
8. Cavallini, G., M. Landredi, M. Lodi, M. Govoni and M. Pampolini. 1987. "Detection and Measurement of a Cellular Immune-Reactivity Towards Polyester and Polytetrafluoroethylene Grafts", *Acta. Chir. Scand.*, 153:179–184.
9. Miller, K. M. and J. M. Anderson. 1988. "Human Monocyte/Macrophage Activation and Interleukin 1 Generation by Biomedical Polymers", *J. Biomed. Mat. Res.*, 22:713–731.
10. Merhi, Y., R. Roy, R. Guidoin, J. Hébert, W. Mourad and S. BenSlimane. 1989. "Cellular Reactions to Polyester Arterial Prostheses Impregnated with Cross-Linked Albumin: *in vivo* Studies in Mice", *Biomaterials*, 10:56–58.
11. Elves, M. W. 1981. "Immunological Aspects of Biomaterials", in *Fundamental Aspects of Biocompatibility, Vol. II*. D. F. Williams, ed. Liverpool, England: CRC Press, p. 159.
12. Mizel, S. B., J. J. Oppenheim and D. L. Rosenstreich. 1978. "Characterization of Lymphocyte-Activating Factor (LAF) Produced by a Macrophage Cell Line, P33D. Biochemical Characterization of LAF Induced by Activated T Cells and LPS", *J. Immunol.*, 120:1504–1512.
13. Lattime, E. C., S. Gillis, C. Davis, O. Stuttman. 1981. "Interleukin 2 Production in the Syngeneic Mixed Lymphocyte Reaction", *Eur. J. Immunol*, 11:67–78.
14. Anderson, J. M., R. E. Marchant, S. Suzuki, K. Phus, C. Hamlin, A. Rabinovitch and A. Hiltner. 1984. "*In*

vivo Biocompatibility Studies. IV. Biomer® and the Acute Inflammatory Response", in *Polyurethanes in Biomedical Engineering*. H. Planck, ed. Amsterdam: Elsevier, p. 143.

15. Eriksson, A. S., L. M. Bjurstein, L. E. Ericson and P. Thomsen. 1988. "Hollow Implants in Soft Tissues Allowing Quantitative Studies of Cells and Fluid at the Implant Interface", *Biomaterials*, 9:86–90.

16. DeBakey, M. E., G. L. Jordan, J. P. Abbott, B. Halpert and R. M. O'Neal. 1965. "The Fate of Dacron Vascular Grafts", *Arch. Surg.*, 89:757–782.

17. Bhuta, I. and R. Dorrouch. 1981. "Non-Infectious Fluid Collection Around Velour Dacron Grafts: Possible Allergic Reaction", *South Med J.*, 74:870–872.

18. Schaffer, C. J. and J. M. Giordiano. 1981. "Reaction to Dacron Velour Bypass Grafts", *Vasc. Surg.*, 15:114–116.

19. Anderson, J. M., K. W. Bennett and J. M. Johnson. 1988. "The Pathology and Healing Responses of Expanded Polytetrafluoroethylene Vascular Access Grafts", in *Vascular Access Surgery, 2nd Edition*. S. E. Wilson, ed., Year Book Medical Publishers Inc., p. 213.

20. DeWeese, J. A. and R. M. Green. 1980. "Anastomotic Neointimal Fibrous Hyperplasia", in *Complications in Vascular Surgery*, V. M. Bernhard and J. A. Towne, eds. New York: Grune and Stratton, pp. 153–165.

21. Tilney, N. L., T. B. Strom and J. W. Kupiec-Weglinski. 1987. "Humoral and Cellular Mechanisms in Acute Allograft Injury", *J. Pediat.*, 111:1000–1003.

22. Mason, D. 1988. "The Roles of T Cell Subpopulations in Allograft Rejection", *Transplant. Proc.*, 20:239–242.

23. Lafrenière-Gagnon, D., R. Guidoin, P. E. Roy, L. Martin, Y. Douville and P. M. Bernard. 1990. "Etude Morphométrique de la Cicatrisation d'une Prothèse Artérielle en Polyester Traitée Avec un Plasma de Fluoroéthylène et Implantée chez le Chien", *Rev. Europ. Tech. Biomed.*, 11:300–309.

24. Guzman, R., D. Lafreniére-Gagnon, N. Chakfe, G. Avril, P. Roy, G. Laroche, P. E. Roy, C. Rouleau, J. F. Girard, Y. Douville, H. P. Noel and R. Guidoin. "Early Experience with the Atrium Plasma TFE Graft: A Clinical and Pathologic Study", (manuscript in preparation).

24

The Atrium Plasma TFE® Arterial Prosthesis: Physical and Chemical Characterization

ROBERT GUIDOIN*,1
MARTIN KING**
MARIE THERRIEN*
ROYSTON PAYNTER†
SOPHIE SIMONEAU*
ELISABETH DEBILLE*
LUC TREMBLAY*
DENIS BOYER*
FRANCIS GILL*

ABSTRACT: The technique of plasma coating emerged in the seventies as a novel and versatile approach to modifying the surface chemistry of a wide range of materials. Chawla developed plasma polymerized silicone coatings and Garfinkle and Hoffman demonstrated that polyester vascular prostheses treated with tetrafluoroethylene plasma yield dramatic improvements in the resistance to thrombus formation and emboli.

Atrium Medical Corporation has produced a Plasma TFE® tubular woven polyester blood conduit, whose internal surface has been treated with fluoropolymer. The absence of crimps and the inclusion of a helically wound external support suggests that this device heralds a new generation of woven polyester vascular prostheses. This study reports the results of an *in vitro* evaluation of this new product.

A unique feature of the Plasma TFE® graft is that it contains texturized yarns in the warp direction and flat multifilament yarns in the weft direction. Such a mixture is not usually found in commercial prostheses, and results in the graft's unique characteristic of expanding at low pressures of less than 50mm Hg, and then exhibiting minimal increases in diameter at internal pressures above 80 mm Hg. Because of the absence of crimps, the elongation of this graft is about half the value for the Woven DeBakey Soft, the least extensible commercial woven control. While the bursting strength is comparable to other woven prostheses, the average water permeability value of 180 ml/cm²/min/120 mm Hg is considerably higher than

the value of 100 quoted in the manufacturer's literature. The suture retention strength results highlight the high frequency of prosthesis rather than the suture breaks and indicate that the suture retention performance can be improved by cutting with a cautery instead of scissors. Surface analysis by ESCA, solvent extraction and differential dyeing demonstrate that the flow surface of the prosthesis contains a non-uniform plasma coating and a high level of extractable contaminants.

INTRODUCTION

The technique of plasma coating emerged in the seventies as a novel and versatile approach to modifying the surface chemistry of a wide range of different materials [1–5]. An abundance of applications has developed [6] in the electronics, metal processing, paper, plastics, textiles and medical products industries where, for example, the technique is used to prepare substrates for liquid crystal displays [7], to reduce corrosion and lubricate metal and plastic surfaces [8], to improve adhesion and printability of paper and plastics [9], to improve the oil and water resistance of textiles [10], to seal membranes and polymer surfaces against leachables [11,12], to insulate neurological electrodes [13,14], and to bond molecules such as heparin [15] and albumin [16,17] to biomaterials so as to improve their blood compatibility [2]. This last application has been described by Chawla, who developed plasma polymerized silicone coatings [18–20], and by Garfinkle and Hoffman [21–24] who demonstrated that polyester vascular prostheses treated with tetrafluoroethylene plasma yield dramatic improvements in the resistance to formation of thrombi and emboli.

Commercialization of this development in the field of arterial prostheses has been undertaken by Atrium Medical Corporation (Hollis, New Hampshire, U.S.A.). It has produced a Plasma TFE® synthetic

¹Correspondence: Dr. Robert Guidoin, Ph.D., Biomaterials Institute, Room Fl-304, St-François d'Assise Hospital, 10 de l'Espinay, Quebec City, QC GIL 3L5, Canada.

* Faculty of Medicine, Laval University and Biomaterials Institute, St-François d'Assise Hospital, Quebec City, Canada
** Clothing and Textiles, University of Manitoba, Winnipeg, Manitoba, Canada
† INRS-Energie, Varennes, Quebec, Canada

artery in which a tubular woven polyester substrate has been surface-treated with fluoropolymer. This novel approach to altering the hemocompatibility of a traditionally highly thrombogenic material has provided Atrium with the opportunity to redesign the form and structure of the woven polyester graft. The absence of crimps and the inclusion of a helically wound external support suggests that this device heralds in a new generation of woven polyester vascular prostheses.

The importance and impact of this development demand a systematic and detailed *in vitro* and *in vivo* evaluation. This paper serves as the first in a series to characterize the properties and performance of this prosthesis. The focus of this chapter is confined to describing the structure, mechanical properties and surface chemistry of the virgin graft. Comparisons will be made with other commerical woven prostheses that are widely used in clinical practice.

THEORETICAL CONSIDERATIONS

Plasma Polymerization

The aim of this technique is to bond a polymer derived from a gaseous "monomer" onto the surface of another material. In this way, the surface properties of the "plasma-polymer" created may be substituted for those of the substrate material. In particular, much research has been directed towards the use of fluorocarbon monomers, since fluorocarbon polymers have desirable low surface energies but cannot be readily graft-polymerized onto other materials. This technique can deposit and chemically bond a uniform, pinhole-free layer of plasma-polymer onto the surface of the substrate. Typical layer thicknesses are in the range of 100–500 Å, although much thicker layers can also be produced.

Apparatus

Various types of reactors have been used for plasma polymerization, some with electrodes mounted inside the chamber, others with electrodes outside. The objective is to couple electrical energy into the gaseous monomer surrounding the substrate. The resulting plasma is comprised of electrons, ions (mostly positively charged), excited molecules, free radicals and ultraviolet photons; it can also produce excited states such as radicals at the substrate surface, through absorption of energetic photons or through energetic particle impact.

Energy is normally supplied from a high-frequency generator and applied to the gas through a pair of plate electrodes (capacitive coupling) or a coil (inductive coupling). The electromagnetic energy reflected from the plasma is monitored and minimized by impedance matching; 13.56 MHz is one of several frequencies available for plasma chemical applications, since it has been authorized for industrial uses other than

communications. The pressure of the gas can be as high as several torr, but 0.2–0.5 torr is the typical working range. The power input is usually between 10 and 100 W, and the time of treatment can vary from seconds to many minutes, depending upon the desired layer thickness.

Polymerization Conditions

The reaction conditions may be characterized by the parameter W/FM, where W = applied power, F = flow rate and M = molecular weight of the gaseous monomer. If the plasma polymerization proceeds in a closed system, the pressure will fall as monomer is consumed. Therefore, one generally uses a steady supply (F) of monomer, while simultaneously removing the gaseous reaction products via a vacuum pump.

Another important variable is the position of the substrate relative to the discharge plates or coil. The reactivity of the gas also has an effect. These factors may combine to produce a highly uniform film strongly bonded to the substrate. Each reactor may be configured differently depending on the size, shape and type of substrate. On account of the large number of variables, each specific application must be investigated and optimized separately.

Polymerization Mechanism

Contrary to conventional free radical polymerization, where one initiates the formation of an orderly chain molecule on a small number of free radical types, plasma polymerization involves the random combination and agglomeration of free radicals. The "polymer" produced is therefore highly cross-linked, and may be considered devoid of any regular repeat unit and structurally unlike any conventional polymer. For example, conventional PTFE is entirely composed of CF_2 repeat units, but the plasma polymer of perfluoroethylene contains CF_3, CF_2, CF, $C-C$ and other functional groups and an overall F/C ratio 2. Unlike the "conventional" route, even saturated molecules, such as C_2F_6, are capable of being polymerized using the plasma technique. What is common to all plasma polymers is that they are highly cross-linked and tend to retain a high residual level of free radicals. The extreme reactivity of the plasma environment provides a means of bonding to virtually any substrate material. However, when the plasma polymer is deposited under conditions leading to high internal stresses, subsequent cracking and peeling of the film may result.

MATERIALS AND METHODS

Graft Selection

Samples of Atrium Plasma TFE® arterial prostheses, as manufactured by Atrium Medical Corporation (Hollis, New Hampshire, U.S.A.), were used in this study. The straight model with 8 mm internal diameter was chosen. It contains a woven polyethylene terephthalate polyester substrate, an external helically-wound polypropylene monofilament support, no crimps, and a surface coating of a tetrafluoroethylene plasma polymer.

Four woven polyester prostheses were selected as the controls. They were the Cooley Low Porosity, Cooley Verisoft (Meadox Medicals Inc., Oakland, New Jersey, U.S.A.), Woven DeBakey Soft (Bard Cardiosurgery Division, C.R. Bard Inc., Billerica, MA, U.S.A.) and Woven Vascutek (Vascutek Ltd., Inchinnan, Scotland, U.K.) grafts. They represent commercial products that are widely accepted and used in clinical practice.

Fabric and Yarn Characteristics

Fabric Structure and Fibre Morphology

The specimens of Atrium Plasma TFE® grafts were exposed to osmium tetroxide vapors and metallized with gold-palladium to improve their conduction and to facilitate observation in a Jeol JSM 35CF scanning electron microscope at a 15 kV accelerating voltage. The control grafts were also examined at the same accelerating voltage.

Porosity

Porosity, which is to be distinguished from water permeability, refers to the proportion of void space or pores within the boundary of a solid material compared to its total volume [25]. Values, usually expressed in percent, can vary theoretically from 0%, for a solid plastic membrane or sheet without pores, to 100% for all air and no solid material. The following equation was used to calculate porosity values, P, for the five prostheses in the study [26].

$$P = 100 \left[1 - \frac{M}{1000 \, hdg} \right]$$

where

M = mass per unit area of prosthesis wall (g/m²)
h = thickness of prosthesis wall (mm)
d_f = density of polyester fibres (g/cm³)

The mass per unit area, thickness and density values were measured using standard methods [25,27,28].

Woven Fabric Count

The tightness of a woven structure is characterized by the frequency of yarns lying in both directions. By viewing the prostheses flattened between glass slides through an optical stereoscopic microscope at 20 times magnification, the number of warp yarns (ends) per cm width and the number of weft yarns (picks) per cm length were counted for each sample.

Filament Diameter

Individual filaments were removed from the prostheses, and the diameter of 20 filaments selected at random from each type of yarn was measured using an optical microscope at 400 times magnification with a micrometer eyepiece previously calibrated against a stage micrometer.

Nominal Linear Density

The size or coarseness of a yarn is measured in units of mass per unit length. The higher the value in decitex (decigrams per kilometer), the thicker or coarser the yarn. Having measured the average filament diameter, D (in μm), and counted the number of filaments in the yarn, n, and assuming the filaments have circular cross section then the yarn's nominal linear density is estimated by:

$$\text{Nominal linear density (dtex)} \cong \frac{ndg\pi}{100} \left[\frac{D}{2} \right]^2$$

These calculated values were confirmed by gravimetric measurements on a known straightened length of yarn exceeding 1 meter, removed from each direction of the prostheses and extended on a crimp tester to remove any residual crimp.

Physical Properties

Water Permeability

This property, often mistakenly referred to as "water porosity" in the medical literature, represents the rate of flow of water through the wall of the dry prosthesis mounted in a flat condition with the crimps removed [29]. Values were obtained following the standard method [27], except that the volume of water that passed through the prosthesis wall under an applied head of pressure (120 mm Hg) was collected and measured for each of the first 5 minutes of the test [25]. An additional series of measurements was performed on the Plasma TFE® prosthesis under applied longitudinal tensions of 100 g, 200 g and 500 g since the manufacturer recommends implanting this prosthesis in a stretched condition. These loads correspond to lengthwise elongations of approximately 5%, 10% and 25% respectively.

Bursting Strength

Measurements of bursting strength were carried out using a Hoffman-Turner probe tester in a compression cell mounted on an Instron Model 1130 tensile tester [27]. Five specimens of each prosthesis were clamped over an 8.1 mm diameter hole using a rubber O-ring measuring 12.6 mm in diameter. A 6.4 mm diameter cylindrical probe with a hemispherical end was forced through each clamped specimen at a constant rate of

100 mm/min. The maximum force was recorded in newtons.

Suture Retention Strength

Suture retention strength measurements of the grafts were also made using an Instron Model 1130 tensile tester with a crosshead speed of 100 mm/min [27,30]. The specimens were cut in the form of a square (15 mm × 15 mm) with one corner bevelled at 45°. Tests were conducted on each specimen at 45°, parallel and perpendicular to the longitudinal axis of the prosthesis. A purpose-built pair of clamps was used to hold each test specimen in the tester and provide a groove to allow a 4-0 stainless steel suture to pass through the wall of the prosthesis exactly 2 mm from the cut edge. The force required to pull the suture from the graft was measured in newtons and averaged over the 5 specimens tested for each prosthesis. Because the Atrium company recommends cutting the Plasma TFE® prosthesis with a hot cautery, two series of suture tearing strength measurement were undertaken, one cutting with the cautery supplied by the manufacturer, the other with scissors.

Dilation

The propensity of the grafts to dilate under static internal pressure was measured by the Optiddiac system [28]. This instrument permits a tubular prosthesis to be mounted over a tubular latex membrane and to be held between two clamps, one of which is fixed and supplies the air pressure, while the other, running on a low-friction track, applies a constant longitudinal tension of 115 g to the specimen. As the air pressure was increased from 0 to 340 mm Hg (0 to 45 kPa) the increase in diameter was measured to the nearest 0.1 mm using a cathetometer. After repeating the test, the average increase in diameter of the graft was calculated at 120 mm Hg (16 kPa), the standard pressure recommended for measuring the internal diameter of vascular prostheses. The whole procedure was repeated with a longitudinal tension of 454 g: this tension approximates the recommended load applied to woven prostheses when measuring the usable length according to the ANSI/AAMI standard method [27].

Elongation

The ability of the grafts to stretch longitudinally was measured using an Instron Model 1130 tensile tester. Five specimens of each tubular graft were clamped and extended by the crosshead moving at a speed of 100 mm/min. Following five preconditioning loading/unloading cycles between 0 and 480 g so as to establish a more stable hysteresis curve, the amount of elongation was recorded for a loading cycle up to 454 g (1 lb). This load approximates that recommended in the standard for measuring the usable length of woven vascular prostheses [27].

Chemical Properties

Surface Chemistry

The prostheses, as received, were cut into coupons for evaluation by X-ray photoelectron spectroscopy, otherwise referred to as XPS or ESCA. The spectra were obtained on an ESCA Lab MK2 made by VG Scientific featuring a Mg Kα beam. The survey scans were recorded to identify the levels of various contaminants. Then, high resolution scans were made of the carbon 1s peak [31].

The carbon 1s peak was resolved into its component peaks: carbon bonded to carbon and hydrogen (C–C); carbon bonded to one oxygen atom (C–O); carbon bonded to two oxygen atoms (O–C=O); and finally carbon bonded to fluorine, which was resolved into CF, CF_2 and CF_3 peaks.

Level of Extractables

The quantification of extractable finishes and contaminants present on the surface of the virgin Atrium and two Cooley prostheses was undertaken using standard procedures established for textile products [32]. Three 2.5 gram specimens of each prosthesis were exposed to a series of multiple quantitative extractions in a Soxhlet apparatus using at least 5 syphoning cycles with each of 5 different solvents. The sequence of solvents in increasing order of polarity was: hexane, 1,1,1-trichloroethane, methanol, water and 0.1N hydrochloric acid. The mass of each extract was determined indirectly by measuring the mass of each dried specimen to the nearest 0.01 mg before and after each extraction. The level of extractables was expressed as a percentage of the mass of the original specimen.

Because initial extraction results suggested that the extractables were not distributed evenly either along the surface of any one Atrium prosthesis or between different prostheses, further extractions were undertaken on small 0.5 g sections cut from three different places along the length of two virgin grafts. The same standard procedure of multiple sequential extractions was used.

In order to assess how much of the extractable material on the virgin Atrium prosthesis was surface soil and aqueous-soluble compounds, an additional duplicate set of extractions was performed on 0.5 g sections cut from adjacent locations along the two grafts. This second series of specimens had been previously cleaned in a solution of sodium bicarbonate at a boil, followed by treatment in sodium hypochlorite bleach solution at room temperature, then rinsed and dried.

Differential Dyeing

In order to assess the distribution and uniformity of the plasma TFE coating on the internal and external surfaces of the Atrium prosthesis, a novel vapour-phase differential dyeing technique was used to stain the polyester fibres [33]. Because the dyestuffs used have a negligible affinity for fluorocarbons, it was believed that this technique could provide clear visual evidence of the chemical nature of the prosthetic surfaces, i.e., whether they were 100% fluorocarbon, 100% polyester or a combination of the two.

Specimens of approximately 2 grams were cut from three different locations along the length of two virgin Atrium prostheses. Each specimen was divided into 2 equal parts, one for dyeing as received, the other for dyeing after cleaning in sodium bicarbonate and bleach as described in the previous section. The specimens together with 100% polyester and fluorocarbon controls were immersed for 5 minutes at room temperature in a dye solution containing 20 g/l Celliton Blue FFR and 20 g/l Celliton Scarlet B disperse dyes (BASF Canada Inc., Montreal, QC). The surface dye was removed by 3 passes through a padder mangle and then the specimens were dried in a hot air oven at 105°C. When dry, the specimens were suspended for 1 minute in an enclosed chamber containing the vapours from boiling a 20/1 mixture of trichloroethylene/ methyl salicylate at 82°C. Any remaining surface dye was removed by rinsing in hot water and scouring with a non-ionic detergent at 50°C for 10 minutes.

The dried specimens were photographed and, following removal of the intensely stained external polypropylene monofilament, the lightness values of their internal and external surfaces were measured on a Hunterlab Tristimulus Colorimeter, Model D25M/L-9 [34]. By operating in a Judd-Hunter Lab scale mode, the L (or lightness) values provided a relative index of the total amount of reflected visible light from each surface on a continuum from theoretically total black (0%) to theoretically pure white (100%). Since the dyes chosen for this experiment selectively stain polyester rather than fluorocarbon surfaces, we believe that the lightness scale we have developed provides a relative quantitative index of the fluorocarbon/polyester character of the prosthetic surface: the higher the lightness value, the less staining and the higher the fluorocarbon content; the lower the lightness value, the more staining and the higher the polyester content. Lightness values were measured on the internal and external surfaces of the dyed 100% fluorocarbon and polyester controls as well as the dyed Atrium grafts before and after cleaning.

RESULTS

Fabric and Yarn Characteristics

The internal and external surfaces of the Atrium Plasma TFE® and the Cooley Low Porosity prostheses are shown in Figures 1, 2, 3 and 4, respectively. The identical 1/1 plain woven fabric construction is self evident. It is common to all five samples. A unique feature of the Plasma TFE® graft is that it contains both texturized and flat multifilament yarns.

Such a mixture of multifilament yarns was not found in any of the four controls (Table 1). Another concern was the level of visible contamination on the internal surface of the Plasma TFE® prosthesis. The extent and concentration of foreign material observed was much higher internally than on the external surface or on the surfaces of any of the four controls.

Details of the fabric structure and yarn characteristics are listed in Table 1. Although the Plasma TFE® prosthesis has an almost square woven construction (i.e., similar ends/cm to picks/cm), which is different from those of the other prostheses, in other respects, that is in terms of thickness, mass per unit area, porosity as well as the nominal linear density of the yarns, the Plasma TFE® graft is remarkably similar to those of the Cooley Verisoft, Woven DeBakey Soft and Woven Vascutek devices. (Note that the Cooley Low Porosity prosthesis has a tighter construction than the other four.)

The significant and uniquely different yarn property found with the Plasma TFE® is the fineness of the filaments in both the warp and weft yarns. An average filament diameter of 9 m means that the cross-sectional area of the filaments is so small that about twice the number of filaments are required in the yarn bundle (i.e., 216 compared to 108) in order to achieve a similar yarn linear density and strength as in the four controls.

Water Permeability

The means and standard deviations of the volumes of water collected during the first minute of the test are listed in Table 2. Also, the mean values over the 5 minutes of the test are plotted in Figure 5. These results show that the water permeability of the Plasma TFE® prosthesis when elongated to 5–10% does not decrease much over time, and is similar to that of the Cooley Verisoft and Woven DeBakey Soft grafts. The Cooley Low Porosity and Woven Vascutek have significantly lower values.

The water permeability value of 180 ± 18 ml/cm²/min 120 mm Hg is however considerably higher than the average value of 100 ml/cm²/min 120 mm Hg quoted in the manufacturer's literature accompanying the prosthesis. As can be seen from Table 2, increasing the tension up to 200 g has no influence on the water permeability behaviour. Only above 200 g (e.g., at 500 g) is the water permeability significantly reduced. Note that the Plasma TFE® prosthesis behaves differently when the external support is removed. The results presented in Table 2 clearly demonstrate how the water permeability of the woven textile structure is reduced as the applied longitudinal tension increases.

Bursting Strength

The mean and standard deviations of the bursting strength results are presented in Table 3. They demon-

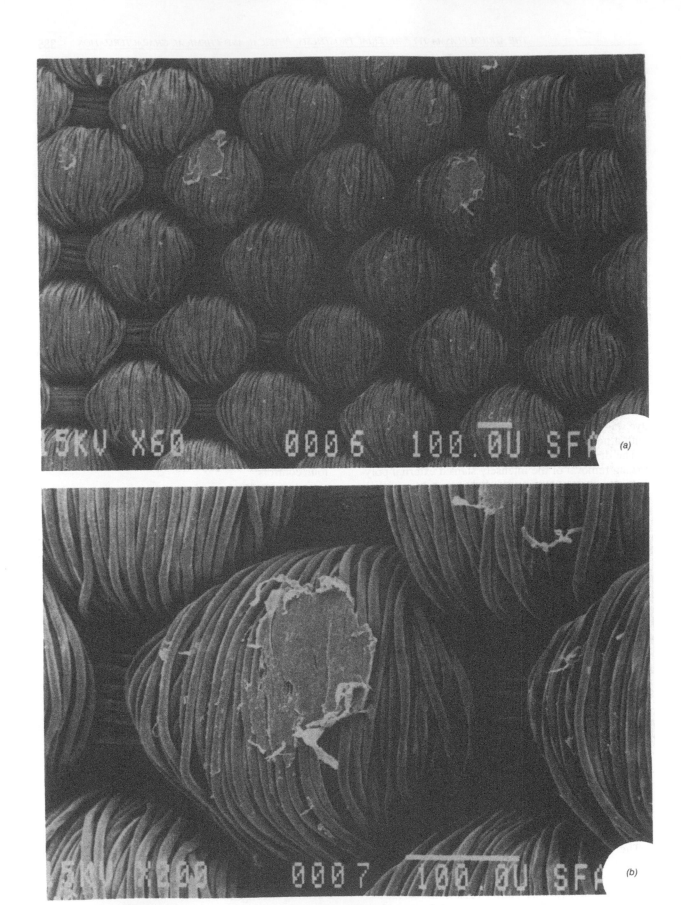

(a)

(b)

Figure 1. SEM photomicrographs of the internal surface of the virgin Atrium Plasma TFE® prosthesis.

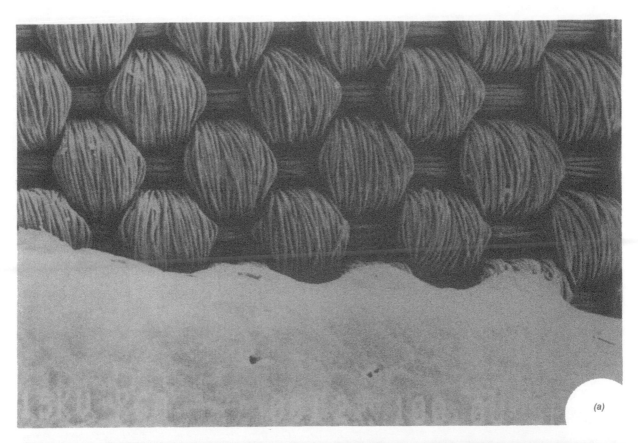

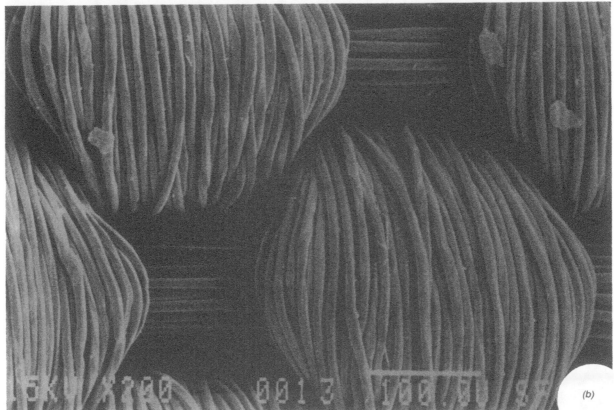

Figure 2. SEM photomicrographs of the external surface of the virgin Atrium Plasma TFE® prosthesis.

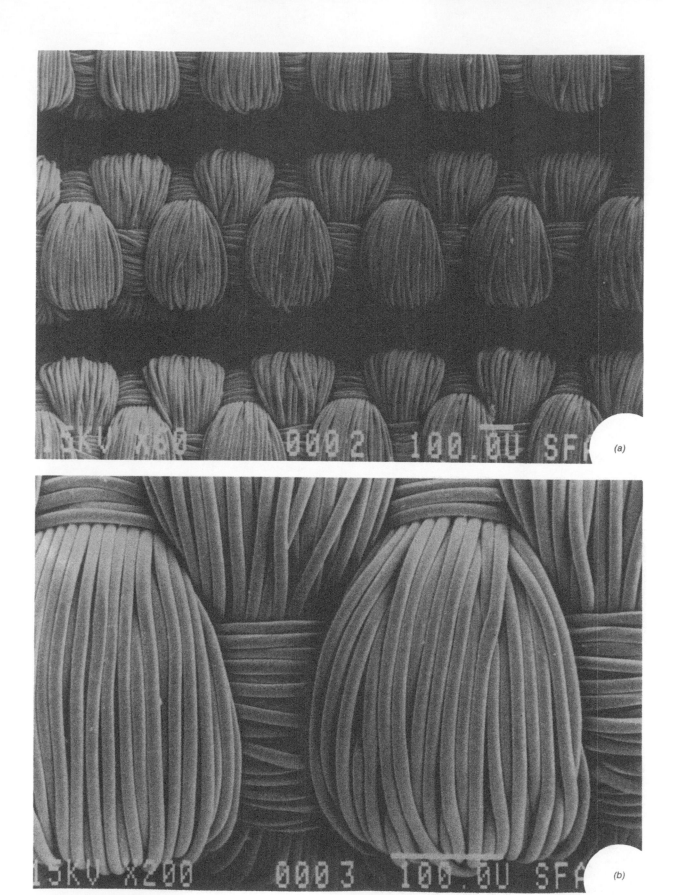

(a)

(b)

Figure 3. SEM photomicrographs of the internal surface of the Cooley Low Porosity prosthesis.

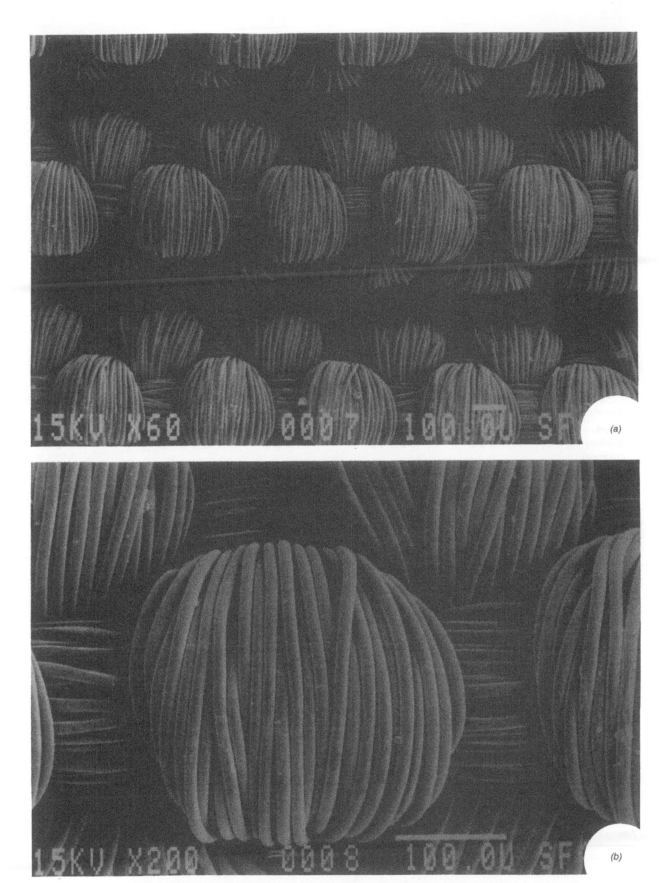

(a)

(b)

Figure 4. SEM photomicrographs of the external surface of the Cooley Low Porosity prosthesis.

Table 1. Fabric structure and yarn characteristics.

	Atrium Plasma TFE	Cooley Low Porosity	Cooley Verisoft	Woven DeBakey Soft	Woven Vascutek
Manufacturer	Atrium Medical Corporation	Meadox Medicals Inc.	Meadox Medicals Inc.	Bard Cardiosurgery	Vascutek
Type	Woven	Woven	Woven	Woven	Woven
Fabric construction	1/1 plain weave	1/1 plain weave	1/1 plain weave	1/1 plain weave	1/1 plain weave
Thickness (mm)	0.30*	0.26	0.27	0.26	0.29
Mass per unit area (g/m^2)	172*	169	152	154	175
Porosity (%)	58.4	52.9	59.2	57.1	56.3
Woven fabric count (ends/cm, picks/cm)	46/43	63/41	58/35	52/32	56/30
Type of multi-filament yarn (warp/weft)	texturized/flat	flat/flat	flat/flat	texturized/ texturized	texturized/ texturized
Nominal linear density (dtex)	180/112	190/100	190/100	170/170	180/90
Approximate filament count	216/96	108/54	108/54	108/108	100/50
Filament diameter (microns)	9.0 ± 0.7/ 10.6 ± 0.3	12.9 ± 0.3/ 13.3 ± 0.6	13.0 ± 0.5/ 13.3 ± 0.5	11.6 ± 1.1/ 12.5 ± 1.2	12.8 ± 1.2/ 13.2 ± 0.5
Delusterant level	semi-dull	semi-dull	semi-dull	bright	semi-dull

*Without support.

Table 2. Water permeability results.

Prosthesis	Applied Tension	Volume of Water Collected during First Minute (ml) Mean ± Standard Deviation	
Atrium Plasma TFE	100 g + 200 g tension	180 ±	18
Cooley Low Porosity	crimps removed	56 ±	6
Cooley Verisoft	crimps removed	181 ±	21
Woven DeBakey Soft	crimps removed	216 ±	38
Woven Vascutek	crimps removed	89 ±	7

Prosthesis	Applied Tension	Mean Volume of Water Collected during First Minute (ml)	
		With Support	Without Support
Atrium Plasma TFE	no tension	182	350
Atrium Plasma TFE	100 g tension	176	206
Atrium Plasma TFE	200 g tension	190	192
Atrium Plasma TFE	500 g tension	50	83

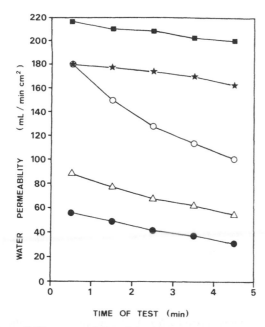

Figure 5. Water permeability of the different prostheses over the 5 minutes of the test (★ Atrium Plasma TFE; ● Cooley Low Porosity; ○ Cooley Verisoft; ■ DeBakey Soft Woven; △ Woven Vascutek.

direction are subdivided into two means and standard deviations (where appropriate) depending on whether it was the prosthesis or suture that broke during the test. The overall mean values for each prosthesis, regardless of the type of failure, have been plotted in Figures 7 and 8.

The mean suture retention strength values from the cautery cut specimens fall in a narrow range between 28.3 and 34.3 N, regardless of the type of prosthesis or the direction of pull, except for the Plasma TFE® prosthesis tested in the perpendicular direction. Its mean value of 25.4 N is marginally lower than the rest. The other unique finding regarding this device was the high frequency (87%) of prosthesis breaks compared to the four control grafts (0–20%), which usually failed due to the suture breaking (Table 4A).

When cutting with scissors, the range of mean suture retention strengths widened with values ranging between 22.5 and 34.2 N (Figure 8). Also, the frequency of prosthesis breaks increased for all grafts, with the Plasma TFE® prosthesis reaching 100%, i.e., never experiencing a suture break. The mean strength for the Plasma TFE® graft in the perpendicular direction of 22.7 N was again among the lowest values recorded.

strate that the bursting strength of the Atrium Plasma TFE® prosthesis is similar to those of the Cooley Low Porosity, Cooley Verisoft and Woven Vascutek controls (Figure 6). Note that the Woven DeBakey Soft prosthesis is significantly stronger, due no doubt to its heavier weft yarn (see Table 1). The high degree of variation found with the Plasma TFE® graft is due in part to the presence of the external support which was not always located in the same position with respect to the probe during the test. However, the contribution of the external support towards the overall bursting strength of the prosthesis is comparatively small, if not negligible. Testing of the graft with and without its external support resulted in no significant difference in mean bursting strength.

Suture Retention Strength

The suture retention strength results are listed in Tables 4A and 4B. Note that the results from each

Dilation

The dilation results presented in Table 5 show that all the prostheses tested exhibited minimal increases in diameter of less than 1% at internal pressures of 120 mm Hg. In fact, when tested at 454 g longitudinal tension, no discernible change in diameter was observed for any of the models. Figure 9 illustrates the increases in diameter over the whole range of internal pressures tested at an applied longitudinal tension of 115 g. Note that the Atrium Plasma TFE® prosthesis is unique in dilating rapidly at low pressures (i.e., less than 50 mm Hg) due, no doubt, to the use of a texturized yarn in the warp direction.

Elongation

The elongation results presented in Table 6 show clearly the significantly lower value for the Atrium Plasma TFE® prosthesis compared with the other four

Table 3. Bursting strength results.

Prosthesis	Bursting Force Mean ± Standard Deviation (newtons)	Minimum Value (newtons)	Maximum Value (newtons)
Atrium Plasma TFE®			
with support	222.1 ± 49.5	165.7	288.6
support removed	217.5 ± 34.6	172.0	260.0
Cooley Low Porosity	236.6 ± 7.7	227.9	242.3
Cooley Verisoft	211.2 ± 13.7	195.5	220.6
Woven DeBakey Soft	366.3 ± 7.7	357.4	371.1
Woven Vascutek	208.9 ± 0.8	208.3	209.8

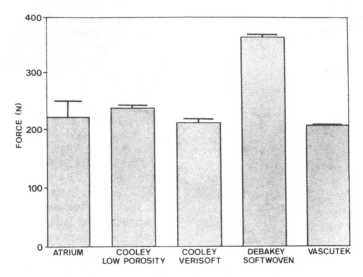

Figure 6. Bursting strengths of the different prostheses.

woven models tested. At both applied tensions reported, the Atrium graft stretched by about half the amount of the next least extensible prosthesis, namely the Woven DeBakey Soft. The implications of this behaviour are discussed later.

Surface Chemistry

The results of the ESCA survey scans tabulated in Table 7 show that the general level of surface contamination of the five prostheses is low except for the Cooley Low Porosity and the external support of the Atrium Plasma TFE® graft, both of which exhibit sig-

nificant levels (over 2%) of silicon, presumably incorporated into a surface lubricant. The presence of the plasma fluoropolymer coating on the Atrium product is evident by the 23–29% fluorine content observed, which was accompanied by a corresponding reduction in the levels of carbon and oxygen. Of additional significance are the variations found between the internal surface, the external textile surface and surface of the external support. The differences of 10%, 6% and 16% for carbon, oxygen and fluorine respectively are real and not due to instrumental errors, and reflect significant differences in chemistry between the three surfaces, with less fluoropolymer present on the ex-

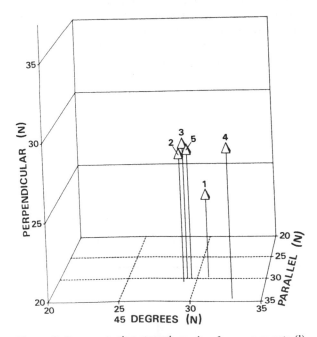

Figure 7. Suture retention strength results after cautery cut: (1) Atrium Plasma TFE; (2) Cooley Low Porosity; (3) Cooley Verisoft; (4) DeBakey Soft Woven; (5) Woven Vascutek.

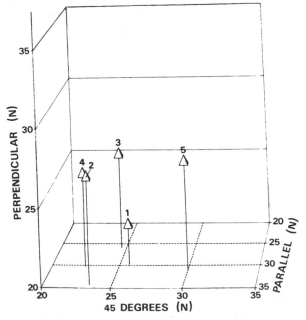

Figure 8. Suture retention strength results after scissors cut: (1) Atrium Plasma TFE; (2) Cooley Low Porosity; (3) Cooley Verisoft; (4) DeBakey Soft Woven; (5) Woven Vascutek.

Table 4A. Results of suture retention strength testing—cautery cut.

| Prosthesis | Parallel Direction | | Perpendicular Direction | | 45° Direction | | Frequency of Prosthesis Breaks (%) |
	Suture Break (newtons)	Prosthesis Break (newtons)	Suture Break (newtons)	Prosthesis Break (newtons)	Suture Break (newtons)	Prosthesis Break (newtons)	
Atrium Plasma TFE	—	29.6 ± 3.1 100%	—	25.4 ± 0.9 100%	31.5 ± 4.1 40%	30.3 ± 1.4 60%	87
Cooley Low Porosity	30.7 ± 0.5 100%	—	28.3 ± 0.6 100%	—	29.1 ± 1.4 100%	—	0
Cooley Verisoft	31.1 ± 0.5 80%	25.7 20%	29.7 ± 1.5 80%	25.4 20%	29.7 ± 1.3 80%	27.5 20%	20
Woven DeBakey Soft	34.3 ± 0.5 100%	—	29.8 ± 3.4 80%	28.1 20%	32.9 ± 0.8 100%	—	7
Woven Vascutek	30.8 ± 1.1 80%	26.6 20%	28.4 ± 1.4 100%	—	29.6 ± 1.6 100%	—	7

Table 4B. Results of suture retention strength testing—scissors cut.

| Prosthesis | Parallel Direction | | Perpendicular Direction | | 45° Direction | | Frequency of Prosthesis Breaks (%) |
	Suture Break (newtons)	Prosthesis Break (newtons)	Suture Break (newtons)	Prosthesis Break (newtons)	Suture Break (newtons)	Prosthesis Break (newtons)	
Atrium Plasma TFE	—	29.7 ± 3.5 100%	—	22.7 ± 2.7 100%	—	25.7 ± 3.8 100%	100
Cooley Low Porosity	34.2 ± 0.6 100%	—	28.4 ± 0.1 40%	25.9 ± 1.7 60%	29.8 ± 0.4 40%	19.1 ± 4.8 60%	40
Cooley Verisoft	30.1 ± 1.6 60%	19.6 ± 6.2 40%	27.0 ± 0.3 80%	23.5 20%	27.6 ± 0.5 60%	20.0 ± 0.3 40%	30
Woven DeBakey Soft	30.2 ± 0.6 100%	—	26.5 ± 0.1 40%	25.9 ± 0.4 60%	27.8 20%	21.2 ± 4.6 80%	47
Woven Vascutek	31.1 ± 0.3 100%	—	27.5 ± 0.3 60%	26.6 ± 0.4 40%	30.8 ± 1.1 80%	26.6 20%	20

Table 5. Dilation results—increase in diameter at 120 mm Hg (%).

Longitudinal Tension	Atrium Plasma TFE	Cooley Low Porosity	Cooley Verisoft	Woven DeBakey Soft	Woven Vascutek
115 g	0.8	0.0	0.2	0.2	0.5
454 g	0.0	0.0	0.0	0.0	0.0

Table 6. Elongation results—increase in length (%).

Longitudinal Tension	Atrium Plasma TFE	Cooley Low Porosity	Cooley Verisoft	Woven DeBakey Soft	Woven Vascutek
115 g	7.9	17.7	45.8	16.4	18.9
454 g	22.1	60.7	108.4	43.8	45.5

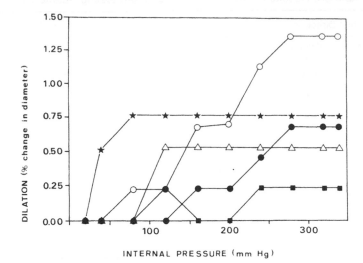

Figure 9. Dilation of virgin prostheses under static internal pressure at a longitudinal tension of 115 g (★ Atrium Plasma TFE; ● Cooley Low Porosity; ○ Cooley Verisoft; ■ DeBakey Soft Woven; △ Woven Vascutek).

ternal support than on the internal surface or on the external textile surface. Such differences are even more clearly presented in Table 8 which lists the relative components within the carbon 1s peaks. The differences between the internal and external surfaces of the Atrium Plasma TFE® prosthesis are greater for the carbon–carbon and carbon–oxygen bonds than for any of the four polyester controls. In addition, the relative proportions of carbon–fluorine bonding are so varied that it is evident that the plasma fluoropolymer coatings on the three surfaces of the Atrium product have significantly different chemical structures and functional groups.

Level of Extractables

The mean results presented in Table 9 show that there are considerably more extractable contaminants

on the surface of the Atrium prosthesis than on the four polyester grafts. Of particular significance is the fact that the Atrium graft yielded a much larger amount of extractables with non-polar solvents. This suggests that the surfaces of the Atrium graft contain more oils, waxes, softeners, silicones or unfixed oligomers than the polyester prostheses.

Table 10 presents the means and standard errors of the extractions performed on two different Atrium prostheses in triplicate. While the within-prosthesis variability lies at about 10%, the results between prostheses vary considerably. Statistical analysis of the data using a t-distribution found significant differences at the 99% confidence interval between the grafts for the total level of extractables and for each individual solvent except for water.

A comparison of the means and standard errors of the virgin and cleaned prostheses is shown in Table 11.

Table 7. Results of ESCA survey scans.

Prosthesis	Surface	%C	%N	%O	%F	%Si	%Na	%Ca	%Mg	%K	%P	%S	%Cl
Atrium	Internal	60	0.5	9.7	30	—	—	—	—	—	—	—	0.2
Plasma	External[1]	65	0.5	7.4	23	2.3	0.8	0.1	—	—	—	0.6	0.3
TFE	External[2]	55	0.7	3.8	39	0.7	0.3	—	—	—	—	0.2	0.3
Cooley Low	Internal	79	—	19	—	2.3	—	—	—	—	—	—	—
Porosity	External	79	0.5	18	—	2.7	—	—	—	—	—	—	—
Cooley	Internal	77	—	23	—	—	0.2	—	—	—	—	—	—
Verisoft	External	75	1.1	22	—	0.8	0.6	—	—	—	—	0.2	0.1
Woven	Internal	77	—	23	—	—	—	0.1	—	—	—	—	0.2
DeBakey Soft	External	76	—	24	—	1.1	—	—	—	—	—	—	0.6
Vascutek	Internal	85	—	15	—	0.4	—	—	—	—	—	—	—
	External	85	—	15	0.3	0.5	—	—	—	—	—	0.1	—

[1]Measurement includes the external support.
[2]Measurement excludes the external support.

Table 8. ESCA results—resolution of carbon 1s peak.

| Prosthesis | Surface | % Carbon 1s | | | | | | |
		C—C	C—O	O=C—O	C=O C—CF	CF	CF$_2$	CF$_3$
Atrium Plasma TFE	Internal	34	19	11	8	9	11	8
	External[1]	53	23	6	3	4	6	5
	External[2]	27	7	—	15	17	22	13
Cooley Low Porosity	Internal	75	15	10	—	—	—	—
	External	81	12	8	—	—	—	—
Cooley Verisoft	Internal	72	14	13	—	—	—	—
	External	72	13	15	—	—	—	—
Woven DeBakey Soft	Internal	68	16	15	—	—	—	—
	External	69	15	16	—	—	—	—
Vascutek	Internal	76	12	11	—	—	—	—
	External	84	7	8	—	—	—	—

[1]Measurement includes the external support.
[2]Measurement excludes the external support.

Table 9. Level of extractables.

Loss of Mass in Each Sequential Extraction (%)	Atrium Plasma TFE	Cooley Low Porosity	Cooley Verisoft	Woven DeBakey Soft	Woven Vascutek
Hexane	0.81	0.10	0.10	0.08	0.26
1,1,1-Trichloroethane	0.27	0	0	0	0
Methanol	0.20	0.12	0.10	0.22	0.11
Water	0.30	0.03	0.05	0.02	0
0.1N Hydrochloric acid	0.15	0.07	0	0.13	0.12
TOTAL	1.73	0.32	0.25	0.45	0.49

Table 10. Variation in extractables within and between atrium prostheses.

Loss of Mass in Each Sequential Extraction (%)	Atrium Plasma TFE #1	Atrium Plasma TFE #2	Observed t Statistic
Hexane	0.71 ± 0.08	1.12 ± 0.12	3.43*
1,1,1-Trichloroethane	0.67 ± 0.03	0.05 ± 0.02	4.41*
Methanol	0.06 ± 0.02	0.42 ± 0.06	4.06*
Water	0.36 ± 0.06	0.30 ± 0.02	1.60
0.1N Hydrochloric acid	0.00 ± 0.00	0.31 ± 0.00	4.41*
TOTAL	1.82 ± 0.04	2.20 ± 0.11	3.63*

*Significantly different at confidence interval of $p < 0.01$.

Table 11. Level of extractables from virgin and cleaned atrium prostheses.

Loss of Mass in Each Sequential Extraction (%)	Virgin Atrium Plasma TFE	Cleaned Atrium Plasma TFE	Observed t Statistic
Hexane	0.92 ± 0.11	0.86 ± 0.07	0.87
1,1,1-Trichloroethane	0.36 ± 0.13	0.44 ± 0.12	0.87
Methanol	0.24 ± 0.08	0.21 ± 0.06	0.57
Water	0.33 ± 0.03	0.39 ± 0.08	1.31
0.1N Hydrochloric acid	0.16 ± 0.07	0.33 ± 0.09	2.67
TOTAL	2.01 ± 0.09	2.24 ± 0.14	2.44

No significant differences observed at confidence interval of $p < 0.01$.

The cleaning procedure appears to have had no significant effect (at 99% confidence interval) on the total individual levels of extractables.

Differential Dyeing

The lightness of the dyed plasma TFE coated prostheses lies in between the hardly stained 100% fluorocarbon material and the heavily stained 100% polyester sample. The numerical lightness values are reported in Table 12. Note that the lightness values for the two Atrium samples (24–27%) lie midway between those of the 100% fluorocarbon (32%) and the 100% polyester (21%) surfaces. This confirms that the chemistry of the Atrium surface, as seen by the dyestuffs, is not pure fluorocarbon but a combination of the two polymers in approximately equal proportions.

Note the high variability of the lightness values for the virgin Atrium prosthesis. This variability can be seen both between samples, in terms of the large difference between means, and within the same sample, in terms of the high standard deviations between the three specimens of the same sample. This suggests that the fluorocarbon surface has not been uniformly applied.

When comparing the lightness values of the dyed internal and external surfaces of the Atrium grafts, it will be seen in Table 12 that the external surface is invariably lighter (i.e., it has a higher lightness value). This indicates that the external surface has a higher fluorocarbon content than the internal surface, which provides even more evidence to support our claim that the fluorocarbon layer has been applied in a non-uniform manner.

Note that the cleaning process has reduced the lightness of three of the four dyed Atrium surfaces. More dyestuff penetrating the cleaned surface means that the dyestuffs saw more polyester after cleaning than before on the virgin Atrium prosthesis. One explanation of this phenomenon is that the cleaning procedure used in our laboratory was responsible for removing some of the fluorocarbon coating.

DISCUSSION

This new Atrium Plasma TFE® prosthesis presents several novel features and makes a number of innovative claims [35]. Let us address each of these in turn.

Absence of Crimps

For many years the crimps or corrugations of textile vascular prostheses have been criticized for their contribution to non-laminar flow and impaired healing characteristics. Consequently, a non-crimped device has potential advantages as a static blood conduit. However, previous clinical experience and animal studies have demonstrated that, in addition to preventing kinking, the crimps provide superior longitudinal compliance (ease of elongation) and facilitate surgical installation under controlled tension [36]. Hence with its limited degree of elongation (Table 6), the Atrium device is likely to be associated with high stress concentrations along the suture line, which in clinical terms predispose the prosthesis to the formation of anastomotic false aneurysms. It is noteworthy that the inventors of the Atrium device recognize the need for some compliance by stating that preferably the product elongates 20–70% [35]. One wonders about the clinical implications of this statement, given that 22% elongation is achieved only at tensions in excess of 450 g. Are such longitudinal tensions surgically practical?

External Support

With the absence of crimps, it is clearly desirable to incorporate a rigid external support to prevent kinking provided it does not compromise other properties of the prosthesis. While the external support of the Atrium graft controls the extent of dilation (Figure 6), previous animal and retrieval studies have found non-uniform healing under and between external spiral monofilaments, have identified difficulties at installa-

Table 12. Lightness measurements of dyed atrium and control prostheses.

Sample of Prosthesis	Surface of Prosthesis	Virgin Prosthesis (%)	Cleaned Prosthesis (%)
100% fluorocarbon	Internal	32.4 ± 0.4*	—
"Edwards" PTFE	External	32.0 ± 0.5	—
Atrium	Internal	26.5 ± 1.0	24.9 ± 0.6
# 1687306	External	27.7 ± 1.5	26.6 ± 0.4
Atrium	Internal	24.3 ± 0.3	24.3 ± 0.3
# 1887166	External	25.8 ± 1.3	25.1 ± 0.4
100% polyester	Internal	21.8 ± 0.1	—
Bard "Bionit"	External	21.0 ± 0.1	—

*Mean ± standard deviation of 3 specimens.

tion because of the need to remove the support near the anastomosis, and have observed abrasion damage to the textile structure due to rubbing of the cut end of the rigid monofilament *in vivo* [36,37]. Note that removal of the support alters the water permeability properties of the graft, which in turn may affect the healing behaviour near the anastomosis.

TFE Plasma Coating

The incorporation of a smooth, clean, uniform fluorocarbon coating has significant advantages for a polyester vascular prosthesis since it renders the luminal surface non-thrombogenic, enhancing blood compatibility and reducing the chance of embolism formation [35]. Nevertheless, the ESCA and differential dyeing results from this study suggest that the plasma coatings on the Atrium products sampled were neither uniform in thickness or in chemistry, nor did they meet the specifications claimed by the manufacturer [35]. A F/C ratio greater than 0.9 and ideally in the range 1.5–1.9 is required to confer non-thrombogenic properties to the luminal surface, yet none of our ESCA measurements have found F/C ratios greater than 0.5 on the internal surface (Table 7). On the other hand, our observations of F/C ratios in the range 0.4–0.7 on the external surface are compatible with the anticipated value of about 0.5 preferred by the manufacturer [35].

In view of the fact that the lightness of the Plasma TFE coated prosthesis lies between that of the pure polyester and pure fluorocarbon controls (Figure 7), it is evident that the disperse dyes see neither a pure polyester nor a pure fluorocarbon surface, but instead a modified polyester surface with reduced dye diffusion properties. The reduction in lightness observed with the cleaned and dyed specimens suggests that the cleaning treatment has either reduced the thickness of the fluorocarbon coating, or increased its diffusivity to small molecules, or both.

Fine Filaments

Because the bending properties of one-dimensional materials vary with the fourth power of their thickness, it is inevitable that the use of thinner (or finer) polyester filaments will produce a softer, more flexible textile structure, with the potential for easier handling and suturing characteristics. However, from a practical point of view, finer filaments are more susceptible to damage and surgical trauma and contribute to lower suture retention strength (Tables 4A and 4B). For these reasons, it is of interest to note that the manufacturer of the Atrium prosthesis has compromised the original preferred specification of a very fine 5–7 micron diameter for the warp filaments. The diameters of the warp filaments sampled in this study fell in the range of 8.3–9.7 microns (Table 1).

Dissimilar Warp and Weft Yarns

The use of a texturized warp yarn and a flat weft yarn has created a number of problems. Firstly, it has contributed to an inherent variability in the woven structure as seen by the high variations in strength and water permeability results. Secondly, it has made the water permeability properties dependent on the level of applied tension, with values below 100 ml/cm²/min 120 mm Hg achieved only at tensions in excess of 200 g. Is this feasible tension to be applied at the time of implantation? Thirdly, it has increased the likelihood of yarn slippage in the weft direction which leads to lower suture retention strength in the perpendicular direction. Cautery cutting is required in order to minimize this problem.

Visible and Extractable Contaminants

SEM observations, particularly of the internal surface of the Atrium prosthesis, indicate an unacceptable level of contamination. Its location suggests that it originated from the mandrel inserted inside the prosthesis at the time of winding the external support during manufacture. Such contaminating particles are likely to be incorporated into the internal capsule and exacerbate the tissue reaction during the healing process.

High levels of extractable materials ranging from 1.7 to 2.2% of the original weight of the virgin Atrium graft have been measured. The largest component is of a non-polar character, suggesting the presence of loosely attached TFE oligomers on the surface. The actual concentration of extractables varies considerably between different virgin grafts. This non-uniformity is no doubt due to a lack of control over the plasma polymerization conditions, and does not appear to be rectified by a simple cleaning procedure in aqueous media. An organic solvent cleaning system may be found more efficacious.

CONCLUSION

Because of the inherent weaknesses identified in this study, it is believed that there is sufficient evidence to indicate that this novel design of prosthesis might lead to complications *in vivo*. Investigations in animals and carefully controlled clinical trials are therefore mandatory prior to determining whether or not this device should be recommended for clinical use.

ACKNOWLEDGEMENTS

This work has been supported by Supplies and Services Canada, Health and Welfare Canada, the Medical Research Council of Canada and Hôpital St-

François d'Assise, Québec. The technical assistance of Brigitta Badour, Jacques Bastien, Suzanne Bourassa, Eden Campbell, Marielle Corriveau, Karen Horth and Nicole Massicotte was greatly appreciated. We extend our gratitude to Drs. M. R. Wertheimer, Claude Poirier, Gérard Roy, Denis Gagnon, Susan Turnbull, Yvan Douville, Alain Adnot, Paul Roy, Camille Gosselin, Attar Chawla, Pierre Blais and Sami Mohanna for their encouragement and guidance.

REFERENCES

1. Washo, R. D. 1976. "Surface Property Characterization of Plasma Polymerized Tetrafluoroethylene Deposits", *J. Macromol. Sci. Chem.*, A10:559–566.

2. Yasuda H., M. O. Bumgarner and R. G. Mason. 1976. "Lindholm Blood Coagulation Test Values of Some Glow Discharge Polymer Surfaces", *Biomat. Med. Dev. Art. Org.*, 4:307–321.

3. Yasuda, H., H. C. Marsh, S. Brandt and C. N. Reilley. 1977. "ESCA Studies of Polymer Surfaces Treated by Plasma", *J. Polym. Sc. (Polym. Chem. Ed.)*, 15:991–1019.

4. Yasuda, H., T. S. Hsu, E. S. Brandt and C. N. Reilly. 1978. "Some Aspects of Plasma Polymerization of Fluorine-Containing Organic Compounds. II. Comparison of Ethylene and Tetrafluoroethylene", *J. Polym. Sci. (Polym. Chem. Ed.)*, 16:415–425.

5. Yasuda, H. 1976. "Plasma Modification of Polymers", *J. Macromol. Sci. Chem.*, A10:383–420.

6. Yasuda, H. 1981. "Glow Discharge Polymerization", *J. Polym. Sci. (Macromol. Rev.)*, 16:199–293.

7. Nakajima, K., A. T. Bell, M. Shen and M. M. Millard. 1979. "Plasma Polymerization of Tetrafluoroethylene", *J. Appl. Polym. Sci.*, 23:2627–2637.

8. O'Kane, D. F. and D. W. Rice. 1976. "Preparation and Characterization of Glow-Discharge Fluorocarbon-Type Polymers", *J. Macromol. Sci. Chem.*, A10:567–577.

9. Anderson, H. R., Jr., F. M. Fowkes and F. H. Hielscher. 1976. "Electron Donor-Acceptor Properties of Thris Polymer Films on Silicon. II. Tetrafluoroethylene Polymerized by RF Glow Discharge Techniques", *J. Polym. Sc.*, 14:879–895.

10. Pender, M. R., M. Shen, A. T. Bell and M. Millard. 1979. "ESCA Characterization of Plasma Polymerized Fluorocarbons", in *Plasma Polymerization*. M. Shen, A. T. Bell, eds. Washington, D.C.: Am. Chem. Soc. Symposium No. 108, pp. 147–162.

11. Heffernan, P. J., K. Yanaglhara, Y. Matsuzawa, E. E. Hennecke, E. W. Hellmuth and H. Yasuda. 1984. "Preparation and Characterization of Composite Hollow Fiber Reverse Osmosis Membranes by Plasma Polymerization. 1. Design of Plasma Reactor and Operational Parameters", *Ind. Eng. Chem. Prod. Res. Dev.*, 23:153–162.

12. Matsuzawa, Y. and H. Yasuda. 1984. "Preparation and Characterization of Composite Hollow Fiber Reverse Osmosis Membranes by Plasma Polymerization. 2. Reproductibility of the Plasma Polymerization Process and Durability of the Resulting Coated Membrane", *Ind. Eng. Chem. Prod. Res. Dev.*, 23:163–167.

13. Cannon, J. G., R. O. Dillon, R. F. Bunshah, P. H. Crandall and A. M. Dymond. 1980. "Synthesis of a Fine Neurological Electrode by Plasma Polymerization Processing", *J. Biomed. Mater. Res.*, 14:279–288.

14. Nichols, M. F., A. W. Hahn, W. J. James, A. K. Sharma and H. K. Yasuda. 1981. "Cyclic Voltammetry for the Study of Polymer Film Adhesion to Platinum Neurological Electrodes", *Biomaterials*, 2:161–165.

15. Hollahan, J. R., B. B. Stafford, R. D. Falls and S. T. Payne. 1969. "Attachment of Amino Groups to Polymer Surfaces by Radiofrequency Plasma", *J. Appl. Polym. Sc.*, 13:807–816.

16. Sipehia, R. and A. S. Chawla. 1982. "Albuminated Polymer Surfaces for Biomedical Application", *Biomat. Med. Dev. Art. Org.*, 10:229–246.

17. Sipehia, R., A. S. Chawla and T. M. S. Chang. 1986. "Enhanced Albumin Binding to Polypropylene Beads Via Anhydrous Ammonia Gaseous Plasma", *Biomaterials*, 7:471–473.

18. Chawla, A. S. 1979. "Use of Plasma Polymerization for Preparing Silicone-Coated Membranes for Possible Use in Blood Oxygenators", *Art. Org.*, 3:92–96.

19. Chawla, A. S. 1979. "Preparation of Silicone Coated Biomaterials Using Plasma Polymerizations and Their Preliminary Evaluations", *Trans. Am. Soc. Artif. Int. Org.*, 25:287–293.

20. Chawla, A. S. 1982. "Toxicity Evaluation of a Novel Filler Free Silicone Rubber Biomaterial by Cell Culture Techniques", *J. Biomed. Mater. Res.*, 16:501–508.

21. Hoffman, A. S. 1984. "Ionizing Radiation and Gas Plasma (or Glow) Discharge Treatments for Preparation of Novel Polymeric Biomaterials", *Adv. Polym. Sc.*, 57:141–157.

22. Hoffman, A. S., B. D. Ratner, A. Garfinkle, T. A. Horbett, L. O. Reynolds and S. R. Hanson. 1986. "The Small Diameter Vascular Graft. A Challenging Biomaterials Problem", *Mat. Res. Soc. Symp.*, 55:3–17.

23. Hoffman, A. S., B. D. Ratner, A. M. Garfinkle, L. O. Reynolds, T. A. Horbett and S. R. Hanson. 1986. "The Importance of Vascular Graft Surface Composition as Demonstrated by a New Gas Discharge Treatment for Small Diameter Grafts", *ASTM STP 898*, Philadelphia: ASTM, pp. 137–155.

24. Garfinkle, A. M., A. S. Hoffman, B. D. Ratner, L. O. Reynolds and S. R. Hanson. 1984. "Effects of a Tetrafluoroethylene Glow Discharge on Patency of Small Diameter Dacron Vascular Grafts", *Trans. Amer. Soc. Artif. Int. Org.*, 30:432–439.

25. Guidoin, R., M. King, D. Marceau, A. Cardou, D. De la Faye, J. M. Legendre and P. Blais. 1987. "Textile Arterial Prostheses: Is Water Permeability Equivalent to Porosity?" *J. Biomed. Mater. Res.*, 21:65–87.

26. Guidoin, R. G., M. King, M. Marois, L. Martin. D. Marceau, R. Hood and R. Maini. 1986. "New Polyester Arterial Prostheses from Great Britain: An *in vitro* and *in vivo* Evaluation", *Ann. Biomed. Eng.*, 14:351–367.

27. 1986. National Standard for Vascular Graft Prostheses, ANSI/AAMI VP20 1986, Association for Advancement of Medical Instrumentation, Arlington, VA.

28. Marceau, D., A. Cardou, R. Guidoin, C. Gosselin and M. King. 1982. "Etude de la Déformation Circonféren-

tielle des Prothéses Artérielles en Polytétrafluoro-éthyléne", *Rev. Europ. Biotech. Med.*, 4:114.

29. Buxton, B. F., D. C. Wukasch, C. Martin, W. J. Liebig, G. L. Hallman and D. A. Cooley. 1973. "Practical Considerations in Fabric and Vascular Grafts. Introduction of a New Bifurcated Graft", *Am. J. Surg.*, 125:288–293.

30. Dumont, H. Manuscript in preparation.

31. Paynter, R. W., M. W. King, R. G. Guidoin and T. J. Rao. 1989. "The Surface Composition of Commercial Polyester Arterial Prostheses. An XPS Study", *Int. J. Art. Org.*, 12:189–194.

32. 1988. Identification of Finishes in Textiles, ANSI/AATCC Test Method 94-1987. 1988. *AATCC Technical Manual*, American Association of Textile Chemists and Colorists, Research Triangle Park, NC, pp. 136–142.

33. Blackburn, D. 1979. "Dyeing of Secondary Acetate and Triacetate Fibres", in *The Dyeing of Synthetic-Polymer and Acetate Fibres*, D. M. Nunn, ed. Bradford, UD: Dyers Company, p. 126.

34. Hunt, R. W. G. 1971. "Color Measurement", *Review of Progress in Coloration and Related Topics*, 2:11–19.

35. U.S. Patent 4,652,263.

36. King, M. W., R. Guidoin, K. Gunasekera, L. Martin, M. Marois, P. Blais, J. M. Maarek and C. Gosselin. 1984. "An Evaluation of Czechoslovakian Polyester Arterial Prostheses", *ASAIO J.*, 7:114–133.

37. Chakfe, N., C. Chaput, Y. Marois and R. Guidoin. 1989. "Etude *in vivo* de Trois Prothèses Artérielles en Polyester Comportant un Support Externe", *Comptes Rendus du 10ieme Congrès Annuel de la Société Canadienne des Biomatériaux, Montreal, QC, June 7–9*.

25

Clinical Application of Antithrombogenic Hydrogel with Long Polyethylene Oxide Chains

SHOJI NAGAOKA* [1]
AKIMASA NAKA**

ABSTRACT: Thirty cases of clinical testing on the PVC drain tubes coated by a hydrophilic copolymer with long polyethylene oxide chains (PEO-COAT® drain tube) were carried out. As controls, non-coated PVC drain tubes were used. Thrombogenesis was observed in 24 out of 30 non-coated PVC drain tubes (80%) and only in 4 out of 30 PEO-COAT® drain tubes (13%). The PEO-COAT® drain tube significantly suppressed the absorption of plasma proteins and adhesion of platelets. The excellent antithrombogenic property of the hydrophilic polymer with long polyethylene oxide chains, which has been suggested by *in vitro* and *in vivo* experiments, was evidenced here clinically.

INTRODUCTION

Thrombogenesis on the surface of artificial materials is triggered by the adsorption to the surface of an artificial material of plasma proteins or platelets and their damage thereon. Therefore, in order to prepare an antithrombogenic surface without using physiologically active substances such as heparin, it is desirable to reduce the interaction between blood constituents and the surface of an artificial material.

Hydrogel with long polyethylene oxide chains is known to show a superior long-lasting antithrombogenicity. This effect is due to the long polyethylene oxide chains with a degree of polymerization of about 100 existing on the surface [1-4].

Spectrophotometric observations, mainly by ESCA or NMR under a hydrated condition, have shown that polyethylene oxide chains are projected from a hydrated surface and are vigorously moving with coordinated water. This thermal mobility of polyethylene oxide chains is much greater than that of other hydrophilic or water-soluble polymers such as polyvinylpyrrolidone, polyhydroxyethylmethacrylate or polyacrylamide [3].

Kinetically, the process whereby plasma protein interacts with and is irreversibly adsorbed onto the surface of a material to form a foothold for platelet adhesion, is largely influenced by the staying time on the surface. On the surface of a polyethylene oxide (PEO)-coated material, micro-flows of water are induced by the above-mentioned movements of hydrated PEO chains, and plasma protein is prevented from staying on the surface, hence the adsorption is inhibited. This is the molecular-level reproduction of the function of the cilia which exists on some mucosal epithelia of the living body and has a very high mobility. Thus, the PEO chain possesses the property which may be called a "molecular cilia". Figure 1 schematically illustrates this function of PEO [3].

On the other hand, the drain tubes which are used for surgical therapies for digestive tracts, i.e., for the drainage of bleeding from lesions, necrotic tissues, exudates, etc., are conventionally made from polyvinylchloride, silicon, latex, etc. These tubes, however, have to be retained often for a long time, and thrombogenesis is clearly observed in some cases, resulting in reduced efficiency of drainage.

In this chapter, the results of clinical evaluation of the drain tube coated with PEO-containing hydrogel (PEO-COAT® drain tube) are presented.

MATERIALS AND METHODS

Preparation of PEO-COAT® Drain Tube

Materials

(1) Material A: the hydrophilic graft copolymer (PEO) [1] made from polyvinylchloride (A, 40%) and methoxypolyethyleneglycol methacrylate (B,

[1]Author to whom all correspondence should be addressed.

* Basic Research Laboratories, Toray Industries, Inc. 1111, Tebiro, Kamakura 248, Japan

** Second Department of Surgery, Nagoya University School of Medicine, Nagoya, Japan

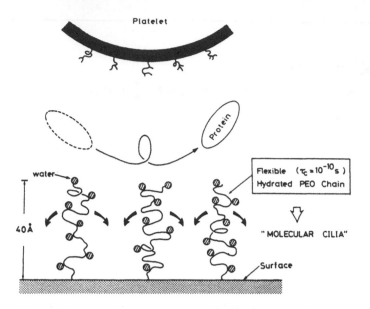

Figure 1. Schematic representation of the interaction between blood components and hydrated PEO chains on the surface. The rapid movement of the long PEO chains influences the micro-hemodynamics at the blood material interface more effectively than do the short PEO chains.

60%, the chain length of polyethylene glycol is ca. 100)

(2) Material B: the soft polyvinylchloride (PVC) made from polyvinylchloride (a) and a plasticizer (b), a:b = 100:70 (w/w)

Preparation Procedures

The inside and outside of the tube made from material B (20–60 cm in length, 3–15 mm in outer diameter and 2–12 mm in inner diameter) were coated with material A to be a thickness of 10–20 μm by means of the solvent cast method using THF. If necessary, 1–10 side pores were made. The tip of each tube was variously shaped depending upon purpose.

Safety Test

The safety of PEO-COAT® drain tube was tested for the following items according to safety standards: (1) quality, (2) physical properties, (3) exudates and (4) sterility.

Table 1. Indwelling time of PEO-COAT® tube and thrombus formation.

Indwelling Time	No. of Cases	No. of Thrombosed Cases	% Thrombosed Cases
1–4 days	9	1	11.1
5–8 days	15	2	13.3
9–12 days	6	1	16.6
Total	30	4	13.3

Clinical Evaluation

The PEO-COAT® drain tube is for drainage after digestive tract surgery. All tubes used were sterilized with ethylene oxide gas and tightly closed in sterile bags until use. The tubes were inserted into appropriate places for individual surgeries, and the excretion through each tube was absorbed by gauze.

Complications caused by the retention of the tube were assessed from the fever, infection and bleeding trends. To judge the formation of thrombi, the inside and outside of the tube were carefully observed with the naked eye on tube withdrawal. To examine the hematological effects of drain tubes, a general hematological test was carried out to determine the numbers of erythrocytes, leukocytes and platelets, the amount of hemoglobin, the hematocrit value, etc., a blood-coagulation function test was used to determine the amount of fibrinogen, etc., a liver function test was used concerning the levels of S-GOT, S-GPT, LDH and bilirubin, and an electrolyte test on the levels of Na, K and Cl was carried out.

Results and Discussion

Safety Assessment

Materials used for clinical experiments fulfilled all safety standards.

Clinical Evaluation

A total of 30 cases, 14 men and 16 women, 27–70 years old, average age = 55.1, were used for the

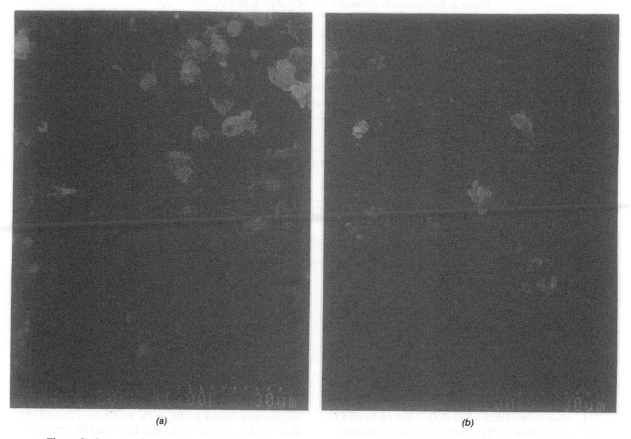

(a)   (b)

Figure 2. Scanning electron microscopical view of the drain tube inner surfaces in case 3: (a) PVC and (b) PEO-COAT®.

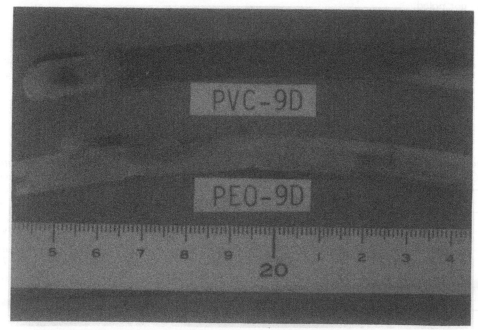

Figure 3. Macroscopical view of the drain tubes in case 3. Upper: PVC, lower: PEO-COAT.

Table 2. Comparison between PEO-COAT® and PVC drain tubes.

Case	Disease	Period of Tube Retention (days)	Site of Tube Insertion	State of Thrombogenesis	
				PEO-COAT®	PVC
1	Metastatic liver cancer	7	Under the right diaphragm	Absent	Some present near side pores
2	Cancer of pancreas	10	Winslow's foramen	Absent	Present, but relatively few
3	Primary liver cancer	9	Under the right diaphragm	Absent	Present, remained even after washing with physiological saline
14	Intra-hepatic calculus	10	Dorsal side of cut surface of the liver	Some present	Present
29	Liver cancer	7	Under the right diaphragm	Absent	Some present

PEO-COAT® drain tube test. The tube was used for drainage of the fluid and pus excreted from the abdominal and thoracic cavities. The period of tube retention ranged from 1 day to 12 days with an average of 5.6. Neither complications nor large changes in blood characteristics due to tube retention were observed. Thrombogenesis was observed in 24 out of 30 PVC drain tubes (80%) and only 4 out of 30 PEO-COAT® drain tubes (13%). These cases with thrombogenesis were examined further.

The indwelling periods of tube in individual cases are shown in Table 1, but a positive correlation between the indwelling time and the incidence of thrombogenesis was not noted.

Table 2 shows the result of comparison between non-coated PVC tube (control tube) and PEO-COAT® drain tube as regards thrombogenesis in 5 out of the 30 cases tested. The control tube generated thrombi in all 5 cases, while PEO-COAT® did so only in 1 case out of 5. Moreover, the thrombi generated on PEO-COAT® were mild, i.e., small in volume and easily soluble.

Table 3. Amount of blood components deposited on PVC and PEO-COAT® drain tubes.

Case	PVC	PEO-COAT®
1	25.6 μg/cm²	1.3 μg/cm²
2	15.5	1.8
3	30.2	1.6
14	24.9	3.2
29	18.0	2.0
Average ± SD	22.8 ± 6.0 μg/cm²	2.0 ± 0.7 μg/cm²

Figure 2 shows the electron micrographs of the insides of drain tubes in case 3. The appearances of drain tubes observed by the naked eye are shown in Figure 3.

Table 3 lists the amounts of blood constituents which adhered to the region without apparent thrombus in these 5 cases. The adhesion of blood constituents was found to be very small in PEO-COAT® drain tube. Thus, the excellent antithrombogenic property of the hydrogel with long PEO chain, which had been suggested by *in vitro* and *in vivo* experiments, was evidenced here clinically as well.

CONCLUSION

Clinical tests on the drain tube having a polyethylene oxide long chain (PEO-COAT® drain tube) were carried out, and its safety and excellent antithrombogenicity were confirmed.

REFERENCES

1. Nagaoka, S. 1984. *Polymers as Biomaterials*. S. W. Shalaby et al., eds. New York, NY: Plenum Press, pp. 361–374.
2. Mori, Y. and S. Nagaoka. 1982. "A New Antithrombogenic Material with Long Polyethyleneoxide Chains", *Trans. Am. Soc. Artif. Intern Organs*, 28:459–463.
3. Nagaoka, S. 1988. "Hydrated Dynamic Surface", *Trans. Am. Soc. Intern. Organs*, 10:76–78.
4. Nakao, A. and S. Nagaoka. 1987. "Hemocompatibility of Hydrogel with Polyethyleneoxide Chains", *J. Biomat. Appl.*, 2:219–234.

26

Woven Velour Polyester Arterial Grafts with Polypropylene Wrap: *In vivo* Evaluation

NABIL CHAKFE*
CYRIL CHAPUT*
YVAN DOUVILLE*
DENIS BOYER*
YVES MAROIS*
MARIE THERRIEN*
PAUL-EMILE ROY*
ROBERT GUIDOIN*.1

ABSTRACT: During the last three decades, polyester arterial grafts have been widely accepted as substitutes for large- and medium-caliber arteries. Because of their handling characteristics and their healing properties, knitted polyester grafts are preferred for peripheral surgery. On the other hand, the woven grafts are the substitute of choice in surgery of the thoracic aorta and ruptured abdominal aortic aneurysms, owing to their mechanical stability. Moreover, they are capable of preventing blood seepage through the wall even in patients who are heparinized, and consequently the graft need not require preclotting. However, because of their tight structure, poor handling characteristics and limited encapsulation, the woven grafts are infrequently implanted for other vascular repairs.

In an attempt to overcome these deficiencies, new prototypes of woven polyester grafts have been developed with two novel design features: a velour effect on the outer surface to promote tissue infiltration, and a polypropylene spiral filament wrap thermally bonded on the outside of the graft to prevent fraying at cut ends. Two prototypes of this device with nominal water permeability of 200 ml/cm²/min (LP, low-porosity prototype) and 1000 ml/cm²/min (HP, high-porosity prototype) were developed.

These two prototypes have been evaluated as thoraco-abdominal bypass grafts in the dog for preestablished durations of 4 hours to 6 months in order to investigate their healing characteristics and their mechanical stability. The new textile design appears to offer significantly improved tissue infiltration and intimal attachment properties in both devices.

Woven grafts of such design compare favorably to any knitted graft commercially available. The LP prototype appears to be more stable and resistant to fraying. It is preferred to the HP prototype, which proved to be less resistant to suture pullout.

INTRODUCTION

Polyester (Dacron®) arterial prostheses have been widely accepted as substitutes for large- and medium-caliber arteries during the last three decades. Tight-woven and warp-knit structures have demonstrated an outstanding *in vivo* endurance. The main advantage of a tightly woven structure is its ability to control and limit blood seepage through the prosthetic wall because of the low water permeability of the products, usually below 200 ml/cm²/min [1]. This is of particular importance during cardiovascular surgery, when systemic heparinization is mandatory during extra-corporeal circulation. Nevertheless, the use and the long-term fate of woven textile grafts appear to be limited by several shortcomings. The woven grafts are stiffer than knitted ones, and handling is more difficult for the surgeon. Woven grafts also have a propensity to fray when cut at 45°, and their healing capacity is limited [2], owing to the poor attachment of the pseudointima to the fabric surface. Woven Dacron grafts are generally considered to be the substitute of choice only in the surgery of the thoracic aorta, where blood seepage through the wall must be prevented.

In an attempt to overcome these deficiencies, engineers at IMPRA, Inc., Tempe, Arizona, have developed two new prototypes of woven polyester prostheses incorporating novel design features. The engineers created a velour effect at the external fabric surface in the hope that this rougher, more permeable surface would promote tissue infiltration, hence improving intimal attachment and graft healing. In addition, they added a thermally bonded, spiralled poly-

1Correspondence: Dr. Robert Guidoin, Ph.D., Biomaterials Institute, Room Fl-304, St-François d'Assise Hospital, 10 de l'Espinay, Quebec City, QC GlL 3L5, Canada.

*Department of Surgery, Laval University, Biomaterials Institute, St-François d'Assise Hospital and Department of Surgery, St. Sacrement Hospital, Quebec City, Canada

propylene filament around the outside of the prosthesis to prevent fraying at cut ends.

Two prototypes of this device have been developed: a LP product (Low-Porosity model) with a nominal water permeability of 200 ml/cm²/min and a HP product (High-Porosity model) with a nominal permeability of 1000 ml/cm²/min. The LP graft is available commercially as the IMPRA PolyPlus® 200; the HP Graft is not yet commercially available. As part of the ongoing evaluation of these grafts to determine their potential benefits for the patients and the surgeons, we hereby report their *in vivo* evaluation.

In this chapter, the healing characteristics and the alteration in mechanical properties of these two new prototypes are investigated. The grafts were implanted as thoraco-abdominal bypasses for scheduled periods ranging from 4 hours to 6 months.

MATERIALS AND METHODS

Graft Selection

Two prototypes, manufactured by IMPRA, Inc., Tempe, Arizona, U.S.A., and distributed in Canada by Pramel, Inc., Longueuil, Quebec, were selected for this investigation (Figures 1 and 2). The LP product with a nominal water permeability of 200 ml/cm²/min was identified as the Low-Porosity prototype, while the HP product with a 1000 ml/cm²/min nominal permeability, was referred to as the High-Porosity prototype. The size and style used was the 8 mm diameter straight prosthesis. A detailed description of the two grafts is given elsewhere [3].

Animal Selection, Hematological Tests and Statistical Analysis

Adult mongrel dogs, preferably females weighing between 15 and 25 kilos, were selected according to the Canadian Council on Animal Care Regulations. In addition to routine hematological tests (i.e., hemoglobin, hematocrit, platelet count, WBC and RBC), blood samples were also characterized by platelet aggregation analysis and thromboelastography. In order to summarize all these parameters and their distributions and to exhibit the pattern of each individual against the group within a global approach, we performed a principal component analysis [4] of both series of dogs implanted for each variable, with the same graft type studied together for the first investigation. A multivariate analysis of variance [5] was done where necessary. This approach was selected to better verify the homogeneity among the two groups for all variables. Hence, the verification may help in discussing the performance of both prototypes evaluated in this study and each individual.

Graft Implantation

The protocol for a thoraco-abdominal bypass, originally described by McCune [6] and now widely accepted [7,8], was followed. A series of implantations was performed so as to evaluate the grafts after seven different predetermined periods of: 4 hours, 1 and 2 days, 1 week, 1, 3 and 6 months.

Prior to surgery, the dogs fasted overnight. They were then anaesthetized with 30 mg/kg of intravenous sodium pentothal (Abbott Labs., Toronto, Ontario, Canada), intubated and mechanically ventilated. Complementary fluothane anaesthesia was given as needed. The abdomen and left hemithorax were shaved and the skin was prepared with chlorexidine gluconate (Hibitane®, Ayerst, Montreal, Quebec, Canada). The abdominal aorta was mobilized from the renal arteries to the aortic trifurcation through a midline lower abdominal incision. The thoracic aorta was isolated by means of a left thoracotomy through the 8th intercostal space. The HP grafts were preclotted according to the protocol described by Sauvage and Yates [9] while the LP grafts were not preclotted. The animals were given 1 mg/kg intravenous heparin (Allen and Hanburys, Glaxo Canada Ltd., Toronto, Ontario, Canada) at least 5 minutes before vascular clamping. The distal anastomosis was then performed in an end-to-side manner between the prosthesis and the infrarenal aorta. The graft was tunnelled in the retroperitoneal, retropleural space. The thoracic aorta was clamped and sectioned after distal ligation and the proximal end-to-end anastomosis was completed. All anastomoses used a continuous 5/0 suture of polypropylene monofilament (Prolene®, Ethicon Sutures Ltd., Peterborough, Ontario, Canada). The rate of blood flow in the graft and the distal abdominal aorta ranged between 1500 and 2000 ml/min and between 150 and 200 ml/min, respectively, ensuring adequate perfusion of the kidneys [8]. The abdomen and thorax were closed in layers using 1 and 2/0 polypropylene monofilament sutures.

The animals were returned to their cages and fed an unrestricted standard diet. All received injectable Garamycin® (Schering Corp. Ltd., Pointe-Claire, Quebec, Canada) intravenously at the time of anaesthesia and 15,000 units of prolonged-effect antibiotics (Penlong 5, Rogar STB Inc., Montreal, Quebec, Canada).

Immediately before the scheduled sacrifice, an angiography was performed on the dogs with grafts implanted for 3 and 6 months using Renograffin® (Squibb Canada Inc., Montreal, Quebec, Canada) as the contrast medium.

For explantation of the prostheses, the dogs were returned to the operating room, anaesthetized and given intravenous heparin (0.5 mg/kg) to minimize the post-mortem thrombotic deposits on the graft. The grafts were removed by a thoraco-abdominal approach. Both kidneys were also removed to assess the extent of possible embolization.

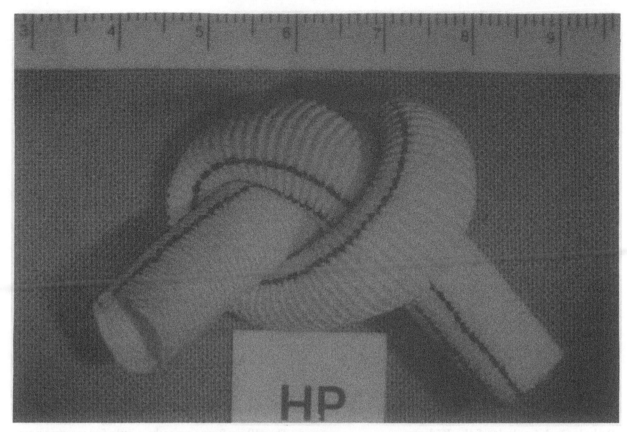

Figure 1. Virgin HP prototype.

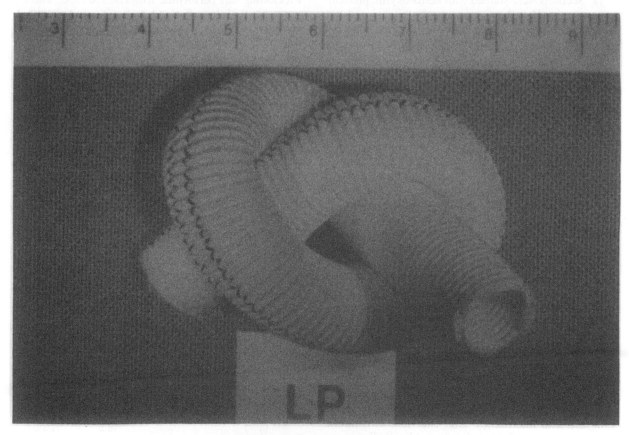

Figure 2. Virgin LP prototype.

Pathologic Analysis of the Implants

The grafts were opened longitudinally, after which they were carefully rinsed and photographed with a Tessovar macrophotography optical system (Carl Zeiss, Oberkochen, Germany) to assess the macroscopic findings. Pathological analysis was conducted on the two anastomotic sections and on another section removed from the middle of the graft. Each of these three specimens was divided into two parts for the following analysis.

The first part was fixed in a 2% isotonic buffered glutaraldehyde solution, rinsed in distilled water and post-fixed in osmium tetroxide. Drying was completed by immersion in a series of aqueous ethanol solutions of increasing concentration, followed by critical point drying using liquid CO_2 as the transfer medium. The specimens were then coated with gold-palladium and examined in a Jeol JSM 35CF scanning electron microscope (Soquelec, Montreal, Quebec, Canada) at a 15 kV accelerating voltage.

The second part was fixed in a 10% solution of formalin and 5 μm thick sections were cut and stained as follows: Weigert, Masson trichrome, Brown and Brenn, and Dahl.

Pathological Analysis of the Kidneys

Representative samples were taken from both kidneys. Sections were stained with hematoxylin, phloxin and safranin (H.P.S.) and systematically screened for evidence of infarcts which might have been caused by circulating microemboli dislodged from the prosthetic wall.

Textile Investigation

The remaining segments from each graft were cleaned to remove the residual tissue by boiling in a 5% sodium carbonate solution. They were then immersed in commercial bleach at room temperature, followed by exhaustive washing with distilled water and air drying. This treatment has been previously shown not to cause any significant change in the properties of polyester fabrics such as stitch density, bursting strength and fiber morphology [10].

The tightness of a woven structure is characterized by the frequency of yarns lying in both directions. By viewing the prostheses flattened between glass slides through an optical stereoscopic microscope at 20 times magnification, the number of warp yarns (ends) per cm width and the number of weft yarns (picks) per cm length were counted for each sample on 3 segments of the graft labelled proximal, central and distal according to their origin. The results were compared with the woven fabric count of the virgin grafts.

The structure and morphology of the Dacron fibers and the polypropylene wrap were evaluated by scanning electron microscopy after exposure to osmium tetroxide vapor and coating with gold-palladium.

X-ray Photoelectron Spectroscopy for Chemical Analysis (ESCA)

ESCA was performed on virgin specimens, on cleaned virgin specimens and on specimens of grafts explanted at 3 and 6 months to evaluate chemical degradation or adsorption of the polyester. The samples were investigated in an ESCA Lab MK2 (Vg Scientific) featuring a Mgkα beam at Laval University. The survey scans were recorded for subsequent identification of the levels of different contaminants.

RESULTS

Hematological Characterization

The principal components did not bring out outliers. No overall difference was found between the two groups of dogs by multivariate analysis of variance except the white blood cell count which was significantly higher by 30% in the IMPRA LP group (Table 1).

Implantation and Follow-up

The HP graft was smooth; a little fraying was noted at the edge of the section before anastomosis. It was, however, not sufficient to justify the use of cautery. Preclotting was performed with relative ease. The LP graft was slightly stiffer and no fraying was observed. In both prostheses, surgical handling was good and difference in the length of time for implantation was not significant (LP: 32.57 ± 4.53 min vs. HP:

Table 1. Means of variables for each type of graft.

	HP Prototype	LP Prototype
Hemoglobin (g/100 ml)	17.3571	15.9286
Hematocrit (%)	49.7143	51.7143
Leukocytes (n/mm³)	9742.9	13928.6
Glycemia (moles/P)	52.25	47.60
Platelets (n/mm³)	359000	355286
Hemochron (s)	172.429	163.833
Platelet aggregation		
time of latence (s)	1.76	0.74
aggregation rate (%)	21.6	34.0
rate/time (%/mn)	1.45667	3.40000
TEG (RWB: Recalcified whole blood)		
R (mm)	11.8571	13.7857
K (mm)	22.5000	27.3571
AM (mm)	47.8571	35.2857
EMX	100.714	59.429
IPT	5.42000	3.09429
TEG (PPP: Poor platelet plasma)		
R (mm)	6.75	11.00
K (mm)	111.0	10.5
AM (mm)	18.5	28.0

Table 2. Characteristics of the HP prototype at retrieval.

Characteristics	Duration						
	4 Hours	1 Day	2 Days	1 Week	1 Month	3 Months	6 Months
Graft structure	straight	bent	bent	straight	bent	straight	straight
External capsule formation	absent	absent	absent	absent	thick	thick	thick
Internal capsule formation	absent	absent	absent	thin	thin	thick smooth	thick smooth
Flow surface color	red	red/white	red/white	white	white	white	white
Thrombus-free surface %	100%	100%	97%	95%	100%	100%	100%

28.71 ± 3.19 mn). Upon release of the blood flow, seepage through the wall was minimal for all grafts.

The operations were uneventful. All dogs survived and were sacrificed according to the predetermined schedule. The angiographies performed just before the sacrifice of those dogs implanted for 3 and 6 months showed that the grafts had remained patent with excellent runoff. No unusual bending, kinking or dilatation was observed in any of the prostheses.

Patency and Macroscopic Observations

The explanted grafts were evaluated in terms of patency, naked-eye observation of healing characteristics and thrombus-free surface (Tables 2 and 3, Figures 3 and 4). Observations can be summarized as follows:

- *HP prototype:* all the grafts were patent at the time of explantation. Three grafts were bent in the area of the retrodiaphragmatic tunnel at 24 hours, 48 hours and 1 month as a result of the location of the tunnel. A thick external capsule was observed from 1 to 6 months. On the other hand, the internal capsule was thin at 1 week and became thicker at 3 and 6 months. Some cracks were observed at 3 months.
- *LP prototype:* all the grafts were patent at the time of explantation. The graft explanted at 4 hours was partially thrombosed. Two grafts were slightly bent in the area of the retro-

diaphragmatic tunnel after 48 hours and 1 month as a result of the surgical technique. A thick external capsule was observed from 1 to 6 months. The internal capsule was very thin at 1 week, thick at 1 month, very thick from 1 to 6 months.

Histopathological Study

- *HP prototype:* histopathological examination of the grafts retrieved after implanted 4, 24 and 48 hours revealed thrombus formation between the crimps with the presence of fibrin entrapping blood cells. Fibrin was also present between the polyester yarns, mainly due to preclotting. At 1 week, the thrombi were more organized and a fibrin network associated with inflammatory cells was observed on the external portion of the graft. The formation of a thin, generally smooth, internal capsule was noted at 1 month, and was partially covered by endothelial-like cells (Figure 5). At the proximal anastomosis, a thick fibrous external capsule originating from the host artery was observed. An intense inflammatory reaction surrounding the polyester yarns and the presence of foreign body giant cells were noted. At 3 months, the internal capsule which was partially covered by endothelial-like cells became thicker. However, the polyester fibers were surrounded by the collagenous capsule.

Table 3. Characteristics of the LP prototype at retrieval.

Characteristics	Duration						
	4 Hours	1 Day	2 Days	1 Week	1 Month	3 Months	6 Months
Graft structure	straight	straight	bent	straight	bent	straight	straight
External capsule formation	absent	absent	absent	absent	very thick	thick	thick
Internal capsule formation	absent	absent	absent	very thin	thin	thick	thick smooth
Flow surface color	white	white	white	white	white	white	white
Thrombus-free surface %	85%	100%	100%	100%	100%	100%	100%

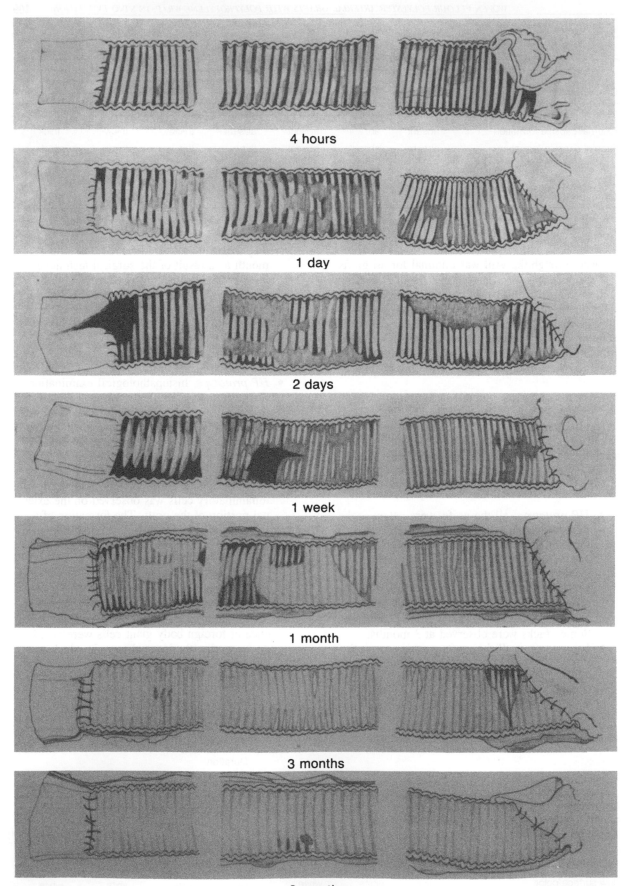

Figure 3. Photograph showing healing sequence of the HP prototype.

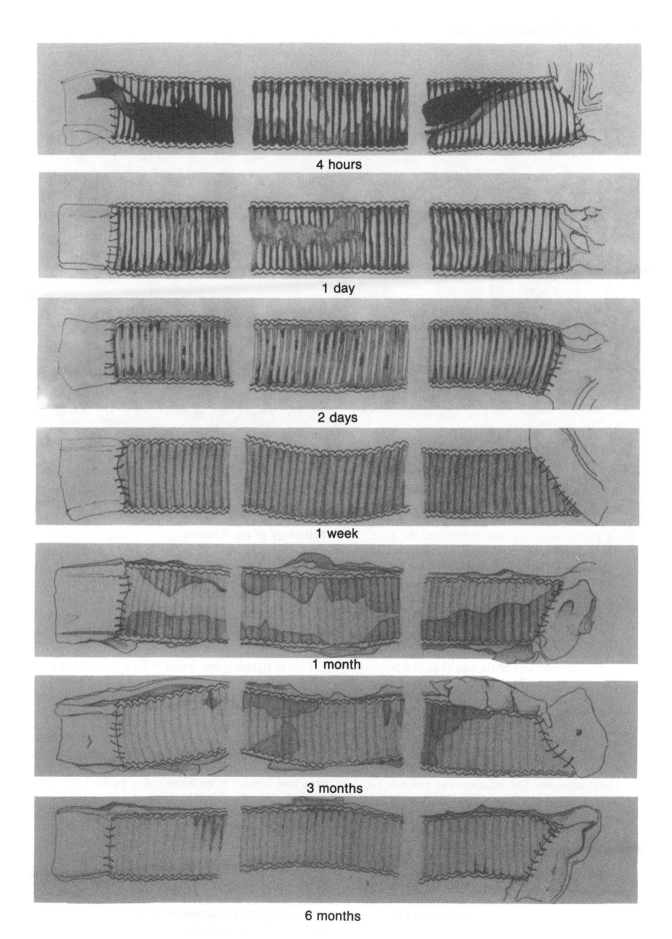

Figure 4. Photograph showing healing sequence of the LP prototype.

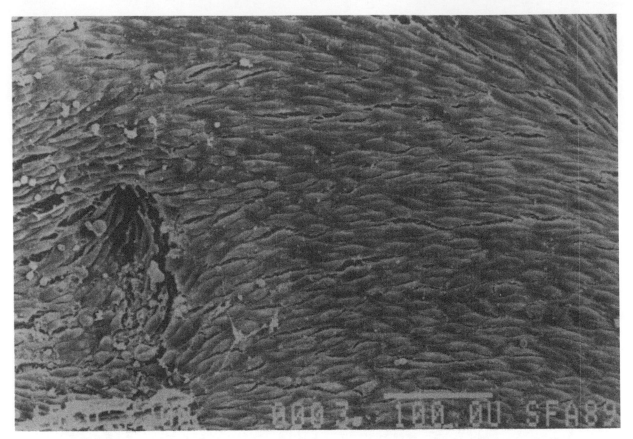

Figure 5. HP prototype at 1 month, SEM (×200), endothelial-like cells covering near the proximal anastomosis.

A granulomatous tissue surrounded the graft. At 6 months, the thickness of the internal capsule increased. A sparse but more regular neoendothelium covered the entire graft (Figure 6) and vasa-vasorum was observed (Figure 7). Moreover, the external capsule revealed a granulomatous tissue associated with a sclerotic hyperplasia in contact with the polyester yarns.

- *LP prototype:* less fibrin was observed between the yarns in the first 3 periods (Figure 8). At 1 week, there were some endothelial-like cells near the proximal anastomosis of the graft (Figure 9). At 1 month, both the external and internal capsules were thick and collagen was found in the valleys of the crimps. The interstitial zone was invaded only in the proximal segment. The inflammatory reaction was more significant than in the HP prototype. At 3 (Figures 10 and 11) and 6 months (Figures 12 and 13), there was a thick external and internal capsule, the latter being notably thinner than in the HP prototype. The collagen matrix was fairly smooth with a sparse neoendothelium covering the entire graft. No calcification and no bacteria were observed with the Dahl and Brenn and Brown stains in any of the prostheses.

Pathology of the Kidneys

Except for a few isolated areas with inflammatory changes, the explanted kidneys from all the animals had a normal microscopic appearance with no evidence of infarcts caused by embolization.

Textile Examination

Loss of tightness was found in both models but was not considered to be significant. This was estimated to be about 10% for the LP prototype and slightly less for the HP prototype. Neither model showed any significant variation with time (Table 4).

Scanning electron microscopy study of the cleaned specimens did not reveal any broken filaments in either model at any time of implantation. The woven structure seemed to be more stable in the LP prototype (Figure 14). After 1 month of implantation, the specimens of both prototypes were difficult to clean. Adherent tissue residues were observed on the surface of the yarns. No fraying was noted on the anastomotic lines; however, stretched weft yarns by the suture thread were observed in the HP prototype at 3 months (Figure 15). Alterations of the polypropylene wrap were observed in both prostheses from 1 week, when it was found to be detached from the yarns and broken in some areas (Figure 16).

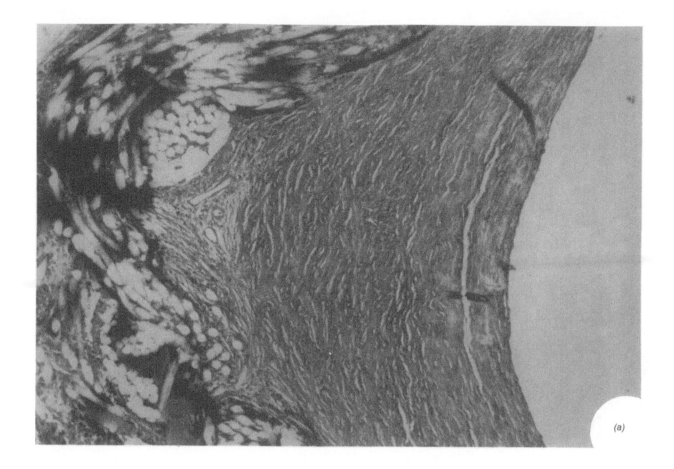

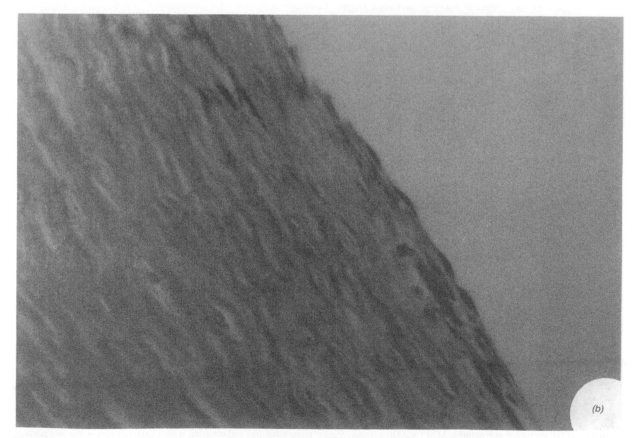

Figure 6. HP prototype at 6 months: (a) Weigert stain (× 100), thick collagenous internal capsule compressing the polyester fibers; (b) Masson Trichrome stain (× 400), collagenous internal capsule with endothelial-like cells near the proximal anastomosis.

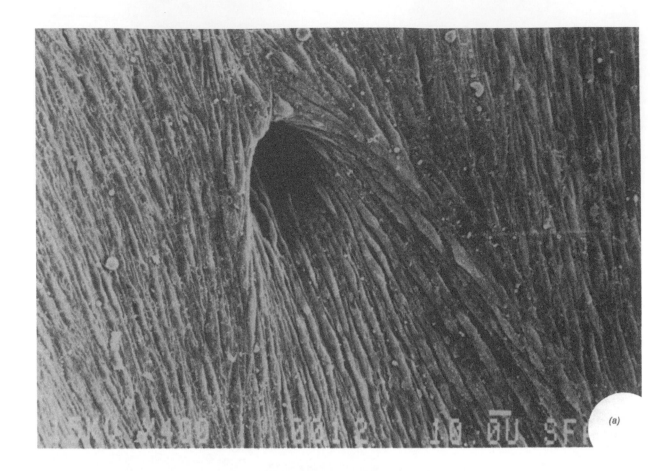

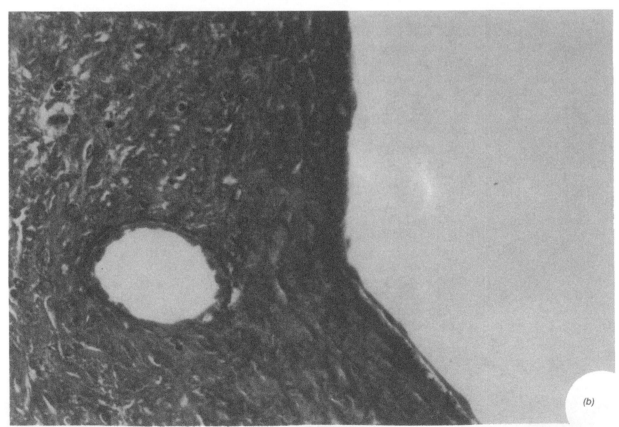

Figure 7. (a) HP prototype at 6 months, SEM (×200), smooth, regular endothelial-like cell covering with a vasa-vasorum in the mid portion of the graft; (b) Weigert stain (×400), thick regular internal capsule with a vasa-vasorum and endothelial-like cells near the proximal anastomosis.

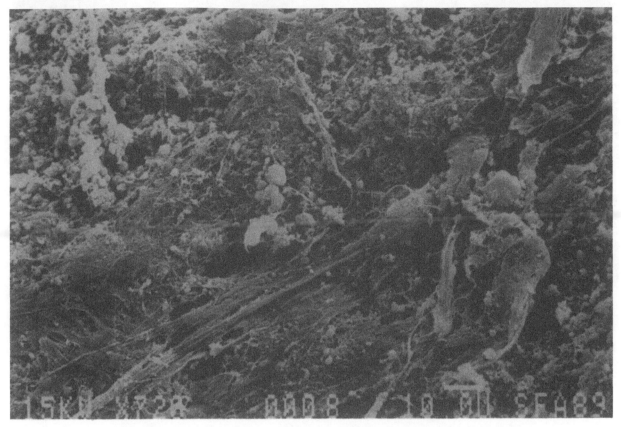

Figure 8. LP prototype at 24 hours, SEM (× 720), bulky fibrin with entrapped blood cells.

X-ray Photoelectron Spectroscopy for Chemical Analysis

No modifications of the spectra were noted after cleaning. The C-rate increased while the O-rate decreased on the explanted graft spectra (Table 5). Two hypotheses may be put forward to account for this: the polyethylene terephthalate chains might have been broken resulting in a release of oxygen, or the polyester surface might have been contaminated by a carbon-rich component. We believe the first hypothesis is doubtful and that the adherent film observed on the surface of the yarns of the two prototypes after cleaning can explain these results.

DISCUSSION

Prior to deciding whether or not to use a new prosthesis, the surgeon must feel confident about its ease of handling and suturability, and must be able to compare its structural features, its ease of installation, its healing characteristics and its *in vivo* durability against existing devices. Any new device should meet the needs of both surgeon and patient.

The initial reaction to handling these grafts was the observation that they are stiffer than knitted grafts,

particularly the LP prototype. However, during implantations, handling and suturability were considered to be very easy for woven grafts. The time of implantation was a little longer for the LP prototype, and cutting the HP prototype was performed carefully because a tendency for fraying was noted at its cut ends.

Table 4. Loss of tightness of the HP and LP prototypes with duration of implantation. Percentage of the virgin values (ends · cm⁻¹/picks · cm⁻¹).

		Average %
HP Prototype	4 hours	11/7.7
	1 day	6.6/5
	2 days	11/0
	1 week	13.3/0
	1 month	11/2.7
	3 months	11/2.7
	6 months	13.3/5
LP Prototype	4 hours	9/6.6
	1 day	9/6.6
	2 days	12/10
	1 week	12/3.3
	1 month	9/6.6
	3 months	9/6.6
	6 months	5.5/3.3

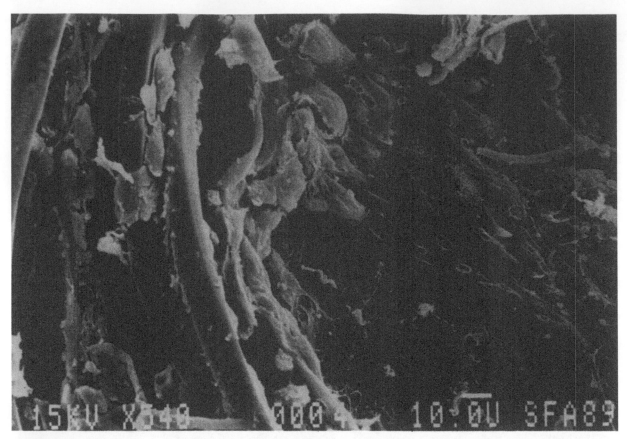

Figure 9. LP prototype at 1 week, SEM (×540), note the extent of the endothelial-like cells near the proximal anastomosis.

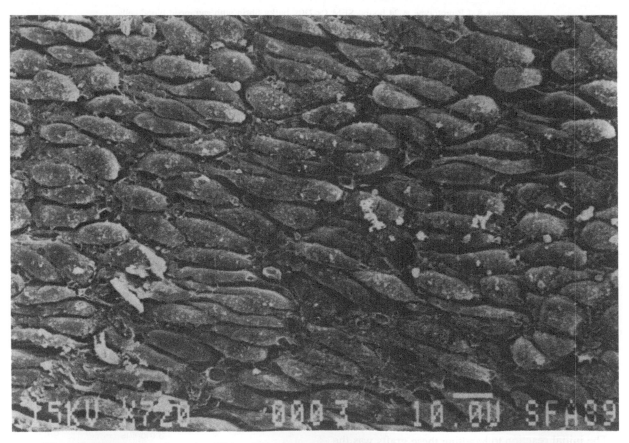

Figure 10. LP prototype at 3 months, SEM (×720), regular endothelial-like cells covering near the proximal anastomosis.

416

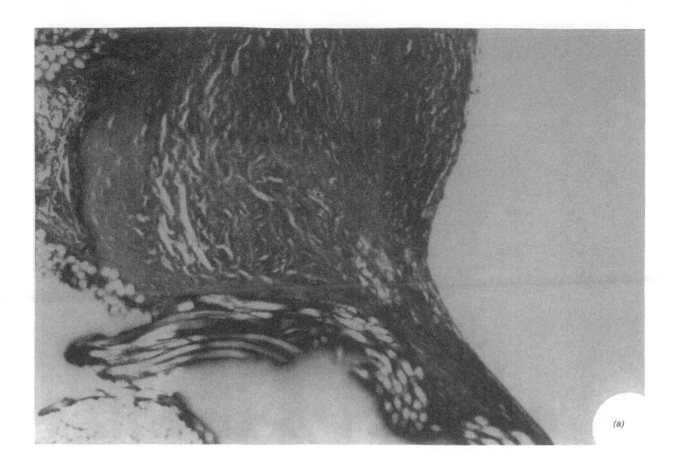

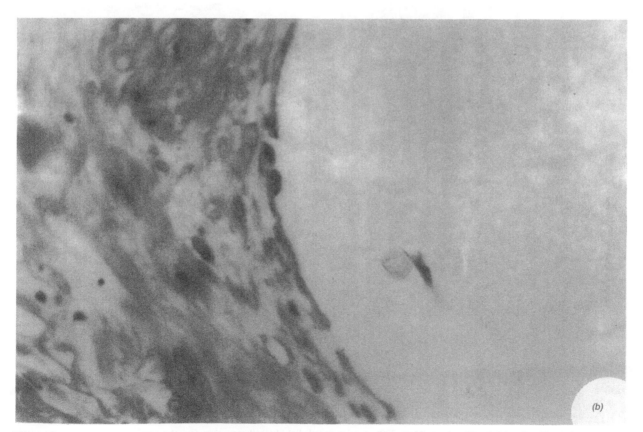

Figure 11. LP prototype at 3 months in the mid portion of the graft: (a) Weigert stain ($\times$ 100), thin internal capsule on the top of the crimps; (b) Masson Trichrome stain ($\times$400), endothelial-like cells.

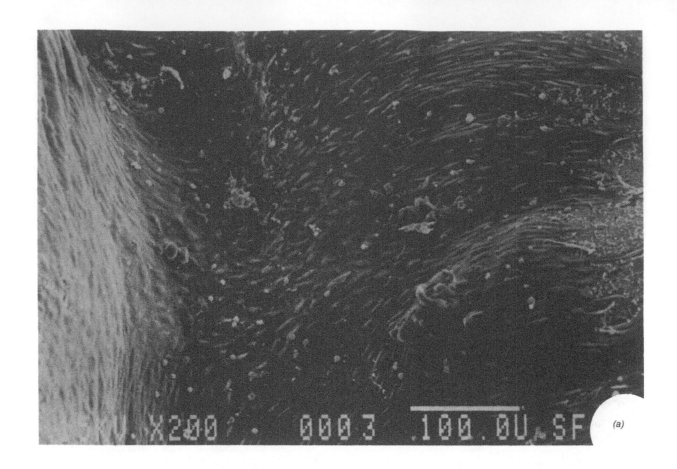

(a)

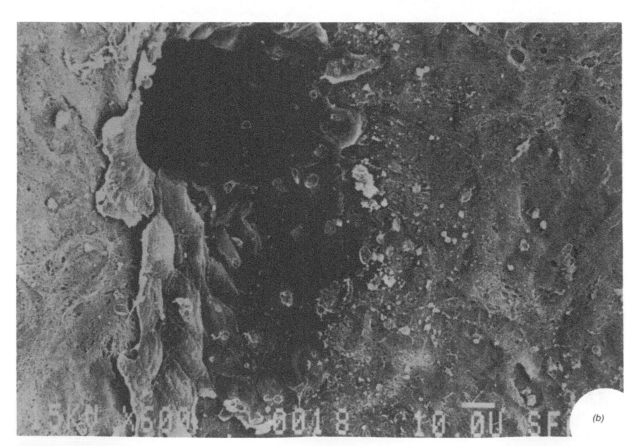

(b)

Figure 12. LP prototype at 6 months: (a) SEM (×200), regular endothelial-like cells covering near the proximal anastomosis; (b) SEM (×600), a vasa-vasorum in the mid portion of the graft.

418

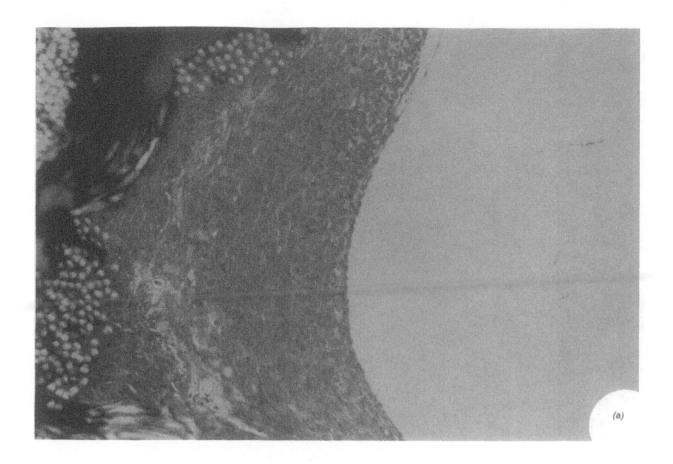

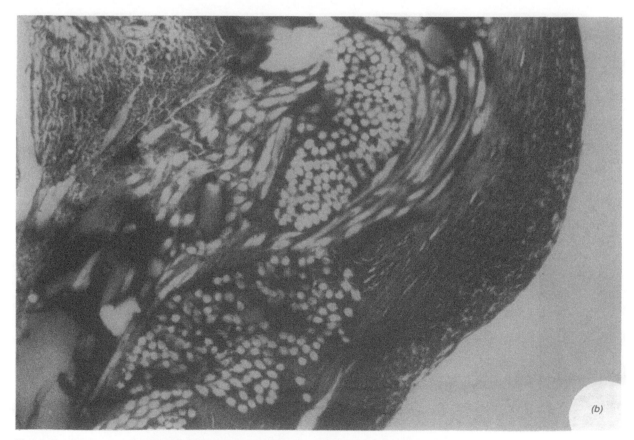

Figure 13. LP prototype at 6 months in the mid portion of the graft: (a) Weigert stain ($\times$ 100), good internal and external capsules; (b) Masson Trichrome stain ($\times$ 100), regular internal capsule with a fragile endothelial-like cell covering.

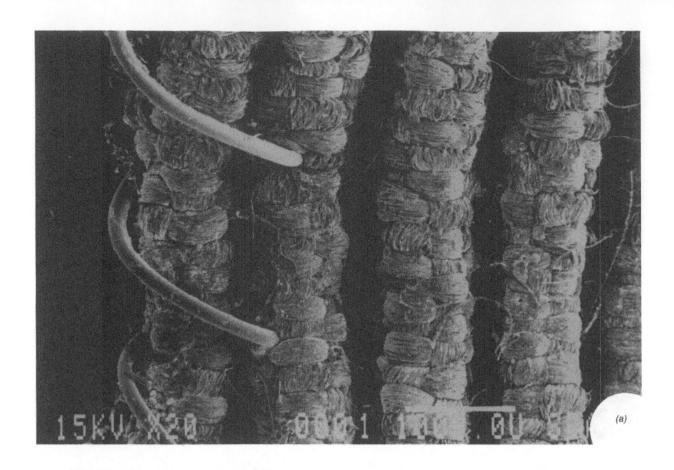

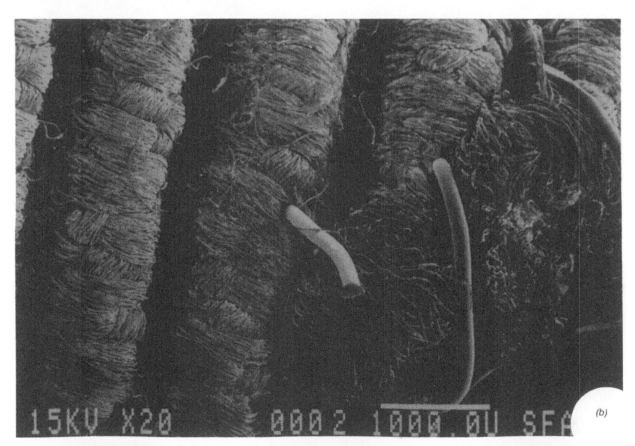

Figure 14. Cleaned LP prototype at 3 months: (a) proximal anastomosis, inner surface, SEM (×20); (b) distal anastomosis, outer surface, SEM (×20).

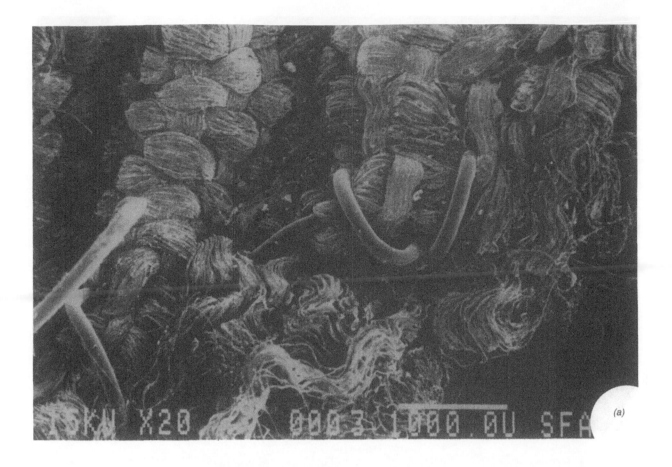

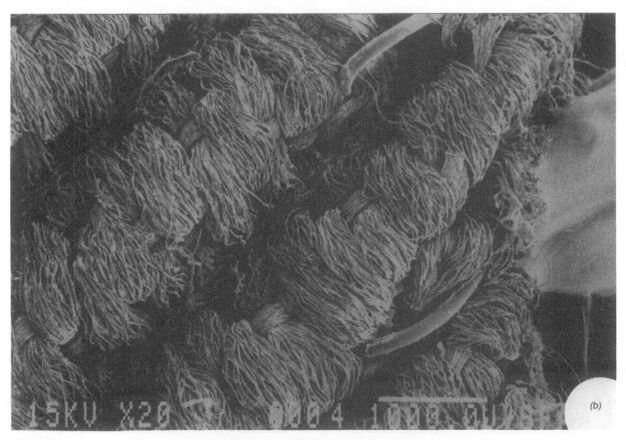

Figure 15. Cleaned HP prototype at 3 months, distal anastomosis: (a) SEM (×20), inner surface, some weft yarns are pulled out by the suture thread; (b) SEM (×20), outer surface. The polypropylene wrap monofilament is broken in some areas.

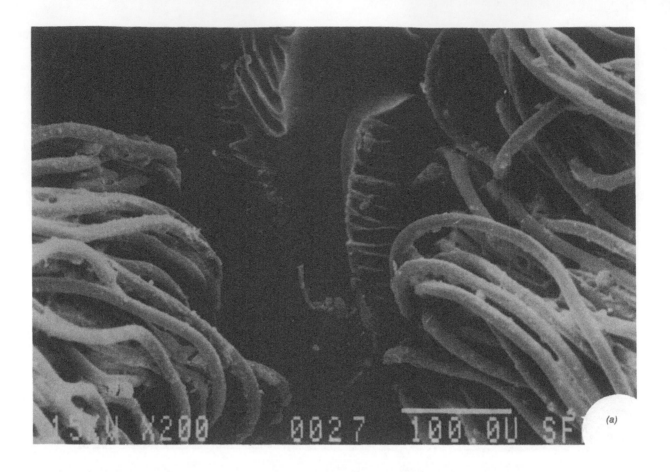

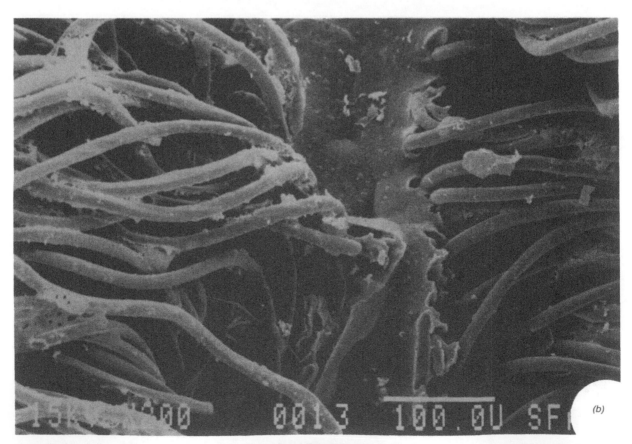

Figure 16. Cleaned HP prototype at 3 months, SEM (×200), the polypropylene wrap monofilament is detached from the yarns.

Table 5. Apparent surface composition of prostheses.

Prosthesis	Surface	C	N	O	Na	Cl	Si	S	F	Mg	Fe	Ca	Al
Virgin LP prototype	Internal	74	—	26	—	0.2	0.5	—	—	—	—	—	—
	External	75	—	22	0.5	1	0.5	—	0.4	—	—	—	—
Virgin and cleaned	Internal	77	—	22	—	0.6	0.4	—	—	—	—	—	—
	External	76	—	19	0.6	2	—	—	2	—	—	—	—
Explanted at 3 months	Internal	88	—	9	0.3	2	—	—	—	0.6	—	—	—
	External	87	—	10	0.8	2	—	—	—	—	—	—	—
Virgin LP prototype	Internal	75	—	25	—	—	—	—	—	—	—	—	—
	External	73	—	25	0.7	0.7	0.1	0.3	—	—	—	—	—
Virgin and cleaned	Internal	76	—	24	0.1	0.6	—	—	—	—	—	0.2	—
	External	75	—	22	0.6	1	—	—	0.7	—	—	0.2	—
Explanted at 6 months	Internal	87	—	11	—	3	—	—	—	—	—	—	—
	External	85	—	11	0.7	3	—	—	—	1	—	—	—
Virgin HP prototype	Internal	74	—	24	0.7	0.3	—	0.3	—	—	—	—	—
	External	76	—	22	1	1	0.3	0.4	—	—	—	—	—
Virgin and cleaned	Internal	75	—	23	0.2	—	0.4	1	—	—	—	—	—
	External	75	—	20	1	2	0.3	—	1	0.6	0.1	—	—
Explanted at 3 months	Internal	88	—	10	—	2	—	—	—	0.4	—	—	—
	External	90	—	9	—	1	—	—	—	0.7	—	—	—
Virgin HP prototype	Internal	74	—	25	0.5	0.2	—	0.2	—	—	—	—	—
	External	75	—	23	0.6	1	0.4	0.1	—	—	—	—	—
Virgin and cleaned	Internal	75	—	23	0.4	0.8	0.2	—	—	0.6	—	—	—
	External	70	—	20	0.8	2	0.6	0.3	2	2	—	0.2	0.8
Explanted at 6 months	Internal	87	0.4	10	0.2	2	—	—	—	—	—	—	—
	External	87	—	11	0.3	2	—	—	—	—	—	0.1	—

The thoraco-abdominal bypass in the dog is now widely accepted as a good model for the *in vivo* evaluation of vascular grafts. The use of segments longer than the thoracic or abdominal aorta alone reflect more closely the experience in humans [11]. Short segments are covered early by endothelial-like cells originating from the anastomoses. Long segments permit a better evaluation of the healing sequence since the endothelialization is not likely to cover the graft entirely. Implantation of a long segment approximates more accurately the actual clinical situation. It also permits textile and mechanical investigations since more material is available. Moreover, dogs have a healing sequence closely related to that of man [12]. In addition, with thoraco-abdominal bypass, any problem of distal embolization can be evaluated since the flow in the abdominal aorta is retrograde and involves 80% of the flow originating from the thoracic aorta. Since the blood flow to the kidneys is supplied by the graft, any emboli which are formed in the graft will be trapped in the kidneys because of their terminal vascularization.

Preclotting was easily performed in the HP graft and there was no blood seepage through the LP graft even though it was not preclotted. It is recommended that for woven prostheses with water permeability of less than 350 ml/cm²/min preclotting is not required [13]. If the use of the LP graft is contemplated for peripheral vascular reconstruction, preclotting will not be necessary unless the patient is heparinized.

The sequence of healing observed was grossly similar in these two grafts. The rate of healing was at least as good as knitted porous [11,14,15] or woven polyester prostheses [16] where endothelial-like cells are usually observed at only 3 months. A marked fibrous infiltration was observed between the yarns of the IMPRA HP. Grafts with such good tissue incorporation are probably more resistant to deformation and to infection than grafts with bare fibers.

The LP prototype woven structure seemed to be more stable and more resistant to fraying. The goal of reducing fraying at cut ends and thereby improving the suture retention strength of these prostheses, by the polypropylene filament bonded at the base of the crimps, appeared to be important at implantation and for short-term implantation. Its usefulness decreases as the healing progresses and the graft is incorporated in a fibrous capsule. Even if this polypropylene filament breaks, the graft performance is not affected since it is wound externally. Polypropylene is known not to cause any foreign body response. For this reason, it is the suture of choice in peripheral vascular surgery using vein grafts.

In conclusion, the new textile design embodied in these two models of woven vascular prostheses appears to offer a significant improvement in tissue infiltration and intimal attachment. No difference in healing was noted between the two models, and we therefore conclude that the LP prosthesis must be preferred because of its better stability.

ACKNOWLEDGEMENTS

This work has been supported by the Medical Research Council of Canada, Pramel, Inc. (Longueuil, Quebec, Canada) and IMPRA, Inc. (Tempe, Arizona, U.S.A.). The sutures were kindly provided by Ethicon, the antibiotics by Schering and the heparin by Glaxo. The technical assistance of J. Bastien, J. Boulet, K. Horth, L. Martin, N. Massicotte and G. Mongrain is much appreciated. We extend our gratitude to A. Adnot, C. Gosselin, H. Green, L. Vermilya, J. B. Sinnott, J. Pratte, L. Dadgar, T. How and I. Niggerbrugge for their help and guidance.

REFERENCES

1. Guidoin, R., M. King, D. Marceau, A. Cardou, D. De la Faye, J. M. Legendre and P. Blais. 1987. "Textile Arterial Prostheses: Is Water Permeability Equivalent to Porosity?" *J. Biomed. Mat. Res.*, 21:65–87.

2. Couture, J., R. Guidoin, M. King and M. Marois. 1984. "Textile Teflon Arterial Prostheses: How Successful Are They?" *Can. J. Surg.*, 27:575–582.

3. Guidoin, R., M. King, M. Therrien, Y. Douville, E. Debille, D. Boyer, S. Simoneau and L. Tremblay. "Woven Velour Polyester Arterial Grafts with a Polypropylene Wrap: A Cosmetic Change or Improved Design" (manuscript in preparation).

4. 1985. *SAS® User's Guide: Statistics, Version 5 Edition*. Cary, NC: SAS Institute Inc., pp. 621–637.

5. 1985. *SAS® User's Guide: Statistics, Version 5 Edition*. Cary, NC: SAS Institute Inc., pp. 113–138, 421–437.

6. McCune, W. S. and W. Blades. 1954. "The Viability of Long Blood Vessel Grafts", *Ann. Surg.*, 134:769–781.

7. Burkel, W. E., D. W. Winter, J. W. Ford, R. H. Kahn, L. M. Graham and J. C. Stanley. 1981. "Sequential Studies of Healing in Endothelial Seeded Vascular Prostheses: Histological and Ultrastructure Characteristics of Graft Incorporation", *J. Surg. Res.*, 30: 305–324.

8. Goëau-Brissonnière O., R. Guidoin, M. Marois, B. Boyce, J. C. Pechère, P. Blais, H. P. Noël and C. Gosselin. 1981. "Thoraco-Abdominal Bypass as a Method of Evaluating Vascular Grafts in the Dog", *Biomat. Med. Dev. Art. Org.*, 9:195–212.

9. Yates, S. G., A. A. B. Barros D'Sa, K. Berger, L. G. Fernandez, S. J. Wood, E. A. Rittenhouse, C. C. Davis, P. B. Mansfield and L. R. Sauvage. 1978. "The Preclotting of Porous Arterial Prostheses", *Ann. Surg.*, 188:611–622.

10. Guidoin, R., M. King, P. Blais, M. Marois, C. Gosselin, P. Roy, R. Courbier, M. David and H. P. Noël. 1981. "A Biological and Structural Evaluation of Retrieved Dacron Arterial Prostheses", in *Implant Retrieval: Material and Biological Analysis*. A. Weinstein, D. Gibbons, S. Brown and W. Ruff, eds. Washington: NBS Publication, pp. 29–129.

11. King, M. W., R. Guidoin, K. Gunasekera, L. Martin, M. Marois, P. Blais, J. M. Maarek and C. Gosselin, 1984. "An Evaluation of Czechoslovakian Polyester Arterial Prostheses", *ASAIO J.*, 7:114–133.

12. Sauvage, L. R., K. E. Berger, S. J. Wood, S. G. Yates, J. C. Smith and P. B. Mansfield. 1974. "Interspecies Healing of Porous Arterial Prostheses. Observations, 1960 to 1974", *Arch. Surg.*, 109:698–705.

13. King M. W., R. G. Guidoin, K. R. Gunasekera and C. Gosselin. 1983. "Designing Polyester Vascular Prostheses for the Future", *Med. Prog. Technol.*, 9:217–226.

14. Torché, D., J. Lacombe, M. King, R. Guidoin, D. Boyer, D. Marceau, Y. Marois and E. Debille. 1989. "An Arterial Prosthesis from Argentina: The Barone Microvelour® Arterial Graft", *J. Biomat. Applic.*, 3: 427–453.

15. Guidoin, R. G., M. King, M. Marois, L. Martin, D. Marceau, R. Hood and R. Maini. 1986. "New Polyester Arterial Prostheses from Great Britain: An *in vitro* and *in vivo* Evaluation", *Ann. Biomed. Eng.*, 14:351–367.

16. Stewart, G. J., N. Essa, K. H. I. Chang and F. A. Reichle. 1975. "A Scanning and Transmission Electron Microscope Study of the Luminal Coating on Dacron Prostheses in the Canine Thoracic Aorta", *J. Lab. Clin. Med.*, 85:208–226.

27

Vascular Prostheses from Polyurethanes: Methods for Fabrication and Evaluation

RAJAGOPAL R. KOWLIGI, Ph.D.*
ROBERT W. CALCOTTE, M.S.*

ABSTRACT: Excellent physical properties and blood compatibility characteristics have made polyurethanes a promising biomaterial for the manufacture of vascular grafts, especially those of 6 mm ID or less. In this chapter, published and patented methods for graft manufacture and testing are reviewed briefly. In addition, methods developed by the authors are described in detail. Results of experiments on the ability to control graft characteristics by altering the fabrication process are also presented. Some in vivo results of these grafts are also discussed with respect to the identification of principal failure modes.

INTRODUCTION

In spite of the fact that artificial vascular materials were introduced in 1952 [1], a small diameter graft less than 5 mm internal diameter is still not successful clinically. The worldwide potential for a 5 mm or less ID graft is about 1.28 million units by 1990 [2]. Solution to the problem of inferior patency of small diameter vascular grafts is thought to require: (1) the development of prostheses whose mechanical properties (elasticity, limpness and ability to conform to its surroundings) match those of the replaced vessel [3–8]; (2) a biocompatible material [9]; and importantly, (3) minimization of tissue response observed at graft-host vessel anastomoses [10–13]. Medical grade polyurethanes, in general, have material properties that meet many of the above requirements.

It is the purpose of this chapter to review the methods for fabrication and testing of the polyurethane-based vascular grafts. Published methods are discussed with respect to their advantages and disadvantages. Methods developed by the authors, specifically for small diameter prostheses fabrication and

testing, are described in detail. Also, results from the in vivo implantation experiments of the grafts made from the spray coating method are discussed with respect to some of the failure modes.

POLYURETHANES IN MEDICAL APPLICATIONS

Polyurethane copolymers are generally composed of short, alternating blocks of soft and hard segment units. The soft segment (SS) is typically a polyester-, polyether-, or a polyalkyl-diol (e.g., polytetramethylene oxide). The hard segment (HS) is formed by polymerization of either an aliphatic or aromatic diisocyanate with a chain extender (diamine or glycol). The resulting product containing the urethane or urea linkage, is copolymerized with the SS to produce a variety of polyurethane formulations [14]. It is projected that about 40 million pounds of polyurethane formulations will be used in medical products in 1992, as compared to about 25 million pounds in 1986. The usage is expected to grow at the rate of 6–8 percent every year [15]. Several medical grade polyurethanes are available commercially (Table 1).

ADVANTAGES OF POLYURETHANES

When compared to other commercial plastics, polyurethanes are outstanding in strength, flexibility and fatigue resistance. They can be cast at only slightly elevated temperatures (compared to room temperature) and are relatively biocompatible [16]. Thrombogenicity of the blood contact surface of polyurethane devices can be reduced by a variety of surface modification techniques, such as imparting negative charges [17,18], covalent bonding of anticoagulants and antiplatelet agents on the blood contact surface [19], and radiation grafting to modify polymer

*IMPRA, Inc., 1625 W. 3rd Street, Tempe, AZ 85281

Table 1. Sources of medical grade polyurethanes.

Trade Name	Manufacturer	Characteristics
Pellethane	Dow Chemical Co. Midland, MI	Linear, segmented aromatic, polyether-based, ethylene diamine extended
Biomer	Ethicon, Inc. Somerville, NJ	Linear, segmented aromatic, polyether-based, butanediol extended
Cardiothane	Kontron Cardiovascular Inc., Everett, MA	Cross-linked aromatic, polyether-based urethane-silicone copolymer
Tecoflex	Thermedics, Inc. Waltham, MA	Linear, segmented aliphatic polyether-based butanediol extended
Surethane	Cardiac Control Systems, Inc., Palm Coast, FL	Segmented polyether urethane, similar to Biomer
Bioflex	Mentor Corporation Goleta, CA	Aromatic, polyether urea urethane, ethylene diamine extended, and combined with silicone dioxide and polydimethyl siloxane
Rimplast	Petrarch Systems Bristol, PA	Silicone aliphatic urethanes, based on Tecoflex aliphatic PBT ethers
BPS-215M	MERCOR, Inc. Berkeley, CA	Polyurethane urea elastomer
Toyobo	Toyobo Co. Osaka, Japan	Proprietary polyether urethanes containing different soft segment molecular weights. Similar to Biomer in properties

surface [20]. Their elastic nature allows for design of vascular grafts with greater mechanical similarity to natural vessels than those made with ePTFE or Dacron [21]. Because of these characteristics, polyurethanes are widely used in the manufacture of medical devices (Table 2).

DEGRADATION OF POLYURETHANES

There has been increasing concern over the degradation of certain polyurethanes upon implantation. This phenomenon has been primarily observed in pacemaker lead wire coatings where material degradation, cracking, calcification, etc., may have con-

Table 2. Application of polyurethanes in medical devices.

- Lead wire coatings for pacemakers
- Acute implantable devices such as hemodialysis catheters
- Temporary and permanent artificial hearts
- In blood dialyzers to bind together bundles of hollow fibers
- Tissue adhesives, wound dressings and denture materials
- Vascular grafts primarily 6 mm ID or less

tributed to a small number of device failures [22,23]. However, these degradation reactions are localized primarily in the upper 10–20 micrometer thickness [23]. In vascular graft applications, the main problems are related to the stress on the polymer material at the host–graft anastomosis, and blood–material interactions. The test geometry is also an important factor that should be considered in evaluating the degradation rate of the polymer. Many polymers are subjected to attack by oxygen and water when they are put into use [24]. Oxidation typically is a chain scission process, which results in carbon–carbon bonds, peroxide bonds, etc. Although any carbon–hydrogen bond may be attacked, positions that are adjacent to double bonds or ether linkages are most vulnerable. Severity of the oxidative effects on polymers depends on the physiological environment. In some of the first commercial urethane foams (1950s), it was found that the urea, urethane and aliphatic ester groups were easily hydrolyzed, the rate increasing with pH above 7.0.

Purely mechanical agents of degradation include the effect of solvents on macroscopic dimensions of the polymer. Solvents may extract portions of polymer systems, e.g., additives and low molecular weight fractions. Other degradative mechanisms are: chain scission, depolymerization, cross-linking, bond changes and side group changes. It has also been suggested that degradation of certain types of polyurethanes releases carcinogenic agents that have produced tumors in animals [25]. However, there is no conclusive evidence that these degradation products cause systemic toxicity in animals.

MANUFACTURE OF POLYURETHANE VASCULAR GRAFTS

Vascular grafts from polyurethanes have been produced by several techniques [26-38], some of which are briefly described in Table 3. Many of these procedures have been patented, and current status is not known. However, it is a well-known fact that none of these methods have produced a clinically acceptable graft from polyurethanes.

We have recently described a novel and unique method for manufacturing small diameter vascular grafts [39]. In this method, known as the Flotation-Precipitation (FP) method, a polymer solution of known concentration is sprayed onto a flowing water surface. The polymer precipitates out of the solution and is transferred to a rotating mandrel lying flush with the flowing surface. These precipitated polymer particles form multilayers of randomly oriented fibers resulting in a porous tube that can be used as a blood conduit.

The fabrication apparatus includes a metal lathe, a rectangular water bath, a syringe pump and an ultrasonic spray nozzle (Figure 1). A standard 5 inch metal lathe (Sears Roebuck and Co.) was modified by removing the original motor and replacing it with two DC motors. One motor controls the mandrel rotation speed and the other controls the lateral movement of the water bath-spray nozzle assembly. The spray nozzle can be positioned at a specified point above the water surface and at a specified distance from the mandrel by a clamp attached to the water bath. This assembly is mounted on the lathe stand that travels parallel to the mandrel. The ultrasonic nozzle (Sono-Tek Corp., Poughkeepsie, NY, Model PT-100) generates a spray by atomizing the polymer solution at the nozzle tip. The atomizing capability is determined by the oscillation frequency of the nozzle tip [40]. This complete fabrication assembly is contained in a fume hood to allow removal of toxic or flammable gases. Suitable polymers for this method must precipitate on contact with the non-solvent (water). We used Surethane (Cardiac Control Systems, Palm Coast, FL), a segmented polyether polyurethane, dissolved in dimethyl-acetamide (DMAC). Important fabrication variables are listed in Table 4.

METHODS FOR VASCULAR GRAFT TESTING

There is a large body of published literature on the development of methods for the physical, chemical and morphologic evaluation of vascular grafts. Test segments for these methods included PTFE or Dacron

Table 3. Methods for the fabrication of polyurethane vascular grafts.

Description	Reference
Application of composite materials technology to produce a four-layered, laminated tube from a segmented polyurethane. Authors claim that graft has anisotropic properties similar to the native vessels.	[26]
Urethane copolymer solution coated onto glass mandrels and then immersed in water to extract the solvent and to precipitate the copolymer into a uniform coating. Properties changed depending on the number of coatings applied.	[27]
Polymer solution is ejected from a syringe into an electrostatic field between a steel mandrel and the syringe. Fibers formed from the solution are collected on the rotating mandrel and eventually build up to form a porous tube.	[28]
A concentrated polymer solution is forced out of an orifice under high pressure forming a fiber, which is wound on a rotating mandrel. After several passes, a porous tube results.	[29]
Precursor skeletal materials (sea urchin spine) shaped to the desired cylindrical configuration are dipped into the polymer solution, whereupon the polymer infiltrates the microporous structure of the cylinder wall. It is then dipped into another solution which dissolves the cylindrical mold leaving a polymer replica tube for use as a graft.	[30]
Single fibers having a sticky surface are sprayed onto a rod to form a tube. The fibers can be applied in selected directions to produce a graft into the wall of which connective tissue cannot grow. Non-kinking, compliant grafts can be provided.	[31]
This method consists of extrusion of polymer solution into a former which is then dipped in a non-solvent bath to produce a foamy polyurethane tube on the former (mandrel).	[32]
A liquid polymer spray, generated by mixing polymer solution and an inert gas in a spray nozzle, is directed onto a rotating mandrel mounted on a lathe. After an appropriate number of passes, the wet tube is dried and slipped off the mandrel for use as a graft.	[33]

Table 4. Primary fabrication process variables.

• Polymer Solution Concentration (g/dl)	2–6%
• Polymer Solution Flow Rate (ml/min)	0.40–2.50
• Mandrel Rotation (rpm)	50–500
• Nozzle Traverse Speed (cm/s)	0.05–0.5
• Number of Layers (or wall thickness)	5–30

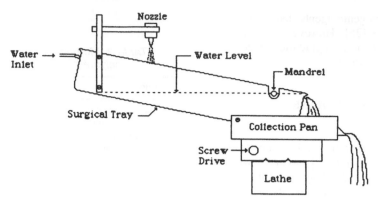

Figure 1. Schematic diagram of the precipitation–flotation method.

or Polyurethane grafts. Table 5 lists most of the graft properties measured along with the references. This list does not include methods for *in vitro* protein adsorption and *in vivo* evaluation, which are beyond the scope of this chapter. Methods used in our experiments are described in the following sections.

Surface and Wall Morphology

For wall morphology studies, circular cross sections were cut and mounted on standard aluminum stubs using superglue (cyanoacrylic). Surface morphology was studied by cutting semi-circular sections and mounting them with the surface of interest facing upward. The samples were sputter-coated with gold-palladium in a DSM-5 module positioned inside a Denton vacuum evaporator and observed using a JSM-35 (JEOL) scanning electron microscope.

Compliance

Graft compliance is a measure of its capacity to increase in volume under the influence of a given internal pressure [45]. Most published values of compliance are of the passive component (function of the tube dimensions and the wall properties) of *in vivo* arterial compliance, since the measurement of the active component (function of the vasoactive substances present in the circulating blood, muscular tone of the wall, pulse rate, age and the pulsatile component of the blood pressure) is very difficult. We designed and built an isotonic/isometric bi-axial testing apparatus [41] to measure the graft compliance, a brief description of which follows.

The experimental setup (Figure 2) consists of a temperature-controlled water bath, in which a stainless steel container is partially submerged. The container is filled with physiological salt solution and holds the graft or arterial specimen and its measurement apparatus. The specimen is mounted on grooved pin connectors between two stainless steel cantilever arms (A, B). The external diameter of the test segment is measured with a thin stainless steel cantilever leaf, to which two semiconductor strain gages are attached. A Statham P23dB pressure transducer is connected in-line for pressure measurements. As the pressure is cycled between 0–200 mm Hg, external diameter and the pressure are simultaneously recorded,

Table 5. Methods for vascular graft testing.

Graft Property	References
Compliance, elasticity, flow in grafts	[5,41–44]
Stress–strain, stress relaxation, creep	[3,5,26,45–48]
Fatigue resistance	[5,48–50]
Porosity	[45,47,48,51,52]
Water entry pressure	[47,53]
Burst strength	[3,45,47,51]
Suture retention strength, suture pullout	[3,45–47,51]
Anastomotic leak rate	[45,47,51]
Kink resistance	[45]
Surface characterization	
• SEM	[45,49,54,55]
• ESCA, FTIR	[45,56–59]
• critical surface tension	[49]

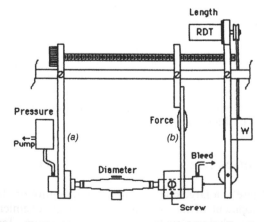

Figure 2. Compliance measurement apparatus. A, B cantilever beams.

from which compliance values are calculated at 100 mm Hg.

Compliance information can also be derived from the stress–strain relationship of a ring segment. In this experiment, a 3 mm graft ring segment is mounted between two hooks on an Instron materials testing machine. The ring segment is strained at a rate of 1 cm/min until it breaks. The load is plotted as a function of strain on a standard XY-plotter. Compliance is then calculated from the equation:

$$C = 1/E(p) = 1/[E(t) * w/r(i)] \qquad (1)$$

where $E(t)$ and $E(p)$ are the elastic moduli in the tangential and radial directions, respectively [45]. The wall thickness (w) and internal radius [$r(i)$] of the graft are known. $E(t)$ can be found by the relation:

$$E(t) = F/(A * e) \qquad (2)$$

where the force (F) and strain (e) are obtained from the load–strain information and the cross-sectional area (A) is obtained by the equation:

$$A = 2 * W(\text{at rest}) * \text{segment length} \qquad (3)$$

Permeability and Water Entry Pressure

Water permeability is often used to obtain a measure of the graft's porosity. It is commonly measured at 100–120 mm Hg, which is considered to be the mean arterial pressure for most humans. In our experiments, a graft segment is mounted on the setup shown in Figure 3, by tying it between two hollow grooved pin connectors, one attached to a stopcock and another attached to a syringe pump through a pressure transducer [53]. A balance scale weighs the collected water. Air is removed from the system by bleeding the line and graft through the stopcock. The line is then closed and the pressure increased until water appears on the outside surface for the first time. This pressure is recorded as the Water Entry Pressure (WEP). After stabilizing the pressure for 100 mm Hg, a beaker is placed under the graft to collect the water for one minute. The weight change in the beaker in one minute gives the water flow rate. Permeability is then calculated from the volume rate of flow and the graft dimensions and is expressed in ml/min/sq cm.

Burst Strength

The ability of grafts to withstand high physiologic pressures is linked to prevention of late failure due to aneurysmal dilatation. Thus it is an important design parameter and is commonly reported for commercial vascular grafts. Test segments (taken from spray coating method) of known dimensions were connected to a syringe pump through rigid tubing connectors and pressurized with distilled water. Decrease in volume of the water in the syringe was taken as equal to the in-

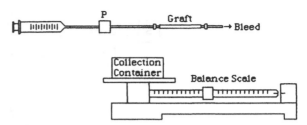

Figure 3. Schematic diagram of the apparatus for measuring the water permeability.

crease in volume of the graft. The volume changes are sufficiently slow that the increase in internal pressure can be obtained from the equilibrium relationship $(P0/V0) = (P1/V1)$, where $P0,V0$ are the initial pressure and initial volume, and $P1,V1$ are the pressure and volume, respectively, at the point of burst.

Kink Resistance

The phenomenon of kinking, seen in vascular grafts positioned across joints such as elbow and knee, is similar to the buckling phenomenon that occurs in thin-walled cylinders subjected to either an axial compressive load or bending [45]. Resistance to kinking may be expressed in several ways: the bending stress required to produce kinking of samples, the angle formed by the two segments of the tube after buckling occurred, or the radius of curvature of a cylindrical tube, on which the graft kinks when it is wrapped around it. We expressed the kink resistance in terms of the angle at which the graft kinks, which is measured with a specially designed kink tester (Figure 4) and by measuring the radius of curvature.

In the kink tester, the graft ends are connected to one port each of two three-way stopcocks. These are mounted in specially designed bearings that enable the stopcocks to rotate freely in the horizontal plane. The stationary bearing A is fixed to the frame of the setup, while the movable bearing B is mounted on the shaft of a motorized screw drive. This bearing can move toward or away from the fixed bearing at controlled speeds, the distance travelled being measured by a linear displacement transducer (L) attached to it. The inlet port of the stationary stopcock is connected to the syringe pump, with a pressure transducer connected in-line to measure the graft internal pressure. The linear transducer and the pressure transducer are both connected to an XY-plotter (Model 700, Allen Datagraph, Inc., Salem, NH).

In a typical experiment, pressure and the distance between the two ends of the graft are recorded on the plotter as the bearing spacing is reduced at a preset speed. When the graft kinks, the pressure suddenly rises, a fact which is indicated on the plotter. The distance between graft ends and the lengths of the graft segments are measured. Kink angle is then deter-

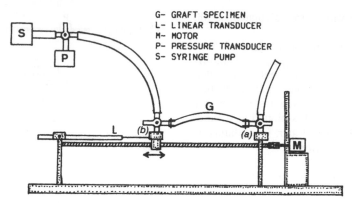

Figure 4. Schematic diagram of the kink measurement apparatus: (a) stationary bearing, (b) moving bearing.

mined from a triangle formed by the graft segments and the end-to-end distance using the law of cosines.

Resistance to kinking was also measured by wrapping a graft segment of known length around various sized cylindrical tubes until the test segment kinks. Kink resistance is then inversely related to the radius of curvature [53]. A typical setup might include ten cylinders ranging in size from 1 cm to 10 cm in diameter. Experiments were carried out with test segments 3–4 mm ID and 8 cm long.

Suture Retention Strength

Ability of the graft wall to retain the sutures is important in preventing the failure of grafts by aneurysmal dilatation and rupture. The wall should be sufficiently elastic to close the suture holes after the suture passes through. Randomly selected graft samples of 4 mm ID were tested by this method. Six to eight sutures (4–0 silk) were driven through the test segment (spray-coated grafts) approximately 1.0 mm from its end. The other end of the graft is clamped to a stand and progressively increasing weights up to 600 grams were added to the gathered ends of the suture. Observations were made for cracks, tears and stretches at the suture locations.

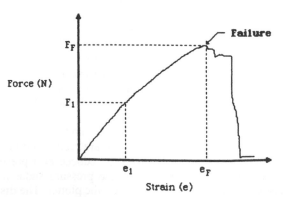

Figure 5. A typical force-extension curve obtained from the stress–strain experiments.

Suture retention strength was also measured on a materials testing machine. For our experiments [53], an Instron Model 1000 material testing machine equipped with a 5 kg load cell was used. A graft segment (FP method) of approximately 3 cm is sutured at two points, 1 mm from one end. The suture is then tied in a loop and mounted in a hook which is connected to the mobile mounting block. Then the non-sutured end of the segment is mounted into a stationary mounting block on the Instron keeping the length of the test segment constant. A strain rate of 1 cm/min was used for all measurements. The load is measured as a function of strain and plotted on a standard XY-plotter until failure occurs at one or more of the suture locations (Figure 5).

Fatigue Testing

One cause of arterial graft failure is the loss of strength of the polymeric material due, especially, to the continued pulsatile stress at the suture locations [50]. Based on a normal heart rate of 72 beats per minute, synthetic grafts should withstand at least 200 million pulsatile cycles over a five year period. The principal components of the fatigue tester (Figure 6) are a custom designed cam drive (D) to generate an arterial pressure waveform, a metal bar (C) with a freely rotating, adjustable fulcrum (F), a variable speed DC motor, a special sample holder, a liquid bath to immerse the sample for purpose of temperature control and a cam follower (G) fixed on a metal bar [45]. The specimen holder is fixed to the base inside the water bath and is stationary. One end of the graft (A) is tied to the circular end of the holder by suture, while a known number of suture holes are passed through the graft at the other end. The sutures are then connected to the hook of a calibrated spring (B) which in turn is connected by a 2–0 Prolene suture to the metal bar. The motor and the cam are positioned in such a way as to provide continuous contact to the cam follower. The waveform frequency (motor r.p.m.) is adjustable as is the waveform amplitude (fulcrum position). An appropriately sized metal ring

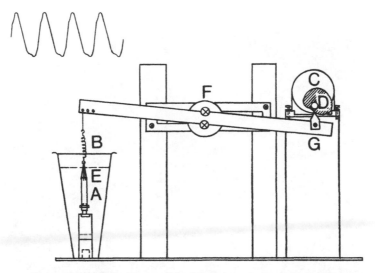

Figure 6. Schematic diagram of the fatigue tester (see text for details).

(E) is positioned between the sutures to keep the graft end from collapsing during the experiment.

In vivo Evaluation

The objective of the *in vivo* study was to evaluate the importance of surface texture and compliance mismatch on the biologic response near the anastomotic regions [45]. Vascular prostheses made from the spray-coating method [33], were implanted in the femoral arteries of dogs (six 3 mm ID and nine 4 mm ID, 4.5 cm long grafts) for four weeks. Bilateral implantation of the graft segments was carried out with the anastomotic location of smooth inner surfaces reversed on the contralateral side. Artery-to-graft compliance ratios ranged from 1.3 to 10.3. At the end of four weeks, they were perfusion-fixed and analyzed by histologic and microscopic methods to detail the events occurring near the anastomotic regions.

RESULTS

Surface and Wall Morphology

A scanning electron micrograph of a typical graft cross section from the spray-coating method is shown in Figure 7. The pores are closed celled and the wall is non-permeable to fluids. Characteristics of the grafts from the FP method are shown in Figures 8–11. These grafts can be made as permeable as desired by adjusting the fabrication process. Pore and fiber size along with their distribution and orientation, and polymer layer interconnections varied with fabrication conditions. All grafts were composed of either interconnected polymer fibers or a combination of interconnected polymer fibers and polymer film. Cross-sectional views of most graft walls showed pore sizes

ranging from 10 micrometers to 1.5 mm across the largest dimension (Figures 8,9). Pores were generally long and narrow with the long axes oriented circumferentially. The distribution of large and small pores varied widely, with inter-connections between individual fiber layers ranging from thick and dense to thin and fibrous. Inside surface patterns generally consisted of focal areas of precipitated film with a minimum number of individual fibers and no preferred fiber orientation (Figure 10). The outer wall structure consisted of large fiber bundles oriented axially, the small fibers oriented circumferentially and interconnecting the fiber bundles (Figure 11).

Compliance

Grafts of varying dimensions and physical characteristics were fabricated from three polyurethanes of interest (Pellethane, Cardiothane, and Tecoflex) using the spray coating method. Test samples made from similar fabrication conditions were selected for comparing their compliances. Tecoflex 80A had the highest compliance (0.37 ± 0.11 %/kPa) for the polymers in question, and was selected for further evaluation.

The compliance values of a set of grafts fabricated from the flotation method are shown in Table 6. All

Table 6. Mechanical properties of grafts made by flotation method.

Graft	Wall Thickness (cm)	Compliance (%/kPa)	Kink Radius (cm)
1	0.065	0.374	2.00
2	0.085	0.281	2.00
3	0.100	0.321	1.30
4	0.110	0.272	1.05
5	0.130	0.321	0.70

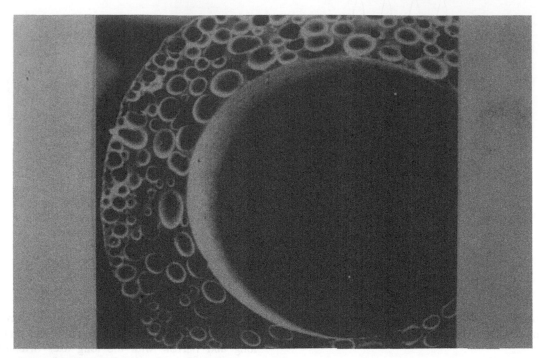

Figure 7. Scanning electron micrograph (SEM) of the cross section of a graft made from the spray-coating method (original mag. ×20).

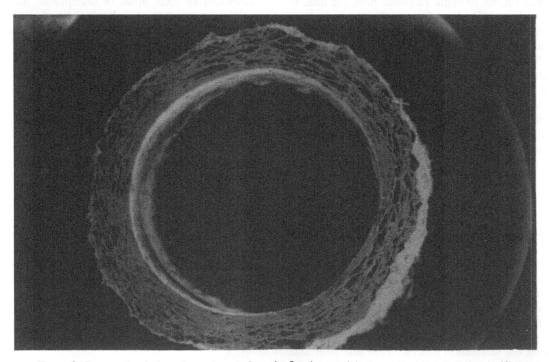

Figure 8. Cross-sectional view of a graft made from the flotation–precipitation method (original mag. ×14).

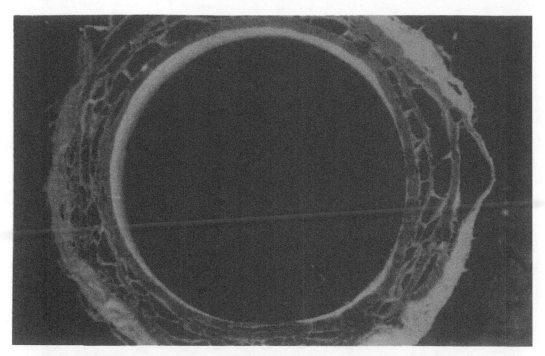

Figure 9. Cross-sectional view of another graft made from the flotation–precipitation method (original mag. × 18).

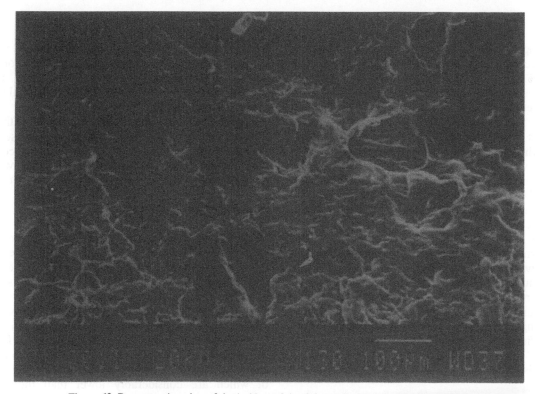

Figure 10. Representative view of the inside surface of the grafts from the flotation method.

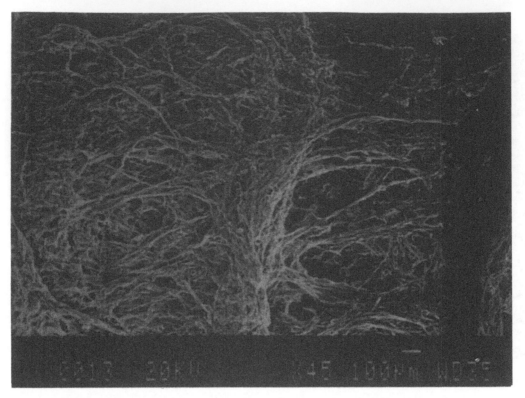

Figure 11. Representative view of the outside surface of the grafts from the flotation method.

values reported are based on a single test. Typical compliance values for these grafts varied from 0.243 to 0.752 %/kPa.

Burst Strength

Analysis of the test results (using grafts from the spray-coating method) showed that the grafts did not burst even when the initial volume increased from 0.2 ml to 11.0 ml. The resulting internal pressure was 5.04 + 0.96 MPa ($n = 3$) at maximum filling, compared to an initial pressure of 0.1 MPa. The shape of the graft did change from a cylinder to an ellipsoid at maximum filling. The graft wall underwent permanent deformation following pressure relief, when the pressure was held at this high value for more than 10–15 minutes. The data suggested that these grafts will not develop aneurysms at normal pressurization, at least during the initial period after implantation. Burst strength measurements were not made on grafts from the flotation method.

Kink Resistance

Preliminary results (grafts from the spray-coating method) suggest that increasing the radius-to-wall thickness ratio from 6 to 15 did not affect the kink angle by more than 1 degree. The speed at which the graft was bent had no effect on the kink angle, at least in the range of speeds investigated (less than 10

cm/min). Similarly, length of the specimen and internal pressure had only a small influence. These observations suggest that the kink resistance (89–91 deg.) may be constant for a particular type of material used in the graft fabrication.

The kink resistance for grafts fabricated with the flotation method is shown in Table 6. In this case, the kink resistance is represented by the radius of curvature where kinking occurred. Kink resistance values for this method varied between 0.50 to 5.00 cm.

Suture Retention Strength

Under microscopic view ($10 \times$), no cracks or tears were observed (grafts from the spray-coating method) at the suture locations, even at forces of up to 8.0 N. When forces of above 4.0 N were applied, suture holes stretched but never exceeded 1 mm in diameter. The shape of the holes under maximum load was elliptical, but closed back when the load was released. It is known that the physiological axial stretch forces in human femoral arteries are of the order 1.5 to 2.0 N and less than 3 N in canine carotid arteries [51], both of which are considerably lower than the above values.

Results of a typical suture retention test series for grafts from the flotation method are shown in Table 7. The suture holes did not break for these grafts until they were elongated more than 19% of the original length. Suture retention values varied between 1.66 to

Table 7. Physical properties for varying wall thickness flotation method (n = 1).

Graft	Wall Thickness (cm)	Suture Retention (N)	% Elong. at Suture Hole Failure	Water Permeability (ml/min/cm sq.)
1	0.065	2.541	93	0.570
2	0.085	2.315	25	0.544
3	0.100	3.605	73	0.380
4	0.110	3.178	19	0.340
5	0.130	3.968	66	0.101

4.40 N and percent elongation at failure varied up to 132% of the resting length.

Fatigue Testing of Grafts

To test the fatigue tester, an experiment was performed under the following conditions: (a) cycling rate 72 beats per minute at room temperature, (b) net axial force 2.7 newtons and (c) six 4-0 suture holes, located 3 mm from the graft end. The experiment continued for 2.2 million cycles, at which point the suture thread failed. The arterial blood pressure waveform was consistent and the instrument is suitable for *in vitro* testing. Currently, additional improvements are being made to provide automatic level control of the saline in the bath and regulation of the bath temperature, respectively. No further data is available at the time of writing this report.

Water Permeability

Water permeability values for grafts fabricated with the flotation method are listed in Table 7. These results show an inverse relationship between wall thickness and water permeability. Permeability values for this method varied between 0 to 16.45 ml/min/sq cm depending on the fabrication conditions. Grafts made from the spray-coating method are not permeable to water or fluids.

In vivo Testing

Most grafts (spray-coating method) had thrombosed at four weeks. Thrombus appeared to initiate in the host vessel (Figure 12) and progressed into the graft but it did not adhere to the graft surface. Absence of the endothelial layer on the arterial surface next to the

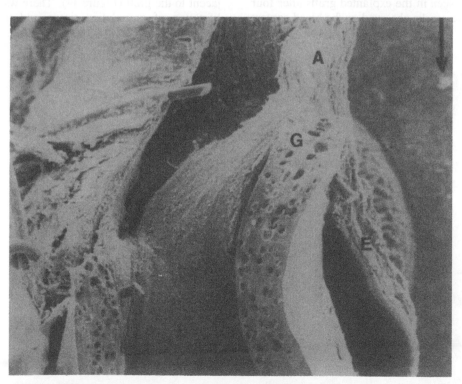

Figure 12. SEM showing the apparent origin of thrombosis from the damaged vessel wall (Dog 5, right proximal anastomosis). The adventitia of the vessel wall can be seen to proliferate into the external capsule. G—graft wall, A—artery wall, L—lumen, E—external capsule. Arrow indicates the flow direction (mag. ×22).

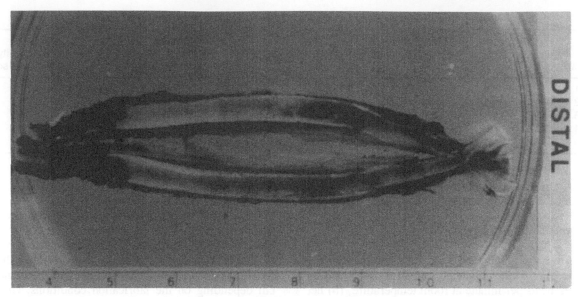

Figure 13. Gross photograph of a patent graft (Dog 4, right side), at 4 weeks. Smooth surface located at the proximal anastomosis.

prosthesis was common in all occluded grafts. In the one patent graft, the smooth surface had no visible adhering thrombus while the rough surface contained micro-thrombi adhering to the surface (Figure 13). No endothelialization of grafts was seen at any of the anastomotic sites, but the native vessel had an intact endothelium adjacent to the graft. No infiltration into wall pores was seen in the explanted grafts after four weeks, nor were cracks observed on the blood contact surface.

Data on compliance matching showed that the 3 mm ID grafts had better matching than the 4 mm ID grafts. Macroscopically, the lumen of 3 mm grafts had less thrombus compared to the 4 mm grafts. The fibrous connective tissue capsule, mainly composed of fibroblasts oriented parallel to the length of the graft, originated from the adventitia of the vessel adjacent to the graft (Figure 14). There was a local proliferation of granulation tissue and fibrosis at the anastomotic site. There was also a similar reaction

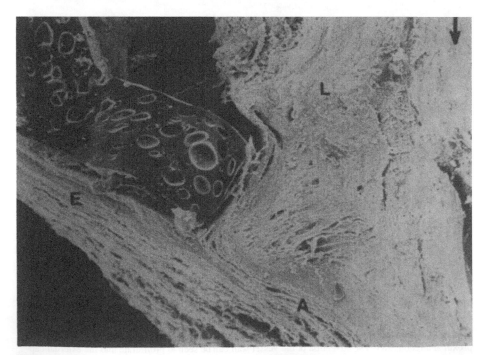

Figure 14. SEM showing the splitting of vessel wall at the anastomotic site (Dog 1, left distal). The adventitia is continuous with the external capsule. G—graft wall, E—external capsule, A—artery wall, L—lumen. Arrow indicates flow direction (mag. ×40).

along the outside of the prosthesis. However, there was no regeneration of smooth muscle or elastin (Figure 15).

DISCUSSION

We fabricated a large number of grafts (3–6 mm ID) from both the spray coating and the FP methods for the purposes of the development of physical, morphological evaluation and *in vivo* testing. However, only the grafts from the spray coating method were used in the *in vivo* evaluation.

The principal difference in grafts from the spray-coating method and other techniques is that the majority of wall pores are not interconnected in the radial direction, i.e., they are closed-celled (Figure 7). Totally or partially closed cell pores are useful for retention of the compliance of vascular grafts, as they do not allow tissue ingrowth and fluid transfer. In contrast, the FP method produces grafts with varying permeabilities as desired. Since both of these methods are based on the same apparatus, it is possible to design graft walls with open-celled and closed-celled pores which may be useful in some situations. Inside surfaces can be made smooth and non-porous, or fibrous and permeable.

In vitro Evaluation

Grafts from both spray-coating and FP methods were evaluated. For spray-coating grafts, tests in-

dicated that some of the graft properties compared favorably with those of the native vessels. These grafts are strong and elastic in nature and their properties could be varied considerably [45].

A number of 3 mm and 4 mm ID grafts were fabricated using the FP method by isolating one fabrication variable in a given experiment. The fabrication variables of interest are listed in Table 4. Results are discussed with regard to the relation between the graft characteristics and the primary fabrication variables (e.g., concentration, wall thickness and flow rate).

Polymer particle size and density on the water surface varied significantly with a change in flow rate. At low flow rates, the volume of solution per unit time at the nozzle tip was low, causing the solution to be completely atomized. This created very small and well-distributed polymer particles on the water surface, resulting in a uniform but scattered distribution of polymer fibers on the mandrel. These grafts consisted of thin layers and inconsistent interconnections between the layers. Higher flow rates introduced large amounts of film and large polymer particles on the water surface which subsequently produced grafts with thick layers and solid layer interconnections.

The effects of changing wall thickness on the permeability of grafts made from solutions of 3% and 4% concentration (w/v) are shown in Figure 16. Permeability decreased slightly with increasing wall thickness for 3% grafts. Although 4% grafts had higher permeabilities, they did not exhibit a uniform change with wall thickness, due to the difficulty in controlling the fiber organization during fabrication. Precipitated film connecting the large precipitating

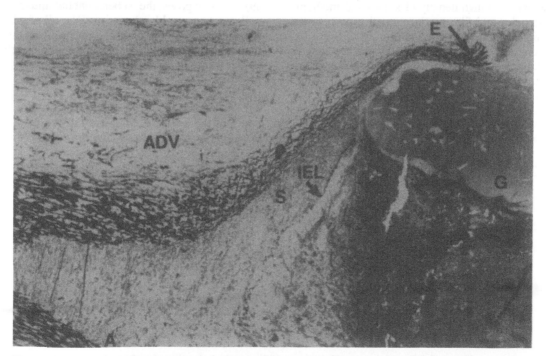

Figure 15. Histologic section of a proximal anastomosis (Dog 13, right side) showing the lack of regeneration of elastin fibers (E), at 4 weeks. Smooth muscle can also be seen on one side (SMC). G—graft wall, ADV-adventitia, A—artery wall, L—lumen. Verhoff's elastic stain (mag. ×60).

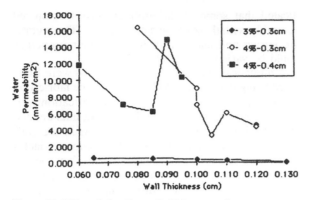

Figure 16. Effect of changing wall thickness on the water permeability, for grafts made from flotation method.

droplets was virtually absent for the 4% solution, resulting in rough and porous surface layers. The 3% solution gave a mixture of film and medium-sized droplets on the flowing surface, resulting in smoother and less porous surface layers on the graft. Because the 4% solution formed a relatively low density of large polymer droplets on the water surface, the subsequent distribution of fibers on the mandrel contained large gaps between fibers. When examined under a scanning electron microscope, 4% grafts showed areas with large pores and weak layer interconnections throughout the cross section. This caused considerable variations in the wall thickness throughout each graft (Figure 8). Electron micrographs of the 3% grafts showed more frequent, solid interconnections between layers and smaller pores. This was consistent with the polymer layer formation on the water surface, where a high density of small- and medium-sized particles and film produce small gaps between accumulated fibers on the mandrel.

One physical property affected by the changes in wall thickness and solution concentration is kink resistance. Figure 17 illustrates the effect of these fabrication variables on kink resistance. It appears that kink resistance increases with increasing wall thickness and decreasing concentration for a given ID. Grafts with thicker walls and lower solution concen-

tration (3%) had fewer weak areas because of uniform fiber distribution, which resulted in a higher kink resistance than the 4% grafts. As previously mentioned (Figure 8) it is thought that inconsistent wall structures may have contributed to the reduction of kink resistance for the 4% grafts.

In examining grafts fabricated with various solution flow rates, we found that low flow rates enhanced many of the desired graft properties. The properties affected by the solution flow rate are the kink resistance, suture retention strength and percent elongation at suture failure. Grafts fabricated with lower flow rates resulted in improved kink resistance and exhibited higher suture retention strength and percent elongation at failure, than grafts made with higher flow rates (Figure 18).

A summary of the relationships between fabrication conditions and physical properties is shown in Table 8. This table can be used as a guide in altering the fabrication variables for the purpose of obtaining desired physical properties.

In vivo Evaluation

The poor performance of the grafts (spray-coating method) in this study can be attributed to one or more of the following causes: (1) surgical trauma to the host vessel at the time of implantation, exposing the thrombus-inducing components to blood, (2) blood flow disturbances at the host–graft interface caused by inversion and eversion of the graft ends, and (3) compliance mismatch.

Damage to the internal elastic lamina was observed in focal areas near the anastomotic regions (Figure 19). This exposes the subendothelial muscular and collagen fibers to blood components, all of which are potent accelerators of platelet activation and the coagulation cascade [60]. This phenomena is clearly seen at four weeks in Figure 20, which shows fibrous tissue growing out from muscular and collagenous layers of the vessel wall.

Eversion and inversion of graft ends can occur as a result of the suture technique used, the ratio of wall thickness to graft diameter and the degree of spatula-

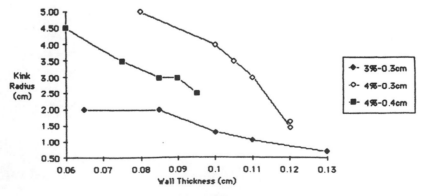

Figure 17. Effect of changing fabrication conditions on the kink radius of grafts made from flotation method.

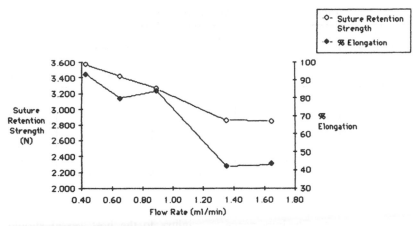

Figure 18. Effect of changing solution flow rates on the graft properties for grafts made from the flotation method.

tion employed in completing the anastomosis. The wall thickness to graft ID ratio varied between 0.07–0.13, compared to values between 0.12–0.33 for native arteries [45]. When suture ends are tied together after the anastomosis is completed, the resulting knots could have brought about the graft inversion or eversion.

Compliance matching between artery and the grafts for 4 mm ID grafts, was worse than for 3 mm ID grafts (student's t-test for difference between means, $p < 0.01$) [45]. Also, the patent graft pair had compli-

ance matching values better than the values seen in other 4 mm grafts. These observations suggest that closer matching of compliances may improve graft patency. Many workers have similarly reported that the graft patency may be a function of the mechanical compliance matching [4,6,7,10].

Of the three native vessel components, only the fibroblasts in the adventitial layer proliferated from both the proximal and distal anastomoses forming a fibrous tissue encapsulation (collar) on the graft surface. However, smooth muscle, elastin and the inter-

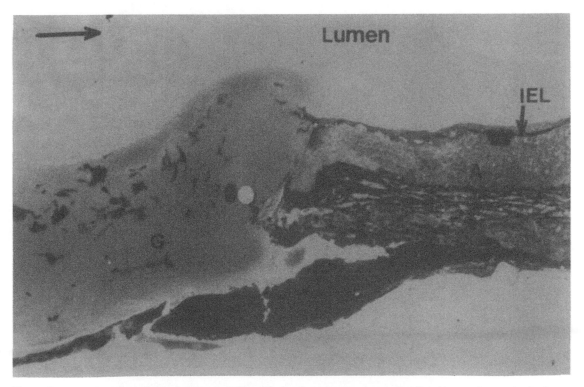

Figure 19. Histologic section of a distal anastomosis (Dog 12), showing damage to the vessel wall architecture 3 days after implantation. G—graft wall, L—lumen, IEL—internal elastic lamina, A—artery wall. Arrow indicates flow direction. Verhoff's elastic stain (mag. ×20).

Table 8. Input variable effects on graft properties.

Desired Properties \ Input Variables	Wall Thickness	Concen-tration	Polymer Flow Rate	Nozzle Traverse Speed	RPM
↑ Permeability	↓	↑	↓	↑	↑
↓ Kink Radius	↑	↓	↓	NR	↑
↑ Suture Retention	↑	↓	↓	NR	NR
↑ % Elongation	NR	NR	↓	NR	NR
↑ Compliance	NR	↑	NR	NR	↑

NR—no relationship determined.

nal elastic lamina did not regenerate. The importance of this observation in relation to prosthetic graft patency is not known.

CONCLUSIONS

We have presented a detailed description of the manufacture and testing methods for vascular grafts from polyurethanes. Grafts from both the spray-coating method and the FP method were characterized in detail. Results indicated that both grafts have some properties similar to those of native vessels. *In vivo* evaluation of the spray-coated grafts suggested that reducing compliance mismatch and minimizing injury to the host vessel should lead to improved patency. It is hoped that a combination of the two fabrication methods presented here will result in a successful, small diameter vascular prosthesis.

ACKNOWLEDGEMENTS

The authors would like to thank the Biomedical Engineering program (Drs. R. C. Eberhart and W. W. von Maltzahn) at the University of Texas at Arlington/University of Texas Southwestern Medical School where most of the work presented here was carried out. Additional thanks to Michelle Lauchner for her secretarial assistance.

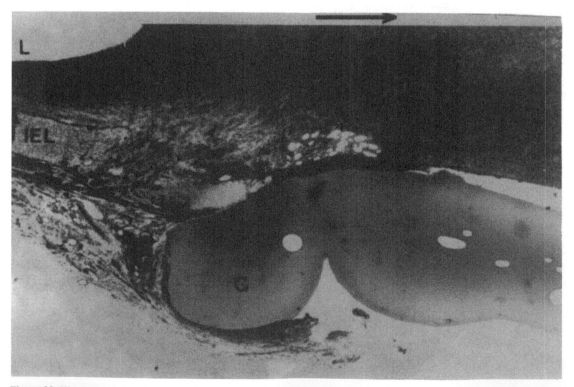

Figure 20. Histologic section of a proximal anastomosis (Dog 6) at 4 weeks, showing clearly the origin of thrombosis from the damaged internal elastic lamina. G—graft wall, L—lumen, IEL—internal elastic lamina, A—artery wall. Verhoff's elastic stain (mag. ×60).

REFERENCES

1. Voorhees, A. B., A. Jaretski and A. H. Blakemore. 1952. "The Use of Tubes Constructed with Vinyon 'N' Cloth in Bridging Arterial Grafts", *Ann. Surg.*, 135:332–336.

2. ———. 1988. *Biomed. Bus. Intl.*, 11(11):173.

3. Pourdeyhimi, B. and D. Wagner. 1986. "On the Correlation between the Failure of Vascular Grafts and Their Structural and Material Properties", *J. Biomed. Mat. Res.*, 20:375–409.

4. Clark, R. E., S. Apostolou and J. L. Kardos. 1976. "Mismatch of Mechanical Properties as a Cause of Arterial Prosthesis Thrombosis", *Surgical Forum*, 27:208.

5. Hasegawa, M. and T. Azuma. 1979. "Mechanical Properties of Synthetic Arterial Grafts", *J. Biomech.*, 12:509–517.

6. White, R., L. Goldberg, F. Hirose, et al. 1983. "Effect of Healing on Small Internal Diameter Graft Compliance", *Biomat., Med. Dev., Art. Org.*, 11(1):21–29.

7. Mehigan, D. G., B. Fitzpatrick, H. L. Browne and D. J. Bouchier-Hayes. 1985. "Is Compliance Mismatch the Major Cause of Anastomotic Arterial Aneurysms?", *J. Cardiovasc. Surg.*, 26:147–150.

8. Kinley, C. E., P. E. Paasche, A. S. MacDonald, A. E. Marble and E. R. Gozna. 1974. "Stress at Vascular Anastomoses in Relation to Host Artery: Synthetic Graft Diameter", *Can. J. Surg.*, 17:74–76.

9. Munro, M. S., R. C. Eberhart, N. J. Maki, B. E. Brink and W. J. Fry. 1983. "Thromboresistant Alkyl Derivatized Polyurethanes", *ASAIO Trans.*, 6(2):65–75.

10. Pomposelli, F., F. Schoen, R. Cohen, D. O'Leary, W. R. Johnson and P. N. Madras. 1984. "Conformational Stress and Anastomotic Hyperplasia", *J. Vasc. Surg.*, 1(4):525–535.

11. Sottiurai, V. S., J. S. T. Yao, W. R. Flinn and R. C. Batson. 1983. "Intimal Hyperplasia and Neointima: An Ultrastructural Analysis of Thrombosed Grafts in Humans", *Surgery*, 93:809.

12. Logerfo, F. W., W. C. Quist, M. D. Novak, H. M. Crayshaw and C. C. Haudenschild. 1983. "Downstream Anastomotic Hyperplasia: A Mechanism of Failure in Dacron Arterial Grafts", *Ann. Surg.*, 197(4):479.

13. DeWeese, J. A. 1978. "Anastomotic Intimal Hyperplasia", in *Vascular Grafts*. P. N. Sawyer and M. J. Kaplitt, eds. New York, NY: Appleton-Century-Crofts.

14. Lelah, M. D. and S. L. Cooper. 1986. *Polyurethanes in Medicine*. Boca Raton, FL: CRC Press, Inc., pp. 87–109.

15. ———. 1988. *Med. Dev. & Diag. Ind.*, 10(11):34.

16. Oertel, G. 1985. *Polyurethane Handbook*. New York, NY: Hanser Publishers, p. 29.

17. Kim, S. W. and J. Feijen. 1986. "Surface Modification of Polymers for Improved Blood Compatibility", *CRC Reviews in Blood Compatibility*, 1(3):229–259.

18. Eloy, R., J. Belleville, M. C. Rissoan and J. Baguet. 1988. "Heparinization of Medical Grade Polyurethanes", *J. Biomat. App.*, 2:475–519.

19. Ito, Y. 1987. "Antithrombogenic Heparin-Bound Polyurethanes", *J. Biomat. App.*, 2:235–265.

20. Jansen, B. 1987. "Chemical Modification of Polyurethanes by Radiation Induced Grafting", *J. Biomat. App.*, 1:502–532.

21. Cronenwett, J. L. and G. B. Zelenok. 1982. "Alternative Small Arterial Grafts", in *Biological and Synthetic Vascular Prostheses*. J. C. Stanley, ed. New York, NY: Grune and Stratton, pp. 595–620.

22. Stokes, K., A. Coury and P. Urbanski. 1987. "Auto-Oxidative Degradation of Implanted Polyether Polyurethane Devices", *J. Biomat. App.*, 1:411–448.

23. Thoma, R. J. 1987. "Poly(urethane) Reactivity with Metal-Ion in Calcification and ESC", *J. Biomat. App.*, 1:449–486.

24. Rodriguez, F. 1970. *Principles of Polymer Systems*. New York, NY: McGraw Hill Company, pp. 270–298.

25. Autian, J. 1979. "Toxicology of Degradation Products of Plastics", in *Corrosion and Degradation of Implant Materials*, ASTM STP 684. B. C. Syrett and A. Acharya, eds. American Society for Testing and Materials, pp. 5–19.

26. Kardos, J. L., B. S. Mehta, S. F. Apostolou, C. Thies and R. E. Clark. 1974. "Design, Fabrication and Testing of Prosthetic Blood Vessels", *Biomat., Med. Dev., Art. Org.*, 2(4):387–396.

27. Lyman, D. J. and F. J. Fazzio. U. S. Patent No. 4,173,689 issued on November 6, 1979.

28. How, T. V. U. S. Patent No. 4,552,707 issued on November 12, 1985.

29. Wong, E. W. C. U. S. Patent No. 4,475,972 issued on October 9, 1984.

30. White, R. A., E. W. White and R. J. Nelson. 1979. "Uniform Microporous Biomaterials Prepared by the Replamineform Technique", *Biomat., Med. Dev., Art. Org.*, 7(1):127–132.

31. Planck, H. and P. Ehrler. U. S. Patent No. 4,474,630 issued on October 2, 1984.

32. Charlesworth, D., E. T. White and S. Kent. U. K. Patent No. 2,130,521B issued on December 11, 1985.

33. Kowligi, R. R., W. W. von Maltzahn and R. C. Eberhart. 1985. "Manufacture and Evaluation of Small Diameter Vascular Grafts", in *Biomedical Engineering IV: Recent Developments*. B. W. Sauer, ed. New York, NY: Pergamon Press, pp. 245–248.

34. Hess, F., C. Jerusalem and B. Braun. 1983. "A Fibrous Polyurethane Micro Vascular Prosthesis", *J. Cardiovasc. Surg.*, 24:509–515.

35. Cahalan, P. T., C. M. Holmblad, R. W. Pike, Jr. and E. M. Schultz. U. S. Patent No. 4,605,406 issued on August 12, 1986.

36. Gogolewski, S. and A. J. Pennings. 1984. "Compliant, Degradable Vascular Prosthesis", in *Polyurethanes in Biomedical Engineering*. H. Planck, et al., eds. Amsterdam, Netherlands: Elsevier Science Publishers, pp. 279–285.

37. Dryer, B., T. Akutsu and W. J. Kolff. 1960. "Aortic Grafts of Polyurethane in Dogs", *J. Physiol.*, 15:18–22.

38. Hughes, H. C. U. S. Patent No. 4,728,328 issued on March 1, 1988.

39. Kowligi, R. R., W. W. von Maltzahn and R. C. Eberhart. 1988. "Synthetic Vascular Graft Fabrication by a Flotation-Precipitation Method", *ASAIO Trans.*, 14:800–804.

40. Product Information Booklet, Sonotek Corp., Poughkeepsie, New York, 12601.

41. von Maltzahn, W. W., R. R. Kowligi and R. W. Calcote. 1986. "Apparatus for Isometric and Isotonic Tests on Arterial Segments", *Proceedings of the 8th Annual IEEE/EMB Society, Fort Worth, Texas, November 7-10*, p. 1658.

42. Megerman, J. and W. M. Abbott. 1983. "Compliance in Vascular Grafts", in *Vascular Grafting*. C. Wright, ed. Boston, MA: John Wright-PSB, Inc., pp. 344–364.

43. Kowligi, R. R., W. W. von Maltzahn and R. C. Eberhart. 1986. "Small Diameter Vascular Grafts: Physical Property Evaluation", in *Biomedical Engineering V. Recent Developments*. S. Saha, ed. New York, NY: Pergamon Press, p. 125.

44. Karino, T., M. Motomiya and H. L. Goldsmith. 1982. "Flow Patterns in Model and Natural Vessels", in *Biological and Synthetic Vascular Prosthesis*. J. C. Stanley, ed. New York, NY: Grune and Stratton, pp. 153–178.

45. Kowligi, R. R. 1988. "Fabrication, Characterization and *in vivo* Evaluation of a New Type of Small Diameter Vascular Graft", Ph.D. dissertation. The University of Texas at Arlington, May 1988.

46. Boyce, B. 1982. "Physical Characteristics of Expanded Polytetrafluoroethylene Grafts", in *Biological and Synthetic Vascular Prostheses*. J. C. Stanley, ed. New York, NY: Grune and Stratton, pp. 553–561.

47. McClurken, M. E., J. M. McHaney and W. M. Colone. 1986. "Physical Properties and Test Methods for Expanded Polytetrafluoroethylene (PTFE) Grafts", in *Vascular Graft Update: Safety and Performance*. ASTM STP 898. H. E. Kambic, A. Kantrowitz and P. Sung, eds. Philadelphia, PA: American Society for Testing and Materials, pp. 82–94.

48. Edwards, W. S., R. Snyder, K. M. Botzko and J. Larkin. 1982. "Physical Design and Durability of Vascular Grafts", in *Biological and Synthetic Vascular Prostheses*. J. C. Stanley, ed. New York, NY: Grune and Stratton, pp. 179–188.

49. Baier, R. E. 1982. "Physical Chemistry of Blood–Surface Interface", in *Biological and Synthetic Vascular Prostheses*. J. C. Stanley, ed. New York, NY: Grune and Stratton, pp. 83–99.

50. White, K. A., R. S. Ward and J. S. Riffle. 1985. "Comparison of Aromatic and Aliphatic Polyetherurethanes for Biomedical Use: II. Results of Accelerated Biaxial Flex Testing at 37°C", *11th Annual Meeting Soc. Biomat., San Diego, CA. April 25-28*, p. 57.

51. Weinberg, S. L., G. B. Cipoletti and R. J. Turner. 1982. "Human Umbilical Veins: Physical Evaluation Criteria", in *Biological and Synthetic Vascular Prostheses*. J. C. Stanley, ed. New York, NY: Grune and Stratton, pp. 433–444.

52. ——. 1986. American National Standard for Vascular Graft Prostheses. Arlington, Virginia Association for the Advancement of Medical Instrumentation.

53. Calcote, R. W. 1989. "The Identification of Process Control Variables for the Fabrication of Small Diameter Vascular Grafts", M.S. Thesis, The University of Texas at Arlington, May.

54. Eberhart, R. C., M. E. Lynch and F. H. Bilge, et al. 1982. "Protein Adsorption on Polymers: Visualization, Study of Fluid Shear and Roughness Effects and Methods to Enhance Albumin Binding", *Advances in Chemistry Series*, No. 199, pp. 293–315.

55. Beahan, P. and D. Hull. 1982. "A Study of the Interface between a Fibrous Polyurethane Arterial Prosthesis and Natural Tissue", *J. Biomed. Mat. Res.*, 16:827–838.

56. Grobe, III, G. L., J. A. Gardella, Jr. and W. L. Hopson, et al. 1987. "Angular Dependent ESCA and Infrared Studies of Segmented Polyurethanes", *J. Biomed. Mat. Res.*, 21:211–229.

57. Ratner, B. D., S. C. Yoon, A. Kaul and R. Rahman. 1984. "Control of Polyurethane Surface Structure by Synthesis and Additives: Implications for Blood Interactions", in *Polyurethanes in Biomedical Engineering*. H. Planck et al., eds. Amsterdam, Holland: Elsevier Science Publishers, pp. 213–229.

58. Ratner, B. D. 1983. "Surface Characterization of Biomaterials by Electron Spectroscopy for Chemical Analysis", *Annals of Biomed. Eng.*, 11:313–336.

59. Martz, H., G. Beaudoin, R. Paynter, M. King, D. Marceau and R. Guidoin. 1987. "Physicochemical Characterization of a Hydrophilic Microporous Polyurethane Vascular Graft", *J. Biomed. Mat. Res.*, 21:399–412.

60. W. J. Williams, E. Beutler, A. J. Erslev and M. A. Lichtman, eds. 1983. *Hematology, 3rd Ed*. New York, NY: McGraw Hill Book Company, p. 1279.

28

Antithrombogenic pO₂ Sensor for Continuous Intravascular Oxygen Monitoring

SHOJI NAGAOKA, Ph.D.*
MASATO MIKAMI*
YOSHIHIRO SHIMIZU*

ABSTRACT: An antithrombogenic pO₂ sensor (An-thron® pO₂ sensor) was produced by coating a hydropholic heparinized polymer (Anthron) on an etched epoxy composite, ultra-microelectrode (microhole electrode). From the *in vitro* tests, both the response time and stability were satisfactory under the conditions of a 20 μm thickness of Anthron coating and a depth up to 100 μm for the microhole.

Additionally, results of *in vivo* tests without systemic heparinization demonstrated that a stable real-time measurement of the intravascular pO₂ value was possible for a long period without thrombus formation or adhesion of blood components on the electrode surface of the Anthron pO₂ sensor. Moreover, the measured data agreed with those from the blood gas analyzer.

Due to the thick thrombus formation on the electrode surface, the control (non-coated) sensor was unable to measure the intravascular pO₂, even for a short period of time.

INTRODUCTION

Measurements of the information from the living body are important for clinical and medical treatment; consequently, a continuous monitoring sensor that is safe and highly reliable is required. In particular, in the clinical tradition, blood gas levels are very important. Monitoring the oxygen partial pressure (pO₂) of the artery shows the state of the respiratory function and is considered to be a powerful means of predicting medical treatment for the functional impediment, determining the cause of it, selecting suitable medical treatments, and evaluating the efficiency of them [1,2].

At the present time, there are three types of apparatuses available for the purposes listed above: 1) the

blood gas analyzer (Auto analyzer) using a polarographic type oxygen electrode, 2) the percutaneous sensor which measures oxygen concentration from the skin surface, and 3) the oximetry which can measure the degree of oxygen saturation by utilizing an optical method. However, the monitoring can only be carried out intermittently, or the information at local parts cannot be obtained. Thus, they are not satisfactory for clinical demands. For this reason, the development of a catheter-type invasive sensor has been attempted [3,4]. However, many problems remain, such as the size or shape of the sensor, the deterioration of the sensor function due to thrombus formation or the adhesion of proteins, and the necessary revisions on the measurement deviation (drift). In view of the above factors, a hydrophilic heparinized polymer, Anthron, demonstrating excellent antithrombogenicity for long periods (due to continuous release of heparin from its surface into the bloodstream) [5–7] is combined with a solid-state, polarographic oxygen sensor, composed of the etched epoxy composite ultra-microelectrode arrays, and is applied to the development of a safe and highly reliable electrochemical sensor for continuous intravascular oxygen monitoring.

EXPERIMENTAL

Fabrication of Microhole Electrodes

The concept of a microhole array with the resulting cylindrical well controlling diffusion has been demonstrated [8].

A bundle of one thousand filaments of high-strength carbon fibers (Torayca T-300, 1 K, diameter 6.93 μm) was pulled through a resin bath of polymeric binder material consisting of 97 parts epoxy (Chissonox 221, Yuka Shell, Tokyo, unless otherwise stated) and 3 parts BF-monoethylamine. The resin-impregnated fibers were wound onto a wooden spool. The impregnated yarn was then cured in an air-heated dryer at

*Medical Devices & Diagnostics Dept., Toray Industries, Inc. Head Office: 2-1, Nihonbashi-muromachi 2-chome, Chuo-ku, Tokyo 103, Japan

103°C for 30 minutes. A needle-type composite was obtained.

This composite was placed into a mixed solution containing acetone/propanol (1/1) to remove contamination from the surface, cut into a 5–11 mm length, and one end of the cut composite was tied around a lead wire. This was coated with a conductive adhesive (silver paste) and hardened at 100°C for 30 minutes. The component was then combined with a 19 Gauge polyurethane catheter, and after that, the tip of the component was polished to a mirror surface.

After polishing, the component was rinsed with de-ionized water and carefully wiped. Diameters of the microelectrode arrays were 0.3 mm for one thousand pieces of fibers. The polished section was immersed in a 2 mM sulfuric acid solution containing 0.2 M sodium sulfate and anodically etched at a constant current greater than 800 mA per cm. The depth of the etching was nearly proportional to the amount of charge added, and the limit of etching was about 500 μm. The depths of the microholes were measured by an optical microscope or a scanning electron microscope. After standing at −0.6 V (vs. SCE) for one hour, it was plated with platinum in the usual manner (plating liquid was purchased from Tanaka Kikinzoku, Tokyo). Scanning electron micrographs of the

cross-sectioned view of the microhole showing the etched carbon fiber surface revealed that the thickness of the platinum layer on the etched carbon fibers was about 0.5 μm and the layer was uniform (Figure 1).

Anthron Coating

Figure 2 shows a schematic representation of heparinized hydrophilic polymer, Anthron. Prior to the heparinization, a quaternary graft polymer was dissolved in 5% concentration THF, coated by the solvent cast method on the sensor (made in the previous section), and dried at 60°C. The thickness of the polymer coating was about 20 μm. After drying, the sensor was immersed in an aqueous solution containing 2 wt% heparin at 60°C for 24 hours, and heparinized. Thus, an antithrombogenic electrochemical sensor for intravascular oxygen monitoring (Anthron pO_2 sensor) was obtained. The control pO_2 sensor used was not coated with Anthron.

Electro-Chemical Measurements

The pO_2 sensor and a reference Ag/AgCl electrode were inserted into a tube in which a physiological saline solution was circulated at a constant flow rate at

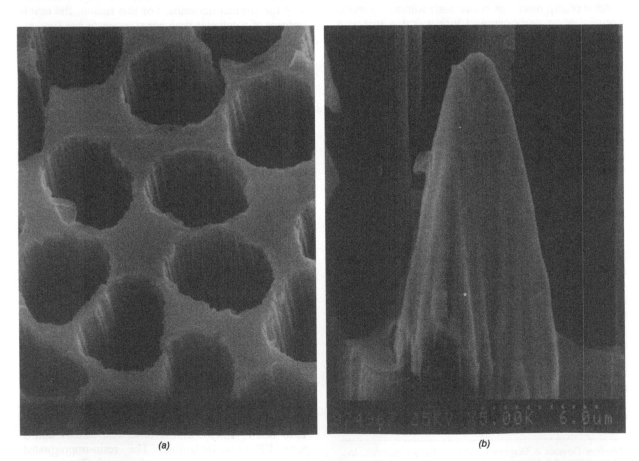

(a)   *(b)*

Figure 1. Scanning electron micrographs of a microhole electrode: (a) the surface of a microhole electrode; (b) a cross-sectioned view of a microhole showing the platinized carbon fiber.

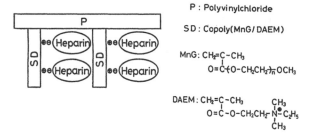

P : Polyvinylchloride

S D : Copoly(MnG/DAEM)

MnG: $CH_2=C-CH_3$
        $O=C(O-CH_2CH_2)_{\overline{n}}OCH_3$

DAEM: $CH_2=C-CH_3$ CH_3
          $O=C-O-CH_2CH_2-\overset{\bullet}{N}-C_2H_5$
                                      CH_3

Figure 2. Schematic representation of the heparinized hydrophilic polymer, Anthron.

37°C. The applied voltage between the two electrodes was 0.6 volts. After the output became stable, the flow rate was varied. During this time, the output was recorded and the effect of the flow rate on the output was investigated. The response time (t_{90}) was defined as the time it took to reach 90 percent of the steady state current between an air-sparged solution and a nitrogen-sparged solution.

Animal Experiments

Rabbits weighing 2–3 kg were used. Under general anesthesia, the pO₂ sensor was inserted by the cut-down method from the femoral artery and placed into the descending aorta. The reference electrode (Ag/AgCl electrode) was wrapped with gauze soaked in physiological saline solution, placed in the abdominal subcutaneous, and the pO₂ in the artery was measured when the potential between the two electrodes was ap-

plied at 0.6 volts. Additionally, a sampling of arterial blood was conducted, and the pO₂ was measured separately using a blood gas analyzer.

After two days of measurements, sodium heparin (200 ug/kg) was given to the animal intravenously. The animal was killed by acute exsanguination from the right femoral artery. The aorta from the ascending to abdominal region was exposed by a long median thoracoabdominal incision and opened longitudinally. The thrombus formation on the pO₂ sensor was observed by scanning electron microscopy (SEM). Specimens for SEM observation were fixed with 1% glutaraldehyde in 0.2M phosphate buffer, pH 7.4, and stained with a 1% OsO₄ solution. Specimens were dehydrated in a graded series of ethanols and amylacetate, then critical-point dried with carbon dioxide and spattered with gold palladium. The examination was performed with a JSM-50A SEM (JEOL, accelerating voltage: 15 kV).

RESULTS AND DISCUSSION

Flow Dependence and Response Time of Anthron pO₂ Sensor

Figure 3 shows the flow dependence of the measured electric current values (relative values) of the sensors before and after Anthron coatings, and the microhole's depths of the sensors were 50, 100 and 200 μm. If the depth of the microhole is larger than 100 μm for the Anthron-coated sensor, it was confirmed that the flow rate variation shows less than

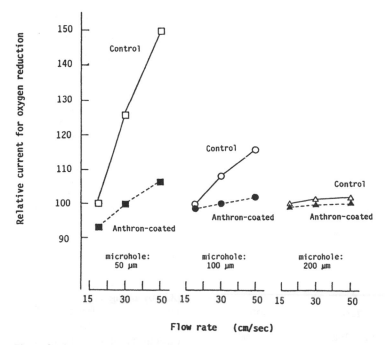

Figure 3. Flow dependence of the current for oxygen reduction (relative value) in a physiological saline solution at 37°C for control and Anthron-coated pO₂ sensor with a microhole depth of 50, 100 and 200 μm.

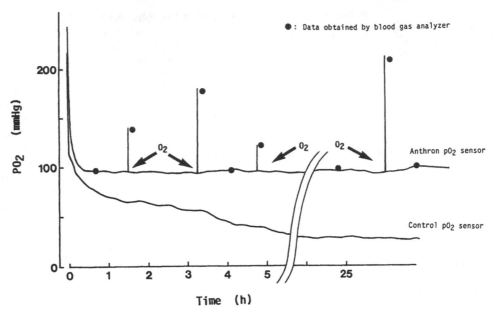

Figure 4. A typical registration period, demonstrating tracings from a control and Anthron pO₂ sensor. The arrows indicate increase of oxygen administration by the respirator.

2–3% experimental error. In addition, from the separate experiments, it has been shown that the measured electric current values were not influenced by the flow directions (parallel or counter-current) at all for the Anthron-coated sensor with microholes having 100 μm depth. Morita et al. reported that it is necessary that the microhole depth for the microhole electrode sensor (the control sensor) should require more than 200 μm to obtain a stable electric current which is not affected by the flow rate [8].

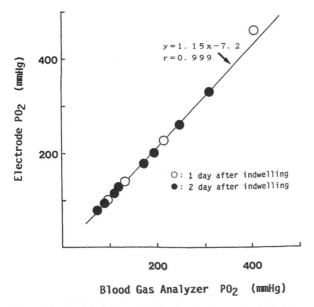

Figure 5. Comparison of pO₂ values obtained by Anthron pO₂ sensor (Electrode pO₂) and blood gas analyzer.

As shown in Figure 3, it was clarified that by using the Anthron coating, a sensor with a microhole depth of 100 μm has a stability equivalent to that of the non-Anthron-coated control sensor with a microhole depth as deep as 200 μm. However, in the sensor with no microhole (the depth is 0 μm), even if coated with Anthron, the measured electric current values have time variation (drift) and function is not stabilized.

These results suggest that even though coated with Anthron, the microhole is effective and necessary to decrease the effect of the flow rate on the electric current and to stabilize it.

Anthron pO₂ sensor catheters with microhole depths of 0, 50, 100 and 200 μm were made and the results of the response times are shown in Table 1. As the depth of the microhole increases, the response time becomes longer. In a clinical setting, the necessary response time is within 30 seconds [9]. The response time of the Anthron pO₂ sensor with a microhole depth of 100 μm is 25.3 seconds, so this requirement is fully satisfied.

From the above results, the Anthron pO₂ sensor with a microhole depth of 100 μm was confirmed to satisfy the stability and response time necessary for clinical use.

Animal Experiments of Anthron pO₂ Sensor

Figure 4 shows the measured values of the arterial pO₂ by using control and Anthron pO₂ sensors in *in vivo* tests as a function of time and compares them with those obtained from the blood gas analyzer. The directional arrows show the oxygen inspiration by using the respirator. The control (non-coated) pO₂ sensor took longer than one hour for stabilization from

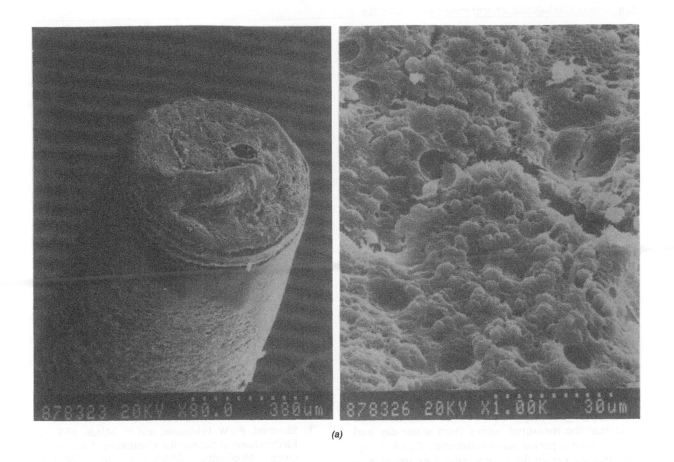

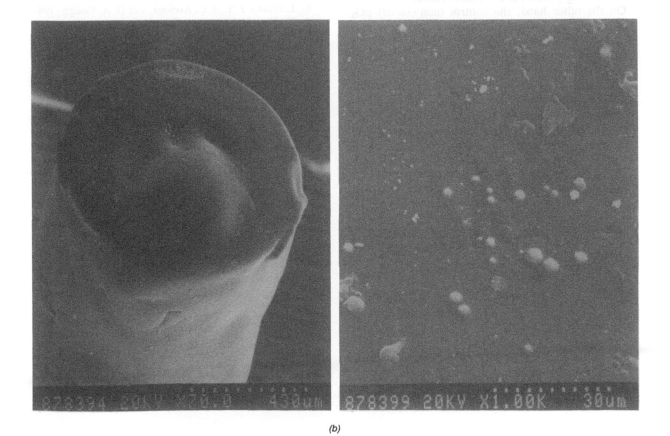

Figure 6. Scanning electron micrographs of the electrode surface after a 2 day *in vivo* test: (a) control pO_2 sensor; (b) Anthron sensor.

Table 1. Observed response times (t_{90}) of Anthron pO_2 sensor.

h^*	(μm)	0	70	100	200
t_{90}	(sec)	15.0	17.0	25.3	47.9

*h is depth of microhole.

starting the measurement and the measurement became impossible because there was no response with respect to the oxygen concentration variation within a few hours. On the other hand, the Anthron pO_2 sensor was stabilized within about 30 minutes, and there was good response with respect to the oxygen concentration variation when the oxygen was inspired. In addition, the measured values (ca. 100 mmHg) of the arterial pO_2 for the self respiration were in agreement with the literature data reported [1]. This measured value was remarkably equivalent to those obtained from the blood gas analyzer. Figure 5 shows the detailed relationship of pO_2 measured by the blood gas analyzer and by the Anthron pO_2 sensor. The two data indicate a linear relationship and the coefficient of correlation, r is 0.999, therefore the two data have a remarkably good equivalence. Furthermore, it was clear that the measured values from a one-day and from a two-day period are not different. This fact suggests that the sensor does not require the correction of drift for long periods and remains stable.

On the other hand, the control (non-coated) pO_2 sensors always presented a marked drift towards falsely low pO_2 values shortly after their insertion into the arterial circulation.

A scanning electron micrograph for the tip of the sensing part is shown in Figure 6. A thick thrombus layer was formed on the sensing part of the control (non-coated) pO_2 sensor tip, which prevents the diffusion of blood oxygen to the electrode surface, and deteriorates the stability and response time of the sensor remarkably.

On the other hand, at the tip of the Anthron pO_2 sensor, the formation of thrombus was hardly recognizable. For this reason, the stability in the living body is excellent and, at the same time, even the initial period responding time (25.3 sec) of the *in vitro* tests is slightly delayed compared to the control (non-

coated) pO_2 senosr (20.1 sec), the function of sensor remained stable for a long period.

CONCLUSION

Using a microhole electrode which is coated with hydrophilic heparinized polymer (Anthron), it was possible to measure the intravascular pO_2 stability for a long period of time in *in vivo* tests without systemic heparinization.

The result is explained by the fact that thrombus formation and the adhesion of blood components on the electrode surface affect the oxygen diffusion to the electrode and deteriorate the function of pO_2 sensor. The Anthron coating is able to suppress these phenomena.

REFERENCES

1. Goeckenjan, G. 1979. "Continuous Measurement of Arterial pO_2", *Biotelemetry Patient Monitg.*, 6:51.
2. Hagihara, B., F. Ishibashi, and T. Sugimoto. 1981. "Intravascular Oxygen Monitoring with a Polarographic Oxygen Cathode", *J. Biomed. Eng.*, 3:9.
3. Eberhard, P., W. Fehlmann, and W. Mindt. 1979. "An Electrochemical Sensor for Continuous Intravascular Oxygen Monitoring", *Biotelemetry Patient Monitg.*, 6:16.
4. Lucisano, J. Y., J. C. Armour, and D. A. Gough. 1987. "*In Vitro* Stability of an Oxygen Sensor", *Anal. Chem.*, 59:736.
5. Mori, Y. and S. Nagaoka. 1978. "The Effect of Released Heparin from the Heparinized Hydrophilic Polymer on the Process of Thrombus Formation", *Trans. Am. Soc. Artif. Intern. Organs*, 24:736
6. Nagaoka, S. and Y. Noishiki. 1989. "Development of Anthron, an Antithrombogenic Coating for Angiographic Catheters", *J. Biomaterials Applications*, 4:3.
7. Nagaoka, S., M. Mikami, and Y. Noishiki. 1989. "Evaluation of Antithrombogenic Thermodilution Catheter", *J. Biomaterials Applications*, 4:22.
8. Morita, K. and Y. Shimizu. 1989. "Microhole Array for Oxygen Electrode", *Anal. Chem.*, 61:159.
9. Buttner, W. 1979. "Practical Experiences with the Routine Application of the Intravascular pO_2 Probe", *Biotelemetry Patient Monitg.*, 6:44.

29

Woven Velour Polyester Arterial Grafts with Polypropylene Wrap: A Cosmetic Change or Improved Design?

ROBERT GUIDOIN*,1
MARTIN KING**
MARIE THERRIEN*
YVAN DOUVILLE*
ELISABETH DEBILLE*
DENIS BOYER*
SOPHIE SIMONEAU*
LUC TREMBLAY*

ABSTRACT: Over the last 30 years since the development of the first woven and knitted polyester arterial grafts, the technology has moved through a number of generations to new and specialized variants, each claiming to have improved handling and healing characteristics or greater durability when implanted in specific sites.

In an attempt to overcome the difficulties of tissue infiltration experienced by woven prostheses, several models of "woven velour" grafts have recently emerged as novel hybrids between the woven and knitted velour structures. Two new prototype woven velour prostheses of different water permeabilities (LP, low-porosity and HP, high-porosity) with an externally wound polypropylene monofilament wrap, were exposed to a series of in vitro tests with the objective of assessing their novel structures, physical properties and surface chemistry, and to compare them against five other commercial woven prostheses.

The LP graft appears to have a strong and stable structure with superior suture retention strength in all three directions, and water permeability near that of the Meadox Woven Double Velour graft. On the other hand, the HP graft has excessively high water permeability for a woven graft, low suture retention strength, and low bursting strength. This evidence suggests that the clinical use of these grafts as vascular substitutes would appear to be safe for the LP but not necessarily so for the HP.

1Correspondence: Dr. Robert Guidoin, Ph.D., Biomaterials Institute, Room Fl-304, St-François d'Assise Hospital, 10 de l'Espinay, Quebec City, QC GlL 3L5, Canada.

*Department of Surgery, Laval University, Biomaterials Institute, St. François d'Assise Hospital and Department of Surgery, St. Sacrement Hospital, Quebec City, Canada

**Visiting Professor, permanent address: Clothing and Textiles, Faculty of Human Ecology, The University of Manitoba, Winnipeg, MB R3T 2N2, Canada

INTRODUCTION

Polyester (Dacron®) and polytetrafluoroethylene (Teflon®) arterial prostheses have emerged as the most stable and durable synthetic blood conduits. They have demonstrated their ability to resist major changes in dimensions during prolonged in vivo implantation [1,2]. Nowadays, polytetrafluoroethylene grafts are only available as microporous tubes [3]. On the other hand, the polyester grafts are only available in textile form.

Currently, there are six types of commercial Dacron® textile grafts, namely the woven, woven velour, knitted, knitted velour, externally supported and impregnated types [4]. In spite of a number of developments in the field of vascular surgery over recent years, the woven polyester graft remains the first choice of many vascular surgeons for the replacement of large- and medium-caliber arteries, for the resection of aneurysms, and sometimes for the treatment of atherosclerotic occlusive disease [5]. The main advantage of using the woven type is clearly recognized: its tightly woven structure readily controls and limits the amount of blood that seeps through the prosthetic wall. This advantage is of particular importance during certain cardiovascular procedures such as ruptured aneurysms, or major thoraco-abdominal repairs when systemic heparinization is frequently required [6]. Nevertheless, the long-term fate of woven textile grafts appears to have two major shortcomings; namely, their propensity to fray when cut and their limited healing capacity [7]. This latter limitation appears to be related to the poor attachment of the pseudo-intima to the smooth, and relatively impermeable fabric surface.

In an attempt to overcome these deficiencies, researchers at IMPRA, Inc., Tempe, Arizona, have developed two new woven prototype polyester prostheses with two novel design features. Firstly, they have used a satin weave to create an external velour effect at the fabric surface. It is claimed that this rougher, more permeable surface will encourage tissue infiltration and hence improve intimal attachment and the graft's ability to heal. The second feature involves the addition of a fine polypropylene monofilament that is wrapped spirally around the outside of the prosthesis and thermally bonded at the base of the crimps. It is believed that by holding the filaments in place, this spiral wrap will reduce the degree of fraying at cut ends and improve the suture retention strength of the graft.

Two versions of this device have been developed; an LP product (low-porosity model) with a nominal water permeability of 200 ml/cm²/min and an HP product (high-porosity model) with a nominal water permeability of 1000 ml/cm²/min. The LP graft is available commercially as the IMPRA PolyPLUS 200®; the HP graft is not commercially available. It is proposed that the importance of these developments be evaluated and the performance of these two models be compared using systematic and standardized *in vitro* and *in vivo* protocols. This chapter describes the structure, physical properties and surface chemistry of the virgin grafts and compares them to a number of other commercial woven polyester arterial prostheses.

MATERIALS AND METHODS

Graft Selection

Two models, manufactured by IMPRA, Inc., Tempe, Arizona, U.S.A., were made available for this investigation. The LP product with a nominal water permeability of 200 ml/cm²/min, was identified as the low-porosity model, while the HP product with 1000 ml/cm²/min nominal water permeability was referred to as the high-porosity model. They were compared with six other woven devices which are commercially available; namely, the Cooley Verisoft® and Woven Double Velour® (Meadox Medicals Inc., Oakland, NJ, U.S.A.), the Woven DeBakey Soft® (Bard Cardiosurgery Division, Billerica, MA, U.S.A.), the Woven Vascutek® (Vascutek Ltd., Inchinnan, U.K.), and the Ochsner 200® and Ochsner 500® prostheses (Intervascular Inc., Clearwater, FL, U.S.A.).

Fabric and Yarn Characteristics

Fabric and Yarn Structure

The specimens were exposed to osmium tetroxide vapor and metallized with gold-palladium to improve their conduction and facilitate observation of the fabric and yarn structures and the surface morphology of the filaments in a Jeol JSM 35CF scanning electron microscope at a 15 kV accelerating voltage. These observations provided information about the type of weave and the type of yarn, as well as details of the woven designs, which are presented as point diagrams and cross-sectional diagrams showing the sequence of yarn interlacements.

Woven Fabric Count

The tightness of a woven structure is measured by the frequency of yarns lying in both directions. By viewing the prostheses flattened between glass slides through an optical stereoscopic microscope at 20 times magnification, the number of warp yarns (ends per cm width) and the number of weft yarns (picks per cm length) were counted for each sample.

Porosity

Porosity, which is to be distinguished from water permeability, refers to the proportion of void space or pores within the boundary of a solid material compared to its total volume [8]. Values, usually expressed in percent, can vary theoretically from 0%, for a solid plastic membrane or sheet without pores, to 100%, for all air and no solid material. The following equation was used to calculate porosity values, P, for the eight prostheses in the study [9]:

$$P = 100\left[1 - \frac{M}{100hd_f}\right]$$

where M = mass per unit area of prosthesis wall (g/m²), h = thickness of prosthesis wall (mm), d_f = density of polyester filaments (g/cm³). Values for the mass per unit area and the thickness were measured using standard methods [10]. The density of the polyester filaments was assumed to be 1.38 g/cm³, as reported in the literature [11].

Filament Diameter

Individual filaments were removed from the prostheses, and the diameters of 20 specimens selected at random from each type of yarn were measured using an optical microscope at 400 times magnification with a micrometer eyepiece previously calibrated against a stage micrometer. The level of delusterant particles incorporated into the filaments during manufacture was also observed using light field microscopy.

Nominal Linear Density

The coarseness of a yarn is measured in units of mass per unit length. The higher the value in decitex (decigrams per kilometer), the thicker or coarser the yarn. Having measured the average filament diameter, D, in μm, and counted the number of filaments in the yarn, n, and assuming that the filaments have a circular cross section, then the yarn's nominal linear density is estimated by:

$$\text{Nominal linear density (dtex)} \cong \frac{n\pi d_f}{100}\left[\frac{D}{2}\right]^2$$

These calculated values were confirmed by gravimetric measurements on known straightened lengths of yarn exceeding 1 meter removed from each direction of the prostheses and extended on a crimp tester to remove the residual crimp.

Physical Properties

Water Permeability

This property, often mistakenly referred to as "water porosity" in the medical literature, represents the rate of flow of water through the wall of the dry prosthesis mounted in a flat condition with the crimps removed [12]. Values were obtained following the standard method [10], except that the volume of water that passed through a 1 cm² area of the prosthesis wall under an applied pressure gradient of 16 kPa (120 mm Hg) was collected and measured for each of the first 5 minutes of the test [8].

Bursting Strength

Measurements of bursting strength were carried out using a Hoffman-Turner mini-probe tester in a compression cell mounted on an Instron Model 1130 tensile tester [10]. Five specimens of each prosthesis were clamped over an 8.1 mm diameter hole using a rubber O-ring measuring 12.6 mm in diameter. A 6.4 mm diameter cylindrical probe with a hemispherical end was forced through each clamped specimen at a constant rate of 100 mm/min. The maximum force was recorded in newtons.

Dilation

The propensity of the grafts to dilate under static internal pressure was measured by the Optiddiac system [13]. This instrument permits a tubular prosthesis to be mounted over a tubular latex membrane and to be held between two clamps, one of which is fixed and supplies air pressure, while the other, running on a low-friction track, applies a constant longitudinal tension of either 113 g (0.25 lb) or 454 g (1 lb) to the specimen. As the air pressure was increased from 0 to 45 kPa (0 to 340 mm Hg), the increase in diameter was measured to the nearest 0.1 mm using a cathetometer. After repeating the test, the average increase in diameter of the graft was calculated at the 16 kPa (120 mm Hg) level, the standard pressure recommended for measuring the internal diameter of vascular prostheses.

Elongation

The ability of the grafts to stretch longitudinally was measured using an Instron Model 1130 tensile tester. Five specimens of each tubular graft were clamped and extended by the cross-head moving at a speed of 100 mm/min. Following five pre-conditioning loading/unloading cycles between 0 and 480 g so as to establish a more stable hysteresis curve, the amount of elongation was recorded for a loading cycle up to 454 g (1 lb). This load approximates that recommended in the standard for measuring the usable length of woven vascular prostheses [10].

Suture Retention Strength

Suture retention strength measurements of the grafts were also made using an Instron Model 1130 tensile tester with a cross-head speed of 100 mm/min [10,14]. The specimens were cut with scissors or with a cautery to form squares (15 mm × 15 mm) with one corner bevelled at 45°. Tests were conducted on each specimen at 45°, parallel and perpendicular to the longitudinal axis of the prosthesis. A specially constructed pair of clamps was used to hold each test specimen in the tester. They are provided with a groove to allow a 4–0 stainless steel suture to pass through the wall of the prosthesis exactly 2 mm from the cut edge. The force required to pull the suture from the graft was measured in newtons and the average for 5 specimens from each prosthesis was calculated.

Chemical Properties

Surface Chemistry

The prostheses, as received, were cut into coupons so that their surface chemistry could be evaluated by X-ray photoelectron spectroscopy, otherwise referred to as ESCA. The spectra were obtained on a Lab MK2 made by Vg Scientific featuring a MgKα beam. Survey scans were recorded to identify the levels of various contaminants. Then, high resolution scans were made of the carbon 1s and the oxygen 1s peaks [15]. Each of these peaks was resolved into its components, namely, carbon bound to (a) carbon and hydrogen (C−C), (b) one oxygen atom (C−O), (c) two oxygen atoms (O−C=O), and oxygen bonded to (d) one carbon atom (C−O) and (e) one oxygen and one carbon atom (O−C=O).

Level of Extractables

The identification of extractable finishes and contaminants present on the surface of the prostheses as received were undertaken using established standard procedures for textile products [16]. From each prosthesis, samples approximately 5 grams in weight were exposed to a series of multiple quantitative extractions with different solvents using 5 solvent cycles in a Soxhlet apparatus. The sequence of solvents in increasing order of polarity was as follows: hexane, 1,1,1-trichloroethane, methanol, water and 0.1N hydrochloric acid. The mass of each extract was determined gravimetrically following evaporation of the respective solvents to dryness, and the level of extractable material was expressed as a percentage of the mass of the original sample.

RESULTS

Fabric and Yarn Characteristics

Woven Design

Details of the woven fabric structures of the two prototypes under evaluation and six control grafts are presented in Table 1. Photomicrographs of the internal and external surfaces of the virgin prostheses can be seen in Figures 1–8. Point diagrams of the woven designs and cross-sectional views of successive warp yarns of four of the different structures are presented in Figures 9–12. Figure 13 illustrates the type of weave found in the two Ochsner prostheses.

It is noteworthy that the two prototype grafts have woven structures that contain alternating satin and plain interlacements similar to the Woven Double Velour prosthesis. However, that is as far as the similarity goes. While the Woven Double Velour has a 6/4 satin weave with the 6 pick floats on the external surface and the 4 pick floats on the internal surface (Figures 4 and 12), the prototype grafts have a 3/1 satin weave. Consequently, the 3 pick floats are present only on the external surface [Figures 1(b), 2(b), 9(b) and 10(b)], and the internal surface maintains an appearance similar to the 1/1 plain weave of the Cooley Verisoft, the Woven DeBakey Soft and the Woven Vascutek [Figures 1(a), 2(a), 3, 5, 6].

In fact, the two prototype grafts have virtually identical woven designs. The only difference found is the reversed order for the third and fourth ends (Figures 9 and 10), but this is of no significance. Both can be described as having a woven external velour structure. This is different from all the control grafts including the Ochsner prostheses which contain a pair of leno warp yarns every seventh and eighth end (Figures 7, 8 and 13). These two crossing ends are referred to as the "standard" warp, which is never raised during weaving, and the "doup" warp, which is raised for every pick, alternating first to the left and then to the right of the "standard" warp. Leno weaves are less likely to fray than plain or satin weaves. Consequently it was thought that the inclusion of this weave in a vascular prosthesis might lead to improvements in suture retention strength.

Polypropylene Wrap

The presence of the external polypropylene wrap can be seen in Figures 1 and 2. This spirally wound monofilament which measured about 100 µm in diameter (similar to a 5/0 suture), appears to have been thermally bonded to the external surface during the crimping stage of production.

Fabric Structure

Table 1 lists the major fabric characteristics. It shows that the two prototype grafts are unique because their walls are thicker and heavier (higher mass per unit area) than any of the six controls. Comparison of the woven fabric counts points to an identical number of ends per cm for the LP prototype and the Woven Double Velour grafts. With fewer picks per cm, one might assume that the LP prototype would be lighter and thinner than the Meadox Medicals Velour prosthesis. This is not the case because of the use of coarser (higher linear density) warp and weft yarns.

Table 1. Characteristics of the woven fabric structure.

	IMPRA Low Porosity	IMPRA High Porosity	Meadox Cooley Verisoft	Meadox Woven Double Velour	Bard Woven DeBakey Soft	Woven Vascutek	Inter-Vascular Ochsner 200	Inter-Vascular Ochsner 500
Type of weave(s)	3/1 satin + 1/1 plain	3/1 satin + 1/1 plain	1/1 plain	6/4 satin + 1/1 plain	1/1 plain	1/1 plain	1/1 plain + leno	1/1 plain + leno
Ends per cm								
—satin	36	32	0	36	0	0	0	0
—plain	36	32	58	36	52	56	42	42
—leno	0	0	0	0	0	0	14	14
—total	72	64	58	72	52	56	56	56
Picks per cm	29	25	35	38	32	30	21	21
Mass per unit area (g/m²)	273*	186*	152	184	154	175	185	142
Thickness (mm)	0.51	0.43	0.27	0.32	0.26	0.29	0.32	0.26
Porosity (%)	61.2	68.7	59.2	58.3	57.1	56.3	58.6	60.6

*Including polypropylene wrap.

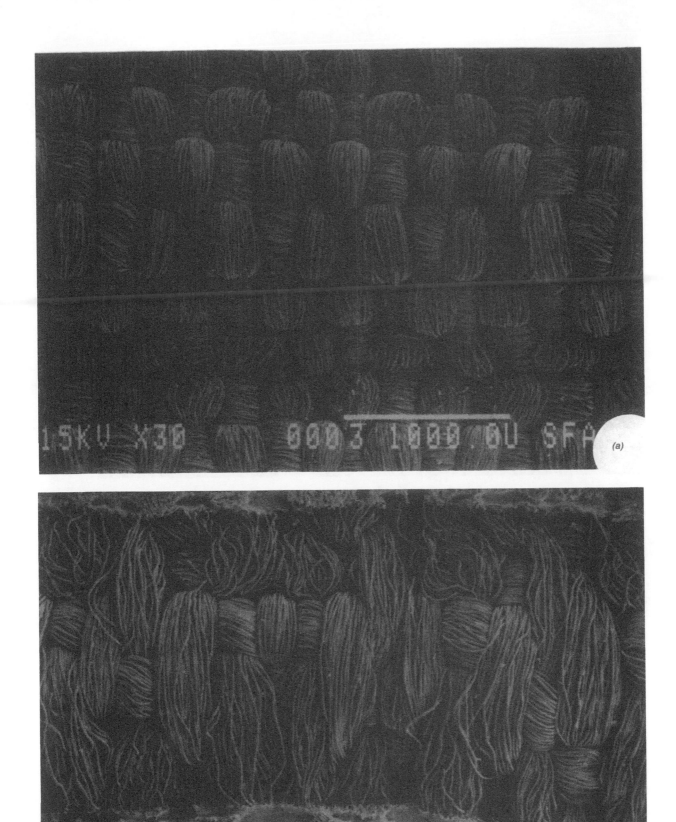

Figure 1. Photomicrographs of IMPRA LP graft: (a) internal surface; (b) external surface with polypropylene wrap.

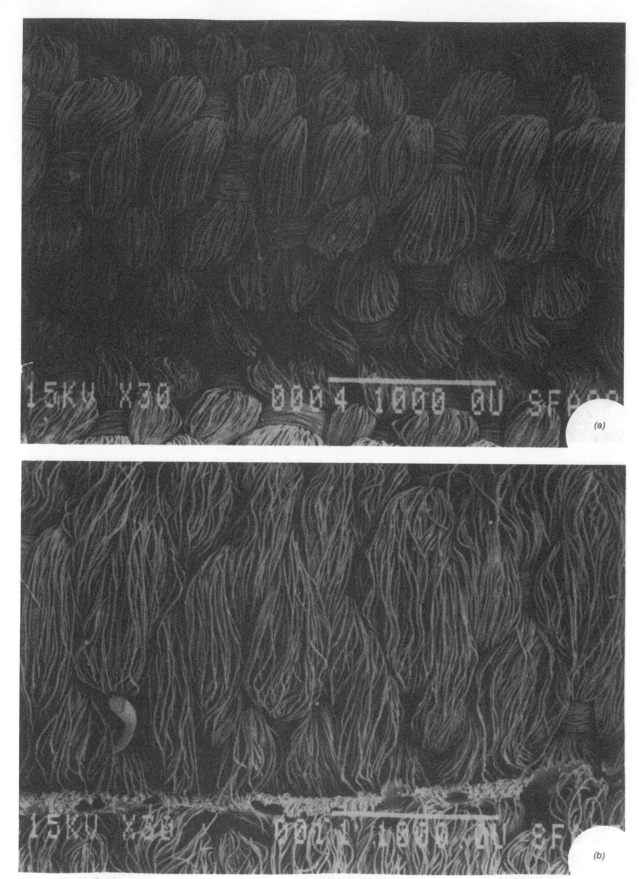

Figure 2. Photomicrographs of IMPRA HP graft: (a) internal surface; (b) external surface with polypropylene wrap.

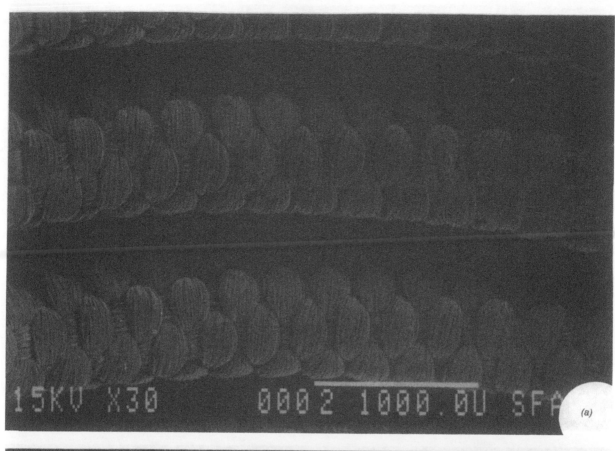

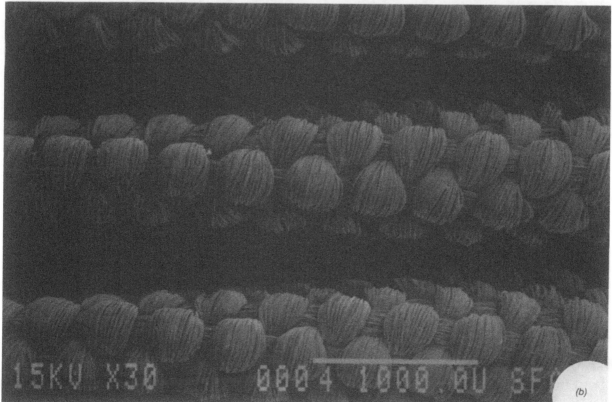

Figure 3. Photomicrographs of Meadox Cooley Verisoft graft: (a) internal surface; (b) external surface.

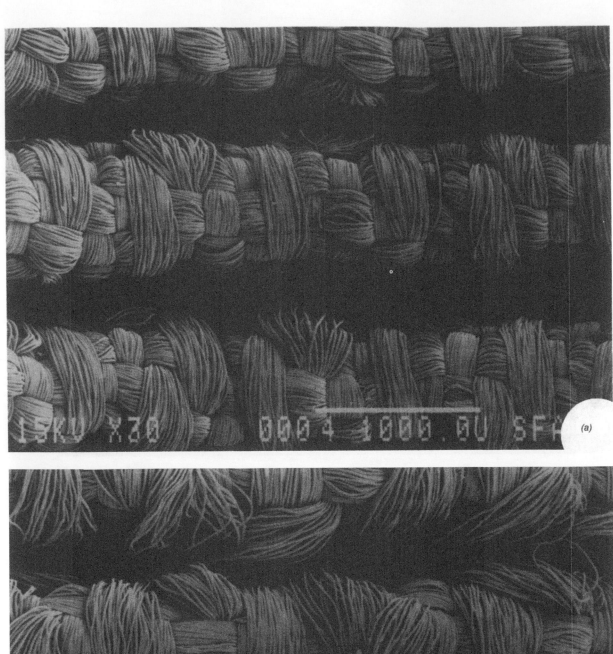

Figure 4. Photomicrographs of Meadox Woven Double Velour graft: (a) internal surface; (b) external surface.

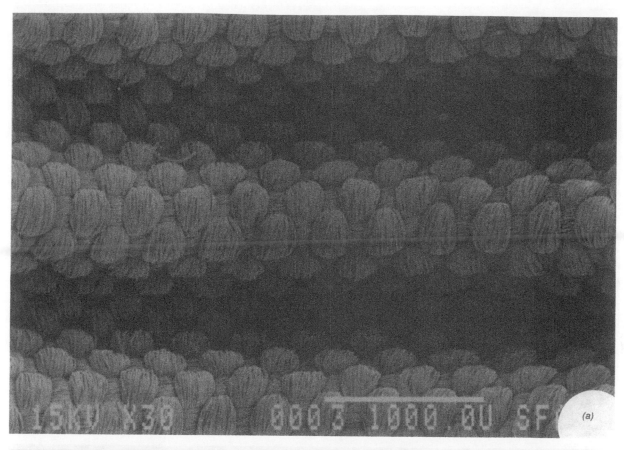

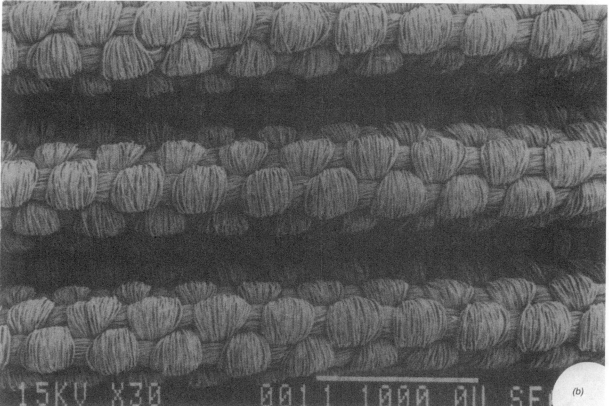

Figure 5. Photomicrographs of Bard Woven DeBakey Soft graft: (a) internal surface; (b) external surface.

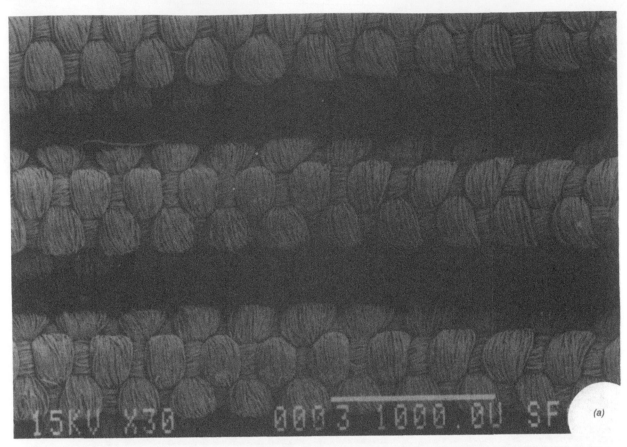

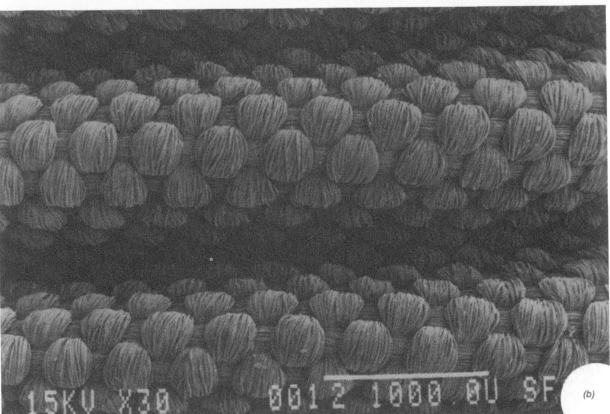

Figure 6. Photomicrographs of Woven Vascutek graft: (a) internal surface; (b) external surface.

458

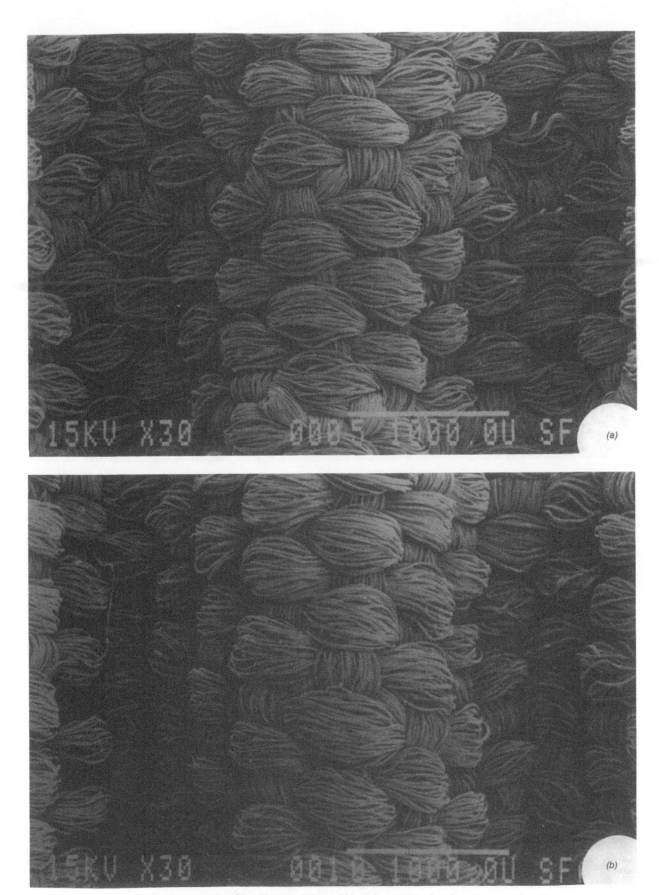

Figure 7. Photomicrographs of InterVascular Ochsner 200 graft: (a) internal surface; (b) external surface.

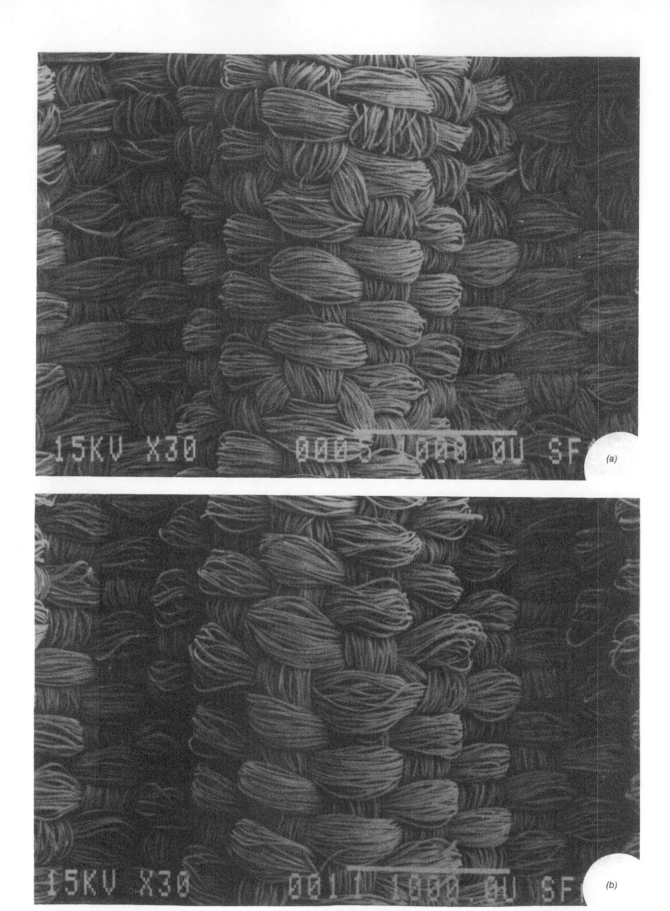

(a)

(b)

Figure 8. Photomicrographs of InterVascular Ochsner 500 graft: (a) internal surface; (b) external surface.

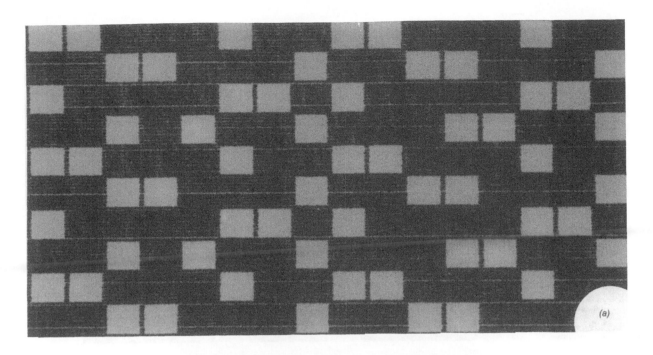

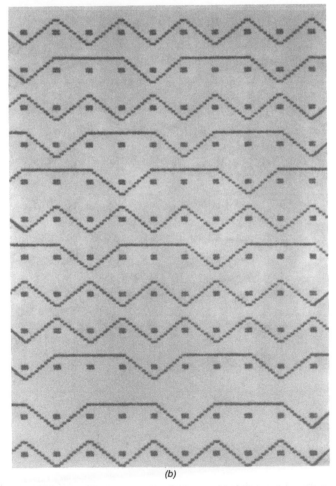

Figure 9. IMPRA LP graft. (a) Point diagram showing sequence of interlacements of 16 warp ends (black) and 10 picks (white) in a paired 3/1 satin and 1/1 plain weave. (b) Cross-sectional views of same 16 warp ends showing sequence of plain and satin interlacements.

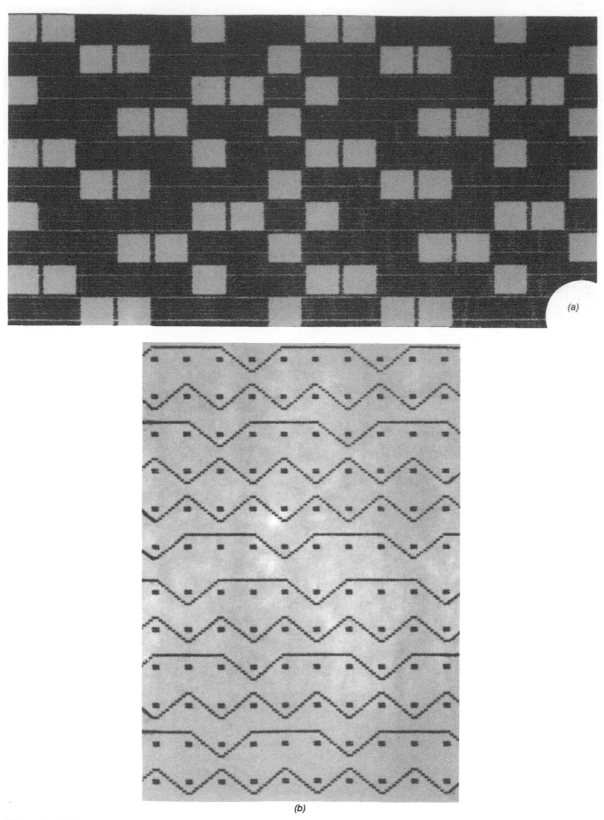

Figure 10. IMPRA HP graft. (a) Point diagram showing the sequence of interlacements of 16 warp ends (black) and 10 picks (white) in a paired 3/1 satin and 1/1 plain weave. (b) Cross-sectional views of same 16 warp ends showing sequence of plain and satin interlacements.

462

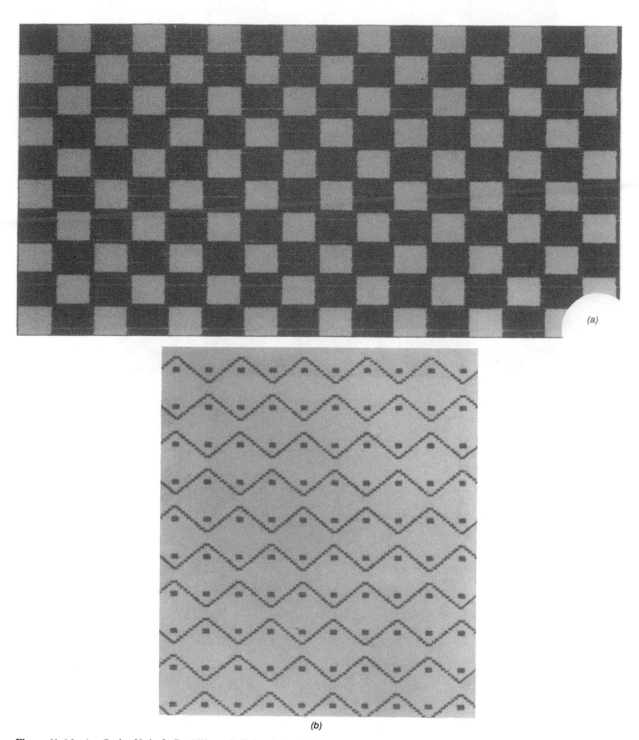

(a)

(b)

Figure 11. Meadox Cooley Verisoft, Bard Woven DeBakey Soft and Woven Vascutek grafts. (a) Point diagram showing sequence of interlacements of 16 warp ends (black) and 10 picks (white) in a 1/1 plain weave. (b) Cross-sectional views of same 16 warp ends showing the sequence of plain weave interlacements.

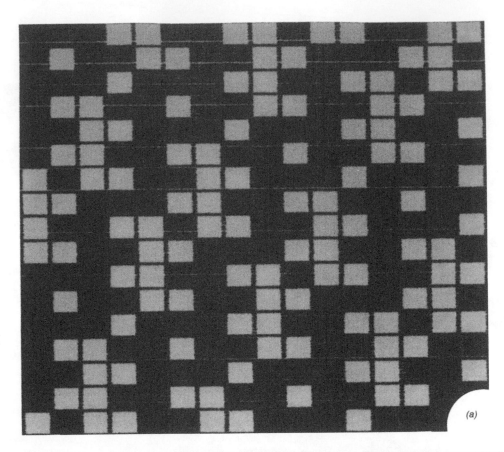

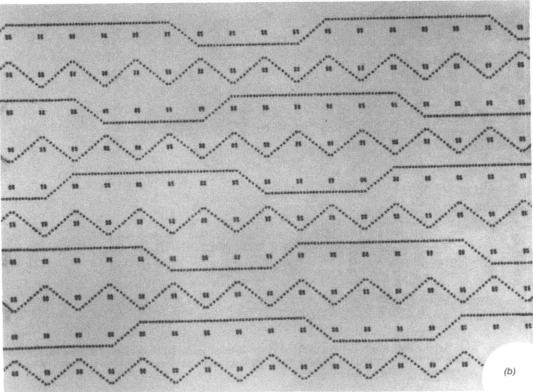

Figure 12. Meadox Woven Double Velour graft. (a) Point diagram showing sequence of interlacements of 16 warp ends (black) and 17 picks (white) in an alternating 6/4 satin and 1/1 plain weave. (b) Cross-sectional views of first 10 warp ends from left showing sequence of satin and plain interlacements.

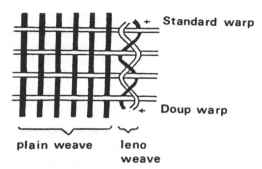

Figure 13. Diagram of InterVascular Ochsner 200 and Ochsner 500 weave showing one repeat of 1/1 plain weave (6 ends) and leno weave (2 crossing ends).

Yarn Characteristics

Table 2 shows that IMPRA have used texturized polyester yarns with similar filament diameter, delusterant level and filament count as Meadox Medicals. The main difference between their products, in addition to the different woven designs, is the different linear densities of the yarns and the woven pick counts. The weft yarn in the LP prototype is about three times as coarse as that of the HP prototype, Cooley Verisoft, Woven Double Velour and Woven Vascutek devices. This accounts for the thicker and heavier wall. In contrast, the low pick count (25

picks/cm) combined with the fine linear density of the weft yarn (105 dtex) explains why the HP prototype graft has a significantly higher porosity than any of the seven other grafts tested.

The yarns used to weave the Vascutek and Ochsner grafts appear to originate from a different source. They are spun using 50 and 34 hole spinnerets, respectively. In addition, the diameter of the Ochsner filaments is significantly larger than those of the other six prostheses.

Physical Properties

Water Permeability

The mean volumes of water collected over the first 5 minutes of the test for five different specimens have been plotted in Figure 14. While the equation of each curve can be calculated so that the theoretical value of the virgin material (at zero time) can be extrapolated, the means and standard deviations quoted in Table 3 correspond to the water permeability during the first minute of the test.

With a value of 905 ml/min/cm², the HP prototype graft has the highest water permeability for any existing woven polyester prosthesis [8]. A value of 312 ml/min/cm² for the LP prototype graft is higher than most of the controls. The Ochsner 500® has a water permeability of 530 ± 109 ml/min/cm². Other cur-

Table 2. Yarn characteristics.

	IMPRA Low Porosity	IMPRA High Porosity	Meadox Cooley Verisoft	Meadox Woven Double Velour	Bard Woven DeBakey Soft	Woven Vascutek	Inter-Vascular Ochsner 200	Inter-Vascular Ochsner 500
Type of multifilament yarn								
—warp, plain	texturized	texturized	flat	flat	texturized	texturized	texturized	texturized
—warp, satin/leno	texturized	texturized	—	texturized	—	—	texturized	texturized
—weft	texturized	texturized	flat	flat + texturized	texturized	texturized	texturized	texturized
Nominal linear density (dtex)								
—warp, plain	210	210	190	105	170	180	285	190
—warp, satin/leno	210	210	—	120	—	—	95	95
—weft	315	105	100	105 + 120	170	90	190	190
Filament count								
—warp, plain	108	108	108	54	108	100	102	68
—warp, satin/leno	108	108	—	54	—	—	34	34
—weft	162	54	54	54 + 54	108	50	68	68
Filament diameter (μm)								
—warp, plain	13.2 ± 0.6	12.8 ± 0.6	13.0 ± 0.5	13.5 ± 0.7	11.6 ± 1.1	12.8 ± 1.2	16.4 ± 1.4	16.8 ± 1.9
—warp, satin/leno	13.9 ± 0.6	13.2 ± 0.8	—	14.4 ± 0.6	—	—	16.5 ± 2.3	16.3 ± 1.5
—weft	13.8 ± 0.7	13.7 ± 0.6	13.3 ± 0.5	{ 13.5 ± 0.8 / 14.4 ± 0.4	12.5 ± 1.2	13.2 ± 0.5	17.2 ± 1.9	15.8 ± 0.6
Delusterant level								
—warp, plain	semi-dull	semi-dull	semi-dull	semi-dull	bright	semi-dull	semi-dull	semi-dull
—warp, satin/leno	semi-dull	semi-dull	—	semi-dull	—	—	semi-dull	semi-dull
—weft	semi-dull	semi-dull	semi-dull	{ semi-dull / semi-dull	bright	semi-dull	semi-dull	semi-dull

WATER PERMEABILITY
FOR EACH MODEL

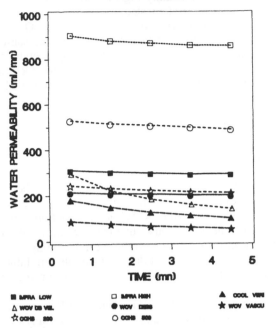

Figure 14. Mean volume of water collected during first 5 minutes of water permeability test.

rent commercial polyester woven prostheses with either a regular plain weave or a low-porosity plain weave have water permeability values of less than 250 and 100 ml/min/cm², respectively [8].

Bursting Strength

The mean and standard deviation for each prosthesis is tabulated in Table 3 and illustrated in Figure 15. The two prototype grafts give the highest and lowest bursting strengths respectively of all 8 types tested.

This is a reflection on the size and hence the strength of the weft yarns. The coarse 315 dtex weft yarn in the LP prototype provides a superior bursting strength of 454 N, whereas the fine 105 dtex yarn in the HP prototype can only support 187 N.

Dilation

The average increases in external diameter associated with increasing the internal pressure of the grafts under 113 g and 454 g tension are plotted in Figures 16 and 17. The mean values at 120 mm Hg are listed in Table 3. None of the prostheses tested exceeded 2.2% dilation, which is consistent with woven grafts and significantly less than the results observed with knitted grafts [17].

Elongation

Table 3 and Figure 18 show the relative amounts of elongation experienced by the different grafts under 454 g (1 lb) longitudinal tension. Despite the inclusion of the external polypropylene wrap, both prototype prostheses elongated readily giving mean values of 88 and 126%. Only the Cooley Verisoft with 108% elongated in the same range.

Suture Retention Strength

The results are listed in Tables 4 and 5. Note that they are subdivided into two means and standard deviations (where applicable) depending on whether the suture or the prosthesis broke during the test. The overall mean values for each prosthesis cut with scissors, regardless of the type of failure, are plotted in Figure 19. Those where grafts were cut with a cautery are plotted in Figure 20. The use of a cautery did not significantly change the suture retention strength of any of the grafts.

The LP prototype prosthesis supported the highest

Table 3. Physical properties.

Property	Units	IMPRA Low Porosity	IMPRA High Porosity	Meadox Cooley Verisoft	Meadox Woven Double Velour	Bard Woven DeBakey Soft	Woven Vascutek	Inter-Vascular Ochsner 200	Inter-Vascular Ochsner 500
Water permeability	ml/min/cm²	312 ± 15	905 ± 67	181 ± 21	395 ± 18	216 ± 38	89 ± 7	245 ± 42	530 ± 109
Bursting strength	N	454 ± 13	187 ± 17	211 ± 13	276 ± 4	366 ± 8	209 ± 1	268 ± 20	259 ± 8
Dilation at 120 mm Hg & 113 g tension	%	0.5	1.9	0.2	2.0	0.2	0.5	0.5	1.2
Dilation at 120 mm Hg & 454 g tension	%	0	2.2	0	0	0	0.4	0.5	1.5
Elongation at 454 g tension	%	88	126	108	75	44	46	40	37

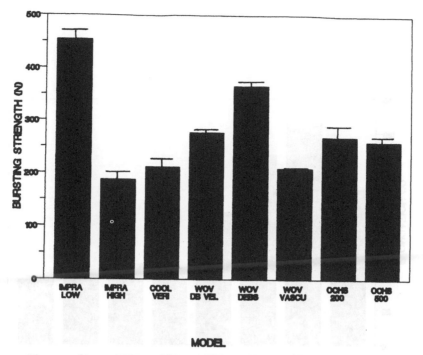

Figure 15. Bursting strength results.

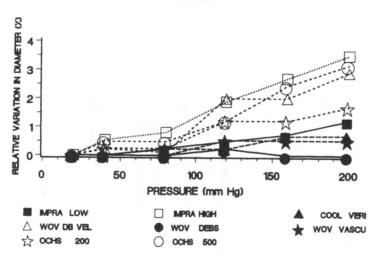

Figure 16. Dilation results (T = 113 g).

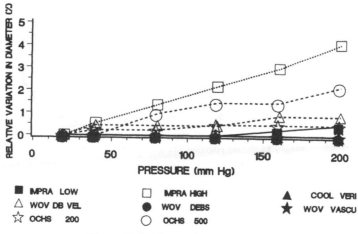

Figure 17. Dilation results (T = 454 g).

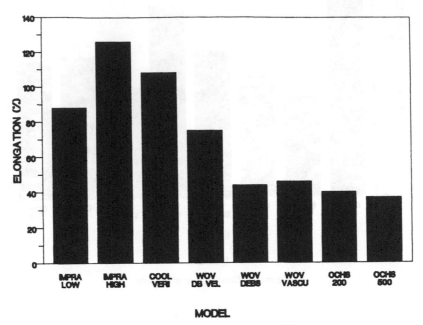

Figure 18. Elongation results (T = 454 g).

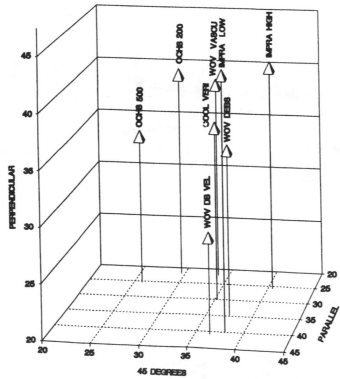

Figure 19. Suture retention strength results (scissors cut).

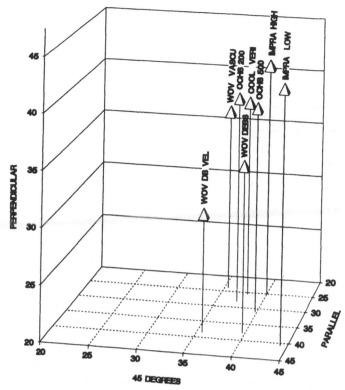

Figure 20. Suture retention strength results (cautery cut).

suture retention strength with an overall mean value for all 3 directions in excess of 40 N. In addition, only 17% of the failures were due to that of the prosthesis. Another graft that gave a superior performance was the Bard Woven DeBakey Soft. Its mean suture retention strength values were above 34.7 N in all 3 directions with or without a cautery. The HP prototype gave a result of only 25.4 N in the parallel direction.

Only the Ochsner 200 prosthesis gave an even worse performance.

Chemical Properties

Surface Chemistry

The results of the ESCA survey scans (Table 6) show that the level of contaminants was greater on the

Table 4. Suture retention strength (scissors).

Prosthesis	Parallel Direction		Perpendicular Direction		45° Direction		Frequency of Prosthesis Breaks (%)
	Suture Break (N)	Prosthesis Break (N)	Suture Break (N)	Prosthesis Break (N)	Suture Break (N)	Prosthesis Break (N)	
IMPRA Low Porosity	39.7 ± 1.6 80%	40.3 20%	42.8 ± 2.9 100%	—	40.6 ± 2.7 60%	34.2 ± 3.5 40%	20
IMPRA High Porosity	39.4 20%	22.3 ± 4.7 80%	40.7 ± 1.4 · 100%	—	40.2 ± 0.3 80%	41.6 20%	33
Meadox Cooley Verisoft	—	29.9 ± 3.2 100%	36.8 20%	35.7 ± 1.5 80%	—	35.2 ± 3.7 100%	93
Meadox Woven Double Velour	40.9 ± 1.8 100%	—	—	28.6 ± 2.3 100%	38.3 ± 0.5 60%	34.0 ± 0.8 40%	47
Bard Woven DeBakey Soft	—	34.8 ± 1.8 100%	37.8 ± 1.7 40%	33.2 ± 1.2 60%	—	37.5 ± 4.4 100%	87
Woven Vascutek	40.0 ± 0.1 40%	38.2 ± 2.5 60%	—	30.7 ± 6.1 100%	38.5 ± 0.1 40%	31.8 ± 10.7 60%	73
InterVascular Ochsner 200	—	21.9 ± 5.9 100%	39.4 ± 7.9 80%	38.6 20%	42.2 20%	26.4 ± 8.6 80%	67
InterVascular Ochsner 500	—	25.5 ± 3.3 100%	39.2 20%	32.6 ± 2.7 80%	—	25.9 ± 6.6 100%	93

Table 5. Suture retention strength (cautery).

Prosthesis	Parallel Direction		Perpendicular Direction		45° Direction		Frequency of Prosthesis Breaks (%)
	Suture Break (N)	Prosthesis Break (N)	Suture Break (N)	Prosthesis Break (N)	Suture Break (N)	Prosthesis Break (N)	
IMPRA Low Porosity	43.6 ± 2.5 60%	36.3 ± 1.1 40%	42.5 ± 2.9 100%	—	44.3 ± 1.5 100%	—	13
IMPRA High Porosity	—	25.1 ± 5.4 100%	41.3 ± 3.1 100%	—	40.8 ± 3.8 60%	38.9 ± 1.5 40%	47
Meadox Cooley Verisoft	—	25.6 ± 1.8 100%	36.8 ± 1.1 40%	38.4 ± 0.8 60%	41.1 ± 3.0 40%	35.8 ± 1.3 60%	73
Meadox Woven Double Velour	42.0 20%	37.7 ± 3.8 80%	—	30.5 ± 2.4 100%	37.6 ± 0.8 80%	27.4 20%	67
Bard Woven DeBakey Soft	39.1 ± 0.5 40%	37.0 ± 3.9 60%	—	34.8 ± 2.7 100%	40.1 ± 1.1 60%	39.1 ± 3.4 40%	67
Woven Vascutek	—	24.0 ± 3.5 100%	37.1 ± 0.2 60%	35.6 ± 1.8 40%	36.8 ± 1.1 40%	34.5 ± 2.6 60%	67
InterVascular Ochsner 200	—	28.2 ± 1.6 100%	38.7 ± 2.8 100%	—	38.3 ± 0.9 60%	35.6 ± 2.1 40%	47
InterVascular Ochsner 500	—	31.0 ± 1.4 100%	38.0 ± 1.1 80%	40.3 20%	39.8 ± 1.5 100%	—	40

Table 6. ESCA survey scans.

Prosthesis	Surface	C (%)	N (%)	O (%)	F (%)	Si (%)	Na (%)	Ca (%)	Mg (%)	K (%)	P (%)	S (%)	Cl (%)
IMPRA Low Porosity	Internal	73.7	—	24.7	—	1.6	—	—	—	—	—	—	—
	External	70.7	0.4	23.3	—	2.9	1.0	—	—	—	—	—	1.7
IMPRA High Porosity	Internal	75.9	—	23.0	—	0.8	0.2	—	—	—	—	—	—
	External	80.0	—	16.2	—	0.7	0.7	—	—	—	—	—	2.2
Meadox Cooley Verisoft	Internal	77.1	—	22.6	—	—	0.2	—	—	—	—	—	—
	External	75.4	1.1	21.8	—	0.8	0.6	—	—	—	—	0.2	0.1
Meadox Woven Double Velour	Internal	73.9	—	25.3	—	0.5	0.3	—	—	—	—	—	—
	External	70.9	0.4	26.1	—	1.5	1.1	—	—	—	—	—	—
Bard Woven DeBakey Soft	Internal	81.2	—	18.6	—	0.2	—	—	—	—	—	—	—
	External	79.4	0.4	19.1	—	0.2	—	—	—	—	—	0.2	0.6
Woven Vascutek	Internal	85.6	—	13.6	0.5	0.3	—	—	—	—	—	—	—
	External	87.2	—	12.0	—	0.6	0.2	—	—	—	—	—	—
InterVascular Ochsner 200	Internal	75.8	—	24.0	—	—	—	—	—	—	—	0.2	—
	External	73.5	0.4	24.6	—	1.2	0.2	—	—	—	—	—	—
InterVascular Ochsner 500	Internal	74.8	1.2	23.2	—	0.6	0.1	—	—	—	—	0.1	—
	External	74.5	0.9	23.7	—	0.7	0.2	—	—	—	—	—	—

external surface than on the internal one for all the prostheses tested. In addition, the presence of unexpectedly high levels of chlorine on the external surfaces of the prototypes cannot be readily explained.

The main difference in surface chemistry between the LP prototype and the 6 controls was that the LP contained fewer $C-C$ bonds and more $C-O$ bonds. This was observed by resolving the carbon 1s peaks (Table 7).

Level of Extractables

While the prototypes and the controls contain certain surface contaminants, the results in Table 8 show that neither prototype model has an unacceptable level of extractables in the five solvents used. Note that all prostheses tested had similar low levels of extractables. The two Ochsner prostheses have more contaminants which are soluble in polar solvents, suggesting the presence of cellulose reactants, starches, polyvinyl alcohol or inorganic salts.

Additional extractions involving the IMPRA prototypes with and without their external wrap demonstrated a slightly larger percent of extractables was obtained in grafts without a wrap, indicating that the wrap itself did not contribute to the level of surface contamination.

DISCUSSION

The results of this study will be discussed under the following six headings.

Hemostasis

The essential feature and most valuable advantage of all woven prostheses over knitted devices has been their ability to control blood loss and prevent blood seepage through the wall even under systemic heparinization or abnormalities associated with a patient's coagulation mechanism. While the exact nature of the relationship between blood permeability and water permeability is not yet understood [9], empirical evidence suggests that in most normal clinical situations preclotting should not be necessary when the water permeability of the prosthesis lies below 350 ml per cm² per minute [18]. With a water permeability of over 900 ml per cm² per minute, it is evident that the HP graft cannot be used without preclotting. Indeed, because of its unique structure, namely a low pick count, a fine weft yarn and a 3/1 satin rather than a simple plain weave, the HP graft has the highest water permeability value ever observed in a commercial woven prosthesis [19]. Since this value is closer to those of warp-knitted designs [8], the graft cannot be recommended for applications where blood loss is critical.

In contrast, the use of a coarser weft yarn and a higher pick count has ensured a lower water permeability of only 312 ml per cm² per minute for the LP graft. While being higher than both the nominal value of 200 claimed by the manufacturer and the values for the four LP control grafts, namely the Cooley Verisoft (180), Woven Ochsner 200 (240), Woven Debakey Soft (215) and the Woven Vascutek (90), it does lie in the expected range of 50–350 ml per cm² per minute for woven prostheses [18], which suggests that the LP graft might have clinical applications in the thoracoabdominal cavity.

Healing Characteristics

It is widely accepted that an external velour surface facilitates preclotting and improves the attachment of

Table 7. Resolved ESCA spectra of carbon 1s and oxygen 1s peaks.

Prosthesis	Surface	Carbon 1s Peak (%)			Oxygen 1s Peak (%)	
		C—C	C—O	O—C=O	C—O	O—C=O
IMPRA Low Porosity	Internal	61.7	24.6	13.7	61.2	38.8
	External	66.0	23.4	10.6	64.5	35.5
IMPRA High Porosity	Internal	68.8	19.9	11.3	61.3	38.7
	External	76.3	16.7	7.0	63.1	36.9
Meadox Cooley Verisoft	Internal	71.8	13.0	15.1	50.4	49.5
	External	72.3	14.3	13.4	56.8	43.2
Meadox Woven Double Velour	Internal	72.3	12.1	15.6	54.1	45.9
	External	67.0	16.5	16.5	54.7	45.3
Bard Woven DeBakey Soft	Internal	79.5	10.5	10.0	52.0	48.0
	External	80.3	10.5	9.2	63.2	36.8
Woven Vascutek	Internal	85.9	7.2	6.9	61.2	38.8
	External	87.2	6.6	6.2	63.6	36.4
InterVascular Ochsner 200	Internal	74.9	13.4	11.6	77.9	22.1
	External	69.9	19.2	10.9	78.0	22.0
InterVascular Ochsner 500	Internal	70.2	18.8	11.0	74.0	26.0
	External	76.3	13.2	10.5	76.4	23.6

Table 8. Level of extractables.

Prosthesis	Type of Solvent (%)					Total (%)
	Hexane	III Trichloroethane	Methanol	Water	0.1N HCl	
IMPRA Low Porosity	0.1	0.1	0.1	0.1	0.1	0.5
IMPRA High Porosity	0.1	0	0.1	0.1	0.1	0.4
Meadox Cooley Verisoft	0.1	0	0.1	0	0.1	0.3
Meadox Woven Double Velour	0.1	0	0.1	0.1	0.1	0.4
Bard Woven DeBakey Soft	0.1	0	0.2	0	0.1	0.4
Woven Vascutek	0.3	0	0.1	0	0.1	0.5
InterVascular Ochsner 200	0	0.1	0	0.3	0	0.4
InterVascular Ochsner 500	0.1	0.1	0	0.2	0.2	0.6

the external capsule to the outer wall [20]. However, the desirability of an equivalent velour feature internally has been questioned by the observation that, in both clinical settings [7] and in animal trials [21,22], velour flow surfaces are associated with the development of a thicker inner capsule and a higher incidence of stenosis. Consequently, an external velour graft is generally considered more efficacious than an internal velour or double velour structure. The use of texturized yarns in the prototype grafts, similar to those found in the Woven DeBakey Soft and Woven Vascutek prostheses, provides a rough luminal surface with a "plain weave" appearance, without the excessive filamentous velour effect. Due to the fact that their porosity values are high for woven prostheses, it is anticipated that the prototype grafts will provide improved attachment of the external capsule and equivalent attachment of the inner capsule when compared to the *in vivo* healing performance of the DeBakey and Vascutek controls.

Propensity to Fray

A major limitation of all woven prostheses is their propensity to fray when cut, especially at an angle, which can lead to suture pull-out and dehiscence *in vivo*. The results from the suture retention strength test provide an indicator of the likelihood of this problem occurring in three different directions: parallel, perpendicular, and at 45° to the axis of the prosthesis. It is believed that the use of coarser weft yarns in the LP prototype (315 dtex) and in the Woven Double Velour (225 dtex) grafts are primarily responsible for providing superior suture retention strengths in the parallel direction. In comparison, the finer weft yarns in the HP (105 dtex) and the Cooley Verisoft (100 dtex)

are much easier to shift, which can lead to frequent prosthesis failures and lower suture retention strengths when tested in the parallel direction.

It is also noteworthy that the results from the two Ochsner grafts cut with scissors were among the lowest of all the prostheses tested. Clearly the inclusion of a leno weave every seventh and eighth end (i.e., every 1.4 mm) does provide adequate suture retention for a 2 mm bite when tested in the perpendicular direction. The leno structure prevents any shifting of the warp yarns. However, in the parallel and 45° angle directions, the situation is totally different as there are only 4 picks (21 picks per cm) between the cut edge and the suture in a 2 mm bite. Under low loads the cut leno ends fray back, unless cut with a cautery, giving unacceptably low suture retention values. The use of either thinner filaments (e.g., 13.5 μm rather than 16.5 μm), or a higher pick count, or both, would assist in improving the interfibre friction and interyarn cohesion and hence increase the overall suture retention strength.

Effect of External Wrap

The addition of an external spirally wound support or wrap has been a feature of commercially produced prostheses from Vascutek and Atrium Inc., U.S.A. and from Czechoslovakia [20,23,24], as well as other manufacturers. The use of an adherent, rigid supporting coil reduces the incidence of kinking and graft closure and has resulted in improved patency for axillo-femoral and femoro-popliteal bypasses [20]. The experience with a non-adherent external coil has been less favorable. We have found during animal studies that the loose cut end of a rigid coil near the anastomosis results in abrasive damage to the underlying textile filaments [23]. The effect of the much finer flexible polypropylene coil attached to the two prototype grafts is therefore of interest. The addition of this external wrap does not appear to have affected the water permeability, bursting strength, dilation and elongation results to any major extent. The external surface chemistry is not altered by the addition of the wrap. It does appear to contribute to a higher suture retention strength in the perpendicular and 45° angle directions. This is because the adhering wrap holds the filaments in adjacent warp yarns together so that they cannot easily be shifted in the circumferential direction by the pull of a suture. Note that this does not apply when sutures are pulled in the parallel direction. Because the wrap does not hold adjacent weft picks together, weft yarns, and particularly fine weft yarns as in the HP prototype, shift and break prematurely resulting in a low suture strength in the parallel direction.

Surface Contaminants

Total levels of extractables are similar to previous values obtained with other commercial polyester vascular prostheses [25]. The largest extractable component was obtained in the hexane fraction. This suggests that the surfaces of the grafts contain oils, waxes and/or silicones which are no doubt incorporated during the manufacturing processes.

The presence of chlorine on the external surfaces of the two prototype grafts is possibly due to residual chlorinated hydrocarbons used as a cleaning solvent during manufacture [26]. The unusually high level of silicon on the LP prosthesis suggests that it has been exposed to surface contamination such as the use of talc to facilitate the wearing gloves by operators during manufacture.

Importance of the Physical Properties

The three most important elements for a successful operation are the ability of the patient to heal, the surgical technique, and the physical characteristics of the prosthesis. Among these, the last one is often underestimated. We do believe that strength and resistance to elongation and dilation are of paramount importance for the long-term durability of an arterial bypass. In the past, we have proposed [18] that the minimum linear density of yarns should be more than 68 decitex in grafts 8 mm and less in diameter, 88 decitex in grafts between 8 and 12 mm, and 110 decitex in grafts more than 12 mm in diameter. The yarns in the prototypes analyzed are above these minimum values.

The woven construction of the LP prototype does not exhibit high deformability in either the longitudinal or the radial direction. It is a great advantage that the effective diameter of the prothesis under pressure is close to the nominal diameter, in order to prevent *in vivo* break-up, damage or rupture of both internal and external capsules. This can lead to the accumulation of thrombotic material likely to facilitate occlusion and bacteremic colonization.

CONCLUSIONS

On account of its coarse weft yarn and novel external woven velour design, the LP graft is a heavy, thick, strong and stable vascular prosthesis. With a water permeability value lying between that of the Meadox Woven Double Velour and the Bard Woven DeBakey Soft grafts, and with a superior suture retention strength in all three directions, the LP graft has the potential to provide an attractive clinical alternative to other woven prostheses. Cytotoxicity tests and animal trials are recommended to assess its healing capacity.

In view of its excessively high porosity and water permeability, low bursting strength, low parallel suture retention strength and ease of dilatation, the HP prototype graft cannot be considered a viable candidate for wide clinical use.

ACKNOWLEDGEMENTS

This work has been supported by the Medical Research Council of Canada, Pramel Inc., Longueuil, QC, Canada and IMPRA Inc., Tempe, AZ, U.S.A. The technical assistance of B. Badour, J. Bastien, S. Bourassa, K. Horth and N. Massicotte has been much appreciated. We extend our gratitude to S. Turnbull, D. Marceau, C. Gosselin, H. Green, L. Vermilya, J. B. Sinnott, T. How, J. Pratte and I. Niggerbrugge for their help and guidance.

REFERENCES

1. Snyder, R. W., B. Tenney and R. Guidoin. 1986. "Strength and Endurance of Vascular Grafts", in *Vascular Graft Update: Safety and Performance*, ASTM STP 898. H. E. Kambic, A. Kantrowitz and P. E. Sung, eds. Philadelphia, PA: American Society for Testing and Materials, pp. 108–121.

2. Guidoin, R., A. R. Downs, X. Barral, M. Marois, P. E. Roy, M. King and C. Gosselin. 1986. "Anastomotic False Aneurysms with Aortic Dacron Graft after Twenty-Five Years", *Ann. Vasc. Surg.*, 1:369–373.

3. McClurken, M. E., J. M. McHaney and W. M. Colone. 1986. "Physical Properties and Test Methods for Expanded Polytetrafluoroethylene (PTFE) Grafts", in *Vascular Graft Update: Safety and Performance*, ASTM STP 898. H. E. Kambic, A. Kantrowitz and P. Sung, eds. Philadelphia, PA: American Society for Testing and Materials, pp. 82–94.

4. Guidoin, R., J. Couture, F. Assayed and C. Gosselin. 1988. "New Frontiers in Vascular Grafting", *Int. Surg.*, 73:241–249.

5. Mathisen, S. R., H. D. Wu, L. R. Sauvage, Y. Usui

and M. W. Walker. 1986. "An Experimental Study of Eight Current Arterial Prostheses", *J. Vasc. Surg.*, 4:33–41.

6. Sauvage, L. R., J. C. Smith, C. C. Davis, E. A. Rittenhouse, D. F. Hall and P. B. Mansfield. 1986. "Dacron Arterial Grafts: Comparative Structures and Basis for Successful Use of Current Prostheses", in *Vascular Graft Update: Safety and Performance*, ASTM STP 898. H. E. Kambic, A. Kantrowitz and P. Sung, eds. Philadelphia, PA: American Society for Testing and Materials, pp. 16–24.

7. Guidoin, R., M. King, P. Blais, M. Marois, C. Gosselin, P. Roy, R. Courbier, M. David and H. P. Noël. 1981. "A Biological and Structural Evaluation of Retrieved Dacron Arterial Prostheses", in *Implant Retrieval: Material and Biological Analysis*. A. Weinstein, D. Gibbons, S. Brown and W. Ruff, eds. Washington, DC: NBS Special Publication 601, National Bureau of Standards, pp. 29–129.

8. Guidoin, R., M. King, D. Marceau, A. Cardou, D. De la Faye, J. M. Legendre and P. Blais. 1987. "Textile Arterial Prostheses: Is Water Permeability Equivalent to Porosity?" *J. Biomed. Mater. Res.*, 21:65–87.

9. Guidoin, R. G., M. King, M. Marois, L. Martin, D. Marceau, R. Hood and R. Maini. 1986. "New Polyester Arterial Prostheses from Great Britain: An *in vitro* and *in vivo* Evaluation", *Ann. Biomed. Eng.*, 14:351–367.

10. 1986. *National Standard for Vascular Graft Prostheses*, ANSI/AAMI VP20-1986. Association for Advancement of Medical Instrumentation, Arlington, VA.

11. 1985. *Identification of Textile Materials, 5th Edition*, Textile Institute, Manchester, UK.

12. Buxton, B. F., D. C. Wukasch, C. Martin, W. J. Liebig, G. L. Hallman and D. A. Cooley. 1973. "Practical Considerations in Fabric and Vascular Grafts. Introduction of a New Bifurcated Graft", *Am. J. Surg.*, 125:288–293.

13. Marceau D., A. Cardou, R. Guidoin, C. Gosselin and M. King. 1982. "Etude de la Déformation Circonférentielle des Prothèses Artérielles en Polytétrafluoroéthylène", *Rev. Europ. Biotech. Med.*, 4:114–116.

14. Dumont, H., R. Guidoin, S. Simoneau, M. Therrien, D. Boyer, T. J. Rao and D. Marceau. "Suture Pull-Out Strength of Textile Polyester Arterial Prostheses: Clinical Significance of the Proposed Standards" (manuscript in preparation).

15. Paynter, R. W., M. W. King, R. G. Guidoin and T. J. Rao. 1989. "The Surface Composition of Commercial Polyester Arterial Prostheses. An XPS Study", *Int. J. Artif. Org.*, 12:189–194.

16. American Association of Textile Chemists and Colorists. 1988. "Finishes in Textiles—Identification, Test Method 94-1987", *Technical Manual, AATCC*, Research Triangle Park, NC.

17. Debille, E. 1989. "Dilatability and Stretching Characteristics of Polyester Arterial Prostheses. Evaluation of the Elastic Behaviour", M.Sc. Thesis, Laval University.

18. King M. W., R. G. Guidoin, K. R. Gunasekera and C. Gosselin. 1983. "Designing Polyester Vascular Prostheses for the Future", *Med. Prog. Technol.*, 9:217–226.

19. Guidoin, R., M. King, C. Gosselin, P. Blais, K. Gunasekera, M. Marois and A. Cardou. 1982. "Les Prothèses Artérielles en Polyester", *Europ. Rev. Biomed. Tech.*, 4:13–25.

20. Sauvage, L. R., J. C. Smith, C. C. Davis, E. A. Rittenhouse, D. G. Hall and P. B. Mansfield. 1986. "Dacron Arterial Grafts: Comparative Structures and Basis for Successful Use of Current Prostheses", in *Vascular Graft Update: Safety and Performance*, ASTM STP 898. H. E. Kambic, A. Kantrowitz and P. Sung, eds. Philadelphia, PA: American Society for Testing and Materials, pp. 16–24.

21. H. D. Wu, M. Zammit, L. R. Sauvage and M. D. Streicher. 1985. "Influence of Inner Wall Filamentousness on the Performance of Small and Large Caliber Arterial Grafts", *J. Vasc. Surg.*, 2:255–262.

22. Guidoin, R., C. Gosselin, L. Martin, M. Marois, F. Laroche, M. King, K. Gunasekera, D. Domurado, M. F. Sigot-Luizard and P. Blais. 1983. "Polyester Prostheses as Substitutes in the Thoracic Aorta of Dogs. I. Evaluation of Commercial Prostheses", *J. Biomed. Mater. Res.*, 17:1049–1077.

23. King, M. W., R. Guidoin, K. Gunasekera, L. Martin, M. Marois, P. Blais, J. M. Maarek and C. Gosselin. 1984. "An Evaluation of Czechoslovakian Polyester Arterial Prostheses", *J. ASAIO*, 7:114–133.

24. Guidoin, R., M. King, M. Therrien, R. Paynter, S. Simoneau, E. Debille, L. Tremblay, D. Boyer and F. Gill. "The Atrium Plasma TFE Arterial Prosthesis: Physical and Chemical Characterization" (manuscript in preparation).

25. Torché D., R. Guidoin, D. Boyer, D. Marceau, Y. Marois, E. Debille, J. Lacombe and M. King. 1989. "An Arterial Prosthesis From Argentina: The Barone Microvelour® Arterial Graft", *J. Biomat. Appl.*, 3:427–453.

26. King, M., P. Blais, R. Guidoin, E. Prowse, M. Marois, C. Gosselin and H. P. Noël. 1981. "Polyethylene terephthalate (Dacron®) Vascular Prostheses—Material and Fabric Construction Aspects", in *Biocompatibility of Clinical Implant Materials, Vol. 2*. D. F. Williams, ed. Boca Raton, FL: CRC Press, pp. 177–207.

30

Newly Developed Hydrophilic Slippery Surface for Medical Application

SHOJI NAGAOKA*
RYOJIRO AKASHI*

ABSTRACT: This chapter describes the development of a hydrophilic polymer surface exhibiting excellent slipperiness properties when in contact with water or physiological fluid, due to the reaction of epoxy containing poly(vinyl pyrrolidone) with the polyamino compound formed on the surface of the substrate.

Epoxy containing poly(vinyl pyrrolidone) was obtained by the copolymerization of vinyl pyrrolidone as a hydrophilic component, glycidyl acrylate as a binding component to the substrate, and vinyl acetate to preserve the strength of the coating layer.

The slipperiness of the surface depends on the molecular weight of the coated hydrophilic copolymer. It was demonstrated that a molecular weight of 400,000 or more is essential to achieve excellent slipperiness.

Polyurethane catheters, both with and without the hydrophilic slippery coating, were evaluated for slipperiness and blood compatibility using rabbit models. In the case of coated catheters, no lesions of the intima of the blood vessels and no thrombus formation on the surface of the catheter were observed. However, the non-coated catheters injured the intima of the blood vessels, and severe thrombus formation was found on their surfaces.

INTRODUCTION

Surface slipperiness is required for medical devices such as catheters or guide wires that are inserted into blood vessels, the urethra, or other parts of the body which have mucous membranes. Unless these devices have good slipperiness, their introduction into the body is not only accompanied by pain, but there is also a danger of damage to the mucous membranes or the intima of the blood vessels. This may lead to infectious diseases or mural thrombus formation [1–4].

Several methods of achieving good slipperiness on surfaces are known. A particularly effective method is one that uses a coating with a hydrophilic polymer. This method involves binding the hydrophilic polymer, including an active hydrogen group (top coat) with polyisocyanate groups, which are coated on the substrate (undercoat) by covalent bonds. However, since such isocyanate groups are highly reactive, they become easily inactivated when exposed to the moisture in air. For this reason, there are problems with the stability of the coatings. Another problem involves the poor, anti-hydrolytic characteristics of the formed chemical bond, which result in low durability of the slipperiness *in vivo*.

We have developed an epoxy group containing hydrophilic copolymers that form stable, covalent bonds with substrate amino groups. The epoxy group is stable in a normal atmosphere, unlike the isocyanate groups.

The hydrophilic component of epoxy-containing hydrophilic polymer (top coat) was biocompatible vinylpyrrolidone. Polyamino compounds, which can be obtained by the hydrolysis of polyisocyanate under special conditions, were used as an undercoat.

This report describes the formation of a surface with excellent slipperiness when in contact with water or physiological fluid and its evaluation both *in vitro* and *in vivo*.

EXPERIMENTAL

Polymer Synthesis

The molecular design of the hydrophilic polymer is indicated by (1) the introduction of a binding site (epoxy group) to an amino group, (2) the need for durability against water or physical friction, and (3) high molecular weight.

*Medical Devices and Diagnostics Dept., Toray Industries, Inc. Head Office 2-1, Nihonbashi-muromachi 2-chome, Chuo-ku, Tokyo 103, Japan

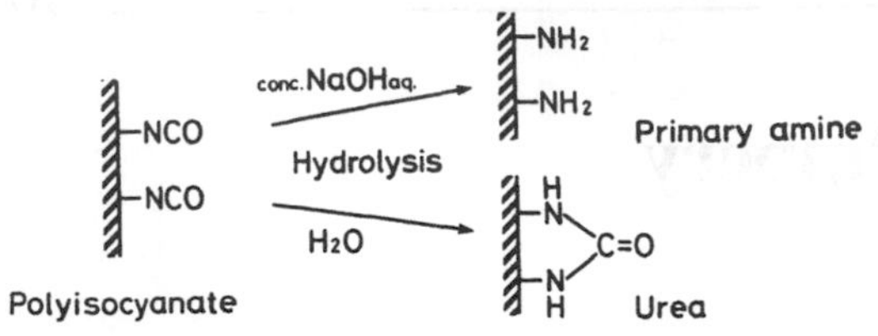

Figure 1. Reaction scheme for the hydrolysis of polyisocyanate.

Regarding item (1), we have examined glycidyl acrylate (GA). With respect to item (2), which will be described in more detail hereafter, it became clear that sufficient durability against water or physical friction cannot be obtained with only NVP and GA; a hydrophobic component is needed. As the hydrophobic component, we selected vinyl acetate (VAc) with a suitable molecular reactivity ratio with NVP. Item (3) is required to obtain sufficient slipperiness.

Water-soluble polymer, present as a trace in water, reduces the friction coefficient on the surface of the wall. This phenomenon is widely known as the "Toms effect" [5]. Although this effect has not been explained well enough from the viewpoint of the molecular level, it is understood that a polymer with a high molecular weight is effective. A similar effect is expected when water-soluble polymer is bound loosely on the substrate in a semi-soluble, diffused structure.

The synthesis of the polymer was based on these design parameters. The polymerization was conducted in a deaeration flask, and for the initiator, azo-bisdimethyl valeronitrile (V-65) was used. The molecular weight of the polymer was measured by GPC (Waters GPC-244) using polystyrene standard.

Coating of the Polyisocyanate and Its Hydrolysis

A 20 cm polyurethane (Pellethane:Tecoflex) tube, with an outer diameter of 0.8 mm, was soaked in a 4%

polyisocyanate (Trimethylol propane/Tolyrene diisocyanate adduct: isocyanate content 13.2 wt%, Nippon Polyurethane Co.) solution of methyl ethyl ketone for 1 min. Then, it was pulled slowly up and dried for 10 min. in a dry nitrogen stream at a temperature of 40°C. The polyisocyanate is highly compatible with the substrate and never peels off from the substrate.

Hydrolysis of isocyanate by water is commonly used to form amino groups, but there is the possibility of a side reaction of the remaining free isocyanate with the amino group to create urea. In order to prevent this, it is recommended that the reaction be carried out in an alkaline water of high concentration at a low temperature [6]. Consequently, 0.1–3.0 N NaOH aq. was used as the hydrolysis medium. After soaking the polyisocyanate-coated polyurethane tubes for a specific amount of time at 20°C, they were rinsed with distilled water for 3 hours and dried in vacuum. Figure 1 shows the scheme of the reaction.

Coating of the Hydrophilic Polymer and Its Reaction with the Polyamine Undercoat

After hydrolysis, the test specimen was dipped in a 4% chloroform solution of the hydrophilic copolymer mentioned before, and slowly pulled up, dried and coated. Then it was heated at 90°C in air for 3 hours to react the epoxy groups with the amino groups. The relatively high temperature and long reaction time were attributable to the lower reactivity of the formed aromatic amines in comparison with the aliphatic amines. The hydrophilic copolymer which was not bound with the polyamine undercoat was extracted by washing in distilled water at 70°C for 3 hours. Figure 2 shows the schematic representation of the reaction.

Next, a test of the durability of the coating layer was performed. The test specimen was boiled for 2 hours and squeezed twice between wet pig skins under a

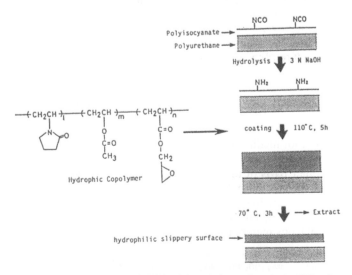

Figure 2. Schematic representation of the reaction to form hydrophilic slippery surface.

compression of 10 g/cm². The change of the static friction coefficient was then measured.

Measurement of the Static Friction Coefficient (Slipperiness)

After the durability test mentioned above, the catheter was cut to a length of 5 cm and fixed on a glass plate as shown in Figure 3. Then, the catheter was wet with physiological saline solution and a weight (100 g, coated with collagen and wet with the same fluid), was placed on the other end of the catheter. One end of the glass plate was gradually inclined in order to obtain the initial inclination angle required for the weight to begin slipping. The static friction coefficient (u) was calculated according to the formula: $u = \tan \theta$.

Animal Experiment

Rabbits weighing 2–3 kg were used. Under general anesthesia (pentobarbitol sodium), a control polyurethane catheter and a polyurethane catheter with the hydrophilic surface (10 cm in length) were inserted into the femoral arteries of the same rabbit.

Then, the catheters were inserted an additional 5 cm and pulled back to the original position while lightly rubbing against the intima of the blood vessels. The procedures were repeated three times with both catheters.

After 3 hours indwelling, the blood vessel was excised along the longitudinal axis. The catheters were removed and thrombus formation on the surface of the tip of the catheter was fixed by the usual method and studied with the Hitachi S-800 scanning electron microscope. At the same time, 5 cm of the blood vessels from the inserted parts of the catheters were excised and histological sections of the inner surfaces were prepared. After staining with hematoxylin-eosin, the sections were observed by optical microscope.

RESULTS AND DISCUSSION

Polymerization of Hydrophilic Polymer

Table 1 shows the relationship between polymerization conditions and the resulting molecular weight of its obtained polymer. It was found that the obtained molecular weight was 125,000–761,000, depending on the polymerization conditions. As shown in the kinetics of radical polymerization, the molecular weight of the obtained polymer depends mainly upon the concentration of the initiator and monomers.

Molecular weight of the hydrophilic polymer became higher with a low concentration of the initiator and high concentration of monomers. Nevertheless, if the concentration of monomers became too high, gel formation occurred and the obtained

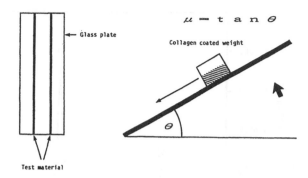

Figure 3. Evaluation method for the slipperiness of the surface.

polymer could not be dissolved. Run 4 is one of the most desirable polymerization conditions, and the molecular weight of the obtained polymer was 5.9 × 10⁵. The polymer obtained in Run 5 was too viscous and it was difficult to coat smoothly.

The optimum polymerization conditions mentioned above were used for synthesis of the hydrophilic polymer with various compositions. Table 2 shows the compositions of polymerization. If was found that a high yield of soluble polymers was obtained with every composition except Run 8. Therefore, the content of GA was fixed to 5 wt%. In addition, NMR measurement using JEOL FX-100 spectrometer made clear that the composition of the obtained polymer was roughly identical with feeded monomer composition.

Hydrolysis of Polyisocyanate and Reaction with Hydrophilic Polymer

Figure 4 shows the spectrum of FT-IR (Shimazu FT-IR 4200) of the surface of the polyurethane coated by polyisocyanate before and after hydrolysis (3 N, NaOH aq., 20°C, 3 min). Isocyanate groups (2260

Table 1. *The relationship between polymerization conditions and the molecular weight of the obtained polymer.*

Run	Monomer* (g)	Solvent** (g)	V-65 (mg)	Yield (%)	Mw × 10⁵
1	20	20	2	70	1.25
2	20	10	2	90	2.60
3	20	5	2	90	5.14
4	20	4	2	90	5.90
5	20	2	2	90	7.61
6	20	0	2	90	Gel
7	20	4	10	90	2.51
8	20	4	6	90	4.50
9	20	4	4	90	5.49
10	20	4	1	70	4.75

*NVP/VAc/GA = 85/10/5 (wt/wt)
**Isopropanol
Polymerization period: 3 days
Temperature: 40°C

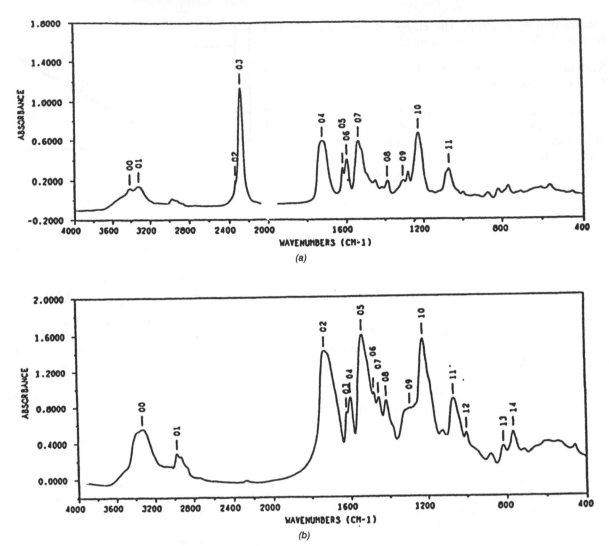

Figure 4. Change of FT-IR spectra accompanied by the hydrolysis of polyisocyanate (a) before hydrolysis and (b) after hydrolysis with 3N NaOll aq.

cm^{-1}) disappeared completely and amino groups (3250 and 3367 cm^{-1}) increased after hydrolysis with NaOH aq.

Figure 5 shows the change in the slipperiness of the surface, which consists of the hydrophilic polymer (NVP/VAc/GA=85/10/5, Mw = 590,000) and the aminated surface formed by the hydrolysis of polyisocyanate under various conditions. The concentration of NaOH and the time of hydrolysis were changed independently. The slipperiness was measured after the durability test.

It is not possible to obtain sufficient slipperiness with 0.1 N NaOH aq. because of the formation of urea as a side reaction. But with 1 to 3 N NaOH aq., the optimal conditions for achieving excellent slipperiness, even after the durability test, were found. One of the optimal amination conditions for binding the hydrophilic polymer was to hydrolyze the polyisocy-

anate surface with 3 N NaOH aq. for 3 to 5 minutes at room temperature. However, the durability decreased and the friction coefficient increased sharply under the conditions of higher alkaline concentration or longer time. These conditions may hydrolyze the substrate, including the thin polyamine layer.

Under scanning electron microscopy, the thickness of the hydrophilic slippery surface was found to be approximatley 2 μm after the durability test. This is clearly thicker than the end-to-end distance of a polymer with a molecular weight of 590,000.

Consequently, it was suggested that the hydrophilic slippery surface was bound by the reaction between epoxy groups and amino groups at the boundary layer, but the upper hydrophilic layer was rendered insoluble by the reaction between the remaining epoxy groups (cross-linking or polymerization) to form a loose layer with high water content.

Table 2. Hydrophilic polymers with various compositions.

Run	NVP (wt%)	VAC (wt%)	GA (wt%)	Yield (%)
1	95	0	5	90
2	85	10	5	90
3	80	15	5	90
4	75	20	5	90
5	70	25	5	90
6	65	30	5	90
7	89	10	1	90
8	90	0	10	Gel

Polymerization conditions: monomers:20 g, iso-ProH:4 g, V-65:0.002 g
Polymerization period: 3 days
Temperature: 40°C

Effect of the Molecular Weight of the Hydrophilic Copolymer on the Slipperiness

Figure 6 shows the slipperiness of the polyurethane catheter fixed on the glass plate (as shown in Figure 3), coated and bound with the hydrophilic copolymer [NVP/VAc/GA = 85/10/5 (wt/wt)] having a different molecular weight. The static friction coefficient was dramatically decreased with the increase of the molecular weight of the hydrophilic polymer up to 400,000. The static friction coefficient of an uncoated (control) polyurethane catheter was 0.32 ± 0.02 ($n = 5$). The polyurethane catheter coated with hydrophilic poly(hydroxyethyl methacrylate) showed a friction coefficient of 0.18 ± 0.02 ($n = 5$). This slipperiness is still not enough for both the mucous membrane and maneuverability of medical devices. The dotted line ($\mu = 0.035$) indicates the static friction coefficient of the polyurethane catheter coated with non-bonded poly vinylpyrrolidone (GAF, Mw = 400,000) solubilized in water. This slippery surface does not injure the mucous membrane or blood vessel. But of course, this slipperiness dissipated in a short while due to the washing-off of the poly vinylpyrrolidone from the surface. As shown in this figure, a molecular weight for the hydrophilic copolymer of at least 400,000 is necessary to obtain excellent slipperiness when in contact with water or physiological fluid.

As mentioned previously, the dependency of the "Toms effect" on the molecular weight of the added polymer has not been sufficiently explained. Nevertheless, it was profoundly interesting that the similar molecular weight effect was observed in semi-soluble and diffused polymers covalently bound to the substrate.

Effect of the Chemical Composition of the Hydrophilic Polymer on the Durability of Slipperiness

Figure 7 shows the relationship between the content of VAc in the hydrophilic polymer and the durability

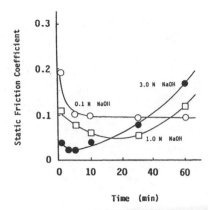

Figure 5. Effect of hydrolysis conditions of polyisocyanate on the slipperiness of the surface. Hydrophilic polymer; NVP/VAc/GA = 85/10/5 (wt/wt), Mw = 590,000.

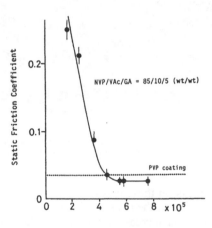

Figure 6. Effect of molecular weight of the hydrophilic polymer on the slipperiness of the surface. Mean ± SD ($n = 5$).

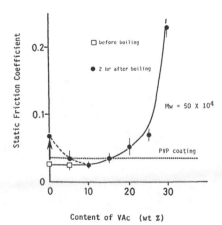

Figure 7. Effect of hydrophilic polymer composition on the slipperiness of the surface. Mean ± SD ($n = 5$).

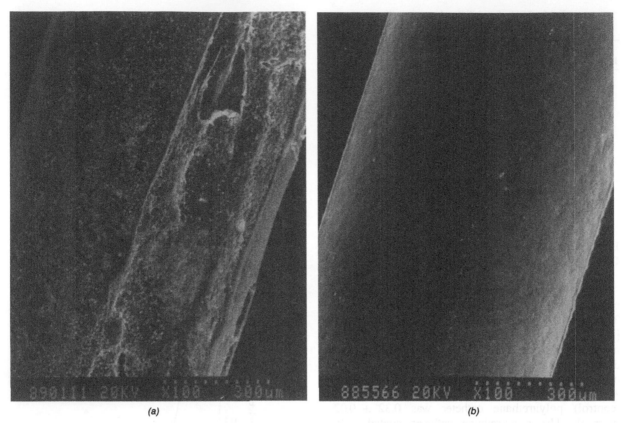

Figure 8. Scanning electron micrographs of the surface of the catheter after indwelling for 3 hours: (a) polyurethane catheter (non-coated), (b) polyurethane catheter with hydrophilic slippery surface.

of slipperiness. In these cases, the content of GA was kept at 5 wt%. As the content of NVP was increased, the slipperiness increased, but, unless hydrophobic monomer (VAc) was copolymerized with 10 wt% or more, it was not possible to obtain sufficient durability, and the slipperiness deteriorated easily (□→● in Figure 7).

These results suggest that the durability is closely correlated to the mechanical strength of the hydrophilic copolymer, and is essential to copolymerize the hydrophobic monomer (VAc) with NVP and GA to make the hydrophilic slippery layer tough against boiling water or physical friction.

However, if the content of VAc was over 10 wt%,

lesions

endothelial cell layer

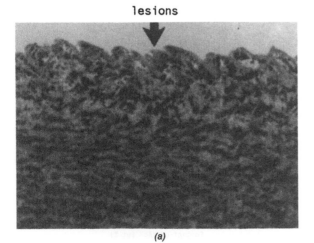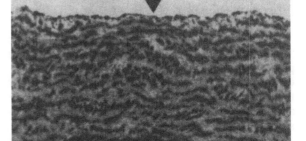

Figure 9. Histological observation of the mural section of the blood vessel after catheter manipulation (stained by hematoxylin-eosine). (a) Polyurethane catheter (non-coated); catheter-induced lesions were clearly observed and endothelial cell layer had fallen off. (b) Polyurethane catheter with hydrophilic slippery surface; no lesions were observed and the endothelial cells formed normal monolayer.

the sufficient hydrophilicity of the copolymer was lost and the slipperiness deteriorated.

As is explained above, the optimal chemical composition was determined to be NVP/VAc/GA = 85/10/5 (wt/wt).

In Vivo Experiments

The insertion and the manipulation of the polyurethane catheter with a hydrophilic slippery surface were much easier than those of the non-coated polyurethane catheter in the femoral artery. Nearly no friction was felt between the catheter and blood vessel in the case of the coated catheter.

Figure 8 shows the scanning electron micrographs of the surfaces of the tip of the catheters after 3 hours indwelling in the femoral artery of the rabbit. The non-coated polyurethane catheter was covered with thrombus composed of a fibrin network, erythrocyte, leucocyte, and platelets (a). In contrast, the polyurethane catheter with the hydrophilic slippery surface showed no thrombus formation or adhesion of blood components (b).

Figure 9 shows histological photomicrographs of cross sections of the femoral arteries that were rubbed with the catheters. In the case of the non-coated polyurethane catheter, intima of the femoral artery was destroyed. There were neither endothelial cells nor an internal elastic membrane. These were obviously catheter-induced lesions.

On the contrary, in the case of the polyurethane catheter with the hydrophilic slippery surface, no lesions were observed and the endothelial cell layer was not damaged.

CONCLUSION

A new hydrophilic slippery surface for medical use has been developed by binding a hydrophilic polymer (top coat) to the polyamino compound (undercoat) formed on the substrate. The hydrophilic copolymer was composed of vinylpyrrolidone, vinyl acetate, and glycydil acrylate. The polyamino compound was obtained by the hydrolysis of polyisocyanate with NaOH of high concentration.

Slipperiness when in contact with water or physiological fluid depends upon the molecular weight of the hydrophilic polymer. To obtain excellent slipperiness, it was essential for the hydrophilic copolymer to have a molecular weight larger than 400,000. The durability of the slipperiness was closely correlated to the mechanical strength of the hydrophilic copolymer, and the addition of hydrophobic vinyl acetate was essential to prevent the deterioration of the slipperiness.

The polyurethane catheter with the hydrophilic slippery surface was easy to insert and did not damage the blood vessel during manipulation and, furthermore, showed excellent blood compatibility.

REFERENCES

1. Ducatman, B. S., J. C. McMichan, and W. D. Edwards. 1985. "Catheter-Induced Lesions of the Right Side of the Heart", *JAMA*, 253:791–795.

2. Ford, S. E. and P. N. Manley. 1982. "Indwelling Cardiac Catheters: An Autopsy Study of Associated Endocardial Lesions", *Arch. Pathol. Lab. Med.*, 106: 314–317.

3. Lange, H. W., C. A. Galliani, and J. E. Edwards. 1983. "Local Complications Associated with Indwelling Swan-Ganz Catheters: Autopsy Study of 36 Patients", *Am. J. Cardiol.*, 52:1108–1111.

4. Lazarus, H. M., J. N. Lowder, and R. H. Herzig. 1983. "Occlusion and Infection in Broviac Catheters During Intensive Cancer Therapy", *Cancer*, 52:23–48.

5. Kohn, M. C. 1973. "Energy Stage in Drag-Reducing Polymer Solutions", *J. Polym. Sci., Polym. Phys. Ed.*, 11:2339–2356.

6. Tanaka, H. 1976. "Hydrolysis of Polyisocyanate", *Bull. Chem. Soc. Japan.*, 49:2821–2823.

31

Endothelial Cell Seeding of Prosthetic Vascular Grafts—Current Status

STEVEN P. SCHMIDT, Ph.D.*,1
WILLIAM V. SHARP, M.D.*
M. MICHELLE EVANCHO, B.S.*
SHARON O. MEERBAUM, B.S.*

ABSTRACT: Endothelial cell seeding (ECS) is the research technology that has developed over the past decade in an effort to create a more biological blood/surface lining on vascular prostheses and thus hopefully a more successful artificial vascular graft in terms of longevity of performance. Since endothelial cells are nature's natural cellular lining of all blood vessels and the chambers of the heart, the ultimate goal of the research is to promote the attachment and reproduction of endothelial cells transplanted from a natural source of these cells in a patient onto a synthetic vascular graft material implanted as a bypass graft in the same patient. The research effort has inherently interested and involved basic scientists as well as clinical researchers in the medical sciences and surgeons. The research efforts have contributed significantly to the understanding of basic endothelial cell functions and blood/surface interactions. This chapter summarizes the historical development of the science of endothelial cell seeding and highlights those areas of research requiring additional investigations. The chapter concludes with the current status of ECS in patients undergoing peripheral revascularization procedures and the possibility of genetically manipulating seeded endothelial cells to produce novel gene products.

INTRODUCTION

The availability of artificial vascular prostheses has been, in large measure, responsible for the evolution and maturation of vascular surgery. The motivation for synthetic vascular graft development probably arose in the frustration of attempts to treat expanding abdominal aortic aneurysms in the 1940s and 1950s.

Voorhees et al. [1] are generally credited with the original publication that led to the hypothesis that synthetic fabrics formed as tubular prostheses could replace diseased natural blood vessels. The clinical evaluation of this hypothesis was reported by Blakemore and Voorhees in 1954 [2]. Upon publication of this article, it became clear that synthetic materials could serve as arterial conduits, and investigators embarked upon the task of discovering the best synthetic material from which vascular grafts could be fabricated.

In spite of the lack of careful, systematic science during the past 30 years of artificial graft development, satisfactory synthetic prostheses such as Dacron and Teflon have been introduced into the armamentarium of the vascular surgeon. These have provided improved life styles and longevities for patients with vascular disease. Szilagyi [3] reviewed the development of arterial substitutes in a 1978 publication and stated that the grafts that have been developed were designed to mimic the most simple function of human arteries—serving as a mechanical conduit—with virtually no regard for the biologic properties of the arterial wall. Thus, the technical achievements and practical successes of artificial vascular grafting have occurred in spite of an incomplete understanding of the complex interactions of blood components with either natural or synthetic vascular walls. Nevertheless, the collective experience of vascular surgeons has been that when these artificial vascular grafts are placed in high-flow, low-resistance locations such as the aortoiliac position, graft patencies and durabilities remain excellent for as long as 10 years post-implantation. When placed in low-flow, small-diameter circulations, however, the failure rates of synthetic vascular grafts are unacceptable. The patency rate of Dacron grafts placed below the inguinal ligament at 8 years is only 10% [4]. Likewise, the patency rate for polytetrafluoroethylene (PTFE or Teflon) grafts implanted for femorodistal reconstructions is only approximately 20% at three years [5]. These data em-

1Author to whom correspondence should be addressed.

*Vascular Research Lab & Department of Surgery, Akron City Hospital, 525 East Market Street, Akron, OH 44309

phasize the limitations of knowledge and technology in developing improved small-diameter vascular prostheses.

Coincident with the development of synthetic materials that were appropriate as arterial substitutes was the evolution of the use of transplanted autogenous veins as vascular grafts in the arterial circulation. It was 100 years ago that Glück [6] descibed the use of an autogenous vein as an arterial conduit to restore circulation through a carotid artery. In 1916 Bernheim [7] described the use of autologous saphenous vein in the reconstruction of peripheral arteries in a patient with a popliteal artery aneurysm. Nearly five decades passed before surgeons embraced the approach of vascular bypass using autologous saphenous veins. The first successful reports of saphenous vein use in femoropopliteal bypass grafting appeared in 1949 [8], for use in renal occlusive disease in 1962 [9] and in coronary artery bypass in 1973 [10]. It is beyond the scope of this paper to review the remarkable contributions of saphenous vein bypass grafting in peripheral vascular and cardiothoracic surgery. It remains true today, however, that the saphenous vein is the "gold standard" for reconstructive surgery of medium and small-diameter arteries and the bypass graft against which all other biologic and synthetic grafts are compared. The limitations of the saphenous vein as a bypass graft are being recognized, however. One-quarter to one-third of saphenous vein bypass grafts deteriorate, as assessed by histology, in the relatively higher flows and pressures of the arterial circulation [11]. Recently, myocardial revascularization using the internal mammary artery has gained support. Long-term patency and patient survival are superior in those patients receiving internal mammary bypass grafts compared with those receiving saphenous vein bypasses [12] presumably because the internal mammary artery is more physiologic than the saphenous vein when implanted in the coronary circulation.

It is thus obvious that in spite of their advantages as small- and medium-diameter arterial replacements, autogenous vein grafts are not the ideal vascular grafts in and of themselves. In addition, in many patients autogenous veins may be diseased and not suitable for use as bypass grafts. In all patients, "nonessential" veins available for use as bypass grafts are limited. The debate continues as to how patients with bypassable diseases should be surgically managed [13]. Thus the need for a successful artificial bypass graft to replace small and medium-diameter blood vessels remains an important issue in vascular surgery.

Some researchers in the field of artificial vascular graft development, recognizing the failure of current synthetic grafts to perform satisfactorily in circulations with small-diameter vessels, have directed their efforts toward novel polymers with mechanical properties more similar to native blood vessels than those currently available. Other investigators have sought to modify the surface properties of synthetic grafts pharmacologically, such as with heparin bonding or radio

frequency glow discharge (RFGD). A third approach has been to try to understand better the cellular and humoral events occurring at both the blood/natural vessel interface as well as the blood/synthetic vessel interface. It is within the framework of this third approach that endothelial cell seeding (ECS) of artificial vascular grafts has evolved as an approach to the problems of small-diameter vascular grafting.

One of the early assumptions for the superiority of saphenous vein grafts compared to synthetic grafts in peripheral vascular surgery was the presence of an intact endothelium on the luminal surfaces of the saphenous vein grafts. Under *in vivo* conditions of normal circulatory physiology, endothelial cells (EC) are the most nonthrombogenic cells known. It has been known from research experiments that synthetic vascular grafts implanted in animals endothelialize, in time, along their entire lengths. This endothelialization occurs only in the anastomotic regions of human vascular grafts, however. The logical assumption of researchers was therefore to improve graft performance by promoting the endothelialization of the entire length of synthetic grafts implanted in humans by seeding EC onto their luminal surfaces. It is the purpose of this chapter to summarize the evolution of research in the field of ECS from early studies through the current status of ongoing clinical trials throughout the world.

HISTORICAL PERSPECTIVE

Endothelial cell seeding of prosthetic vascular grafts was made technically possible as a consequence of advancements in the derivation and *in vitro* cultivation of vascular EC. Jaffe et al. [14] first described in 1973 the isolation and culture of human umbilical vein EC by collagenase digestion of the luminal surfaces of umbilical veins. An early attempt to develop blood-compatible interfaces on prosthetic vascular graft materials was described by Burkel and Kahn in 1977 [15]. These investigators seeded a variety of cell types including EC onto microfiber scaffolds lining nonporous vascular prostheses *in vitro*. On the materials that were evaluated, endothelial cell coverage ranged from 28–94%. These authors concluded, however, that although endothelium represented the most theoretically advantageous lining of vascular prostheses because of its inherent blood compatibility, the relatively slow replication of these cells limited their usefulness when seeded onto grafts.

Malcolm Herring, M.D., is generally recognized as the "father" of ECS as a result of his 1978 publication [16]. This landmark report described the derivation of canine venous EC from external jugular veins by mechanical disruption of the cells from the luminal surfaces of the veins using a steel wool pledget. These cells were subsequently mixed with whole blood used to preclot porous 6 mm internal diameter (i.d.) Dacron prostheses and the grafts were implanted in the infrarenal aorta. The grafts were evaluated at 4 weeks postoperatively. The mean thrombus-free surface area of seeded grafts was 76% compared to 22% for nonseeded grafts and the glistening luminal surface of seeded grafts histologically resembled endothelium. This report was rapidly followed by two publications from the same group which documented the existence of Weibel-Palade bodies (the ultrastructural hallmark of endothelium) on seeded graft linings (17) and confirmed the positive identification of endothelium lining prosthetic grafts by immunoflourescent staining for Factor-VIII-related antigen (18). These authors also studied the proliferation of seeded EC on 14 different designs of prosthetic grafts including Dacrons, Teflon, Orlon and polyurethane-backed graft (19). The latter study concluded that weft-knit Dacron grafts were most suitable for ECS and that it was difficult for cellular elements to adhere to Teflon.

Utilizing enzymatic techniques for the harvest of EC from canine external jugular veins, Graham et al. [20,21] contributed significantly to the development of the technology of ECS with two reports in 1980. These authors derived EC by sequential incubations of the vein luminal surfaces in trypsin and collagenase. In one experiment these enzymatically-harvested EC were seeded immediately following their derivation onto 6 mm double velour Dacron thoracoabdominal bypass grafts [20]. In the second experiment the canine venous EC were cultured *in vitro* following their enzymatic derivation for 14 days prior to their seeding onto 6 mm Dacron thoracoabdominal bypass grafts [21]. This study introduced the option of tissue culture of EC prior to graft seeding. In both studies endothelial cell coverage of the luminal surfaces of the grafts exceeded 80% at 4 weeks postoperatively. These early studies of both Herring and Graham guided the subsequent efforts of researchers in the field of ECS.

The next stage of the research effort involved evaluating the efficacy of ECS in performances of small-caliber vascular grafts (4 mm i.d.). The pioneering research of Herring and Graham had evaluated 6 mm i.d. vascular grafts seeded with EC. These grafts were implanted in high-flow and -pressure circulations as infrarenal aortic grafts or thoracoabdominal bypass grafts. In these circulations, under the evaluated rheologic conditions, even nonseeded prosthetic grafts could be expected to remain patent and to develop a relatively nonthrombogenic pseudointima. In contrast, because small-diameter vascular grafts may be of greatest utility in situations of low-flow circulation, ECS may theoretically offer its greatest advantage in preventing thrombosis. In 1982 we reported our early data evaluating 4 mm double velour Dacron (Microvel) grafts in the canine carotid artery model [22]. In that year also Stanley et al. [23] described an experiment in which 10 cm lengths of 4 mm i.d. endothelial cell seeded and nonseeded externally supported knitted Dacron grafts were evaluated as bilateral iliofemoral bypasses. In our study the mean

patency of successfully seeded grafts was 100% at week 4 postoperatively and mean thrombus free surface area was 80% by 4 weeks postoperatively. In contrast the thrombus free surface area of nonseeded grafts was only 18%. Photomicrographs of representative grafts from this study are illustrated in Figure 1. In the Stanley study 73% of the seeded grafts were patent at the time of harvest; patency in nonseeded grafts was 27%. Both studies concluded that EC surfaced on the grafts within 2–4 weeks postoperatively and created a confluent monolayer of endothelium.

Further data from our laboratory confirmed the theoretical advantages of ECS in maintaining small-diameter vascular graft patency during conditions of acute reduction in blood flow through the graft [24,25]. In these studies we seeded 6 cm lengths of 4 mm i.d. Dacron double-velour grafts with enzymatically-derived EC, waited for postoperative maturation of the neointima, and then acutely reduced blood flow for 4 hours through each seeded graft and its contralateral nonseeded control. All seeded grafts remained patent during the controlled low flows; in contrast, 50% of the nonseeded grafts thrombosed during low flow when the experiment was performed at three weeks postoperatively and 25% at 5 weeks postoperatively. Blood flows returned to near-initial levels following the experimental period of low flow in seeded grafts but remained depressed in the non-seeded controls. This experiment generated the objective data proving that endothelial cell seeded grafts did indeed outperform nonseeded grafts under conditions of low flows similar to the circulatory conditions of poor runoff in peripheral bypass grafting.

Graham et al. [26] also reported in 1982 the successful seeding of expanded polytetrafluoroethylene (ePTFE, Teflon) prostheses in the canine model. This study was important in advancing the technology of ECS to the prosthetic graft material that is preferred by many vascular surgeons because of its handling characteristics and resistance to infection. Subsequent studies have suggested that the endothelium-lined inner capsule which matures in endothelial cell seeded PTFE grafts is thinner than that in Dacron grafts, which may be of long-term benefit to the performance of the graft [27]. Photomicrographs of seeded and nonseeded PTFE grafts from some of our previous studies are shown in Figure 2.

Many investigators have conducted experiments to identify the biologic and physiologic mechanisms by which ECS might improve vascular graft performance. Sharefkin et al. [28] performed platelet survival studies in dogs with seeded and unseeded thoracoabdominal grafts using indium-111-oxine labeled platelets. The research concluded that when ECS was technically successful, the degree of platelet interaction with Dacron vascular prostheses was reduced and a normal platelet survival time was restored. Clagett et al. [29] reported the parallel between platelet serotonin levels (a monitor of platelet release) and the normalization of platelet survival times in dogs with en-

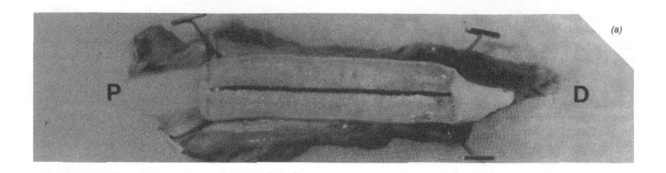

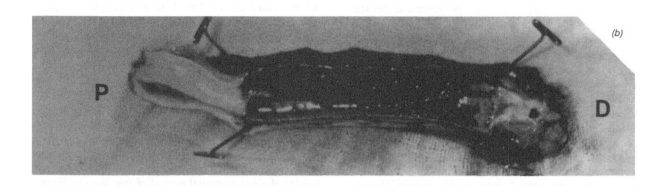

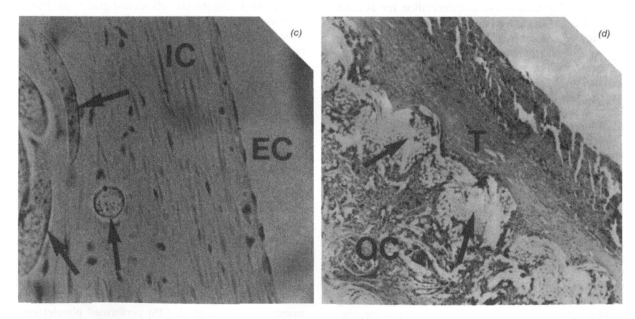

Figure 1. (a) 6-cm length of endothelial cell seeded Dacron vascular graft harvested after 4 weeks implantation in a canine carotid artery. The luminal surface of the graft is 100% thrombus-free and the neoendothelium imparts a glistening surface to the graft. P = proximal end of the graft; D = distal end of the graft. (b) 6-cm length of nonseeded Dacron vascular graft harvested from a canine carotid artery after 4 weeks implantation. Although this graft remained patent, the luminal surface was completely covered by red thrombus. P = proximal end of the graft; D = distal end of the graft. (c) Histologic section of an endothelial cell seeded Dacron vascular graft with the nuclei of endothelial cells (EC) resting upon the graft's internal capsule (IC) which is composed of myofibroblastic and smooth muscle cells. Sections through the Dacron fibers are shown with the arrows. (d) Histologic section of a nonseeded Dacron graft demonstrating the luminal–graft interface of thrombus (T) resting upon the Dacron fibers (arrows); OC = outer capsule of the graft.

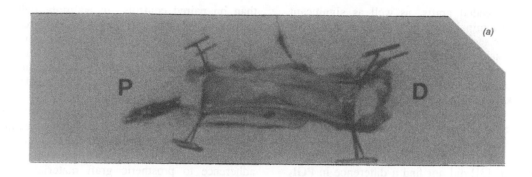

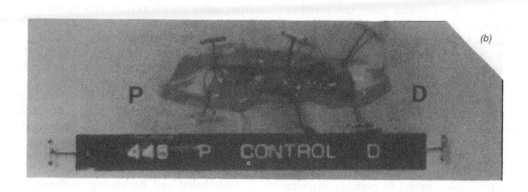

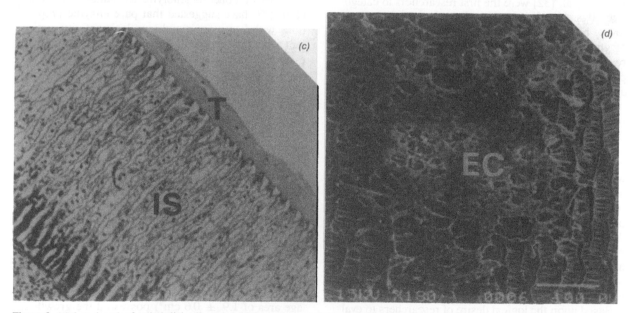

Figure 2. (a) 6-cm length of endothelial cell seeded PTFE vascular graft harvested after 4 weeks implantation in a canine carotid artery. The luminal surface of the graft is virtually thrombus-free. P = proximal end of the graft; D = distal end of the graft. (b) 6-cm length of nonseeded PTFE vascular graft harvested from a canine carotid artery after 4 weeks implantation. Although patent, the luminal surface of this PTFE graft was occupied by a pseudointima of thrombus and trapped blood cells. P = proximal end of the graft; D = distal end of the graft. (c) Histologic section of nonseeded PTFE graft with thrombus (T) at the interface between the graft and lumen. The nuclei of cells can be seen in the internodal spaces (IS) of this PTFE graft. (d) Scanning electron micrograph of a mass of endothelial cells (EC) surfacing upon the luminal surface of this PTFE graft. The raised portions of the cells are the cell nuclei.

dothelial cell seeded grafts, as well as significant differences in luminal surface production of 6-keto-$PGF_{1\alpha}$ between seeded and nonseeded grafts. 6-keto-$PGF_{1\alpha}$ is the stable hydrolysis product of prostacyclin (PGI_2), a prostaglandin synthesized from arachidonic acid in EC and the most potent biologic antithrombogenic agent known. Other investigators have also studied the prostaglandin biochemistry of seeded and nonseeded vascular grafts. We reported [30] that EC seeded onto vascular grafts do indeed synthesize PGI_2 but at levels significantly less than native artery.

Sicard et al. [31] did not find a difference in PGI_2 levels between seeded and nonseeded vascular grafts, but did report that seeding lessened thromboxane A_2 production by the walls of seeded grafts compared to nonseeded controls. Thromboxane A_2 (TXA_2) is synthesized from arachidonic acid primarily in platelets and is a potent platelet aggregator. The suggestion was thus that an alteration in the ratio between PGI_2 and TXA_2 may then be responsible for the reduction in platelet deposition upon seeded grafts, which ultimately translates into enhanced longer-term graft patency. The specific effects and consequences of ECS upon the prostaglandin biochemistry of vascular grafts remain controversial, however, and the subject of ongoing research.

The use of the canine model to evaluate vascular graft performances has been controversial among researchers. While it has been known for many years that dogs are hypercoagulable compared to humans, Kaplan et al. [32] were the first researchers to categorize dogs according to their thrombotic potentials as low or high responders. In their study the patency rate of grafts implanted in the carotid circulation of low responders was 100% at 3 weeks postimplantation; patency of grafts in high responders not treated with antiplatelet medications was 10%. High responders treated with antiplatelet medications had graft patency rates of 100%. We evaluated the efficacy of a variety of medications in combination with ECS upon the performance of both Dacron and PTFE vascular grafts in canines [33,34]. In our study, grafts that were seeded with EC and implanted in dogs receiving antiplatelet medications performed better than respective controls, even though many of the antiplatelet drugs completely eliminated PGI_2 synthesis by the seeded grafts through inhibition of the endothelial cell cyclooxygenase enzyme. These studies thus suggested that high levels of PGI_2 were not necessary to maintain high thrombus-free surface areas on seeded grafts in antiplatelet medicated dogs.

Based upon the logical desire of researchers to evaluate the efficacy of endothelial cell seeded grafts in humans, researchers at Tufts New England Medical Center first evaluated endothelial cell seeded grafts in baboons as an alternative to dogs [35]. Although there were no differences in patencies between the seeded and control grafts in this study, in which 5 cm lengths of 4 mm i.d. Dacron grafts were evaluated, platelet accumulation on seeded grafts was significantly less than on paired controls. In addition, cells on the luminal surfaces of the seeded grafts were identified as EC based upon morphologic and immunohistochemical characteristics. Although the limitations of these animal models are understood, the dog and baboon remain the choices of animal models for investigators researching ECS.

In order for ECS to be clinically practical and embraced by vascular surgeons as a viable treatment option, researchers realized that improvements in the efficiencies of cell harvest from donor vessels and cell adherence to prosthetic graft materials would be needed. These needs were emphasized when Roseman et al. [36] described the efficiency of harvest of EC from native vessels as only 15% of the available cells. In addition, these authors reported that only 19.8% of the cells harvested from canine external jugular veins actually adhered to porous PTFE grafts after seeding and that cell losses continued for up to 24 hours following restoration of blood flow through the grafts. Assuming the lack of an alternative source of endothelium in human clinical vascular graft seeding, technicians would have to harvest EC from short lengths of autogenous veins not otherwise usable as bypass conduits, and thus the number of cells potentially available is limited.

Endothelial cell harvesting inefficiencies may be attributed to inherent variabilities of crude bacterial collagenase preparations derived from *Clostridium histolyticum*. These preparations contain varying amounts of noncollagenolytic substances. Sharefkin et al. [37] have suggested that pure enzyme preparations with basement membrane lysis activity equivalent to that of crude collagenase preparations are necessary for the reliable enzymatic harvest of EC that must accompany the clinical implementation of the technique. Those research laboratories which have been most successful in harvesting EC have defined lots of collagenase with high levels of activity from manufacturers rather than using collagenase from various manufacturing lots. It must be emphasized, however, that the upper limit of efficiency of harvest of EC from donor veins may ultimately depend upon the patient's age and health status. Thus, even with optimal harvesting efficiencies, sufficient numbers of EC may not be available from veins to adequately seed long lengths of graft and subsequently cover the luminal surface of the graft with endothelium in short postoperative times. Watkins et al. [38] did demonstrate that the EC available from adult human (mean age 55.8 ± 9.8 years) saphenous vein segments (average area of 1.9 ± 0.6 cm^2) possessed the growth capacity *in vitro* to cover the luminal areas of vascular prostheses commonly used in peripheral vascular surgery. However, in their study, cells harvested from 10 of the 53 vein segments processed did not grow in culture. This supports the suggestion that factors other than collagenase, both biologic and technical, may be important in endothelial cell derivation for vascular graft seeding.

In addition to investigating the inefficiencies of cell harvest, researchers have also addressed the problem of increasing the number of EC retained on the prosthetic graft after seeding. Because Dacron grafts are porous, the method of seeding EC has been to mix the inoculum of cells with the whole blood used to preclot the interstices of the graft. This technique presumably harbors the EC within the graft wall as well as on the luminal surface. Using indium-111-oxine labeled EC Sharefkin et al. [39] estimated that 75% of EC seeded onto Dacron grafts remain attached. Commercially available PTFE grafts, on the other hand, are described as microporous with mean internodal distances of 30 μ, and are not preclotted by the surgeon prior to implantation. In addition, the luminal surfaces of PTFE grafts are hydrophobic. Thus, it is not surprising that adherence of seeded cells to native PTFE is poor. Williams et al. [40] reported experiments evaluating the compatibility of adult human EC derived from iliac veins with both Dacron and PTFE *in vitro*. Their study concluded that essentially no EC adhered to untreated grafts. In contrast, endothelial cell adherence increased dramatically on grafts treated with extracellular matrix, plasma or fibronectin. The effect of fibronectin upon endothelial cell attachment to prosthetic vascular grafts has received considerable attention. Fibronectin is an adhesive glycoprotein which is a part of the natural basement membrane upon which EC attach *in vivo*. The combination of fibronectin-coating on polystyrene and addition of endothelial cell growth factors to the culture media made possible significant advances in the ability of tissue culturists to grow and passage EC *in vitro* and justified the interest in fibronectin as a vascular graft coating.

Ramalanjaona et al. [41,42] studied endothelial cell adherance and retention on fibronectin-coated PTFE grafts using indium-111-oxine labeled EC. Twice as many cells adhered to fibronectin-coated PTFE grafts compared to uncoated grafts, and the loss of cells from the graft following restoration of blood flow was reduced. These authors also reported the methodology by which fibronectin could be coated onto PTFE grafts to create a stable bond during pulsatile flow. In their animal studies, however, pretreatment of the experimental animals with antiplatelet agents was required to maintain graft patencies since fibronectin-coating also increased platelet accumulation on the luminal surfaces of the grafts. In addition to the above studies, Kesler et al. [43] described *in vitro* studies in which fibronectin enhanced the strength of attachment of EC to both PTFE and polyester elastomer. Seeger and Klingman [44] corroborated this enhancement of fibronectin-coating in the retention of seeded EC upon PTFE.

Our own experience with fibronectin-coated grafts is that although fibronectin enhances cell retention on both plain and carbon-coated PTFE grafts compared with tissue culture media-coated grafts, there is no advantage of fibronectin-coating over autologous serum

[45]. In our subsequent studies with PTFE, therefore, we have chosen to suspend the inoculum of seeding cells in either the recipient's plasma or serum and to bathe the luminal surface of the PTFE with this cell suspension, or forcefully inject the serum/cell suspension through the internodal spaces of the graft. The issue of fibronectin-coating or of graft precoating with any other adhesive protein remains largely unresolved, however.

In addition to precoating PTFE grafts to enhance adherence of EC, researchers have investigated the effects of modification of graft internodal distances or porosities upon the development of the neointima in seeded grafts. We investigated three designs of ePTFE with mean internodal distances of 28, 40 and 52 μ in a 1988 report [46] in which these grafts were seeded with venous EC and implanted in the carotid arteries of dogs. We concluded that grafts with mean internodal distances of 40 μ were most successful in maintaining patencies and thrombus-free surface areas while promoting controlled inner capsule healing. Likewise, Kempczinski et al. [47] have reported excellent results seeding a highly porous (mean internodal distance 45 μ), unreinforced PTFE prosthesis. Commercially-available PTFE prostheses have mean internodal distances of approximately 30 μ and the internodal spaces remain filled with air when implanted clinically by vascular surgeons. By slightly expanding these internodal spaces and inoculating the cells into the internodal spaces suspended in serum or plasma, it has been assumed that more cells can be retained within the structure of the graft than is possible with surface seeding alone and that controlled ingrowth through the graft from the external capsule can proceed at a rate sufficient to establish a supporting subendothelium for the seeded cells to mature upon. In contrast to the support for this hypothesis from these two reports, Lindbald et al. [48] recently reported that altering graft internodal distances did not cause significant changes in attachment to PTFE grafts. Thus, the data and conclusions from porosity studies are equivocal and futher investigation of the attachment of EC to materials of differing porosities is certainly warranted.

The theoretical importance of complete graft endothelialization prior to implantation has prompted several reports of *in vitro* graft endothelialization. The experience from the animal research studies has been that luminal surfacing of the seeded cells may require 2–4 weeks for complete endothelialization in the postoperative period. During this time of evolution of the neointima, the graft remains highly thrombogenic and small-diameter grafts may occlude in experimental animals and humans unless antiplatelet drugs are administered. Certainly endothelialization of the graft luminal surface at the time of implantation would reduce the thrombotic potential of the graft in the early postoperative period. This endothelialization would have to occur *in vitro*. Foxall et al. [49] studied the attachment and growth of adult human EC on

PTFE and Dacron *in vitro*. Comparative studies were performed on grafts pretreated with collagen-fibronectin and on untreated grafts. On the treated PTFE, seeded cells formed a confluent monolayer in culture in nine days. Coverage of treated Dacron at nine days after seeding was poorer and cells did not attach nor grow on untreated grafts.

Sentissi et al. [50] investigated the adherence of bovine aortic endothelial cells to PTFE grafts pretreated with a collagen-fibronectin coating under conditions of low (25 ml/min) and high (200 ml/min) flow rates *in vitro*. The study concluded that the collagen-fibronectin coating promoted the attachment and adherence of these cells with minimal loss of cells during flow. The design of this study included a two week static incubation of the seeded cells on the prosthetic graft material prior to 60 minutes of flow. In similar studies using human umbilical vein EC, Anderson et al. [51] concluded that immediate confluent endothelial cell coverage required seeding at least 5×10^5 cells/cm^2 with subsequent incubation for at least 15 minutes in complete culture medium on grafts pretreated with collagen. Under these conditions cell spreading occurred within several hours.

Additional studies from this laboratory [52,53] have shown that confluent and durable endothelial cell monolayers can be established on prosthetic grafts within two hours. The minimum number of human umbilical vein EC required to achieve confluence was 1.4×10^5 cells/cm^2 of graft and confluence was achieved following two hours of *in vitro* perfusion with culture media at a rate of 15 ml/min. The cells were seeded onto prosthetic grafts that had been precoated with collagen type I. Established monolayers of EC maintained confluency even when flow rates through the grafts were maintained at 100 ml/min. These preformed confluent endothelial cell monolayers eliminated almost completely platelet deposition when the grafts were inserted as extension segments into arteriovenous silicone rubber shunts in baboons. Thus it does appear that under conditions of relatively low-flow *in vitro* perfusion, preformed confluent monolayers can theoretically be established on vascular grafts in a timely manner. However, the effects of *in vitro* environments upon vascular EC may be detrimental. The potential for both genotypic and phenotypic changes of EC in culture exists and many clinicians are opposed to subjecting the harvested cells to culture in undefined media-containing serum. While most surgeons would probably accept 2 hours as a reasonable time to achieve confluence based upon the potential advantages conferred to the graft by complete endothelialization, any additional time added to a surgical protocol for bypass grafting may be met with resistance.

Recognizing the limited availability of donor cells from available autologous veins for clinical graft seeding, the need for relatively high seeding densities to achieve rapid endothelialization, the need for enhancement of cell attachment by adhesive proteins and the potential disadvantages of tissue culture and *in vitro* perfusion to enhance cell spreading to achieve confluency, researchers have turned their attention to alternate sources of cells for graft seeding. In 1984 researchers reported significant coverage of Dacron grafts seeded with peritoneal mesothelial cells at the time of graft implantation in dogs [54]. A follow-up study demonstrated that these grafts seeded with mesothelial cells released more prostacyclin than unseeded grafts [55]. We have been most impressed, however, with the ongoing efforts to derive EC from the microvessels of human fat for graft seeding. Jarrell et al. first reported in 1986 their technique to derive microvascular EC from human perinephric and omental fat [56]. They reported the method of enzymatic harvest of the EC using collagenase and the purification of the isolated cells with a Percoll gradient. Their reported technique resulted in $1.25 \pm 0.45 \times 10^6$ cells/gram of fat processed. These EC firmly adhered to plasma-coated Dacron grafts and were resistant to shear-induced stresses. The immediately obvious advantage of endothelial cell derivation from fat is that all patients requiring bypass surgery will have stores of fat which could theoretically be obtained by liposuction. The large number of cells that can be obtained per gram of fat processed makes saturation density seeding, or "sodding", as the process is referred to by Jarrell and his colleagues, a possibility, even in the long lengths of graft often required for peripheral vascular bypasses. In addition, these investigators have reported the firm adherence of these cells to plasma-coated Dacron within 10 minutes and amnion-collagen-coated Dacron in 30 minutes [57]. Complete graft coverage occurred on the amnion-collagen-coated Dacron that resembled normal vessel wall morphology at 30 minutes after sodding.

Several investigators have seeded synthetic grafts with microvascular EC which were evaluated in animal models. Pearce et al. [58] initially reported the successful seeding of 60 μ pore-size PTFE grafts with microvascular EC derived from omentum. Patency of seeded grafts was 58%. We seeded 4 mm Dacron grafts with EC derived from the microvessels of omental fat and implanted the grafts in the canine arteries of dogs for 5 weeks [59]. The mean patencies of both the seeded and nonseeded grafts in our study was 89%. However, the mean thrombus-free surface area of the seeded grafts was 95%, differing significantly from that of nonseeded grafts, which was 43%, implying a beneficial effect of the seeded microvascular cells.

We have also seeded microvascular EC onto PTFE grafts that were evaluated in canine carotid arteries. In these short-term studies the patencies and thrombus-free surface areas of seeded grafts were good. However, the inner capsules of the seeded PTFE grafts were thicker than those in grafts from previous experiments in which the PTFE grafts had been seeded with venous endothelium. This thickness presumably resulted from the presence of many contaminating cells in addition to EC in the seeding inoculum. In their studies comparing the performances of grafts seeded with EC from the microvessels of fat and from the jugular vein, Sterpetti et al. [60] concluded the technique of deriving EC from fat needed refinement in order to reduce the occurrence of contaminating cells. Recognizing this need for ongoing refinements we remain excited over the potential of derivation of EC from microvessels as an alternative to venous EC for graft seeding, and as a development which could be embraced by vascular surgeons to move ECS into the clinical arena.

Because of the reported successes of ECS in lessening the thrombogenicity of arterial conduits, several researchers have investigated the effect of ECS upon the performance of venous prostheses. Prostheses are rarely used in the venous circulation because the low venous blood flows through these highly thrombogenic grafts can result in rapid occlusions. The results of ECS in the venous circulation have been less positive than those in the arterial circulation. Plate et al. [61] reported that early patency rates did not benefit from ECS of iliocaval grafts and that both seeded and nonseeded grafts developed endothelial linings in this model. Herring et al. [62] also reported no benefit of ECS in improving early patencies of ePTFE inferior vena cava replacements. In contrast, Köveker et al. [63] recently reported that ECS enhanced endothelialization on synthetic vena cava grafts and improved their thromboresistance. Additional studies need to be performed to determine the efficacy of ECS in enhancing venous prosthetic graft performance.

A persistent problem that has plagued researchers in the field of ECS is the confirmation that the cells which are seeded are truly the precursors of EC that ultimately form the neoendothelium on the graft. The suggestion has often been made that the technique of ECS might provide the stimulus for spontaneous endothelialization. Hollier et al. [64] seeded EC enzymatically derived from the jugular veins of female pigs onto thoracoabdominal bypass grafts implanted in male pig littermates. At 4 weeks postoperatively, the seeded grafts were endothelialized but chromosome analysis revealed surface endothelium that originated from the male host rather than from the female donor. The pig may not have been a good model for this study, however, as synthetic grafts rapidly endothelialize in the pig by 4 weeks post-implantation even when the grafts are not seeded.

In studies comparing homologous and autologous seeding of ePTFE arterial-venous prostheses in dogs, grafts seeded with large numbers of homologous EC generated mid-graft endothelial cell linings [65]. In a similar study, nonautologous ECS in combination with immunosuppression therapy resulted in an endothelial lining comprised primarily of host cells, thus suggesting that nonautologous seeding may indeed induce host EC to form a graft neointima [66]. Clowes et al. [67] have suggested that endothelial cells lining graft luminal surfaces may originate from the

transmural ingrowth of capillaries through graft pores. In contrast, data have recently become available that do confirm that the EC on harvested, seeded grafts originated from the seeding inoculum [68]. These data resulted from gene transfer studies. It is clear from the above examples that although almost all investigators concur on the existence of endothelium on seeded vascular grafts, the origin of the luminal EC remains controversial.

The technology of ECS has evolved in time coincident with major advances in the understanding of endothelial cell biology. The endothelial monolayer is a dynamic tissue with a repertoire of functions that have been largely unappreciated. Specific anticoagulant mechanisms exhibited by EC include the production of heparin-like glycosaminoglycans, prostacyclin production, plasminogen activator production and expression of thrombomodulin. These normal anticoagulant properties of the vascular endothelium argue in favor of seeding or promoting the growth of an endothelial lining on the lumen of prostheses. In addition to these anticoagulant properties, however, it is now also appreciated that EC may function under certain conditions to promote coagulation. Procoagulant products of EC include tissue factor, von Willenbrand factor, plasminogen activator inhibitor, thrombospondin and collagens [69]. These procoagulant functions of EC are useful physiologically, but may be undesirable in terms of vascular graft performance. It is probable that the techniques for deriving EC for vascular graft seeding, the process of seeding the graft, and the evolution of the seeded graft *in vivo* may induce responses in EC that are different from the functions of unperturbed cells. It can be theorized that the balance between anti- and procoagulant properties of EC ultimately dictates the thrombotic potential of the graft. It is clear that the focus in the evaluation of vascular graft performance must shift to include critical evaluation of the functional status of the EC at the blood/material interface.

CLINICAL STUDIES

The first clinical trial of ECS of vascular prostheses was reported by Herring et al. [70] in 1984. In their study, grafts were implanted in 161 patients. Grafts were seeded with EC mechanically harvested from adjacent subcutaneous veins in the leg. The study concluded that ECS improved graft patency rates but that the results were worse if the patient was a smoker. Herring et al. [71] updated the data from this study in a 1987 report. Seeded Dacron graft patency was superior to nonseeded patency between the first and second postoperative years, but not statistically significant. Seeded graft patency at 7 years was 30.8%; patency was 37.1% in nonseeded grafts. Smoking adversely affected seeded graft patency. Herring et al. [71] also reported results of a second clinical trial in which PTFE grafts were seeded with EC. At two years, patency of seeded PTFE grafts averaged 73.9%, which was not significantly different from patency of vein grafts in a concurrent patient population (84.6%). The PTFE grafts were seeded with cells derived from collagenase treatment of external jugular vein segments from each patient. Herring, et al. [72] were able to confirm extensive endothelialization of a seeded PTFE graft by histological observations in a patient at the 90th postoperative day.

Zilla et al. [73] also reported results from a series of 18 patients undergoing femoropopliteal bypass. PTFE grafts were seeded with EC derived from the external jugular vein in 9 of the patients. An average of 3.1×10^3 cells/cm² were seeded. Patients were monitored by a battery of platelet function studies as well as by a measure of the uptake of indium-111-oxine labeled platelets. On the basis of these follow-ups the degree of endothelialization in the seeded grafts was postulated as only minor. The authors emphasized a particular concern of all investigators designing clinical trials of endothelial cell seeded grafts—the need for direct biopsy of the graft in order to determine the degree of endothelialization. Results from additional clinical trials of endothelial cell seeded grafts have been reported from the University of Göteborg, Sweden [74]. These authors seeded one limb of Dacron aortic bifurcation grafts with EC derived from distal saphenous vein segments. The contralateral limb of each graft was nonseeded. Platelets from each patient were labeled with indium-111-oxine and platelet accumulations on each limb of the grafts were measured at 1 and 4 months postoperatively. The report concluded that there was a significant reduction in the accumulation of labeled platelets on the limbs of the grafts seeded with venous EC.

It is very difficult to design a clinical trial to evaluate ECS of vascular prostheses in humans. We received permission from our hospital's Institutional Review Board (IRB) to conduct a limited study to address some of the technical and logistical problems of transferring the technology of ECS from the laboratory to the clinical setting. Since January, 1987, 20 patients have undergone peripheral vascular reconstructions at Akron City Hospital in which 6 mm i.d. Gore-Tex PTFE grafts were seeded with EC. The results of the study were reported at a recent symposium [75]. In designing a clinical trial of ECS, investigators must first address the issue of the appropriate population in which the grafts can be evaluated. If one selects, for example, the population of patients requiring femoro-popliteal bypass surgery, should ECS be limited to those procedures in which the distal anastomosis is above the knee? If below-the-knee procedures are included, should the patients be randomized according to the number of runoff vessels into the legs and feet? Are the benefits of ECS well enough documented to randomize all patients requiring the surgery, regardless of the presence or absence of a suitable saphenous vein? Since the saphenous vein remains the "gold standard" against which all other vascular grafts, both natural and prosthetic, are compared, should the experiment be designed with saphenous vein grafts as the control grafts or with nonseeded prosthetic grafts of the same design, as the control? Would it be ethical to implant a nonseeded prosthetic graft in a patient that possessed a suitable saphenous vein?

In our preliminary study the surgeries were all leg-saving procedures in patients that did not have available autologous veins to use as bypass grafts. These patients were the "worst-case scenarios" of all patients that would potentially receive endothelial cell seeded grafts in peripheral vascular reconstructions. All of the procedures required below-the-knee distal graft anastomoses and the runoff conditions ranged between one and three vessels. An additional decision of importance in designing a clinical trial of ECS is the origin of the seeded cells—e.g., venous vs. microvascular origin? Because of our experience with microvascular EC derived from fat, we chose, in our study, to derive the seeding cells from masses of abdominal fat to assure large numbers of cells for seeding. For most of the patients in our study the initial procedure was to remove a large mass of anterior wall abdominal fat through a small incision. The mass of fat was subsequently divided and all large vessels and visible connective tissues were dissected from the sample. "Clean" fat samples were minced using two scalpels until the sample reached "cream of wheat" consistency. Subsequently the EC were harvested enzymatically using collagenase. In several patients, fat samples were derived by liposuction. This technique finely minces the fat, thus exposing more surface area to collagenase action, and our harvest of EC from these patients was greater than from the manual mincing technique. In our study the mean number of cells obtained per gram of fat was 6.83×10^5 and the mean number of cells seeded per graft was 8.04×10^6. Based upon these numbers, the seeding density averaged 4.41×10^4 cells/cm² for a 50 cm length of 6 mm internal diameter vascular graft.

In clinical studies, decisions must be reached regarding graft pretreatment, seeding methodology and *in vitro* incubation prior to surgical implantation. In our study all cells were seeded immediately onto the prosthetic grafts prior to implantation—there was no period of *in vitro* culture. The seeding cells were mixed with the patient's plasma and plasma/cell suspension was injected into the lumen and through the internodal spaces of the PTFE grafts. The grafts had not been precoated with specific adhesive proteins. Finally there exist the complicated issues of patient follow-up and proving that graft performance has indeed been enhanced as a result of ECS. In order to directly demonstrate the existence of EC on the graft's luminal lining, a biopsy should ideally be performed at a site removed from either anastomosis. The occurrence of EC could then be documented by histologic and/or electron microscopic studies. However, the functional status of the cells, if identified, would be very difficult to ascertain. Most centers have relied upon platelet-labeling as an indirect statement of the efficacy of ECS. Presumably fewer platelets accumulate on endothelial cell seeded grafts. However, we have had difficulty with patient compliance in returning to our institution for platelet scans and the results we have obtained have not been particularly diagnostic.

The surgeon is ultimately concerned with patency of the graft. Our data to date, from this preliminary series of patients, is that 70% of the grafts remain patent with the longest graft following 18 months. Other centers are currently conducting clinical trials, so additional data will be forthcoming regarding the performance of endothelial cell seeded grafts. At least two studies have been approved by the FDA that involve devices generically known as endothelial cell seeding kits. These kits are designed for general marketing to vascular surgeons. Our perspective has been somewhat more conservative, perhaps. We feel that if ECS does prove beneficial to vascular graft performance, specialized centers for ECS could be developed with appropriate technicians and equipment to ensure quality control. However, the data will dictate the approach and the ultimate fate of the promising technology of ECS.

Regardless of the ultimate fate of ECS in clinical bypass surgery, the technology has spawned a number of important directions that may, in addition, profoundly affect patient care. Most notable is the recent report that EC may be manipulated genetically, with the potential to therapeutically deliver many gene products directly into the vasculature [76]. Genetically engineered EC could be introduced to the recipient on seeded vascular grafts. Thus endothelial cells seeded on vascular grafts may play an important role in gene therapy not previously conceived.

REFERENCES

1. Voorhees, A. B., A. Jaretski and A. H. Blakemore. 1952. "The Use of Tubes Constructed from Vinyon 'N' Cloth in Bridging Arterial Defects", *Annals of Surgery*, 135:332.

2. Blakemore, A. and A. B. Voorhees. 1954. "The Use of Tube Constructed of Vinyon 'N' Cloth in Bridging Arterial Defects: Experimental and Clinical", *Annals of Surgery*, 140:324.

3. Szilagy, D. E. 1978. "Perspectives in Vascular Grafting", in *Vascular Grafts*. P. N. Sawyer and M. J. Kaplitt, eds. P23, Appleton, Century, Crofts.

4. Darling, R. C. and R. R. Linton. 1972. "Durability of Femoropopliteal Reconstruction", *American Journal of Surgery*, 123:472.

5. Bergen, J. J., F. J. Veith, V. M. Bernhard, J. S. T. Yao, W. R. Flinn, S. K. Gupta, L. A. Scher, R. H. Samson and J. B. Towne. 1982. "Randomization of Autogenous Vein and Polytetrafluoroethylene Grafts in Femorodistal Reconstructions", *Surgery*, 92:921.

6. Glück, T. 1898. "Die Moderne Chirugie des Circulation Sapparates", *Berl. Klin.*, 70:1.

7. Bernheim, B. M. 1916. "The Ideal Operation for Aneurysm of the Extremity. Report of a Case", *Bulletin of Johns Hopkins Hospital*, 27:93.

8. Kunkin, J. 1949. "Le Traitement de L'arterite Obliterante par la Greffe Veineuse", *Arch. Mal. Coeur.*, 42:371.

9. Stewart, B. H., M. S. DeWeese, J. Conway and R. J. Correa, Jr. 1962. "Renal Hypertension: An Appraisal of Diagnostic Studies and of Direct Operative Treatment", *Archives of Surgery*, 85:617.

10. Garrett, H. E., E. W. Dennis and M. E. DeBakey. 1973. "Aortocoronary Bypass with Saphenous Vein Graft. Seven Year Follow-up", *JAMA*, 223:792.

11. Szilagyi, D. E., J. P. Elliott and J. H. Hageman. 1973. "Biologic Fate of Autogenous Vein Implants as Arterial Substitutes: Clinical, Angiographic and Histopathologic Observations in Femoropopliteal Operations for Atherosclerosis", *Annals of Surgery*, 178:232.

12. Grondin, C. M., L. Campeau, J. Lesperance, M. Enjalbert and M. G. Bourassa. 1984. "Comparison of Late Changes in Internal Mammary Artery and Saphenous Vein Grafts in Two Consecutive Series of Patients 10 Years after Operation", *Circulation*, 70(Suppl 1):208.

13. Quinones-Baldrich, W. J., R. W. Busuttil, J. D. Baker, C. L. Vescera, S. S. Ahn, H. I. Machleder and W. S. Moore. 1988. "Is the Preferential Use of Polytetrafluoroethylene Grafts for Femoropopliteal Bypass Justified?" *Journal of Vascular Surgery*, 8:219.

14. Jaffe, E. D., R. L. Nachman, G. Becker and C. R. Minick. 1973. "Culture of Human Endothelial Cells Derived from Umbilical Veins", *Journal of Clinical Investigation*, 52:2745.

15. Burkel, W. E. and R. H. Kahn. 1977. "Cell-Lined, Nonwoven Microfiber Scaffolds as a Blood Interface", *Annals of the New York Academy of Science*, 283:419.

16. Herring, M., A. Gardner and J. Glover. 1978. "A Single-Staged Technique for Seeding Vascular Grafts with Autogenous Endothelium", *Surgery*, 84:498.

17. Herring, M. B., R. Dilley, R. A. Jersild, Jr., L. Boxer, A. Gardner and J. Glover. 1979. "Seeding Arterial Prostheses with Vascular Endothelium. The Nature of the Lining", *Annals of Surgery*, 190:84.

18. Dilley, R., M. Herring, L. Boxer, A. Gardner and J. Glover. 1979. "Immunofluorescent Staining for Factor VIII Related Antigen", *Journal of Surgical Research*, 27:149.

19. Herring, M., A. Gardner and J. Glover. 1979. "Seeding Endothelium onto Canine Arterial Prostheses. The Effects of Graft Design", *Archives of Surgery*, 114:679.

20. Graham, L. M., W. E. Burkel, J. W. Ford, D. W. Vinter, R. H. Kahn and J. C. Stanley. 1980. "Immediate Seeding of Enzymatically Derived Endothelium in Dacron Vascular Grafts. Early Experimental Studies with Autologous Canine Cells", *Archives of Surgery*, 115:1289.

21. Graham, L. M., D. W. Vinter, J. W. Ford, R. H. Kahn, W. E. Burkel and J. C. Stanley. 1980. "Endothelial Cell Seeding of Prosthetic Vascular Grafts. Early Experimental Studies with Cultured Autologous Canine Endothelium", *Archives of Surgery*, 115:929.

22. Belden, T. A., S. P. Schmidt, L. J. Falkow and W. V. Sharp. 1982. "Endothelial Cell Seeding of Small-Diameter Vascular Grafts", *Transactions American Society for Artificial Internal Organs*, 28:173.

23. Stanley, J. C., W. E. Burkel, J. W. Ford, D. W. Vinter, R. H. Kahn, W. M. Whitehouse, Jr. and L. M. Graham. 1982. "Enhanced Patency of Small-Diameter, Externally Supported Dacron Iliofemoral Grafts Seeded with Endothelial Cells", *Surgery*, 92:994.

24. Hunter, T. J., S. P. Schmidt, W. V. Sharp and G. S. Malindzak. 1983. "Controlled Flow Studies in 4 mm Endothelialized Dacron Grafts", *Transactions American Society for Artificial Internal Organs*, 29:177.

25. Schmidt, S. P., T. J. Hunter, W. V. Sharp, G. S. Malindzak and M. M. Evancho. 1984. "Endothelial Cell-Seeded Four-Millimeter Dacron Vascular Grafts: Effects of Blood Flow Manipulation through the Grafts", *Journal of Vascular Surgery*, 1:434.

26. Graham, L. M., W. E. Burkel, J. W. Ford, D. W. Vinter, R. H. Kahn and J. C. Stanley. 1982. "Expanded Polytetrafluoroethylene Vascular Prostheses Seeded with Enzymatically Derived and Cultured Canine Endothelial Cells", *Surgery*, 91:550.

27. Herring, M., S. Baughman, J. Glover, K. Kisler, J. Joseph, J. Campbell, R. Dilley, A. Evan and A. Gardner. 1984. "Endothelial Seeding of Dacron and Polytetrafluoroethylene Grafts: The Cellular Events of Healing", *Surgery*, 96:745.

28. Sharefkin, J. B., C. Latker, M. Smith, D. Cruess, G. P. Clagett and N. M. Rich. 1982. "Early Normalization of Platelet Survival by Endothelial Seeding of Dacron Arterial Prostheses in Dogs", *Surgery*, 92:385.

29. Clagett, G. P., W. E. Burkel, J. B. Sharefkin, J. W. Ford, H. Hufnagel, D. W. Vinter, R. H. Kahn, L. M. Graham and J. C. Stanley. 1982. "Antithrombotic Character of Canine Endothelial Cell-Seeded Arterial Prostheses", *Surgical Forum*, 33:471.

30. Sharp, W. V., S. P. Schmidt and D. L. Donovan. 1986. "Prostaglandin Biochemistry of Seeded Endothelial Cells on Dacron Prostheses", *Journal of Vascular Surgery*, 3:256.

31. Sicard, G. A., B. T. Allen, J. A. Long, M. J. Welch, A. Griffin, R. E. Clark and C. B. Anderson. 1984. "Prostaglandin Production and Platelet Reactivity of Small-Diameter Grafts", *Journal of Vascular Surgery*, 1:744.

32. Kaplan, S., K. F. Marcoe, L. R. Sauvage, M. Zammit, H.-D. Wu, S. R. Mathisen and M. W. Walker. 1986. "The Effect of Predetermined Thrombotic Potential of the Recipient on Small-Caliber Graft Performance", *Journal of Vascular Surgery*, 3:311.

33. Schmidt, S. P., T. J. Hunter, L. J. Falkow, M. M. Evancho and W. V. Sharp. 1985. "Effects of Antiplatelet Agents in Combination with Endothelial Cell Seeding on Small Diameter Dacron Vascular Graft Performance in the Canine Carotid Artery Model", *Journal of Vascular Surgery*, 2:898.

34. Hirko, M. K., S. P. Schmidt, M. M. Evancho, W. V. Sharp and D. L. Donovan. 1987. "Endothelial Cell Seeding Improves 4 mm PTFE Vascular Graft Performance in Antiplatelet Medicated Dogs", *Artery*, 14:137.

35. Shepard, A. D., J. Eldrup-Jorgenson, E. M. Keough, T. F. Foxall, K. Ramberg, R. J. Connolly, W. C. Mackey, V. Gavris, K. R. Auger, P. Libby, T. F. O'Donnell and A. D. Callow. 1986. "Endothelial Cell Seeding of Small-Caliber Synthetic Grafts in the Baboon", *Surgery*, 99:318.

36. Rosenman, J. E., R. F. Kempczinski, W. H. Pearce and E. B. Silberstein. 1985. "Kinetics of Endothelial Cell Seeding", *Journal of Vascular Surgery*, 2:778.

37. Sharefkin, J. B., H. E. Van Wart, D. F. Cruess, R. A. Albus and E. M. Levine. 1986. "Adult Human Endothelial Cell Enzymatic Harvesting", *Journal of Vascular Surgery*, 4:567.

38. Watkins, M. T., J. B. Sharefkin, R. Zajtchuk, T. M. Maciag, P. A. D'Amore, U. S. Ryan, H. Van Wart and N. M. Rich. 1984. "Adult Human Saphenous Vein Endothelial Cells: Assessment of Their Reproductive Capacity for Use in Endothelial Seeding of Vascular Prostheses", *Journal of Surgical Research*, 36:588.

39. Sharefkin, J. B., C. Lather, M. Smith and N. M. Rich. 1983. "Endothelial Cell Labeling with ¹¹¹Indium-Oxine as a Marker of Cell Attachment to Bioprosthetic Surfaces", *Journal of Biomedical Material Research*, 17:345.

40. Williams, S. K., B. E. Jarrell, L. Friend H. S. Radomski, R. A. Carabasi, E. Koolpe, S. N. Mueller, S. C. Thornton, T. Marinucci and E. Levine. 1985. "Adult Human Endothelial Cell Compatibility with Prosthetic Graft Material", *Journal of Surgical Research*, 38:618.

41. Ramalanjaona, G., R. F. Kempczinski, J. E. Rosenman, E. C. Douville and E. B. Silberstein. 1986. "The Effect of Fibronectin Coating on Endothelial Cell Kinetics in Polytetrafluoroethylene Grafts", *Journal of Vascular Surgery*, 3:264.

42. Ramalanjaona, G. R., R. F. Kempczinski, J. D. Ogle and E. B. Silberstein. 1986. "Fibronectin Coating of an Experimental PTFE Vascular Prosthesis", *Journal of Surgical Research*, 41:479.

43. Kesler, K. A., M. B. Herring, M. P. Arnold, J. L. Glover, H-M. Park, M. N. Helmus and P. J. Bendick. 1986. "Enhanced Strength of Endothelial Attachment on Polyester Elastomer and Polytetrafluoroethylene Graft Surfaces with Fibronectin Substrate", *Journal of Vascular Surgery*, 3:58.

44. Seeger, J. M. and N. Klingman. 1985. "Improved Endothelial Cell Seeding with Cultured Cells and Fibronectin-Coated Grafts", *Journal of Surgical Research*, 38:641.

45. Schmidt, S. P., K. L. Boyd, T. R. Pippert, S. A. Hite, M. M. Evancho and W. V. Sharp. 1987. "Endothelial Cell Seeding of Ultralow Temperature Carbon-Coated Polytetrafluoroethylene Grafts", in *Endothelialization of Vascular Grafts*. P. Zilla, R. Fasol, M. Deutsch, eds. Basel: Karger, pp. 145–159.

46. Boyd, K. L., S. Schmidt, T. R. Pippert, S. A. Hite and W. V. Sharp. 1988. "The Effects of Pore Size and Endothelial Cell Seeding Upon the Performance of Small-Diameter ePTFE Vascular Grafts Under Controlled Flow Conditions", *Journal of Biomedical Material Research*, 22:163.

47. Kempczinski, R. F., J. E. Rosenman, W. H. Pearce, L. R. Roedersheimer, Y. Berlatzky and G. Ramalanjaona. 1985. "Endothelial Cell Seeding of a New PTFE Vascular Prosthesis", *Journal of Vascular Surgery*, 2:424.

48. Lindbald, B., S. W. Wright and R. L. Sell. 1987. "Alternative Techniques of Seeding Cultured Endothelial Cells to ePTFE Grafts of Different Diameters, Porosities and Surfaces", *Journal of Biomedical Material Research*, 21:1013.

49. Foxall, T. L., K. R. Auger, A. D. Callow and P. Libby. 1986. "Adult Human Endothelial Cell Coverage of Small-Caliber Dacron and Polytetrafluoroethylene Vascular Prostheses *in vitro*", *Journal of Surgical Research*, 41:158.

50. Sentissi, J. M., K. Ramberg, T. F. O'Donnell, Jr., R. J. Connolly and A. D. Callow. 1986. "The Effect of Flow on Vascular Endothelial Cells Grown in Tissue Culture on Polytetrafluoroethylene Grafts", *Surgery*, 99:337.

51. Anderson, J. S., T. M. Price, S. R. Hanson and L. A. Harker. 1987. "*In vitro* Endothelialization of Small-Caliber Vascular Grafts", *Surgery*, 101:577.

52. Schneider, P. A., S. R. Hanson, T. M. Price and L. A. Harker. 1988. "Durability of Confluent Endothelial Cell Monolayers on Small-Caliber Vascular Prostheses *in vitro*", *Surgery*, 103:456

53. Schneider, P. A., S. R. Hanson, T. M. Price and L. A. Harker. 1988. "Preformed Confluent Endothelial Cell Monolayers Prevent Early Platelet Deposition on Vascular Prostheses in Baboons", *Journal of Vascular Surgery*, 8:229.

54. Clarke, J. M. F., R. M. Pittilo, L. J. Nicholson, N. Woolf and A. Marston. 1984. "Seeding Dacron Arterial Prostheses with Peritoneal Mesothelial Cells: A Preliminary Morphological Study", *British Journal of Surgery*, 71:492.

55. Bull, H. A., R. M. Pittilo, J. Drury, J. G. Pollock, J. M. F. Clarke, N. Woolf, A. Marston and S. J. Machin. 1988. "Effects of Autologous Mesothelial Cell Seeding on Prostacyclin Production within Dacron Arterial Prostheses", *British Journal of Surgery*, 75:671.

56. Jarrell, B. E., S. K. Williams, G. Stokes, F. A. Hubbard, R. A. Carabasi, E. Koolpe, D. Greener, K. Pratt, M. J. Moritz, J. Radomski and L. Speicher. 1986. "Use of Freshly Isolated Capillary Endothelial Cells for the Immediate Establishment of a Monolayer on a Vascular Graft at Surgery", *Surgery*, 100:392.

57. Jarrell, B. E., S. K. Williams, L. Solomon, L. Speicher, E. Koolpe, J. Radomski, R. A. Carabasi, D. Greener and F. E. Rosato. 1986. "Use of an Endothelial Monolayer on a Vascular Graft Prior to Implantation", *Annals of Surgery*, 203:671.

58. Pearce, W. H., R. B. Rutherford, T. A. Whitehill, C. Rosales, K. P. Bell, A. Patt and G. Ramalanjaona. 1987. "Successful Endothelial Seeding with Omentally Derived Microvascular Endothelial Cells", *Journal of Vascular Surgery*, 5:203.

59. Schmidt, S. P., N. Monajjem, M. M. Evancho, T. R. Pippert and W. V. Sharp. 1988. "Microvascular Endothelial Cell Seeding of Small-Diameter Dacron Vascular Grafts", *Journal of Investigative Surgery*, 1:35.

60. Sterpetti, A. V., W. J. Hunter, R. D. Schultz, J. T. Sugimoto, E. A. Blair, K. Hacker, P. Chasan and J. Valentine. 1988. "Seeding with Endothelial Cells Derived from the Microvessels of the Omentum and from the Jugular Vein", *Journal of Vascular Surgery*, 7:677.

61. Plate, G., L. H. Hollier, R. J. Fowl, J. R. Sande and M. P. Kaye. 1984. "Endothelial Seeding of Venous Prostheses", *Surgery*, 96:929.

62. Herring, M., A. Gardner, P. Peigh, D. Madison, S. Baughman, J. Brown and J. Glover. 1984. "Patency in Canine Inferior Vena Cava Grafting: Effects of Graft Material, Size, and Endothelial Seeding", *Journal of Vascular Surgery*, 1:877.

63. Köveker, G. B., W. E. Burkel, L. M. Graham, T. W. Wakefield and J. C. Stanley. 1988. "Endothelial Cell Seeding of Expanded Polytetrafluoroethylene Vena Cava Conduits: Effects on Luminal Production of Prostacyclin, Platelet Adherence, and Fibrinogen Accumulation", *Journal of Vascular Surgery*, 7:600.

64. Hollier, L. H., R. J. Fowl, R. C. Pennell, C. F. Heck, K. A. H. Winter, D. N. Fass and M. P. Kaye. 1986. "Are Seeded Endothelial Cells the Origin of Neointima on Prosthetic Vascular Grafts?" *Journal of Vascular Surgery*, 3:65.

65. Zamora, J. L., L. T. Navarro, C. L. Ives, D. G. Weilbaecher, Z. R. Gao and G. P. Noon. 1986. "Seeding of Arteriovenous Prostheses with Homologous Endothelium", *Journal of Vascular Surgery*, 3:860.

66. Wakefield, T. W., E. M. Earley, T. E. Brothers, W. E. Burkel, L. M. Graham, R. D. Fessler, N. Saenz, R. M. Sell and J. C. Stanley. 1988. "Karyotype Analysis of Cell Sex to Determine the Source of Vascular Graft Luminal Linings Following Autologous and Nonautologous Endothelial Cell Seeding", *Transactions American Society of Artificial Internal Organs*, 34:864.

67. Clowes, A. W., M. M. Clowes, T. R. Kirkman and M. A. Reidy. 1986. "Capillary Endothelium Can Substitute for Arterial Endothelium in Healing Arterial Replacements", *Federation Proceedings*, 45:473.

68. Callow, A. D., R. Nitzberg, P. Libby, R. Connolly, K. Gould, L. Birinyi, J. Wilson and R. Mulligan. 1989. "Confirmation by Gene Transfer Technology of the Origin of the Endothelial Cells on Harvested Seeded Vascular Grafts", Abstract, Submitted to the American Surgical Association.

69. Libby, P., L. K. Birinyi and A. D. Callow. 1987. "Functions of Endothelial Cells Related to Seeding of Vascular Prostheses: The Unanswered Questions", in *Endothelial Cell Seeding in Vascular Surgery*. M. Herring and J. D. Glover, eds. Orlando: Grune & Stratton, pp. 17–35.

70. Herring, M., A. Gardner and J. Glover. 1984. "Seeding Human Arterial Prostheses with Mechanically Derived Endothelium. The Detrimental Effect of Smoking", *Journal of Vascular Surgery*, 1:279.

71. Herring, M. B., R. S. Compton, A. L. Gardner and D. R. Le Grand. 1987. "Clinical Experiences with Endothelial Seeding in Indianapolis", in *Endothelialization of Vascular Grafts*. P. Zilla, R. Fasol and M. Deutsch, eds. Basel: Karger, pp. 218–224.

72. Herring, M., S. Baughman and J. Glover. 1985. "Endothelium Develops on Seeded Human Arterial Prosthesis: A Brief Clinical Note", *Journal of Vascular Surgery*, 2:727.

73. Zilla, P., R. Fasol, M. Deutsch, T. Fischlein, E. Minar, A. Hammerle, O. Krupicka and M. Kadletz.

1987. "Endothelial Cell Seeding of Polytetrafluoroethylene Vascular Grafts in Humans: A Preliminary Report", *Journal of Vascular Surgery*, 6:535.

74. Risberg, B., P. Ortenwall, H. Wadenvik and J. Kutti. 1987. "Endothelial Cell Seeding: Experience and First Clinical Results in Göteborg", in *Endothelialization of Vascular Grafts*. P. Zilla, R. Fasol and M. Deutsch, eds. Basel: Karger, pp. 225–232.

75. Sharp, W. V., S. P. Schmidt, S. O. Meerbaum and T. R. Pippert. "Derivation of Human Microvascular Endothelial Cells for Prosthetic Graft Seeding", presented at *The Third Annual Symposium on Endothelial Seeding, October 20–21, 1988, Indianapolis, Indiana*.

76. Zweibel, J. A., S. M. Freeman, P. W. Kantoff, K. Cornetta, U. S. Ryan and W. F. Anderson. 1989. "High-Level Recombinant Gene Expression in Rabbit Endothelial Cells Transduced by Retroviral Vectors", *Science*, 243:220.

Part 5

ORTHOPEDIC APPLICATIONS

32

Carbon-Reinforced Composites in Orthopedic Surgery

P. CHRISTEL, M.D., Ph.D.*
L. CLAES, Ph.D.**
S. A. BROWN, Ph.D.†

ABSTRACT: This chapter reviews the current state of the art of the use of Carbon-Fiber-Reinforced Composites in orthopedic surgery. Carbon-Fiber-Reinforced Carbon (CFRC), Carbon-Fiber-Reinforced Polysulfone (CFRPS) and Carbon-Fiber-Reinforced Polyaryl Ether Ether Ketones (CFRPEEK) are successively considered for total hip replacement and internal fixation. Manufacturing processes, mechanical performances, and biological properties of these composites are reviewed according to the data of the scientific literature and the experience of the authors.

INTRODUCTION

One of the major unsolved problems in orthopedic surgery is the mismatch existing between bone and implant stiffness. Ceramics and metals are at least 10 to 40 times stiffer than human cortical bone. In the load-sharing between the implant and bone, the amount of stress carried by each of them is directly related to their stiffness. Bone thus becomes insufficiently loaded, and its adaptive remodeling leads to cortical thinning and increased porosity.

Matching bone and implant stiffnesses should limit the so-called stress shielding. In this respect, the use of low-stiffness materials appears quite interesting; however, low strength associated with the low stiffness of traditional materials usually impairs their potential use in human clinical situations.

The concept of using composite materials for or-

thopedic implants finds its origin in the fact that this category of material can exhibit simultaneously high strength and low rigidity. Many composites have mechanical strength sufficient to withstand the repetitive physiological load needed in the human body; moreover, their properties can be strengthened in preferential directions and adapted to the loading conditions. Among all the available composites, the carbon-fiber-reinforced ones (CFR) have been studied extensively either as CFR-resins or CFR-carbon (CFRC) because of their excellent mechanical properties.

This chapter will review the research and development associated with the use of CFR-composite materials for hip prosthesis and for osteosynthesis. It is the result of an international collaborative work, and a particular focus will be made on the following materials: CFRC by P. Christel, CFR-polysulfone (CFRPS) by L. Claes, and the promising CFR-polyaryl ether ether ketones (CFRPEEK) by S. Brown.

CARBON-FIBER-REINFORCED COMPOSITES FOR TOTAL HIP REPLACEMENT

Manufacturing Processes of CFRC

Basically CFRC materials are a class of composites made of carbon fibers embedded within a carbon matrix. Although the material is made entirely of carbon, there are several categories of carbon fibers, carbon matrices, and manufacturing processes [1–4]. This explains why there are many different types of CFRC with different properties.

Carbon Fibers Arrangement for CFRC

Carbon fibers are generally obtained by pyrolysis of organic fibers like polyacrylonitrile (PAN) or rayon fibers. When prepared from PAN precursor, the process involves three steps: stretching of molecular

* Laboratoire de Rechérche Orthopedique, Faculté de Médecine Lariboisiére Saint-Louis, Université Paris 7, 10 Avenue de Verdun, F-75010, Paris, France
** Sektion für Unfallchirurgische, Forschung und Biomechanik, Ulm University, Oberer, Eselberg 7, D-7900 Ulm, Germany
† Dept. of Biomedical Engineering, Case Western Reserve University, Cleveland, OH 44106

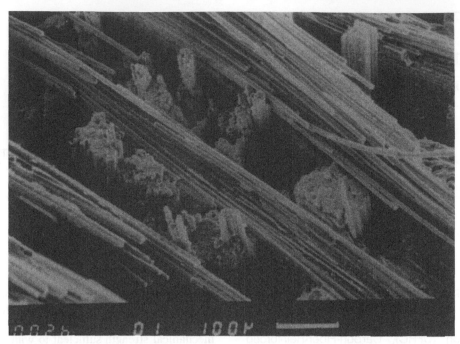

Figure 1. Fractography of 2-D reinforcement of a CFRC composite before CVI as shown by SEM. The braided laminates are oriented at 90°.

chains, stabilization with spared oxidation at a temperature of 200 to 350°C, and carbonization at temperatures of about 1400°C to obtain high tensile-strength fibers, or an additional heat treatment up to 2600°C, yielding high-modulus fibers. The fibers, which have a 7-μm diameter, may be obtained with various cross sections, surface roughnesses and microporosities to modulate their adhesion to the matrix. Usually the fibers are coated with an organic resin, called sizing agent, which disappears during the heating necessary to the manufacturing process. Before infiltration with the carbon matrix, fibers can be woven to form braids or tissue fabrics (Figure 1). Their orientation in the fabric layer may be uni-, bi-, tri-, or multiaxial. In bulk composites, the fibers may also have a directional arrangement in from one to six directions.

With PAN, three categories of carbon fibers may be obtained: high-modulus (HM), high-tensile-strength (HT), and intermediate fibers. In the process used for the manufacturing of the stem of the hip prosthesis described in this chapter, the intermediate fibers are obtained by pyrolysis of a PAN thick cloth precursor resulting in a carbon cloth, where the characteristics of the individual carbon fibers cannot be measured accurately. This cloth is a homogeneous needled three-dimensional structure formed of superposed layers of fibrous material [5]. This uniformity is accomplished by first superposing layers of a fibrous material in sheet form onto a support, and subsequently needling each new layer onto the preceding ones as it is superposed until the required thickness is reached. The distance between the support and the needles is then modified at each superposition of a new layer, to keep a substantially constant needling depth, right through the entire needling of the stack of layers. The support is formed of a material that permits the needles to penetrate it so that the initial layers of material are needled with the same needle penetration as later layers. The support and needles are moved apart as each new layer is superposed, by a distance equal to the thickness of a needled layer. Thus, the needling is performed with a uniform density throughout the whole thickness of the structure (Figures 2 and 3). The process is applicable both in the manufacture of three-dimensional structures formed with superposed flat sheets of fibrous material, and the manufacture of three-dimensional structures of revolution. After the last layer has been stacked and needled, finishing needling steps are carried out, with the distance between the support and the needles being modified after each finishing needling step, so that the needling density inside the upper layers is substantially equal to that in the other layers. For the final layers, the needling rate is reduced to compensate for the lessened clogging of the needle in having fewer layers to penetrate.

The sheet of fibrous material can be supplied in different forms, depending on the application. The fibrous material may be partly constituted of a layer of discontinuous fibers obtained by carding (card webs), or of a layer of continuous fibers obtained by criss-crossing unidirectional webs of continuous yarns or tows followed by low-density needling (pre-needling) of the layer together as shown in Figure 4. When greater mechanical strength is required, the fibrous layer is made by at least one woven layer which can be either a complex constituted by a fabric of continuous or discontinuous fibers (satin or plain weave type) as shown on Figures 4(a) and 4(b) or a fabric on its own, constituted by yarns in the warp direction and by a roving in the weft direction [Figure 4(c)].

Carbon Matrix for CFRC

There are several ways to obtain a carbon matrix. Accordingly, the resulting matrix structure can range from carbon to graphite, depending on the matrix precursors, the processing conditions, and the heat treatment.

The Chemical Vapor Infiltration Process (CVI)

This process is based on the diffusion of a carbon-bearing gas within the porous substrate. The quality of the matrix depends on temperature, pressure, flow rate, substrate density, and area. Among the various CVI processes available, the most widely used are the isothermal and the temperature gradient processes. In the isothermal process, the substrate is heated by an induction-heated susceptor and the hydrocarbon gas is converted into carbon when contacting the substrate. As a result, there is an overcrusting of the substrate surface which needs to be machined away after each infiltration cycle. Multiple cycles are necessary to achieve maximum density. In general, the infiltration lasts at least 2000 hr, resulting in composites with over 99% pure carbon, and a residual open porosity ~7–10% (Figure 5). Pores have a tunnel morphology. The matrix has the organized structure of pyrolytic carbon made of microcrystallites having a turbostratic arrangement. This is the process which is used for the manufacturing of the CFRC hip prosthesis described here.

The temperature gradient process permits continuous infiltration with shorter deposition times but is limited to single-item infiltration. The inner side of the substrate is in direct contact with a hot mandrel, its outer surface being exposed to a cool environment. Carbon deposition starts in the depth of the substrate and progresses radially as the densified parts of the substrate become inductively heated.

Liquid Impregnation Technique (LIT)

With this process, the porous substrate is impregnated with liquid organic precursors and densification is achieved through recarbonization cycles. The applied pressure for impregnation varies up to 100 MPa depending on the precursor material. The impregnation step can last up to 20 hr. Recarbonization is obtained by heating the material between 1000 and 2800°C. Densification cycles are repeated 4 to 12 times depending on the sample thickness and required final porosity. The conversion of the organic precursor into carbon can be responsible for fiber damage

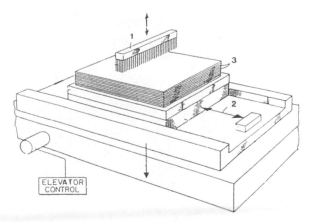

Figure 2. Schematic diagram illustrating the manufacturing process of three-dimensional structures by needling of flat layers. 1, needle board submitted to a vertical reciprocating motion; 2, platen reciprocally driven in motion with respect to the support table; 3, needled sheets.

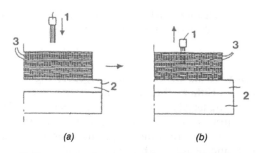

Figure 3. Cross-sectional views of different stages in the production of a structure with the process illustrated on Figure 2. (a) and (b) show the needles respectively in high and low positions. The needles penetrate into the texture through a depth equal to several times the thickness of a needled sheet. When the thickness of the structure increases, the needle board goes up in order to maintain a constant needling density.

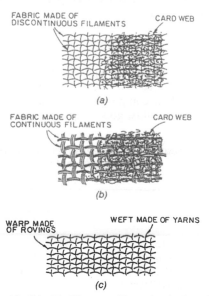

Figure 4. (a), (b), (c). Diagrams illustrating various forms of fibrous material which can be used for carrying out the manufacturing process (see text).

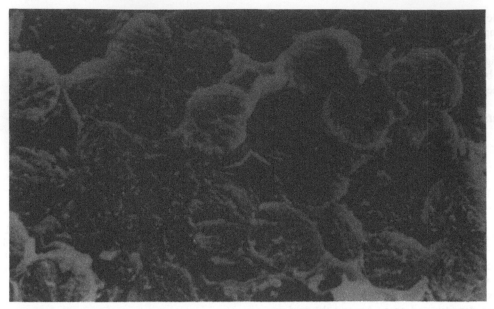

Figure 5. Unidirectional CVI-CFRC composite. Voids between braided fibers have been filled by infiltration at high temperature with dense pyrolytic carbon. Small residual pores are visible.

secondary to the matrix shrinkage occurring during pyrolysis. Either thermosetting resins or thermoplastic materials can be used as precursors. The thermosetting resins carbonize in a nongraphitizable solid carbon, whereas thermoplastic materials result in a liquid-phase carbonization ending in soft graphitizable carbons. If pitches are used as matrix precursors, elemental sulfur needs to be added to obtain high carbon yields [1,2]. This manufacturing process is employed at a lower cost than the CVI. However, the matrix has a vitreous structure and retains the original impurities included in the pitch. The final composite has an internal closed porosity with prestressed fibers [3,4].

CFRC Materials Properties

Specific biomechanical requirements for orthopedic applications have led to the development of a new generation of carbon composites with high mechanical strength, low modulus, good toughness, and excellent fatigue behavior. The measurements carried out on 2- and 3-axial CFRC, obtained by LIT using an organic resin as matrix precursor, have demonstrated similar properties (Table 1). This may be explained by the material's defects related to this particular type of processing. For CVI-CFRC, within a given dimensional arrangement, the fiber type (HM or HT) and, to a lesser extent, density, can influence the composite properties. Table 1 also contains comparison of the properties of three types of CVI-CFRC. B1 type 1 had a reinforcement built from a HT fiber cloth woven with 1000 dry filaments yarn fitted on a bidirectional orthogonal arrangement, whereas B1 type 3 had a reinforcement built from a cloth with 3000 filaments. B4 was made of the multidirectional intermediate fiber cloth obtained by needling of superposed layers of fibrous material as described above.

It is difficult to compare CVI-CFRC fatigue characteristics to those of LIT-CFRC where the fatigue limits are 65 to 70% of the static strength [6]. These materials have been tested by investigators using

Table 1. Comparative mechanical properties of 2- and 3-axial CFRC-LIT [6] with CVI-CFRC having different structures [14,28]. The values given for CVI-CFRC were obtained for a load applied parallel to the laminates.

	LIT-CFRC		CVI-CFRC		
	2-Axial	3-Axial	B1-Type 1	B1-Type 3	3 B4
Shear strength (MN/mm²)	31.1	29.9	15–32	10–15	23–30
Twist angle to failure (°)	12.3	9.7	—	—	—
Shear modulus (GN/mm²)	2.6	3.1	—	—	—
Bending strength (MN/mm²)	248	283	500–600	450–640	200–240
Strain to failure (%)	1.5	1.6	1	1	0.8
Bending modulus (GN/mm²)	43.7	42.9	50–58	55	33–39

different methods, numbers of specimens, and sample geometries. However, in all cases the Woelher curves are comparable to those of isotropic pyrolytic carbon [7]. It should be pointed out that although the two components of CFRC are intrinsically brittle, they exhibit a pseudoplastic behavior and do not fail catastrophically in the physiological temperature range. The degree of pseudoplasticity varies according to the type of carbon fibers, the characteristics of the reinforcement, and the manufacturing process [6]. However, CFRC cannot be deformed and adapted to bone contour during surgery which limits its use as internal fixation plates.

Evaluation of CFRC Biocompatibility

Studies of the biocompatibility of CFRC for orthopedic applications have been closely related to the end use. The materials have been tested under bulk and particulate forms, in bone, in soft tissues, and intra-articularly.

Subchronic Studies

Intramuscular acute and subchronic implantations of bulk CFRC lead to a benign fibrous encapsulation of the implants. Particles migrating from the implants may cause a local inflammatory reaction related to the intensity of particle release [8]. The use of a pyrolitic carbon coating on the implant surface has been shown to slow down and limit particle migration from the CFRC compact material. All the published results [9–12] have shown that CFRC is well accepted by connective tissues, provided the intrinsic cohesion of the composite is adequate to avoid excessive production of particles. CFRC cylinders implanted transversally in sheep femur have shown osseointegration (Figure 6), with cortical bone in direct contact with the implant surface, and no fibrous membrane detectable at the bone–implant interface, using optical microscope observation [13]. Bone was able to grow in the material pores and was able to remodel as demonstrated by double fluorochrome labelling [14,15]. However, as these results were obtained in a nonfunctionally loaded situation, these results cannot be extrapolated to functioning implants where bending, shear, and torsion loads occur.

A material in bulk form may yield little or only mild biological response, whereas tissue response in the testing of particulate material may be severe [16]. In this prospect, CFRC particles have been implanted in animals in many different sites: subcutaneous, intramuscular, intramedullary, intra-articular, and intravenous [8,9,12,17,21]. The particles appeared to be eliminated through lymphatic routes, as well as hematogeneously, and collected in the parenchymal organs. Small carbon particles were usually located within macrophages or giant cells whereas bigger particles were observed extracellularly. Carbon fibers injected in rabbits' knee joints, for up to one year, did not in-

duce histological cartilage degeneration or modification of its mechanical properties [19]. In intramedullary site, up to 12 weeks in the rat, the observed foreign body reaction has been minimal, with little induced fibrosis [10]. Carbon particles were found embedded within newly-formed bone. Few carbon fragments were observed in lungs, liver, spleen, and kidneys without foreign body reaction. All the investigators have concluded the absence of adverse tissue reaction to implanted carbon particles, as is the case in the well-documented tissue reaction to carbon dust in human patients [17,18,22]. The fibrogenic response to CFRC particles has always been found small, and decreases with time (Figures 7 and 8).

Long-Term Studies

The primary aim of these studies is to investigate the potential carcinogenic ability of CFRC. Accordingly, administration of the test agent must closely simulate the one by which human exposure occurs [23]. Few published studies are currently available. Strand and powdered forms of AS 3000 nonbraided carbon fibers (Grafil, Courtauld) have been implanted in muscles and around the femur in hind legs of adult Wistar rats up to 18 months [24]. In no case has death been related to the presence of the foreign material. The tissue reaction has always been observed to be minimal, with few giant cells. The fibers were coated with epithelioid cells. Many carbon particles were observed in the interstitium, with some in the phagocytic cells and the lymphatic capillaries. However, in this study, the organs were not examined and the carbon fibers were not characterized for their length distribution. Although the Wistar rat rarely survives longer than 2 years, the 18-month duration of this experiment was short, compared to the 24–30 months normally recommended for this kind of chronic study [25,26].

Regarding the carcinogenicity of other fibers, dimensional characteristics of carbon filaments appear far from the carcinogenic ones. Asbestos fibers are known to induce pleural tumors when their size is in the range of 0.25 μm in diameter and greater than 8 μm in length [27]. Carbon fibers are 7 μm in diameter and never split longitudinally producing thicker particles rather than thinner ones. Nevertheless, the extrapolation of the results of carcinogenic studies carried out in rodents to predict human hazard is always difficult, as is their interpretation. The results depend on many parameters such as species, strain, route of exposure, doses, age at inception of test, and duration of observation.

CFRC Hip Stems

The CFRC hip stem described herein was manufactured by CVI and coated with dense pyrolytic carbon. B1 types 1 and 3 as well as B4 structures were used. Three stem sizes, having the Müller straight design,

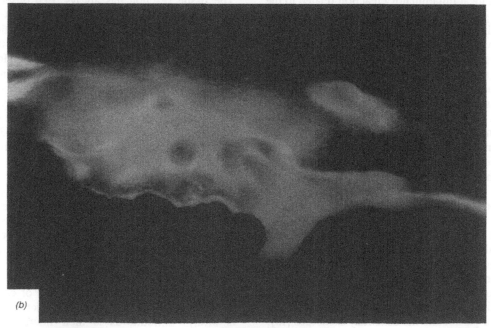

Figure 6. CFRC–bone interface in a transcortical plug model in sheep femur. The implant, inserted for 6 months, was coated with dense pyrolytic carbon. (a) Paragon staining, ×20. At the optical level, there is a direct bone-implant contact with bone growing in a material's pore. (b) Double tetracycline labelling demonstrates active bone remodeling in the material's pore.

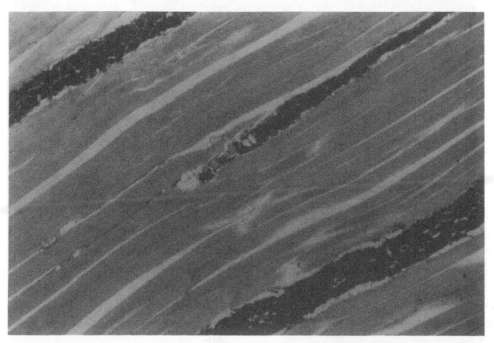

Figure 7. Histology of rabbit muscle implanted with carbon particles for 16 weeks. The particles are packed between the muscles fiber without sign of adverse tissue reaction (Van Gieson staining, ×300).

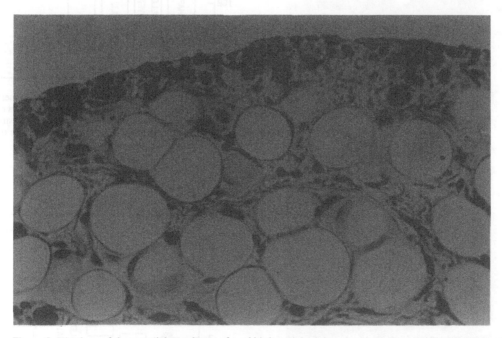

Figure 8. Histology of the synovial membrane of a rabbit knee joint injected with carbon particles one week before. Particles are concentrated in the superficial layer of the synovium with a macrophagic reaction. No strong foreign body reaction is visible (Giemsa staining, ×100).

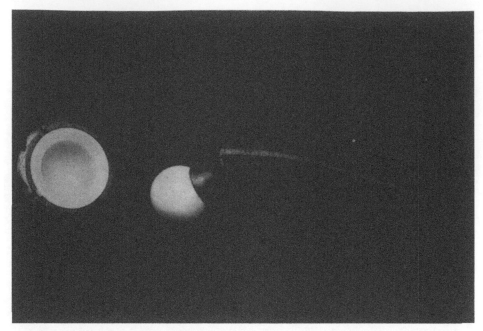

Figure 9. CVI-CFRC total hip prosthesis with alumina head and CFRC-backed UHMWPE cup.

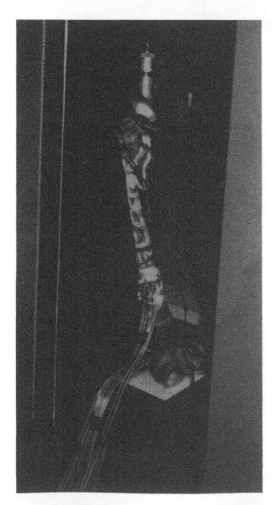

Figure 10. Experimental setup used to measure the stress distribution over the implanted CFRC stem. The femur was also fitted with strain gauges in order to study the modifications of its strain pattern after prosthesis implantation.

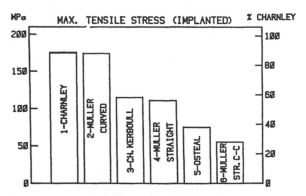

Figure 11. Comparative maximum tensile stresses measured on the lateral stem aspects. The values are expressed in MPa on the left ordinates and in percentage of the maximum tensile stress recorded on the standard Charnley stem on the right ordinates (CH Kerboull is an oversized Charnley stem made in 316L).

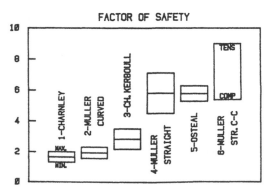

Figure 12. Factors of safety in bending calculated for each tested stem. For metal alloy stems, minimum and maximum values were computed according to the available values of the alloys' fatigue strength. For CFRC values are given in relation with the maximum tensile and compressive stresses recorded on the composite stem.

were available (Figure 9). The mechanical performances of these stems have been evaluated through static and fatigue tests.

Static Testing

Resistance to fatigue is one of the first criteria to consider when designing a femoral stem for THR. Accordingly, stress analysis, in relation with material and implant design, is necessary to perform. Comparative stress distribution was conducted on several common prostheses having various cross sections and made of different materials [29,30]. 316L stainless-steel (Charnley), HS21 cobalt-chromium (standard Müller), Ti6Al4V titanium alloy (Osteal), MP35N cobalt-nickel alloy (Müller straight) and CFRC stems were fitted with strain gauges distributed all along their lateral and medial aspects. They were cemented into fresh human cadaver femurs and physiologically loaded up to 3000 N (Figure 10). The following parameters were calculated from the gauges' outputs: maximum tensile stress, maximum stress gradient, and bending factor of safety (ratio of the fatigue strength to the maximum tensile stress) [28]. Regardless of stem type, the typical stress distribution exhibited a bell-shaped curve. For HS21 and 316L stems, the larger stems resulted in lower stresses and higher factors of safety (Figures 11 and 12). The factor of safety was increased even further when using super alloys such as MP35N and Ti6Al4V. The CFRC stem exhibited lower stresses resulting in a bending safety factor close to MP35N. CFRC composite allowed the use of larger and stronger stems without the extra penalty of a high rigidity [29,30].

Fatigue Testing

The fatigue tests were conducted according to the configuration recommended in ISO TC 150 SC4 GT1 N1, with a 2 mm/min loading rate at a 10 Hz frequency. The median axis of the prosthesis, as defined in ISO 7206/1, was tilted at 25° to the vertical in the ML plane. No inclination was given in the AP plane. The fatigue test consisted of applying a series of compressive cycles varying between 800 and 8,000 N during the first 5×10^6 cycles and between 1,000 and 10,000 N during the following 2.5×10^6 cycles. The load was applied through a polyethylene cone resulting in an annular contact with the prosthesis head; the stem was immersed in a Ringer's solution maintained at room teperature. After the 7.5×10^6 cycles were completed, the stems were statically loaded at rupture. No stem broke during the fatigue test and the comparison of the static strength values after fatigue, with those obtained on similar stems without fatigue, did not show any significant influence of the fatigue process on the static stem strength which was approximately 15×10^3 N [28,31].

Finite Element Analysis

CFRC being highly anisotropic, simple models cannot predict the mechanical behavior of these composites. Purposely, a 3-D finite-element model (FEM), taking into account the local anisotropic elastic stiffness, has been used to analyse the stem stress-distribution. Due to a plane symmetry, the mesh has been generated only on the half stem-thickness with 20-node volume elements (Figure 13). The shape of the volume elements has taken into account the stem curvatures and 21 integrating points for the accuracy of the calculations (file no. 21 in the MARC code library on UNIVAC 1100/80). The final model has been made of 78 volume elements representing more than 500 nodes [28,31]. The fatigue test configuration previously described was modelled. The embedment was considered perfect with no deformation and loading was simulated with a nodal force applied through the center of the prosthesis head. The material had three different Young's moduli, shear moduli, Poisson's ratios, and different compressive and interlaminate shear strengths according to the direction of loading with regard to the laminates. The stresses were calculated in the planes of maximum and minimum stress within the stem, both in the plane of symmetry and in the perpendicular planes. The computed static strength of the stem was estimated at 8,700 N whereas, in the meantime, the fracture load was ex-

FINITE ELEMENT MESH
H010 TYPE III

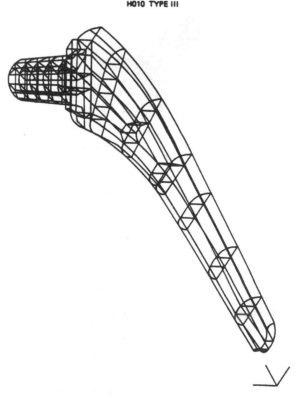

Figure 13. 3-D model used for the finite element analysis.

perimentally measured at 13,000 N. This difference could be related to nonlinear phenomena occurring in the composite when stresses close to the fracture strength are not taken into account in the FEM. The maximum stresses were located on the medial side of the prosthesis neck subjected to compression, where the fracture occurred during destructive testing (Figure 14).

A human clinical trial was started several years ago in France on a limited number of patients using the previously described stem design. The low radiodensity of CFRC, 500 Hansfield units, allowed investigators to perform a radiological follow-up using CT scan to monitor the bone–stem interface. No material-related complications have been observed [28].

Other CFR Materials for Total Hip Replacement

A press-fit CFR-PSF femoral stem has been designed to be evaluated in the dog [32]. It contained a core of unidirectional carbon/polysulfone composite enveloped with a bidirectional 45° braided layer composed of carbon/polysulfone composite covering the core and all encased in an outer coating of pure polysulfone. The implant was shaped and sized to match the contours of the medullary canal of the proximal

DISPLACED POSITION PLOTS X10
LOAD : 6400 N
(25° PHYSIOLOGICAL CONFIGURATION)
H010 TYPE III

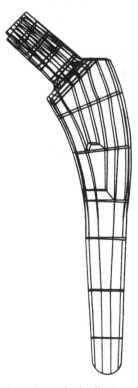

Figure 14. Stem deformation under loading as calculated from the FEM. The maximum deformation stands in the prosthesis neck.

femur of a greyhound. The implant geometry was such that the naturally occurring internal cancellous structures of the proximal femur would be preserved and participate in load transfer from the implant to the bone. After sacrifice between 1 and 24 months, all the stems were found well-fixed and functioning. All implants maintained their structural integrity and constructive bone remodelling was demonstrated by radiographs and CT scan. Both bone and fibrous tissue, containing few inflammatory cells, were found at the bone–implant interface. No mechanical properties of this particular composite have been given. Bulk polysulfone has a well-established biocompatibility [33], but it has been reported to fracture at relatively low tensile stress in a lipid-containing environment [34]. At stress levels attainable in composite THR femoral components, it has been shown that annealed polysulfone exhibited environment stress crazing and eventual fracture when exposed to lipid-containing tissues [35]. This phenomenon may be a cause of concern for the use of polysulfone in permanent implants.

CARBON-FIBER-REINFORCED COMPOSITES FOR FRACTURE FIXATION

The internal fixation of diaphyseal fractures by bone plates is a well-recognized treatment. However, stabilizing bone by rigid fixation plates leads to stress protection of bone. This effect may cause bone loss and a decrease of bone strength [36]. Many investigators have shown that the degree of stress protection depends on the rigidity of the plates [36–40]. CFR plates have been used for less-rigid fixation because of their low modulus of elasticity. Other advantages of this material are its radiolucency, which is important for fracture repair, for example in tumor patients, and its low specific weight, which is also interesting for external fixation applications. Figure 15 shows the ASIF external fixateur with two CFR-epoxy tubes in a model for the stabilization of tibial fractures. For this application, a unidirectional fiber orientation is often used to get a high bending stiffness and thus a high stability of the osteosynthesis.

For the first time, a CFR-PMMA plate was used by Akeson and Woo in 1975 [41,42] in order to study the influence of low-rigidity plate on bone remodelling. In the following years similar investigations on CFR-epoxy resin plates were performed by Bradley et al. [43] and on CFRC plates by Claes et al. [44]. Partially resorbable composite plates were made of carbon fibers and degradable polylactic acid [45]. The advantage of such a material would be a reduction in plate stiffness during the healing time of the fracture. This would gradually increase the stress on the healing tissue and decrease the stress-shielding effect. However, an unsolved problem seems to be related to the tissue reaction to the remaining carbon fiber bundles which do not resorb. All composites were made of various structures from commercially available pre-pegs or carbon fiber cloth. They differed in fiber orientation and volume content. The strength of the composite is dependent on the material, the fiber volume content and the fiber orientation [43,45–48]. Epoxy resin, as matrix material, showed the highest strength, followed by polysulfone and pure carbon, whereas polylactic acid exhibited the lowest values [45,47–49]. Composites made in sandwich-structure demonstrate high bending and tensile strength, comparable to stainless steel, but a torsional strength still low because of their inherent limited interlaminar shear strengths [47,48]. The bending stiffness of the composite plates was approximately a third of the stiffness of comparable stainless steel plates [40,41,43,44,50]. Using less rigid composite plates, significantly lower stress protection effects on bone could be measured [44]. Figure 16 shows the strain distribution, which is proportional to stress, measured over the surface of a sheep metatarsus after application of either a 6 mm 316L stainless steel or a CFRC plate with a constant bending moment of 7.5 Nm [44]. Secondary to stress shielding, a stress reduction of the bone could be demonstrated for both plates; however, this effect was higher for the stiffer steel plate than for the less rigid composite plate. The effect was more pronounced directly beneath the plate but was also observed on the cortex opposite to the plate.

Comparative animal experiments with composite and metal plates demonstrated that the stiffer metal plates led to a higher transient osteoporosis than the less rigid composite plates [42,44,51]. The CFR-epoxy plates have been used in clinical investigations [52]. Besides a lower stress-protection, the less rigid fixation plates were used to potentially stimulate more callus formation by higher micromovements in the fracture gap [52]. However, the clinical use was limited because the straight composite plates could not be bent and twisted at surgery to adapt them to the outer shape of the bone.

Carbon-Fiber-Reinforced-Polysulfone Composite for Internal Fixation

Internal Fixation Plates

As it can be adapted to bone surface at surgery, polysulfone, a thermoplastic material, was used as a matrix material for bone plates [45,51]. By heating CFRPS composites above 230°C the plates can be deformed. A necessary requirement is an equal distribution of the temperature and pressure all over the composite during the hot forming process. For this purpose a special hot bending apparatus was developed [45]. This system contained an electric oven, with adjustable temperature, and a special bending press which allows the surface shape of the bone to be duplicated by a template and a pin board [45]. The plate can be deformed in one compression step after 7 minutes of heating and can be used 2 minutes later, after cooling down to room temperature. The motion

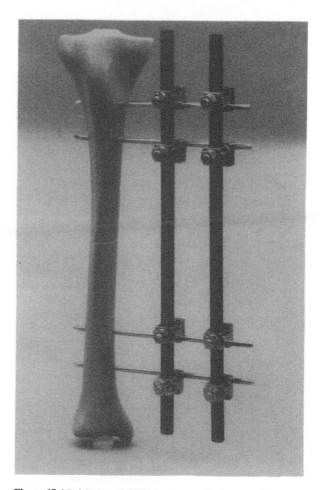

Figure 15. Model of an external fixation application at a tibial fracture with rods made of carbon-fiber-reinforced epoxy.

of the laminates relative to each other during this bending process reduces the bending strength of the plates by about 25% (Figure 17). Deforming plates without holes affects the strength significantly less (about 10%). This strength reduction can probably be reduced by a higher compression force applied during the bending process.

From a biomechanical point of view, a bone plate must have a sufficient bending and torsional stiffness at the fracture site but it should have a low axial stiffness to avoid stress protection [39]. By a tailor-made fiber-reinforcement and a special design of the outer shape of the plate, such special plate properties can be achieved [50]. Figure 18(a) shows a CFR-polysulfone (CFRPS) plate with a thickness of 5 mm in the center and 2.5 mm at both ends which stabilizes a metatarsal fracture of a sheep. The special design of the plate results in a higher stiffness in the center and lower stiffness at the end. In addition to the geometrical factor, the modulus of elasticity was varied over the plate's cross section by selecting different fiber orientations (±45 degree cloth in combination with unidirectional, UD, fibers).

Two different types of plates were made. Type A

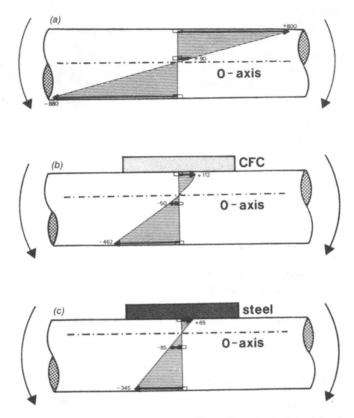

Figure 16. The stress protection effect of bone plates: strain (proportional to stress) at the bone surface under a constant bending moment. (a) Bone without plate; (b) bone with CFC plate; (c) bone with stainless steel plate.

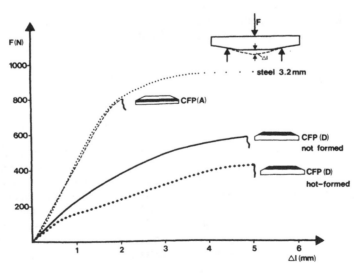

Figure 17. Force–deflection diagram of a standard stainless steel plate, two composite plates with various reinforcements (type A and type D) and a composite plate (type D) after hot forming at 230°C.

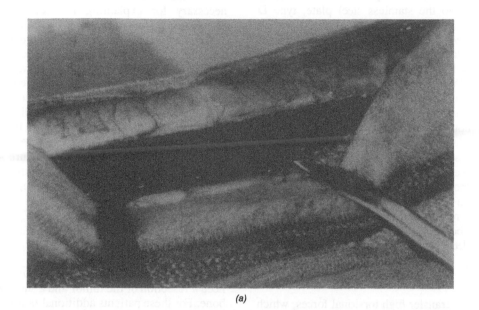

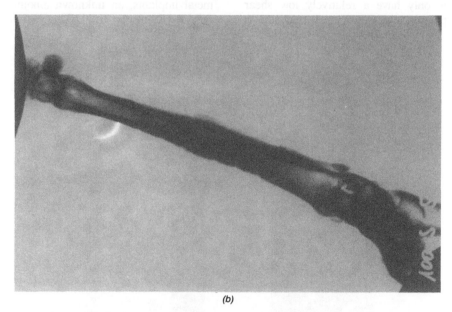

Figure 18. (a) Stabilizing of a metatarsal fracture of a sheep by a 6 hole carbon fiber reinforced polysulfone plate with screws made of the same material. (b) X-ray of the sheep metatarsal 8 weeks after stabilization by a radiolucent composite plate and composite screws.

had the unidirectional fiber fraction in the middle third and type D in the upper third of the cross section. Figure 17 shows the bending stiffness of these two plates in comparison to a standard 3.2 mm stainless steel plate. Whereas type A had a bending stiffness similar to the stainless steel plate, type D showed only about half the bending stiffness. During an axial tensile test of the plates, the surface strain at the bottom surface in the middle of the plate was measured using strain gauges. The results at a 100 N force showed 35 mm/m for the 316L stainless steel plate and 375 mm/m for the type D composite plate.

The comparison of bending stiffness and axial stiffness for both types of plates demonstrates the effect of a special design of the composite plate. The bending stiffness of the type D plate in comparison to the stainless steel plate is only reduced by a factor of two, whereas the axial stiffness of the composite plate is more than ten times lower than that of the stainless steel plate. Therefore the biomechanical requirement for a moderate bending stiffness but low axial stiffness could be fulfilled.

CFRPS Screws

Screws have to transfer high torsional forces, which produce high shear stress in the implant. Because CFR composites only have a relatively low shear strength in comparison to stainless steel, steel screws cannot be copied in composite material without considerably lower mechanical properties.

Because of the micro-rough and structured surface of machined composite screws and the good integration of this material in bone, a high removal torque is necessary for explanting the screw after several months. In animal experiments with composite plates and composite 3.5 mm screws (Figure 18) the screws could not be removed after 24 weeks. The screw heads broke when using a screw driver for removal. The design of special composite screws is therefore necessary and the composite properties must be considered. The thread geometry as well as the ratio of outer diameter to core diameter have to be modified. Special 6 mm and 4.5 mm O.D. screws were developed for the spine as shown in Figure 4. However these screws were designed for tumor operations where the screws act as permanent implants which do not have to be removed.

Radiolucent CFRPS Implants for Bone-Tumor Surgery

Pathological fractures caused by bone tumors often need a resection of the tumor and a stabilization of the bone. For these patients additional radiotherapy of the operated area often has to be done. Using standard metal implants, an unknown amount of radiation is reflected from the metal. This makes the calculation

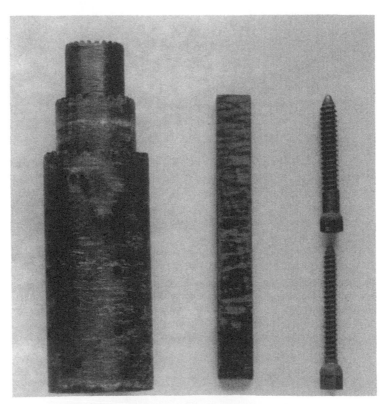

Figure 19. Implant set made of carbon-fiber-reinforced-polysulfone for the stabilization of spinal defects after tumor resection. Tubes in three diameters, plate and screws.

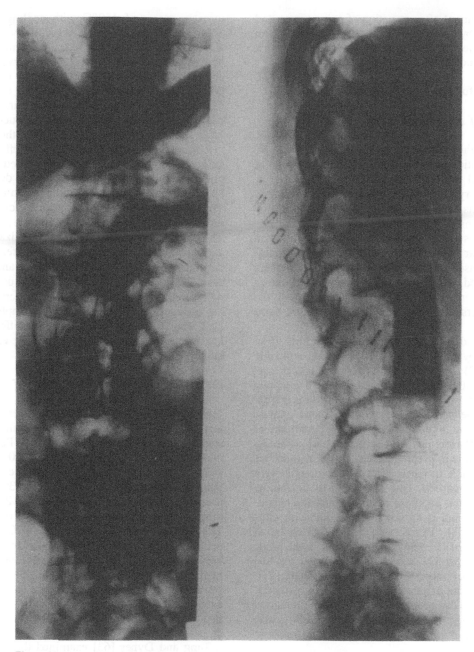

Figure 20. X-ray of the operated spine with an implanted tube for segmental replacement, plate and screw for stabilization. The radiopaque area is caused by bone cement which is filled in the center of the tube.

of the radiation dose very difficult. A great advantage of the composite implant is its radiolucency, so the previous effect does not occur. Thus it is much easier to control the radiological development of metastases and to use other diagnostic methods without reflection problems like the CT scan. For a first clinical application, a special set of implants was developed for spine tumor operations. It contains CFRPS plates, 6 mm and 4.5 mm screws and tubes for the segment replacement made of the same material (Figure 19). The plates were 5 × 12 mm in cross section and 300 mm long. They can be cut intraoperatively to the neces-

sary length and the holes for the screws can be drilled where necessary. By this intraoperative procedure the distances of the screw holes can be optimally adapted to the individual distances of the spinal segment of each patient. Sawing the tube allows the adaptation of the implant to the shape of the defect caused by the tumor resection. The implants can be stabilized by the special screws.

In the past two years, several patients have been operated on with composite plates with good results [53] and three patients have been treated with the complete implant set in the last few months. Figure 20 shows an

X-ray of a patient after resection of spine tumor and stabilization by plate, screws and tube. The shadow in the spinal defect is caused by the bone cement which filled the center of the composite tube.

CFRPEEK for Internal Fixation Devices

Properties of Neat PEEK

Polyaryl-ether-ether-ketones (PEEK) are made by the condensation polymerization of alkali bisphenates and activated aromatic dihalides [54,55]. However, due to their crystallinity, PEEKs are very insoluble in most solvents, so that during polymerization the growing chains precipitate and growth is stopped. Using solvents such as methylene chloride resulted in low molecular weights. It was not until 1969 when liquid HF was used that high molecular weight polymers were prepared. The use by ICI of phenyl sulphone as a solvent at temperatures up to 335°C resulted in the high polymers that have been offered for sale since 1982 [54].

Several grades of the neat PEEK resin have been developed by ICI chemicals. Injection-moldable PEEK (450G) is available with chopped glass or carbon fibers; 450CA30 is reinforced with 30% chopped carbon fiber. The continuous carbon fiber/PEEK composite referred to as Aromatic Polymer Composite (APC-2) and is reinforced with 61% by volume of unidirectional Hercules AS4 (unsized) carbon fibers. This is available in prepreg sheets. PEEK composites are also available in fabric form as a comingled yarn of PEEK and carbon. Due in part to its crystalline nature, PEEK has excellent environmental and chemical resistance and is known to be insoluble in most solvents [56–58]. PEEK also has extremely good hydrolysis resistance. Soaking injection mold grade PEEK (450G) for 322 days at 100°C in water resulted in a decrease of only 5% in the tensile strength [57]. It is also resistant to hard radiation (X, beta, gamma). No breakdown has been observed at gamma radiation exposures below 1,000 Mrad [55,56]. PEEK is also reported to have an indefinite shelf life [56].

Crystallinity of Neat PEEK

PEEK is a highly aromatic semicrystalline thermoplastic with a melting temperature of 334°C and a glass transition temperature of 145°C. The maximum crystallinity is in the range of 48% although 33% crystallinity is more common [59]. The optimum temperature range for crystallization from the melt is 180–320°C, with spherulitic radii in the range of 12.7–21.9 μm for temperatures of 240 and 287°C respectively [55]. The density of the noncrystalline and crystalline phases as determined by X-ray diffraction are 1.2626 g/cm^3 and 1.4006 gm/cm^3, respectively [60]. The degree of crystallinity is very dependent on the cooling rate from the melt. Seferis [60] used a specially designed mold which could operate at tempera-

tures in excess of 450°C with cooling rates up to 3000°C/min. A maximum crystallinity of 33% was achieved at a cooling rate of 0.6–6°C/min. A plateau between 60 and 1800°C/min was observed with 24% crystallinity. With a rapid quench in excess of 6000°C/min, the crystallinity dropped to below 5%. The results also indicated that there can be a significant skin-core effect with molded products, with surfaces showing lower crystallinity than the bulk.

Annealing can also have significant effects on crystallinity. Ostberg and Seferis [61] started with a neat polymer (450G) with a crystal volume determined to be 1.8% using the density gradient technique (DTG). The crystallinity of samples annealed for one hour at 210°C and 310°C were 22% and 32.6%, respectively. They observed that the induced crystallization may be a consequence of changes in crystal perfection that occur during the first few minutes of the annealing process. When crystallinity was measured using differential scanning calorimetry (DSC), the crystallinity of the as-received 210°C and 310°C samples was 11.1, 28.2, and 32.3%, respectively. This difference at the low levels was attributed to annealing effects of the DSC melting method [61].

Crystallinity of Carbon Composites of PEEK

The presence of carbon fiber has been shown to affect the crystallization of PEEK. Lee and Porter [62] studied the crystallinity of a neat PEEK matrix material (Mn = 14,100, Mw = 38,600) and the effects of unsized Thornel 300 PAN carbon fibers. Samples were held for various times at 390°C without pressure, followed by compression at 2 MPa for 30 minutes, and then cooling at either 7 or 0.6°C/min. The samples were quenched from 270°C to room temperature. Their results demonstrated reduced nucleation density with increasing melt time. Increasing fiber content resulted in crystallization at a lower supercooling, suggesting that fibers act as nucleation agents. All PEEK samples with carbon fibers exhibited a higher nucleation density than neat PEEK with an equivalent thermal history.

Tung and Dynes [63] examined the crystallization of APC-2 samples heated to 400°C for 10–15 min and then cooled at slow (1.5–5°C/min), fast (70°C/min) and very fast (2500°C/min) rates. At the high quench rates, very little time was allowed for small crystallites to grow in size and perfection. Spherulite size ranged from 25 μm at the slow rate, to 8 μm at the fast rate. The degree of crystallinity ranged from 50% to 33%. The slow cooling rate samples also demonstrated the formation of transcrystalline regions where the crystals nucleate perpendicular to the fibers.

The crystallinity of APC-2 and two "non-optimised" carbon fiber/PEEK composites was investigated by Peacock et al. [58]. They observed crystallite spherulite growth directly on the carbon fibers. The nucleation was more frequent with the HS4 fibers, with nucleation points typically 5 μm apart. The transverse flexural strength of the APC-2 was 152 MPa, compared to 54 and 76 for the other two composites. Examination of the fracture surfaces revealed the AS4 fibers of the APC-2 to be well coated with matrix, whereas the other composites showed bare fibers revealing that failure had occurred at the fiber–matrix interface. Their study demonstrated the importance of the optimisation of the fiber–matrix interface that had been achieved with APC-2.

Mechanical Properties of Neat PEEK

All grades of PEEK are tough, strong, have excellent fatigue resistance [56,59] and have excellent load-bearing properties over long periods [56]. Some mechanical properties are listed in Table 2 [64]. The properties are influenced by the crystallinity of PEEK. For instance the temperature and cooling rates for optimal crystallinity can be modified for specific processes such as injection-molding or extrusion. In the study by Seferis [60] the mechanical properties of specimens with a range of crystallinity of 10–33% was studied. The tensile strength of these samples ranged from 70–100 MPa, with the strain to failure decreasing from 33% to 8% with increasing crystallinity.

Mechanical Properties of Chopped Fiber-Reinforced PEEK

From the discussion above, it should be obvious that the mechanical properties of injection mold grade 30% chopped carbon-fiber-reinforced PEEK (450CA30) will depend on the degree of crystallinity resulting from the processing conditions. The data from ICI [64] for tensile and flexural strength are given in Tables 2 and 3. The effects of processing were observed in studies by Brown et al. [65,66], as shown in Table 4, in which as-received flexural testing bars had strengths ranging from 272 to 317 MPa. The mechanical properties of the molded material will be significantly affected by the resulting orientation of the fibers after processing. Although the ideal molding of a chopped 30% fiber-reinforced plate would be the random distribution of the carbon fibers, this is not technically feasible, or theoretically possible for injection molding. Jones, Leach and Moore [59] have indicated that there is a certain degree of anisotropy for all injection-molded bars, the extent of which is influenced by molding thickness and gate geometry [55]. A diverging flow field is produced from injection molding. The fibers in the skin regions (surfaces of the mold) are predominantly aligned along the principle flow direction while the core fibers are transversely aligned. Injection molded disks rotated and tested every 10 degrees showed a range of flexural stiffness from 10 to 33 GPa [59]. Although the flexural properties should be dominated by the skin, the data has revealed that the strength of CFRPEEK is dominated by the fibers aligned 90 degrees in the

Table 2. Tensile properties of neat PEEK (450G), and chopped carbon-fiber-reinforced PEEK (450CA30), and continuous carbon fiber composites (APC-2) [64].

	Strength (MPa)	Strain (%)	Modulus (GPa)
450G	93	50	3.6
450CA30	208	1.3	13
APC-2 1	2130	1.45	134
APC-2 t	80	1.00	8.9
APC-2 +45	300	17.2	19.2

Table 3. Flexural properties of PEEK and carbon composites [64].

	Strength (MPa)	Strain (%)	Modulus (GPa)
450G	170	—	3.6
450CA30	318	—	13.0
APC-2 1	1880	—	121
APC-2 t	137	—	8.9

Table 4. Flexural properties of 30% chopped fiber CFRPEEK before and after oven heating (O-heat) and 6 degrees contouring [65], and specimens as-received, after heating with the quartz IR heater, and after heating and contouring to 8 degrees [66].

	Strength (MPa)	Strain (%)	Modulus (GPa)
Oven heat:			
As received	272(19)	2.13(.1)	15.6(2)
Contour	277(11)	2.27(.2)	15.1(1)
IR heat:			
As received	317(4)	2.32(.09)	18.3(.4)
Heat only	332(4)*	2.31(.06)	19.1(.3)
Contour	314(6)	2.14(.10)	18.6(.4)

*Indicates statistically significant difference from as-received.

Table 5. Flexural properties of continuous carbon fiber, 61% v/v APC-2 and hybrid comingled yarn PEEK composites [68].

	Strength (MPa)	Strain (%)	Modulus (GPa)
APC-2	2200	1.78	123
Fiber hybrid	2160	1.65	131
Cloth hybrid	855	1.49	57

core. Therefore a unique property value for stiffness or strength will not exist.

Besides acting as a nucleating agent for crystallinity, fibers will also affect crack propagation. Fatigue crack propagation studies of chopped glass and carbon-reinforced specimens were conducted by Freidrich et al. [67] to study the effects of reinforcement on crack propogation. They observed that the fracture characteristics were dominated by fiber–matrix separation and that propagation was along the interfaces of the fibers if they were parallel to the crack direction, or through the matrix if perpendicular. For a given stress intensity, cracks in glass-reinforced composites propagated less than half as fast as in neat PEEK samples. In the case of carbon composites, crack propagation was 1 to 2 orders of magnitude less than in neat PEEK. The domination of the fiber-matrix bonding of the CFRPEEK resulted in deviation in crack direction. This resulted in difficulties in crack length measurements and calculation of fracture toughness. Similar increases in fatigue strength of carbon versus glass-reinforced PEEK composites have been reported by Jones et al. [59].

Mechanical Properties of Continuous Carbon Fiber Composites

As with the chopped fiber composites, continuous fiber composite mechanical properties will depend on processing conditions and the resultant crystallinity. Properties also depend on fiber orientation. As shown in Table 2, the tensile strength of APC-2 is 2130 MPa in the longitudinal direction, but only 80 MPa in the transverse direction. The +45 degree laminate is reported to have a strength of 300 MPa [64]. Comparable differences in tensile moduli are seen. Similar differences between longitudinal and transverse strength results with flexural testing are also seen in Table 3. The flexural strength of APC-2 is given as 1880 and 137 MPa, in the longitudinal and transverse directions, respectively. The processing technique used by Huettner and Weiss [68] resulted in a flexural strength of 2200 MPa, as shown in Table 5. Hybrid composites made with HS-4 fibers comingled PEEK had comparable properties. The cloth hybrid strength and modulus were considerably less. However, the cloth composite would not have the directional sensitivity of the parallel fiber composites.

Biological Suitability of CFRPEEK

There are three aspects of the biological suitability of CFRPEEK. From the environmental point of view, does the chemical stability data discussed imply stability *in vivo*, i.e., are there any adverse effects on the material due to implantation? Similarly, are there any adverse effects of PEEK on the biological media, i.e., is it biocompatible? Finally, do CFRPEEK composites have mechanical properties appropriate for implant applications? Being a relatively new material,

the data on these subjects are as yet quite limited. The question of material degradation has been addressed in two studies of the chopped fiber composite. Williams et al. [69] measured the flexural strength of neat and CFRPEEK after 2 months in saline at 37°C and 80°C, and after 2 or 6 months in the subcutaneous space of rabbits. Brown et al. [65] measured flexural strength and fracture toughness before and after exposure to saline for 3 weeks at 37°C. In all cases there were no significant changes in mechanical properties. Although the numbers are not sufficient for statistical analysis, a similar lack of *in vivo* degradation of CFRPEEK plates used for fracture fixation has been reported by Jockisch et al. [70].

The biological response to CFRPEEK has been studied *in vitro* with direct contact cell culture by Wenz et al. [71]. No cytotoxic response was observed. The *in vivo* response to specimens implanted in muscle have been studied in rats [69] and in rabbits [70]. These studies have demonstrated a normal inflammatory response to surgical trauma, and the development of a benign fibrous capsule. Fat deposits were observed in the early response and some persisted up to 30 weeks. However, the significance of this observation is not known. The tissue response to carbon fiber and composite debris has been described as minimal in these studies. Similar minimal tissue response to wear debris was observed in tissues around fracture-fixation plates [70].

The issue of mechanical properties depends on the particular application. For prosthetic joint replacement, the strength of APC-2 is more than adequate. For fracture fixation applications the issue is twofold. First, can a low-modulus material be fabricated to avoid stress-shielding effects? The answer to this question is yes. The second question pertains to the specific application of the composite material for fracture-fixation plates. This application requires that the plates be contourable to fit the contours of the bone. The work by Brown et al. [65,66] has been directed to this question. Several methods of heating and contouring chopped fiber CFRPEEK have been investigated. Flexural test specimens (6.2 mm thick) were heated, bent with a 3-point plate bending device, and cooled. The bars were then heated, straightened and cooled a second time for flexural testing. As shown in Table 4, heating in an oven and contouring produced no significant changes in mechanical properties [65]. The data in Table 4 also show that heating with radiant heat from infrared lamps resulted in an increase in strength [66]. This could be due to annealing and an increase in surface crystallinity. Multiple IR heating and bending cycles have produced no measurable changes in the mechanical properties of the CFRPEEK.

CONCLUSIONS

From the information contained in this chapter, it appears that CFR-composites have a potential for use in orthopedic surgery. CVI-CFRC exhibits both static and dynamic mechanical properties suitable for THR. Biocompatibility evaluations of CFRC show neither short- nor long-term adverse tissue response. An implant with appropriate elastic properties provides the possibility for the natural bone remodelling to occur, enhancing implant stability.

CFRPS, a thermoplastic composite used as internal fixation plate, can be simply deformed by heating, during surgery, to be adapted to the antomical shape of the bone surface. In animals, the use of such plates leads to a significant reduction in the bone stress-shielding when compared to metal plates.

PEEK is a semicrystalline high-performance polymer with a high degree of temperature and chemical stability. Reinforcing PEEK with carbon results in an increase in the crystallinity of the matrix demonstrating a synergistic reaction. The CFRPEEK composites have high strength and stability. As much of the data presented demonstrate, the exact mechanical properties depend on processing history and resultant crystallinity. Preliminary biological testing data indicate a high potential for CFRPEEK for implant applications.

REFERENCES

1. Fitzer E., W. Huettner and L. M. Manocha. 1980. *Carbon*, 18:291–295.

2. Fitzer, E., K. H. Geigl and W. Huettner. 1980. *Carbon*, 18:265–270.

3. Fritz, W., W. Huettner and G. Hartwig, 1979. In *Non-Metallic Materials and Composites at Low Temperature*. New York: Plenum Press, pp. 245–266.

4. Loll, P., P. Delhaes, A. Pacault and A. Pierre. 1977. *Carbon*, 15:383–390.

5. U. S. Patent No. 4,790,052. Dec. 13, 1988. Process for Manufacturing Homogeneously Needled Three-Dimensional Structures of Fibrous Materials.

6. Huettner, W. and K. J. Huettinger. 1984. In *The Cementless Fixation of Hip Endoprostheses*. Berlin: Morsher Ed, Springer Verlag, pp. 81–94.

7. Shim, H. S. 1984. *Biomat. Med. Dev. Art. Org.*, 2:55–60.

8. Christel, P. S., B. Buttazzoni, J. L. Leray and C. Morin. 1982. In *Biomaterials*. G. Winter, D. Gibbons and H. Plenk, Jr., eds. New York: Wiley, pp. 87–96.

9. Helbing, G., D. Wolter, R. Neugebauer and J. Coldewey. 1977. *Trans. 3rd Annu. Meet. Soc. Biomaterials, New Orleans, LA*, p. 151.

10. Neugebauer, R., G. Helbing, D. Wolter, W. Mohr and G. Gistinger, G. 1981. *Biomaterials*, 2:182–184.

11. Wolter, D., C. Burri, G. Helbing, W. Mohr and A. Ruter. 1978. *Arch. Orthop. Traum. Surg.*, 91:19–29.

12. Christel, P., M. Homerin and A. Dryll. 1984. *Trans. 2nd World Congr. Biomaterials, Washington, D.C.*, p. 72.

13. Leclercq, S., P. Christel, A. Meunier, P. Dallant, G. Guillemin and L. Sedel. 1986. *Trans. 12th Annu. Meet. Soc. Biomaterials, Minneapolis, Minnesota*, p. 104.

14. Christel, P. S. 1986. *CRC Crit. Rev. Biocompatibility*, 2:189–218.

15. Christel, P. S., A. Meunier, J. M. Dorlot, J. M. Crolet, J. Witvoet, L. Sedel and P. Boutin. 1988. In *Bioceramics: Material Characteristics Versus in vivo Behavior*. P. Ducheyne and J. E. Lemons, eds. *Ann. New York Acad. Sci.*, 253:234–256.

16. Willert, H. C. and M. Semlitsch. 1976. In *Biocompatibility of Implant Materials*. D. F. Williams, ed. London: Sector Publ., pp. 39–59.

17. Helbing, G., D. Wolter, R. Neugebauer and J. Coldewey. 1977. *Trans. 3rd Annu. Meet. Soc. Biomaterials, New Orleans, LA*, p. 144.

18. Helbing, G., C. Burri, W. Mohr, R. Neugebauer and D. Wolter. 1980. In *Evaluation of Biomaterials*. G. D. Winter, J. L. Leray and K. de Groot, eds. Chichester: J. Wiley & Sons, p. 373–380.

19. Parsons, R., S. Byhani, H. Alexander and A. B. Weiss. 1983. *Trans. Orthop. Res. Soc.*, 8:9.

20. Wolter, D., E. Fitzer, G. Helbing and J. Coldewey. 1977. *Trans. 3rd Annu. Meet. Soc. Biomaterials, New Orleans, LA*, p. 119.

21. Forster, I. W., Z. A. Ralis, B. McKibbin and D. H. R. Jenkins. 1978. *Clin. Orthop.*, 131:299–305.

22. Holt, P. F. and M. Horne. 1978. *Environ. Res.*, 17:276–283.

23. Page, N. P. 1977. *J. Environ. Pathol. Toxicol.*, 1:161–164.

24. Tayton, K., G. Phillips and Z. Ralis. 1982. *J. Bone Joint Surg.*, 64B:112–114.

25. Support Document Test Data Development Standards: Chronic Health Effects, Toxic Substances, Control Act Section 4, Doc. No EPA 560/11-79-001, Health Review Division. Office of Toxic Substances, Environmental Protection Agency, Washington, D. C. 1979.

26. Oppenheimer, B. S., E. T. Oppenheimer, A. P. Stout, M. Willhite and I. Danishefsky. 1958. *Cancer*, 11:204–207.

27. Wagner, J. C. and G. Berry. 1969. *Br. J. Cancer*, 23:567–572.

28. Christel, P. S., A. Meunier, S. Leclercq, P. Bouquet and B. Buttazzoni. 1987. *J. Biomed. Mater. Res.*, 21:191–218.

29. Meunier, A., P. S. Christel and L. Sedel. 1989. In *Bioceramics*. H. Oonishi, H. Aoki and K. Sawai, eds. Tokyo: Ishiyaku EuroAmerica Inc., 1:347–352.

30. Meunier, A., P. Christel and L. Sedel. 1989. In *Interfaces in Medicine and Mechanics*. K. R. Williams and T. H. J. Lesser, eds. Trowbridge: Dotesios Printers Ltd., pp. 215–226.

31. Christel, P. S. 1985. In *Biomechanics: Current Interdisciplinary Research*. E. Schneider and S. M. Perren, eds. Dordrecht: Martinus Nijhoff, pp. 61–72.

32. Magee, F. P., A. M. Weinstein, J. A. Longo, J. B. Koeneman and R. A. Yapp. 1988. *Clin. Orthop.*, 235:237–252.

33. Spector, M., R. J. Davis, E. M. Lunceford and S. L. Harmon. 1983. *Clin. Orthop.*, 176:34–42.

34. Union Carbide Europe S. A. 1982. *UDEL Polysulfone: Chemical and Solvent Resistance, Geneva*, p. 17.

35. Asgian, C. M., L. N. Gilbertson, R. D. Blessing and

R. D. Crowinshield. 1989. *Trans. 15th Annu. Meet. Soc. Biomaterials, Lake Buena Vista, FL*, p. 17.

36. Woo SL-Y, K. S. Lothringer, W. H. Akeson, R. D. Coutts, Y. K. Woo, B. R. Simon and M. A. Gomez. 1984. *J. Orthop. Res., 1:431–449*.

37. Claes, L., U. Palme, E. Palme and U. Kirschbaum. 1982. In *Biomechanics: Principles and Applications*. R. Huiskes, D. van Campen and J. de Wijn. The Hague: Martinus Nijhoff, pp. 325–330.

38. Tonino, A. J., C. L. Davidson, P. J. Klopper and L. A. Linclau. 1976. *J. Bone Joint Surg.*, 58B:197–202.

39. Moyen, B., P. Lahey, E. Weinberg and W. Harris. 1978. *J. Bone Joint Surg.*, 60A:940–946.

40. Claes, L. 1989. *J. Orthop. Res*, 7:170–177.

41. Akeson, W. H., SL-Y Woo, R. D. Coutts, J. W. Matthews, M. Gonsalves and D. Amiel. 1975. *Calcif. Tissue Res.*, 19:27–37.

42. Woo, SL-Y, W. H. Akeson, R. D. Coutts, L. Rutherford, D. Doty, G. F. Jemmot and D. Amiel. 1976. *J. Bone Joint Surg. (Am.)*, 58:190–195.

43. Bradley, G. W., G. B. McKenna, H. K. Dunn, A. Daniels and W. O. Statton. 1979. *J. Bone Joint Surg. (Am.)*, 61:866–872.

44. Claes, L., L. Kinzl and R. Neugebauer. 1981. *Biomed. Tech.*, 26:66–71.

45. Claes, L. 1988. In *Hefte zur Unfallheilkunde*. Berlin, Heidelberg, Heft 200, New York: Springer Verlag, pp. 625–633.

46. Rumelhart, C., P. Comtet, B. Moyen and B. Buttazzoni. 1985. In *Biomechanics: Current Interdisciplinary Research*. S. M. Perren and E. Schneider, eds. Dordrecht: Martinus Nijhoff, pp. 159–165.

47. Fitzer, E. and W. Hüttner. 1979. *Carbon*, 18:383–387.

48. Claes, L., W. Hüttner and R. Weiss. 1986. In *Biological and Biomechanical Performance of Biomaterials*. P. Christel, A. Meunier and A. J. C. Lee, eds. Amsterdam: Elsevier Science Publishers, pp. 81–86.

49. Parsons, J. R., H. Alexander, S. F. Corcoran, J. Korluk and A. B. Weiss. 1979. *Trans. 11th Internat. Biomaterials Symposium*, 3:105.

50. Claes, L. and C. H. Etter. 1985. In *Entwicklungstendenzen bei Implantatwerkstoffen*. G. Friedbold, ed. Berlin: Deutscher Verband für Materialprüfung, Arbeitskreis Implantate, pp. 83–96.

51. Claes, L. and C. H. Etter. 1985. In *Bio-Medical Engineering, 1st International Conference*, 17/1–17/6.

52. Tayton, L., C. Johnson-Nurse and B. McKibbin. 1982. *J. Bone Joint Surg. (Br.)*, 64:105–111.

53. Burri, C., L. Claes and O. Wörsdörfer. 1986. *Unfallchirurg*, 89:528–532.

54. Attwood, T. E., P. C. Dawson, J. L. Freeman, L. R. J. Hoy, J. B. Rose and P. A. Staniland. 1981. *Polymer*, 22:1096–1103.

55. Nguyen, H. X. and H. Ishida. 1987. *Poly Comp.*, 8:57–73.

56. Searle, O. B. and R. H. Pfeiffer. 1985. *Poly. Eng. and Sci.*, 25:474–476.

57. Cogswell, F. N. and M. Hopprich. 1983. *Composites*, 14:251–253.

58. Peacock, J. A., B. Fife, E. Nield and C. Y. Barlow. 1986. In *Composite Interfaces*. H. Isida and J. L. Koenig, eds. Amsterdam: Elsevier, pp. 143–146.

59. Jones, D. P., D. C. Leach. and D. R. Moore. 1985. *Polymer*, 26:1385–1393.

60. Seferis, J. C. 1986. *Polymer Composites*, 7(3):158–169.

61. Ostberg, G. M. K. and J. C. Seferis. 1987. *J. Appl. Poly. Sci.*, 33:29–39.

62. Lee, Y. and R. S. Porter. 1986. *Poly. Eng. & Sci.*, 26:633–639.

63. Tung, C. M. and P. J. Dynes. 1987. *J. Appl. Poly. Sci.*, 33:505–520.

64. ICI. Victrex PEEK and Fiberite APC-2 Technical Data Sheets.

65. Brown, S. A., R. S. Hastings, J. J. Mason and A. Moet. 1990. *Biomaterials*, 11:541–547.

66. Brown, S. A., J. J. Mason, K. A. Jockisch, R. S. Hastings and A. Moet. 1990. *Adv. Biomaterials 9*. G. Heimke, U. Soltesz and A. J. C. Lee, eds. Amsterdam: Elsevier, pp. 123–128.

67. Friedrich, K., R. Walter, H. Voss and J. Karger-Kocsis. 1986. *Composites*, 17:205–216.

68. Huettner, W. and R. Weiss. In *Carbon Fibers and Filaments*. J. L. Figueiredo, ed. Kluwer (in press).

69. Williams, D. F., A. McNamara and R. M. Turner. 1987. *J. Mat. Sci. Let.*, 6:188–190.

70. Jockisch, K., S. A. Brown, K. Merritt and A. Moet. 1989. *Trans. Soc. for Biomaterials*, 12:13.

71. Wenz, L. M., K. Merritt, S. A. Brown and A. Moet. 1990. *J. Biomed Mater. Res.*, 24:207–215.

33

Reproduction in a Polymer Composite of Some Mechanical Features of Tendons and Ligaments

MANUEL MONLEÓN PRADAS*
RICARDO DÍAZ CALLEJA*

ABSTRACT: This study presents a composite material made out of a rubbery polymer matrix reinforced by bundles of a highly crystalline polymeric fibre. The composite has a structure similar to parallel-fibred collagenous tissues, and it reproduces the typical nonlinear viscoelastic behaviour met in tendons and ligaments. To a certain extent, it even reproduces the same deformation mechanism responsible for the mechanical behaviour of those tissues. The polymers employed are biocompatible, so that the results can be of use in the design of tendon and ligamentous prosthesis.

INTRODUCTION. THE HAND TENDON: STRUCTURE AND FUNCTION AS RELATED TO ITS MECHANICAL BEHAVIOUR

The tendon is a part of a *biomechanical chain* comprising the muscle, the bone and itself. Far from being a passive element, it reveals a dynamical adaptative behaviour to face external actions [1]. Its composition and structure provide the tissue with the most adequate mechanical behaviour to fulfill its functions. Among these, the load-bearing function is most widely recognized. But this main function is accompanied by other no less important ones, such as certain kinematical and damping features.

From the point of view of their composition, tendons (as well as many other living tissues) are *composite materials*. Their overall mechanical behaviour is thus determined by the properties of the components, their relative amounts, and their geometrical disposition [2]. Collagen is the main component of

tendons and also of ligaments. It constitutes up to 96% of the tendon's dry weight. This macromolecular assemblage has a highly crystalline nature, because of its hierarchical structure starting at the level of microfibrils and leading to the tendinous units in a way which is well understood [3]. The macroscopic collagen bundles are aligned in parallel and show an undulated geometry. They are immersed in the so-called *ground substance*, a complex made out of elastine and mucopolysaccharide hydrogel.

There is an intimate connection between morphology and function in tendons (and also in ligaments). The unidirectionally arranged, undulated collagen bundles cause a progressive transition between states of stretching of the specimen with different numbers of effectively loaded bundles, determining a J-shaped convex stress-strain curve. It is remarkable that most common engineering materials exhibit a concave stress-strain relationship. This property of collagenous tissues is very important in explaining their toughness and shock-damping features [4]. The presence of an initial low-modulus region allows the tissue to deform in this range with a very low value of strain energy, thus explaining the greater toughness of the biological tissues when compared to engineering materials with fracture work of the same order of magnitude.

In the sense just described, one can speak of a *damping* function of the tissue constituting tendons and ligaments. The main function is, of course, the *transmission of force* between muscle and bone, and as a specific feature of this last, one must also point out the *kinematical aspect:* in order to assure that the muscle works always in traction, the tendons (at least those of the hand) must be able to bend around certain articulation bones. Finally, thanks to their viscoelastic behaviour, tendons and ligaments *relax* a certain amount of the initial stress corresponding to a fixed imposed strain. In this sense their behaviour is adaptive.

*Laboratory of Thermodynamics and Physical Chemistry, Universidad Politécnica, P.O. Box 22012, 46071 Valencia, Spain

CONCEPT OF THE POLYMER COMPOSITE

Any proposal of an artificial organ must satisfy certain obvious requisites. Among the most important are those of *biocompatibility, morphology* and *functional adaptation.*

In the case of tendons and ligaments the *morphological* requirements are in principle easy to fulfill, as long as they are basically cylindrical organs whose length predominates over their transverse dimensions. These characteristics are reproducible in artificial systems with different solutions.

The critical test of a proposed prosthesis is its functional adaptation, that is, the degree to which the functions of the tissue are reproduced by the artificial member. In this respect, an "artificial tendon" should (1) possess the same flexibility as the natural tissue in order to bend around the articulations and assure the application of the load to the muscle always in the mode of a traction, (2) have analogous mechanical strength levels and be light, (3) possess the same extensibility and be capable of restoring the initial rest length, avoiding permanent deformations which could destabilize the biomechanical chain, (4) reproduce in its behaviour the characteristic form of the stress-strain curve which is responsible for the damping properties of the tissue, and, finally, (5) assure time invariance of the mechanical properties.

The conjunction of all these properties is almost impossible to meet in a single pure material. A *multi-component structure* has therefore been explored; in particular, a *polymeric matrix unidirectionally reinforced by continuous fibres with crimped rest geometry.* As a matrix we have employed an amorphous, rubbery (at human body temperature) polymer: both poly(methyl acrylate) and poly(ethyl acrylate) — which from now on are respectively labelled PMA and PEA — have been tried. The reinforcing elements are fibre bundles of the highly crystalline polymer poly-(p-phenylene terephtalamide) — from now on, PPTA — known commercially as Kevlar-49. The individual fibre has a very small diameter and its rest configuration has the form of a sinusoidal wave.

This structure and the underlying geometry immediately confer the composite with the following properties: (a) high strength with low weight; (b) maximum effectiveness in the reinforcing effect: the use of continuous and unidirectionally disposed fibres avoids the stress concentrations associated with short fibre reinforcement; (c) continuous fibre reinforcement also eliminates one of the dangers of the use of filled plastics in prosthetics: the partial liberation of the filler in the living tissue; (d) the composite bars have a negligible bending resistance, because of the small diameter of the fibres and the fact that the matrix has a rubbery nature; they can easily circumvent the natural pulleys of articulation bones; (e) the composite recovers completely its original length after the cessation of the applied load, because of the restoring force of the matrix, thus preventing perma-

nent deformations in the fibre bundles; (f) neither highly crystalline polymers nor amorphous polymers in their rubbery state present the phenomenon of *physical aging* (the isothermal approach to their state of stable thermodynamical equilibrium), implying dimensional changes, see [5], so the mechanical properties as well as the dimensions of the composite bar can be safely regarded as stable in time; (g) finally, due to the geometry of its internal structure and the general characteristics of polymer behaviour, the composite behaves viscoelastically and develops its modulus when it is stretched, thus reproducing the typical nonlinear viscoelastic behaviour that confers load-bearing collagenous tissue with its most important features (see next section for proof).

The *biocompatibility* of the polymers of the acrylic family is an established fact, and they find application not only as cements and prosthetic replacements for hard tissues, but also increasingly of soft tissues [6–10]. Not so ample is the experience with PPTA, but it is nevertheless encouraging: not only has its good *biocompatibility* been reported, but also its property of stimulating the ingrowth of connective tissue between the fibre net [11]. This fact could provide a firm basis for the solution of the problem of anchorage to the muscle.

EXPERIMENTAL

Several samples of PMA and PEA reinforced by PPTA fibre bundles were prepared. The source of the PPTA bundles was commercial Kevlar-49, which gave them a planar sinusoidal wave form, as described in [12]. A monomer of methyl and ethyl acrylate was poured in a special mould, where the fibre bundles had been previously arranged with the desired pre-stretch. The resulting samples were in the form of little bars, suited for the creep apparatus. Polymerization was then carried out in an oven at the adequate temperatures, and the samples were then stored *in vacuo* until their weight remained constant (for more details see [12]).

The samples were subjected to different creep tests in an apparatus designed by us and described in [13]. During all the tests the temperature was kept constant at 36°C. After each test the sample was left to recover its original length. No permanent deformation was ever observed for the strain and loading ranges to which the samples were subjected.

The matrix polymer was removed from both ends of each sample so that the fibre bundles could be directly clamped. This fact not only assures that the clamped cross sections remain fixed during the creep of the specimen, but also provides to a certain extent a method to achieve similar anchorage conditions to those which are met in the case of the collagen fibre bundles of the tendon, whose ingrowth at the distal and proximal ends into the tissue of muscle and bone (see [14,15]) keeps them fixed during the deformation.

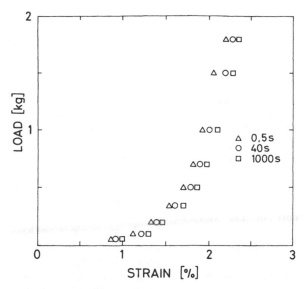

Figure 1. Isocrone creep curves at the time instants 0.5 s, 40 s and 1000 s for sample (C1).

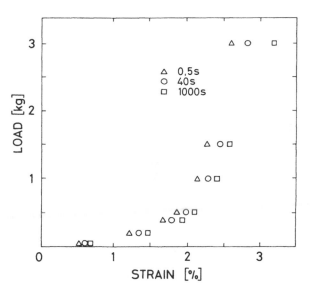

Figure 2. Isocrone creep curves at the time instants 0.5 s, 40 s and 1000 s for sample (C2).

We report here results obtained on four samples with the following composition: sample (C1) consisted in PEA reinforced by *one* PPTA fibre bundle; (C2) was PEA reinforced by *two* PPTA fibre bundles; (C3) was PEA with *three* bundles; and (C4) consisted in PMA reinforced with *one* PPTA bundle. Each fibre bundle had approximately 700 fibres and a weight per unit of its crimped initial length (before prestretching it) of 0.122 mg/mm (see [12]).

Information about the tests done on the flexor tendon samples, which provided the results cited below, can be also found in [13].

RESULTS AND DISCUSSION

Figures 1 to 4 show the isocrone creep curves of the samples (C1) to (C4) respectively. Of interest to us here are the following facts.

First of all, the curves show clearly the two regions of behaviour typical of collagenous tissues: an initial low modulus "toe" region followed by a progressive increase in modulus up to a "linear" stress-strain characteristic. The time evolution of these curves is also clearly seen.

Table 1. Values of the slope of the linear part of the isocrones 0.5 and 1000 seconds and its relative time variation calculated as [E(0.5 s)–E(1000)]E(0.5 s).

Sample	E(0.5 s) [kg/%]	E(1000 s) [kg/%]	△ [%]
(C1)	2.9	2.6	10.3
(C2)	4.2	2.5	40.5
(C3)	4.2	2.6	38.1
(C4)	3.8	3.2	15.8

Secondly, the approximate values of load at which the transition between both regions takes place is in the range 0.6–0.9 kg independent of the strain amplitude of the "toe" region. In [13] the interval of 0.5–0.8 kg was found for five samples of flexor tendons of the hand. There, values of strain for the "toe" region of the tendons were seen to lie between 1.0% and 1.9%.

Table 1 gives the percentage of the time variation of the linear modulus as calculated from the experimental values for the linear part of each isocrone. In tendons these values lie in the range between 11.7% and 26.6%, see [13]. As was noted in [12], the change of this value with the number of bundles in the composite sample can be due to the fact that in a single bundle

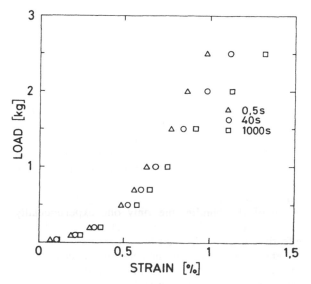

Figure 3. Isocrone creep curves at the time instants 0.5 s, 40 s and 1000 s for sample (C3).

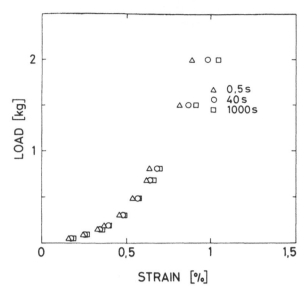

Figure 4. Isocrone creep curves at the time instants 0.5 s, 40 s and 1000 s for sample (C4).

the fibres are more tightly packed than in the complex formed by several bundles.

In [12] and [13] the creep behaviour of the tendon and composite samples was studied with the aim finding a suitable constitutive equation to describe it. Such a model was proposed and its material functions were calculated from the results of experimental tests. The accuracy of the model was tested by comparing the behaviour predicted by the constitutive equation against the results of several multiple step creep tests. The qualitative features of the constitutive equation imply that the deformation mechanism responsible for the observable behaviour must be that of the sequential stretching of the bundle of fibres, even for the low modulus part of the curve. In the case of tendons, this interpretation can be further supported by the observation made in [16] that fibrillar creep starts as early as 0.1 seconds after the application of load, matrix creep occupying the previous time instants. In our present case, PMA as well as PEA are, at human body temperature, rubbery polymers of very low modulus, so that very low loads and very early instants of time would be needed to register the transition or matrix creep. This fact is confirmed by measurements by us on samples of pure PMA and PEA [17]. In this sense, the deformation mechanism of the tendon and of our composite samples is the same: creep of the matrix extended to a time instant earlier than 0.5 seconds, followed by the fibrillar creep of the bundle, the only one experimentally observed from 0.5 s on, with increasing number of effective fibers as the load level is raised.

Other points related to the constitutive behaviour of the composite samples of less interest for our present purpose were discussed in [12].

CONCLUSIONS

The composite system studied bears some points of *structural similitude* with the tissue of tendons and ligaments. Firstly, in both cases we are dealing with macromoleculr systems with a highly crystalline fibrous component (collagen in the case of tendons and ligaments, PPTA in the composites) embedded in an amorphous matrix (the mucopolysaccharide complex of the ground substance on the one hand and PEA or PMA on the other). Secondly, in both systems matrix and fibres play the same mechanical role: fibres are the load-bearing elements, whereas the matrix amalgamates the fibre complex and provides part of the restoring force. Thirdly, a global mechanical behaviour with a characteristic initial low-modulus region followed by a linear higher-modulus region is in both cases achieved through the same mechanism of the sequential stretching of initially crimped fibre bundles. Finally, both the biological tissue and the artificial system reveal an anelastic, viscoelastic, mechanical behaviour, with delayed response to changes in the applied actions. The latter two features provide the tissue with stress relaxation and shock-absorbing properties.

It is possible, in sum, to combine biocompatible polymers so as to reproduce qualitatively and quantitatively the main features of the behaviour of collagenous tissues, and moreover to satisfy not only overall strength requirements, but also energetic (damping and stress relaxing) ones akin to those of the biological tissue.

Interesting to point out is also the fact that the method employed here to fabricate the composite samples allows in principle the possibility of varying the amplitude of the initial "toe" region as well as the final value of the linear modulus, by varying the initial prestretch and the number of fibres. This means that it could be possible to comply with the individual characteristics of specific tendons and ligaments present in the body.

ACKNOWLEDGEMENTS

The partial support of the CAICYT through grant no. 0654/81 is thankfully acknowledged.

REFERENCES

1. Fernandez, F. M. 1983. "Le Complexe Os-Tendon-Muscle Consideré Comme Entité Biomécanique", *Acta Orthop. Belg.*, 49:13–29.

2. Crisp, J. 1972. "Properties of Tendon and Skin", in *Biomechanics, Its Foundations and Objectives*, Fung, Perrone, Anliker, eds. Prentice Hall, pp. 141–171.

3. Baer, E., L. Gathercole and A. Keller. 1974. "Structure

Hierarchies in Tendon Collagen: An Interim Summary", *Proc. Colston Conf.*, Dept. of Physics, University of Bristol.

4. Gordon, J. 1980. "Biomechanics: The Last Stronghold of Vitalism", *The Mechanical Properties of Biological Materials* (several contributors). Cambridge University Press, pp. 1–11.

5. Struik, L. 1978. *Physical Aging in Amorphous Polymers and Other Materials*. Elsevier.

6. Ducheyne, P., G. van der Perre and A. Aubert, eds. 1984. *Biomaterials and Biomechanics*. Elsevier.

7. Winter, G., J. Leray and K. de Groot, eds. 1980. *Evaluation of Biomaterials*. J. Wiley.

8. Goldberg, E. and A. Nakajima. 1980. *Biomedical Polymers*. Academic Press.

9. Refojo, M. 1975. "Materials for Use in the Eye", in *Polymers in Medicine and Surgery*. Kronental, Oser, Martin, eds. Plenum Press.

10. Kumakura, M. and I. Kaetsu. 1983. "Hydrophilic Polymeric Membranes Obtained by Radiation-Cast Copolymerization of Ethyl Acrylate with Various Monomers," *J. Mater. Sci.*, 18:1335–1340.

11. Claes et al. 1984. "Animal Experiments for Comparison of Various Alloplastic Materials in Ligament Replacement", in *Biomaterials and Biomechanics*. Ducheyne et al., eds. Elsevier.

12. Monleón, M. and R. Díaz. 1989. "A Kind of Extensible, Modulus Developing Polymer Composite", *Composite Sci. & Technol*, 36:227–241.

13. Monleón, M. and R. Díaz. 1989. "Nonlinear Viscoelastic Behaviour of the Flexor Tendon of the Human Hand", *J. of Biomechanics*, 23:773–781.

14. Hanak, H. and P. Bock. 1971. "Die Feinstruktur der Muskel-Sehnen-Verbindung von Skellett- und Herzmuskel", *J. Ultrastruct. Res.*, 36:68–85.

15. Cooper, R. and S. Misol. 1970. "Tendon and Ligament Insertion. A Light and Electron Microscopy Study", *J. Bone Jt. Surg.*, 52A:1–20.

16. Goldstein, S., et al. 1987. "Analysis of Cumulative Strain in Tendons and Tendon Sheaths", *J. of Biomechanics*, 20:1–6.

17. Monleón, M. 1988. "Mecánica de los Tejidos Colaginosos Humanos y de los Polímeros Enfibrados, en Vistas a la Sustitución Protésica de Tendones y Ligamentos", Dr. Eng. Sci. Thesis, Universidad Politécnica de Valencia.

Part 6

PHARMACEUTICAL APPLICATIONS

34

Skin Permeation Enhancers for Improved Transdermal Drug Delivery

BRUCE J. AUNGST, Ph.D.*

ABSTRACT: Transdermal dosage forms provide controlled drug dosing through the skin from bandage-like delivery systems. This method of drug delivery can provide certain medical advantages for many drugs. The skin is a very good barrier preventing the absorption of such foreign substances; therefore, most drugs don't diffuse through it rapidly enough for ordinary formulations to be administered transdermally. Skin permeation enhancers increase skin permeability and may make it feasible to deliver many more drugs transdermally. In addition, they may be useful for improving the efficacy of poorly permeating, topically acting drugs. The literature on skin permeation enhancers is reviewed, with particular emphasis on structure/activity relationships, mechanisms of enhancing skin permeability, and toxicity of skin permeation enhancing agents. Although this summary may not enable one to predict how to effectively and safely enhance transdermal or dermal delivery for some given drug, it should provide an understanding of the studies that are important to reaching such a target. As an introduction, the properties of skin as a barrier and the pathways of transport across the skin are discussed.

INTRODUCTION

Rationale for Transdermal Delivery of Drugs

Transdermal drug delivery refers to the method of delivering therapeutic drug doses through the skin to treat diseases for which systemic drug absorption is required. Although this concept has probably been used for a very long time, the technology to control the dose and dosing rate, and to package the dose into bandage-like patches has only recently been developed and applied. Because the few products that have been introduced have been fairly successful commercially, the interest in transdermal drug delivery has continued to grow.

When transdermal delivery is compared to other routes of administration it is apparent that for many drugs it offers a means of improving therapy. Some of the most important potential benefits of transdermal delivery are listed in Table 1. These can be further illustrated using as examples the drugs that are presently available as products or are in development. The first transdermal patch introduced to the market was the scopolamine system (Transderm Scop, Ciba-Geigy) developed by the Alza Corporation. This system is used for prevention of motion sickness. It offers the benefits of efficacy equal to intramuscular therapy, while the incidence of side effects is greatly reduced [1]. Scopolamine's effects, both pharmacologic and toxic, are proportional to its plasma concentrations. The scopolamine patch was designed to produce constant plasma concentrations at levels above the minimum effective concentration, but below those at which side effects occur.

Nitroglycerin is a good example of a drug which is metabolized very rapidly, and which consequently has a very short systemic half-life. In addition, oral nitroglycerin doses are generally ineffective because of extensive presystemic metabolism by the gut and/or liver. By administering the drug transdermally, plasma nitroglycerin concentrations can be sustained for 24 hours with the convenience of once-a-day dosing. Several forms of transdermal nitroglycerin have become available and are commonly used for prophylaxis of angina attacks.

Estradiol is also subject to presystemic metabolism when administered orally. Although oral estradiol provides effective estrogen replacement therapy, one of the products of presystemic metabolism, estrone, is pharmacologically active and has been implicated as having adverse effects on the liver. The relative estrone and estradiol plasma concentrations are more

*DuPont Merck Pharmaceutical Co., P.O. Box 80400, Wilmington, DE 19880-0400

Table 1. Potential medical advantages provided by administering a drug transdermally, and examples of drugs for which these apply.

Transdermal Can Provide	Potential Medical Advantage	Example
Controlled release and absorption	Plasma concentrations can be maintained relatively constant. Side effects can be avoided and the pharmacologic effect maintained.	Scopolamine Clonidine Testosterone
Avoidance of gastrointestinal tract	Avoids unpredictable absorption for drugs metabolized by intestines and liver. Avoids gastric irritation. Avoids bad taste.	Nitroglycerin Estradiol Testosterone Nicotine
Once-a-day or less frequent dosing	More convenient dosing regimen for drugs with short half-lives. Improved patient compliance.	Nitroglycerin Scopolamine

similar to physiological levels after transdermal dosing than after oral dosing, thus providing a potentially greater safety margin [2].

Limitations

If one surveys the available transdermal products with regard to the doses administered (summarized in Table 2), it is readily apparent that for each product the doses are fairly low. This is also true for most of the drugs being developed as transdermal delivery systems, but not yet commercially available. A major factor limiting the success of transdermal drug delivery is the impermeable nature of the skin. Because the skin is inherently impermeable, the doses that can be administered through it, using a reasonable surface area, are low. The limiting dose is generally ≤ 10 mg/day. Drugs that have relatively good skin permeability properties, such as nitroglycerin and nicotine, can be administered trandermally at slightly higher doses. But many drugs are not effective at doses of 10 mg/day, and thus appear to be excluded from consideration for transdermal systems. Many others permeate skin poorly, and even though they are very potent they cannot be delivered through normal skin at rates equivalent to therapeutic doses. For many of these drugs, however, there appear to be very logical medical advantages to transdermal dosing. These potential medical advantages and the possibility that offering those advantages would capture the market for those drugs have driven research in the area of manipulating skin permeability, so that those drugs that cannot be delivered through normal skin at sufficient rates might be formulated into transdermal systems.

Skin permeation rates are dependent on a number of factors, and can be manipulated in a number of ways. Among these are alteration of the drug's solubility or concentration in the vehicle, its partition coefficient, the solvent used as the vehicle, or the site and species from which the skin is derived. These areas will not be covered in this review. The other variable, and the focus of this report, is the diffusivity of the skin. Several techniques have been successfully used to increase the skin diffusivity. Two of these are iontophoresis and phonophoresis, in which drugs are driven through the skin by applied energy in the forms, respectively, of an electric current and sound. The third technique, and the subject of this review, is the use of chemical agents to temporarily increase skin permeability so that the absorption of a co-applied drug can be increased. These chemical agents, when used for this purpose, are referred to as permeation enhancers, penetration enhancers, or absorption promoters. As this research area is reviewed it is important to remember that the objective is to *temporarily* increase skin permeability. An increase in skin permeability associated with skin toxicity would usually not be acceptable clinically.

THE BARRIER

Structure and Composition of Skin

The skin is inherently a relatively impermeable membrane. This property serves its purposes of shielding the body from the environment, keeping potential toxins out, and regulating the escape of water. Human skin is structured in several layers, the major divisions being the dermis, or underlying layer, and the epidermis, or outermost layer. The very outermost layer of the epidermis is comprised of dead cells which are tightly packed together in a lipoidal matrix. This layer is called the stratum corneum. It is generally regarded as the least permeable layer of skin, and therefore it is almost always the rate-limiting barrier for drug absorption.

The stratum corneum is formed as cells of the underlying viable epidermis differentiate. During this process the shape of the cells changes from round to flat. Lamellar granules appear within the cells and then migrate to the cell membrane and fuse with it, extruding their contents of lipids to the intercellular space. The interior of the cells become filled with keratin and other matrix proteins, and the organelles are broken down. The various layers of the epidermis represent the various stages of differentiation, terminating in a stratum corneum which is continuously sloughed off and replaced from underneath.

The stratum corneum on most of the body is usually 15 to 20 cell layers thick. The cells are extremely elongated and flattened. The proteins within the cells, keratin and others, are arranged in fibrils and appear to attach to desmosomes, which may bridge the gaps between cells. Rather than a usual lipid bilayer membrane, the boundary of the cells of the stratum corneum consists of an envelope of cross-linked proteins and hydroxyceramides. The intercellular lipid matrix is arranged in lamellar sheets, a result of fusion of the extruded contents of the lamellar granules. The lamellar appearance probably represents alternating bilayers of lipid polar groups and hydrophobic tails, which interdigitate to form a tightly packed matrix [3]. As in lipid bilayer membranes, the intercellular stratum corneum lipids can form a structured matrix by the alignment of the various hydrophobic tails. The composition of the stratum corneum lipids is summarized in Table 3. The hydrophobic tails of these various lipids are predominantly chains of 16 or 18 carbon atoms, except the ceramides, which have a good proportion of 22 carbon and 26 carbon hydrophobic tails [5].

Pathways of Absorption

The pathways of absorption can be classified either anatomically or according to models based on the physico-chemical properties of diffusion and the diffusing substances. Both of these approaches may be useful when examining the mechanisms of permeation enhancement. However, the components of the models, which usually have separate polar and non-polar pathways, may or may not have anatomical correlates.

Anatomically, substances can cross the stratum corneum barrier via three routes.

(1) Appendages—Diffusion or bulk fluid flow through sweat glands (pores) and along hair follicles and sebaceous glands.

(2) Paracellular—Diffusion along the circuitous pathways around the cells of the stratum corneum.

(3) Transcellular—Diffusion across the cell envelopes and intracellular spaces.

Scheuplein [6] examined the potential contribution of the appendages to drug diffusion through skin using a mathematical analysis based on relative surface areas and diffusivities. He concluded that because the appendages make up only 1/1000th of the total surface area, for permeable substances they probably contribute little to the total diffusion at steady-state. However, it was also pointed out that the appendages could contribute more immediately after a substance is applied to skin, or could be effective for very poorly permeating substances. Only recently was it verified that the appendages probably can contribute to permeation.

Table 2. Drugs presently available in transdermal dosage forms and the range of doses available.

	Range of Available Doses
Scopolamine	0.5 mg/3 days
Nitroglycerin	2.5–15 mg/day
Estradiol	0.05–0.1 mg/day
Clonidine	0.1–0.3 mg/day

Keister and Kasting [7] derived diffusion equations with which the fractional contribution of the appendages could be estimated utilizing *in vitro* skin permeation data. With ibuprofen at pH 7.4 (ionized), the appendages accounted for about 25% of the total flux at steady-state. Kao et al. [8] showed that the permeation rates for benzo[a]pyrene and testosterone through skin of various species of mice correlated with the density of skin appendages, and examination by fluorescence miscroscopy revealed fluorescent areas correlating with the follicular ducts and sebaceous glands. They concluded that for testosterone, which permeated skin fairly rapidly, the appendages contributed relatively little to total diffusion, but for benzo[a]pyrene, which permeated much slower, the appendages contributed significantly.

Histochemical techniques have also been used to try to ascertain the relative contributions of the transcellular and paracellular routes of skin permeation. In a study by Nemanic and Elias [9], butanol was applied to mouse and human stratum corneum and allowed to penetrate 5 minutes to 2 hours, after which it could be visualized after *in situ* precipitation with osmium vapor. It was mostly deposited in the intercellular spaces, suggesting a predominance of paracellular diffusion. Similarly, Bodde et al. [10] applied mercuric chloride to human skin *in vitro* and after various periods of penetration precipitated it as mercuric sulfate. These investigators concluded that for this substance the paracellular route of permeation dominates, although after longer exposure times the stratum corneum cells began to take up the marker. In contrast, Scheuplein and Blank [11] concluded that in the cases of water and polar alcohols transcellular diffusion must predominate, based on a physico-

Table 3. Lipid composition of human stratum corneum (adapted from Reference [4]).

	% by Weight
Triglycerides	25
Fatty acids	19
Ceramides	18
Sterols (unesterified)	14
Sterol/wax esters	5
n-Alkanes	6
Squalane	5
Polar lipids	5
Cholesterol sulfate	<2

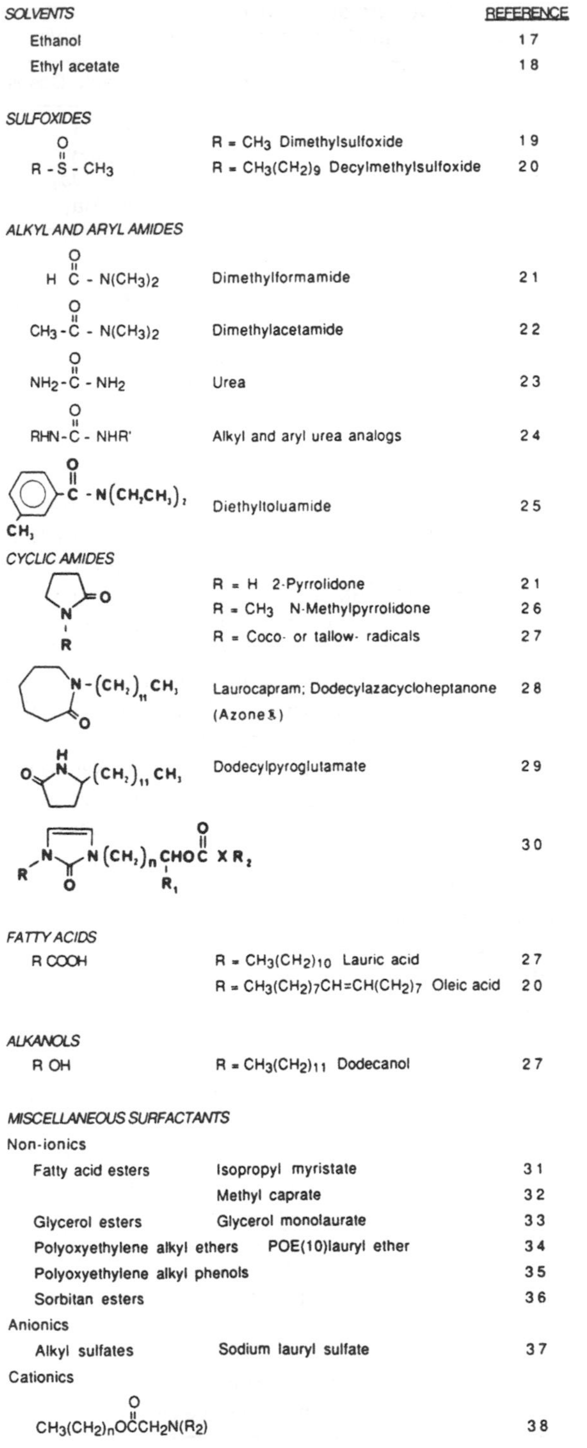

SOLVENTS   <u>REFERENCE</u>

Ethanol   17

Ethyl acetate   18

SULFOXIDES

O
‖
R - S - CH₃   R = CH₃ Dimethylsulfoxide   19
                     R = CH₃(CH₂)₉ Decylmethylsulfoxide   20

ALKYL AND ARYL AMIDES

O
‖
H C - N(CH₃)₂   Dimethylformamide   21

O
‖
CH₃-C - N(CH₃)₂   Dimethylacetamide   22

O
‖
NH₂-C - NH₂   Urea   23

O
‖
RHN-C - NHR'   Alkyl and aryl urea analogs   24

O
‖
⬡ C - N(CH₂CH₃)₂   Diethyltoluamide   25
CH₃

CYCLIC AMIDES

⬠=O   R = H   2-Pyrrolidone   21
 N   R = CH₃ N-Methylpyrrolidone   26
 R   R = Coco- or tallow- radicals   27

N-(CH₂)₁₁CH₃   Laurocapram; Dodecylazacycloheptanone   28
   O   (Azone®)

O=⬠(CH₂)₁₁CH₃ H   Dodecylpyroglutamate   29

N⬠N (CH₂)ₙCHOC X R₂ [structure]   30
R O   R₁

FATTY ACIDS

R COOH   R = CH₃(CH₂)₁₀ Lauric acid   27
                     R = CH₃(CH₂)₇CH=CH(CH₂)₇ Oleic acid   20

ALKANOLS

R OH   R = CH₃(CH₂)₁₁ Dodecanol   27

MISCELLANEOUS SURFACTANTS
Non-ionics
  Fatty acid esters   Isopropyl myristate   31
                         Methyl caprate   32
  Glycerol esters   Glycerol monolaurate   33
  Polyoxyethylene alkyl ethers   POE(10)lauryl ether 34
  Polyoxyethylene alkyl phenols   35
  Sorbitan esters   36
Anionics
  Alkyl sulfates   Sodium lauryl sulfate   37
Cationics
           O
           ‖
  CH₃(CH₂)ₙOCCH₂N(R₂)   38

Figure 1. General classification of skin permeation enhancers, and representative compounds and references.

chemical analysis of the diffusion characteristics of these compounds and on the volume of the intercellular spaces (estimated to be 5%) relative to the total stratum corneum volume.

Since it has proven difficult to definitively characterize the anatomical routes of skin permeation, simplified models of the barrier structure have been developed based on permeability data of various com-

pounds. A general feature of such models is the inclusion of non-polar and polar routes of permeation. Evidence supporting a non-polar or lipid route includes the following. (1) Skin or stratum corneum permeability has been correlated with drug lipophilicity in several studies using various drugs with no structural similarity [12] or within a series of structural homologs [13]. (2) Regional differences in skin permeability have been inversely correlated with stratum corneum lipid content, and were not related to the number of cell layers or the thickness of the stratum corneum [14]. Regulation of stratum corneum permeability by the lipids within it implies that the route of permeation is through the lipids. It is reasonable to assume that the lipid or non-polar route of skin diffusion models is in reality the intercellular lipids.

The correlation between skin permeation and lipophilicity has not always held true. For example, there was no correlation between ether/water partition coefficients and permeability coefficients within a group of hydrophilic compounds [15]. Ionized compounds have also been observed to permeate skin [16], and these would not be expected to diffuse through a lipophilic membrane or lipid channels. There is therefore evidence to support inclusion in the models of a pathway by which polar compounds diffuse through skin. Unlike the lipid pathway, however, there is no evidence to imply an anatomical correlate for the polar pathway. It could be associated with the appendages, hydrated intracellular or cell envelope proteins, or aqueous channels through the lipophilic bilayers of the intracellular spaces.

PERMEATION ENHANCEMENT

There have been a large number of publications in which one or more chemicals have been shown to increase the permeability of skin to drugs. Three important criteria should be considered in collectively evaluating these works, and in addressing the needs for the future.

- Structure/effect relationships—Ideally one would like to be able to predict how to safely promote absorption through skin for some given drug. Presently this cannot be done *a priori*. Development of some general structure/effect relationships should be useful as a foundation for understanding and eventually predicting the actions of transdermal absorption promoters.
- Mechanisms—An understanding of the mechanisms of action of various compounds or classes could enable the identification or design of more effective or safer permeation enhancers.
- Toxicity—If any skin permeation enhancer is to be used clinically it will have to be proven to be safe. Irritation and sensitization potential must be evaluated. These critical criteria prob-

ably will limit the usefulness of most of the compounds to be discussed, although in many cases they have not yet been thoroughly evaluated.

Structure/Effect Relationships

Most of the compounds that have been shown to increase skin permeability generally fall into one of the categories listed in Figure 1. The figure also includes representative references in which the effects of some of these compounds have been reported.

Several structure/effect relationships that seem to occur consistently can be proposed.

Some permeation enhancers act as solvents. This is based primarily on the fact that they increase skin permeation only when applied at high concentrations. In addition to ethanol and ethyl acetate, the other categories also include dimethylsulfoxide, dimethylformamide, dimethylacetamide, 2-pyrrolidone, and N-methylpyrrolidone, which probably can be considered as solvents. In fact, they are often used as solvents for both polar and non-polar solutes. It can therefore be imagined that these materials readily penetrate the stratum corneum and in high enough concentrations they dissolve or loosen the packed lipids or proteins that constitute the barrier.

The structures of most others have a hydrophobic tail and a polar functional group. Because of this, many of these compounds are amphiphilic; they have a certain affinity for both polar and non-polar solvents.

The optimum number of carbon atoms for aliphatic side chains is 10–14. This characteristic appears to hold true for each of the structural classes, with few exceptions. An example of data showing the chain length dependence of skin permeation enhancement with saturated fatty acids and alkanols is given in Figure 2. Similar results have also been reported with polyoxyethylene alkyl ether non-ionic surfactants [39], alkyl methyl sulfoxides [40], and 1-alkyl- or 1-alkenylazacycloalkanones [41]. The reasons for these chain length dependencies are not known.

Several studies have also shown that with fatty acids and fatty alcohols, the effects of the agents on skin permeation are greater when the hydrophobic tail is unsaturated. The data in Figure 3 illustrate this. Compounds in the other categories have generally not had unsaturated side chains, so it is not known whether this property would also apply to those types of compounds.

The polar functional group may have structural diversity. For the most part, the classification of compounds listed as in Figure 1 was based on the differences of the polar functional groups. What properties differentiate effective permeation enhancers from ineffective compounds? One distinguishing feature could be the relative hydrophobicity or hydrophilicity of the compound. To evaluate this we previously determined the effects on human skin of a series of compounds having different hydrophilic

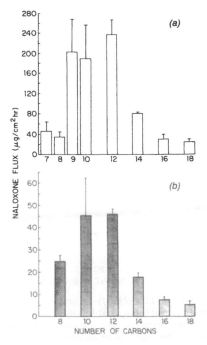

Figure 2. Effect of chain length of fatty acids (a) or fatty alcohols (b) on *in vitro* human skin permeation rates for naloxone. Vehicles contained 10% enhancer in propylene glycol saturated with naloxone base (from Reference [27]).

functional groups, but each having a dodecyl side chain. The permeant was naloxone and the vehicle was propylene glycol. As shown in Figure 4, the most effective adjuvants were the least hydrophilic ones, using the hydrophil–lipophil balance (HLB) values as an index of relative hydrophilicity. The dependence of efficacy on hydrophobicity could be related to the degree of skin permeation of the permeation enhancers. Other chemical properties of the polar functional group probably also contribute to the effectiveness of compounds as permeation enhancers. For example, hydrogen bonding tendencies could be important determinants of how the agents interact with

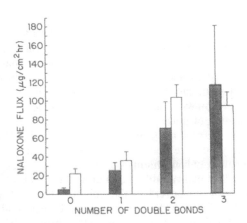

Figure 3. Comparison of the effectiveness of saturated and unsaturated C_{18} fatty acids (open bars) and fatty alcohols (closed bars) as permeation enhancers for naloxone. Experiments were as described for Figure 2 (from Reference [27]).

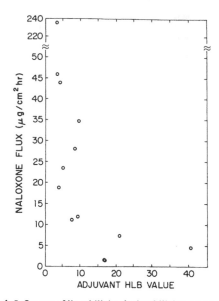

Figure 4. Influence of lipophilicity–hydrophilicity, as measured by the hydrophil–lipophil balance (HLB) values, on efficacy as human skin permeation enhancers. The enhancers each had a laurate hydrophobic tail, but various polar functional groups. Vehicles contained 10% enhancer in propylene glycol, saturated with naloxone base (from Reference [27]).

skin lipids, proteins, or water. Agents in the various categories of permeation enhancers probably function at least in part through different mechanisms. Because these agents often have identical hydrophobic side chains these mechanistic differences must be related to the different polar functional groups. Proposed mechanisms will be discussed in a subsequent section.

Drug/Vehicle/Enhancer Interactions

Skin permeation enhancers affect the permeation rates of individual drugs differently, and their effects are also highly dependent on the vehicle in which the drug and enhancer are dissolved. The former point was clearly illustrated in the work of Yamada and Uda [42], which is summarized in Table 4. The range of enhancement attained by including oleic acid in propylene glycol vehicles ranged from 2.6-fold for oxendolone to 90-fold for indomethacin. The variance of effects of particular permeation enhancers may be related to the routes by which a drug diffuses through normal skin, and the extent of enhancement of that route or routes. Some enhancers seem to promote permeation of polar compounds while others seem to promote permeation of non-polar compounds. This is probably because they have different mechanisms of permeation enhancement.

An additional variable modulating the effects of skin permeation enhancers is the vehicle. The data presented in Table 5 demonstrate this. Lauric acid increased naloxone permeation rates through human skin 150-fold when propylene glycol was the vehicle, but only 2.6-fold with isopropyl myristate as the vehi-

cle. In contrast, sodium lauryl sulfate was hardly effective as a permeation enhancer when propylene glycol was used as the vehicle, but was much more effective when mineral oil was the vehicle. One reason the vehicle plays such an important role is that it affects the skin permeation of the permeation-enhancing agent. Several studies have shown that the magnitude of skin permeation enhancement is related to the skin permeation of the enhancing agent.

Proposed Mechanisms

Before discussing the mechanisms of permeation enhancement, it should be useful to review the pathways of permeation and the methods used to evaluate the mechanisms of permeation enhancement. Summarizing from a previous section, anatomically the routes of skin permeation are transcellular, paracellular, and through the appendages. The intercellular spaces are filled with compact lamellae composed of lipids, and the intracellular volume is primarily filled with cross-linked proteins. These materials present the barriers to permeation. Skin permeation has also been modeled, and the models generally have consisted of separate polar and non-polar routes. The non-polar route is probably in reality the paracellular route, whereas the polar route has no definite anatomical correlate. Skin permeation enhancement can be similarly modeled to ascertain whether the polar or non-polar routes are affected, and this can be used to build an information base to help understand the mechanisms of permeation enhancement.

Other tools that have been used to provide valuable information regarding mechanisms are the methods of physical characterization of treated stratum corneum using differential scanning calorimetry (DSC) and infrared spectroscopy. DSC measures the heat flow associated with physical changes, such as the melting of a solid, as a material is subjected to temperature changes. Examination of isolated and specially hydrated stratum corneum by several investigators us-

Table 4. Skin permeation enhancement for various drugs with 10% oleic acid in propylene glycol. Groups of 3 rats were dosed transdermally using either the vehicle with enhancer (E) or a control vehicle of propylene glycol (C), and the area under the plasma drug concentration vs. time curve (AUC) was measured. E_{AUC}/C_{AUC} represents the enhancement factor. Adapted from Reference [42].

Drug	Dose	E_{AUC}/C_{AUC}
4-(4-Methylbenzoyl)-1-indanecarboxylic acid	5 mg	49.8
Diazepam	5 mg	6.7
Indomethacin	5 mg	90.2
Nifedipine	3 mg	3.5
Oxendolone	10 mg	2.6
Protirelin tartrate	0.8 mg	6.8

ing DSC has usually shown 4 endothermic transitions as temperature was increased from 25°C to 105°C. Typical transition temperatures are 35°, 65°, 80°, and 95°. These have been postulated to be associated, respectively, with changes in loosely associated lipids, intercellular lipids, a lipid–protein complex associated with the cell membrane, and intracellular proteins [43]. Although other investigators may have slightly different transition temperatures, it is fairly clear that the lower transition temperatures reflect skin lipids, and the highest transition temperature reflects skin proteins. It is therefore possible using DSC to evaluate whether skin permeation enhancers affect skin lipids or proteins.

Infrared spectroscopy has been used to measure changes in the carbon–hydrogen (C–H) stretching vibrations of stratum corneum lipids as a function of temperature. Thermally induced changes result in a frequency shift and broadening of the C–H stretching absorbances, and because these changes suggest increased motional freedom of the lipid hydrophobic tails they have been referred to as increased lipid fluidity.

We shall consider skin permeation enhancement mechanisms according to the classification of compounds in Figure 1.

Solvents

These are liquids that only affect skin permeability at high concentrations and are often used as chemical solvents. Ethanol and ethyl acetate were listed in the solvent category in Figure 1, but other compounds in the other categories share the aforementioned properties. Ethanol at concentrations of 25% to 50% appears to create solvent-filled channels in the stratum corneum allowing increased permeability, especially for polar compounds [17]. Permeation enhancement with ethanol was correlated with the skin permeation rate of ethanol, and this was consistent with ethanol increasing the drug solubility in the skin [44]. At 75% and 100% concentrations, permeability increases were irreversible, suggesting lipid extraction or irreversible protein conformation changes [17]. The mechanisms of ethyl acetate and other similar alkyl

ester solvents are not known, but in one report these were much more effective than ethanol in increasing skin permeability [18].

Sulfoxides

Dimethylsulfoxide only increases skin permeability at high ($\geq 50\%$) concentrations. It was proposed that three mechanisms contribute to the permeation enhancing effects: solvation and elution of stratum corneum lipids, conformational changes of stratum corneum proteins, and delamination as a result of the movements of dimethylsulfoxide and water across the stratum corneum [37,45]. Using DSC, dimethylsulfoxide was shown to alter the high transition temperature lipoprotein and intracellular protein peaks [46]. Barry [47] claimed that dimethylsulfoxide also affects stratum corneum lipids, based on DSC results, and he proposed that it displaces water associated with the polar functional groups of lipids, resulting in increased lipid fluidity. Decylmethylsulfoxide, in contrast to dimethylsulfoxide, is an effective skin permeation enhancer at low (e.g., 1%) concentrations. Conformational changes of skin proteins were demonstrated for both dimethylsulfoxide and decylmethylsulfoxide using infrared spectroscopy [48]. Decylmethylsulfoxide preferentially enhanced the permeability of polar compounds [49], consistent with relatively small changes in lipid peaks on DSC [47].

Alkyl and Aryl Amines

Dimethylformamide (DMF) and dimethylacetamide (DMA) appear to have properties and mechanisms similar to dimethylsulfoxide [37,47]. The effects of diethyltoluamide (DEET) on skin permeation rates were also attributed primarily to its solvency properties in that it permeated skin rapidly, increasing the thermodynamic activity of the drug in the vehicle remaining on the skin, and increasing drug solubility in the stratum corneum [50]. Similar to other solvents, DMF, DMA, and DEET affect skin permeability only at high concentrations. The mechanism of effect of urea on skin has not been studied. Urea de-

Table 5. *Effects of lauric acid, lauryl alcohol, and sodium lauryl sulfate on naloxone permeation rates through human skin* in vitro *using various vehicles containing 10% permeation enhancer and naloxone in excess of saturated solubility. From Reference [27].*

Vehicle	Naloxone flux (μg/cm² hr)			
	No Enhancer	Lauric Acid	Lauryl Alcohol	Na Lauryl Sulfate
Propylene glycol	1.6 ± 0.4	235.2 ± 29.9	45.8 ± 2.4	4.6 ± 0.9
Isopropanol	16.6 ± 4.7	160.6 ± 60.0	28.4 ± 11.8	31.5 ± 19.8
Polyethylene glycol 400	1.8 ± 0.6	46.1 ± 25.3	12.2 ± 5.4	1.6 ± 0.5
Mineral oil	1.3 ± 0.3	18.8 ± 6.4	11.1 ± 2.7	42.6 ± 32.3
Isopropyl myristate	7.7 ± 0.1	20.0 ± 3.0		

rivatives with long hydrophobic tails were more potent skin permeation enhancers than urea, and this was related to their higher partition coefficients and retention in and disruption of the stratum corneum [24].

Cyclic Amides

N-methylpyrrolidone and 2-pyrrolidone are also similar to solvents, altering skin permeability only at high concentrations. Like dimethylsulfoxide, these agents may displace the water associated with stratum corneum proteins or polar head groups of lipids, and preferentially increase permeability of polar compounds [21,47]. As in the other classes, pyrrolidone derivatives with a long hydrocarbon tail are much more potent skin permeation enhancers. Laurocapram (Azone®) is probably the most frequently studied skin permeation enhancer. DSC showed that laurocapram affected stratum corneum lipids, but not proteins [47]. Microscopic examination of stratum corneum using a method in which mercury permeates skin and then is precipitated showed that laurocapram enhanced diffusion through the paracellular route [10]. Other investigators who applied neat laurocapram to skin have suggested that laurocapram also affects stratum corneum proteins (by DSC examination) and that this may increase permeation of polar compounds [51]. Another effect of laurocapram is to increase the skin permeation rate of the co-applied solvent, which can increase partitioning of the drug into skin or allow the solvent to have a greater disrupting effect on the stratum corneum [52,53].

Fatty Acids

Most evidence indicates that fatty acids disrupt the packed structure of lipids in the intercellular spaces of the stratum corneum and thereby increase skin permeability. Golden et al. [54] presented convincing support of this hypothesis by directly correlating increased permeability with quantified changes (by DSC and infrared spectroscopy) in stratum corneum lipids after treatment with various fatty acids. Fatty acids increased permeation of both polar and nonpolar compounds [42,55]. In addition to disrupting the packed structure of stratum corneum lipids, fatty acids may increase skin permeability by enhancing skin permeation of the solvent [56] and by forming more lipophilic ion pairs with cationic drugs [57].

Alkanols

Few studies have addressed the mechanisms by which alkanols affect skin permeability.

Miscellaneous Surfactants

Because this category represents a collection of diverse agents differing in their chemical properties, they cannot be collectively categorized according to their mechanisms of effect on skin permeability. A few can serve as examples, however. Walters [34] examined the effects of various non-ionic surfactants and concluded that they could increase the fluidity of and eventually solubilize and elute skin lipids, as well as disrupt intracellular protein structure. Polyoxyethylene[10]lauryl ether preferentially enhanced the permeation of ionized species of nicotinic acid [58]. Scheuplein and Ross [37] reported that the effects of sodium laurate and sodium lauryl sulfate included protein denaturation, membrane expansion, and loss of water binding capacity. In the DSC experiments of Barry [47] both protein and lipid components of skin were affected by 1% sodium lauryl sulfate solutions.

TOXICITY ISSUES

Many of the agents that have been reported to have skin permeation enhancing effects will never be used in marketed products for that purpose because they cause skin toxicity. A fundamental presupposition of enhancing skin permeation is that it must be done without causing skin toxicity. Thorough skin toxicity testing has not been done for most permeation enhancers, or the information is not yet available to the public. Of course, these compounds would also have to be systemically non-toxic.

Skin toxicity is usually manifested as either irritant contact dermatitis or contact sensitization. An irritant contact dermatitis response is that which may occur after a single application. The overt symptoms are localized redness (erythema) and swelling (edema) at the site of exposure. A sensitization reaction involves a specific immunological response to an agent applied to the skin after previous systemic or topical exposure. Initial toxicity testing generally involves evaluating

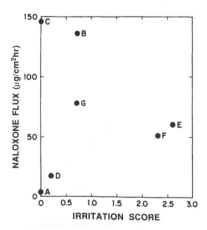

Figure 5. Relationship between enhancement of naloxone flux with various fatty acids and primary skin irritation indices for those vehicles. Vehicles: A—propylene glycol (PG), B—10% lauric acid in PG, C—10% neodecanoic acid in PG, D—10% stearic acid in PG, E—10% isostearic acid (C16 branched) in PG, F—10% oleic acid in PG, G—10% elaidic acid in PG (from Reference [60]).

Table 6. Representative patents in select categories of skin permeation enhancers.

Enhancer	Drug	Vehicle	U.S. Patent # (year)	Assignee
Sulfoxides				
Dimethylsulfoxide	Not specified	Not specified	3511554 (1970) 3711602 (1973)	Crown Zellerbach
Aliphatic sulfoxides	Antimicrobials Sunscreens, others Anticholinergics	Not specified	3527664 (1970) 3903256 (1975) 3953599 (1976)	Proctor & Gamble
Cyclic Amides				
2-Pyrrolidone, C1–C4 Pyrrolidones	Griseofulvin Theophylline Lincomycin	Not specified	3932653 (1976) 3957994 (1976) 3969516 (1976)	Nelson Research
Various alkyl cyclic amides (including laurocapram)	Not specified	Not specified	3989816 (1976) 4316893 (1982) 4405616 (1983) 4562075 (1985)	Nelson Research
Laurocapram	Not specified	C3–C4 diols, pyrrolidones	4557934 (1985)	Proctor & Gamble
Fatty Acids				
Oleic acid	Corticosteroids	C3–C4 diols	4552872 (1985)	Proctor & Gamble
C8–C15 Fatty acids	Opioids	Propylene glycol	4626539 (1986)	DuPont
C5–C20 Fatty acids	Molsidomine	Not specified	4731241 (1988)	Takeda
Oleic acid	Not specified	Ethyl hexanediol	4764381 (1988)	Key
Linoleic acid	Diltiazem	Propylene glycol	4777047 (1988)	Godecke

the potential of a compound to cause irritant contact dermatitis. This is usually done in rabbits, because this is a sensitive animal model, and erythema and edema are measured. Histological examination of the skin may also be performed.

Toxicity is a result of alteration in, or damage to viable cells (viable epidermis and dermis). Permeation enhancement is an effect on the stratum corneum. Is permeation enhancement associated with toxicity? This is a question that must be addressed whenever considering the clinical application of a permeation enhancer. However, there have been only a few published studies attempting to answer it. A series of cyclic amides (N-alkylazacycloheptan-2-one derivatives) were tested for permeation enhancing activity and toxicity to skin cells *in vitro* [59]. In this case there was a correlation between permeation enhancing activity and toxicity. There was also a good correlation between permeation enhancement and primary skin irritation in rabbits with a series of 1-alkyl- or 1-alkenylazacycloalkanones [41]. However, another report [60] showed that it may be possible to separate toxic and permeation enhancing effects. A series of fatty acid isomers were evaluated with regard to how much they increased permeation of naloxone through human skin *in vitro* and how irritating they were in a primary irritation test in rabbits. As shown in Figure 5, although there was again a trend for effective permeation enhancers to be irritating, one fatty acid was a very effective permeation enhancer and was non-irritating.

Are there then certain mechanisms of permeation enhancement that are not necessarily associated with toxicity? Proposed mechanisms of skin permeation enhancement include disrupting the packed structure of intercellular lipids, altering the conformation of stratum corneum proteins, extraction of lipids or proteins, and loosening the water structure or displacing it with another solvent. Do these cause toxicity? Generally, we don't know. However, toxicity might be related to the reversibility of enhancing effects. Some mechanisms would intuitively appear to be reversible, and possibly non-toxic, and others would appear to be irreversible and with greater potential for toxicity. For example, extraction of lipids and proteins would be a relatively irreversible effect. Various non-ionic and ionic surfactants may extract lipids or proteins, and these have usually been irritating (see review by Bodde et al. [61]). Fluidization of intercellular lipids or disruption of stratum corneum water might intuitively appear to be more transient effects, and possibly also less toxic. This remains to be proven though.

PATENTS

A brief discussion of patents in the area of skin permeation enhancers should be useful to those wishing to commercialize a product utilizing such agents. In this case only U.S. patents will be considered. The use of some compounds, such as laurocapram, as permeation enhancers would seem to be well protected by patents. This would especially be true for novel compounds designed specifically for the purpose of improving some aspect of skin permeation. In other cases, known "off-the-shelf" compounds were shown to be effective as permeation enhancers and that use was patented. Because the effects of specific compounds on permeation of specific drugs is usually not predictable *a priori*, and is highly dependent on the solvent, there have been numerous patents allowed on compositions of specific combinations of drug, enhancer, and vehicle. Table 6 lists examples of some patents in selected categories of permeation enhancers, illustrating how claims range in scope from narrow to broad coverage. In addition, systems controlling the release of the permeation enhancer have also been patented.

REFERENCES

1. Shaw, J. E. and S. K. Chandrasekaran. 1978. "Controlled Topical Delivery of Drugs for Systemic Action", *Drug Metab. Rev.*, 3:223–233.

2. Powers, M. S., L. Schenkel, P. E. Darley, W. R. Good, J. C. Balestra and V. A. Place. 1985. "Pharmacokinetics and Pharmacodynamics of Transdermal Dosage Forms of 17β-Estradiol: Comparison with Conventional Oral Estrogens Used for Hormone Replacement", *Am. J. Obstet. Gynecol.*, 152:1099–1106.

3. Swatzendruber, D. C., P. W. Wertz, D. J. Kitko, K. C. Madison and D. T. Downing. 1989. "Molecular Models of the Intercellular Lipid Lamellae in Mammalian Stratum Corneum", *J. Invest. Dermatol.*, 92:251–257.

4. Lampe, M. A., M. L. Williams and P. M. Elias. 1983. "Human Epidermal Lipids: Characterization and Modulations during Differentiation", *J. Lipid Res.*, 24:131–140.

5. Elias, P. M. 1988. "Structure and Function of the Stratum Corneum Permeability Barrier", *Drug Develop. Res.*, 13:97–105.

6. Scheuplein, R. J. 1967. "Mechanisms of Percutaneous Absorption II. Transient Diffusion and the Relative Importance of Various Routes of Skin Penetration", *J. Invest. Dermatol.*, 48:79–88.

7. Keister, J. C. and G. B. Kasting. 1986. "The Use of Transient Diffusion to Investigate Transport Pathways through Skin", *J. Contr. Rel.*, 4:111–117.

8. Kao, J., J. Hall, and G. Helman. 1988. "*In vitro* Percutaneous Absorption in Mouse Skin: Influence on Skin Appendages", *Toxicol. Appl. Pharmacol.*, 94:93–103.

9. Nemanic, M. K. and P. M. Elias. 1980. "*In situ* Precipitation: A Novel Cytochemical Technique for Visualization of Permeability Pathways in Mammalian Stratum Corneum", *J. Histochem. Cytochem.*, 28:573–578.

10. Bodde, H. E., M. A. M. Kruithof, J. Brussee and H. K. Koerten. 1989. "Visualisation of Normal and Enhanced HgCL₂ Transport through Human Skin *in vitro*", *Int. J. Pharmaceut.*, 53:13–24.

11. Scheuplein, R. J. and I. H. Blank. 1971. "Permeability of the Skin", *Physiol. Rev.*, 51:702–747.

12. Michaels, A. S., S. K. Chandrasekaran and J. E. Shaw. 1975. "Drug Permeation through Human Skin: Theory and *in vitro* Experimental Measurement", *Amer. Inst. Chem. Eng. J.*, 21:985–996.

13. Anderson, B. D. and P. V. Raykar. 1989. "Solute Structure-Permeability Relationships in Human Stratum Corneum", *J. Invest. Dermatol.*, 93:280–286.

14. Elias, P. M., E. R. Cooper, A. Korc and B. E. Brown. 1981. "Percutaneous Transport in Relation to Stratum Corneum Structure and Lipid Composition", *J. Invest. Dermatol.*, 76:297–301.

15. Ackermann, C. and G. L. Flynn. 1987. "Ether-Water Partitioning and Permeability through Nude Mouse Skin *in vitro*. I. Urea, Thiourea, Glycerol and Glucose", *Int. J. Pharmaceut.*, 36:61–66.

16. Swarbrick, J., G. Lee, J. Brom and N. P. Gensmantel. 1984. "Drug Permeation through Human Skin II: Permeability of Ionizable Compounds", *J. Pharm. Sci.*, 73:1352–1355.

17. Ghanem, A. H., H. Mahmoud, W. I. Higuchi, U. D. Rohr, S. Borsadia, P. Liu, J. L. Fox, and W. R. Good. 1987. "The Effects of Ethanol on the Transport of β-Estradiol and Other Permeants in Hairless Mouse Skin. II. A New Quantitative Approach", *J. Contr. Rel.*, 6:75–83.

18. Catz, P. and D. R. Friend. 1989. "Alkyl Esters as Skin Permeation Enhancers for Indomethacin", *Int. J. Pharmaceut.*, 55:17–23.

19. Kligman, A. M. 1965. "Topical Pharmacology and Toxicology of Dimethyl Sulfoxide—Part 1", *J. Amer. Med. Assoc.*, 193:796–804.

20. Cooper, E. R. 1984. "Increased Skin Permeability for Lipophilic Molecules", *J. Pharm. Sci.*, 73:1153–1156.

21. Southwell, D. and B. W. Barry. 1983. "Penetration Enhancers for Human Skin: Mode of Action of 2-pyrrolidone and Dimethylformamide on Partition and Diffusion of Model Compounds Water, n-Alcohols, and Caffeine", *J. Invest. Dermatol.*, 80:507–514.

22. Akerman, B., G. Haegerstam, B. G. Pring and R. Sandberg. 1979. "Penetration Enhancers and Other Factors Governing Percutaneous Local Anaesthesia with Lidocaine", *Acta Pharmacol. Toxicol.*, 45:58–65.

23. Beastall, J., R. H. Guy, J. Hadgraft and I. Wilding. 1986. "The Influence of Urea on Percutaneous Absorption", *Pharmaceut. Res.*, 3:294–296.

24. Williams, A. C. and B. W. Barry. 1989. "Urea Analogues in Propylene Glycol as Penetration Enhancers in Human Skin", *Int. J. Pharmaceut.*, 56:43–50.

25. Windheuser, J. J., J. L. Haslam, L. Caldwell and R. D. Shaffer. 1982. "The Use of N,N-Diethyl-m-Toluamide to Enhance Dermal and Transdermal Delivery of Drugs", *J. Pharm. Sci.*, 71:1211–1213.

26. Akhter, S. A. and B. W. Barry. 1985. "Absorption through Human Skin of Ibuprofen and Flurbiprofen; Effect of Dose Variation, Deposited Drug Films, Occlusion and the Penetration Enhancer N-Methyl-2-Pyrrolidone", *J. Pharm. Pharmacol.*, 37:27–37.

27. Aungst, B. J., N. J. Rogers and E. Shefter. 1986. "Enhancement of Naloxone Penetration through Human Skin *in vitro* Using Fatty Acids, Fatty Alcohols, Surfactants, Sulfoxides, and Amides", *Int. J. Pharmaceut.*, 33:225–234.

28. Stoughton, R. B. and W. O. McClure. 1983. "Azone®: A New Non-Toxic Enhancer of Cutaneous Penetration", *Drug Develop. Ind. Pharm.*, 9:725–744.

29. Priborsky, J., K. Takayama, T. Nagai, D. Waitzova, J. Elis, Y. Makino and Y. Suzuki. 1988. "Comparison of Penetration-Enhancing Ability of Laurocapram, N-Methyl-2-Pyrrolidone and Dodecyl-L-Pyroglutamate", *Pharm. Weekbl. [Sci.]*, 10:189–192.

30. Wong, O., N. Tsuzuki, B. Nghiem, J. Kuehnhoff, T. Itoh, K. Masaki, J. Huntington, R. Konishi, J. H. Rytting, and T. Higuchi. 1989. "Unsaturated Cyclic Ureas as New Non-Toxic Biodegradable Transdermal Penetration Enhancers. II. Evaluation Study", *Int. J. Pharmaceut.*, 52:191–202.

31. Sato, K., K. Sugibayashi and Y. Morimoto. 1988. "Effect and Mode of Action of Aliphatic Esters on the *in vitro* Skin Permeation of Nicorandil", *Int. J. Pharmaceut.*, 43:31–40.

32. Chukwumerije, O., R. A. Nash, J. R. Matias and N. Orentreich. 1989. "Studies on the Efficacy of Methyl Esters of n-Alkyl Fatty Acids as Penetration Enhancers", *J. Invest. Dermatol.*, 93:349–352.

33. Franz, J. M., A. Gaillard, H. I. Maibach and A. Schweitzer. 1981. "Percutaneous Absorption of Griseofulvin and Proquazone in the Rat and in Isolated Human Skin", *Arch. Dermatol. Res.*, 271:275–282.

34. Walters, K. A., M. Walker and O. Olejnik. 1988. "Non-Ionic Surfactant Effects on Hairless Mouse Skin Permeability Characteristics", *J. Pharm. Pharmacol.*, 40:525–529.

35. Dalvi, U. G. and J. L. Zatz. 1981. "Effect of Non-Ionic Surfactants on Penetration of Dissolved Benzocaine through Hairless Mouse Skin", *J. Soc. Cosmet. Chem.*, 32:87–94.

36. Sarpotdar, P. P. and J. L. Zatz. 1986. "Evaluation of Penetration Enhancement of Lidocaine by Nonionic Surfactants through Hairless Mouse Skin In Vitro", *J. Pharm. Sci.*, 75:176–181.

37. Scheuplein, R. and L. Ross. 1970. "Effects of Surfactants and Solvents on the Permeability of Epidermis", *J. Soc. Cosmet. Chem.*, 21:853–873.

38. Wong, O., J. Huntington, T. Nishihata and J. H. Rytting. 1989. "New Alkyl N,N-Dialkyl-Substituted Amino Acetates as Transdermal Penetration Enhancers", *Pharmaceut. Res.*, 6:286–295.

39. Walters, K. A., and O. Olejnik. 1983. "Effects of Nonionic Surfactants on the Hairless Mouse Skin Penetration of Methyl Nicotinate", *J. Pharm. Pharmacol.*, 35 (Suppl.):75P.

40. Sekura, D. L. and J. Scala. 1972. "The Percutaneous Absorption of Alkyl Methyl Sulfoxides", in *Pharmacology and the Skin*. W. Montagna, E. J. Van Scott, and R. B. Stoughton, eds. New York, NY: Appleton-Century-Crofts, pp. 257–269.

41. Okamoto, H., M. Hashida and H. Sezaki. 1988. "Structure-Activity Relationship of 1-Alkyl- or 1-Alkenylazacycloalkanone Derivatives as Percutaneous Penetration Enhancers", *J. Pharm. Sci.*, 77:418–424.

42. Yamada, M. and Y. Uda. 1987. "Enhancement of Percutaneous Absorption of Molsidomine", *Chem. Pharm. Bull.*, 35:3390–3398.

43. Golden, G. M., D. B. Guzek, R. R. Harris, J. E. McKie and R. O. Potts. 1986. "Lipid Thermotropic Transitions in Human Stratum Corneum", *J. Invest. Dermatol.*, 86:255–259.

44. Berner, B., G. C. Mazzenga, J. H. Otte, R. J. Steffens, R.-H. Juang and C. D. Ebert. 1989. "Ethanol:Water Mutually Enhanced Transdermal Therapeutic System II. Skin Permeation of Ethanol and Nitroglycerin", *J. Pharm. Sci.*, 78:402–407.

45. Kurihara-Bergstrom, T., G. L. Flynn and W. I. Higuchi. 1986. "Physicochemical Study of Percutaneous Absorption Enhancement by Dimethyl Sulfoxide: Kinetic and Thermodynamic Determinants of Dimethyl Sulfoxide Mediated Mass Transfer of Alkanols", *J. Pharm. Sci.*, 75:479–486.

46. Khan, Z. U. and I. W. Kellaway. 1989. "Differential Scanning Calorimetry of Dimethylsulphoxide-Treated Human Stratum Corneum", *Int. J. Pharmaceut.*, 55:129–134.

47. Barry, B. W. 1987. "Mode of Action of Penetration Enhancers in Human Skin", *J. Contr. Rel.*, 6:85–97.

48. Oertel, R. P. 1977. "Protein Conformational Changes Induced in Human Stratum Corneum by Organic Sulfoxides: An Infrared Spectroscopic Investigation", *Biopolymers*, 16:2329–2345.

49. Barry, B. W. and S. L. Bennett. 1987. "Effect of Penetration Enhancers on the Permeation of Mannitol, Hydrocortisone and Progesterone through Human Skin", *J. Pharm. Pharmacol.*, 39:535–546.

50. Kondo, S., T. Mizuno and I. Sugimoto. 1988. "Effects of Penetration Enhancers on Percutaneous Absorption of Nifedipine. Comparison between DEET and Azone", *J. Pharmacobio-Dyn.*, 11:88–94.

51. Lambert, W. J., W. I. Huguchi, K. Knutson, and S. L. Krill. 1989. "Dose-Dependent Enhancement Effects of Azone on Skin Permeability", *Pharm. Res.*, 6:798–803.

52. Ito, Y., T. Ogiso and M. Iwaki. 1988. "Thermodynamic Study on Enhancement of Percutaneous Penetration of Drugs by Azone®", *J. Pharmacobio-Dyn.*, 11:749–757.

53. Mahjour, M., B. E. Mauser and M. B. Fawzi. 1989. "Skin Permeation Enhancement Effects of Linoleic Acid and Azone on Narcotic Analgesics", *Int. J. Pharmaceut.*, 56:1–11.

54. Golden, G. M., J. E. McKie and R. O. Potts. 1987. "Role of Stratum Corneum Lipid Fluidity in Transdermal Drug Flux", *J. Pharm. Sci.*, 76:25–28.

55. Bennett, S. L. and B. W. Barry. 1985. "Effectiveness of Skin Penetration Enhancers Propylene Glycol, Azone, Decylmethylsulphoxide and Oleic Acid with Model Polar (Mannitol) and Nonpolar (Hydrocortisone) Penetrants", *J. Pharm. Pharmacol.*, 37 (Suppl):84P.

56. Yamada, M., Y. Uda and Y. Tanigawara. 1987. "Mechanisms of Enhancement of Percutaneous Absorption of Molsidomine by Oleic Acid", *Chem. Pharm. Bull.*, 35:3399–3406.

57. Green, P. G., J. Hadgraft, and G. Ridout. 1989. "Enhanced *in vitro* Skin Permeation of Cationic Drugs", *Pharm. Res.*, 6:628–632.

58. Walters, K. A., O. Olejnik and S. Harris. 1984. "Influence of Nonionic Surfactant on the Permeation of

Ionized Molecules through Hairless Mouse Skin'', *J. Pharm. Pharmacol.*, 36 (Suppl.):78P.

59. Ponec, M., M. Haverkort, Y. L. Soei, J. Kempenaar, J. Brussee and H. Bodde. 1989. "Toxicity Screening of N-Alkylazacycloheptan-2-One Derivatives in Cultured Human Skin Cells: Structure-Toxicity Relationships'', *J. Pharm. Sci.*, 78:738–741.

60. Aungst, B. J. 1989. "Structure/Effect Studies of Fatty Acid Isomers as Skin Penetration Enhancers and Skin Irritants'', *Pharm. Res.*, 6:244–247.

61. Bodde, H. E., J. Verhoeven and L. M. J. van Driel. 1989. "The Skin Compliance of Transdermal Drug Delivery Systems'', *Crit. Rev. Ther. Carrier Sys.*, 6:87–115.

35

Oligomeric Prodrugs

P. FERRUTI*
E. RANUCCI*

ABSTRACT: A prodrug is defined as a substance that, though inactive per se, once administered gives rise to the active drug as a consequence of chemical transformation occurring within the body. The aim of this chapter is to give a comprehensive survey of oligomeric prodrugs containing oligomeric, micromolecular and polymeric promoieties. The main structural peculiarities of the latter are the size, which is larger, and their functionality, which is usually multiple. To this purpose the chapter has been divided into four parts. The first deals with the basic definitions of prodrugs, oligomers and polymers. The second section discusses general concepts, especially in relation with the rationale of the prodrug approach and the relevant properties of oligomeric prodrugs. The third section deals with the synthetic strategies which can be utilized for obtaining oligomeric prodrugs. The fourth section is a critical review of the oligomeric prodrugs described so far with the literature. This chapter provides a comprehensive overview of oligomeric prodrugs containing oligomeric promoieties.

BASIC DEFINITIONS AND SCOPE

Prodrugs

It is commonly agreed that a prodrug is defined as a substance that, though inactive per se, once administered gives rise to the active drug as a consequence of chemical transformation occurring within the body [1]. The term was first proposed by Albert [2], who suggested the prodrug approach in order to modify temporarily the physico-chemical properties of drugs to increase their usefulness.

Typically, a prodrug is obtained by the attachment of a chemical entity, the promoiety, to the parent drug. Thus, a prodrug is composed of two parts, the drug moiety and the promoiety, connected by a chemical bond that has been purposely designed to be cleaved at a useful rate after administration. It is somewhat controversial whether a salt between an ionic drug and a counterion (playing in this case the role of promoiety) still falls within the concept of prodrug. Even if this opinion has been sustained [3], we prefer to consider ionic derivatives of drugs as outside the scope of this chapter.

Oligomers and Polymers

According to the Union of Pure and Applied Chemistry (I.U.P.A.C.) [4], an oligomer is defined as a substance composed of molecules containing a few of one or more species of atoms, or groups of atoms, repetitively linked to each other. These atoms or groups of atoms are called constitutional units.

On the other hand, a polymer is most obviously defined as a substance composed of molecules containing "many" constitutional units repetitively linked to each other. It follows that there is not a sharp boundary between the concepts of polymer and oligomer.

The above oligomer definition is completed by the IUPAC with the further statement that the physical properties of an oligomer vary perceivably with the removal or addition of one or a few of the constitutional units to its molecules. As a rule, it is not so for a polymer. This additional statement is probably the most meaningful conceivable differentiation between oligomers and polymers, but is not absolute, because ultimately it depends on the resolution power of our analytical instruments.

For the purpose of this article, we have chosen to consider an oligomer as a substance whose molecules contain between 3 and 50 constitutional units, and which weighs no more than 5×10^3. For the sake of

*Dipartimento di Ingegneria Meccanica, dell'Università di Brescia, Via D. Valotti, 9 25060 Brescia, Italy

simplicity, and somewhat at the expense of precision, polymers and oligomers when reckoned with together will be collectively referred to as macromolecules.

It should be noted that none of the above definitions makes any reference to polydispersity. Therefore, the above figures refer to average values, as is usual in polymer chemistry. In case of oligomers, however, truly monodisperse samples are in some cases available.

Oligomeric and Polymeric Prodrugs

Following the definitions of prodrugs and oligomers and polymers described previously, an oligomeric or polymeric prodrug is defined as an oligomer or polymer, pharmacologically inactive per se, which once administered undergoes within the body a chemical transformation giving rise to the active drug.

Two main categories of oligomeric and polymeric prodrugs can be defined [5]:

(a) One or more drug moieties are attached to a macromolecular promoiety. The release occurs independently of a degradation of the main backbone, which may or may not take place on time by a different process.

(b) The drug moieties are a part of the macromolecular backbone. The release of the drug takes place through a degradation process by which the entire prodrug molecule breaks down into fragments.

Category (a) may be subdivided. The drug moieties can be attached to the macromolecular promoiety either along the main chain, as side substituents (a-1), or just at one or both ends (a-2). The above is best clarified in Table 1.

While polymeric prodrugs of category (a) usually belong to subcategory a-1, rather than a-2, oligomeric prodrugs may belong to both. The reason is that when the molecular weight of the promoiety is too high, at-taching drug moieties only at its ends would result in a loading of active species too low to be therapeutically meaningful. It is not so in the case of oligomers.

The aim of this chapter is to give a comprehensive survey of oligomeric prodrugs containing oligomeric promoieties. Consequently, prodrugs of category (b) will not be considered in detail. Emphasis will be laid on basic chemical work as well as on the examples of oligomeric prodrugs already described in the literature. It is our hope to provide the reader with a helpful base for further creative work in this promising area of research.

GENERAL CONCEPTS

Rationale of the Prodrug Approach

It is common knowledge that the vast majority of the new molecules with an established therapeutic potential prepared in research laboratories are dropped before reaching the medical practice. Leaving apart any business-related consideration, this is mostly due to some drawback in one of the various phases normally encountered in the process of drug development. This is also the reason why an otherwise useful drug is often abandoned or replaced by others after years of use.

The above phases have been defined as the pharmaceutical, pharmacokinetic, and pharmacodynamic ones [6]. The first is the phase of development occurring between the identification of the potential drug, and its incorporation into a delivery system. The second is the phase involving the study of adsorption, distribution, metabolism and excretion of the drug. The third is the phase related to the drug-receptor interaction. Since it is not likely that the prodrug approach may be useful in this phase, we shall not deal with it any further.

Table 1. Main categories of oligomeric prodrugs.

Code	Structure and Reactions Leading to the Drug Release[a]		
a-1	A—(C)$_{\overline{n-a}}$(X)$_{\overline{a}}$B $\mid$ Y $\mid$ (D)	$\longrightarrow$	A—(C)$_{\overline{n-a}}$(X)$_{\overline{a}}$B + $(n-a)$D $\mid$ Y
b-1	A—(C)$_n$—YD	$\longrightarrow$	A—(C)$_n$—Y + D
b	A—(D)$_{\overline{n-a}}$(X)$_{\overline{a}}$B	$\longrightarrow$	$(n-a)$D + aX + (A,B)[b]

[a]n = Polymerization degree.
A,B = Terminal groups (may be H).
D = Drug moiety & free drug.
X = Subsidiary unit often introduced for solubilizing purposes.
C = Constitutional unit.
Y = Connection cleavable in the body fluids, often including a spacer whose function is to facilitate cleavage. Structural changes in both D and Y after cleaving are not indicated.
[b]Compounds, if any, deriving from terminal groups. If these are a part of D or X, they remain attached to them.

In all phases there are requirements to be fulfilled by the candidate drug. To better elucidate this concept, the term "barrier to drug development" has been proposed by Stella [1]. These barriers should not be confused with physiological barriers, such as the blood–brain barrier, which, however, may constitute a "barrier" in Stella's sense.

Several of the above barriers can be easily recognized. In the pharmaceutical phase, for instance, the candidate drug may have problems of odour, taste, pain upon injection, or gastric irritation. It may also have problems of chemical stability, solubility, compoundability into dosage form, etc.

In the pharmacokinetic phase, the candidate drug may be incompletely adsorbed across physiological barriers, or too rapidly excreted, or pre-systemically metabolized in the gastrointestinal (G.I.) tract, the liver, etc. It may be localized at a place different from the one where its action is needed, possibly exerting adverse effects at the same level. Its rate of action onset may be unfavorable, etc.

It may be observed that all the above barriers, including those concerning adsorption, excretion, and metabolism, are related to the physico-chemical properties of the candidate drug. It follows that, in the attempt to overcome one or more barriers, the prodrug approach is generally correct. In some cases, it is the only conceivable approach.

Oligomeric versus Both Polymeric and Micromolecular Prodrugs

We have chosen the term "micromolecular" to indicate prodrugs whose promoiety is neither polymeric nor oligomeric. Looking for a distinction between micromolecular and polymeric promoieties, the main structural peculiarities of the latter are their size, which is larger, and their functionality, which is usually multiple. The latter point is better elucidated by comparing a macromolecular promoiety to a rope carrying many clothes-hangers. It was by considering polymeric promoieties that complex systems containing the drug moieties, solubilizing units, spacing arms, and homing devices for specific targeting were first conceived [7], and then realized [8–10].

It is apparent that oligomeric prodrugs are in several aspects intermediate between polymeric and micromolecular prodrugs. Therefore, we should question whether there is any reason to treat them separately, and what the rationale is for selecting oligomeric systems within the prodrug approach.

Relevant Differences between Polymeric and Micromolecular Promoieties

To give an answer to the above questions, it may be useful to recall some substantial behavioural differences between polymeric and non-polymeric compounds in biological environments, and to relate them to the barriers to drug development as described previously.

(1) A polymer is non-volatile, i.e., it has a negligible vapour pressure. Thus, a polymeric promoiety is ideal for masking evil odours.

(2) A polymeric promoiety has a high "sheltering" potential. Thus, it may be very effective in lowering, or eliminating, bad tastes, pain upon injection, gastric irritation, and pre-systemic metabolism.

(3) As pointed out above, a promoiety may carry several functional groups. Consequently, it may be purpose-tailored to have a high solubilizing power in water, or just in aqueous acidic or alkaline media. It may be made more hydrophilic, lipophilic, or amphiphilic. It may carry directing groups. It may have the drug moieties attached in different ways, through different spacing arms, thus graduating the release of the drug, and/or having the drug released at a particular level, e.g., inside cells.

Thus, polymeric promoieties have a very high and often unique potential for overcoming such pharmaceutical and pharmacodynamic barriers as solubility, compoundability, unfavourable rate of onset, low duration of action, wrong localization within the body, etc.

(4) A high molecular weight polymer is poorly or not at all adsorbed upon oral administration unless previously degraded [11]. This means that a polymeric prodrug, as such, rarely crosses the G.I. walls in substantial amounts. The active drug, to be adsorbed, must be released at the same level. Thus, polymeric promoieties are not recommended for overcoming a barrier connected with incomplete adsorption of the drug itself through the G.I. tract.

(5) A high molecular weight polymer injected into a living organism suffers practically no elimination through the usual excretion routes. Elimination takes place only when the molecular weight is below a certain threshold depending upon the structure [11–13], at a rate increasing, the other conditions being equal, by decreasing the molecular weight. Thus, polymeric promoieties appear quite effective in overcoming the barrier of a too-rapid excretion, but may have serious problems in being themselves eliminated after the detachment of the drug molecules.

Oligomeric Promoieties and Prodrugs

It is apparent that polymeric prodrugs, attractive as they are, may have serious shortcomings. On the other hand, micromolecular prodrugs may have a too-limited scope. Oligomeric prodrugs are, in principle, able to couple the higher potential of the polymeric prodrugs with the lack of systemic problems of the micromolecular ones.

To the point, it may be worthwhile to summarize some relevant considerations, both structural and physiological, regarding oligomers as promoieties.

First of all, starting from oligomers functionalized only at their ends it is possible to obtain prodrugs of Cat. a-2 with a reasonable loading of drug moieties. This means that it is possible to utilize as promoieties oligomers whose constitutional units, though endowed with the desired physico-chemical properties, do not carry drug-binding sites, as for instance poly-(ethyleneglycols). Furthermore, in many end-functionalized oligomers, the reactivity of a chemical function attached to the end of a flexible chain can be more predictable than that of the same function attached as side substituent to a high molecular weight polymer. With the possible exception of oligomers with a very low degree of polymerization, the reactivity of a chemical function attached at the end of a chain is in fact practically independent of the length of the segment to which it is attached. This is based on known theoretical calculations for polycondensation and stepwise addition processes [14].

Oligomers can be eliminated from the body through the usual excretion routes irrespective of any biodegradability question. We may go further, stating that a non-toxic, non-degradable oligomer is, in principle, safer than a degradable promoiety of whatever size, since problems arising from the possible toxicity of metabolites are not to be encountered.

Oligomeric prodrugs can in principle be adsorbed orally or transdermally. Moreover, with low molecular weight amphiphilic oligomers it is possible to prepare prodrugs with increased bioavailability, at least after oral administration, as if the oligomeric promoiety exerted a transport effect [15–17]. Oligomeric promoieties, in fact, may offer unique possibilities for obtaining prodrugs with an optimal hydrophilic/hydrophobic balance (e.g., with amphiphilic properties) coupled with low melting point, good overall solubility and limited molecular mass. Let us consider, for instance, an oligomeric drug of category a-2, whose general structure is: $A[C]_n YD$ (see Table 1). Provided, as is often the case, that we master the oligomerization process, it is sufficient to vary n until reaching the desired properties. This goal can be achieved however large, insoluble, high-melting, hydrophobic or hydrophilic the drug residue may be. It should be mentioned that amphiphilic molecules, i.e., those molecules characterized by affinity for both fatty phases and aqueous phases, are in principle the best candidates to traverse physiological multilayer barriers, such as the skin [18].

The transport properties are adversely affected by the molecular mass as well as by the melting point [18]. However, in oligomeric prodrugs the polymerization degree needs not to be large (it is often be-

tween 4 and 10) and both oligomers and their adducts most often either have very low melting points, or do not crystallize at all.

Many of the above potentialities are shared to some extent by micromolecular, but not by polymeric ones. On the other hand, most advantages of the latter, and particularly those reported previously under headings (1), (2), and (3), may be shared by oligomeric promoieties. Sustained activity on time may also be achieved, and to some extent modulated (along with the physico-chemical properties of the prodrug) by varying the polymerization degree [15,16].

Thus, a rationale for selecting oligomeric prodrugs as a distinct region within the more general prodrug approach exists, even if so far, the potentialities of oligomers as promoieties do not seem to have been sufficiently exploited. It is our opinion, however, that much of the work which has been carried out on this subject has not yet appeared in the literature.

SYNTHESIS OF OLIGOMERIC PRODRUGS

Synthetic Strategies

As pointed out previously, the oligomeric prodrugs considered in this chapter belong to two main categories, referred to in Table 1 as a-1 and a-2, respectively. These will be treated separately.

Synthesis of Oligomeric Prodrugs of Cat. a-1

As pointed out in Table 1, oligomeric prodrugs of this category have the general structure

$$A \left[\begin{matrix} C \\ | \\ Y \\ | \\ D \end{matrix} \right]_{n-a} \left[X \right]_a B$$

which reduces to

$$A \left[\begin{matrix} C \\ | \\ Y \\ | \\ D \end{matrix} \right]_n B$$

when no other constitutional units are present.

To synthesize such a structure, two main strategies (α) and (β) can be conceived. The first one involves the preparation and oligomerization of a monomer containing the drug as side substituent. The second one involes the preparation of an oligomer carrying chemical functions able to react selectively with suitable functional groups present in the drug molecule [19-20]. Both strategies are best clarified by the following examples, concerning esters of a hydroxylated drug with an oligomer of acrylic acid:

$$(\alpha) \quad DOH + CH_2=CHCOZ \longrightarrow DOCOCH=CH_2 + ZH$$
$$(I) \qquad (II) \qquad\qquad (III)$$

(III) + Initiator + Chain Transfer Agent
(see Promoiety-Forming a-1 Oligomers of Polyvinylic Structure)

$$\longrightarrow A\left[\begin{array}{c} CH_2-CH \\ | \\ CO \\ | \\ OO \end{array}\right]_n B$$
$$(IV)$$

where (I) is a hydroxyl-containing drug, (II) is an activated derivative of acrylic acid, where Z stands for the leaving group, (III) is the acrylic ester of (I), and (IV) if the final oligomeric prodrug in which A, B, D and *n* have the same meaning as in Table 1.

$$(\beta)\ a)\ \ CH_2=CH + INITIATOR + CHAIN\ TRANSFER\ AGENT \longrightarrow$$
$$\begin{array}{c} | \\ CO \\ | \\ OH \end{array}$$
$$(V)$$

$$\longrightarrow A\left[\begin{array}{c} CH_2-CH \\ | \\ CO \\ | \\ OH \end{array}\right]_n B$$
$$(VI)$$

$$b)\ (VI)\ +\ ACTIVATING\ AGENT \longrightarrow A\left[\begin{array}{c} CH-CH \\ | \\ CO \\ | \\ Z \end{array}\right]_n B$$
$$(VII)$$

$$c)\ (VII)\ +\ (I) \longrightarrow (IV)\ +\ ZH$$

where (I) and (IV) are the same as in example (a), and (VI) and (VII) are an oligomer of acrylic acid and its activated derivative. The strategy (α) allows us, in principle, to avoid any trouble connected with an incomplete coupling reaction. In front of this, strategy (β) has two important advantages: (1) any interaction which may occur during polymerization between the growing radicals (or ions), the initiator, or the chain-transfer agent, and the chemical functional groups present in the drug molecule, such as for instance unsaturated structures, is avoided; (2) a single activated oligomer may be used to prepare many oligomeric prodrugs, by simply treating the oligomer with the different drugs, provided they bear suitable binding functions.

Synthesis of Oligomeric Prodrugs of Cat. a-2

While in the case of oligomeric prodrugs of Cat. a-1 there was a choice between two different synthetic strategies (α) and (β), in the case of oligomeric prodrugs of Cat. a-2 the only meaningful strategy is the latter. In other words, the preparation of a-2 oligomeric prodrugs usually involves a coupling reaction between the drug and pre-synthesized oligomers suitably functionalized at one or both ends:

$$Z(C)_nZ + 2DZ' \longrightarrow D(C)_nD + 2\ ZZ'$$

where C and D have the same meaning as in Table 1, and Z and Z^1 are the leaving moieties of the oligomer and the drug, respectively. In most cases, one of the two is H.

Conclusive Remarks

Most a-1, and all a-2 oligomeric prodrugs described in the literature have been prepared by route β. Therefore, the synthesis of the functional oligomers corresponding to both categories of oligomeric prodrugs will be reviewed in detail.

A preliminary distinction should be made in both cases, between polyvinylic oligomers on one side, and polycondensation stepwise polyaddition, and ring-opening polymerization oligomers, whose chain structures cannot be brought under a common definition, on the other side. The first ones will be collectively considered. The second ones will be considered individually. Among promoiety-forming non-polyvinylic oligomers of Cat. a-2, polyethyleneglycols will be considered separately.

Promoiety-Forming a-1 Oligomers

Promoiety-Forming a-1 Oligomers of Polyvinylic Structure

The vast majority of polyvinylic polymers and oligomers may be represented as follows

$$A\left[\begin{array}{c} R \\ | \\ CH_2-C \\ | \\ R^1 \end{array}\right]_n B$$

where A, B and *n* have the same meaning as in Table 1, R is most often H or CH_3, and R^1 is a variable chemical group. These macromolecules are obtained by polymerization of the corresponding vinyl monomers, $CH_2=C\begin{smallmatrix}R\\|\\R^1\end{smallmatrix}$ with ionic or radical systems.

IONIC SYSTEMS

Ionic polymerizations are seldom used with monomers carrying reactive side functions, because most catalysts, being themselves extremely reactive, are not compatible with the presence of reactive functions. On the other hand, reactive functions are needed in the constitutional units of promoiety-forming a-1 oligomers.

A recent "living" cationic polymerization system, however, appears to give interesting results in this respect [21]. This system is based on the HI/I^2 catalytic couple, and allows the synthesis of low molecular weight, narrowly distributed products starting from monomers of vinyl ether structure, carrying side groups able to yield the desired functions, namely carboxy-, amino-, and hydroxy-groups, by further reaction.

a) $CH_2=CH$ + $HI \cdot I_2$ $\longrightarrow$ CH_3-CH $I....I_2$ (with $\delta+$ $\delta-$)
   (I)   (II)

b) (II) + (I) $\xrightarrow{n\ steps}$ $CH_3-CH\left[CH_2-CH\right]_n CH_2-CH$ $I....I_2$ ($\delta+$ $\delta-$)

This system is "living" because there is no termination, unless a foreign reactive substance is introduced as terminator. While anionic "living" systems were discovered long ago [22], cationic living systems are a recent acquisition. A synthetic advantage of living systems is that n is simply determined by the monomer/catalyst ratio, and the molecular weight distribution is narrow, following Poisson's law [22].

RADICAL SYSTEMS

Most of the promoiety-forming oligomers and polymers described in the literature are obtained by radical polymerization.

The commonly accepted pattern of radical polymerization is the following [23]:

(1) Production of primary radicals:
    (various means) $\longrightarrow R^\cdot$

(2) Initiation: $R^\cdot + M \longrightarrow RM^\cdot\ (=M_1^\cdot)$

(3) Propagation: $M_n^\cdot + M \longrightarrow M_{n+1}^\cdot$

(4) Termination: (a) $M_n^\cdot + M_m^\cdot \longrightarrow M_{n+m}$
                  (b) $M_n^\cdot + M_m^\cdot \longrightarrow M_n + M_m$

where $R^\cdot$ = radical; $M_n^\cdot$ = growing radical containing n units; M_n = "dead" polymer containing n units.

A fifth elementary reaction, the chain transfer, may take place. In radical polymerizations, a chain transfer reaction is generally defined as a reaction of the growing radical with a substance T, resulting in a "dead" polymer molecule, and a new radical species derived from T [24,25]:

(5) $M_n^\cdot + T \longrightarrow M_n + T^\cdot$

If the constant of the reaction (3) is k_P, and that of reaction (5) is K_T, a chain transfer constant C_T is defined as [25]:

$$C_T = k_t/k_p \tag{1}$$

More plainly, a chain transfer reaction takes place when a growing radical reacts with the variable substance acting as chain transfer agent, breaking it into two fragments, one of which remains attached to the growing end, which "dies", while the other gives rise to a new radical:

....$CH_2-CH^\cdot$ + $A-B$ $\longrightarrow$ ....CH_2-C-A + $B^\cdot$

(A-B = T)

In many cases A is H, or halogen. This reaction may occur with variable frequency, either with a normal component of a polymerizing system, such as monomer, initiator, already formed polymer, and solvent, or with a substance introduced purposely.

The newly formed radical $B^\cdot$ may or may not be able to react with the monomer, re-initiating the polymerization process. In the latter case, the reaction equals in practice a termination reaction and is regarded as a special case, not considered here any further. In the former case, and if the reinitiation process is not too slow, the net effect of the reaction (apart from the case of chain transfer to polymer) is to break down the average size of the macromolecules produced, introducing in a part of them fragments of the chain transfer agent.

When the chain transfer agent is present in sufficient amount, and is highly reactive, virtually all the macromolecules produced start with one fragment of chain transfer agent, and terminate with the other, so that the polymerization reaction, in this case usually referred to as "telomerization", takes the following form:

$n\ M$ + $A-B$ $\longrightarrow$ $A[M]_n B$

with n usually low.

The close correspondence between the above structure and those shown in Table 1 is immediately apparent. The use of telomerizing agents is in fact one of the main routes for the preparation of promoiety forming oligomers.

The kinetics of chain transfer have received much attention since the beginning of polymer science [25,26]. They have been recently reviewed by Farina [24]. Telomerization kinetics differs from that of normal polymerization. In particular, the value of K_T may depend on the degree of polymerization [24]. The point has been widely investigated because product distribution is very sensitive to the value of C_T. If we consider C_n as the transfer constant relative to the growing radical with polymerization degree n, the results of a huge number of telomerization reactions have shown that transfer radicals contain polar atoms (e.g., CCl_3), C_1, C_2 and some of the higher terms differ from each other and from the limiting value C_T observed in polymerizations. For other telogens, and especially for thiols, the effect is much lower and can be considered within the experimental error [24]. An extensive study centered on telomerization kinetics has been undertaken by Pietrasanta, Bauduin, Boutevin, and others who have the production of promoiety-forming oligomers as one of their aims [27–33].

To discuss in detail the large amount of work done on this subject would be outside the scope of this chapter, and only a few generalizations useful to give practical guidelines will be made here. By taking into account a single value of C_T, the average degree of polymerization $\bar{n}$ is given by the well-known Mayo equation [25]

$$\frac{1}{\bar{n}} = \frac{1}{\bar{n}_o} + C_T \frac{[T]}{[M]} \qquad (2)$$

where $\bar{n}_o$ refers to a polymerization run under the same conditions but in the absence of T. When the chain transfer reaction to T strongly predominates, i.e., when $1/\bar{n}_o$ is negligible, Equation (2) reduces to

$$\frac{1}{\bar{n}} = C_T \frac{[T]}{[M]} \text{ or } \bar{n} = \frac{1}{C_T} \frac{[M]}{[T]} \qquad (3)$$

By increasing the monomer's conversion (i.e., the product's yield), $[M]/[T]$ increases for $C_T > 1$, and decreases for $C_T < 1$. Only when $C_T = 1$, does $[M]/[T]$ remain constant on time during polymerization. This means that, according to Equations (2) and (3), $\bar{n}$ increases or decreases, respectively, as polymerization proceeds, remaining constant only for $C_T = 1$.

If $[T_o]/[M_o]$ and $\bar{n}_o$ are the initial chain-transfer agent/monomer ratio and the average polymerization degree; $[M]/[T]$ and $\bar{n}_t$ are the same entities at the time t; and Y_t is the total monomer conversion $(M_o - M_t)/(M_o)$ at the same time (i.e., the product's yield), it can be demonstrated [24] that:

$$\frac{[T]_t}{[M]_t} = \frac{[T_o]}{[M_o]} (1 - Y_t)^{c_T-1} \qquad (4)$$

Consequently, after Equation (3):

$$\bar{n}_t = \frac{1}{C_t} \frac{[M_o]}{[C_o]} (1 - Y_t)^{(1-c_T)} \qquad (5)$$

Being, after Equation (3):

$$\bar{n}_o = \frac{1}{C_T} \frac{M_o}{T_o},$$

$$\frac{\bar{n}_t}{\bar{n}_o} = (1 - Y_t)^{(1-c_T)} \qquad (6)$$

From a practical standpoint, Equation (6) indicates that it is not convenient to use monomer/chain transfer

agent combinations with $C_T \gg 1$, since even at moderate yields the polymerization degree is rapidly increasing as a consequence of preferential transfer agent consumption. This results in a very broad polydispersity, and even in a bimodal molecular weight distribution.

The increase of $\bar{n}$ versus Y is not so rapid when $1 < C_T < 2$, and the reaction is not pushed over 60% yield. The same consideration applies to the decrease of $\bar{n}$ versus Y with $C_T < 1$. Better results are in many cases obtained when $C_T \neq 1$ by running the reaction not in batch, but with delayed addition techniques.

We need not review here all the methods which have been described for determining C_T values, for which the reader should refer to the literature [24–33]. It may suffice to report here that from the literature data, and our own experience, acrylic monomers and primary mercaptans very often form quite amenable systems, C_T being not far from 1, and often slightly lower. Good results have also been obtained with the same monomers and halogenated compounds, if the polymerization is run with redox catalysts [28].

Table 2 collects several examples of promoiety-forming polyvinylic oligomers of Cat. a-1. The selection has been made on the basis of their potential utility. Both "primary" oligomers (e.g., directly obtained from the monomers) and "secondary" ones (e.g., obtained by chemical modification of the former) are reported. Some products obtained by functionalization of oligomeric dienes prepared by ionic initiators have also been added.

Non-Polyvinylic Promoiety-Forming a-1 Oligomers

Under this heading we collect all promoiety-forming a-1 oligomers whose structure is not non-polyvinylic. We have considered promoiety-forming oligomers, both those claimed to have been synthesized with this purpose, and those which in our opinion deserve attention in the same respect. It may be observed that most polycondensation- and stepwise-addition polymers studied as promoieties [5] contain hydrolyzable bonds in their main chain. Consequently, many of them are expected to be degradable in the body fluids, giving off in most cases safe degradation products. Thus, one of the main limitations in the use of polymeric prodrugs, the elimination of polymeric residues, is not applicable to their case. This is perhaps the reason why little attention has been paid to using oligomers of the same structure as promoieties, even if they often appear to be easily available from a synthetic point of view.

We have resolved to report here some of the polymers to which the above observation applies. The selection has been made on the basis of their novelty, their potential interest, and the ease with which oligomers instead of polymers could presumably be prepared, or are commercially available. The main reason, in the authors' opinion, why these oligomers

No.	Structure	n[b]	Synthetic Method[c]	Ref.
1	$Cl[CHCH_2]_n CCl_3$ [d] with COOH	2–50	T. Acrylic acid, Fe^{3+}/ benzoin (redox), CCl_4	[34] [36] [37] [42]
2	$Cl[CHCH_2]_{n-a}[CHCH_2]_a CCl_3$ with COCl, COOH	=	M. 1, $SOCl_2$	[35] [42]
3	$Cl[\ldots]_{n-a}[CHCH_2]_a CCl_3$ (lactone), COOH	=	M. 1, $(CH_3CO)_2O$	[35] [42]
4	$Cl[CHCH_2]_{n-a}[CHCH_2]_a CCl_3$ with $C=O$, O, phenyl-NO_2, COOH	≅ 20	M. 1, HO—⟨⟩—NO_2, DCCI	[35] [37]
5	$Cl[CHCH_2]_n CCl_3$ with CHO		T. Acrolein, Fe^{+3}/ benzoin (redox), CCl_4	
6	$C_4H_9[CH_2 CHCHCH_2]_n H$ with R, OH	many	M. Polybutadiene[e] (R = H), or polyisoprene[e] (R=CH_3)	[38] [39]
7	$C_4H_9[CH_2 CHCHCH_2]_n H$ with R, OCCl, O	many	M. 6, $COCl_2$	[38]
8	$Cl[CH-CH_2]_n CCl_3$ with $CH_2 NH_2$	≅ 20	M. Poly(acrylonitrile)[f], B_2H_6	[37]
9	$H[CHCH_2]_n P(OC_2H_5)_2$ with OH, O	≅ 35	M. Poly(vinylacetate)[g]	[41]
10	$H[CH-CH_2]_n [CHCH_2]_a P(OC_2H_5)_2$ with OCH_2CH_2OH, OH, O	=	M. 9, CH_2-CH_2 (epoxide), OH^-	[41]
11	$CH_3 O[CH_2 C]_n H$ with CH_3, COOH	3	M. Poly(methylmethacrylate)[h]	[43] [44]
12	$CH_3 O[CH_2 C]_n H$ with CH_3, COCl	=	M. 11, $SOCl_2$	[43]

Table 2 (continued).

No.	Structure	n[b]	Synthetic Method[c]	Ref.
13	CH$_2$O(CH$_2$C(CH$_3$)(CO)(NHCHCOOH)(R))$_n$H	=	M. 11, OCN-CHCOOH; with R 12, H$_2$NCHCOOH with R	[43]
14	CH$_3$O(CH$_2$C(CH$_3$)(CH$_2$OH))$_n$H	=	M. Poly(methylmethacrylate)[h], LiAlH$_4$	[43] [44]
15	CH$_3$O(CH$_2$C(CH$_3$)(CH$_2$OCCl, ‖O))$_n$H	=	M. 14, COCl$_2$	[45]
16	CH$_3$O(CH$_2$C(CH$_3$)(CH$_2$O-C=O-NH(CH$_2$)$_5$CHNH$_2$-COOH))$_n$H		M. 15, α-NH$_2$- and COOH-protected lysine, then cleavage of protecting groups.	[46]
17	C$_{10}$H$_{22}$S(CHCH$_2$(C=O)(NHCH$_2$COOH))$_n$H	3–13	T. Acryloylglycine[i], AIBN, 1-decanethiol	[33]
18	CH$_3$(CHCH$_2$(O(CH$_2$)$_3$COOH))$_n$H	8–50	M. CH$_3$(CH-CH$_2$(CH$_2$CH(COOEt)$_2$))$_n$H[i], OH$^-$, then H$^+$	[21]
19	CH$_3$(CHCH$_2$(OCH$_2$CH$_2$OH))$_n$H	=	M. CH$_3$(CHCH$_2$(O(CH$_2$)$_2$OSiMe$_2$R))$_n$H[i] H$^+$ or F$^-$	[21]
20	CH$_3$(CHCH$_2$(OCH$_2$CH$_2$NH$_2$))$_n$H	=	M. CH$_3$(CHCH$_2$(OCH$_2$CH$_2$-phthalimide))$_n$H[i], hydrazine.	[21]
21	(CHCH$_2$(Si(CH$_3$)$_2$(CH$_2$)$_3$NHCO-))$_n$	4–10	See footnote i of Table 10	—

[a] Including oligomers of conjugated dienes.
[b] Average polymerization degree.
[c] T = telomerization; M = modifying reaction. The substances after T are, in order, the monomer, the catalyst, and the telomerizing (=chain transfer) agent. The substances after M are, in order, the starting oligomer, referred to with its Systemic No. if already present in this table, and the reagent(s).
[d] The same oligomer with other terminal groups also described in Reference [36].
[e] Prepared according to Swarč et al. [40].
[f] Prepared as No. 1, by substituting acrylonitrile for acrylic acid.
[g] Preparation method not fully described.
[h] Prepared according to Reference [44].
[i] Oligo(N-acryloylpeptide)s of different structures also described in Reference [33].

Table 3. Non-polyvinylic promoiety-forming oligomers of Cat. a-1.

No.	Common Name	Structure	n^a	Ref.
1	Poly(aspartic acid)	$\left[\begin{array}{c}O \\ \parallel \\ CHCNH \\ \mid \\ CH_2 \\ \mid \\ COOH\end{array}\right]_n$	Various	Comm.
2	Poly(glutamic acid)	$\left[\begin{array}{c}O \\ \parallel \\ CHCNH \\ \mid \\ (CH_2)_2 \\ \mid \\ COOH\end{array}\right]_n$	Various	Comm.
3	Poly(α,β-2-hydroxyethyl-aspartamide)	$\left[\begin{array}{c}O \\ \parallel \\ CHCNH \\ \mid \\ CH_2 \\ \mid \\ CONHCH_2CH_2OH\end{array}\right]_n$	Various	[47–49][b]
4	Poly[α-(2-hydroxyethyl-L-glutamine]	$\left[\begin{array}{c}O \\ \parallel \\ CHCNH \\ \mid \\ (CH_2)_2 \\ \mid \\ CONHCH_2CH_2OH\end{array}\right]_n$	Various	[50][b]
5	Poly[α-2-hydroxypropyl-L-glutamine]	$\left[\begin{array}{c}O \\ \parallel \\ CHCNH \\ \mid \\ (CH_2)_2 \\ \mid \\ CONHCHCH_2OH \\ \mid \\ CH_3\end{array}\right]_n$	Various	[50][b]
6	Poly(α-malic)	$\left[\begin{array}{c}O \\ \parallel \\ OCCH \\ \mid \\ CH_2 \\ \mid \\ COOH\end{array}\right]_n$	<10–30	[51,52]
7	Poly(β-malic)	$\left[\begin{array}{c}O \\ \parallel \\ OCCHCH_2 \\ \mid \\ COOH\end{array}\right]$	30–>300	[52–55]

548

Table 3 (continued).

No.	Common Name	Structure	n^a	Ref.

8   Poly(α,β-malic acid)

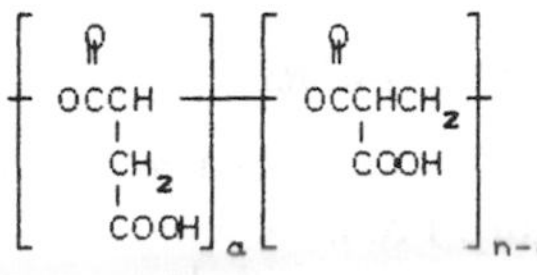

$$\left[\begin{array}{c} O \\ \parallel \\ OCCH \\ | \\ CH_2 \\ | \\ COOH \end{array}\right]_a \left[\begin{array}{c} O \\ \parallel \\ OCCHCH_2 \\ | \\ COOH \end{array}\right]_{n-a}$$

< 10 [56]

9   Poly(ethyleneimine)

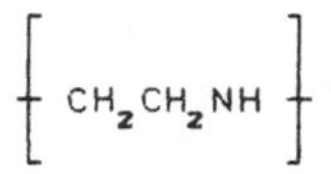

$$\left[CH_2CH_2NH \right]$$

Various   Comm.

10   Poly(ethyleneimine) modified with acrylic acid

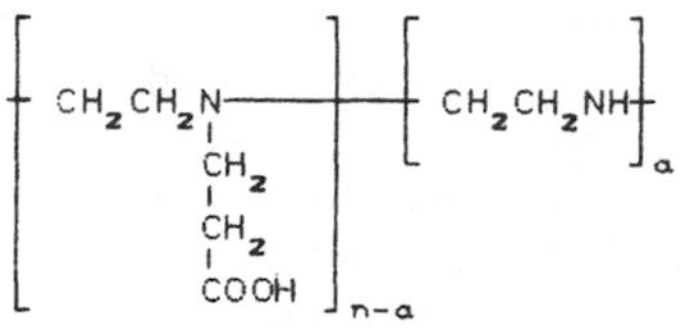

$$\left[\begin{array}{c} CH_2CH_2N \\ | \\ CH_2 \\ | \\ CH_2 \\ | \\ COOH \end{array}\right]_{n-a} \left[CH_2CH_2NH \right]_a$$

Various   [57]

11   Poly(dimethylsiloxane)s

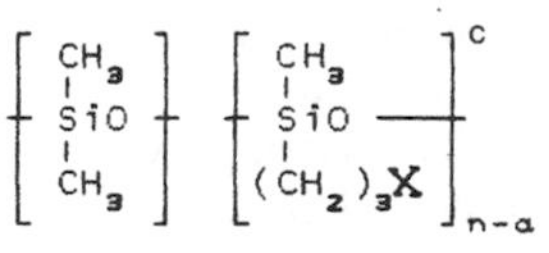

$$\left[\begin{array}{c} CH_3 \\ | \\ SiO \\ | \\ CH_3 \end{array}\right] \left[\begin{array}{c} CH_3 \\ | \\ SiO \\ | \\ (CH_2)_3X \end{array}\right]^c_{n-a}$$

$1-7$ [58]

12   Poly(amidoamine)s

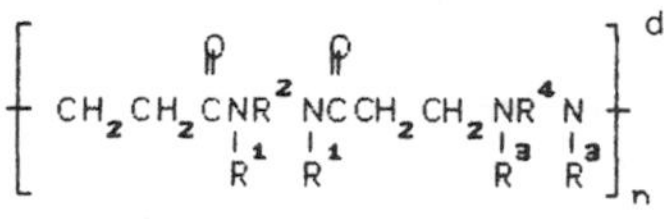

$$\left[\begin{array}{c} O \quad\quad O \\ \parallel \quad\quad \parallel \\ CH_2CH_2CNR^2NCCH_2CH_2NR^4N \\ | \quad | \quad\quad\quad | \quad | \\ R^1 \quad R^1 \quad\quad R^3 \quad R^3 \end{array}\right]^d_n$$

or

$$\left[\begin{array}{c} O \quad\quad O \\ \parallel \quad\quad \parallel \\ CH_2CH_2CNR^2NCCH_2CH_2N \\ | \quad | \quad\quad\quad | \\ R^1 \quad R^1 \quad\quad R^3 \end{array}\right]^d_n$$

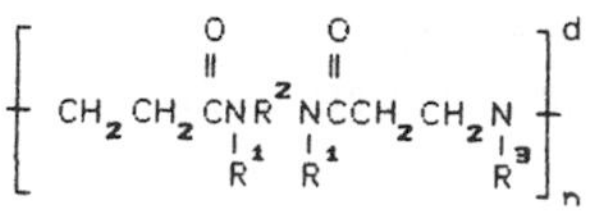

$5-50$ [59]

[a] See footnote (b) of Table 2.
[b] Reference not specifically related to the synthesis of oligomers, which, however, could be obtained if desired.
[c] X = OH, NH_2, COOH.
[d] By using as aminic monomers hydroxyalkylamines and amino acids or peptides, OH and COOH groups can be introduced as side substituents. Several of these products are described in Reference [58], and additional references therein.

549

though biodegradable, should deserve a trial as pro-moieties, is that they could be used to obtain prodrugs exhibiting some of the properties sought in their polymeric counterparts, yet which are suitable for non-traumatic ways of administration.

All the structures of the macromolecular promoiety-forming substances considered in this section are listed in Table 3. Some considerations on each family of macromolecules listed in this table are reported below.

POLY(AMINO ACID)S AND RELATED POLYMERS

Poly(amino acid)s have often been considered as promoiety-forming polymers [5,60,61]. From a chemical standpoint, many amino acid oligomers with low degrees of polymerization and narrow distribution are easily obtainable, and in many cases are commercially available. Poly(amino acid)s, in fact, can be synthesized by polymerization of their N-carboxy-anhydrides with bases, and this process has the characteristics of a "living" system. Nevertheless, very few examples of the use of oligomeric amino acids as promoieties can be found in the literature.

To be used as promoieties, polymeric amino acids must contain functional groups, such as $-OH$, $-COOH$, and $-NH_2$. These reactive groups are protected before preparing and polymerizing the corresponding N-carboxyanhydrides. The protecting groups are removed after polymerization. At this stage, functional groups different from the original ones may be introduced in a single step. Hydroxylated poly(glutamine)s have been prepared in this way [49]. It may be observed that the structurally related poly-D, L-hydroxyethyl aspartamide is obtained by a different process [47,49].

Table 3 lists some poly(amino acid)s which in the authors' opinion might be useful as promoieties in oligomeric form, either as such or as copolymers with more hydrophobic units, such as those deriving from leucine, valine, etc. The potential of such oligomers for preparing prodrugs to be administered orally should be taken into account. We have excluded poly-lysine from Table 3 because it is well known to be very toxic. The authors wonder, however, if the addition of acrylic acid to the pendant amino groups, according to the following scheme:

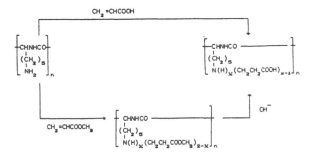

would lead to products with reduced toxicity, hence making them useful for forming promoieties. The

same technique for the same purpose has been applied in the case of poly(ethyleneimine).

POLY(MALIC ACID)

There are two isomers and poly(malic acid),

$$H-(OCHCO)_n^-OH \qquad H-(OCHCH_2CO)_n^-OH$$
$$|\quad\qquad\qquad\qquad\qquad |$$
$$CH_2COOH \qquad\qquad\qquad COOH$$

Poly(α-Malic Acid)   Poly(β-Malic)

Both are being purposely studied as potential polymeric promoieties, combining multifunctionality, water solubility, and biodegradability to form non-toxic products [51,55]. Only recently have they been obtained as high polymers, by ring-opening polymerization of the cyclic anhydrides of their benzyl esters, and then hydrogenolytic cleavage of the benzyl group [55]. We report them here because there are published syntheses of oligomeric products, either by dehydrative polycondensation of α- and β-benzyl malates with carbodiimides [52] (we think that N,N'-carbonyldiimidazole might give better results), or by direct polycondensation of the acids themselves, the latter method resulting in a highly irregular structure [56]. Even the first products obtained by Vert through the ring-opening method might be still defined as oligomers [53,54].

POLY(ETHYLENEIMINE)S

Poly(ethyleneimine)s can be obtained commercially in a wide spectrum of molecular weight fractions, ranging from the dimer to high molecular weight polymers. The commercial polymers are usually highly branched, containing primary as well as tertiary amino groups [62,63], and therefore the structure usually attributed to these products

$$\left[CH_2CH_2NH\right]_n$$

is highly idealized. However, truly linear poly(ethyleneimine)s with molecular weights on the order of a few thousand have been synthesized starting from 2-oxazolines [64].

We report this polymer here because it has been tested as a promoiety, although it was found to be too toxic to be of any utility. However, its toxicity was substantially reduced by introducing pendant carboxyl groups by a Michael type addition of acrylic acid [57].

POLY(DIMETHYLSILOXANE)S

Poly(dimethylsiloxane)s appear to be quite promising candidates for use as promoieties since they are physiologically inert, liposoluble, and endowed with a very low glass transition temperature and a high chain flexibility. They would appear to be the best choices to impart lipid-solubility and permeability through physiological barriers to the exceedingly hydrophilic drugs.

A recent paper published by Bachrach and Zikha [58] is probably the only account on this topic to be found so far in the literature. In this chapter, both polymeric and oligomeric dimethylsiloxane promoieties are described. They were functionalized by first introducing SiH groups into their main chains, and then adding allylic compounds:

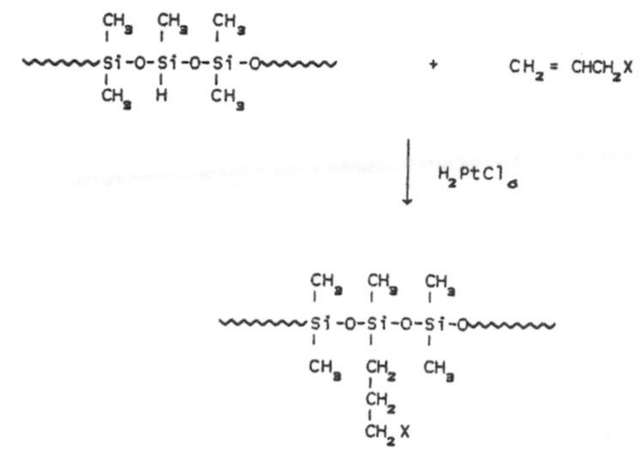

$$X = Br, \; COOSi(CH_3)_3, \; NHSi(CH_3)_3$$

The trimethyl silyl groups were removed in boiling alcohol to give free carboxy- or amino groups. Several drugs were then attached to both functionalized oligomers and polymers.

POLY(AMIDOAMINE)S

Poly(amidoamine)s are regular polymers in which ter-amino and amido groups are regularly arranged along the macromolecular chain [65]. They are obtained by polyaddition of primary monoamines, or bis(secondary amines), to bis-acrylamides:

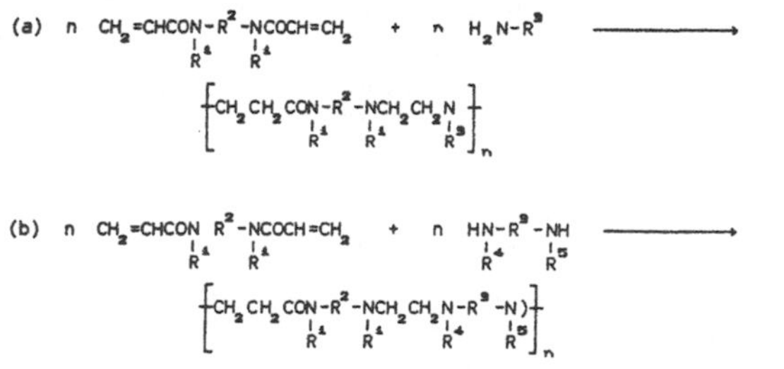

This polymerization reaction has some peculiar features. It takes place readily in water or alcohols, at room temperature, and without added catalysts. The chemistry and the properties of poly(amidoamine)s have been thoroughly reviewed [65].

Poly(amidoamine)s have been studied until recently mostly for their biomedical interest as heparin-complexing agents, leading to heparin-complexing resins [66,67] and heparinizable materials [68–70]. Recently, however, we have started to consider poly-(amidoamine)s as promoieties. Their potential interest in this respect lies in the following combination of properties:

(1) They are usually prepared under very smooth conditions, and a wide variety of structures are easily available.

(2) They are bases of low to medium strength, with sharp basicity constants. It is possible to graduate basicity according to needs. For instance, polymers expected to be fully ionized inside lysosomes, and poorly ionized in the bloodstream, are easily obtainable.

(3) Side functions suitable for binding drug moieties can be easily introduced.

(4) Their polymerization degree can be varied to a considerable extent by simple means, such as the initial comonomer's ratio.

It may be added that some poly(amidoamine) has been shown to be endowed with a significant ability to reduce the size and number of metastases in mice [71]. A preliminary investigation on some poly(amido-amine)s as potential soluble drug carriers is presently being performed [72].

Promoiety-Forming a-2 Oligomers

Promoiety-Forming a-2 Oligomers of Polyvinylic Structure

Both radical and ionic processes can be employed to obtain end-functionalized oligomers of polyvinylic structure.

IONIC PROCESSES

End-functionalized oligomers and low polymers can be obtained by the "living polymer" technique. Anionic living polymers have been described long ago, and have been adequately reviewed [22]. Some relevant features of the living system have been reported previously.

In anionic living polymers, mostly derived from hydrocarbon monomers, the growing end is a carbanion, and reacts as such. Consequently, reactive end-groups can be introduced by reaction with a suitable agent acting as terminator, or "killer", as in the following example, regarding styrene as monomer:

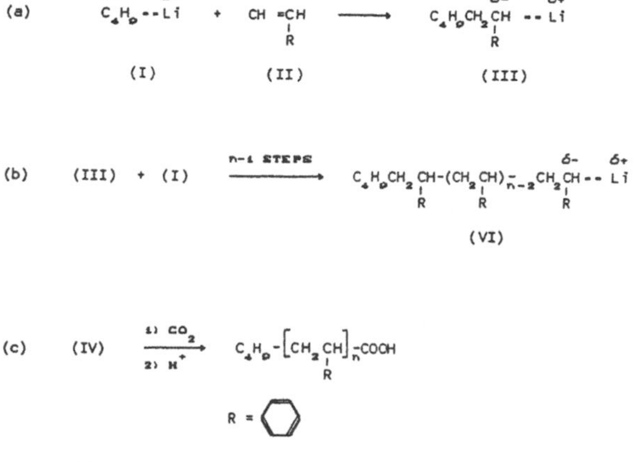

The use of difunctional initiators can lead to α,ω-difunctionalized (telechelic) oligomers.

Despite the large potentials of the above polymerization systems, both theoretical and practical, its scope for preparing oligomeric prodrugs is rather limited, being limited the choice of the monomers to which it applies. However, oligodienes obtained in this way have been used to this purpose (see Table 5).

The same cationic living system mentioned previously can be utilized to produce end-functionalized oligomers of vinyl ethers [21]. Two distinct strategies are available. The first makes use of a functional vinyl ether in step (a) of the scheme reported in the section "Ionic Systems". The second makes use of a functional terminator:

$$\text{\textapprox}CH_2CHI \overset{6+}{\cdots} \overset{6-}{I_2} + :NuX \longrightarrow \text{\textapprox}CH_2CHNu + X^-$$
$$\qquad\qquad OR \qquad\qquad\qquad\qquad\qquad OR$$

Where Nu is a nucleophilic reagent, for instance a malonic ester anion, which can be subsequently transformed into a CH_2COOH group by hydrolysis and decarboxylation [21].

RADICAL PROCESSES

Resuming the discussion on chain transfer reactions in the section on "Promoiety-Forming a-1 Oligomers of Polyvinylic Structure", it is apparent that a telomerization reaction is well suited to obtaining end-functionalized oligomers, if functional chain transfer (telomerizing) agents are employed. In the case of acrylic monomers, and for the same reasons given previously, functional mercaptans can be recommended. Some of these are commercial or are at any rate readily available products, and those which in the

authors' opinion, deserve a particular attention are reported in Table 4.

The above point is better clarified as follows. The oligomerization of an acrylic ester, for example methylacrylate, in presence of a functional mercaptane, for example 2-mercaptoethanol, would take essentially the following course:

Termination of the kinetic chain takes place as in the scheme reported in the aforementioned section. If the transfer reaction (a) is frequent, the number of macromolecules (III) not carrying at both ends fragments of chain transfer agent, in the example H and SCH_2CH_2OH, are negligible.

In case of most non-acrylic monomers, their C_T values with mercaptans, including those reported in Table 4, are very high. As a result, if the polymerization is run in batch, the mercaptan is rapidly consumed and the reaction product, even at moderate yields, contains high molecular weight polymer besides the functionalized oligomer. The latter must be separated by fractionation. This is, for instance, the case of N-vinylpyrrolidinone with 2-mercaptoethanol, and 2-mercaptoacetic acid [73,74].

The telomerization technique offers, in principle, two distinct opportunities. The first one is the possibility of using oligomeric promoieties with a variable combination of physico-chemical properties, owing to the very large number of vinyl monomers available. The second one is the possibility of obtaining oligomers having different types of reactive groups along their main chain, and at their end, by using functional monomers and chain transfer agents with different functionalities. It may be noted that, according to the mechanism of radical polymerization, it is possible to obtain end-functionalized products also starting from initiators able to produce functional primary radicals [75]. However, this method is not recommended for obtaining promoiety-forming oligomers, since from one side the number of easily available functional initiators is not high, and from the other side is not easy to lower the polymerization degree beyond a certain limit by increasing the initiators/monomer ratio without inducing undesirable side reactions.

Table 4. Some functional mercaptans useful as chain-transfer agents in the synthesis of promoiety forming oligomers of Cat. a-2.

Syst. No.	Structure	Commercial Name
1	$HSCH_2CH_2OH$	2-mercaptoethanol
2	$HS-\langle\bigcirc\rangle-OH$	4-hydroxythiophenol
3	$HSCH_2CH_2NH_2$	Cisteamine
4	$HSCH_2COOH$	2-mercaptoacetic acid
5	$HSCH_2CH_2CH_2COOH$	3-mercaptopropionic
6	$HSCHCH_2COOH$ / $COOH$	Thiosuccininic acid
7	$HSCHCH_2COOH$ / NH_2	Cisteine

Several vinyl- and diene-oligomers which either have been used, or in the authors' opinion may be useful for preparing oligomeric prodrugs of Cat. a-2 and listed in Table 5.

Poly(ethyleneglycols)

Among the promoiety-forming oligomers of Cat. a-2, poly(ethyleneglycols) (PEGs):

$$HO-[CH_2CH_2O]_n-H$$

have received the greatest attention so far. They offer, in fact, a unique combination of commercial availability (either as pure compounds ($n < 4$), or as fractions of narrow molecular weight distribution), lack of toxicity [79], end-group reactivity, and amphiphilic properties. The preparation and properties of PEGs will not be discussed here; they have been adequately reviewed [80–82]. The chemistry of PEG has also been excellently reviewed [89]. Star-shaped PEGs, having functionalities of 3 or more, can also be prepared [84].

As such, PEGs can yield ester derivatives of carboxylated drugs through their hydroxyl end-groups. However, a number of other functional groups have been introduced for obtaining new drug-binding or protein-binding derivatives. Most of these are listed in Table 6. In the same table, the synthetic procedures by which they are obtained are outlined. Monoethers of PEGs may constitute an alternative to simple PEGs, providing wider opportunities for obtaining prodrugs with optimal hydrophilic/hydrophobic balance. Many of them are commercially available, especially the monomethylethers, and the monoethers of long-chain hydrocarbons, the latter being sold as non-ionic surfactants (Triton N, Triton X, etc.). However, commercially available PEG monomethylethers (MPEGs) are often impure, the chief impurity being plain PEG. In case of lower molecular weight derivatives, the latter may be selectively extracted by water from chloroform or methylene chloride solutions, since according to our experience the partition coefficients are in favour of water for low molecular weight PEGs, but not for their monomethylethers. This method has been applied also for PEG 2000 ($\bar{n} = \sim 45$)[85], but fails for higher molecular weight derivatives. In this case, chromatographic techniques can be employed [86]. It might be more convenient in some cases to prepare PEG monoethers in the laboratory. The synthesis of PEG monoethers has been reviewed by Harris [89]. PEG monoethers, as well as PEGs, have been further functionalized. The corresponding derivatives are listed in Table 6.

Other Promoiety Forming A-2 Oligomers of Non-Polyvinylic Structure

PEG ANALOGS

Among PEG analogs, poly(1,2-propyleneglycols) (PPGs):

$$HO-\left[CH_2\overset{\overset{\displaystyle CH_3}{|}}{C}HO\right]_n-H$$

are also commercially available. They are much less hydrophilic than PEGs: in fact, PPGs with $n > 10$ are almost insoluble in water. Copolymers PEG/PPG are sold as non-ionic detergents. We think that PPGs used as promoiety-forming oligomers may prove to be more convenient than PEGs in case of hydrophilic drugs [129].

In this respect, other hydroxy-terminated oligomers of similar structure might be considered, such as for instance poly(1,3-propyleneglycol)s,

$$HO-\left[CH_2CH_2CH_2O\right]_n-H$$

which can be prepared by cationic oligomerization of oxetane in the presence of 1,3 propanediol [124].

POLY(2-OXAZOLINE)S

This term refers to the polymerization products of 2-oxazoline and its N-alkyl derivatives, and is rather improper, since these products are in fact linear poly(N-acylethyleimine)s:

When R = H or CH₃, we are in the presence of macromolecular analogs of N,N¹-dimethylformamide (DMF) or N,N¹-dimethylacetamide (DMA), respectively.

The polymerization of 2-oxazolines takes place with electrophilic initiators, such as methyl tosylate [106]. It is a living polymerization system, and narrow molecular weight distribution polymers and oligomers with predetermined size can be obtained:

Termination occurs if nucleophilic reagents are added [125]. If these are functionalized, end-functionalized poly(oxazoline)s result. Furthermore, by using difunctional initiators, poly(oxazoline)s functionalized at both ends can be obtained. Block copolymers with PEG have also been prepared.

In our opinion, end-functionalized poly(oxazoline)s might provide an alternative to PEGs. Besides being straightforwardly prepared, they are water soluble, amphiphilic, and on the whole are endowed with the properties one would expect looking at their micromolecular counterparts, DMF and DMA, which are among the most powerful solvents known. Therefore, they will probably draw attention both for preparing oligomeric prodrugs, and for modifying enzymes, assuming they prove to be toxicologically safe.

Table 5. Promoiety-forming oligomers of Cat. a-2 with a polyvinylic structure.[a]

No.	Structure	n[b]	Synthetic Method[c]	Ref.
1	C_4H_9[CH$_2$C=CHCH$_2$]$_n$CH$_2$CH$_2$OH (R)[d]	$\cong 20$	T. "Living poly(diene)s terminated by $\overset{O}{C H_2-C H_2}$.	[76] [77]
2	HOCH$_2$CH$_2$[CH$_2$C=CHCH$_2$]$_n$CH$_2$CH$_2$OH (R)[d]	$\cong 20$	As above, obtained by dufunctional initiators.	[76] [77]
3	C_4H_9[CH$_2$C=CHCH$_2$]$_n$CH$_2\overset{O}{O}CCl$ (R)	$\cong 20$	M. 1, COCl$_2$	[76]
4	ClCOCH$_2$CH[CH$_2$C=CHCH$_2$]$_n$CH$_2$OCCl (R)[d]	$\cong 20$	M. 2, COCl$_2$	[76]
5	[CH$_2$C=CHCH$_2$]$_n$NHR (CH$_3$)[e]	$\cong 10$	T. Isoprene, LiNHR	[78]
6	R[CH$_2$CH]$_n$COOH (OR)[f]	8–50	T. See the text.	[21]
7	HOOC[CH$_2$CH]$_n$COOH (OR)	8–26	T. See the text.	[21]
8	R[CH$_2$CH]$_n$NH$_2$ (OR)[f]	11–20	T. See the text.	[21]
9	NH$_2$[CH$_2$CH]$_n$NH$_2$ (OR)	13	T. See the text.	[21]
10	H[CH$_2$CH]$_n$CH$_2$CH$_2$OH[g]	5–1000	T. Vinylpyrrolidone, AIBN, HSCH$_2$CH$_2$OH	[73] [74]
11	H[CH$_2$CH]$_n$CH$_2$COOH[g]	5–1000	T. Vinylpyrrolidone, AIBN, HSCH$_2$CH$_2$COOH	[73] [74]

[a] See footnote (a) of Table 2.
[b] See footnote (b) of Table 2.
[c] See footnote (c) of Table 2, with the only difference that T means every type of polymerization.
[d] R = H or CH$_3$
[e] R = CH(CH$_3$)$_2$ and other secondary alkyl groups.
[f] R = H or CH$_3$O.
[g] Highly polydisperse products were obtained, due to the very high C_T's (see the text). Narrowly distributed fractions of $n \cong 10$–30 could be separated from the raw products by chromatographic techniques.

Table 6. Functionalized poly(ethyleneglycols).[a]

No.	End Groups[b]		Synthetic Method[c,d]	Ref.
	F1	F2		
1	OH	Id	Commercial	—
2	OH	OCH_3	Commercial	—
3	$\overset{O}{\overset{\|}{O}}CNH\overset{OH}{\overset{\|}{C}}HCH_2OH$	OCH_3	27, $H_2N\overset{OH}{\overset{\|}{C}}HCH_2OH$	[87]
4	Br, Cl	Id	1, $SOBr_2$, $SOCl_2$	[88–90]
5	As above	OCH_3	2, as above	[91]
6	$CH_3-C_6H_4-SO_3$	Id	1, $CH_3-C_6H_4-SO_2Cl$	[92]
7	As above	OCH_3	2, as above	[93–95]
8	CH_3SO_3	Id	1, CH_3SO_2Cl	[96]
9	NH_2[e]	Id	4, NH_3	[89]
			4, $KOCH_2CH_2NH_2$	[97]
			14, $CH_3COO^-NH_4^+$, $NaCNBH_3$	[98]
10	NH_2	OCH_3	7, K^+ phtalimide, then H_2NNH_2	[93–95]
			5, NaN_3, then H_2/Pd	[88]
11	$NH(CH_2)_6NH_2$	Id	4, $H_2N(CH_2)_6NH_2$ (20-fold excess)	[99]
12	$NH(CH_2)_2NH_2$	Id	4, $H_2N(CH_2)_2NH_2$ (excess)	[100]
13	$O_2CNH(CH_2)_6NH_2$	OCH_3	2, $OCN(CH_2)_6NCO$ (excess), then HCl	[101]
14	OCH_2CHO[f]	Id, OCH_3	1(2), MnO_2	[102,103]
			1(2), $(CH_3)_3COK$, $BrCH_2CH(OEt)_2$, then HCl	[98]
			1(2), $(CH_3)_2SO$ + CH_3COOH	[98]
15	$O\overset{O}{\overset{\|}{C}}NHCH_2CHO$	OCH_3	3, $NaIO_4$	[87]
16	$O-C_6H_4-CHO$	OCH_3	5, $KO-C_6H_4-CHO$	[104,105]
17	OCH_2COOH[g]	Id	1, microbial oxidation	[106]
		Id, OCH_3	1(2), $KMnO_4$	[107]
			1(2), Na/ Naphtalene, $BrCH_2COOEt$, then OH^-	[89,108–111]
			14, H_2O_2	[112]
18	$OOC(CH_2)_2COOH$	Id	1, succinic anhydride, basic catalysts	[88,89 111,113]

(continued)

Table 6 (continued).

No.	End Groups[b]		Synthetic Method[c,d]	Ref.
	F1	F2		
19	OOC(CH$_2$)$_2$COOH	OCH$_3$	2, as above	[89,97, 112]
20	OOC(CH$_2$)$_7$COOH	Id, OCH$_3$	1(2), HOOC(CH$_2$)$_7$COOH, DCCI, pyridine	[99]
21	NHCO(CH$_2$)$_2$COOH	Id, OCH$_3$	9, succinic anhydride	[89,103]
22	OOCCH=CHCOOH	OCH$_3$	2, maleic anhydride, dimethylaminopyridine	[114]
23	(benzene ring) HOOC, COOH; NHCO—COOH; HOOC, COOH	OCH$_3$	5, sodium benzenehexacarboxylate, EDCI	[115]
24	(triazine ring with two Cl) O—	Id, OCH$_3$	1(2), cyanuric chloride	[116]
25	OOCNH(CH$_2$)$_6$NCO	Id, OCH$_3$	1(2), OCN(CH$_2$)$_6$NCO	[88,101, 117]
26	OCOCl	Id, OCH$_3$	1(2), COCl$_2$	[118,119]
27	OCOO—(phenyl)—NO$_2$	OCH$_3$	2, ClCOO—(phenyl)—NO$_2$	[87]
28	OCON (imidazole)	Id	1, CDI	[120]
29	As above	OCH$_3$	2, CDI	[121]
30	OOC(CH$_2$)$_2$COON (succinimide)	OCH$_3$	19, N-hydroxysuccinimide, DCCI	[89,112]
31	OOC(CH$_2$)$_2$CON (imidazole)	Id	18, imidazole, DCCI	[113]
32	OOC(CH$_2$)$_2$CON (benzotriazole)	Id	18, 1-H benzotriazole, DCCI	[113]
33	OCH$_2$CH—CH$_2$ (epoxide)	OR[h]	—[h], epichlorohydrin	[122]

[a]F^1[CH$_2$CH$_2$O]$_n$CH$_2$CH$_2$$F^2$. Only functions suitable for coupling reactions have been considered.

[b]When $F^1 = F^2$, the second entry is Id.

[c]In the order: starting material (as its Syst. No. in this table); functionalizing reagent; other reagents. Acid scavengers and solvents are not indicated.

[d]In principle, any functionalization method described for 1 is also suitable for 2. The reverse may not be true. The distinction has been maintained only when considered opportune.

[e]Many aminated derivatives, usually PEG–PPG copolymers, are sold under the name of "Jeffamines".

[f]The published synthetic methods have been critically reviewed [105].

[g]A dicarboxylated PEG is commercially available (Fluka).

[h]Reaction performed on C$_8$H$_{17}$—(phenyl)—O(CH$_2$CH$_2$O)$_9$CH$_2$CH$_2$OH (Triton X-100).

Several a-2 oligomers other than PEGs which in the Authors' opinion might provide useful promoieties are listed in Table 7, together with further indications on their preparation processes.

Types of Drug–Oligomer Bonds

By definition, the bond between the promoiety and the drug moiety in oligomeric prodrugs must be cleavable in the body environment. Hydrolyzable bonds have been almost exclusively considered even if, in principle, bonds susceptible to reductive cleavage might be used as well. The most common hydrolyzable bonds, namely amidic bonds, peptidic bonds, urethane bonds, carbonate bonds, ester bonds, hydrazone bonds, and imino (Schiff base) bonds, are depicted in Table 8.

The question of the cleavability within the body of the above bonds deserves some comment. It is obvious that cleavage within the body should take place at a rate sufficient to ensure a useful level of the free drug at the side of action. This rate depends primarily on the type of bond, but other factors such as hydrophilicity and sheltering by the promoiety may play a very important role.

To our knowledge, no comprehensive studies have been published on this subject concerning macromolecular prodrugs. From the few data found in the literature, mostly on polymeric prodrugs [129–133], and from our own experience, we may draw the following conclusions:

(1) Because their structures lead to larger sheltering effects, type a-1 oligomeric prodrugs, the other conditions being equal, are expected to be less hydrolyzable than the a-2 ones, unless a sufficiently long spacer has been inserted between oligomer and drug. As regards a-2 oligomeric prodrugs, the discussion on the reactivity of terminal functions reported in the section on "Oligomeric Promoieties and Prodrugs" should include the hydrolysis of drug-oligomer bonds. This means that, in the absence of enzymatic catalysis, they should be hydrolyzed at a rate not very different from that of micromolecular prodrugs of similar structure. When enzymes are involved in cleavages, some retarding effect in comparison with micromolecular analogs may be expected if the structure of the oligomeric promoiety is alien to the body.

(2) Amidic linkages are seldom cleaved at a useful rate, unless the prodrug is internalized by cells and is susceptible to attack by lysosomal enzymes. The same is true for peptidic linkages. In the latter case, this property has been exploited in a sophisticated approach to cancer chemotherapy with polymeric prodrugs able to release the active principle only after being internalized [129,130].

(3) Ester bonds between an oligomeric carboxylated

a-1 promoiety, without spacers, are probably slowly hydrolyzed in the body fluids, especially when the constitutional unit is methacrylic (Nos. 11 and 12 of Table 2). Esters of carboxylated drugs with hydroxylated promoieties are probably more hydrolyzable.

(4) Urethane bonds and carbonate bonds follow qualitatively the same pattern of esters. In many cases, however, a lower rate of hydrolysis may be expected.

(5) Hydrazone bonds and imino bonds are usually rapidly cleaved.

A number of exceptions might be found to the above rules, which are only aimed at providing a rough guide for planning derivatives to be afterwards carefully tested *in vivo*.

Coupling Reactions

It may be observed that many drug-oligomer bonds listed in Table 8 are of the ester and amidic types, obviously involving drugs containing hydroxy, amino, or carboxy groups. These are the most commonly encountered bonds in oligomeric as well as in polymeric and micromolecular prodrugs. The synthetic problems involved in creating these bonds will be discussed in some detail. A few bonds are typical of carbonyl groups, such as the hydrazone-, the imino-, and the acetal groups. They are created according to classical methods of organic chemistry, and no synthetic problems are usually encountered provided the properly functionalized oligomers are available. This point will not be discussed any further.

Coupling Reactions Involving Hydroxylated and Aminated Drugs

Hydroxylated drugs can be bound to oligomers by means of ester or carbonate bonds. In the former case, the oligomer must be carboxylated, and the coupling reaction deserves comments. The "classical" esterification method, i.e., the direct condensation reaction by heating in the presence of acid catalysts:

$$1) \quad RCOOH + DOH \xrightarrow{H^+} RCOOR' + H_2O$$

R = oligomeric residue; DOH = hydroxylated drug

is seldom employed. It should be noticed, in fact, that, after the coupling reaction, it is often difficult to purify the oligomeric prodrug from decomposition or side reaction products. These are likely to occur, since in most oligomer–drug pairs at least one component is not insensitive to the forcing conditions required to drive the esterification reaction near to completion.

The preferred strategy is to prepare first an activated derivative of the carboxylated oligomer, and

Table 7. Non-polyvinylic promoiety-forming oligomers of Cat. a-2 other than PEGs.

No.	Structure	n	Synthetic Method	Ref.
1	HO–[CH$_2$–CH(CH$_3$)O]$_n$–H	many	Commercial.	—
2	HOOC(CH$_2$)$_2$COO–[CH$_2$CH(CH$_3$)O]$_n$–OOC(CH$_2$)$_2$COOH	many	1, succinic anhydride basic catalysts.	[126]
3	(imidazolyl)NOC(CH$_2$)$_2$COO–[CH$_2$CH(CH$_3$)O]$_n$–O(CH$_2$)$_2$CON(imidazolyl)	many	2, imidazole, DCCI.	[126]
4	(benzotriazolyl)NOC(CH$_2$)$_2$COO–[CH$_2$CH(CH$_3$)O]$_n$–O(CH$_2$)$_2$CON(benzotriazolyl)	many	2, DCCI, 1-H benzotriazole.	[126]
5	HOOC(CH$_2$)$_3$COO–[CH$_2$CH(CH$_3$)O]$_n$–OC(CH$_2$)$_3$COOH	many	1, glutaric anhydride, basic catalysts.	[126]
6	(imidazolyl)NOC(CH$_2$)$_3$COO–[CH$_2$CH(CH$_3$)O]$_n$–O(CH$_2$)$_3$CON(imidazolyl)	many	5, then as 3.	[126]
7	(benzotriazolyl)NOC(CH$_2$)$_3$COO–[CH$_2$CH(CH$_3$)O]$_n$–O(CH$_2$)$_3$CON(benzotriazolyl)	many	5, then as 4.	[126]
8	HO–[CH$_2$CH$_2$CH$_2$O]$_n$–H [c]	3–7	Cationic polym. of trimethylene oxide (oxetane) in the presence of 1,3-propanediol.	[124]
9	CH$_3$–[NCH$_2$CH$_2$(C=O, CH$_3$)]$_n$–OOC(CH$_2$)$_3$COOH [c]	10–50	"Living" polym. of 2-methyloxazoline with monofunctional initiators (see the text), then termination with glutaric acid.	[125]

558

Table 7 (continued).

No.	Structure	n	Synthetic Method	Ref.
10	$\left[HOOC(CH_2)_3COO\left[CH_2CH_2\underset{\underset{CH_3}{\overset{C=O}{|}}}{N}\right]_n X \right]_2$ [c,d]	10–50	As above, using difunctional initiators.	[125]
11	$HO(CH_2)_3\left[\underset{CH_3}{\overset{CH_3}{|}}SiO\right]_n\underset{CH_3}{\overset{CH_3}{|}}Si(CH_2)_3OH$	many	$HO\left[\underset{CH_3}{\overset{}{|}}SiO\right]_n H$ + $Cl\underset{CH_3}{\overset{CH_3}{|}}Si(CH_2)_3OOCCH_3$, then OH^-.	[127]
12	$CH_2CHCH_2O(CH_2)_3\left[\underset{CH_3}{\overset{CH_3}{|}}Si\text{-}O\right]_n\underset{CH_3}{\overset{CH_3}{|}}Si(CH_2)_3OCH_2CH\text{-}CH_2$	many	a As above, using $Cl\underset{CH_3}{\overset{CH_3}{|}}Si(CH_2)_3OCH_2CH\text{-}CH_2$	[127]
			b $H\left[\underset{CH_3}{\overset{CH}{|}}SiO\right]_n\underset{CH_3}{\overset{CH_3}{|}}SiH$ + $CH_2=CHCH_2O\text{-}CH\text{-}CH_2$	[128]

[a]See the corresponding footnote of Table 6.

[b]This is the structure popularly attributed to PPG. However, we have gathered NMR evidence that at least in some commercial samples both hydroxyl end groups are secondary, i.e., the real structure of these PPG samples probably is:

$$HOCHCH_2\left[\underset{CH_3}{\overset{CH_3}{|}}CHCH_2\right]_a O \left[CH_2\underset{CH_3}{\overset{}{|}}CHO\right]_b CH_2\underset{CH_3}{\overset{CH_3}{|}}CHOH$$

[c]N-ethyl derivatives also described in the same reference. Other N-alkyl and aryl-derivatives have not been considered.

[d]X = Difunctional initiator's residue.

Table 8. Chemical bonds between drug moiety and promoiety in macromolecular prodrugs.

No.	Name	Structure[a]	Synthetic Method[b]
1	Amide	O‖ MCND | R	O‖ MCX + DNHR
1a	Amide	O‖ MNCD | R	O‖ MNHR + DCX
2	Ester	O‖ MCOD	O‖ MCX + DOH
2a	Ester	O‖ MOCD	O‖ MOH + DCX
3	Urethane	O‖ c MNCOD | R	O‖ MNHR + DOCX
3a	Urethane	O‖ MNCOD | H	MNCO + DOH
4	Carbonate	O‖ MOCOD	O‖ α) MOCX + DOH; O‖ β) MOH + DOCX
5	Urea	O‖ c MNCND | | R R	O‖ MNCX + DNHR | R
5a	Urea	O‖ MNCND c | | H R	MNCO + DNHR
6	Imino	MC=ND | R	MC=O + DNH₂ | R
6a	Imino	MN=CD | R	MNH₂ + DC=O | R
7	Hydrazone	O‖ MCNHN=CD | R	O‖ MCNH=NH₂ + DC=O | R

[a]M = Macromolecular promoiety, D = drug moiety.
[b]X = Leaving group.
[c]R = H or a higher substituent.

then to react it with the drug. The same strategy can be used for creating amidic linkages:

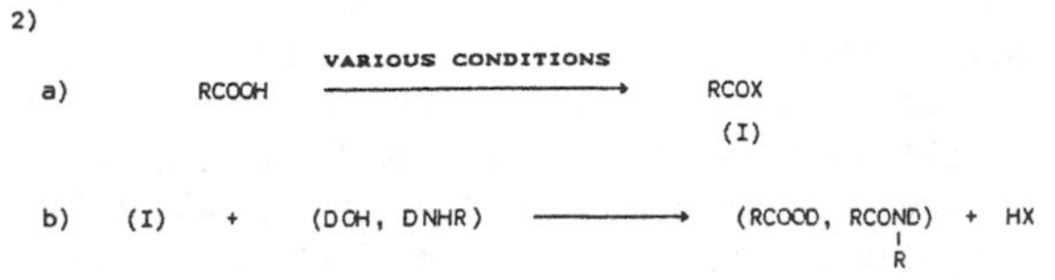

2)

R and D as in the previous case, X = leaving group

Carbonate bonds are usually obtained by first activating a hydroxylated oligomer via chloroformate or imidazolyl formate, and then reacting it with the drug. The reverse method, i.e., the activation of the drug, is less frequently practiced. Urethane bonds with aminated drugs can be obtained by the same derivatives:

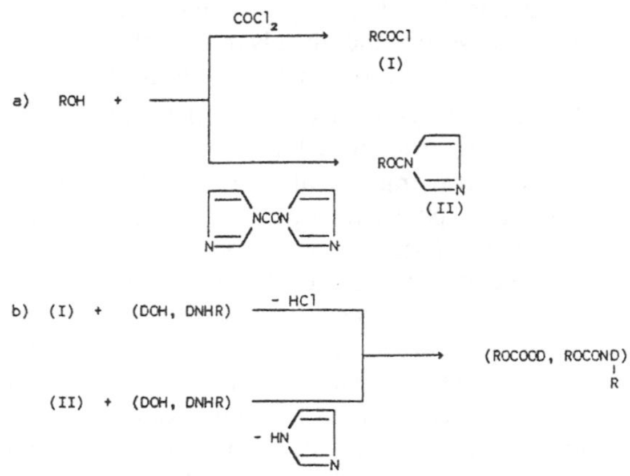

The same bond with hydroxylated drugs can be obtained using an oligomer bearing isocyanate group (e.g., No. 13 of Table 6).

Some oligomeric activated derivatives have been reported in Tables 2, 3, 5, 6, and 7.

Although a detailed discussion on the reactivities of the above derivatives is too cumbersome for the scope of this chapter, a few practical observations can be made. Leaving apart isocyanates, the reactivity of each derivative depends primarily on the nature of its leaving group. The main leaving groups which either have been, or might be involved in the synthesis of oligomeric prodrugs are listed in Table 9, roughly arranged in order of increasing reactivity. It should be considered, however, that steric hindrance reduces reactivity. In the absence of spacing arms, for instance, activated derivatives of poly(methacrylic) acid are much less reactive than their acrylic counterparts [134].

All derivatives of Table 9 react quantitatively under mild conditions with aliphatic and cycloaliphatic primary and secondary amines, giving amido linkages

(urethane in case of imidazolylformates and chloroformates). They also smoothly react with hydrazine [135]. In our experience, 4-nitrophenyl esters, N-hydroxysuccinimmide esters, and benzotriazolides, (Nos. 1, 3, and 4 of Table 9) are the most convenient to use in obtaining amidic linkages, combining reactivity with low sensibility to moisture. The latter property makes it easy to isolate the corresponding activated oligomers.

The first terms of Table 9, as indicated, do not react smoothly with alcohols. Even with the most reactive derivatives other than chlorides, corresponding to leaving groups (Nos. 4–8 of Table 9), nearly quantitative reaction yields are often obtained only by using catalysts, such as triethylamine or, better, 4-dimethyl-

Table 9. Relevant leaving groups in condensation reactions leading to amidic and ester bonds.

No.	Name of the Acyl Derivative	Structure of the Leaving Group
1	4-nitrophenylesters	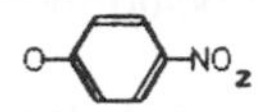
2	2,4,5 trichlorophenyl esters	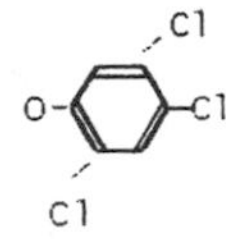
3	N-hydroxysuccinamide esters	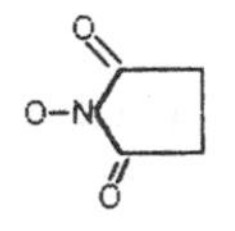
4	Benzotriazolides	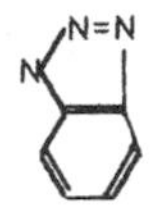
5	N-hydroxybenzotriazolylesters	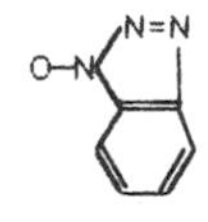
6	N-hydroxyimidazolylesters	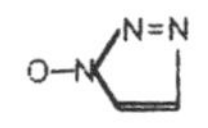
7	Imidazolides and imidazolyl formates	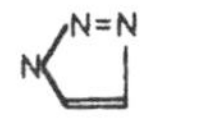
8	Carbodiimides-addition compounds	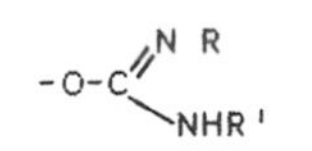
9	Chlorides and chloroformates[a]	C l

[a]Sometimes referred to as chlorocarbonates, especially in older literature.

aminopyridine and related compounds. In case of secondary alcohols, besides using catalysts, it is usually opportune to heat at 50–70°C for several hours or even days. Benzotriazolides usually offer a good compromise between reactivity and ease in handling.

As far as selectivity is concerned, if the coupling reaction is run under mild conditions, only amides (and urethanes) are formed with hydroxylated amines even with fairly reactive derivatives, such as Nos. 4 and 7 of Table 9 [136]. A polymeric benzotriazolide proved to be selective even in the case of a poly-(hydroxylated) compound, in which only one of the hydroxyls was primary, hence more reactive [137]. As a final observation acyl chlorides (No. 9 of Table 9) should be used with precaution. They are poorly compatible with some solvents otherwise useful as reaction media, such as for instance dimethylsulphoxide, and amides. Furthermore, some oligomers are degraded by strong acids, and therefore special care should be devoted to effectively scavenging HCl at every synthetic stage. For instance, PEGs are degraded not only by free HCl, but also by pyridinium hydrochloride [98,138].

Coupling Reactions Involving Carboxylated Drugs

The preferred strategy is usually to activate the carboxy group of the drug, and then to react it with the selected hydroxylated or aminated oligomer. As such, it is simply the reverse of the strategy discussed in the previous section for preparing derivatives of hydroxylated and aminated drugs with carboxylated oligomers, and does not need to be discussed any further in general terms.

The case of drugs bearing both hydroxy and carboxy groups, however, deserves some comment. If an ester bond is desired with a hydroxylated oligomer, it is possible in our experience to take advantage of the fact that, at room temperature and in the absence of catalysts, the carboxy groups usually react rapidly with N,N^1-carbonyldiimidazole, giving imidazolides, while the hydroxy groups react much more slowly with both N,N^1-carbonyldiimidazole and imidazolides. Thus, by using a large excess of oligomer in the second stage, and provided the product can be isolated from byproducts and unreacted oligomer, the reaction can be brought to high yields:

R—OH = hydroxylated oligomer

This method is obviously limited to low molecular weight oligomers. It has proved to be very effective for coupling large, hydrophobic hydroxylated-carboxylated moieties to low molecular weight PEGs [139].

EXAMPLES OF OLIGOMERIC PRODRUGS

Several examples of oligomeric prodrugs of Cats. a-1 and a-2 are listed in Tables 10 and 11, respectively. In the same tables, we have also reported some combinations of oligomers with model compounds, studied to calibrate the synthetic methods. Looking at the literature, it is apparent that oligomeric prodrugs have not yet received all the attention which in our opinion they deserve. We think that this is due to a combination of factors, which can be summarized as follows:

(1) "Traditional" medicinal chemistry is continually producing improved drugs.

(2) Some barriers, e.g., bad odour or bad taste, can be overcome by simple means, such as encapsulation, compounding etc. The use of these techniques is commonplace in pharmaceutical formulations.

(3) Modern drug delivery systems appear quite promising for obtaining prolonged action. They have, however, the disadvantage of needing in most cases to be traumatically inserted.

(4) There is always a considerable inertia involved in developing products which are on the borderline between two traditionally distinct disciplines, in our case pharmacology and macromolecular chemistry. Different ways of thinking, coupled with the human tendency to stick to one's own traditions, are involved. To give an example, pharmacologists are used to dealing with single chemical species, having well-defined molecular weights, melting and/or boiling points, etc. They look with suspicion on the idea of testing polydisperse families of compounds, with *average* molecular weights and no definite physical constants, presented as individual polymeric or oligomeric substances by macromolecular chemists.

In front of these difficulties, some oligomeric prodrugs, when tested *in vivo*, gave excellent results. It would be outside the scope of this chapter to discuss in detail the performances of all of the substances listed in Tables 10 and 11. However, to give an example, we thought it would be interesting to relate here the results obained by us with some PEG derivatives of 4-isobutylphenyl-2-propionic acid (Ibuprofen), a well-known anti-inflammatory drug (No. 17 of Table 10).

Three derivatives were prepared, IBU-1, IBU-2, and IBU-3. IBU-1 was the monoester of tetraethyleneglycol, while IBU-2 and IBU-3 were the diesters of PEG-1000 ($\bar{n} = 21$) and PEG-2000 ($\bar{n} = 45$), respectively. Their synthesis was performed according to the following scheme:

Ibuprofen   Ibuprofen Imidazolide (IBUIM)

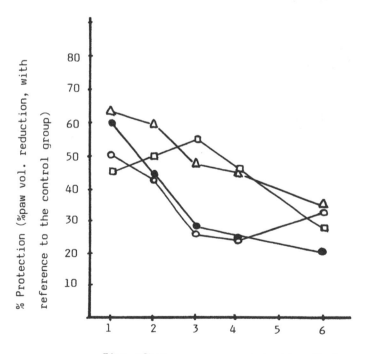

These derivatives were orally administered to fasting rats. Both protection against carrageenan-induced rat paw edema [151] under two different experimental conditions, and plasma levels, were measured. The results are shown in Figures 1-4. Only IBU-1 and IBU-3 are considered in these Figures. IBU-2 always showed an intermediate behaviour.

It may be observed (Figures 1 and 2) that in all cases a more sustained activity on time was achieved. Moreover, in the case of IBU-1 the initial activity was higher than that of equivalent doses of the free drug. This means that the bioavailability was considerably increased. These results were fully confirmed by measuring the blood levels of the drug at different times after administration (Figures 3 and 4). The acute toxicity of all these derivatives was very low, their LD_{50}

being always higher than 2000 mg/kg. Their ulcerogenic potency was somewhat lower than that of free Ibuprofen.

It is open to question why the bioavailability of IBU-1 (see Figure 3) was considerably higher than that of free Ibuprofen. It may consist either in a vehiculating effect by the promoiety across the gastrointestinal walls, leading to faster adsorption, or in a protection against partial inactivation by the liver (first-passing effect), or in a combination of both. At any rate, IBU-1 was adsorbed quickly enough to give an increase of Ibuprofen blood levels faster than that observed after administering the free drug, though needing an intermediate hydrolysis step.

Other hydrophobic acids (for instance No. 24 of Table 11), when bound as monoesters to lower PEGs, behave in the same way [17]. On the other side, it is our opinion that low-molecular weight hydrophobic oligomers would prove quite effective for increasing the bioavailability of hydrophilic drugs.

CONCLUSIONS

Oligomeric prodrugs based on known products may provide in many cases an alternative that is more ap-

Figure 1. ● — Ibuprofen, △ — IBUCOO(CH$_2$CH$_2$O)$_3$CH$_2$CH$_2$OH (IBU-1), □ — IBUCOO(CH$_2$CH$_2$O)$_{20.3}$COIBU (IBU-2), ○ — IBUCOO(CH$_2$CH$_2$O)$_{45}$CO-IBU (IBU-3)

All substances were administered orally at the abscissa times before subplantar injection of carrageenan, in a dose corresponding to 100 mg/kg Ibuprofen, to male and female Wistar rats (12 for every compound and every measurement). Paw volumes were measured 4 hr after carrageenan injection.

Table 10. Oligomeric prodrugs of Cat. a-1.

No.	Drug Linked[a]	Structure[b]	Type of Bond[c] and Synthetic Method	Leaving Group[d,e]	Starting Oligomer Table	No.	Performance[f,g]	Reference
1	Quinine (antimalarial)		4(α)	Cl	2	7	NI	[38]
2	Cholesterol		4(α)	Cl	2	7	—	[38]
3	Testosterone		4(α)	Cl	2	7	NI	[38]
4	Phenylacetic acid (M)		2a	Cl	2	9	—	[41]
5	Indomethacine (antiinflammatory)[h]		2	Cl	2	9	NI	[41,140]
6	As above	As above	2a	Cl	2	10	NI	[41,42]
7	Benzyl alcohol (M)		2	Cl	2	2	—	[34,42,140]
8	N-methylaniline (M)		1	Cl	2	2	NI	[34]

Table 10 (continued).

No.	Drug Linked[a]	Structure[b]	Type of Bond[c] and Synthetic Method	Leaving Group[d,e]	Starting Oligomer		Performance[f,g]	Reference
					Table	No.		
9	As No. 7	As No. 7	1	—	2	3	—	[34]
10	As No. 8	As No. 8	1	—	2	3	—	[34]
11	As No. 7	As No. 7	1	NP	2	4	—	[34]
12	As No. 8	As No. 8	1	NP	2	4	—	[34]
13	4-hydroxyacetanilide	HO-⟨⟩-NHCOCH$_3$	2	OH	2	1	—	[34]
14	Butyl-4-aminobenzoate (anesthetic)[h]	H$_2$N-⟨⟩-COOC$_4$H$_9$	1	DCCI	3	11	NI	[58][i]
15	Procaine (anesthetic)	H$_2$N-⟨⟩-COOCH$_2$CH$_2$N(C$_2$H$_5$)	1	DCCI	3	11	NI	[58]
16	Atropine (anticholinergic)		2	DCCI	3	11	NI	[58]
17	5-Fluorouracile		5a[i]	—	2	21	H, R	[141]
18	D,L-Mexiletine (antiarrhythmic)	H$_2$N(CH$_2$)$_3$O-⟨⟩ (CH$_3$, CH$_3$)	1	—[l]	3	1	H, R	[142]

[a]Common name and pharmacological activity.
[b]An arrow indicates the chemical group involved in binding.
[c]See Table 9. When no other indication is given, the synthetic method is that reported in the same table.
[d]When a condensing agent, as for instance a carbodiimide, is used, it is understood that the leaving group is that deriving from its reaction with the carboxy group involved.
[e]NP = 4-nitrophenoxy; DCCl = dicyclohexylcarbodiimide.
[f]In comparison with the free drug. The entry is omitted when a medl compound is involved.
[g]NI means not indicated by the authors; H = higher activity; P = prolonged activity; R = reduced toxicity; A = higher bioavailability.
[h]Other drugs have been linked to the same oligomers (and polymers) by uncleavable linkages.
[i]Monomer prepared by method 5a, then polymerized by radical initiators.
[l]"Conventional methods."

565

Table 11. Oligomeric prodrugs of Cat. a-2.[a]

No.	Drug Linked[b]	Structure[c]	Type of Bond[d] and Synthetic Method	Leaving Group[e,f]	Starting Oligomer Table	Starting Oligomer No.	Performance[g,h]	Reference
1	Quinine	See Table 10, No. 1.	4(α)	Cl	5	3, 4	NI	[76,143,144]
2	Cholesterol	See Table 10, No. 2.	4(α)	Cl	5	3, 4	—	[76]
3	Testosterone	See Table 10, No. 3.	4(α)	Cl	5	3, 4	P, A	[76,145]
4	Histamine (M)	$H_2NCH_2CH_2$—(imidazole)	3b	Cl	5	3	—	[146]
5	Methanol (M)	C_3OH	2	Im, Bz	6	31, 32	—	[113]
6	Cyclohexanol (M)	(cyclohexyl)—OH	2	Im, Bz	6	31, 32	—	[113]
7	4-Hydroxybenzoic acid (M)	HO—(phenyl)—COOH	2	Im, Bz	6	31, 32	—	[113]
8	Morpholine (M)	O(ring)NH	1	Im, Bz	6	31, 32	—	[113]
9	Piperidine (M)	(piperidinyl)NH	3b	Im	6	28	—	[119]
10	p-Cresol (M)	CH_3—(phenyl)—OH	4	Im	6	28	—	[119]
11	n-Hexanol (M)	$CH_3(CH_2)_5OH$	4	Im	6	28	—	[119]
12	Isopropanol (M)	$(CH_3)_2CHOH$	4	Im	6	28	—	[119]
13	Nicotinic acid (M) (hypolipemizing agent)	(pyridyl)—COOH	2a	Im	6	1, 2	NI	[123]
14	Procaine	See Table 10, No. 15	4(α)	Cl	6	26	—	[147]
15	Atropine	See Table 10, No. 16.	4 3a 3a	Cl	6 6 6	26 25 17	— — —	[148] [88] [88]
16	1-Amphetamine (CNS stimulant)	(phenyl)—CH_2CHCH_3 with NH_2	1		6	18	—	[88]
17	Ibuprofen (antiinflammatory)	$(CH_3)_2CHCH_2$—(phenyl)—$CH(CH_3)COOH$	2a	Im	6	1	I, P, R, A	[16]
18	Penicillin V	HOOC, H_3C, H_3C, S, N, O, NHCOR (penicillin structure)	2a		6	1		[88]

Table 11 (continued).

No.	Drug Linked[b]	Structure[c]	Type of Bond[d] and Synthetic Method	Leaving Group[e,f]	Starting Oligomer Table	No.	Performance[g,h]	Reference
19	Quinidine + spacer (glycine) (antiarrhythmic)		1		6	12		[88]
20	3-(3,17-dihydroxy-1,3,5-esatrien-7α-yl)butanoic acid		1a		6	11		[91]
21	3-oxo-4-androsten-17β-carboxylic acid		1a		6	11		[91]
22	Aspirin (antiinflammatory)		2a	Cl	6	1	I, P	[88]
23	Salicylic acid (antinflammatory)		4	Cl	6	26		[149]
24	Ursodeoxycholic acid (cholagogue)		2a	Im	6	1	P, A	[17]
25	5-Fluorouracil + spacer (anticancer)		2a	NI	6	2	"significant activity"	[150]

[a] As regards PEG derivatives the list is not exhaustive; its aim is merely to show the large potential of this family of oligomers as promoieties. For instance, some derivatives of PEG with biologically active substances, which can be regarded as oligomeric prodrugs, are listed with no references quoted in 1989 SIGMA Catalogue, including No. 17, published by us since 1981 [16].

[b] Common name and pharmacological activity.

[c] An arrow indicates the chemical group involved in binding.

[d] See Table 9. When no other indication is given, the synthetic method is that reported in the same table.

[e] When a condensing agent, as for instance a carbodiimide, is used, it is understood that the leaving group is that deriving from its reaction with the carboxy group involved.

[f] NP = 4-nitrophenoxy; DCCI = dicyclohexylcarbodiimide.

[g] In comparison with the free drug. The entry is omitted when a medl compound is involved.

[h] NI means not indicated by the authors; H = higher activity; P = prolonged activity; R = reduced toxicity; A = higher bioavailability.

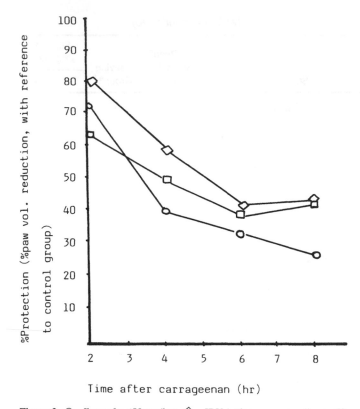

Figure 2. ○ – Ibuprofen (50 mg/kg), ◇ – IBU-1 (dose corresponding to 50 mg/kg Ibuprofen), □ – IBU-1 (dose corresponding to 30 mg/kg Ibuprofen). Substances were administered orally 1 hr before carrageenan injection in 28 male Wistar rats, randomly assigned to times, after carrageenan injection.

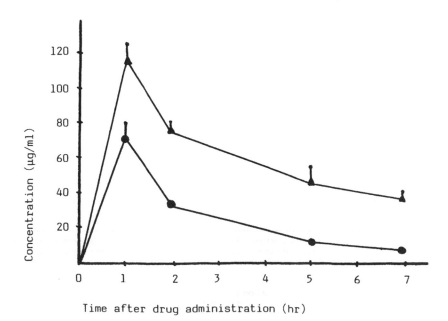

Figure 3. Ibuprofen plasma levels in male Wistar rats, after oral administration of Ibuprofen (●, 58.8 mg/kg), and IBU-1 (▲, dose corresponding to 58.8 mg/kg Ibuprofen).

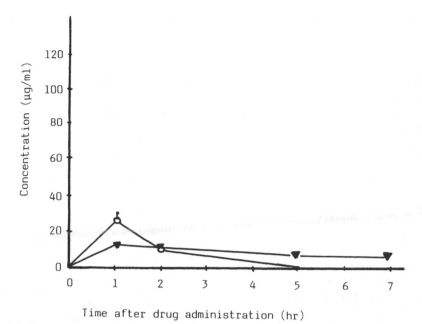

Figure 4. Ibuprofen plasma levels in male Wistar rats, after oral administration of Ibuprofen (○, 19.2 mg/kg), and IBU-3 (▼, dose corresponding to 19.2 mg/kg Ibuprofen).

pealing in terms of cost and probability of success than the search for entirely new drugs. It may be added that while prodrugs are in general justly subject to the same state regulations as new candidate drugs before being introduced into the medical practice, a combination of an already well-characterized drug with a safe promoiety is less likely to pose toxicological problems. Macromolecular chemistry has provided an imposing array of synthetic methods which are still waiting to be fully exploited for preparing oligomeric prodrugs. It has been our aim to provide the reader with a comprehensive survey of the present state of the art on this subject.

REFERENCES

1. Stella, V. J., W. N. A. Charman and V. H. Naringrekar. 1985. *Drugs*, 29:455.
2. Albert, A. 1958. *Nature*, 182:421.
3. Stella, V. 1975. "Prodrugs: An Overview and Definition" in *Pro-Drugs as Novel Drug Delivery Systems*. Hitachi and Stella, eds. Washington, DC: American Chemical Society, pp. 1–115.
4. IUPAC Commission on Macromolecular Nomenclature. 1974. *Pure Appl. Chem.*, 40:479.
5. Ferruti, P. and M. C. Tanzi. 1986. *CRC Critical Reviews in Therapeutic Drug Carrier Systems*, 2:175.
6. Ariens, E. J. and A. M. Simonis. 1974. "Drug Action: Target Tissue Dose Response Relationship and Receptors", in *Pharmacology and Pharmacokinetics*. Torrel et al. eds. New York, NY: Plenum Press, pp. 163–169.
7. Ringsdorf, H. 1975. *J. Polym. Sci. Symp.*, 51:135.
8. Rowland, G. F., G. J. O'Neill and D. A. L. Davies. 1975. *Nature*. London, 255:487.
9. Duncan, R., P. Kopečková-Rejmanová, J. Strohalm, I. Hume, H. C. Cable, J. Pohl, J. B. Lloyd and J. Kopeček. 1987. *Br. J. Cancer*, 55:165.
10. Kopeček, J. and R. Duncan. 1987. *J. Controlled Rel.*, 6:315.
11. Cartlidge, A., R. Duncan, J. B. Lloyd, P. Kopečková-Rejmanová and J. Kopeček. 1987. *J. Controlled Rel.*, 4:253.
12. Seymour, L. W., R. Duncan, J. Strohalm and J. Kopeček. 1987. *J. Biomed. Mat. Res.*, 21:1341.
13. Azori, M., I. Szinai, Z. Veres, J. Pató, L. Ötvös and F. Tüdos. 1986. *Makromol. Chem.*, 187:297.
14. Flory, J. P. 1956. *Principles of Polymer Chemistry*. Ithaca, NY: Cornell University Prep.
15. Ferruti, P., G. C. Scapini, L. Rusconi and M. C. Tanzi. 1984. "New Polymeric and Oligomeric Matrices as Drug Carriers", in *Polymers in Medicine*. E. Chiellini and P. Giusti, eds. Plenum Publishing Corp., pp. 77–95.
16. Cecchi, R., L. Rusconi, M. C. Tanzi, F. Danusso and P. Ferruti. 1981. *J. Med. Chem.*, 24:622.
17. Ghedini, N., P. Ferruti, V. Andrisano, M. R. Cesaroni and G. C. Scapini. 1983. *Synthetic Commun.*, 13:701.
18. Houk, J. and R. H. Guy. 1988. *Chem. Reviews*, 88:455.
19. Ferruti, P. 1975. *Pharmac. Res. Commun.*, 7:1.
20. Ferruti, P. 1977. *Il Farmaco Ed. Sci.*, 33:220.
21. Sawamoto, M., S. Aoshima and T. Higashimura. 1988. *Makromol. Chem. Macromol. Symp.* 13/14:513.
22. Szwarc, M. 1968. "Living Polymers", in *Encyclopedia of Polymer Science and Technology, Vol. 8.* H. Mark and N. G. Gaylord, eds., pp. 303–324.
23. Bamford, C. H. 1985. "Radical Polymerization", in *Encyclopedia of Polymer Science and Engineering*,

Vol. 13. H. F. Mark, N. M. Bikales, G. C. Overerger and G. Menges, eds., pp. 708–852.

24. Farina, M. 1987. *Makromol. Chem. Macromol. Symp.*, 10/11:255.

25. Mayo, F. R. 1943. *J. Am. Chem. Soc.*, 65:2324.

26. Flory, P. J. 1937. *J. Am. Chem. Soc.*, 59:241.

27. Boutevin, B., Y. Piétrasanta and G. Bauduin. 1985. *Makromol. Chem.*, 186:283.

28. Boutevin, B. and Y. Piétrasanta. 1985. *Makromol. Chem.*, 186:817.

29. Boutevin, B. and Y. Piétrasanta. 1985. *Makromol. Chem.*, 186:831.

30. Bauduin, G., B. Boutevin, J. P. Mistral and L. Sarraf. 1985. *Makromol. Chem.*, 186:1445.

31. Boutevin, B. and Y. Piétrasanta. 1985. *Makromol. Chem.*, 186:1457.

32. Boutevin, B., M. Maliszewcz and Y. Piétrasanta. 1985. *Makromol. Chem.*, 186:1467.

33. Pucci, B., E. Guy, F. Vial-Reveillon and A. A. Pavia. 1988. *Eur. Polym. J.*, 24:1077.

34. Bauduin, G., D. Bondon, J. Martel, Y. Piétrasanta and B. Pucci. 1981. *Makromol. Chem.*, 182:773.

35. Bauduin, G., J. M. Bessière, D. Bondon, J. Martel and Y. Piétrasanta. 1982. *Makromol. Chem.*, 183:3491.

36. Bauduin, G., D. Bondon, Y. Piétrasanta, B. Pucci and F. Vial-Reveillon. 1979. *Eur. J. Med. Chem.-Chimica Therapeutica-*, 14:119.

37. Bauduin, G., S. Casadio, Y. Piétrasanta and B. Pucci. 1980. *Chimica e Industria (Milan)*, 62:421.

38. Pinazzi, C. P., A. Menil, J. C. Rabadeux and A. Pleurdeau. 1975. *J. Polymer. Sci.*, (Symposium No. 57):1.

39. Levesque, G. and C. P. Pinazzi. 1971. *Bull. Soc. Chim. Fr.*, p. 1008.

40. Szwarč, M., M. Levy and R. Milkovich. 1956. *J. Amer. Chem. Soc.*, 78:2656.

41. Bauduin, G., J. M. Bessière, D. Bondon, J. Martel and Y. Piétrasanta. 1981. *Makromol. Chem.*, 182:3397.

42. Pinazzi, C., J. C. Rabadeux and A. Pleurdeau. 1977. *J. Polym. Sci., Polym. Chem.*, 15:2909.

43. Laguerre, A., J. C. Rabadeux, H. Gueniffey and C. M. Bruneau. 1987. *Eur. Polym. J.*, 23:851.

44. Volker, Th., A. Neumann and U. Baumann. 1963. *Makromol. Chem.*, 63:182.

45. Laguerre, A., J. C. Rabadeux, H. Gueniffey and C. M. Bruneau. 1985. *Eur. Polym. J.*, 21:349, 619.

46. Laguerre, A., J. C. Rabadeux, H. Gueniffey and C. M. Bruneau. 1987. *Eur. Polym. J.*, 23:113.

47. Kalal, J., J. Drobnick, J. Kopeček and J. Exner. 1978. *Br. Polym. J.*, 10:111.

48. Van Heeawijk, W. A. R., M. E. Eenink, J. Feijen, H. M. Pinedo, J. Lankelma and P. Lelieveld. 1982. "Synthesis and Characterization of Macromolecular Prodrugs of the Antitumor Antibiotic Adriamycin", *Int. Symp. Polymers in Medicine*, Preprint, Porto Cervo, Sardinia, pp. 23.

49. Drobník, J. and F. Rypáček. 1984. *Adv. Polym. Sci.*, 57:1.

50. Rypáček, F., V. Saudek, J. Pytela, V. Skarda. 1985. *Makromol. Chem.*, (Suppl. 9):129.

51. Ouchi, T. and A. Fujino. 1989. *Makromol. Chem.*, 190:1521.

52. Nakashima, R., T. Okauda, M. Okazaki and T. Ouchi. 1977. *Rep. Fac. Eng. Tottori Univ.*, 8:124.

53. Vert, M. and R. W. Leng. 1979. *Polym. Prepr. (Am. Chem. Soc. Div. Polym. Chem.)*, 20:608.

54. Leng, R. W. and M. Vert. 1981. U. S. Patent 4265247, *Chem. Abstr.*, 95:116201g.

55. Johns, D. B., R. Lenz and M. Vert. 1986. *J. Bioact. Compatible Polym.*, 1:47.

56. Otani, N., Y. Kimura and T. Kitao. 1961. *Kobunshi Ronbunshu*, 44:701.

57. Hirano, T., W. Klesse and H. Ringsdorf. 1979. *Makromol. Chem.*, 180:1125.

58. Bachrach, A. and A. Zilkha. 1984. *Eur. Polym. J.*, 20:493.

59. Ferruti, P., M. A. Marchisio and R. Barbucci. 1985. *Polymer*, 26:1336.

60. McCormick-Thomson, L. A. and R. Duncan. 1989. *J. Bioact. Compatible Polym.*, 4:242.

61. Bennett, D. B., N. W. Adams, X. Li, J. Feijen and S. W. Kim. 1988. *J. Bioact. Compatible Polym.*, 3:44.

62. Dick, R. C. and G. E. Ham. 1970. *J. Macromol. Sci.*, A4:1301.

63. Lukovkin, G. M., V. S. Pshezhetsky and G. A. Murtazaeva. 1973. *Europ. Polym. J.*, 9:559.

64. Saegusa, T., H. Ikeda and H. Fujii. 1972. *Polym. J.*, 3:35.

65. Ferruti, P., M. A. Marchisio and R. Barbucci. 1985. *Polymer*, 26:1336.

66. Marchisio, M. A., T. Longo and P. Ferruti. 1973. *Experientia*, 29:93.

67. Marchisio, M. A., P. Ferruti, S. Bertoli, G. Barbiano di Belgiojoso, S. M. Samour and K. D. Wolter. 1988. *Polymers in Medicine III*. C. Magliaresi et al., eds. Amsterdam: Elsevier Science Publishers B.V., pp. 111–120.

68. Ferruti, P., I. Domini, R. Barbucci, M. C. Beni, E. Dispensa, S. Sancasciani, M. A. Marchisio and M. C. Tanzi. 1983. *Biomaterials*, 4:217.

69. Ferruti, P., G. Casini, F. Tempesti, R. Barbucci, R. Mastacchi and M. Sarret. 1985. *Biomaterials*, 5:234.

70. Barbucci, R., G. Casini, P. Ferruti and F. Tempesti. 1985. *Polymer*, 26:1349.

71. Ferruti, P., F. Danusso, G. Franchi, N. Polentarutti and S. Garattini. 1973. *J. Medic. Chem.*, 16:497.

72. Duncan, R., E. Ranucci and P. Ferruti (in preparation).

73. Andreani, F., E. Salatelli and P. Ferruti. 1986. *J. Bioact. Compatible Polym.*, 1:72.

74. Veronese, F., E. Ranucci, P. Ferruti, *J. Bioact. Compatible Polym.* (in press).

75. Heitz, W. 1987. *Makromol. Chem., Macromol. Symp.*, 10/11:297.

76. Pinazzi, C. P., A. Menil and A. Pleurdeau. 1975. *Bull. Soc. Chim. France*, p. 667.

77. Goldberg, E. J. 1962. U. S. Patent 3055952.

78. Nagasaki, Y., A. Higuchi, H. Goan, N. Yoshino and T. Tsuruta. 1989. *Makromol. Chem.*, 190:53.

79. Hunter, C. G., D. E. Stevenson and P. L. Chambers. 1967. *Food. Cosmet. Toxicol.*, 5:195.

80. Stone, F. W. and J. J. Stratta. 1967. "1,2-Epoxide Polymers", in *Encyclopedia of Polymer Science and Technology*. H. F. Mark and N. G. Gaylord, eds. Wiley, New York: Wiley, 6:103–145.

81. Bailey, F. E. and J. V. Koleske. 1976. *Poly(ethylene oxide)*, New York: Academic Press.

82. Powell, G. M. 1980. "Polyethylene Glycol", in *Handbook of Water-Soluble Gums and Resins*. New York: McGraw-Hill, Chapter 18.

83. Harris, J. M. 1985. *J. Macrom. Sci. Rev. Macrom. Chem. Phys.*, C25:325.

84. Gnanou, Y., P. Lutz and P. Rempp. 1988. *Makromol. Chem.*, 189:2885.

85. Toke, L., G. T. Szabno and K. Aranyosi. 1979. *Acta Chim. Acad. Sci. Hung.*, 100:257.

86. Sukata, K. 1983. *Bull. Chem. Soc. Jpn.*, 56:280.

87. Vandoorne, F., J. Loccufier and E. Schacht. 1989. *Makromol. Chem. Rapid Commun.*, 10:271.

88. Zalipsky, S., C. Gilon and A. Zilkha. 1983. *Eur. Polym. J.*, 19:1177.

89. Buckmann, A. F., M. Morr and G. Johansson. 1981. *Makromol. Chem.*, 182:1379.

90. Johansson, G. 1970. *Biochim. Biophys. Acta*, 222:381.

91. Chaabouni, A., P. Hubert, E. Dellacherie and J. Neel. 1978. *Makromol. Chem.*, 179:1135.

92. Simionescu, C. I. and I. Rabia. 1983. *Polym. Bull.*, 10:311.

93. Mutter, M. 1978. *Tetrahedron Lett.*, p. 2839.

94. Geckeler, K. 1979. *Polym. Bull.*, 1:427.

95. Ciuffarin, E., M. Isola and P. Leoni. 1981. *J. Org. Chem.*, 46:3064.

96. Harris, J. M. and M. G. Case. 1983. *J. Org. Chem.*, 48:5390.

97. Kern, W., S. Iwabuchi, H. Sato and V. Bohmer. 1979. *Makromol. Chem.*, 180:2539.

98. Harris, J. M., M. Yalpani, J. M. Van Alstine, E. C. Struck, M. G. Case, M. S. Pale and D. E. Brooks. 1984. *J. Polym. Sci. Polym. Chem.*, 22:341.

99. Johansson, G., R. Gysin and S. D. Flanagan. 1981. *J. Biol. Chem.*, 256:9126.

100. Flanagan, S. D. and S. H. Barondes. 1975. *J. Biol. Chem.*, 250:1484.

101. Okamoto, A., K. Toyoshima and I. Mita. 1983. *Eur. Polym. J.*, 19:314.

102. Royer, G. P., 1977. U. S. Patent 4,002,531. *Chem. Abstr.*, 86:67539b.

103. Boccu, E., R. Lagajolli and F. M. Veronese. 1983. *Z. Naturforsch*, 38c:94.

104. Bayer, E., H. Zheng and K. Geckeler. 1982. *Polym. Bull.*, 8:585.

105. Paley, M. S. and J. M. Harris. 1987. *J. Polym. Sci. Polym. Chem.*, 25:2447.

106. Matsumura, S., N. Yoda and S. Yoshikawa. 1989. *Makromol. Chem. Rapid Commun.*, 10:63.

107. Johansson, G. and A. Hartman. 1974. *Proc. Int. Solvent Extract. Conf., Lyon*, p. 927.

108. Royer, G. P. and G. M. Anatharmaiah. 1979. *J. Am. Chem. Soc.*, 101:3394.

109. Fradet, A. and E. Marechal. 1981. *Polym. Bull.*, 4:205.

110. Geckeler, K. and E. Bayer. 1979. *Polym. Bull.*, 1:691.

111. Geckeler, K. and E. Bayer. 1980. *Polym. Bull.*, 3:347.

112. Veronese, F. M., E. Boccu, O. Schiavon, G. P. Velo, A. Conforti, L. Franco and R. Milanino. 1983. *J. Pharm. Pharmacol.*, 35:757.

113. Ferruti, P., M. C. Tanzi, L. Rusconi and R. Cecchi. 1981. *Makromol. Chem.*, 182:2183.

114. Berlinova, I. V. and I. M. Panayotov. 1987. *Makromol. Chem.*, 188:2141.

115. Leonard, M. and E. Dellacherie. 1988. *Makromol. Chem.*, 189:1809.

116. Abuchowski, A., T. van Es, N. C. Paczuk and F. F. Davis. 1977. *J. Biol. Chem.*, 252:3578.

117. Branstetter, F., H. Schott and E. Bayer. 1974. *Tetrahedron Lett.*, p. 2705.

118. Takerkart, G., E. Segard and M. Monsigny. 1974. *FEBS Lett.*, 24:214.

119. Galin, J. C., P. Rempp and J. Parrod. 1965. *C. R. Acad. Sc. (Paris)*, (t. 206, groupe 7)5558.

120. Tondelli, L., M. Laus, A. S. Angeloni and P. Ferruti. 1985. *J. Controlled Rel.*, 1:251.

121. Beauchamp, C. O., S. L. Gonias, D. P. Menapace and S. V. Pizzo. 1983. *Anal. Biochem.*, 131:25.

122. Pitha, J., K. Kociolek and M. G. Caron. 1979. *Eur. J. Biochem.*, 94:11.

123. Ghedini, N., V. Zecchi, A. Tartarini, G. Scapini, V. Andrisano and P. Ferruti. 1986. *J. Controlled Rel.*, 3:185.

124. Gonzalez, C. C., A. Bello and J. M. Perena. 1989. *Makromol. Chem.*, 190:1217.

125. Miyamoto, M., K. Naka, M. Taokumizu and T. Saegusa. 1989. *Mokromolecules*, 22:1604.

126. Rusconi, L., M. C. Tanzi, C. Zambelli and P. Ferruti. 1982. *Polymer*, 23:1689.

127. Boutevin, B. and B. Youssef. 1989. *Makromol. Chem.*, 190:277.

128. Madec, P. J. and E. Marechal. 1978. *J. Polym. Sci. Polym. Chem.*, 16:3165.

129. Duncan, R., H. C. Cable, J. B. Lloyd, P. Rejmanova and J. Kopeček. 1983. *Makromol. Chem.*, 184:1997.

130. Duncan, R. and J. Kopeček. 1984. *Advances Polymer Sci.*, 57:53.

131. Dumitriu, S., S. Oprea, M. Popa and R. Staicu. 1988. *Chimica Oggi*, 9:59.

132. Pató, J., M. Azori, K. Ulbrich and J. Kopecek. 1984. *Makromol. Chem.*, 185:231.

133. Pató, J., M. Azori, F. Fehérvári, G. P. Aleskiuk and F. Tüdos. 1985. *Makromol. Chem.*, (Suppl. 9):159.

134. Ferruti, P., A. Bettelli and A. Feré. 1972. *Polymer*, 13:462.

135. Ferruti, P., M. C. Tanzi and F. Vaccaroni. 1979. *J. Polym. Sci. Polym. Chem.*, 17:277.

136. Ferruti, P. 1973. "Functionalization of Polymers", in *Reaction on Polymers*. J. A. Moore, ed. Boston, MA: Reidel Publishing, pp. 73–101.

137. Ghedini, N., P. Ferruti, V. Andrisano and G. Scapini. 1983. *Synth. Commun.*, 13:707.

138. Harris, J. M., N. H. Hundley, T. G. Shannon and E. C. Struck. 1982. *J. Org. Chem.*, 47:4789.

139. Ghedini, N., P. Ferruti, V. Andrisano, M. R. Cesaroni and G. Scapini. 1983. *Synthetic Comm.*, 13:701.

140. Bauduin, G., J. Bessière, J. Martel and Y. Piétrasanta. 1984. *Makromol. Chem.*, 185:2361.

141. Ouchi, T., K. Hagita, M. Kwashima, T. Inoi and T. Tashiro. 1988. *J. Controlled Rel.*, 8:141.

142. Ye, Y., Y. Lin, C. Li and L. Xia. 1984. *Bejing Daxue Xuebao, Ziran Kexueban*, 6:59; 1987. *C. Abstr.*, 106:67647d.

143. Pinazzi, C., A. Menil and A. Pleurdeau. 1973. *C. R. Acad. Sc. Paris*, (t277,Série C):89.

144. Pinazzi, C., A. Menil and A. Pleurdeau. 1973. *Bull. Soc. Chim. France*, p. 1345.

145. Pinazzi, G. P., A. Menil, J. C. Rabaudeux and A. Pleurdeau. 1974. *J. Polym. Sci., Polym. Letters*, 12:447.

146. Pinazzi, C., J. C. Rabaudeux and A. Pleurdeau. 1977. *J. Polym. Sci. Polym. Chem.*, 15:1319.

147. Weiner, B. Z. and A. Zilkha. 1973. *J. Med. Chem.*, 16:573.

148. Weiner, B. Z., A. Zilkha, G. Porath and Y. Grunfeld. 1976. *Eur. J. Med. Chem. Chim. Ter.*, 11:525.

149. Weiner, B. Z., A. Havron and A. Zilkha. 1974. *Isr. J. Chem.*, 12:823.

150. Tatsuro, O. 1987. *Baiotekuronoji Kenkyu Hokokusho*, p. 94; 1988, *C. Abstr.*, 109:324c.

151. Winter, C. A., E. A. Risley and G. W. Nuss. 1963. *J. Pharmacol. Exp. Ther.*, 141:369.

36

Polymer Medical Dressings Containing Wound Healing Factors. Clinical Studies with Placental Angiogenic and Growth Factors

H. BURGOS, MPH, Ph.D.*

ABSTRACT: The effects of purified angiogenic and growth factors from human term placenta in polymeric carrier-dressings were studied during the treatment of chronic venous ulcers. Two double-blind initial clinical trials were carried out. Placental factors incorporated in agar-polyacrylamide dressings were used in the first trial for patients with large ulcers requiring hospitalization. Eighteen patients were randomly assigned to receive a maximum of two dressings either containing or not containing these factors. The amount of granulation and epithelial tissue was clinically estimated 48 hours after each dressing application. Patients receiving placental angiogenic and growth factors showed increased granulation and epithelial tissue. Placental factors incorporated in hydroxyethyl cellulose jelly dressings were used in a second trial for patients with small ulcers (less than 30 cm² surface area) not requiring hospitalization.

Sixteen patients were randomly allocated to receive dressings either containing or not containing these factors on an out-patient basis at weekly intervals during 12 weeks, with optional crossover midway through the treatment period. Clinical assessment of effects was carried out at each dressing application, as was measurement of ulcer size at alternate dressing applications. Patients receiving placental angiogenic and growth factors showed a mean percentage reduction of 37.24% in ulcer size. Results obtained in these clinical trials indicate that placental angiogenic and growth factors produce enhanced granulation and epithelial tissue formation and an accelerated rate of healing. They also indicate that polymeric dressings are suitable carriers for biologically active growth factors.

INTRODUCTION

Man has always shown an instinctive urge to cover his wounds for healing and protection purposes. This practice has evolved with time regarding the materials used for dressing and the topical preparations used for healing. That skin wounds need a dressing of some sort or another is an issue on which there is no complete agreement. Many cutaneous wounds, surgical wounds and burns are left exposed to the external environment or, at least, to controlled environmental conditions, and healing does occur under these circumstances [1]. With the introduction of absorbent cotton wool for dressings by Gamgee in 1880 and "tulle-gras" by Lumiere in 1903, the great majority of skin wounds, including burns and ulcers, have been dressed with soft paraffin impregnated gauze (tulle-gras) and absorbent cotton wool supported by a bandage. Antiseptic or bacteriostatic medications have been topically applied to the wound bed prior to dressing, and desloughing preparations have been done when elimination of necrotic tissues has not been previously carried out by surgery.

All wounds in man except the most superficial ones produce scar to some extent [1]. Epithelium grows down into the wound to finally make a continuous epithelial lining over the cut dermis in incised, clean, closed wounds [2] or over the granulation and scar tissue in open wounds [3]. Regeneration of epithelium from the wound edge is accompanied by regeneration from the lining of hair shafts and sweat glands in partial-thickness skin wounds, and healing occurs in about 3 weeks or less [1]. Skin donor sites, irrespective of size, are completely covered by epithelium in about 4 days [2]. On the other hand, epithelium can regenerate only from the wound edge in full thickness skin wounds involving loss of hair shafts and sweat glands [1]. This type of healing is slow in man and, almost invariably, treatment of these wounds calls for skin grafts [4].

*Blond McIndoe Centre for Medical Research, Queen Victoria Hospital, East Grinstead, Sussex, RH19 3DZ, U.K.

In spite of the fact that Robert Liston (1794–1847) covered skin wounds with lint dipped in water (sometimes with added carbolic acid if infection was present or imminent) and kept this dressing damp until improvement of the wound was evident, it was only recently reported that a moist environment enhances epithelialization in partial-thickness excision wounds and that desiccation of the wound surface, which occurs in exposed wounds and wounds covered with conventional dressings, leads to scab formation with substantial loss of superficial tissues [5–9]. Wound dehydration plays an important role in determining the final depth of wound damage [10].

This discovery gave rise to the investigation of new types of dressings that would allow healing of skin wounds under moist conditions. A number of occlusive and semi-occlusive polymer dressings (silicone, polyethylene, polyurethane and hydrogel films, membranes and foams) that would retain moisture at the wound surface and absorb or permeate excess fluid exudate appeared on the market [1,11–14]. The amount of exudate produced in skin wounds, however, all too often is considerable, especially in abraded and granulated wounds. Excessive exudate accumulates under these dressings, in spite of the partial permeability to water and presence of perforations that some of them have, and peripheral leakage of exudate occurs even when adhesive types of dressings are used. The need for frequent dressing changes then becomes imperative as the alternative of dressing perforation or syringe puncture and exudate evacuation has, in practice, limited application. Increased tissue damage under the small holes of perforated plastic film dressings has been reported [15]. This, in addition, may open a port of entry for opportunistic infection.

A new approach in wound healing has been opened with the purification and synthesis of growth-promoting factors that stimulate formation of different types of tissues. It should be possible with these growth factors to produce not only acceleration of healing but also modulation of the rate of healing in wounds [16]. Isolation and purification of angiogenic and growth-promoting factors from human placenta have been carried out [17–19]. Previous studies [20] have shown that polymeric dressings, Geliperm (Geistlich, Wolhunsen, Switzerland), a polyacrylamide-agar membrane dressing, and K-Y lubricant jelly (Johnson & Johnson Ltd., Slough, U.K.), a hydroxyethyl cellulose based gel, were suitable carriers for local administration of placental angiogenic and growth factors (PGFs). Preliminary clinical results indicated that purified PGFs promoted accelerated granulation tissue formation and epithelialization in chronic venous ulcers [20]. Two pilot clinical trials were carried out to study the effect of these factors during the treatment of chronic varicose ulcers. Because of the potential advantages of hydrogel dressings, Geliperm was used as carrier of PGFs for the treatment of large chronic venous ulcers requiring hospitalization. K-Y jelly was used as carrier of PGFs

for the treatment of small ulcers, not requiring hospitalization.

MATERIALS AND METHODS

Isolation and purification of placental angiogenic and growth factors (PGFs) have been previously described in detail by Burgos [17,18]. Briefly, whole human placentae at term, including extra-embryonic membranes and overlying decidua, were collected and homogenized in 0.15 mol/l NaCl buffered with 50 mmol/l Tris/HCl to pH 7.4 (buffered saline) with a commercial blender, and PGFs extracted by glass rod swirling at 4°C. The homogenate was centrifuged to get rid of tissue debris, and the supernatant-containing protein and peptide solutes collected and passed through ionic exchange (DEAE-Sepharose CL6B, Pharmacia U.K.) and gel filtration (Sephacryl S-300, Pharmacia U.K.) chromatography columns. Eluted fractions containing isolated biologically active PGFs were pooled and sterilized by ultrafiltration through molecular membranes of 0.2 μ pore size cutoff. These pools were frozen or lyophilized, and kept at $-20°C$ until use. PGF pools contain angiogenic and mitogenic factors of different molecular weight, including small molecular weight peptides of less than 500 daltons and polypeptides in the region of 18,000 daltons as well as high molecular weight factor–carrier protein complexes over 100,000 daltons [17,18].

Geliperm-dry is a gel made by copolymerizing a mixture of 3.5% methylbisacrylamide and 1% agarose or agar-agar. Once the polymerization process is fully completed, the monomer is eliminated by washing to less than 2 ppm. This constitutes a wet type of Geliperm dressing with a water content of 96–97%. Geliperm-dry is obtained by evaporating the water content at 40°C to 5% level. Geliperm-dry is available as 0.15 mm thick gel sheets measuring 25 × 11 cm, packed in sterile containers. Both components of Geliperm have the capacity to absorb fluids. A sheet of Geliperm-dry absorbs about 28 g-weight of a 0.9% solution of NaCl in 1 hour, the bulk of fluid being absorbed rapidly in the first 10–15 minutes. Reconstituted gel becomes slightly swollen, smooth, pliable and elastic. It allows passage of secretions and proteins but it is impermeable to bacteria because of the degree of cross-linking (Geistlich information). Experimental dressings were prepared by immersing a piece of appropriately-sized Geliperm-dry in a solution containing PGFs (26 μg protein/ml/cm² gel) for 2 hours at room temperature to allow incorporation of PGFs [20]. Control dressings were prepared by immersing the gel in buffered solution without PGFs.

K-Y jelly is made of 5% hydroxyethyl cellulose and 15% glycerin in a phosphate buffer pH 7.1 ± 0.5, giving a viscosity of approximately 500,000 cP (Johnson & Johnson information). Having been modified to contain less water than the standard preparation, it can readily be mixed with solutions of proteins or medications in anhydrous or solution form to give a gel of good consistency for topical application that can easily be washed off body surfaces. It is supplied sterile in sealed tubes. Experimental gel was prepared by mixing K-Y jelly with a solution containing PGFs (26 μg protein/ml final mixture) at a ratio 3:1 (jelly: PGF solution), incorporation of PGFs being immediate [20]. Control gel was prepared with the buffered solution without PGFs.

Patients

Approval for both clinical trials was obtained from the Hospital Ethical Committee. Patients were admitted via out-patient referrals by their general medical practitioners. Written consent for the trial was obtained from the patient in the presence of a third party after full explanation of the procedures and nature of the treatment. Patients with evidence of artheriopathy or aetiology other than venous origin and patients receiving antibiotic therapy were excluded from the trials.

Procedures

On admission, patients were randomly allocated to receive dressings containing PGFs (experimental group) or not containing PGFs (control group) in a double-blind experimental design. Large ulcers, requiring hospitalization, were treated with Geliperm dressings with or without PGFs. Ulcers with a surface area not larger than 30 cm^2 were treated with K-Y gel with or without PGFs. Initial cleansing of the ulcer was carried out with Ringer's solution wash and, if necessary, desloughed with half-strength Eusol B.P. in paraffin emulsion. This was followed by daily washing with Ringer's solution and dressing with paraffin-impregnated gauze (Jelonet, Smith & Nephew, U.K.). A cleansing agent (Aserbine, Bencard, U.K.) was applied, when necessary, until the ulcer was clean and free of pathogens before application of Geliperm dressings. Geliperm dressings with or without PGFs were left for 48 hours. The ulcer was cleaned with Ringer's solution wash, and dressing repeated if no change had occurred in the ulcer bed. Initial cleansing of the ulcer before application of K-Y gel with PGFs or without PGFs was also carried out with Ringer's solution wash and, if necessary, desloughed with half-strength Eusol. No attempt to obtain an ulcer bed free of pathogens before application of K-Y dressings was done, as this trial was carried out on an out-patient basis and, therefore, had only a low chance to maintain sterility. Bacteriological swabs, however, were taken periodically during the entire duration of the trial for monitoring type and degree of microorganism infection.

Following a Ringer's solution wash, K-Y dressings with PGFs or without PGFs were applied once a week up to a total of 12 dressings, in a double-blind crossover design with the option of changing to the other treatment group or remaining in the same group at midway in the treatment period, in accordance with the patient's own judgement. Clinical evaluations were carried out by the same member of the clinical team throughout the entire duration of the studies. These included 35 mm colour photographs taken under standard conditions. Tracing of the ulcer outline on sterile acetate sheet was carried out at alternate K-Y gel applications. These tracings were analysed in an image analyzer (Digiplan, MOP Systems, Model AM03) to measure ulcer areas. All patients, experimental and control, continued to receive adequate treatment, including skin grafts, after the trials. Procedures following the trials were out of the scope of the present studies.

RESULTS

Randomization procedures allocated 11 patients to treatment group A and 7 patients to treatment group B in the first trial using Geliperm gel. Treatment group A corresponded to patients receiving Geliperm dressings containing PGFs (experimental group), and treatment group B corresponded to patients receiving Geliperm dressings not containing PGFs (control group). Table 1 summarizes the main clinical details and results obtained. More females than males entered the trial (2.6:1 ratio). This trend was maintained in the experimental group and in the control group. Higher incidence of ulcers in females has been found in the past [32] and this was not considered unusual. Age was not significantly different between the experimental group and the control group: 63.73 ± 13.78 years (mean $\pm$ standard deviation) in the experimental group and 71.57 ± 8.28 years in the control group. Ulcer duration in the control group was about twice of that in the experimental group (24.57 ± 15.34 years and 11.64 ± 7.35 years respectively). All patients but one (patient number 3) in the experimental group showed increased granulation and epithelialization after one PGF-Geliperm dressing with the exception of patient number 11 who needed 2 dressing applications. None of the patients in the control group showed any change in the ulcer bed, except patient number 12 who presented a marginal increase of granulation without initial epithelialization after 2 dressing applications.

In the second trial using K-Y jelly dressings, 16 patients were randomly assigned to treatment group A (8 patients) and treatment group B (8 patients), and reassigned after 6 dressing applications according to the optional crossover at half-way in the treatment period. This allocated 13 patients to the treatment group A and only 3 patients to the treatment group B in the second half of the studies. The resulting treatment regimens formed 4 groups as follows:

- treatment A followed by treatment A = 7 patients (group AA)

Table 1. Granulation and epithelial tissue in chronic ulcers treated with placental angiogenic and growth factors.

Patient Number	Sex	Age (years)	Before Dressing G*	Before Dressing E**	After 1st Dressing G	After 1st Dressing E	After 2nd Dressing G	After 2nd Dressing E	Ulcer Duration (years)	Cause or Complication and Previous Treatment
Experimental Group										
1	F	42	1	–	3	+			14	Deep venous thrombosis, pernicious anaemia, split skin graft × 5
2	F	62	1	–	2	+			25	Vein injection, veins stripped
3	M	53	1	–	1	–	1	–	18	Deep venous thrombosis, oedema, eczema
6	M	75	1	–	2	+			3	Chronic icthyopia, cellulitis
9	F	74	1–2	–	3	+			17	Rheumatoid arthritis, split skin graft
10	M	54	1	–	2	+			5	Deep venous thrombosis, eczema, vein injection
11	F	44	1	–	1	–	2	+	14	Deep venous thrombosis, split skin graft × 2
13	F	84	1	–	3	+			2	Deep venous thrombosis, phlebitis, vein injection
14	F	66	1	–	2	+			15	Rheumatoid arthritis, chemical sympathectomy, split skin graft
17	F		1	–	1–2	+			11	Veins stripped, pinch graft × 2, split skin graft
18	F	76	1–2	–	2	+			4	Deep venous thrombosis, pinch graft × 3, split skin graft
Control Group										
15	M	64	1	–	1	–	1	–	12	Deep venous thrombosis, pinch graft × 3
4	F	67	1–2	–	1–2	–	1–2	–	11	Diabetes, split skin graft
5	F	64	1	±	1	±	1	±	37	Phlebitis, split skin graft × 2
7	F	68	1	±	1	±	1	±	15	Deep venous thrombosis, pinch graft
8	F	84	1	–	1	–	1	–	53	Veins stripped, split skin graft
12	M	82	1	–	1	–	1–2	–	21	Deep venous thrombosis, veins stripped, split skin graft
16	F	72	1–2	–	1–2	–	1–2	–	23	Deep venous thrombosis, split skin graft × 2

*Granulation: 1, insufficient to allow skin graft; 2, adequate for skin graft; 3, overgranulation.
**Presence of initial epithelialization. +present; – absent; ± marginal.
(Reproduced with permission from Burgos, H. et al., 1989: *J. Roy. Soc. Med.*, 82:598–599.)

Table 2. Baseline demographics of patients with chronic ulcers.

	Treatment Group			
	AA	AB	BA	BB
Number of patients	7	1	6	2
Sex: male	2	0	3	0
female	5	1	3	2
Age (years)	76.86 ± 12.08*	69	58.83 ± 10.65	67.5 ± 7.78
Ulcer duration (years)	18.14 ± 18.87	20	9.33 ± 4.93	1.65 ± 0.49
Initial ulcer size (cm²)	10.31 ± 6.26	3.96	15.23 ± 6.70	3.69 ± 0.50

A = Treated with dressings containing placental growth factors.
B = Treated with dressings not containing placental growth factors.
* = Mean ± standard deviation.

- treatment A followed by treatment B = 1 patient (group AB)
- treatment B followed by treatment A = 6 patients (group BA)
- treatment B followed by treatment B = 2 patients (group BB)

Treatment A corresponded to K-Y dressings containing PGFs (experimental dressings), and treatment B corresponded to K-Y dressings not containing PGFs (control dressings). Baseline demographics for each group are outlined in Table 2. Statistical analyses were confined to groups AA and BA only as numbers of patients in the remaining groups were too small. More females than males also entered this trial (2.2:1 ratio). This trend was maintained in group AA (2.5:1 ratio) but not in group BA (1:1 ratio). No significant difference between these groups was found regarding age and initial ulcer size.

Mean ulcer duration in group AA was about twice of that in group BA. On clinical examination, ulcers appeared to go through an initial period of enlargement, including breakdown of surrounding skin areas, during the first weeks of treatment, before a clear picture of improvement was established in ulcers that continued to heal until the end of the studies. Tables 3 and 4 show the results obtained regarding ulcer size. A mean decrease in ulcer size of 2.97 cm^2 was present in patients of group AA receiving PGF-Geliperm dressings during the entire duration of the study. This corresponds to an overall reduction of 37.24% in ulcer size in group AA.

Reduction in ulcer size was accompanied by a significant increase in granulation and epithelial tissue in 85.7% of the ulcers in group AA. Tables 5 and 6 summarize the results obtained regarding amounts of granulation and epithelial tissue respectively. A significant amount of granulation in group AA was formed over the entire duration of the trial ($x^2 = 7.36$; d.f. = 2; $p > 0.02$) as was a significant amount of epithelial tissue ($x^2 = 10.5$; d.f. = 3; $p > 0.01$).

On the other hand, a mean increase of 11.19 cm^2 in ulcer size was present over the entire duration of the trial in group BA receiving control dressings during the first half of the study followed by experimental dressings after the midway optional crossover. This corresponds to an overall increase of 24.77% ulcer size in group BA. However, highly significant increase in granulation and epithelial tissue was present in 83.3% of the ulcers in group BA during the second part of the study while receiving treatment A (PGF-KY dressings). Significantly more granulation was formed in group BA during treatment A than during treatment B ($x^2 = 10$; d.f. = 2; $p > 0.001$) and significantly more epithelial tissue as well ($x^2 = 5.33$; d.f. = 1; $p > 0.02$). This produced a significant overall increase in granulation ($x^2 = 12$; d.f. = 2; $p > 0.001$) and epithelial tissue ($x^2 = 8.56$; d.f. = 1; $p > 0.001$) during the entire trial duration.

Table 3. Ulcer size in chronic ulcers treated with or without placental growth factors.

Treatment Group	Patient Number	Ulcer Size (cm²) At Baseline	At Crossover	At End Point
AA	1	1.51	0.68	0.00
	16	18.17	12.23	9.93
	14	17.41	47.70	15.60
	9	5.40	2.94	2.92
	3	13.54	3.57	7.58
	6	7.57	5.89	5.27
	8	8.54	4.38	10.08
AB	11	3.96	6.96	5.40
BA	4	7.06	7.14	12.34
	5	15.16	31.09	30.80
	10	27.23	32.84	72.19
	12	16.35	6.42	11.29
	15	13.02	10.56	10.80
	13	12.53	15.30	21.10
BB	2	4.04	2.71	4.38
	7	3.33	3.97	23.77

	Mean ± Standard Deviation		
A	9.51 ± 6.21	10.54 ± 15.40	
B	12.34 ± 7.78	13.75 ± 11.91	
AA	10.31 ± 6.26	11.06 ± 16.56	7.34 ± 5.17
BA	15.23 ± 6.70	17.23 ± 11.85	26.42 ± 23.72

A = Treated with dressings containing placental growth factors.
B = Treated with dressings not containing placental growth factors.

DISCUSSION

The ideal wound dressing has not yet been found. Different types of wounds require different types of dressings. This complicates the search for ideal types of dressings. There are, however, some characteristics that seem to be desirable in all medical dressings. Browne [21] gives a list of desirable features in wound dressings (Table 7). Other characteristics like low cost and relative ease of application may also be considered. The increasing knowledge concerning the physiopathology of skin wounds and mechanisms of wound healing and repair that has accumulated in the last decades has given rise to the search for new types of medical dressings. The contribution made by the background information on biocompatible polymers has been considerable, and so has the study of interactions between biopolymers and proteins, a decisive factor in the development of polymeric dressings carrying biologically active components.

Since the embedding of a drug into an inert porous polymeric matrix was proposed by Higuchi in 1963 [22] immobilization of bioactive components in polymeric carriers for slow and controlled release has been applied successfully in local and systemic drug delivery. Entrapping of protein macromolecules and tumour angiogenic factor in polymer pellets was used by Langer and Folkman [23] to carry out biological

Table 4. Percentage change in ulcer size of chronic ulcers treated with or without placental growth factors.

Treatment Group	Patient Number	% Change Baseline to Crossover	% Change Crossover to End Point	% Change Baseline to End Point
AA	1	−55.0	−100.0	−100.0
	16	−32.7	−18.8	−45.3
	14	+63.5	−67.3	−10.4
	9	−45.5	−00.7	−45.9
	3	−73.6	+52.9	−44.0
	6	−22.2	−10.5	−30.4
	8	−48.7	+56.5	+15.3
AB	11	+43.1	−22.4	+26.6
BA	4	+01.1	+42.1	+42.8
	5	+51.2	−00.9	+50.8
	10	+17.0	+54.5	+62.3
	12	−60.7	+43.1	−30.9
	15	−18.9	+02.3	−17.0
	13	+18.1	+27.5	+40.6
BB	2	−32.9	+38.1	+07.8
	7	+44.2	+74.9	+86.0

	Mean		
A	−21.39		
B	+2.39		
AA	−30.60	−12.56	−37.24
BA	+1.30	+28.10	+24.77

A = Treated with dressings containing placental growth factors.
B = Treated with dressings not containing placental growth factors.
− Indicates reduction in ulcer size.
+ Indicates increase in ulcer size.

assays. Polymers (polyacrylamide, Hydron S, ethylene/vinyl acetate copolymer) were dissolved in appropriate solvents and mixed with macromolecular proteins. The mixture was cast in moulds, and the solvent evaporated. These pellets showed sustained release of macromolecules when implanted in the cornea of rabbits. Burgos [17] immobilized placental angiogenic and growth factors in agar–gelatin matrix contained inside a capsule made of ethylene/vinyl acetate copolymer. Pure gelatin capsules were previously coated with copolymer dissolved in dichloromethane, the solvent evaporated, and the capsule exhaustibly washed of the solvent. The semi-permeability of the thin vinyl polymer capsule made this device able to function as a subcutaneous osmotic pump delivery system for slow and sustained release of growth factors.

The large degree of polymerizability presented by vinyl polymers at low temperature and the low dose of irradiation needed to initiate a chain reaction for polymerization have been used with advantage for immobilization of anticancer drugs, hormones, enzymes and antigens in monolithic devices [24]. Biocomponent and monomer are mixed, and the mixture is then shaped for polymerization in this system. Immobilization of biocomponents by adsorption onto an already fully polymerized carrier calls for less stringent requirements. PGFs exhibit aromatic and hydrophobic interactions with polysaccharide and polyacrylamide gel beds [17,18]. Antibiotics have been immobilized by ionic exchange or covalently coupled on cellulose derivatives in medical bandages [25].

Principles controlling protein adsorption to polymers, and conditions for desorption and release of proteins, are well established, especially with protein-containing buffer systems [26–29]. Protein adsorption to solid surfaces is an inevitable effect for any surface in contact with a protein-containing buffer [27]. Desorption occurs when the surface tension of the buffer decreases to a level between that of the protein and that of the polymeric carrier, the free energy of adhesion becoming positive and the van der Waals interactions between protein and polymer becoming repulsive [28]. Release would then follow by diffusion. Absorption of PGFs by Geliperm-dry was rapid (within 2 hours), and release showed a large burst-effect [20]. This is a characteristic of surface-immobilized biocomponents.

Table 8 shows the release of PGFs incorporated in Geliperm gel. The burst-effect was, undoubtedly, enhanced in these studies because the aqueous phase

Table 5. Amount of granulation in chronic ulcers treated with or without placental growth factors.

Treatment Group	Amount of Granulation Tissue At Baseline	At Crossover	At End Point
A	0.25 ± 0.71*	1.00 ± 0.93	
B	0.00 ± 0.00	0.38 ± 0.74	
AA	0.29 ± 0.76	1.14 ± 0.90	1.43 ± 0.79
BA	0.00 ± 0.00	0.38 ± 0.82	1.00 ± 1.00

A = Treated with dressings containing placental growth factors.
B = Treated with dressings not containing placental growth factors.
* = Mean ± standard deviation.
0 = No granulation tissue.
1 = Some granulation tissue.
2 = Granulation adequate for skin graft.

Table 6. Amount of epithelial tissue in chronic ulcers treated with or without placental growth factors.

Treatment Group	Amount of Epithelium At Baseline	At Crossover	At End Point
A	0.00 ± 0.00*	0.63 ± 0.74	
B	0.00 ± 0.00	0.38 ± 0.52	
AA	0.00 ± 0.00	0.71 ± 0.76	1.14 ± 0.90
BA	0.00 ± 0.00	0.17 ± 0.41	0.38 ± 0.41

A = Treated with dressings containing placental growth factors.
B = Treated with dressings not containing placental growth factors.
* = Mean ± standard deviation.
0 = No epithelium.
1 = Epithelial margin <5 mm.
2 = Epithelial margin >5 mm.

(instead of buffer phase) was used as sink for the released PGFs.

On the other hand, the rate of release of drugs suspended in ointment bases can be regulated by controlling the concentration of the drug, the diffusion coefficient (viscosity) and the solubility of the drug [30]. Concentration and viscosity could easily be changed in PGF-KY gels, but solubility was less amenable to control within the physiological buffer systems used in these preparations. Absorption of PGFs and K-Y jelly was immediate by mixing the components to homogeneity, and release was gradual into the buffer sink [20]. This type of release indicates a greater dissolution of biocomponents in the jelly matrix. Table 9 shows the release of PGFs incorporated in K-Y jelly. Both PGF-Geliperm and PGF-KY dressings would exhibit a slower rate of release into the surface sink presented by a skin ulcer. Sustained release of an active agent from a properly selected material to act as rate-controlling carrier, and release of the active agent at the desired site of activity are the two major purposes of a carrier [31]. Geliperm and K-Y dressings fulfilled these purposes. Evaluation of other characteristics of these dressings was out of the scope of the trials. The results obtained in the present clinical studies point out the potential use that polymer dressings may offer as carriers for biologically active growth factors.

Many preparations have been claimed to speed up healing. That acceleration of healing occurs by the effect of such preparations is very difficult to ascertain. A better management of the wound may account for the enhanced rate of healing found in some cases. Results obtained in the present first clinical trial showed enhanced granulation and accelerated epithelialization in ulcers treated with PGFs. This trend was supported by the results obtained in the second clinical trial. Ulcers treated with PGFs presented increased granulation and epithelial tissue and decreased ulcer size, including complete closure of the ulcer. The consistent trend for ulcers treated with PGFs to decrease in size may well have resulted in complete closure and healing of the ulcer in many patients, had the treatment continued for longer periods of time. Other growth-promoting factors, fibroblast growth factor (FGF), epidermal growth factor (EGF), platelet-derived growth factor (PDGF) etc, also produce acceleration of healing [16,32].

It is clear that clinical use of growth-promoting factors may play an important role in wound healing. There is, however, the need for more studies on the effect of these factors in skin wounds, on dose and frequency of application. Titration of mitogenic activity of PGFs demonstrated a wide range of PGF concentrations expressing biological activity [20]. This gives an ample margin to work out the most appropriate dose to meet individual requirements by varying the concentration of PGFs prior to incorporation in the carrier dressing. There is a need to study the mechanisms of action of these factors, as well as their

Table 7. Desirable features in wound dressings.

1. Should be sterile
2. Should not allow passage of bacteria or support bacterial growth
3. Should provide mechanical protection for the wound
4. Should conform to the contour of the wound
5. Should absorb or transmit wound exudate
6. Should provide a suitable microclimate for healing:
   a) Warmth
   b) Moisture at wound–dressing interface
   c) Access for oxygen
7. Should not fragment or discharge toxic substances into the wound
8. Should not damage or inhibit new tissues developing in the wound. Should not adhere to the wound
9. Should be non-allergic and non-sensitizing
10. Should provide comfort

(Reproduced with permission from Browne, M. K., 1987. *Care, Science and Practice*, 5:13–15.)

Table 8. Release of placental growth factors incorporated in Geliperm.

Time (hours)	% Mitogenic Activity
0	0
1/2	56
1	75
2	88
4	91
8	93
24	98

Pieces of Geliperm membrane containing placental factors were immersed in distilled water at 4°C for increasing periods of time to allow release of factors into the water sink. The liquid was collected, lyophilized and added to 3T3 fibroblast cultures. Mitogenic activity was measured by the amount of 3H-thymidine incorporated into DNA, and calculated as % of total activity released in 48 hours.
(Reproduced with permission from Burgos H., 1987. *Clin. Materials*, 2:133–139; Edward Arnold, Publisher.)

Table 9. Release of placental growth factors incorporated in K-Y jelly.

Time (hours)	Optical Absorbancy at 280 nm			
	4°C		37°C	
	−PGFs	+PGFs	−PGFs	+PGFs
0	.000	.000	.000	.000
1	.024	.049	.024	.083
2	.043	.093	.053	.139
4	.060	.128	.087	.209
8	.084	.180	.122	.296
24	.121	.277	.208	.506

Aliquots of K-Y jelly containing or not containing placental factors were immersed in buffered saline at 4°C and 37°C for increasing periods of time to allow release of factors into the buffer sink. The liquid was collected and optical absorbancy measured at 280 nm.
+PGFs = K-Y jelly containing placental growth factors.
−PGFs = K-Y jelly not containing placental growth factors.
(Reproduced with permission from Burgos, H., 1987. *Clin. Materials*, 2:133–139; Edward Arnold, Publisher.)

additive and/or synergistic effects, so that appropriate mixtures of factors can be prepared in accordance with the type and condition of the wound. A mixture of PGFs rather than just one of the family of placental factors was used in the present studies because previous experimental and clinical results indicated additive and synergistic biological activities of these factors [17,20]. Composition of growth factor mixtures may also be chosen and modified according to especial or specific purposes besides the prime object of healing: enhanced angiogenesis, keratinocyte proliferation, inhibition of fibroblast proliferation and scar formation etc. There are different pathways in wound healing that may be open to modulation by the biological activities of growth factors.

There is, on the other hand, a need for research and development on medical dressings. Advancement in biocompatible polymers and polymer synthesis technology will, no doubt, result in the production of better types of dressings, carriers of growth-promoting factors. Synthetic polymers can theoretically be made to meet any specific characteristic that is required in carrier and delivery devices, while maintaining compatibility with the bioactive agent. Conventional chemical synthesis may, however, produce biomaterials with a limited range of properties that cannot satisfy the demands imposed by ideal types of dressings. Natural polymers may give an alternative approach although these may have to be modified in order to conform with the requirements for medical applications.

On the other hand, a conjugated approach taking advantage of both synthetic and natural polymer systems may be more appropriate for meeting the broad spectrum of characteristics required by ideal wound dressings, carriers of growth-promoting factors. Dressings for the present clinical studies fall under this category. Even more, biodegradable dressings may, in cases, be indicated in wound healing. Amnion epithelium, a biodegradable biological dressing possessing angiogenic factors, has been successfully used in the treatment of chronic ulceration of the legs [33]. In this connection, the large degree of biodegradability exhibited by natural polymers would place them at advantage over synthetic polymers.

On another line of studies, biodegradable polymeric membrane carriers for cultured human epithelium (and also for skin grafts) may overcome the drawbacks of currently used gauze carriers. In addition, growth-promoting factors may be incorporated in biodegradable polymeric membranes carrying cultured epithelium, to enhance angiogenesis of the wound bed on one side and stimulate growth of graft keratinocytes on the other. This may improve the rate of take of cultured skin autografts, currently running at only 30% even after transfer of successfully cultured epithelium [34]. Enhanced angiogenesis and granulation tissue formation and accelerated incorporation of dermis allografts carrying decidua angiogenic factors have been reported by Burgos et al. in experimental skin wounds [35]. This may provide an efficient way of treating wounds with deep loss of tissues, especially burn wounds where angiogenesis is slow to start and slow to proceed [16]. A new era in wound healing is emerging with the use of growth-promoting factors and the aid of biopolymer technology. The initial steps have already been taken.

ACKNOWLEDGEMENTS

This work was supported by grants from the East Grinstead Medical Research Trust and Johnson & Johnson Ltd. Both clinical trials were carried out with the collaboration of Dr. A. Herd, Clinical Research Fellow, and Mr. J. P. Bennett, FRCS, Consultant in Plastic Surgery. The author thanks Mrs. I. Andrews, SRN, for clinical assistance, and Dr. B. Dennis and Miss C. Mulligan, SRN, of Johnson & Johnson for the preparation of protocols, subject records and forms, and statistical analyses.

REFERENCES

1. Lawrence, J. C. 1983. *Wound Healing Symposium*. Oxford: The Medicine Publishing Foundation.
2. Calnan, J. S. 1983. *Wound Healing Symposium*. Oxford: The Medicine Publishing Foundation.
3. Remensnyder, J. P. 1983. *Wound Healing Symposium*. Oxford: The Medicine Publishing Foundation.
4. Casons, J. S. 1983. *Treatment of Burns*. London, England: Chapman and Hall.
5. Winter, G. D. 1962. *Nature*, 193:293–294.
6. Hinman, C. D. and H. Maibach. 1963. *Nature*, 200:377–378.
7. Sharbaugh, R. J., T. S. Harges, and F. A. Wright. 1973. *Amer. Surgeon*, 39:253–256.
8. Bergman, R. B. 1977. *Arch. Chirurg Niederland*, 29:69–72.
9. Thomson, C. W., D. W. Ryan, L. J. Dunkin, M. Smith and M. Marshall. 1980. *Lancet*, i:568–570.
10. Zawacki, B. E. 1974. *Ann. Surg.*, 180:98–102.
11. Groves, A. R. 1983. *Wound Healing Symposium*. Oxford: The Medicine Publishing Foundation.
12. May, S. R. 1983. *Wound Healing Symposium*. Oxford: The Medicine Publishing Foundation.
13. Spector, M., L. Rhinelander and F. Nahai. 1987. *Biomaterials and Clinical Applications*. Amsterdam, Netherlands: Elsevier Science Publishers.
14. Jonkman, M. F., H. J. Meijer, J. W. Leenslag, A. J. Pennings, P. Nieuwenhuis and I. Molenaar. 1987. *Biomaterials and Clinical Applications*. Amsterdam, Netherlands: Elsevier Science Publishers.
15. Winter, G. 1963. *J. Invest. Dermatol.*, 45:299.
16. Hunt, T. K. 1984. *J. Trauma*, 24:S39–S46.
17. Burgos, H. 1983. *Eur. J. Clin. Investig.*, 13:289–296.

18. Burgos, H. 1986. *Eur. J. Clin. Investig.*, 16:486–493.

19. Moscatelli, D. A., M. Presta, P. Mignatti, D. E. Mullins, R. M. Crowe and D. B. Rifkin. 1986. *Anticancer Res.*, 6:861–863.

20. Burgos, H. 1987. *Clinc. Materials*, 2:133–139.

21. Browne, M. K. 1987. *Care, Science and Practice*, 5:13–15.

22. Higuchi, T. 1963. *J. Pharm. Sci.*, 52:1145–1149.

23. Langer, R. and J. Folkman. 1976. *Nature*, 263:797–799.

24. Kaetsu, I. 1983. *Biocompatible Polymers, Metals and Composites*. Lancaster, PA: Technomic Publishing Co., Inc.

25. Simionescu, C. and S. Dumitriu. 1983. *Polymers in Medicine, Biochemical and Pharmacological Applications*. New York, NY and London, England: Plenum Press.

26. Szycher, M. 1983. *Biocompatible Polymers, Metals and Composites*. Lancaster, PA: Technomic Publishing Co., Inc.

27. Brash, J. L. 1983. *Biocompatible Polymers, Metals and Composites*. Lancaster, PA: Technomic Publishing Co., Inc.

28. Neumann, A. W., D. R. Absolom, W. Zingg, C. J. van Oss and D. W. Francis. 1983. *Biocompatible Polymers, Metals and Composites*. Lancaster, PA: Technomic Publishing Co., Inc.

29. Vroman, L. 1983. *Biocompatible Polymers, Metals and Composites*. Lancaster, PA: Technomic Publishing Co., Inc.

30. Higuchi, T. 1961. *J. Pharm. Sci.*, 50:874–875.

31. McRea, J. C. and S. W. Kim. 1983. *Biocompatible Polymers, Metals and Composites*. Lancaster, PA: Technomic Publishing Co., Inc.

32. Brunt, J. V. and A. Klausner. 1988. *Biotechnology*, 6:25–30.

33. Bennett, J. P., R. Matthews and W. P. Faulk. 1980. *Lancet*, i:1153–1156.

34. Eldad, A., A. Burt, J. A. Clarke and B. A. Gusterson. 1987. *Burns*, 13:173–180.

35. Burgos, H., E. S. Lindenbaum, D. Beach, N. G. Maroudas and B. Hirshowitz. 1989. *Burns*, 15:310–314.

37

Studies of Wound Healing and the Effects of Dressings

S. E. BARNETT, CBiol, MIBiol*
S. J. IRVING, BSC, CBiol, MIBiol*

ABSTRACT: The healing of wounds and the use of dressings are so commonplace an occurrence that they are often taken for granted. For most minor injuries there is probably little advantage in sophisticated dressings; however, for satisfactory healing after trauma involving extensive tissue loss, it is now recognised that the right choice of dressing for a particular wound at a particular healing stage is important because of the need to control the microenvironment of the healing wound. The effects of both established and novel dressing types are presented, and compared on a standard wound model, with particular reference to the problem of adhesion.

INTRODUCTION

The ability of the human body to heal its wounds involves its more primitive function of preserving life, and there are many factors both favourable and unfavourable that can influence the series of well-ordered cellular and biochemical events in the repair process.

It is a well-known fact that most wounds, in an otherwise healthy person, will heal naturally without complex intervention, even in the presence of a limited degree of infection. However, from the earliest days of recorded history man has made use of a large variety of substances and methods to dress wounds [1]. The Ebers Papyrus (c. 1550 B.C.), accepted as the oldest complete Egyptian medical treatise, mentions castor oil for application to septic wounds and burns and the use of hartshorn "to drive out painful swellings" [2].

By simple observation, people quickly identified those substances and methods that promoted healing of an injury. The body of knowledge that evolved concerning the efficacy of such dressings would have been passed on to succeeding generations.

This empirical approach to wound management has persisted throughout history, and it was not until the early part of this century that studies were made into the processes occurring within the wound rather than simply the external manifestations. Almost all of these early studies of healing tissues were carried out using experimental animals, particularly small mammals, and the results were accepted as corresponding exactly to the human condition. The failure to appreciate the fact that the resemblance of human skin to that of various breeds of hairless mice and dogs and sparsely haired pigs is only superficial and does not constitute a real similarity has led to disappointing results. If animal skin had been fully studied, it would have been possible to select the right species for specific experimental purposes pertinent to human medicine. Unfortunately, most studies in comparative cutaneous biology are poorly documented and little is known about the skin of some animals. This must then be taken into account in reporting effects of dressings and medicaments since no skin, not even that of great apes, is quite like that of man [3].

The first comprehensive microscopical survey of human wounds and how they compared to wounds in experimental animals was carried out by Hartwell in the 1930s [4]. By comparing human wounds with those studied in dogs, guinea pigs, rabbits and pigs, he showed the marked differences in the mechanisms of healing of both the epithelial and sub-epithelial tissues. He concluded that only in the domestic swine did the histological picture of healing resemble that found in human wounds. Further evidence of this resemblance was provided by the work of Hinman et al. [5] who compared healing in healthy male volunteers with that in pedigree pigs, and the more recent work of Gangjee et al. on percutaneous wound healing [6].

Major use of the pedigree domestic pig for wound healing research was made by the late George Winter

*Department of Research in Plastic Surgery, Regional Plastic, Maxillofacial & Oral Surgery Centre, Mount Vernon Hospital, Northwood, Middlesex, HA6 2RN, U.K.

between 1960 and 1979. He defined the advantages of this animal model over more commonly used species bearing in mind that there were undoubtedly differences in the structure of skin from different areas of the body and other breeds of pig [7]. With these reservations it is possible to compare the skin of the pig and that of man. Winter's studies concerned skin from a single body region, the back, of pedigree Large Whitae pigs.

The thickness of the epidermis and dermis are about the same. In man and the pig there are fewer hair follicles per unit area of skin than in the majority of mammals, and associated with this is a well-developed system of epidermal ridges and a distinct dermal papillary layer. In both man and pig there is a relatively deep layer of fat under the dermis (the superficial fascia of human anatomy) and there is no panniculus carnosus. In neither is the skin very mobile on the underlying structures.

In both porcine and human skin hair replacement occurs independently in individual follicles and not in waves of simultaneous activity, as it does, for instance, in the rat [8] and the mouse [9].

According to Moritz and Henriques [10] the distribution of blood vessels in the skin of the pig is very similar to that in man. Thus, in its basic structure porcine skin is quite similar to human skin. Most of the similarities seem to be due to the fact that in man and the pig, fat rather than fur provides the body's insulation against excessive heat loss.

The main differences between pig skin and human skin lie in the kind of epidermal appendages and structure, and the role of the skin in the regulation of body heat by sweating. Hair follicles in pig skin are much larger than in human skin. The sebaceous glands on the other hand are smaller. Skin from the general body surface of the pig, like that of most mammals, differs from human skin in the presence of many large apocrine glands and the total absence of eccrine glands. Most reports agree that the pig does not regulate body temperature by sweating, as humans do. The function of the apocrine glands is thus unclear.

The skin of the pig is thus considered to resemble the skin of man more closely than that of any other commonly used experimental animal, but it is not identical; porcine and human skin differ significantly when looked at in detail.

Winter developed a number of standard wound models in the domestic pig and described in detail the mechanisms by which they heal [11]. These standard models were also used to test the effects of dressings [12], dressing régimes [13], and other topical treatments [14]. The results of these very fundamental studies gave what is possibly the first truly comparative experimental evidence proving that wounds that are kept moist heal faster than those which suffer dehydration [15]. Much of the recent development in wound dressing design is based upon this understanding [16].

Many classifications of wounds have been made over the years but from a treatment standpoint there are essentially two types of wounds: those which are characterized by loss of tissue and those in which no tissue has been lost [17].

Three stratagems of healing are discerned:

(1) Some of the lost tissue is replaced from the uninjured tissue around the wound, which is stretched into the wound by contraction of the repair tissue.

(2) Some of the lost tissue is replaced by a specific repair tissue. The dermis is incapable of regeneration, and therefore the tissue that repairs the wound originates locally from vascular, loose connective tissue adjacent to the wound.

(3) Some of the lost tissue is truly regenerated, notably the epidermis, and the blood and lymphatic vessels. Nerves and elastic tissue are also replaced to some extent, but skin wounds are basically healed by growth of the epidermis, the blood and lymphatic vessels, and fibrous tissue. The main problems, therefore, are the initiation and control of the growth of epidermal and endothelial cells and fibroblasts.

The primary tactic for the growth of epidermal cells and fibroblasts is cell locomotion. It is believed that loss of contact inhibition starts these cells moving into an adjacent space not populated by homologous cells. Probably the same thing applies to endothelial cells. Movement cannot be sustained for long without replenishment of cell numbers, and sooner or later if a tissue is to grow, cells must reproduce themselves by increased mitotic activity.

Thus, the broad outlines of the healing process are clear. The injury, or loss of cells consequent upon injury, is the primary stimulus to healing. It unlocks basic cell mechanisms—locomotion and cell division—which in the interest of order in the tissues are normally under control of inhibitory mechanisms. Such inhibitory mechanisms, feeding back information about fluctuations in the density of the cell population to the cells concerned, satisfactorily account for normal growth adjustments in the tissues. How far is wound healing to be regarded as an explosive episode of normal growth and how far is it a special process unlike anything that occurs in the tissues from day to day? The situation is clearest in the epidermis where it seems likely that regeneration after injury differs in no essential aspect from the continuous "physiological regeneration" of the epidermis.

EVALUATION OF DRESSINGS—METHODS OF STUDY

Ideally one would like to study the effects of dressings, ointments, and other topical medicaments directly upon wounds in man, and in the last resort a novel treatment will be judged only in the light of extensive clinical experience. In the early stages of investigations into a new dressing, clinical trials may be out of the question or, if done, may yield meagre results because individuals and their wounds vary so much. No two wounds are ever exactly alike, and an enormous effort is required to produce statistically valid results. Mere inspection or photography of wounds gives insufficient information. It may occasionally be possible to obtain biopsies of patients' tissues for microscopic examination, and some useful fundamental observations on the effects of dressings have been obtained this way. Often, however, it is neither practical nor ethical to obtain more than a few biopsies of experimentally treated human wounds. In the face of these difficulties, a suitable wound model is often necessary. A reliable technique is essential and adequate controls should also be included. The test must be appropriate to the intended practical applications and preferably it should yield quantitative data.

The experimental data presented here are based on work carried out using the domestic pig. It is essential to use a healthy uniform breed of animals, and ordinary farm pigs are not satisfactory. Animals are purchased from a pedigree herd and are individually selected on the basis of a healthy appearance and a clean untraumatised skin. They are brought into the animal house and kept in individual pens and acclimatised for three weeks to their accommodation and to handling in order to minimise stress which adversely affects healing [18].

The relatively large size of the pig allows for comparison of up to six wounds treated with an experimental dressing with six wounds as controls on the same animal, at the same time, under identical environmental conditions thus reducing both interanimal variation and the number of animals required. The use of a padded guard prevents accidental damage to the wounds and allows for the use of standard secondary dressings.

For many purposes, a shallow excised wound provides the best opportunity for making meaningful observations on the effects of dressings and medicaments. Epithelization, mainly from the cut ends of hair follicles, is complete in about seven days under normal conditions, which allows a sufficient margin either way to detect acceleration or inhibition of epidermal regeneration brought about by different treatments. Such wounds never become septic, and the basic pattern of healing is well documented. A large surface area of superficial dermis is exposed, allowing gross differences to be recorded when conditions at the wound surface are varied. The wound is equivalent to a Thiersch graft donor site or a graze, and thus has clinical relevance. Incisions are less helpful because when the wound edges are brought close together by sutures new epidermis bridges the narrow gap within 48 hours.

Deep excised wounds and burns pose special problems. Experimentally it is more difficult to produce a standard lesion and consequently the speed of healing is more variable. It has been found that more knowledge can be gained from a qualitative assessment of the stage of healing reached by deep wounds at any given time rather than attempting to produce quantitative data for statistical analysis.

Female Large White pigs weighing about 32 Kg are used. They are anaesthetized with halothane as described by Batchelor [19]. The hair on the back is clipped three days before the start of an experiment and a guard put on. The skin is shaved, washed with Savlon®, rinsed and dried. The positions of the wounds are marked within the area protected by the guard. Using a square template, four shallow incisions are made outlining an area of 2.5 cm². Two sides are aligned in the direction of hair growth. Using a sharp scalpel held horizontally in the plane of the surface and beginning at the dorsal edge, a thin layer of tissue is dissected away. The cut is made about 0.5 mm deep, passing through the papillarly layer of the dermis. This removes all the surface epidermis including the epidermal ridges. The hair follicles are resected through the pilary canal region just above the point where the sebaceous gland opens into the follicle. Slight initial bleeding is quickly followed by the appearance of droplets of straw-coloured fluid on the surface, which coalesce to cover the wound in proteinaceous exudate. The wounds are not swabbed or interfered with in any way. A standard full thickness wound can be produced by excising the skin to a predetermined depth (normally 7–9 mm) within a similar standard area, i.e., 2.5 cm².

Six such wounds spaced about 6 cm apart in two rows of three are made on either side of the midline. The wounds on one side are allocated to the experimental treatment and those on the other side are treated as controls. It is desirable that investigators agree to adopt the same control dressings to facilitate comparisons of results obtained by different laboratories.

The basic standard must be no dressings at all, which is the way healing first evolved. Wounds exposed to the air form a scab and healing takes place beneath this dry crust. Cotton gauze (BPC) has been used as a control because it is a widely used, long-established, standard hospital dressing. On shallow wounds it may be used as a pad of known ply held in place with a circle of adhesive plaster so that the upper surface of the gauze is exposed to the atmosphere.

An early standard for covered wounds was a thin (0.0015″) natural grade polythene film. This contained no additives, was permeable to oxygen, impermeable to water vapour, and gave reproducible results. More recently we have used a clinical equivalent such as Op-Site®.

The evaluation of the effects of a dressing using histological methods requires specimens from a given number of comparable wounds at daily intervals at least until epidermal repair is complete. In practice this means anything from three to eight days in the porcine skin shallow wound model, because using no dressing the wound is fully epithelized between the seventh and eighth day, while under an occlusive film the wound is covered with new epidermis in under four days. Long-term studies to determine the effect, if any, of a dressing on contraction or scar formation may be required, but most dressings are not designed for long-term usage without additional therapy.

Epidermal wound healing may be most accurately measured in serial histological sections. Biopsy specimens are taken with the aid of a template measuring 1.0 cm × 4.5 cm. The specimens extend into the fat under the dermis and encompass the entire width of the wound and some undamaged skin at the margins and are orientated in such a way that the hair follicles are seen in longitudinal section. The tissue is fixed in 10% formal saline and trimmed for histology 24 hours later. A series of 40 sections, each 10 μm thick, cut at 50 μm intervals are stained with Ehrlich's haematoxylin and eosin. The sections are inspected under the microscope at 100× magnification and the wound edge is aligned under a crosswire mounted in the eyepiece. The wound edges are identified by the position of the shallow incisions marked against the template used in making the wounds. The moving stage of the microscope is equipped with a displacement transducer coupled to a computer. The mode of operation is to record the position of the wound edge and then move the stage until the cross-wire aligns with the end of the sheet of epidermis migrating from that edge, and record the measured length. Similarly, the length of each sheet of epidermis regenerating from hair follicles, ducts, glands, etc. is measured. The sum of all measured lengths of new epidermis is expressed as a percentage of the total length of wound surface examined.

A sufficient number of wounds for each treatment must be examined for statistical analysis. Where practical, biopsy specimens should be cut with the dressing in place on the wound surface to avoid damage to the wound during removal of the dressing and to enable the precise relationship between the dressing and the wound to be studied in the microscope.

A number of other methods have been proposed for the measurement of epidermal regeneration. One using donor site type wounds relies on the uptake by dividing cells of tritiated thymidine, which is assayed by scintillation counting [20]. There are two main objections to this method: (1) not all dividing cells in a wound will be epidermal cells; a significant proportion of the radioactive material will be incorporated into endothelial cells of blood vessels and into mononuclear cells and fibroblasts: and (2) the primary tactic of epidermal regeneration is cell movement, not mitosis. The burst of mitosis occurs in the undamaged epidermis at the wound margins and in the outer root sheath of hair follicles, and only later in the new epidermis, which is established on the wound surface following epidermal cell migration.

Another method [21] relies on an optical densitometer to measure the amount of haematoxylin-stained material on the wound surface, based on the assumption that everything coloured by haematoxylin is new epidermal tissue. For most wounds this is not true, and a significant source of error may result from the failure of the apparatus to distinguish between haematoxylin-stained leucocytes, which are normally abundant on a wound surface. This method was developed for use with the suction blister model in which it is claimed that leucocytes are not seen, so the wound is suitable for the study of the effects of drugs on epithelization but not for the study of dressings.

Among the procedures used to evaluate new dressing materials are investigations of skin irritation by patch testing and skin sensitization. Materials that have not been completely characterized toxicologically, or extracts whose chemical composition is not fully known, can be evaluated in animal models [22]. For local and systemic toxicity testing, saline extracts may be injected into mice intravenously, intramuscularly, intraperitoneally, intraocularly or intradermally, the route chosen being dependent on the nature of the material and its intended application. Implantation methods of toxicological testing may also be employed [23].

Some information can be obtained by the histological examination of wounds treated with dressings in the pig. The epidermal cells migrating across the wound, the venules and capillaries exposed in the wound surface, and the leucocytes that arrive in the damaged area, are all sensitive to adverse influences. Toxicity may be revealed by inhibition of epidermal regeneration, death of epidermal cells and the presence of abnormal cellular reactions in the dermis.

MECHANISMS OF WOUND HEALING

Most successful in the comparative assessment of dressing material has been the standard partial-thickness wound. This injury, which is similar to a graft donor site, is capable of rapid and complete remodelling in a relatively short period of time. Re-epithelization of this wound can be quantified and is not complicated by factors such as contraction.

A partial-thickness wound involves complete removal of the epidermis together with the papillary layer of dermis. In order to understand the effect of a dressing on the healing of such a wound, it is first necessary to study the natural healing pattern when the wound is exposed.

The injury causes a local inflammatory response which begins within a few minutes of wounding. Substances released by the injured tissue, e.g. bradykinin and histamine, cause an increase in vascular permeability resulting in an outflow of serous exudate. By 4 hours, a layer of clear exudate can be seen lying above the blood clot on the wound surface (Figure 1). Leucocytes are also released from the capillaries and migrate into the injured area to ingest any foreign material or micro-organisms that may have

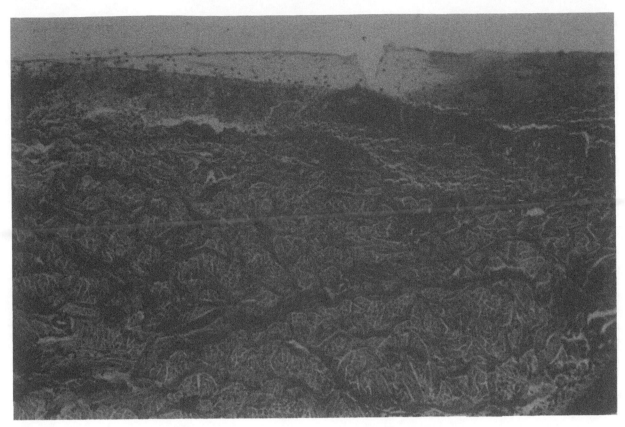

Figure 1. Appearance of a partial-thickness wound at 4 hours showing a clear exudate layer above the blood clot with evenly dispersed leucocytes. H&E × 125

entered the wound. By 8 hours, the leucocytes have formed a layer of cells at the wound surface. The increase in serous exudate within the injured area also causes oedema of the dermal collagen with disruption of the normal "basket weave" pattern of the collagen fibres.

By 24 hours, the acute inflammatory response has subsided and the serous exudate layer has gelled. The exposed surface is dry due to loss of water to the atmosphere (Figure 2). This drying will continue until an equilibrium is reached whereby loss of water by evaporation is balanced by diffusion from the deeper tissues. The plane of equilibrium lies in the dermis below the original wound surface. This dehydration results in scab formation and the fully formed dry scab is composed of both exudate and collagen fibres together with the layer of leucocytes that migrated to the surface within the first few hours (Figure 3). There is no clear line of separation between the skin and the scab; it is integrated with the viable dermal tissue, from which collagen fibres can be seen passing into the dehydrated area. Once scab formation is complete, epidermal regeneration begins. New epidermis migrates from the epidermis at the wound edges, from the outer sheaths of hair follicles within the wound, and from the walls of gland ducts. Thus, the sources of new epidermis are not confined to the wound perimeter, but are evenly scattered throughout the

wound (Figure 4). An increase in the mitotic activity in the basal cell layer within these areas provides the sources of new epidermal cells. In the epidermis surrounding the wound, increased numbers of dividing cells are seen up to 5 mm from the wound edge at 48 hours.

Due to the presence of dehydrated dermal tissue in the scab, epidermis migrates through viable collagen immediately beneath the dried tissue. The epidermis has no blood supply of its own and must remain in contact with viable tissue. This necessitates an initial "burrowing down" by epidermis originating from the wound edges and cleaving of dermal fibrous tissue in its path (Figure 5). Complete epidermal cover is re-established by about 7 days and the scab is shed (Figure 6). Regeneration of new dermal collagen is now seen. This new connective tissue arises from the sub-papillary plexus from which blood vessels grow into the fluid which collects beneath the new maturing epidermis. After 8–12 days this new epidermis enters a hypertrophic stage with prolongations of the epidermis maintaining contact with mature collagen and dividing the developing connective tissue into compartments each containing one or two growing blood vessels and the associated papilla of new connective tissue (Figure 7). Maturation of the new collagen fibres continues, the prolongations of the epidermis reduce and, once remodelled, the skin is fully healed.

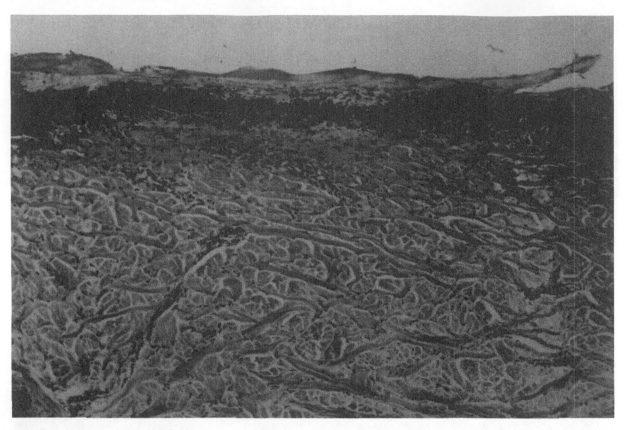

Figure 2. Appearance of a partial-thickness wound at 24 hours showing dehydration of the surface and banding of leucocytes. H&E ×125

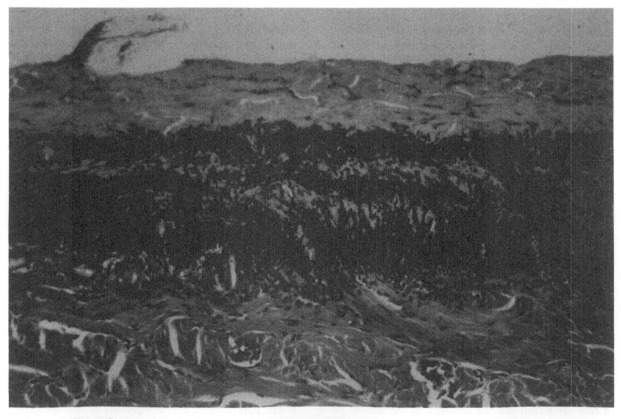

Figure 3. Appearance of normal scab formation in a partial-thickness wound at 3 days. H&E ×200

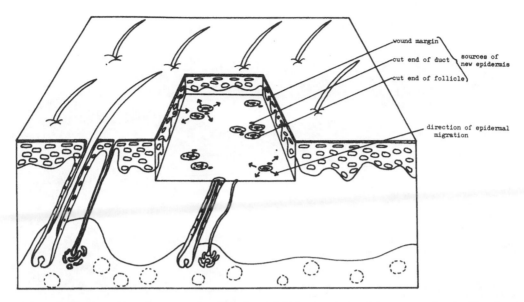

Figure 4. Diagram to show the extent of a standard partial-thickness wound and the sources of new epidermis.

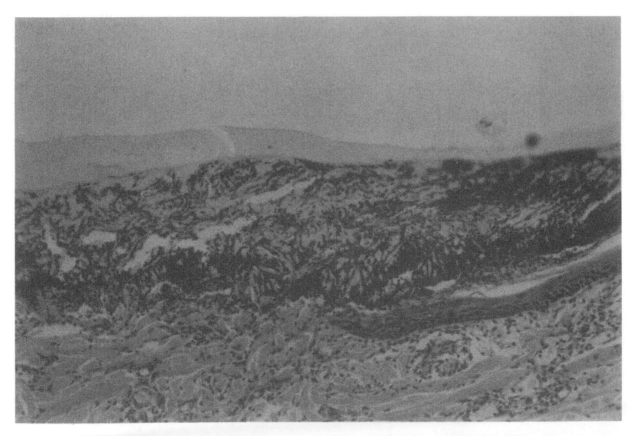

Figure 5. Epidermal migration beneath the scab of a standard partial-thickness wound at 3 days. H&E ×125

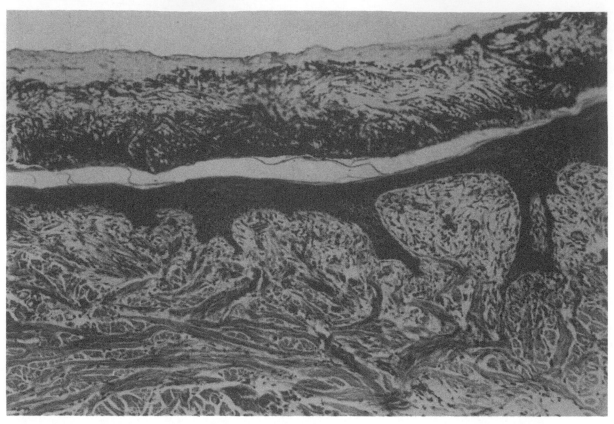

Figure 6. Appearance of a partial-thickness wound at 7 days to show separation of the dehydrated tissue. H&E × 125

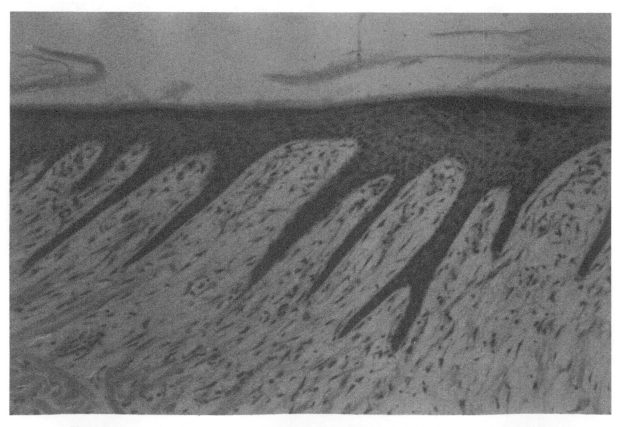

Figure 7. Hypertrophy of new epidermis and connective tissue repair in partial-thickness wound. H&E × 125

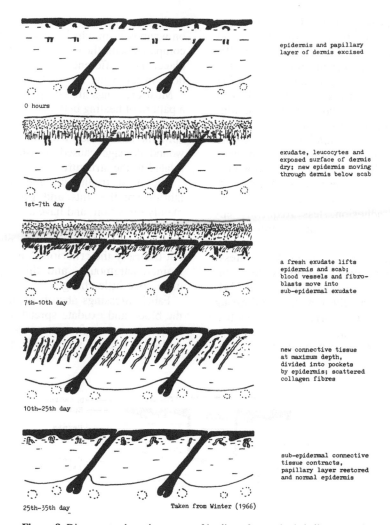

epidermis and papillary
layer of dermis excised

0 hours

exudate, leucocytes and
exposed surface of dermis
dry; new epidermis moving
through dermis below scab

1st-7th day

a fresh exudate lifts
epidermis and scab;
blood vessels and fibro-
blasts move into
sub-epidermal exudate

7th-10th day

new connective tissue
at maximum depth,
divided into pockets
by epidermis; scattered
collagen fibres

10th-25th day

sub-epidermal connective
tissue contracts,
papillary layer restored
and normal epidermis

25th-35th day   Taken from Winter (1966)

Figure 8. Diagram to show the pattern of healing of a standard shallow wound.

This can take up to one month, but once complete it is difficult to distinguish the wound area from normal skin even in histological section.

As stated earlier, only such a superficial wound is capable of rapid and complete remodelling. On shallow wounds, epidermal growth takes place before any new connective tissue is formed (Figure 8). In deeper wounds, growth of epidermis and the repair tissue goes on simultaneously (Figure 9). The deeper damage to the collagen takes months or even years to fully repair, if it ever does. Studies of clean incisions which were sutured immediately after injury show that even after 35 days no collagen continuity had been re-established across the incision line (Figure 10), although no actual loss to tissue was involved and the epidermal integrity would have been regained within hours after injury.

DRESSINGS AND WOUND HEALING

As discussed above, the healing process of a wound is complex, involving a number of interrelated pro-

cesses—clotting, inflammation, cell migration, tissue replacement and fibrosis. Most dressing research has been directed towards providing the ideal environment for these processes to occur naturally. Parallel to this has been the research into dressings which give increased healing rates that may not only give a better quality of wound repair but may also reduce hospitalization times and after-care.

Alongside these considerations is the necessity for specialized wound dressings for particular problems, e.g. pressure sores, leg ulcers, or burns, where healing times may be prolonged. Many workers have described the criteria for the "ideal" dressing, but it must be recognised that many dressings, while being ideal for one type of wound, may be totally unsuitable for another.

One unsatisfactory feature of many commonly used dressings is that they cause fresh damage to the wound when removed because of their adherence to the wound surface. This adhesion is caused by changes in the properties of the proteinaceous exudate which covers the wound surface following an injury. While in fluid form, it causes no problem. It has surfactant properties and readily penetrates among fibres and into any surface irregularities of dressings (Figure 11). As it dries it becomes a powerful glue, binding the dressing into the scab. Removing an adherent dressing before the regenerated epidermis is mature, and when it has acquired an easily ruptured layer of keratin, causes pain and fresh damage to the wound. The practical solution is to prevent dehydration of the exudate at the interface between the dressing and the wound. The length of time the dressing is left on the wound is critical because it is one of the factors which determine how viscous the exudate becomes.

Another cause of adhesion, less frequently encountered, is growth of tissue into a dressing or wound packing.

Adhesion can be measured *in vitro* by drying dressings under carefully controlled conditions of temperature and humidity, against a standard material [24]. These studies, however, merely show that all dressing materials that have any kind of irregular surface texture will key to drying serum.

A more accurate appraisal can be made histolog-

ically by measuring the amount of epidermis present on wounds from which dressings have been removed, compared with those on which the dressing is left in place. The difference gives the amount of damage done in removing the dressing.

Most dressings are composite structures producing a pattern of healing between the two extremes of complete exposure and complete occlusion, in an effort to combine absorbency with moist wound healing. Any wound damage caused on dressing removal can be related to the structure of the dressing.

The most traditional and widely used dressing fabrics are the lints and gauzes. These are based mainly on cotton, and have a long history of use [25]. During the last 40 years, rayon gauze has also been used in conjunction with or in place of cotton gauze, but basically the criterion of high absorbency has remained paramount, and this type of dressing has undergone little change.

Fabric dressings absorb readily, even fiercely, and the blood and exudate spread far along the fibres. A large exposed surface area favours rapid drying and within 24 hours a scab can be formed. The dried ex-

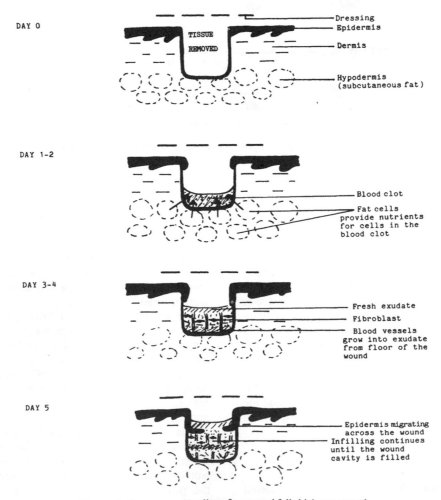

Figure 9. The pattern of healing of a covered full-thickness wound.

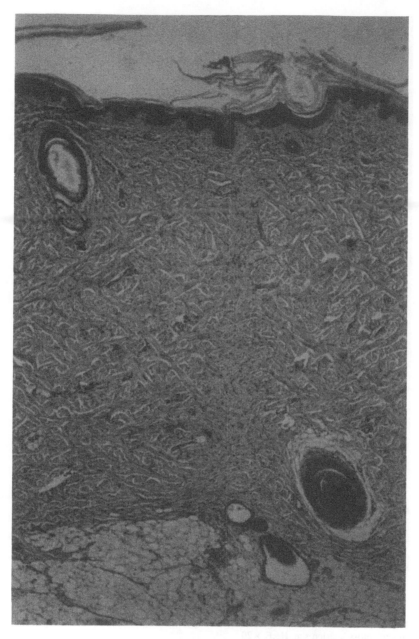

Figure 10a. Appearance of skin at 35 days following an incisional wound. H&E ×20

udate converts the supple fabric to a board-like structure and the inevitable small movements between dressing and wound irritate the tissues and the surrounding skin. A dry dressing does little to relieve pain. A fabric thoroughly incorporated into the scab cannot be removed without damage to the healing tissues.

Although cotton gauze provides a relatively poor environment for healing, it is the standard by which other dressings are judged because it is still widely used as a surgical dressing in hospitals. The continued popularity is partly a matter of tradition, partly a matter of convenience of having one uncomplicated, easily sterilisable, piece of material, that can serve in

the operating theatre and the wards as a swab, a cleansing tissue and a dressing.

Histologically, the amount of dehydration seen under a physically porous, open weave pad (Figure 12) will depend on the amount of exudation from the wound, the bulk of the dressing and the time since wounding occurred. Studies on the standard shallow wound have shown that a pad of 4-ply cotton gauze will allow gross wound dehydration by 3 days, whereas wounds under 12-ply pads, also biopsied at 3 days, demonstrated two conditions for epidermal regeneration: (1) Dehydration of the exudate had occurred, involving the uppermost layer of the dermal collagen (Figure 13). The epidermis had migrated at a

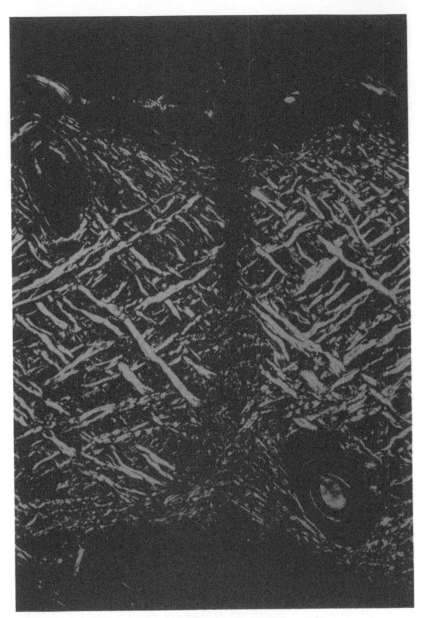

Figure 10b. Area of skin in Figure 10a seen in polarised light—note lack of collagen continuity across incision site. H&E ×20

level beneath this dehydrating layer with epidermal cells having to "cleave" through viable collagen bundles. Hence the resulting rate of epidermal regeneration was slower and the sheet of epidermis thicker in depth. (2) Where dehydration had not occurred so freely, due to dressing thickness, some moist exudate remained at the wound/dressing interface (Figure 14) and epidermal cells could be seen as a thinner sheet of tissue migrating through this moist layer. This resulted in a faster rate of epithelization in these areas.

Cotton gauze removal caused varying amounts of wound disruption, reflecting the differences in healing patterns noted above. If the dressing parted at a level above the leucocytic layer, then little or no epidermal damage occurred. If, however, the wound had suffered greater dehydration, the leucocytic layer was lost with the dressing leaving a completely denuded wound surface, and causing epidermal damage and fresh wound bleeding (Figure 15).

The problems of adhesion with cotton gauze are largely mitigated by the use of paraffin-impregnated gauzes such as tulle gras. Providing sufficient paraffin is applied with the gauze, this remains an effective, cheap dressing, suitable for abrasions and scalds. Its use in deep wounds is to be avoided because of the possibility of paraffin being incorporated into the repair tissue.

In 1956 experiments were carried out be Scales et al. [26] using microporous polyvinylchloride on

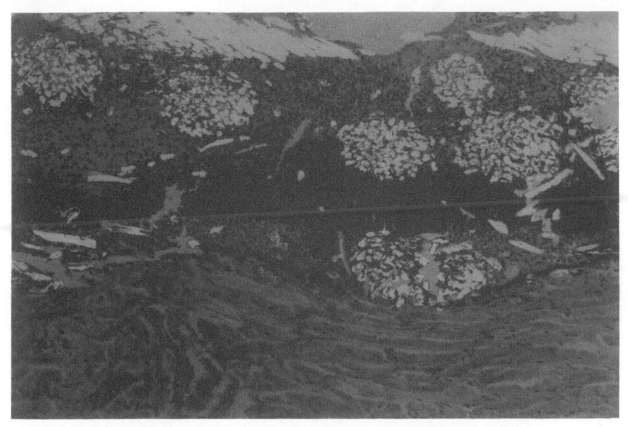

Figure 11. Penetration of an open-weave dressing by exudate and leucocytes at 3 days. Note banding of leucocytes as exudate dries and close contact of dressing fibres to the wound surface. H&E × 125

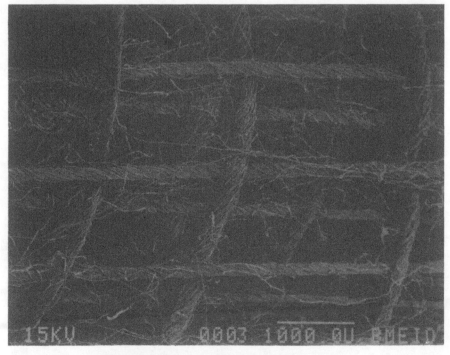

Figure 12. Surface of 12-ply cotton gauze (BPC) dressing.

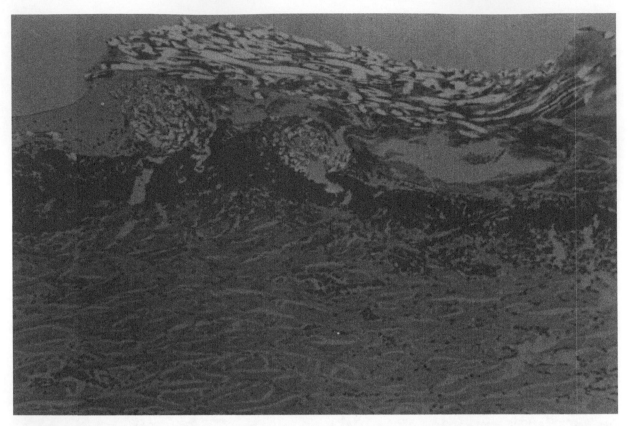

Figure 13. Wound surface appearance under 12-ply cotton gauze at 3 days to show the dehydration, with dressing involvement, and the level of epidermal migration. H&E × 125

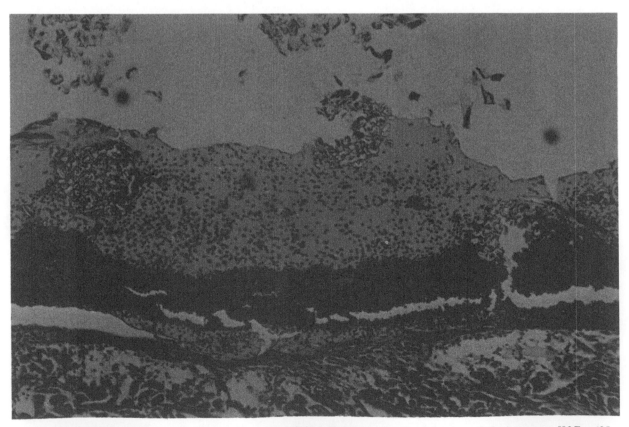

Figure 14. Epidermal healing beneath 12-ply cotton gauze at 3 days. Note layer of moist exudate beneath the leucocytes. H&E × 125

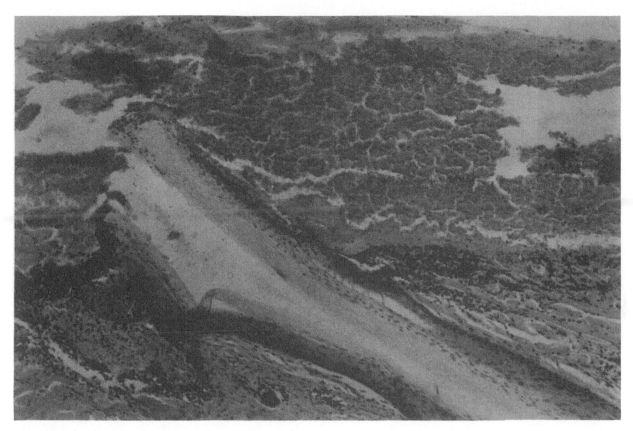

Figure 15. Haemorrhage at wound surface caused by removal of cotton gauze dressing. No epidermal repair from the hair follicle can be seen. H&E × 125

standard shallow wounds in porcine skin. The material has a water vapor permeability of about 2500 g/m²/24 hr. Water vapour loss from the wound surface was restricted sufficiently to ensure that it remained moist and that the regenerating epidermis migrated through a layer of free exudate above the cut surface of the dermis. This dressing is sold complete with a cotton pad as AirStrip®. The development of AirStrip® and similar proprietary dressings such as Band-Aid® were the result of the first recognition that prevention of gross dehydration could improve healing rates and quality of wound care.

The concept of moist wound healing has gradually led to a change in both the methods and products associated with the management of wounds. The traditional acceptance of the absorbent cover, which frequently produces a dry wound surface with problems of adhesion and subsequent secondary trauma, has been replaced by the currently accepted philosophy that a moist wound is a healing wound (Figure 16).

In order to provide absorbency and yet still maintain a moist wound surface, a number of dressings, designed to be non-adherent, have been created, composed of an absorbent pad covered with a perforated film. This film is the wound contact layer. Examples of this type of dressing are Melolin®, Telfa®, Perfron®, and Lotus®.

Melolin® comprises an absorbent cotton and gauze pad faced on one side only with a perforated polyester film (Figure 17). Telfa® is essentially the same, the main differences being that the pad is faced on both sides by the polyester film and the perforations are larger (Figure 18). Telfa® pads are also less bulky than Melolin®. These dressings have been studied in controlled animal trials [27] using porcine skin and the standard shallow wound models. The pattern of repair is similar beneath both, with areas of dehydration and leucocytic concentration, directly related in size and position to the film perforations, being seen on the wound surface at 3 days (Figure 19). The leucocytes were observed to move freely within the exudate beneath the polyester film to the sites of the perforations, where they accumulated due to fluid loss into the bulk of the dressing (Figure 20). The resuling "plug" of leucocytes then acted to reduce further wound dehydration.

On removal of these dressings only a few of these dehydrated areas were left in place (Figure 21). They were mainly lost with the dressing together with the moist, free exudate. Removal of the Telfa® dressings caused more extensive epidermal loss than removal of the Melolin®, although evidence of fresh bleeding was seen with both of these dressings (Figure 22). No adverse cellular effects were noted beneath either of

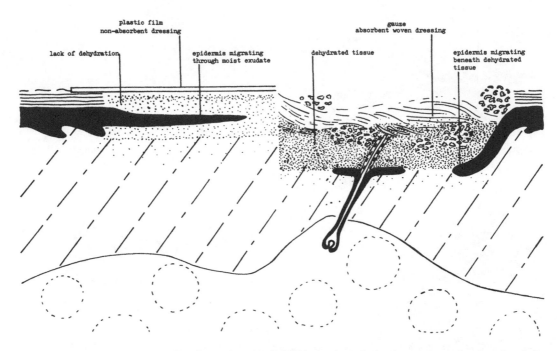

Figure 16. Diagram to show the differences in the epidermal migration beneath absorbent and non-absorbent dressings.

Figure 17. Surface of Melolin® dressing. ×20

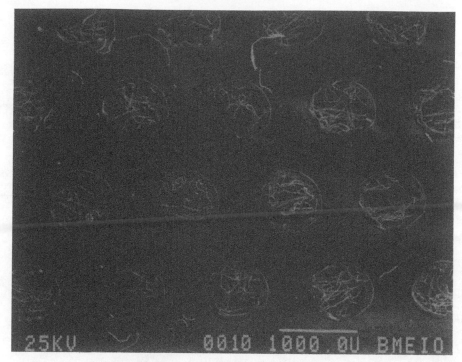

Figure 18. Surface of Telfa® dressing. ×20

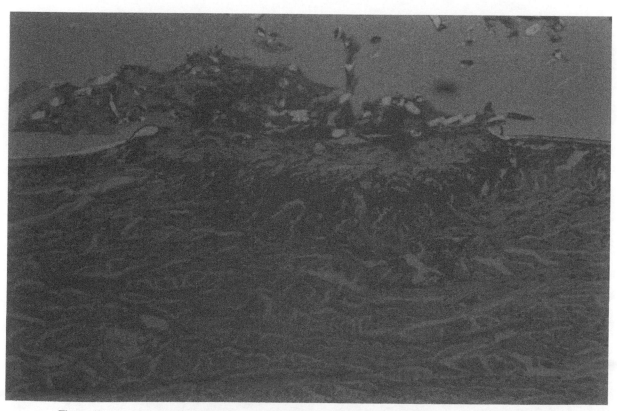

Figure 19. Area of tissue dehydration associated with a film perforation site in Telfa® polyester film. H&E ×125

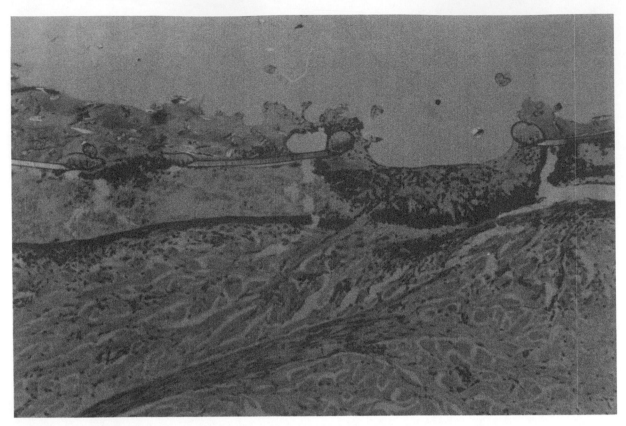

Figure 20. Tissue dehydration and collagen involvement at the site of a perforation in the polyester film cover of a Melolin® dressing. H&E × 125

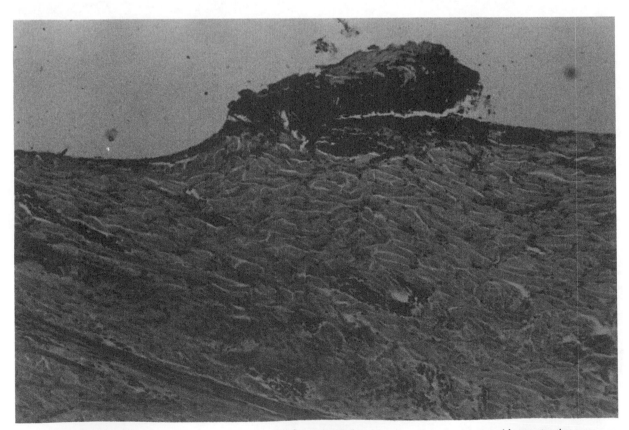

Figure 21. Denuded wound surface following removal of a Telfa® dressing pad at three days. Only the dehydrated leucocytes that were associated with a film perforation remain. H&E × 125

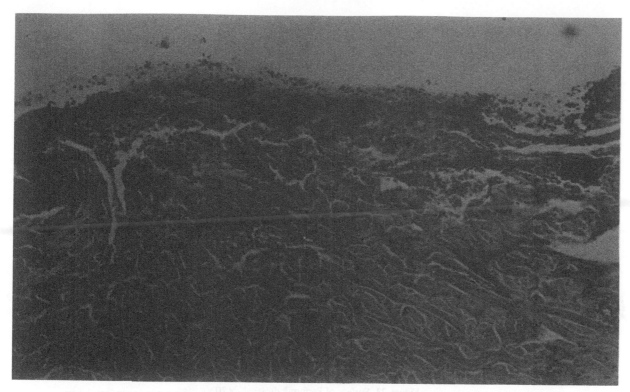

Figure 22. Epidermal damage and haemorrhage caused by removal of a Melolin® dressing at 3 days. H&E × 125

these two dressings. The greater bulk of the Melolin® reduced the incidence of strike-through without noticeable loss of conformability.

Perfron® and Lotus® are also similar to each other in composition. Perfron® dressings are absorbent cotton pads in a sleeve of apertured viscose non-woven fabric coated with polypropylene, while in Lotus® the cotton pad is covered by an apertured non-woven fabric comprising 90% polypropylene and 10 polyamide. The apertures in Perfron® are regularly spaced but not of a uniform size or structure (Figure 23). In the Lotus® pad the surface perforations are well-defined apertures, but are of varying size and distribution (Figure 24). As a result there are similarities in the healing patterns beneath these two dressings when compared with Melolin® and Telfa®. For instance, dehydrated leucocytes and dermal collagen can be seen in relation to the sites of apertures. Elsewhere the wound surface had remained moist (Figure 25).

The effects of removing both Perfron® and Lotus® pads from partial-thickness wounds were comparable. The wounds were denuded of all moist exudate, but the areas of dehydration remained intact on the wound surface. Little epidermal loss was recorded but dressing removal resulted in the rupture of the dermo-epidermal junction (Figure 26), and once the epidermis has been lifted from the underlying dermis it is unlikely to remain viable.

The use of polypropylene is also seen in such dressings as Micropad® and Mesoft®, but in the form of fibres. Micropad® is an absorbed viscose pad heat-

bonded between layers of polypropylene fibres, while Mesoft® is an 8-ply pad of 23.2% polypropylene fibres, 53.3% viscose fibres, and 23.5% resin finish. Micropad® and Mesoft® also differ from the four dressings described above in that they do not have an apertured surface (Figures 27 and 28). Micropad® dressings are compressed pads with little bulk, and this lack of dressing thickness resulted in immediate strike-through by the blood when pads were applied to standard partial-thickness wounds. Despite this, little dehydration of the wound surface was seen at three days in histological sections (Figure 29). Epidermis, one to three cells thick, was migrating through moist exudate over most of the wound surface. Unlike the situation in many other dressings, leucocytes had not penetrated into the Micropad®; the surface polypropylene was porous to exudate only.

On removal of Micropad®, disruption to the wound surface, resulting in some epidermal loss and associated bleeding, was seen only where dehydration had occurred. Where the wound surface was moist the dressing had parted above the regenerating epidermis and below the leucocytic layer (Figure 30).

Mesoft® pads are thicker than Micropad® and did not allow immediate blood strike-through when applied to standard shallow wounds. By three days, however, some degree of strike-through was seen on all the wounds treated. Epidermal regeneration was well advanced by 72 hours under Mesoft®, although the wound surface showed more areas of dehydration than were seen under Micropad®. The epidermis had

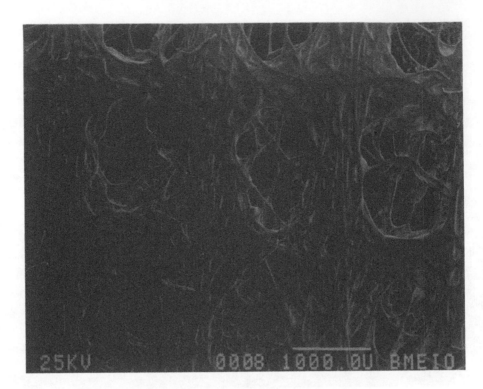

Figure 23. Surface of Perform® dressing. ×20

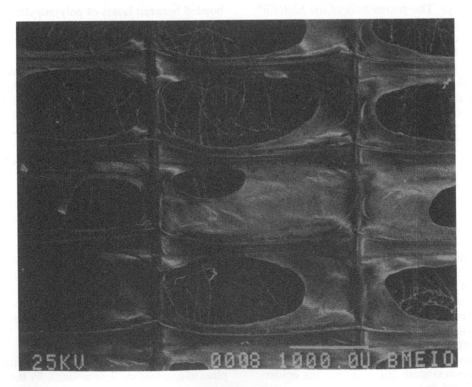

Figure 24. Surface of Lotus® dressing. ×20

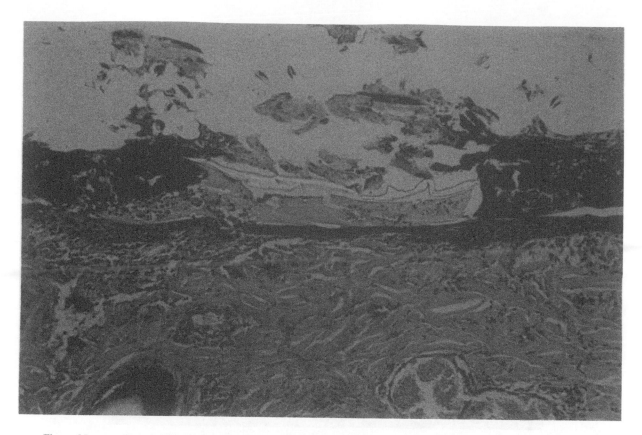

Figure 25. Area of moist exudate and areas of dehydration beneath apertured cover-stock of Lotus® dressing pad. H&E × 125

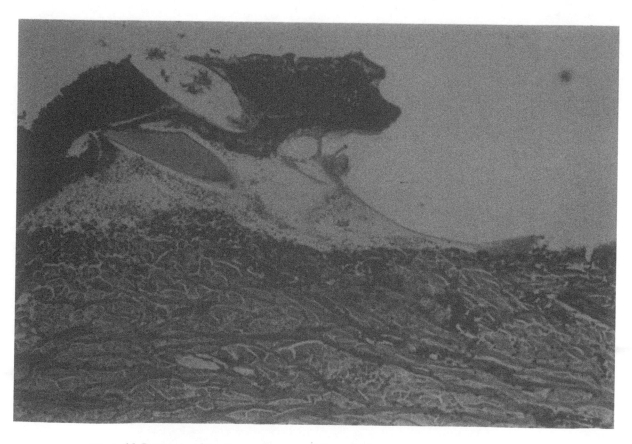

Figure 26. Damage to epidermis caused by removal of Lotus® dressing pad at three days. H&E × 125

Figure 27. Surface of Micropad® dressing. ×20

Figure 28. Surface of Mesoft® dressing. ×20

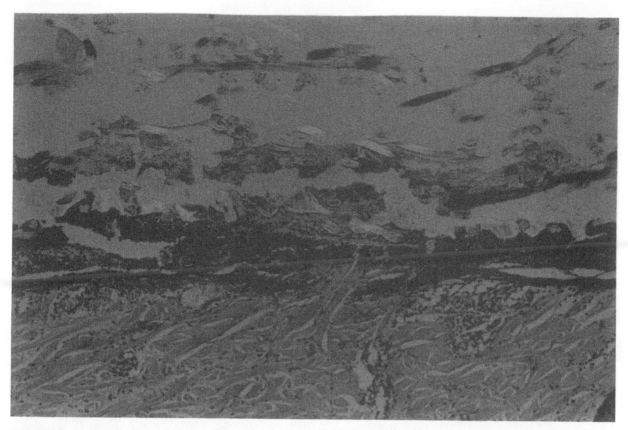

Figure 29. Wound surface at 3 days under Micropad® showing regenerating epidermis beneath cellular exudate. Some dehydration and collagen involvement can also be seen. H&E ×125

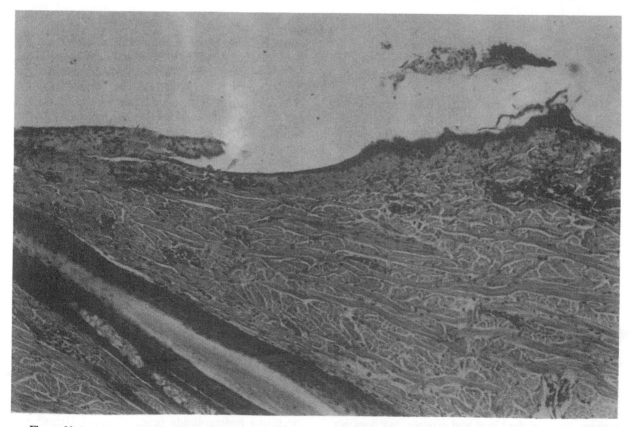

Figure 30. Loss of moist exudate from above the regenerating epidermis following removal of a Micropad® dressing. H&E ×125

605

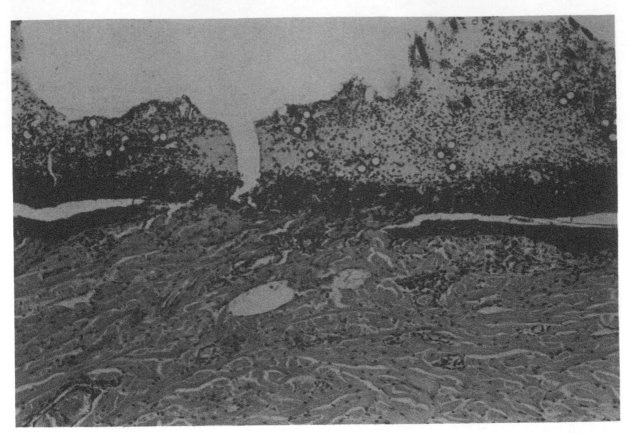

Figure 31. Epidermal migration beneath a Mesoft® dressing at 3 days on a standard partial-thickness wound. H&E × 125

migrated directly beneath the leucocytes as a layer two to four cells thick. The dressing fibres were seen in close contact with the regenerating surface (Figure 31).

Mesoft® dressings were strongly adherent and, at 3 days, it was not possible to remove all pads intact. Dressing fibres remained incorporated in the wound exudate (Figure 32) indicating that the bond between the layers of the dressing was weaker than the adhesion of the dressing to the wound surface. Where the dressing did come away intact it caused little disruption of the regenerating surface, but some areas of fresh haemorrhage were noted.

The proprietary dressings described so far are all examples of different dressing types, but they share the common feature of still being based on an absorbent pad. An initial move from this trend can be seen in the polyurethane foam dressings such as Lyofoam® [28]. Polyurethane foam is normally hydrophobic and, therefore, not intrinsically wettable. It only absorbs by capillary attraction once sufficient pressure has been applied to force blood and serum into the interstices. Lyofoam®, however, is surface treated by applied heat and pressure which not only renders the surface smooth (Figure 33) but also wettable. This surface membrane is found to be absorbent enough to remove much of the blood and exudate, but does not blot the wound surface dry due to the absence of any wicking effect by an absorbent pad [29]. Epidermal

migration takes place in a thin film of fluid above the cut surface of the dermis. Because of the hydrophobic backing, penetration of fluid to the outer surface of the dressing does not ordinarily occur. Numerous white cells are present in the exudate on the wound surface and within the pores of the surface membrane of the dressing (Figure 34) where they act to combat wound infection.

Many dressings have been, and still are, promoted as being the "ideal" dressing but there is growing awareness that not only is there no single dressing suitable for all wounds, but also no one dressing is suitable for the complete management of a single wound. This appreciation of the varying needs of a wound through the varying stages of healing arises from the recognition that the microenvironment, particularly at the wound/dressing interface, can and should be controlled if wound healing is to progress at the optimum level (Figure 35). The concurrent development of alternative technology during the past fifteen years has resulted in the design, development and production of new types of polymer-based wound management products [30].

These new dressings include the semi-occlusive films (e.g., OpSite®, Bioclusive®, and Steridrape®) and hydrogels (e.g., Vigilon® and Geliperm®) and the occlusive hydrocolloids (e.g., Comfeel Ulcus® and Granuflex®).

Semi-occlusive films were originally designed for

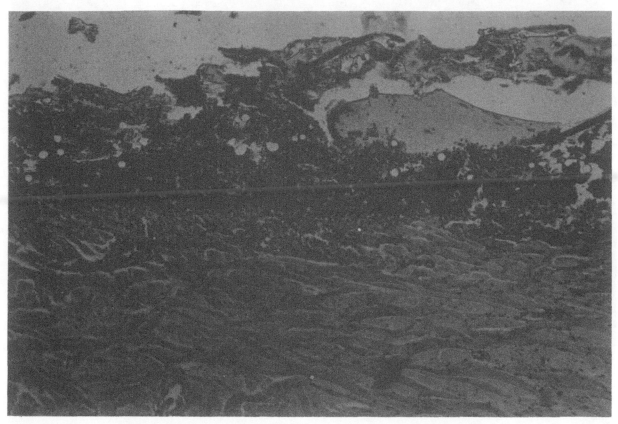

Figure 32. Adherent dressing fibres within the wound exudate after removal of the rest of a Mesoft® dressing pad from the surface of a standard partial-thickness wound. H&E × 125

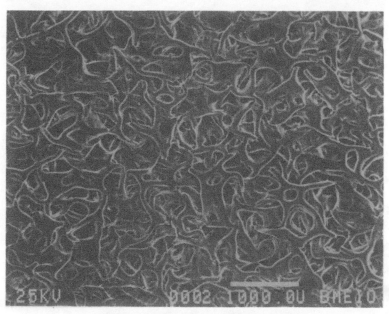

Figure 33. Surface of Lyofoam® dressing. × 20

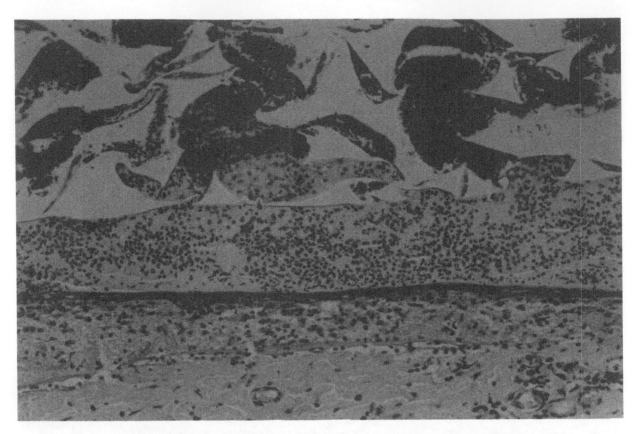

Figure 34. Lyofoam® dressing in place on a standard shallow wound at 3 days. H&E ×125

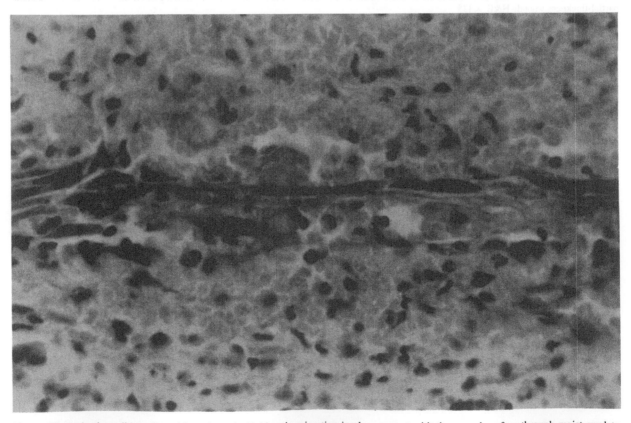

Figure 35. Optimal conditions for epidermal repair. Epidermis migrating in close contact with the wound surface through moist exudate. Leucocytes are evenly dispersed in the exudate and there is no dermal dehydration. H&E ×800

use as adhesive surgical drapes but their potential for use as dressings was soon realised. They are composed of a thin, transparent, polyurethane film spread on one surface with an adhesive which gives adhesion to dry skin and non-adhesion to a wet wound surface. They are highly comformable due to their elastomeric and extensible properties. They are impermeable to water and bacteria but permeable, to varying degrees, to gaseous transfer. An uncovered wound will lose water vapour at the rate of around 6000 g/m²/24 hr depending on site and wound condition. This can be reduced to 2500 g/m²/24 hr or less by the use of a semi-occlusive film. The permeability to oxygen of these films can vary between 4,000 and 10,000 cm³/m²/24 hr at ambient atmospheric pressure depending on the different formulations.

In use the films frequently give a marked reduction in pain response by patients which is presumably due to prevention of dehydration of the neurones.

Because these dressings do not incorporate an absorbent component, exudate from the wound collects beneath the dressing to form a bag of fluid. Using Op-Site® on the standard partial-thickness pig wound it was found that the volume of retained fluid reached a maximum at 3 days, and if dressings were left undisturbed this had reduced, at 5 days, by evaporation through the film to leave a thin layer of gelled exudate on the wound surface. The elasticity of the film allowed it to contract back to conform to the contours of the wound. Buchan et al. [31] studied the wound exudate from human graft donor sites collected under Op-Site® and compared it to the exudate from the pig wounds collected under similar conditions. They concluded that the composition and properties of the pig wound exudate were very similar to those of human wound exudate, with only minor differences. They demonstrated that the wound exudate, under Op-Site®, contains large numbers of actively bactericidal neutrophils, high levels of lysozyme and clinically normal levels of plasma proteins [32]. The exudate is, therefore, actively bactericidal, and should be left undisturbed unless clinical signs of infection indicate the need for topical antibacterial agents.

The histology of standard partial-thickness wounds covered with Op-Site® shows a moderate leucocytic reaction in the exudate layer covering the wound. The regenerating epidermis is seen, in section, as a tongue of epidermal cells moving through the moist exudate either directly upon the dermal fibrous tissue or just above it (Figure 36). Epidermal repair is complete by 5 days and new keratin formation can be seen. Connective tissue repair is evident by 5 days with the ingrowth of new blood vessels and fibroblast infiltration beneath the epidermis. The time scale in human donor sites is slightly different, with epithelization being completed between 5–10 days after wounding.

By not having an absorptive layer this type of dressing has no associated problems of adherence. Epidermis migrating through exudate on the wound surface is, however, still vulnerable to dressing disturbance even if there is no dressing adherence. A suction effect may be produced if a film dressing is removed before the dermo/epidermal junction is established (Figure 37).

Hydrogels are also semi-occlusive and have the absorbent capacity not provided by the semi-permeable films. They are composed of insoluble hydrophilic polymers arranged in a three-dimensional network. They are prepared from a variety of materials including gelatin, polysaccharides, polyacrylamide polymers, and polymers derived from methacrylic esters. Hydrogels currently available include Geliperm® and Vigilon®.

Geliperm® is an elastic gel-film composed of sterile water (96%) bound by a polyacrylamide and agar network [33]. Vigilon® is a colloid in gelatinous form with water (96%) as the dispersion medium and insoluble cross-linked polyethylene oxide (4%). It is centered by a low-density polyethylene net to provide strength [34].

The gels absorb fluid into the polymer matrix and, while this remains unsaturated, they have a water vapour permeability comparable to semi-occlusive films. Once the gel becomes saturated it will allow water transmission. The high moisture content of the gels also allows a dissolved oxygen permeability which is at least equal to that of a film dressing. They also give pain relief on application to a wound not only because of their moisture retention but also because of their effect of cooling the wound and maintaining this lowered temperature for some hours after application.

Because of high water content of these materials and their high gaseous permeability, they can rapidly dry out if not protected. Secondary dressings of an absorptive pad and/or bandage, or periodic re-wetting of the dressing, may be recommended. Vigilon® dressings are faced with an inert polyethylene film to control water vapour transmission.

The histology and standard partial-thickness wounds covered with Vigilon® and Geliperm® show epidermal regeneration occurring within a moist exudate directly over the dermal surface (Figure 38). There has been no dehydration or dermal involvement.

In contrast to the single polymer hydrogels, those products termed hydrocolloids are compound formulations containing not only hydrogels but elastomeric and adhesive components. They are completely occlusive, the exclusive of atmospheric oxygen being to encourage the development of a well-vascularized wound bed. Hydrocolloid dressings currently available include Granuflex®, Dermiflex®, Comfeel® and Tegasorb®. They are based on sodium carboxymethylcellulose, which acts as the primary gelling element and absorbent of the dressing, to which has been added elastomers and other additives. This inner adhesive layer is covered with an impermeable foam outer layer.

Like hydrogels, hydrocolloids will swell in the pres-

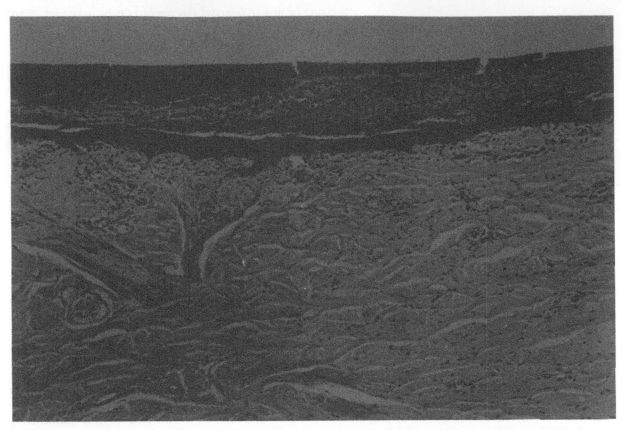

Figure 36. Epidermal regeneration in a partial-thickness wound at 3 days beneath an Op-Site® dressing. H&E × 125

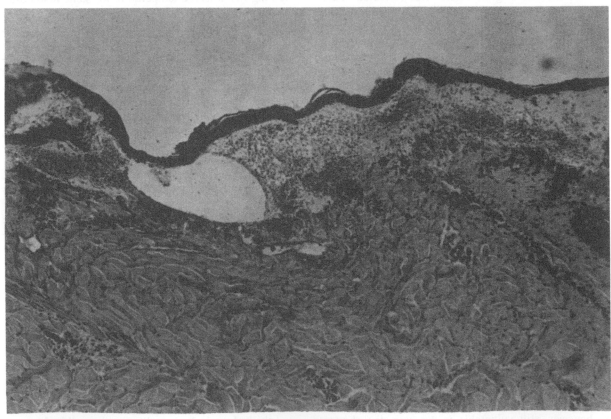

Figure 37. Elevation of epidermis from dermis due to dressing removal. H&E × 125

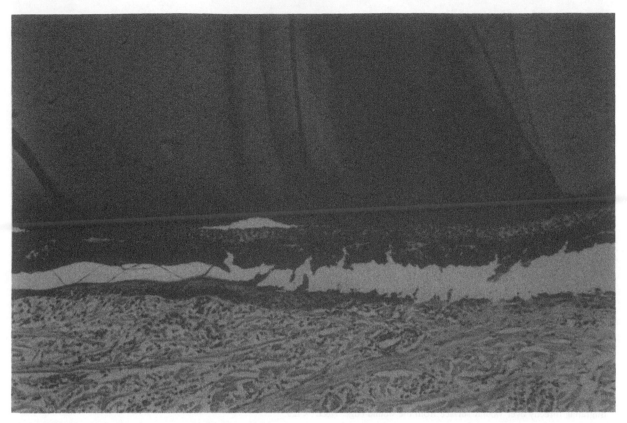

Figure 38. Hydrogel dressing in place on a partial-thickness wound at 3 days. Epidermis can be seen migrating beneath the leucocytic layer (Space between leucocytic layer and epidermis is an artifact of processing). H&E × 125

ence of fluid, but unlike the hydrogels this is not a three-dimensional response of the entire gel. Hydrocolloids swell in a linear fashion with a higher moisture retention at the wound/dressing interface. The gel expands proportional to the amount of exudate available and so fills the wound defect. The presence of the outer foam layer means that a pressure is maintained on the floor of the wound by the swollen gel. Hydrogels remain chemically inert in the presence of wound fluids but hydrocolloids interreact with the exudate. In the case of Granuflex®, which contains a polymer mix of polyisobutylene, gelatin and pectin, the gel degrades to release the available protein and polysaccharides. The resulting colloidal gel absorbs the soluble components from within the serous exudate and also removes bacterial and cellular debris since the white cells remain viable and capable of phagocytosis. Two strains of bacteria that Granuflex® is claimed to be very effective against are *Staph. aureus* and *Pseudomonas aeruginosa* [35].

In clinical use the gel is yellow and may resemble pus and have a characteristic odour. This is easily removed by saline irrigation when the dressing is changed. The mode of action of hydrocolloid dressings makes them particularly suitable for the treatment of ulcers.

The histology of a standard partial-thickness wound at 3 days shows tongues of epidermal tissue 2–5 cells

thick over almost the whole wound surface (Figure 39). This new epidermis was migrating through a layer of moist exudate containing leucocytes, erythrocytes and fibrin. A few vesicles of dressing medicament trapped beneath the migrating epidermal tissue were also noted (Figure 40).

In contrast to the sophisticated technology associated with the polymeric dressing materials, the past decade has also seen an increased interest in the use of "natural" dressings. Such materials often have a long, albeit anecdotal, history of usage but the empirical observations can be explained in the light of greater understanding of the wound healing process. The authors have studied a number of such materials including sphagnum moss [36,37,38] sugar [39] and calcium alginate extracted from seaweed [40].

Sphagnum is the botanical name of the group of mosses which form the basic vegetation of peat bogs scattered across the northern hemisphere (Figure 41). There are many species and varieties but not all are suitable for medical use [41]. Sphagnum has far more medical importance than other mosses mainly because of its great absorbent power (Figure 42) and its slight antiseptic properties [42] and it has a long history of use in wound treatment. One of the earliest documented cases is a Gaelic chronicle of 1014 relating the use of moss to treat the wounded after the battle of Clontarf. Moss was also known to have been

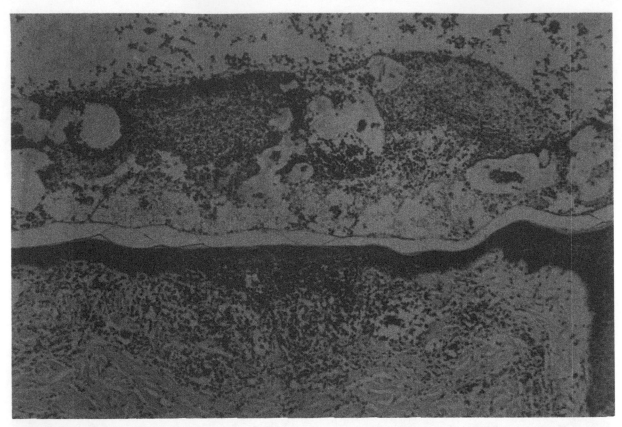

Figure 39. Hydrocolloid dressing in place on a partial-thickness wound at 3 days. Dressing has absorbed exudate and leucocytes. Epidermis is migrating directly over wound surface from the wound edge. H&E × 125

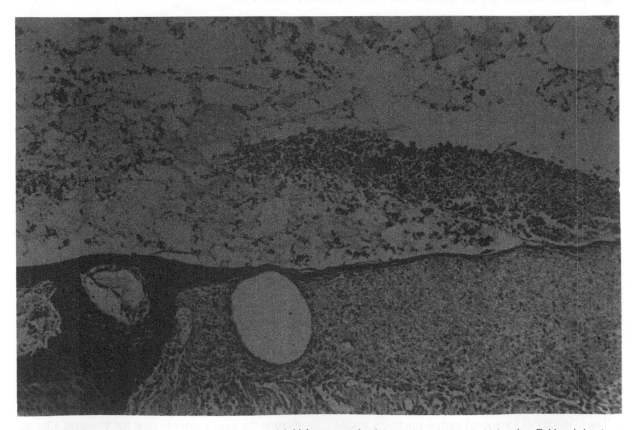

Figure 40. Epidermal migration from a hair follicle on a partial-thickness wound at 3 days under a hydrocolloid dressing. Epidermis is migrating over an exudate/gel layer. Entrapment of the gel has occurred beneath the new tissue. H&E × 125

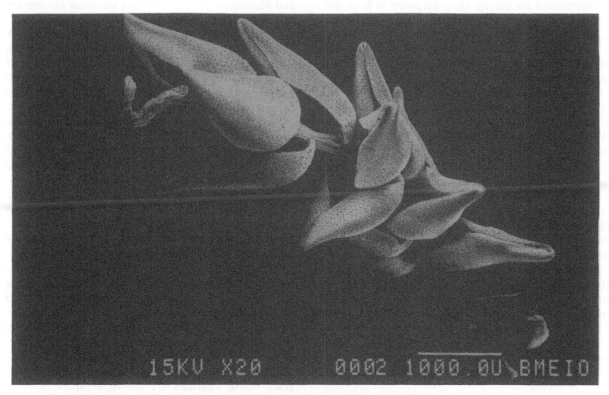

Figure 41. Single stalk of *S. palustre.* ×20

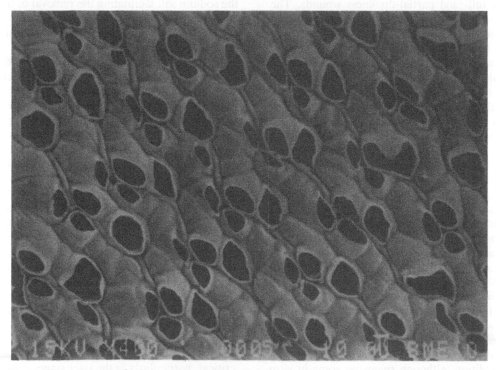

Figure 42. Arrangement of cells in a single sphagnum leaf. Between the network of small elongated chlorophyllose cells are the large, dead and empty hyaline cells, each perforated by pores. It is through these pores that liquids pass into the cells. ×400

recommended for use by army surgeons in both the Napoleonic and Franco-Prussian wars. Scientific studies into the medical use of sphagnum were carried out in Germany in the late 1800s and it was also used extensively as a first aid dressing during the Russian-Japanese war of 1904.

The value of sphagnum as a wound dressing was not generally accepted until World War I, however, when it was of great importance as a cotton substitute [43,44]. Scarce cotton was required for use in explosives and by the end of the war the total British output of sphagnum dressings was around 200,000 per month. The cessation of hostilities in November 1918 brought to a halt the sphagnum industries of Europe and America. During World War II attention was again called to peat moss as a suitable material for surgical dressings but the need for a cotton substitute never became critical.

Sphagnum moss was reported to make a better dressing than cotton [45], its main advantage being (1) moss absorbs liquids more rapidly and in amounts greater than in cotton, (2) sphagnum retains liquids much better, thus reducing the number of times a dressing needs to be changed, (3) liquid is distributed more evenly through the mass of sphagnum and (4) sphagnum dressings are cooler and softer than those made of cotton.

Sphagnum, in both the natural state and in a processed form in a prototype dressing, has been studied on standard full- and partial-thickness wounds. The moss retains a moist wound surface even in the absence of an occlusive cover with exudate and leucocytes being taken into the cells of the moss (Figure 43). No cytotoxic effects were seen and all wounds studied healed without complication. The relatively high cost of moss compared to other materials together with the seasonal variation of its availability have meant that it has not been commercially exploited for use as a dressing. Preliminary studies have shown that sphagnum will respond to hydroponic growth methods and research continues, both in America and the U.K., into its possible use in high-absorption products such as tampons and incontinence pads.

Sugar and sugar-rich compounds such as honey have been used in the treatment of wounds for thousands of years, the earliest documentation relating to the treatment of battle wounds in ancient Egypt around 1700 B.C. Sugar therapy has continued to be used as an aid to wound healing in many areas around the world. It is recognised that there may be problems associated with the application of sugar to an open wound. The absorption of glucose and fructose may lead to metabolic problems particularly in cases of diabetes. In addition, although sugar has some *in vitro* antimicrobial activity, honey can sometimes contain resistant organisms which will infect a previously clean wound.

Two sugar paste formulations have been developed at Northwick Park Hospital, Harrow, England by Seal and Middleton. Both pastes have excellent *in vitro* antimicrobial activity and have provided effective treatment for infected and malodorous wounds [46,47]. A recent study using standard deep wounds in the pig compared the effects of sugar paste with a number of clinical antiseptics often used in conjunction with gauze packing. The consistency of the sugar paste means that it can be moulded and packed into the wound without the need for gauze and the damage caused by repeated changes of wound packing is thus eliminated [48]. The sugar, unlike the gauze, is degradable and does not suppress granulation tissue ingrowth by continual applied pressure. All the antiseptic treatments showed some delay to healing whereas those treated with sugar healed satisfactorily without the need for sterility. Colonization of their surface with bacteria did not impair the formation of collagen tissue nor epidermal migration (Figure 44).

Alginates, derived from the alginic acids of seaweed, are highly absorbent, gel-forming materials with haemostatic properties. Calcium alginate has a well-established history of use in wound dressings, principally in the form of woven or knitted fabrics [49]. More recent developments in the medical uses of alginates have resulted in a non-woven calcium alginate for use as a primary dressing. In contact with body fluids, alginates are known to break down to simple monosaccharide-type residues and be totally absorbed. The wound exudate converts the calcium to the sodium salt facilitating the removal of the dressing by dissolution. Any residual fibres remaining within the wounds are biodegradable thus eliminating the need for complete removal [50].

Groves and Lawrence [51] have shown that significant haemostasis can be obtained when calcium alginate is applied to graft donor sites in the immediate post-surgery phase. Controlled trials on standard wounds in pigs, have shown calcium alginate to be successful in use on partial-thickness wounds both with and without occlusion. Where no additional dressing pad was used to prevent dehydration the mean epidermal regeneration under calcium alginate, at 3 days, was almost double that of the control wounds (54% compared to 28% for wounds with no dressing). When calcium alginate was used with occlusion (Figure 45) the mean rate of epidermal healing was no better than the control, i.e., Op-Site® alone, but the wounds were at a more mature stage of healing by 3 days.

The experiments on full-thickness wounds confirmed earlier findings with alginate; they are efficient haemostatic agents that are well tolerated by the body fluids and cellular components (Figure 46), but when used in cavities, the ratio of alginate to wound fluid is critical, particularly in the later stages of healing. Cellular responses to unwetted calcium alginate may be seen if too great an amount is used.

At present there are two commercially available alginate dressings both presented in the non-woven form. These are Sorbsan®, on which the above cited

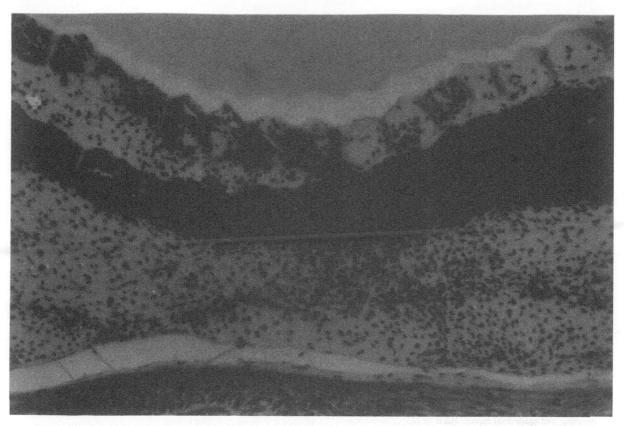

Figure 43. Movement of leucocytes and exudate into sphagnum moss cells on a partial thickness wound at 3 days. H&E ×400

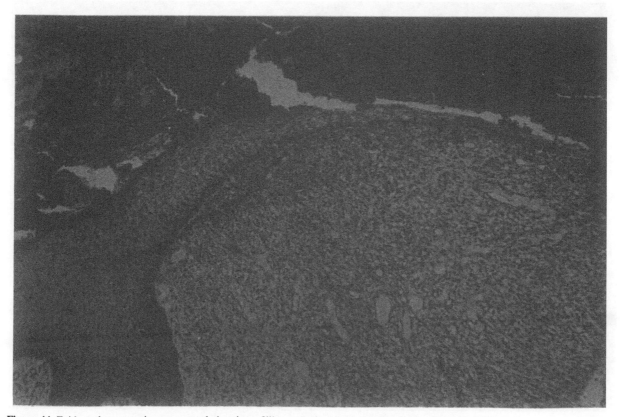

Figure 44. Epidermal regeneration over granulation tissue filling a standard deep wound at 7 days. Wound had been treated with sugar paste. H&E ×125

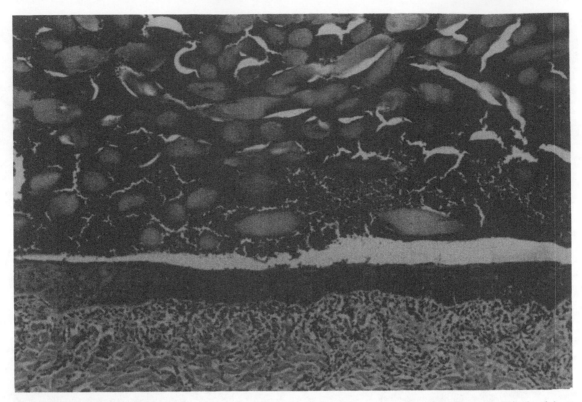

Figure 45. Partial-thickness wound under calcium alginate and Op-Site® at 3 days to show leucocytic dispersal within the alginate dressing and epidermal repair. H&E × 125

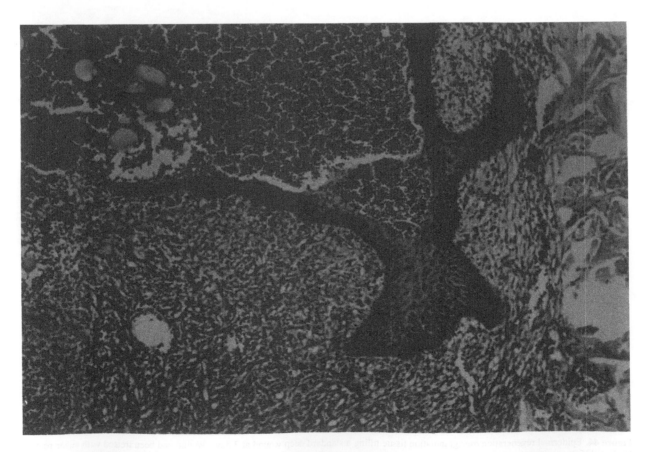

Figure 46. Epidermal repair at the corner of a standard deep wound under calcium alginate at 5 days. H&E × 125

research has been carried out, and Kaltostat®. Although both are based on calcium alginate, the two dressings differ in their physical presentation, their relative sodium and calcium content, and in the proportion of monomeric uronic acids in the polymers. As a consequence of this, the rate of gelling of the alginate and the nature of the resulting gel are different, and this is reflected in the different recommended régimes for the two dressings.

CONCLUSION

The use of a dressing on a wound is so common a practice that the choice of which dressing and the concept of wound management may often take a low priority. It is, however, now recognized that many factors affect the speed and quality of wound repair: extent of trauma, stress, oxygen tension, pH, temperature and vascularization of the wound site and any other medication being administered. In the face of all these possible variables the healing of wounds cannot always be taken for granted. For example, in a pressure sore where a bed of necrotic tissues exists, the surrounding epidermis will regenerate but will not migrate across the lesion to effect a closure.

Given that a potential for healing exists, the microenvironment of a wound can be influenced and controlled by the dressing used. It is the conditions at the wound/dressing interface, e.g., dehydration or lack of dehydration of the wound exudate, which directly influence the rate of epidermal regeneration essential for successful wound healing. These wound/dressing interface conditions are a function of the structure and composition of the wound contact surface of the dressing. With particular reference to the problem of dressing adhesion, the damage caused on dressing removal is not necessarily proportional to the degree of dressing adherence seen. Rather, it is related to dressing construction. Disruption of the repair tissue is related not only to the degree of dehydration at the wound surface but also to the relative maturity of the epidermis and its position within the exudate at the time of dressing removal. Dressings should not, therefore, be regarded as mere wound "lids" to be removed and changed without regard to the underlying tissue. Unless there are other indications, e.g., infection or the need to remove stitches, then dressings should only be changed when appropriate to the wound and not simply as part of an arbitrary dressing régime.

Modern dressings are no longer simply a cover to hide a wound from sight, absorb excess exudate, and keep the wound clean. They have the ability to interact with the wound to provide the optimal conditions for wound healing, and can be specifically prescribed for different wound types.

The microenvironment of the wound can be influenced by a dressing in the following ways:

(1) Humidity levels between wound and dressing

(2) Thermal insulation

(3) Removal of excess exudate

(4) Degree of gaseous exchange

(5) Exclusion of bacteria

(6) Chemical interaction between dressing and wound

(7) Degree of trauma caused on dressing removal

The exact requirements within these categories will vary according to the wound type being treated. In addition, there are specific requirements such as deodourizing, which is provided for by the addition of activated charcoal to many proprietary dressings, or bactericidal activity which is accompanied by the impregnation of dressings with antibiotic agents.

Proper management of any wound, therefore, requires a knowledge of the basic principles of wound healing and bacteriology. Experience gained without prior knowledge of the fundamentals of wound care is often acquired at the expense of the patient. Ambroise Paré, the French military surgeon of the sixteenth century, summed up the available knowledge of fundamental wound healing mechanisms with his famous quotation, "I make the wound and God heals it". Happily now in the twentieth century we are in a much better situation to influence this process beneficially.

REFERENCES

1. Whipple, A. O. 1963. *The Story of Wound Healing and Wound Repair*. Springfield, IL: Charles C. Thomas.

2. Guthrie, D. 1945. *History of Medicine*. London.

3. Montagna, W. and P. F. Parakkal. 1974. *The Structure and Function of Skin*. London, England: Academic Press.

4. Hartwell, S. W. 1955. *The Mechanism of Healing in Human Wounds*. Springfield, IL: Charles C. Thomas.

5. Hinman, C. D., H. I. Maibach, and G. D. Winter. 1963. "Effect of Air Exposure and Occlusion on Experimental Human Skin Wounds", *Nature*, 200: 377–379.

6. Gangjee, T., R. Colaizzo, and A. F. von Recum. 1985. "Species-Related Differences in Percutaneous Wound Healing", *Ann. Biomed. Engineer*, 13:451–467.

7. Winter, G. D. 1966. "A Study of Wound Healing in the Domestic Pig", PhD Thesis, University of London, 73–80.

8. Butcher, E. O. 1934. "The Hair Cycles in the Albino Rat", *Anat. Rec.*, 61:5–19.

9. Dry, F. W. 1926. "The Coat of the Mouse (Mus Musculus)", *J. Genet.*, 16:287–340.

10. Moritz, A. R. and F. C. Henriques. 1947. "Studies of Thermal Injury", *Amer. J. Path.*, 23:695–720.

11. Winter, G. D. 1966. "A Study of Wound Healing in the Domestic Pig", PhD Thesis, University of London, 206–346.

12. Simpson, B. J., and G. D. Winter. 1971. "A Method for Studying the Performance of Dressings Using a Stan-

dard Wound in the Domestic Pig", In *Surgical Dressings and Wound Healing*. K. J. Harkiss, ed. Bradford University Press.

13. Winter, G. D. 1971. "Healing of Skin Wounds and the Influence of Dressings on the Repair Process", In *Surgical Dressings and Wound Healing*. K. J. Harkiss, ed. Bradford University Press.

14. Winter, G. D. and L. Wilson. 1976. "Corticosteroid Induced Atrophy in the Skin of the Domestic Pig", In *Mechanisms of Topical Corticosteroid Activity*. L. C. Wilson, R. Marks, eds. London: Churchill Livingstone.

15. Winter, G. D. 1972. "Epidermal Regeneration Studied in the Domestic Pig", In *Epidermal Wound Healing*. H. I. Maibach, D. T. Rovee, eds. Chicago, IL: Year Book Medical Publishers.

16. Alvarez, O. M., P. M. Mertz, and W. H. Eaglestein. 1983. "The Effect of Occlusive Dressings on Collagen Synthesis and Re-Epithelisation in Superficial Wounds", *J. Surg. Res.*, 35:142–148.

17. Westaby, S. 1985. *Wound Care*. London, England: William Heinemann Medical Books.

18. Winter, G. D. and D. J. D. Perrins. 1970. "Effects of Hyperbaric Oxygen Treatment on Epidermal Regeneration", In *Proc. 4th Inter. Cong. Hyperbaric Med.* I. Wada, I. Iwa, eds. Tokyo, Japan: Igaku Shoin.

19. Batchelor, G. 1988. "The Pig in Wound Healing and Surgical Dressing Research; A Revision and Update", *Animal Technology*, 39:167–170.

20. Salomen, A. 1974. "Quantitative Measurement of Donor Site Epithelisation Comparing Various Dressings", In *International Symposium on Wound Healing*, Erasmus University of Rotterdam, pp. 28–31.

21. Winter, G. D. 1975. "Epidermal Wound Healing", In *Surgical Dressings in the Hospital Environment*. T. D. Turner and K. R. Brain, eds. Surgical Dressing Research Unit, UWIST, Cardiff.

22. Marks, R. 1985. "The Use of Models for the Study of Wound Healing", In *An Environment for Healing: The Role of Occlusion*. T. J. Ryan. ed. International Congress and Symposium Series; 88. Royal Society of Medicine, London.

23. Hicks, R. 1971. "Toxicological Problems of Surgical Dressings Materials", In *Surgical Dressings and Wound Healings*. K. J. Harkiss, ed. Bradford University Press.

24. Scales, J. T. and G. D. Winter. 1961. "The Adhesion of Wound Dressings, An Experimental Study", In *Wound Healing*. D. Slome, ed. Oxford: Pergamon Press.

25. Elliott, I. M. Z. 1964. *A Short History of Surgical Dressings*. London, England: Pharmaceutical Press.

26. Scales, J. T., A. G. Towers, and N. Goodman. 1956. "Development and Evaluation of a Porous Surgical Dressing", *British Medical Journal*, ii:962–980.

27. Varley, S. J., and S. E. Barnett. 1986. "A Study of Wound Dressing Adhesion", *Clinical Materials*, 1:37–57.

28. Hughes, L. E., K. G. Harding, S. Bale, and B. McPake. 1989. "Wound Management in the Community-Comparison of Lyofoam and Melolin", *Care-Science & Practice*, 7:64–67.

29. Winter, G. D. 1975. "Epidermal Wound Healing Under a New Polyurethane Foam (Lyofoam) and Cotton Gauze", *Plast. & Recon. Surg.*, 56:531–537.

30. Turner, T. D. 1985. "Semiocclusive and Occlusive Dressings", In *An Environment for Healing: The Role of Occlusion*. International Congress and Symposium Series; 88. Royal Society of Medicine, London.

31. Buchan, I. A., J. K. Andrews, S. M. Lang, J. G. Boorman, J. V. Harvey Kemble, and B. G. H. Lamberty. 1980. "Clinical and Laboratory Investigation of the Composition and Properties of Human Skin Wound Exudate Under Semi-Permeable Dressings", *Burns*, 7:326–334.

32. Buchan, I. A., J. K. Andrews, and S. M. Lang. 1981. "Laboratory Investigation of the Composition and Properties of Pig Skin Wound Exudate under Op-Site", *Burns*, 8:39–46.

33. Trade Literature, Geistlich-Pharma, Switzerland.

34. Trade Literature, Bard Ltd., Sunderland, England.

35. Trade Literature, Squibb Surgicare Ltd., Hounslow, England.

36. Varley, S. J. and S. E. Barnett. 1987. "Sphagnum Moss and Wound Healing I", *Clinical Rehabilitation*, 1:147–152.

37. Varley, S. J. and S. E. Barnett. 1987. "Sphagnum Moss and Wound Healing II", *Clinical Rehabilitation*, 1:153–160.

38. Irving, S. J., and S. E. Barnett. 1987. "Sphagnum Moss and Wound Healing III", in preparation.

39. Archer, H. G., S. E. Barnett, S. J. Irving, K. R. Middleton, and D. V. Seal. 1989. "A Controlled Model of Moist Wound Healing: Comparison Between Semi-Permeable Film, Antiseptics and Sugar Paste", *J. Exp. Path.*

40. Barnett, S. E. and S. J. Varley. 1987. "The Effects of Calcium Alginate on Wound Healing", *Ann. Roy. Coll. Surg. Eng.*, 69:153–155.

41. Dachnowski-Stokes, A. P. 1942. "Sphagnum Moss for Use in Surgical Dressings", *Scientific Monthly*, 55: 291–292.

42. Nichols, G. E. 1918. "The Sphagnum Moss and Its Use in Surgical Dressings", *Journal N.Y. Botanical Garden*, 19:203–220.

43. Nichols, G. E. 1920. "Sphagnum Moss: War Substitute for Cotton in Absorbent Surgical Dressings", *Smithsonian Institute Annual Report, 1918*, pp. 221–234.

44. Hotson, J. W. 1921. "Sphagnum Used as a Surgical Dressing in Germany During the World War", *Bryologist*, 24:74–78 and 89–96.

45. Porter, J. B. 1918. "Sphagnum Surgical Dressings", *Int. J. Surg.*, 30:129–135.

46. Middleton, K. and D. V. Seal. 1985. "Sugar as an Aid to Wound Healing", *Pharm. J.*, 235:757–758.

47. Middleton, K. and D. V. Seal. 1989. "Development of a Semi-Synthetic Sugar Paste for Promoting Healing of Infected Wounds", In *Pathogenesis of Wound and Biomaterial-Associated Infections*. I. Eliasson, ed. London, England: Springer-Verlag.

48. Barnett, S. E. 1987. "Histology of the Human Pressure Sore", *Care-Science and Practice*, 5:13–18.

49. Blaine, G. 1947. "Experimental Observations on Absorbable Alginate Products in Surgery", *Ann. Surg.*, 125:102–107.

50. Burrow, T. and M. J. Welch. 1983. "The Development and Use of Alginate Fibres in Nonwovens for Medical End-Uses", In *Nonwoven Conference Papers*, G. E. Cusick, ed. UMIST.

51. Groves, A. R. and J. C. Lawrence. 1986. "Alginate Dressing as a Donor Site Haemostat", *Ann. R. Coll. Surg. Engl.*, 68:27–28.

38

Phagocytosis of Polymeric Microspheres

YASUHIKO TABATA, Ph.D.*
YOSHITO IKADA, Ph.D.*

ABSTRACT: One of the important objectives in the current drug therapies is the selective delivery of drugs and diagnostic agents to a specific site or organ in the body, which would result in a reduction of unwanted side effects and adverse reactions. Drug delivery may be achieved with the use of a wide variety of drug carriers including macromolecules and colloidal systems, such as polymeric microspheres, liposomes, and emulsions. However, few investigations have been carried out on the interaction between polymeric microspheres and macrophages (Mø), which are the main cells of mononuclear phagocyte systems directly responsible for the clearance and disposition of the microspheres injected into the body.

This article views the phagocytosis of polymeric microspheres by Mø, focusing the physicochemical characteristics of the microspheres such as their size, surface charge, and surface hydrophobicity. It is demonstrated that the variation of these characteristics leads to a remarkable alteration in the Mø phagocytosis of the microspheres, regardless of the properties constituting the microspheres. The findings will provide information useful for the fate and distribution of the microspheres injected into the body, and a guidance for the development of polymeric microspheres as carriers applicable for drug delivery systems.

INTRODUCTION

Living systems inevitably initiate host defense mechanisms against a foreign substance. Thus, the presence of foreign materials causes acute inflammatory changes, evokes an immune reaction, or is associated with the infiltration of cells, predominantly of the mononuclear phagocyte after an acute inflammatory reaction. It is the macrophage that is the most important cell in the mononuclear phagoctye system (MPS), and that plays a major role in all these kinds of inflammation. Mononuclear phagocytes are all derived from bone marrow precursors, which circulate first as monocytes before entering tissues under physiological or inflammatory conditions, where they mature to macrophages [1]. The epitheloid and inflammatory giant cells, commonly seen in areas of chronic inflammation, are also derived from the macrophage following appropriate environmental stimuli.

The property which most distinctly separates macrophages from other cell types is the avidity with which macrophages ingest a wide variety of substances. The macrophages ingest the substance if it is small enough to be internalized into the phagocytic cells, or they differentiate into multinucleate foreign-body giant cells by their self-fusion if the substance is much larger in size than themselves. Functionally, macrophages are a rather diverse group of cells, operating at many levels in their response to invading foreign materials. Moreover, macrophages are important in the development and regulation of the immune response, together with lymphocytes, since macrophages can behave as accessory cells to facilitate the progression of immune functions, and as suppressor cells, thereby limiting the extent of host responses to a particular stimulus. In addition, macrophages play a role in the host resistance to attacks by parasites, tumors, and a wide variety of microorganisms. During the maturation of these host responses, macrophages respond to mediators released by the other leukocytes, or they themselves release the soluble mediators which have primary or secondary effects on the development of host response patterns.

Polymer materials have been widely used in medicine as artificial organs, surgical devices, and as means to assist drug delivery. Most of them are non-

*Research Center for Medical Polymers and Biomaterials, Kyoto University, 53 Kawahara-cho, Shogoin, Sakyo-ku, Kyoto 606, Japan

toxic, available with a wide variety of properties, and can be readily fabricated into many forms, such as microspheres, fibers, textiles, films, tubes, and molded products. In addition, their surfaces can be modified physically, chemically, and biochemically, in contrast to metals and ceramics. The diversity of their surface properties results in a variety of host response patterns. Since inflammatory responses to polymer materials in the body are inevitable, it is indispensable to investigate interactions between the polymer materials and the living system in order to develop biocompatible polymers which are actually applicable for clinical medicines.

Recently, polymeric microspheres have attracted much attention as carrier matrices for the sustained release of bioactive substances and for targeting therapeutic or diagnostic agents to their site of action. However, when administered into the body, the microspheres inevitably are exposed to attack from host defense systems. This is one of the major problems to be solved, when the more effective use of polymeric microspheres is desired for drug delivery systems. Most types of microspheres tend to be rapidly cleared from body fluids by the cells of the mononuclear phagocyte system (MPS). This has an important consequence, because microspheres can easily be targeted to liver and, to a lesser extent, to spleen and bone marrow. This is advantageous in imaging these organs and in trying to achieve a slow release of carrier-entrapped drugs within these organs. However, if localization of microspheres in other sites is required, their normal rapid MPS-mediated clearance must be prevented.

As macrophages play an important role in MPS-mediated clearance of microspheres in this way, an investigation into the interactions between the microspheres and the macrophage is unavoidable if polymer carriers are to be applicable to the drug delivery systems. If a drug becomes effective only when internalized into phagocytic cells, the drug-microsphere composite must have a size susceptible to phagocytosis and a surface structure which is readily recognized by the cells as a target to ingest. On the other hand, if phagocytosis of the drug must be avoided, the microspheres should have a surface to which the defense system is quite indifferent.

This article describes macrophage phagocytosis of polymeric microspheres for the purpose of gaining a deeper understanding of the polymer interaction with phagocytic cells. The information provided should contribute to the development of polymeric biomaterials, especially polymeric microspheres to be used as carriers applicable for drug delivery systems.

PREPARATION OF POLYMERIC MICROSPHERES

It has been demonstrated that the size and the surface properties of the particles are major factors regulating phagocytosis of the particles [2–6]. How-

ever, the particles employed are mostly limited to commercial latexes, bacteria, pollen, and carbon microspheres. Therefore, it is extremely difficult to study the effects of the size and the particle surface on phagocytosis. To understand the detailed phagocytosis behavior of macrophages (Mø), the use of well-characterized microspheres is highly desirable. In this connection, synthetic polymeric microspheres are the most suited for this purpose, not only because their homogeneous size is widely controlled with ease, but also because they are amenable to the surface modifications through which we can prepare microspheres with different surface natures starting from the same material. Moreover, biodegradable microspheres can also be prepared by selecting appropriate polymer materials.

Monodispersed Polymeric Microspheres

Polymeric microspheres with monodispersed distribution in size are highly preferable for phagocytosis assays, because the size largely governs the phagocytosis of the microspheres by Mø. In addition, the microspheres should be prepared without any surfactants to exclude the influence of the soap molecules adsorbed onto the surface on the phagocytosis of the microspheres.

Polystyrene microspheres, generally called latex, are the particles used most widely in cell biology and most suitable for phagocytosis study, because of their advantage of uniform size, nontoxicity, high stability, and commercial availability in various sizes. For special purposes, monodispersed latex particles can be prepared in the laboratory by using emulsion polymerization with or without surfactants [7–9]. Single-step polymerization yields particles smaller than 5.0 μm [10], while two-step or seed polymerization gives larger grains [11–13].

We have synthesized monodispersed polystyrene microspheres by soap-free emulsion polymerization of styrene at 70°C for 30 hr using potassium persulfate as an initiator [14]. The microspheres of widely different diameters were obtained by changing the monomer and initiator concentrations in the microsphere synthesis. However, it was difficult to prepare monodispersed microspheres with a diameter larger than 2 μm by this method. Much bigger microspheres can be obtained by the use of seeded-growth procedure [9,11–13]. However, in many seeded-growth syntheses, new nucleation frequently occurs leading to a new set of particles and thus to a bimodal, or even broader distribution [15] in addition to the growth of the seed particles.

Microspheres other than polystyrene and with a sharp distribution in size are also available for phagocytosis study. Among them are microspheres prepared from poly(methyl methacrylate) (PMMA), poly(vinyl toluene), and poly(vinyl acetate), but are little used in phagocytosis research. Polyacrolein microspheres were selected as monodispersed microspheres with a large diameter [16] and used to prepare microspheres with a similar surface to polystyrene. When aldehyde groups of the microspheres are reacted with aniline, we can introduce the phenyl groups into the microspheres through Schiff base formation. Phenylation of polyacrolein was followed through a contact angle measurement using polyacrolein films. Moreover, introduction of the phenyl groups onto the surfaces of polyacrolein microspheres can be confirmed by measuring the zeta potential of phenylated microspheres, because it should have a surface almost identical to that of polystyrene microspheres. Any morphological change does not take place during the phenylation reaction. SEM photographs of the phenylated polyacrolein microspheres of different sizes are shown in Figure 1, together with those of polystyrene microspheres. As can be seen, both of the microspheres are almost monodispersed in size, regardless of their diameters.

Surface Modification of Polymeric Microspheres

Phagocytosis of microspheres by Mø is greatly influenced by the physicochemical characteristics of the microsphere surface, especially by the surface charge and the hydrophobicity. Until now, most of the research on phagocytosis has been carried out using

polystyrene latex beads [17–19]. It is, however, very difficult to modify the surface of this particle. Such modifications would provide microspheres having different surface natures but the same microsphere size. The extent of microsphere phagocytosis is supposed to depend on the surface properties if the size is kept constant.

Various monodispersed polymeric microspheres having surface functional groups are prepared [20–23] and the nature and density of the functional groups can be changed by varying the initiator of emulsion polymerization, by copolymerizing with ionic monomers, or by subsequent chemical transformation. Some microspheres have surface functional groups, such as hydroxyl, carboxyl, or amino groups, available to surface modifications of microspheres. For many reactions coupling drugs, including bioactive substances and proteins, to functional microspheres, the common methods are given in Figure 2. These monodispersed functional microspheres have been utilized extensively in therapeutic and diagnostic applications [24], but few investigations have been reported on their application to phagocytosis study.

Cellulose is very useful as the starting material of microspheres for phagocytosis research, because this hydrophilic but water-insoluble polymer can be chemically modified with ease. Cellulose micro-

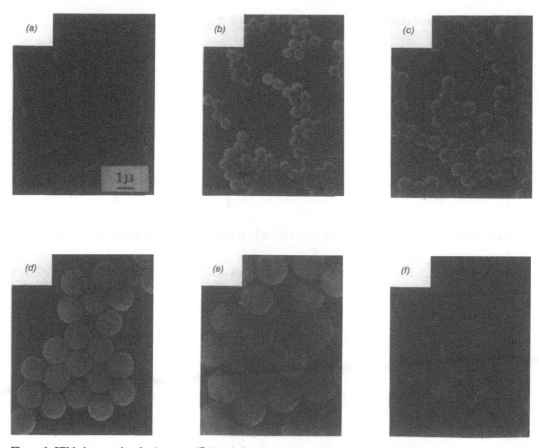

Figure 1. SEM photographs of polystyrene (Pst) and phenylated polyacrolein (PPA) microspheres of different sizes; (a) Pst 0.46 μm, (b) PPA 0.80 μm, (c) Pst 0.91 μm, (d) Pst 1.73 μm, (e) PPA 2.30 μm, and (f) PPA 4.60 μm.

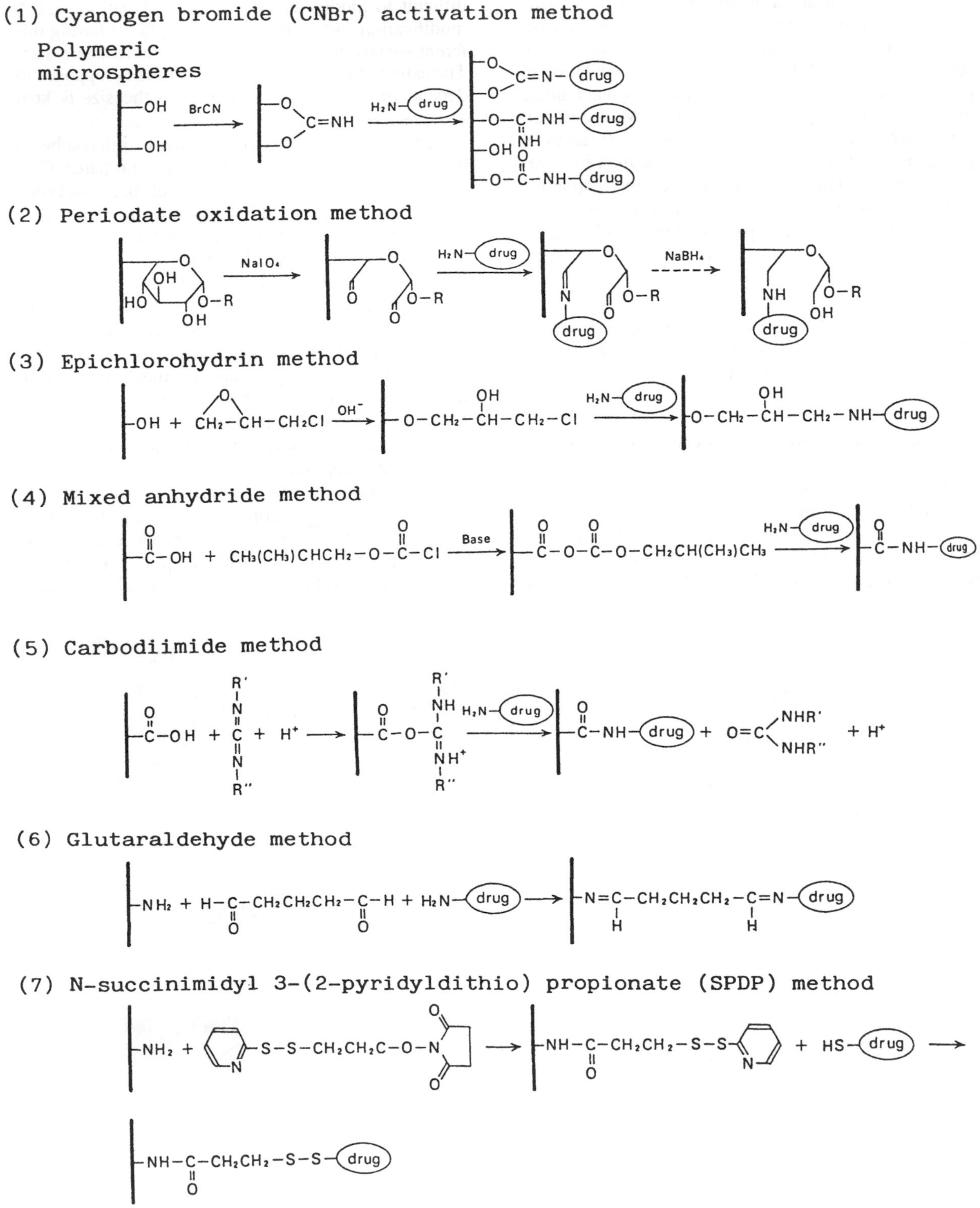
(1) Cyanogen bromide (CNBr) activation method
Polymeric microspheres
BrCN
(2) Periodate oxidation method
NaIO₄
NaBH₄
(3) Epichlorohydrin method
(4) Mixed anhydride method
Base
(5) Carbodiimide method
(6) Glutaraldehyde method
(7) N-succinimidyl 3-(2-pyridyldithio) propionate (SPDP) method

Figure 2. Various coupling methods of drugs to polymer microspheres having surface functional groups. Functional groups of the drugs and microspheres are interchangeable with each other.

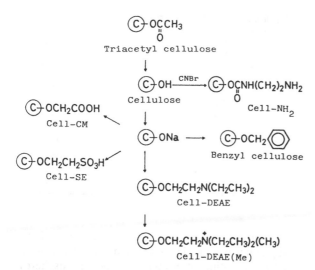

Figure 3. Reaction scheme of chemical modification of cellulose microspheres.

spheres are generally regenerated by the alkaline saponification of the triacetyl cellulose microspheres, which can be prepared by the solvent evaporation method [25] from the O/W emulsion of methylene chloride of triacetyl cellulose. The size of the cellulose microspheres can be changed by the input power of sonication at emulsification. For instance, we can obtain cellulose microspheres with an average diameter of 1.5 μm, which is a size very susceptible to M$\emptyset$ phagocytosis as will be described later.

The resulting cellulose microspheres can be cross-linked with epichlorohydrin [26]. The chemical modification of the cross-linked cellulose micro-

spheres is carried out by etherification of alkali-cellulose [25–28] as shown in Figure 3. Carboxymethyl cellulose (Cell-CM) and sulfoethyl cellulose (Cell-SE) microspheres with negative surfaces can be prepared from the cellulose microspheres. Diethylaminoethyl cellulose (Cell-DEAE) and its quaternary ammonium salt, Cell-DEAE(Me) microspheres with positive surfaces are also obtained by surface modification of cellulose microspheres. Benzyl cellulose microspheres with hydrophobic surfaces are produced by the phenylation of the cellulose microspheres. Primary amino groups (Cell-NH$_2$) can be introduced to the cellulose microspheres using the conventional cyanogen bromide (CNBr) activation method [29].

SEM photographs of different modified cellulose microspheres are shown in Figure 4. All the microspheres are seen to be spherical with diameters of less than 2 μm. No change in the average diameter and aggregation of the microspheres takes place during the reaction of surface modification. Table 1 shows the zeta potential of all the microspheres, determined by electrophoresis, together with their contact angles. This result indicates that anionic and cationic microspheres with the same average diameter but different surface charges and different hydrophobicities can be prepared by this reaction procedure.

The surface hydrophobicity of microspheres is one of the main factors regulating phagocytosis of microspheres by Mo. Microspheres having different hydrophobicities can be prepared by conversion of the hydrophilic surfaces of cellulose microspheres into hydrophobic ones by allowing alkyl amines of different carbon numbers or aromatic and cycloaliphatic

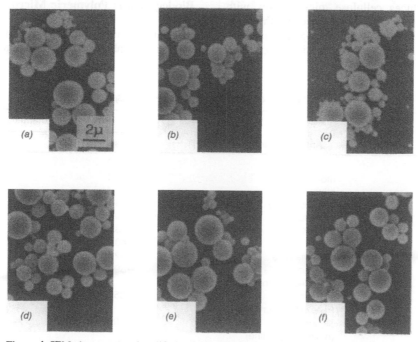

Figure 4. SEM photographs of modified cellulose microspheres; (a) triacetyl cellulose, (b) cellulose, (c) Cell-CM, (d) Cell-SE, (e) Cell-DEAE, and (f) benzyl cellulose microspheres.

Table 1. Zeta potentials and contact angles of modified cellulose microspheres.

Microspheres	Average Diameter (μm)	Zeta Potential (mV)	Contact Angle (deg)
Cellulose	1.5	−2.7	11.9
Cross-linked-cellulose	1.5	−2.7	13.0
Cell-CM	1.5	−17.1	29.4
Cell-SE	1.5	−20.9	25.6
Cell-NH$_2$	1.5	+4.6	28.0
Cell-DEAE	1.5	+14.2	24.5
Cell-DEAE(Me)	1.5	+15.1	28.6
Triacetyl cellulose	1.5	−19.9	33.2
Benzyl cellulose	1.5	−65.2	47.8

amines to link to the cellulose microspheres using the CNBr activation method [30], which is widely used in Sepharose gel preparation for hydrophobic chromatography [31–33]. A similar reaction involving surface modification is applicable to a sizable regenerated cellulose film which may be used as a reference material to estimate the surface reaction much more easily than the tiny cellulose microspheres. The contact angles of the film surfaces increase with reaction time, and become higher as the carbon number of aliphatic amines increases.

The zeta potentials of the microspheres reacted with various amines are given in Table 2, together with those of the films reacted under the same conditions as those for the microspheres. The modified cellulose microspheres have almost the same zeta potentials as the modified cellulose films, clearly indicating that the surfaces of the microspheres are chemically covered with the hydrocarbon chains, similar to the films. SEM observation demonstrated that the surface modification produces cellulose microspheres with graded water wettabilities of the surface and the same size distribution without any morphological change in the microspheres during the modification reaction.

The surface modification of cellulose microspheres with proteins was carried out both by covalent grafting and by precoating of proteins to the microspheres. Grafting reactions of various proteins to the cellulose microspheres can be conducted by the CNBr activation method [29]. The proteins employed are bovine serum albumin (BSA), bovine immunoglobulin (IgG), gelatin (Gel.), tuftsin (Tuft.), and human serum fibronectin (FN). SEM photographs of the protein-grafted cellulose microspheres, which are abbreviated as Cell-g-BSA, Cell-g-IgG, Cell-g-Gel., Cell-g-Tuft., and Cell-g-FN microspheres, respectively, demonstrate no morphological change in the microspheres during the grafting reactions (Figure 5). Besides, to enable the protein precoating of microspheres through adsorption, the hydrophilic cellulose surface was converted to a hydrophobic one (Cell-C$_6$) by allowing n-hexylamine to bind to the cellulose microspheres by the CNBr activation method.

Biodegradable Polymeric Microspheres

Recently, much attention has been paid to polymeric microspheres as carriers applicable to the sus-

Table 2. Zeta potentials of modified cellulose microspheres and films.

Abbreviation	Amines Used	Zeta Potentials (mV) Microspheres	Films
Cell-OH	—	−2.7	−2.6
Cell-C$_1$	methylamine	−7.1	−8.2
Cell-C$_2$	ethylamine	−16.4	−15.0
Cell-C$_3$	n-propylamine	−23.2	−24.2
Cell-C$_4$	n-butylamine	−20.8	−22.7
Cell-C$_6$	n-hexylamine	−33.4	−34.8
Cell-C$_8$	n-octylamine	−40.6	−41.0
Cell-C$_{10}$	n-decylamine	−42.0	−40.0
Cell-C$_{12}$	laurylamine (n-dodecylamine)	−39.0	−41.0
Cell-C$_{16}$	cetylamine (n-hexadecylamine)	−35.0	−34.2
Cell-C$_{18}$	stearylamine (n-octadecylamine)	−30.0	−35.0
Cell-∅	aniline	−65.0	−69.6
Cell-○	cyclohexylamine	−41.7	−40.6

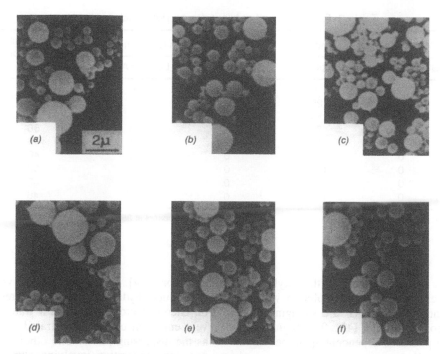

Figure 5. SEM photographs of protein-grafted cellulose microspheres; (a) cellulose, (b) Cell-g-BSA, (c) Cell-g-IgG, (d) Cell-g-FN, (e) Cell-g-Tuft., and (f) Cell-g-Gel. microspheres.

tained release of various drugs and targeting of therapeutic or diagnostic agents to their sites of action. However, when administered into the body, nondegradable polymer microspheres such as polystyrene and modified cellulose microspheres, undergo neither digestion nor metabolization *in vivo*, resulting in a lasting influence on the living environment. Consequently, employment of biodegradable microspheres as carriers for drug delivery systems is preferable in order to avoid accumulation of foreign materials in the body. Biodegradable microspheres can be classified into two categories, synthetic polymeric and protein microspheres, with respect to materials constituting microspheres.

Among many synthetic biodegradable polymers, poly(L-lactic acid) (PLLA), poly(D,L-lactic acid) (PDLLA), poly(glycolic acid) (PGA), and their copolymers (PGLA) are synthetic biodegradable polymers used most extensively in medical applications. Microsphere preparations have been used as carrier materials for the controlled release of a wide variety of drugs [34–40]. All of these polylactides are synthesized by polycondensation of the respective monomer acid or by ring-opening polymerization of the respective lactide. The weight-average molecular weight of polymers can be controlled from 1,000 to 10,000 by changing the extent of reduced pressure in polycondensation. Table 3 indicates that the content of L-lactic acid in PGLA copolymers is almost the same as that in the monomer feed for polymerization [41]. Polymers with higher molecular weights are obtainable by ring-opening polymerization of lactide and/or glycolide which are produced by depolymerization of the corresponding polymers.

PLLA and PGLA microspheres are generally prepared by the solvent evaporation method [42]. The size of the microspheres prepared by the conventional method and widely used as drug release matrices is too large to be ingested by Mø. However, ultrasonication allowed us to reduce the size of the microspheres susceptible to Mø phagocytosis. According to this method, the microspheres' size can be regulated by changing the input power of sonication in emulsification. The polylactide microspheres employed for phagocytosis study are all spherical with a diameter less than 2 μm, regardless of the kind of polymers, as shown in Figure 6.

The *in vitro* release profiles of a fluorescent dye, rhodamine 6GX, from PDLLA and PLLA microspheres of different molecular weights, are shown in Figure 7. It is seen that the rhodamine 6GX is released faster from the PLLA microspheres with the decreasing molecular weight. The release rate of PLLA microspheres is lower than that of PDLLA microspheres in spite of their similar molecular weights, because of differences in crystallizability. The effect of monomer composition on the release profiles of microspheres composed of PGLA with a similar molecular weight is given in Figure 8. The results indicate that the degradation rate of the polylactide microspheres, and thereby the release rate of drugs contained in the microspheres, can be controlled over a wide range by altering the molecular weight and the monomer composition of polymers constituting microspheres [41].

Another kind of synthetic biodegradable microspheres used for Mø phagocytosis is polyalkylcyanoacrylate nanoparticles with a diameter smaller than

Table 3. Preparation of polylactides by polycondensation.

Code	Weight Percent in Monomer		Molar Percent in Copolymer		Monomer Conversion (%)	$\bar{M}w$
	Glycolic Acid	L-Lactic Acid	Glycolic Acid	L-Lactic Acid		
PGA	100	0	100	0	38	3,500[a]
PGLA-1	75	25	78	22	51	3,200[a]
PGLA-2	50	50	57	43	50	2,900
PGLA-3	30	70	32	68	56	3,300
PGLA-4	25	75	29	71	46	2,800
PLLA-1	0	100	0	100	48	3,400
PLLA-2	0	100	0	100	53	8,000
PLLA-3	0	100	0	100	60	13,000
PDLLA	0	100[b]	0	100[b]	46	3,300

[a]Determined by the measurement of intrinsic viscosity in 1,1,1,3,3,3-hexafluoro-2-isopropanol at 25°C.
[b]D,L-lactic acid.

0.3 μm. They are prepared by adding the alkylcyano-acrylate monomers to an aqueous solution with or without surfactants at various pH values ranging from 2 to 4 under vigorous stirring [43]. The degradation rate of the microspheres is dependent upon the length of alkyl chains of alkylcyanoacrylate monomers used and increases with the increasing alkyl chain length.

The protein which is most widely used as a microsphere material is serum albumin from bovine, human, or other appropriate species. There are two basic methods for the production of albumin microspheres. One is either thermal denaturation at an elevated temperature from 95°C to 170°C, or chemical cross-linking in vegetable oil or organic solvent emulsions [44]. The latter method, which is claimed to produce "hydrophilic" microspheres [45], depends on chemical cross-linking in a water-in-organic solvent emulsion using concentrated polymer solutions as the dispersing phase. The other method is simple one-step preparation involving either thermal denaturation of protein aerosol in gas medium [46] or an aerosol step followed by denaturation in oil [47]. The size of the albumin microspheres prepared by these methods ranges from 0.2 to 100 μm in diameter.

Gelatin has been commonly utilized for microencapsulation, such as complex coacervation [48], simple coacervation [49], emulsification [50], and its modified emulsification [51–53]. Since the heat dena-

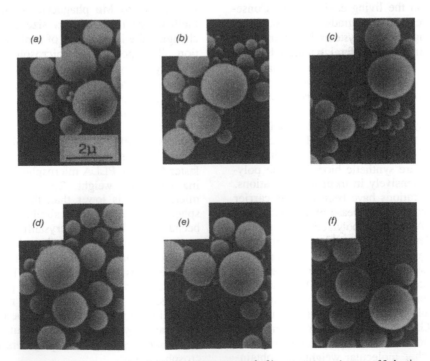

Figure 6. SEM photographs of microspheres composed of homo- and copolymers of L-lactic acid and glycolic acid; (a) PGA, (b) PGLA-1, (c) PGLA-2, (d) PGLA-3, (e) PGLA-4, and (f) PLLA-1 microspheres (see Table 3 concerning the code of microspheres).

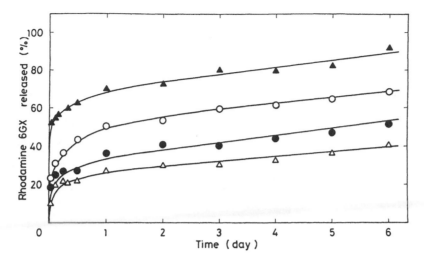

Figure 7. *In vitro* release profiles of rhodamine 6GX from poly(lactic acid) microspheres; (○) PLLA-1, (●) PLLA-2, (△) PLLA-3, and (▲) PDLLA microspheres (see Table 3 concerning the code of microspheres).

turation method described above cannot be applied to the microsphere preparation of gelatin (denatured collagen), the microsphere requires stabilization by chemical cross-linking. Glutaraldehyde is one of the best known cross-linking reagents for proteins, and numerous investigators have reported the cross-linking of collagen with glutaraldehyde [54–56]. Cross-linking of gelatin microspheres is carried out by an addition of glutaraldehyde in the organic phase after generating a water-in-organic solution emulsion to avoid aggregation in the microsphere preparation [57]. Figure 9 shows light micrographs of the resulting gelatin microspheres in a suspension state in phosphate-buffered saline solution (PBS). Clearly, the shape of microspheres is invariably spherical and apparently swollen when the concentration of gelatin and glutaraldehyde is used in microsphere preparations.

In addition, the size can be widely changed without any aggregation of the microspheres by selecting the appropriate input power of sonication in emulsification. Figures 10 and 11 show the degradation of gelatin microspheres and thereby the release of interferon (IFN) from the microspheres, respectively. The degradation of gelatin microspheres can be controlled by changing the extent of cross-linking which can be regulated by the amount of gelatin and glutaraldehyde added to microsphere preparations. This leads to a satisfactory regulation of release rate of IFN contained in the microspheres.

BIOCHEMISTRY OF PHAGOCYTOSIS

The ingestion of foreign materials by cells was first clearly described by Metchnikoff [58] though it had been mentioned by several earlier workers. The term phagocytosis initially meant the ingestion of solid

foreign materials by cells. More recently it has been realized that there are a number of ways in which cells may take in materials. As long ago as 1931, Lewis showed that Mø in tissue culture would take in microscopically visible droplets prepared from the culture fluid. This is so-called pinocytosis. Not long after the introduction of the electron microscope it became apparent that ingestion is also seen for tiny vesicles of 0.1 μm or less in a diameter. This has been given several names, of which perhaps the best is micropinocytosis. The general aspects of the uptake of substances by cells have been reviewed by Jacques [59]. According to that review, Mø are quantitatively superior in endocytic capacity to other types of cells in the body, and it is an assigned task of Mø to ingest a wide variety of substances which have invaded the living system.

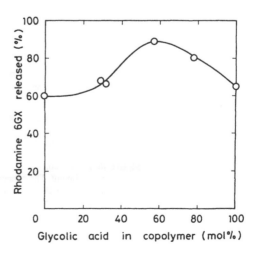

Figure 8. Effect of the monomer composition on release of rhodamine 6GX from the microspheres of PGLA microspheres.

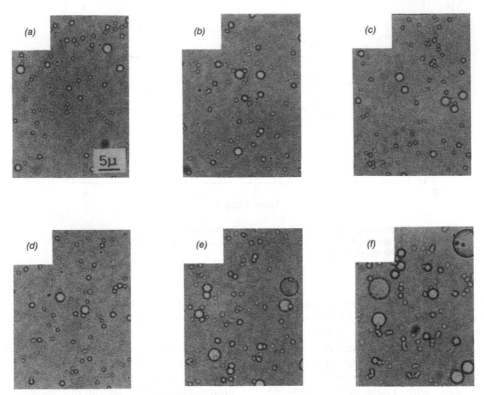

Figure 9. Light microscopic photographs of gelatin microspheres cross-linked with glutaraldehyde in concentrations of 1.33 (a), 0.71 (b), 0.28 (c), 0.14 (d), 0.05 (e), and 0.03 mg/mg gelatin (f).

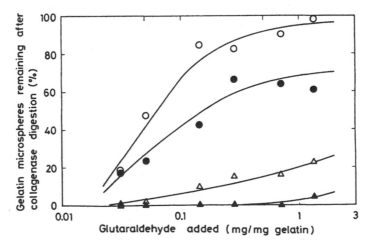

Figure 10. *In vitro* collagenase digestion of gelatin microspheres of different extents of cross-linking. The concentration of gelatin used in microsphere preparations is 10 ($\bigcirc$), 5 ($\bullet$), 2.5 ($\triangle$), and 1 wt% ($\blacktriangle$).

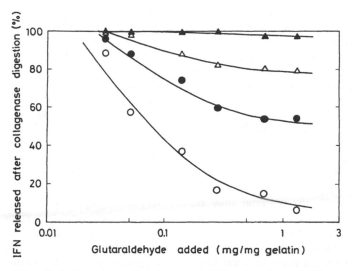

Figure 11. *In vitro* release of interferon from gelatin microspheres of different extents of cross-linking after collagenase digestion for 30 min. The concentration of gelatin used in microsphere preparations is 10 (○), 5 (●), 2.5 (△), and 1 wt% (▲).

Endocytosis is the process of internalizing extracellular materials by an invagination of the plasmalemma through various pathways illustrated in Figure 12. The endocytic activity has always been divided into two categories: phagocytosis, or eating, and pinocytosis, or drinking. The term phagocytosis is used to describe the internalization of large particles, such as those visible by light microscopy, mostly some viruses and bacteria. Uptake occurs by close apposition of a segment of plasma membrane to the particle's surface, excluding most, if not all, of the surrounding fluid. The term pinocytosis is used to describe the vesicular uptake of everything else, including insoluble particles (lipoproteins, ferritin, colloids, immune complex), soluble macromolecules (enzymes, hormones, antibodies, toxins), fluids, and low-molecular-weight

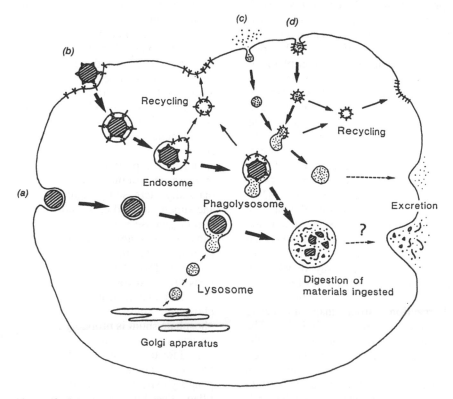

Figure 12. Schematic diagram illustrating various pathways of endocytosis; (a) phagocytosis, (b) receptor-mediated phagocytosis, (c) pinocytosis, and (d) receptor-mediated pinocytosis.

solutes. It is likely that these materials are all interiorized in vesicles with electron-lucent contents, and it is assumed that extracellular fluids are included in the contents. Although these are not identical in cellular processes, they have much in common, such as the requirement for an energy source (ATP) and for physiologic temperature.

The phenomenon of phagocytosis seen in living cells in tissue culture or in a rabbit's ear chamber is dramatic. The Mø which have been moving with flapping ruffles at their leading edge, push out processes towards a particulate substance and rapidly flow around it. The process of ingestion may take only a few minutes. Once ingested, the material may be totally digested, or may persist in the form of an indigestable residue, may actually fill up the cell, and, if toxic, may kill the cell. Another less common form of phagocytosis occurs when the particle is too large for one cell to ingest. In this case, several cells flow around it and form a capsule.

Early literature on phagocytosis was reviewed by Mudd et al. [60], Berry and Spies [61], and Hirsh [62]. The events of phagocytosis are considered to take place in three consecutive stages: attachment, ingestion, and digestion of the particles. The attachment of particles to the plasma membrane is a prerequisite for interiorization and leads to a localized perturbation of the membrane beneath the attachment site. This is characterized morphologically by the aggregation of actin-like filaments, associated with the formation of pseudopods that enclose the particle. However, it is not clear at present how a cell recognizes a particle as being foreign, though the presence of specific surface receptors has been postulated. The membrane of Mø contains the receptors specific for the Fc fragment of IgG and for third component of complements [63,64]. There is no doubt that these receptors mediate the specific binding between Mø and molecules or particles bearing the corresponding ligands.

The phagocytosis of nonantigenic particles, such as latexes and powdered carbons, cannot always be linked with the need for specific receptors or opsonizing factors. The phagocytic cells have on the cell surface a capability to recognize foreign substances by their surface properties. In the beginning of the 1820s, the response of cells to foreign bodies on the basis of surface tension effects was described by Fenn and Mudd [65,66]. Mudd et al. [60] subsequently pointed out the similarity between the way in which a phagocyte spreads on a surface and the way in which it spreads on a particle (phagocytosis). It has been demonstrated that cell attachment to foreign bodies is a physicochemical reaction rather than an active energy-dependent biological reaction [67–70]. The physicochemical reaction may be discussed on the basis of adhesion work of films with cells in water, provided that only dispersive and polar forces are operative in the adhesion phenomena of L cells to conventional polymer films in aqueous media [70]. The attachment of a particle to the cell-bearing surface receptors for ligands on the particle surface gen-

erally occurs independently of temperature [71] and the expenditure of metabolic energy. Rovinovitch [72] demonstrated that the attachment of aldehyde-fixed erythrocytes to Mø was less dependent on temperature and did not require divalent cations or serum, in contrast to ingestion which was reduced at lower temperatures and by some metabolic inhibitors.

Once a particle is attached to a cell surface, the formation of a phagosome is triggered so that the particle is internalized and transported to the inside of the cell membrane [73]. A common feature seems to be that the engulfing plasma membrane which surrounds the particles during their entry to Mø by phagocytosis is very closely apposed to the surface of the particle, so that very little fluid may enter the inside with the particle. For the receptor-mediated phagocytosis, it seems apparent that the receptors on the cell surface successively interact with the ligands disposed around the particles, "zipping" the plasma membrane shut around the particles as summarized by Silverstein et al. [74].

The actual mechanism of the cytoplasmic movements involved in the ingestion phase of phagocytosis is obscure, but the action of the cytoskeleton system is clearly attributed to the ingestion phase [75,76]. The cytoplasm immediately beneath the area of the particle-associated plasma membrane is devoid of organelles, and has been termed the hyaline cortex. It contains a network consisting of actin microfilaments. The actin-binding protein and myosin are also concentrated into this region [77]. When small particles impinge on the surface of Mø, they are swept by active ruffling movements of the cell membrane into vacuoles which then pass deep into the cell. When the size of the materials to be phagocytosed is larger than Mø, the process of the ingestion is somewhat different. Mø become very closely apposed to the foreign substances and adherent to one another by tightly interlocking cell processes. The cytoplasma next to the substances is entirely ectoplasmic and free of organelles, leading to the formation of the hyaline cortex.

During the particle ingestion, phagocytes show an increase in cyanide-insensitive O_2 consumption, a markedly increased production of hydrogen peroxide and superoxide radicals, and stimulation of the oxidation of glucose via the pentose phosphate shunt [78]. Most workers agree that this burst of oxidative activity results from the activation of a plasma-membrane-linked NADH [79] or NADPH [80] oxidase that converts O_2 to hydrogen peroxide via superoxide anions [81], and that hydrogen peroxide drives the hexose phosphate shunt. The stimulation of the pentose phosphate shunt is probably related to the need to synthesize a new cell membrane. Reduced NADP is required for the synthesis of fatty acids which are essential components of the cell membrane required for phagocytosis. This need for NADPH is probably fulfilled, therefore, by the stimulation of the hexose monophosphate shunt.

After ingestion of the vesicle which forms around

the phagocytosed particle, the phagosome fuses with one or more lysosomes to form a secondary lysosome or phagolysosome. The hydrolytic enzymes contained in the lysosome are thus discharged into the enlarged vacuole to degrade the contents. The lysosome is a membranous bag of hydrolytic enzymes to be used for the controlled intracellular digestion of ingested materials. The lysosomal enzymes of Mø have been studied by Cohn and Wiener [82]. Approximately 40 enzymes are now known to be contained in lysosomes. They are all hydrolytic enzymes, including proteases, nucleases, glucosidases, lipases, phospholipases, phosphatases, and sulfatases. In addition, all are acid hydrolases, optimally active near the pH of 5 maintained within this organelle. The newly formed phagosome is acidified rapidly and this process is initiated prior to fusion with lysosomes although the two processes are linked closely in time [83,84]. The acidic environment within phagolysosomes gives rise to the dissociation of ligand-receptor complexes, degradation of ligands and receptors, and retrieval of receptors and membrane constituents by recycling [85].

FACTORS REGULATING PHAGOCYTOSIS

Size of Polymeric Microspheres

The dependence of Mø phagocytosis on the size of microspheres was examined using monodispersed polystyrene and monodispersed phenylated polyacrolein microspheres [14]. There is no straightforward method for evaluating Mø phagocytosis, especially when comparison is to be made using microspheres of different sizes. One may evaluate the extent of phagocytosis by either the number or the volume of the total microspheres which a Mø has phagocytosed. Thus, the number or the volume of the microspheres was measured when a fixed number or a fixed volume per Mø was given.

Figure 13 illustrates the result when the microsphere number is fixed. Clearly, the number of microspheres phagocytosed per Mø has a maximum at a diameter between 1.0 and 2.0 μm, regardless of the presence of fetal calf serum (FCS) in Mø cultures. The effect of FCS addition on Mø phagocytosis will be described later. Besides this, the number of microspheres with a small diameter was larger than that with a larger diameter, when the volume added to Mø was fixed. However, the ratio of the number of phagocytosed microspheres to that of the microspheres added became maximal in a range of diameter between 1.0 and 2.0 μm. Kawaguchi et al. [86] reported that the particles with a diameter between 0.4 and 1.0 μm were the most easily ingested by leukocytes, when the volume added was fixed. Moreover, it was demonstrated that the largest uptake by leukocytes was for the particles with a diameter ranging 0.3 to 2.6 μm [87]. It seems that Mø may have the ability to recognize the size of foreign materials attached to them, but the reason is at present undefined. In addi-

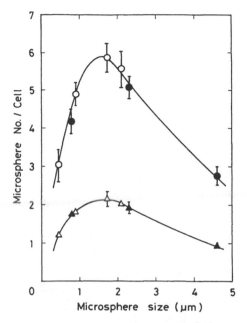

Figure 13. Mø phagocytosis of microspheres with different sizes in the absence (○, ●) and presence (△, ▲) of FCS (open mark, polystyrene microspheres; solid mark, phenylated polyacrolein microspheres).

tion, the polystyrene microspheres with a diameter of 2.1 μm and the phenylated polyacrolein microspheres with a diameter of 2.3 μm were ingested to a similar extent, indicating that Mø phagocytosis was not governed by the bulk property of microspheres, but merely by the surface property of microspheres.

Surface Charge of Polymeric Microspheres

Mø phagocytosis of modified cellulose microspheres with different surface charges was investigated [14] and the time course of phagocytosis in the absence of FCS is shown in Figure 14. The microspheres have the same average diameter of 1.5 μm but different surface charges (Table 1 and Figure 4). Clearly, the number of microspheres phagocytosed by one Mø increases with the incubation time for all the microspheres and is dependent on the surface properties. The hydrophobic microspheres (benzyl cellulose) are the most susceptible to phagocytosis and the nonionic hydrophilic ones (unmodified cellulose) are the least. However, the surface charge of hydrophilic microspheres has a great effect on phagocytosis. The result given in Figure 14 shows that microspheres with cationic surfaces [Cell-DEAE(Me)] are more readily ingested than those with anionic surfaces (Cell-SE). This is, however, not correct, because the surface density differs among microspheres with both cationic and anionic surfaces. In this connection, the zeta potential of every modified cellulose microsphere is employed as a relative measure of the charge density, and the number of microspheres phagocytosed per one Mø was plotted as a function of their zeta potentials in Figure 15. It is seen that the phagocytosis is enhanced as the absolute value of zeta potentials in-

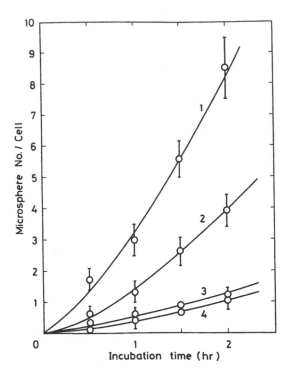

Figure 14. Time course of Mø phagocytosis of modified cellulose microspheres in the absence of FCS; (1) benzylcellulose, (2) Cell-DEAE(Me), (3) cellulose, and (4) Cell-SE microspheres.

creases for both the negatively charged and the positively charged surfaces. It is interesting to point out that the lowest phagocytosis is realized for the surface with a zeta potential of zero. It seems that the negatively charged membrane of Mø and the presence of divalent cations like Ca^{2+} and Mg^{2+} in the culture medium are closely related to the dependence of phagocytosis on the zeta potential of the charged microspheres.

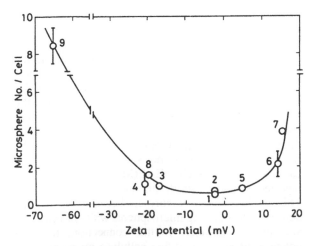

Figure 15. Effect of the surface charge on phagocytosis of modified cellulose microspheres by Mø; (1) Cell-OH, (2) cross-linked Cell-OH, (3) Cell-CM, (4) Cell-SE, (5) Cell-NH₂, (6) Cell-DEAE, (7) Cell-DEAE(Me), (8) triacetyl cellulose, and (9) benzylcellulose microspheres.

Surface Hydrophobicity of Polymeric Microspheres

Most of the investigations on the phagocytosis of foreign particles have demonstrated that the uptake of the particles by the phagocytic cells is largely influenced by the physicochemical properties of the particle surface, especially its hydrophobicity [3,5,6,18, 88–91]. In general, an increase in the hydrophobicity of a particle surface leads to an enhanced uptake, unless the surface is very strongly hydrophobic. Van Oss et al. [88] have shown that bacteria with a higher contact angle than that of neutrophils were readily phagocytosed by them and that those with a lower contact angle were phagocytosed to a much lesser extent by neutrophils. It is likely that phagocytosis of microspheres by Mø takes place through at least two steps, attachment and ingestion, as described earlier. The first event may be dominated by a common physicochemical process, while the second event must involve a series of biological reactions.

The modified cellulose microspheres with different water wettabilities were added to Mø in order to investigate the dependence of Mø phagocytosis on the surface hydrophobicity. Figure 16 indicates that there is definitely an optimal surface hydrophobicity for the microspheres to be phagocytosed. In addition, as shown in Figure 16, the number of biodegradable PLLA and PGLA microspheres phagocytosed also obeys the observed dependence of Mø phagocytosis on microsphere hydrophobicity, indicating that Mø phagocytosis is not governed by the bulk properties of microspheres such as the degradability of microspheres themselves, but by the surface properties of microspheres.

A similar dependence of surface wettability on cell adhesion was also found for the adhesion of bacteria onto flat films of different hydrophobicities [92,93]. The fact strongly indicates that common forces are operative between a cell surface and a synthetic polymer surface, irrespective of the nature of the cells. In the previous work [70], we theoretically evaluated the work of adhesion between two different substances in aqueous media and reached the conclusion that a substance cannot strongly adhere to the opposite substance in aqueous media if one of the surfaces is either extremely hydrophilic (very low contact angle) or extremely hydrophobic (very high contact angle). The result shown in Figure 16 is in good agreement with this theoretical prediction, indicating the similarity between the cell attachment on a substance surface and Mø attachment on a particle for phagocytosis.

Physical phenomena associated with the cell surface, such as cell adhesion and phagocytosis, may be characterized as being dominated by surface free energies, which are the relevant thermodynamic potentials for these processes [6]. The calculation of a change in the free energy of the modified microspheres during phagocytosis demonstrates that phago-

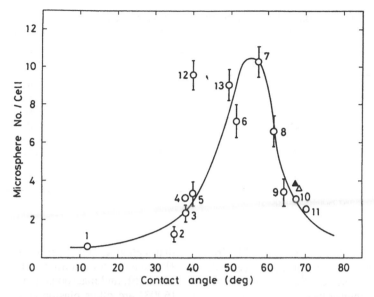

Figure 16. Effect of the contact angle on phagocytosis of modified cellulose microspheres by Mø; (1) Cell-OH, (2) Cell-C_1, (3) Cell-C_2, (4) Cell-C_3, (5) Cell-C_4, (6) Cell-C_6, (7) Cell-C_8, (8) Cell-C_{10}, (9) Cell-C_{12}, (10) Cell-C_{16}, (11) Cell-C_{18}, (12) Cell-$\varnothing$, (13) Cell-$\bigcirc$, ($\triangle$) PLLA, and ($\blacktriangle$) PGLA microspheres (see Table 2 concerning the code of microspheres).

cytosis increases with the increasing negative free energy change, in agreement with the thermodynamic expectation [30]. This indicates that the engulfing process in phagocytosis may essentially be explained by the interfacial free energy effects.

The relationship between phagocytosis of the microspheres and their zeta potentials is shown in Figure 17. Phagocytosis takes place more markedly with the increasing negative zeta potentials of the microsphere surface, suggesting that the interaction of the Mø with the microsphere surface in the cell culture medium is largely governed by electrostatic forces. Divalent cations in the culture medium would be localized between the two substances in order to reduce the free energy of the total system. Also, the addition of EDTA to the system led to a reduction of phagocytosis only in the region of high negative values of zeta potentials of the microspheres. This result implies that bridging is formed between the microspheres and the cells through divalent cationic ions in the culture medium.

It may be concluded that the van der Waals interaction is the most important factor in the attachment of microspheres to Mø followed by the internalization of

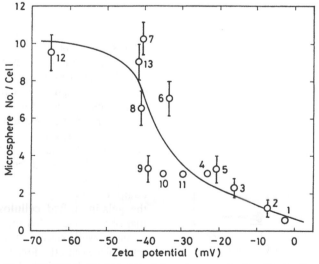

Figure 17. Effect of the zeta potential on phagocytosis of modified cellulose microspheres by Mø (see Figure 16 concerning the numbers in the figure).

Table 4. Phagocytosis of protein-grafted cellulose microspheres by macrophages.

Microspheres	FCS (−)		FCS (+)	
	Microsphere No./Cell	Ratio[a]	Microsphere No./Cell	Ratio[a]
Polystyrene[b]	5.88	14.70	2.16	6.55
Cellulose	0.40	1.00	0.33	1.00
Cell-C$_6$	7.02	17.55	3.57	10.82
Cell-g-BSA	0.25	0.63	0.26	0.79
Cell-g-IgG	9.24	23.15	10.08	30.55
Cell-g-Gel.	7.31	18.28	11.29	34.21
Cell-g-Tuft.	6.71	16.78	6.79	20.58
Cell-g-FN	8.41	21.03	8.71	26.39

[a]Ratio to the number of cellulose microspheres phagocytosed.
[b]Diameter is 1.73 μm.

the microspheres, and that there is an optimal hydrophobicity for the surface of microspheres susceptible to phagocytosis, regardless of the biodegradable nature of microspheres themselves.

Proteins and Other Additives

Mø phagocytosis is greatly affected by the presence of various proteins contained in serum. It is well known that some specific proteins remarkably enhance the phagocytosis of particles. This phenomenon is called opsonization [94,95]. Most popular proteins among those responsible for opsonization, that is, opsonins, are immunological proteins like immunoglobulin G [96,97] and the third component of complements (C3b) [98]. A tetrapeptide "hormone", tuftsin, stimulates phagocytosis by specifically binding to immunoglobulin [99]. In addition, it is known

that methylated albumin [6,100], fibronectin [101,102], Hageman factor (clotting factor XII) [6], fibrinogen or fibrin [6], and macrophage migration inhibition factor [6,103] are other plasma components possessing opsonizing potential.

Table 4 summarizes the results of Mø phagocytosis of cellulose microspheres whose surfaces were grafted with various protein molecules, together with the microspheres not grafted or modified by coupling with a n-hexyl (C$_6$) chain, as well as polystyrene microspheres. In addition, the effect of fetal calf serum (FCS) added to Mø cultures on phagocytosis is also given. Several interesting features can be seen in the results. First, the cellulose microspheres grafted with BSA undergo the least phagocytosis, irrespective of the presence of FCS. The next least phagocytosis is observed for the original microspheres of cellulose. In contrast, the surface modification with C$_6$ chains greatly enhances Mø phagocytosis, almost to a level similar to that of the polystyrene microspheres. Second, the Mø phagocytosis is remarkably accelerated by surface grafting of the cellulose microspheres with proteins other than BSA. Third, an addition of FCS to the culture medium increases the uptake of gelatin-grafted cellulose microspheres to a remarkable extent, whereas added FCS decreases the phagocytosis for microspheres having a hydrophobic surface, such as C$_6$-coupled cellulose and polystyrene microspheres.

The effect of FCS addition can be seen much more distinctly in Figure 18, where the number of microspheres phagocytosed is plotted against the FCS concentration of the medium for some typical microspheres. The results obviously confirm the findings demonstrated in Table 4. Phagocytosis of the original and the BSA-grafted cellulose is insignificant and hardly influenced by the presence of FCS, while the addition of FCS apparently increases phagocytosis for the gelatin-grafted cellulose, in marked contrast to that of the C$_6$-coupled microspheres.

As is well known, protein adsorption generally takes place onto the foreign surfaces, especially when they are moderately hydrophobic. It is likely that protein desorption also depends on the hydrophobicity of the surface to which the protein has been adsorbed.

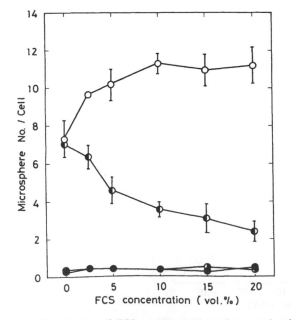

Figure 18. Influence of FCS concentration on phagocytosis of protein-grafted cellulose microspheres by Mø; (○) Cell-g-Gel., (●) Cell-g-BSA, (◐) Cell-OH, and (◑) Cell-C$_6$ microspheres.

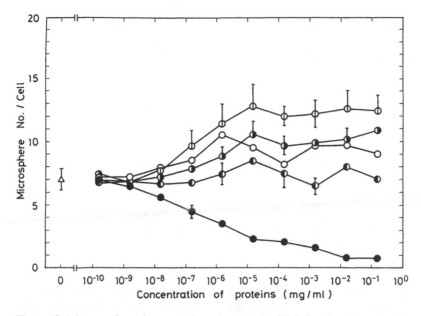

Figure 19. Influence of protein precoated on phagocytosis of Cell-C_6 microspheres by Mø in the absence of FCS; (⦾) IgG, (⦿) FN, (○) Gelatin, (●) BSA, and (△) none.

Presumably, the more strongly the protein is adsorbed, the less readily it may be desorbed. In this connection, the surface of C_6-coupled cellulose microspheres has sufficient hydrophobicity to be strongly absorbed by proteins and to be highly resistant to protein desorption. Figures 19 and 20 show the effect of protein precoating on the Mø phagocytosis of the C_6-coupled cellulose microspheres in the absence and the presence of FCS, respectively. One prominent change is observed for IgG and BSA: the former increases the phagocytosis, while the latter decreases it with the increasing concentration at precoating.

This trend is similar to that found for protein-grafted microspheres, indicating that the proteins must be adsorbed onto the surface of C_6-coupled microspheres, apparently with the firmness of covalent grafts. The other striking finding in Figure 20 is that gelatin precoating remarkably promotes the microsphere's phagocytosis in the presence of FCS, though the precoating with opsonic proteins, such as

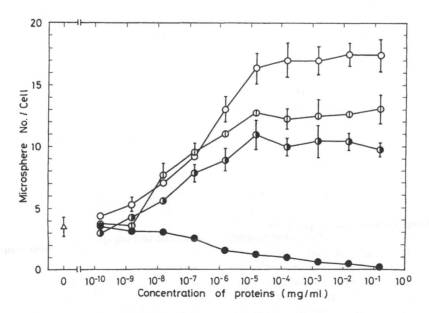

Figure 20. Influence of protein precoated on phagocytosis of Cell-C_6 microspheres by Mø in the presence of FCS; (⦾) IgG, (⦿) FN, (○) gelatin, (●) BSA, and (△) none.

Table 5. Influence of macromolecule precoating of PGLA-2 microspheres on phagocytosis by macrophages.

Macromolecules[a] for Precoating	Contact Angle (deg)	Microsphere No./Cell FCS (−)	Microsphere No./Cell FCS (+)
None	70.9	3.80	2.64
BSA	26.2	1.62	1.30
IgG	24.5	6.20	6.21
FN	21.2	4.48	4.82
Tuftsin	32.4	3.44	3.79
Gelatin	21.3	4.10	9.67
PVA	20.4	0.52	0.42
Dextran	24.4	2.09	1.97
PAAm	25.2	1.30	1.17
PHEG	28.2	2.78	2.52
CMC	24.3	2.42	1.86
PVP	36.4	2.79	2.24

[a]The concentration of macromolecules for precoating is 0.15 mg/ml.

IgG and FN, increases the phagocytosis almost to the level of that without FCS. A similar trend mentioned above was also observed when biodegradable PLLA, PGA, and PGLA microspheres were used for Mø phagocytosis.

The above results can be explained in terms of the surface hydrophobicity of microspheres and opsonization, regardless of the degradability of microspheres themselves. There is no reason to suspect that the resistance of the virgin cellulose microspheres against phagocytosis is due to its low hydrophobicity (high hydrophilicity). BSA has neither the opsonizing ability nor the propensity to alter the hydrophobicity of the cellulose, and consequently does not increase phagocytosis when grafted to the cellulose surface. Polystyrene, C_6-coupled, PLLA, PGLA, and PGA microspheres with very hydrophobic surfaces will be preferably coated by albumin, the most abundant protein in FCS, leading to suppressed phagocytosis, when placed in the medium containing FCS. In addition, Table 5 demonstrates that lowering the hydrophobicity of the microsphere surfaces by precoating with nonproteinaceous macromolecules, such as poly(vinyl alcohol) (PVA), dextran, polyacrylamide (PAAm), poly(N-hydroxyethyl-L-glutamine) (PHEG), carboxymethyl cellulose (CMC), and poly(vinyl pyrrolidone) (PVP), led to a reduction in Mø phagocytosis.

The exceptions are the microspheres modified with gelatin, regardless of the mode of surface binding—that is, either covalently grafting (Table 4) or physical coating (Figure 20). FN and other cell-adhesive proteins contained in serum may primarily be bound to the gelatin microsphere surface due to the bioaffinity of gelatin. Gudwicz et al. [104] and other investigators [105] have demonstrated an enhancement of Mø phagocytosis of gelatin-coated latex particles by an addition of FN to Mø cultures. Consequently, the opsonizing ability of gelatin must be more strongly enhanced in the presence than in the absence of FCS.

In addition to its opsonic ability, gelatin has an inherent propensity for Mø phagocytosis. The high susceptibility of gelatin to ingestion by Mø has been demonstrated for microspheres prepared from gelatin. Gelatin microspheres are readily phagocytosed by Mø (Figure 21) and the Mø phagocytosis takes place independent of the extent of microspheres cross-linking, as shown in Figure 22. However, when the concentration of gelatin and glutaraldehyde in microspheres preparation is low, gelatin microspheres are highly swollen and become large (Figure 9), resulting in a reduction of Mø phagocytosis. Moreover, we succeeded in a very effective delivery of some drugs into Mø using the gelatin microspheres [106,107]. Besides, it is apparent that the FCS addition has no remarkable effect in Mø phagocytosis of the microspheres grafted or precoated with proteins other than gelatin, denoting that these surfaces are not bound by any serum proteins in FCS, in contrast to the microspheres without grafting.

FATE OF POLYMERIC MICROSPHERES IN MACROPHAGE

Uptake of polymeric microspheres by Mø proceeds as shown in Figure 12, regardless of the nature of microsphere matrix, such as its degradability. Thus, polymeric microspheres are ingested by Mø in phagocytic vacuoles (phagosomes) that fuse them with lysosomes to form phagolysosomes, where the ingested microspheres are exposed to an attack by various hydrolytic enzymes of the lysosomes in order to degrade them. However, when the microspheres to be ingested were prepared from nondegradable polystyrene, the resistance of the microspheres to the lysosomal enzymes led to their intact presence within the cells and the lysosomal vesicles without exocytosis [108]. Uptake of biodegradable PGA microspheres within the cytoplasm of Mø was similar to that seen when the polystyrene microspheres were identified in Mø cytoplasm. TEM observation demonstrated incorporation of the phagocytosed microspheres into cytoplasmic phagolysosomes [109].

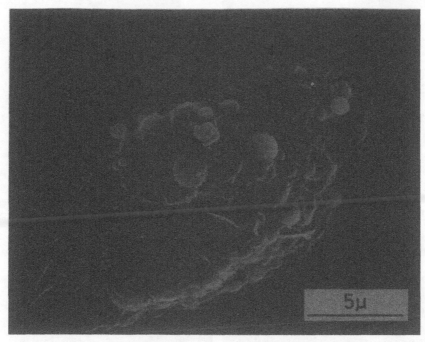

Figure 21. A SEM photograph of Mø with gelatin microspheres ingested.

The use of the Mø culture system is an effective method for studying the process of microsphere phagocytosis, and for evaluating the time course of microsphere degradation in the cells, when combined with electron microscopic techniques. Figure 23 shows SEM photographs of the mode of degradation of PGLA-2 microspheres with the passage of culture time. Figure 23(a) shows the Mø before incubation with the microspheres, and Figures 23(b) to 23(e) show the Mø incubated with the microspheres for 2 hr, 6 hr, 4 days, and 7 days, respectively. It is apparent that the microspheres were well phagocytosed by Mø within 6 hr. Then, the contour of the microspheres in the Mø gradually disappeared with the increasing incubation time. After 7 days, no microspheres were observed in the cells. In addition, phase-contrast microscopic observation more clearly confirmed that the disappearance of PGLA-2 microspheres inside the Mø was not due to exocytosis, but to degradation. On the contrary, microspheres prepared from PLLA-3

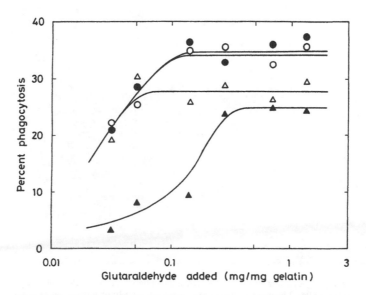

Figure 22. Mø phagocytosis of gelatin microspheres of different extents of cross-linking. The concentration of gelatin used in microsphere preparations is 10 (○), 5 (●), 2.5 (△), and 1 wt% (▲).

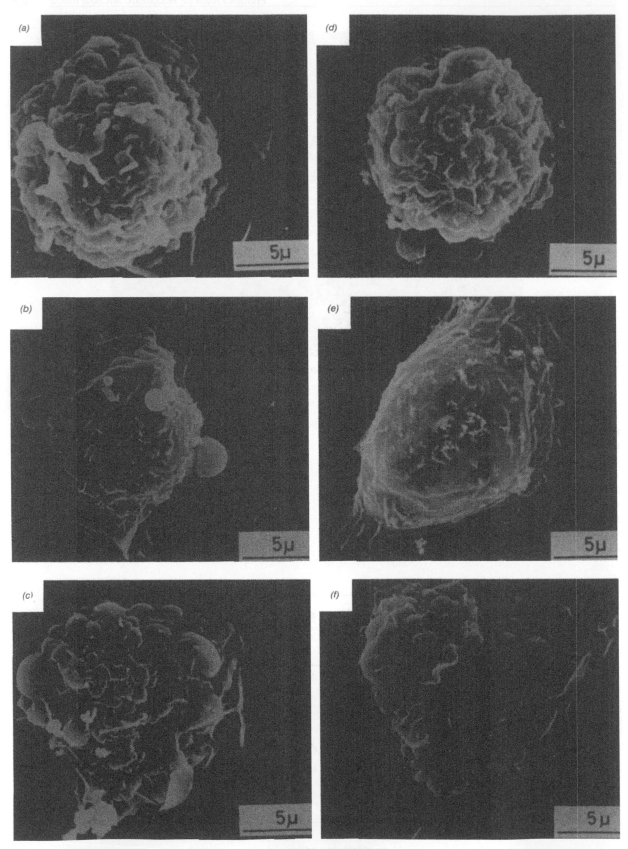

Figure 23. SEM photographs of Mø phagocytosing PGLA and PLLA microspheres; (a) Mø before phagocytosing PGLA microspheres, (b) Mø phagocytosing PGLA microspheres after 2 hr incubation, (c) Mø having completely phagocytosed PGLA microspheres after 6 hr incubation, (d) Mø with the phagocytosing PGLA microspheres gradually being degraded in the interior of the Mø after 4 days incubation, (e) Mø with the entirely degraded PGLA microspheres after 7 days incubation, and (f) Mø with phagocytosed PLLA microspheres after 7 days incubation.

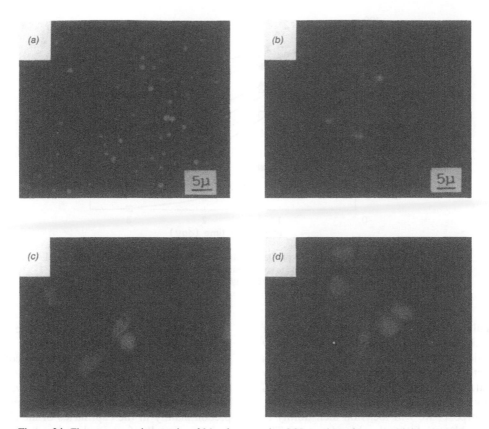

Figure 24. Fluorescence micrographs of Mø phagocytosing PGLA microspheres containing rhodamine 6GX; (a) microspheres containing rhodamine 6GX, (b) Mø having completely phagocytosing PGLA microspheres after 6 hr incubation, (c) Mø with the phagocytosing PGLA microspheres gradually being degraded in the interior of the Mø, leading to slow release of rhodamine 6GX from the microspheres in the cell after 2 days, and (d) Mø with the entirely degraded microspheres after 7 days incubation.

with a weight-average molecular weight higher than that of PGLA, still remained in the cell even after 7 days, as shown in Figure 23(f). The time sequence of rhodamine 6GX release from the PGLA-2 microspheres in Mø was observed by fluorescence microscopy (Figure 24).

As can be seen, the microspheres ingested by Mø were found to have clear contour, and the dye occupied the space inside the cell except for the cell nucleus after 4 hr incubation. The contour of the microspheres within the cell gradually disappeared and the dye in the microspheres diffused all over the internal space of the cell during the incubation time, resulting in the staining of the whole cell by the fluorescent dye. These results indicate that the phagocytosed microspheres were gradually degraded in the interior of Mø during the incubation time, leading to a slow release of the substance incorporated in the microspheres in the cells. The degradation behavior of polylactide microspheres and subsequent release profiles of drugs in Mø could be regulated by changing the molecular properties of PLLA and PGLA constituting microspheres, similarly to those for the microspheres *in vitro* as shown in Figures 7 and 8.

The gelatin microspheres were not degraded by the simple hydrolysis without enzymes, unlike the PLLA and PGLA microspheres, but were digested in Mø after being phagocytosed. The degradation profiles of the microspheres in Mø are shown in Figure 25. It is obvious that the microspheres phagocytosed were gradually degraded in the cells during the incubation time. The rate of degradation could be controlled by changing the extent of cross-linking of the microspheres with glutaraldehyde in the preparation [57], similar to the *in vitro* degradation of the microspheres with collagenase. It may be suggested that the gelatin microspheres ingested are incorporated into cytoplasmic phagolysosomes and subsequently degraded by an attack from lysosomal enzymes.

PHAGOCYTOSIS OF POLYMERIC MICROSPHERES *IN VIVO*

Research concerning Mø phagocytes *in vivo* has generally concentrated on the ability of mononuclear phagocyte system (MPS), such as monocytes, lung, liver, and spleen Mø, to clear substances introduced

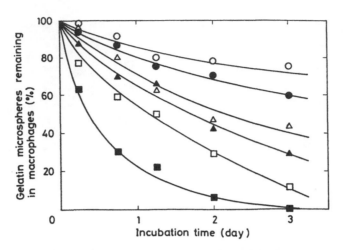

Figure 25. Degradation profiles in Mø of gelatin microspheres cross-linked with glutaraldehyde in concentrations of 1.33 (O), 0.71 (●), 0.28 (△), 0.14 (▲), 0.05 (□), and 0.03 mg/mg gelatin (■).

into the circulation. The *in vivo* fate of most types of polymeric microspheres is profoundly affected by their interaction with the cells of MPS, which has been excellently reviewed by Edman et al. [110] and by Douglas et al. [111]. The cells belonging to the MPS have a variety of important biological functions [112], but for our purpose, we will focus on their ability to remove microspheres from the bloodstream. The natural functions of the MPS cells probably involve the removal of protein aggregates derived from tissue destruction and repair, clearance of senescent erythrocytes, and removal of invading bacteria, fungi, and viruses. However, the MPS cells are also highly efficient in removing foreign particles, including polymeric microspheres, injected for therapeutic and diagnostic purposes. The cells can often take up polymeric microspheres by apparently nonspecific phagocytosis [113].

A variety of methods have been used for microsphere formation including non-degradable polystyrene, poly(methyl methacrylate) (PMMA) and polyacrylamide (PAAm) microspheres, as well as PLLA, PGA, PGLA, polycyanoacrylate, starch, and protein microspheres, which would be more likely to be fully biodegradable [42,110]. Measurable amounts of polystyrene [107] and PAAm microspheres [110] persist in the tissue for many weeks after administration. It seems likely, however, that PGA [108] and protein microspheres [110] may be degraded *in vivo* in a period of days.

Size is one of the important factors influencing the distribution and fate of microspheres after intravenous (i.v.) injection, regardless of the nature of microsphere matrix, such as its degradability. Large microspheres with a diameter larger than about 7 μm are mainly cleared by simple entrapment or filtration, usually in the lung capillary bed [114]. Those below this size but larger than 100 nm will normally pass through the lung without being trapped or taken up by

alveolar Mø, and will accumulate in the liver and the spleen. Some histological studies have revealed that microspheres of 3 to 5 μm were found consistently in vascular channels, Kupffer cells, and the sinusoids of the liver and spleen, and bone marrow with Mø, while the microspheres of 12 μm in a diameter were found predominantly in the capillaries of the alveolar walls and occasionally free in the alveolar lumina in the lung [115–117]. Microspheres smaller than 100 nm have the possibility of leaving the systemic circulation through fenestrations in the cells lining blood vessels. These fenestrations have different sizes depending on the capillary beds. The capillary endothelium of the pancreas, intestines, and kidney has fenestrations of 50–60 nm while that of the liver, spleen, and bone marrow has fenestrations of about 100 nm. There is a suggestion that capillaries in inflammatory regions may have greater permeability [118].

Although alteration of the surface characteristics of polymer microspheres can lead to a significant change in clearance kinetics, eventual uptake by the MPS still usually ensues. The uptake of the microspheres by the Mø residing at liver, spleen, and bone marrow is governed mainly by the physicochemical properties of the microsphere surface, such as the surface charge and hydrophobicity [6,119], similar to the situation observed from *in vitro* experiments. Microspheres with hydrophobic surfaces will be removed from the circulation rapidly, while those with more hydrophilic surfaces would be expected to remain in circulation for longer periods of time [6]. Microspheres with hydrophobic surfaces, such as polystyrene microspheres, are normally taken up by the MPS cells of the liver and spleen after i.v. injection [107,110,111, 119].

This rapid and efficient removal is a result of two interrelated processes. The first is the coating of the microspheres by blood components, such as IgG, complements, and FN (opsonization) that render them recognizable by Mø. The second is the adhesion of the microspheres to the surface of Mø and their subsequent engulfment. In an attempt to avoid the rapid clearance by Mø, the microspheres are often coated wtih hydrophilic macromolecular materials to give a hydrophilic surface. This may give rise to a minimum uptake by Mø. Coating of microspheres with negative and positive macromolecules can also alter organ uptake considerably, as reported by Wilkins and Myers [120], who found that the positively charged gelatin-coated polystyrene microspheres of 1.3 μm diameter accumulated initially in the lung and later in the spleen, while negatively charged gelatin-coated microspheres were found in liver and spleen.

Jeppsson and Rossner [121] and Gery [122] have studied emulsion systems and demonstrated that nonionic surfactants of the Pluronic (Poloxamer) series could modify the kinetics of their clearance. Illum and Davis [123–125] showed that the blood clearance and organ distribution of polystyrene microspheres 1.27 μm and 50 nm in diameter could be altered when Poloxamer 338 and 188 were used as the coating agents. Coating of the microspheres with the surfactant gave rise to a significant increase in the number of microspheres reaching the lung and a corresponding reduction in the quantity reaching the liver. The reduced uptake of the coated microspheres in the liver is related directly to the physicochemical properties of the adsorbed Poloxamer layer. It is known that the complement system is activated when it comes into contact with synthetic polymer surfaces and that certain complement components can be taken up rapidly [126]. Microspheres coated with the complement proteins will be cleared rapidly by liver and spleen. However, the coating of microspheres with Poloxamer 338 reduced or even eliminated the uptake or the opsonic materials, and the subsequent phagocytic engulfment by the Kupffer cells in liver was minimized [125].

Another approach is the incorporation of carbohydrate residues onto the microsphere surfaces. A variety of cells are known to have lectin-like cell surface receptors [127]. It has already been demonstrated that the incorporation of carbohydrate residues into liposomes leads to a change in their clearance characteristics [128–130]. However, such an attempt has not yet been made for polymeric microspheres. In principle, one can introduce onto the microspheres appropriate ligands which recognize cell surface receptors, in order to obtain important changes in the clearance and distribution of the microspheres.

CONCLUSION

One of the important objectives in the current drug therapies is the selective delivery of drugs and diagnostic agents to a specific target site or organ in the body. This would not only lead to a reduction in unwanted side effects and adverse reactions, but could also open up the possibility of using highly toxic substances that cannot be employed at present because of unselective distribution in the body. A good example of the need of drug targeting is in cancer chemotherapy, where agents that show an activity against neoplastic tissues also have a toxic effect on normal tissues. This is because, due to the normal broad tissue distribution of the drug, it will kill off healthy cells as well as cancer cells. It would be of considerable benefit in drug therapy if drug molecules could be targeted to the site where they are regulated, so the amount appearing elsewhere might be minimized.

Selective drug targeting may be achieved by approaches that differ widely and which range from chemical means such as the use of prodrugs, to the use of macromolecules and cells as well as colloidal particles. Different types of colloidal systems, such as liposomes, emulsions, and polymeric microspheres, have been reported in the literature. Colloids have the advantage of being able to entrap relatively large amounts of pharmacological agents, and are relatively easy to prepare. Injection of active agents incorporated in carrier microspheres into the bloodstream has often a great advantage over the injection of the agents themselves. However, once they come in the blood, the fate of any microspheres is determined by the MPS cells which clear such materials rapidly in liver, spleen, or bone marrow. Therefore, it is essential to understand how this clearance is mediated by Mø belonging to the cells of MPS. The understanding will allow manipulation of both microspheres and host so as to enhance or prevent MPS-mediated blood clearance and to achieve its objective of providing tissue selectivity for drug delivery.

This chapter viewed the phagocytosis of polymeric microspheres by Mø from a standpoint of material science, to clarify major factors affecting the clearance and disposal of the microspheres injected into the body. The uptake of the microspheres by Mø is mainly governed by the physicochemical characteristics of the microspheres, especially their size, surface charge, and surface hydrophobicity, regardless of the bulk properties of microspheres themselves, such as their degradability. These results are provided on the basis of *in vitro* experiments and cannot be necessarily extrapolated to the *in vivo* mutual action of the microspheres to Mø. However, they will provide information useful for the fate and distribution of the microspheres injected into the body, and a suggestive hint for the development of polymeric microspheres as carriers applicable for drug delivery systems.

REFERENCES

1. Carr, I. 1973. *The Macrophage: A Review of Ultrastructure and Function*. London and New York: Academic Press.
2. North, R. J. 1970. *Semin. Hematol.*, 7:161.
3. Cohn, Z. A. 1970. *Mononuclear Phagocytes*. R. van

Furth, ed. Oxford, NY: Blackwell Scientific Publications, p. 121.

4. Griffin, F. M., Jr., J. A. Griffin, J. E. Leider and S. C. Silverstein. 1975. *J. Exp. Med.*, 142:1263.

5. Stossel, T. P. 1975. *Semin. Hematol.*, 12:83.

6. van Oss, C. J. 1975. *Phagocytic Engulfment and Cell Adhesiveness*. New York and Basel: Marcel Dekker Inc.

7. Kotera, A., K. Furusawa and Y. Takeda. 1970. *Kolloid-Z. u Z. Polymere*, 239:677.

8. Goodwin, J. W., J. Hearn, C. C. Ho and R. H. Ottewill. 1974. *Colloid and Polym. Sci.*, 252:464.

9. Hearn, J., R. H. Ottewill and J. N. Shaw. 1970. *Br. Polym. J.*, 2:116.

10. Almog, Y., S. Reich and M. Levy. 1982. *Br. Polym. J.*, 14:131.

11. Chung-li, Y., J. W. Goodwin and R. E. Ottewill. 1976. *Prog. Colloid and Polym. Sci.*, 60:173.

12. Goodwin, J. W., R. H. Ottewill, R. Pelton, G. Vianllo and D. E. Yates. 1978. *Br. Polym. J.*, 10:173.

13. Ugelstad, J., K. H. Kaggerund, F. K. Hansen and A. Berge. 1979. *Makrom. Chem.*, 180:737.

14. Tabata, Y. and Y. Ikada. 1988. *Biomaterials*, 9:356.

15. Matsumoto, T., M. Okubo and T. Imai. 1974. *Kobunshi-Ronbunshu*, 31:576.

16. Margel, S. 1985. *Methods Enzymol.*, 112:165.

17. Walter, H., E. J. Krob and R. Garza. 1968. *Biochim. Biophys. Acta*, 165:507.

18. van Oss, C. J. 1978. *Annu. Rev. Microbiol.*, 32:19.

19. Capo, C. P., P. Bongrand, A. M. Benoliel and R. Depieds. 1979. *Immunology*, 36:501.

20. Rembraum, A., S. P. S. Yen, E. Cheong, S. Wallace, R. S. Molday, I. L. Gordon and W. J. Dreyer. 1976. *Macromolecules*, 9:328.

21. Bhattacharyya, B. R. and B. D. Halpern. 1977. *Polymer News*, 4:107.

22. Marumoto, K., T. Suzuta, H. Noguchi and Y. Uchida. 1978. *Polymer*, 19:867.

23. Kawaguchi, H., H. Hoshino, H. Amagasa and Y. Ohtsuka. 1984. *J. Colloid Interface Sci.*, 97:465.

24. Suzuta, T. 1983. *Controlled Drug Delivery, Clinical Applications, Vol. II*. S. D. Bruck, ed. Boca Raton, FL: CRC Press, Inc., p. 149.

25. Matsumoto, K., C. Hirayama and Y. Motozato. 1981. *Chem. Soc. Japan*, 12:1890.

26. Mckelvey, J. B., R. R. Benerite, R. J. Berni and B. G. Burgis. 1963. *J. Appl. Polym. Sci.*, 7:1371.

27. Peterson, E. A., and H. A. Sober. 1956. *Am. Chem. Soc.*, 20:75.

28. Peska, J., J. Stamberg and J. Hradil. 1986. *Angew. Makrom. Chem.*, 53:73.

29. March, S. C., I. Parikh and P. Cuatrecasas. 1974. *Annl. Biochem.*, 60:149.

30. Tabata, Y. and Y. Ikada. 1989. *J. Colloid Interface Sci.*, 127:132.

31. Cuatrecasas, P. 1970. *J. Biol. Chem.*, 245:3059.

32. Er-el, Z., Y. Zeidenzing and S. Stalteil. 1972. *Biochem. Biophys. Res. Commun.*, 49:383.

33. Hofstee, B. H. 1973. *Biochem. Biophys. Res. Commun.*, 50:751.

34. Mason, N., C. Thies and T. J. Cicero. 1976. *J. Pharm. Sci.*, 65:547.

35. Wise, D. E., G. J. McCormick, G. P. Willet and G. C. Anderson. 1976. *Life Sci.*, 19:867.

36. Wakiyama, N., K. Juni, and M. Nakano. 1982. *Chem. Pharm. Bull.*, 30:2621.

37. Beck, L. R., E. F. Charles, Jr., Z. P. Valerie, H. W. Walter and R. T. Thomas. 1983. *Am. J. Obstet. Gynnecol.*, 147:815.

38. Juni, K., J. Ogata, N. Matsui, M. Kokubo and M. Nakano. 1985. *Chem. Pharm. Bull.*, 33:1734.

39. Kwong, A. K., S. Chou, A. M. Sun, M. V. Sefton and M. F. A. Goosen. 1986. *J. Controlled Release*, 4:47.

40. Wada, R., S.-H. Hyon, Y. Ikada, H. Yoshikawa and S. Muranishi. 1988. *J. Bioactive Compatible Polym.*, 3:126.

41. Tabata, Y., and Y. Ikada. 1988. *J. Biomed. Mater. Res.*, 22:837.

42. Beck. L. R., D. R. Cowsar, D. H. Lewis, R. J. Cosgrove, C. T. Riddle and S. L. Epperly. 1979. *Fertil. Steril.*, 31:545.

43. Kreuter, J. 1985. *Methods Enzymol.*, 112:129.

44. Tomlinson, E. and J. J. Burger. 1985. *Methods Enzymol.*, 112:27.

45. Longo, W. E., H. Iwata, T. A. Lindheimer and E. P. Goldberg. 1982. *J. Pharm. Sci.*, 71:1323.

46. Przyborowski, M., E. Lachnik, J. Wiza and I. Licińska. 1982. *Eur. J. Nucl. Med.*, 7:71.

47. Millar, A. M., L. McMillan, W. J. Hannan, P. C. Emmett and R. J. Aitken. 1982. *Int. J. Appl. Radiat. Isot.*, 33:1423.

48. Madan, P. L., L. A. Luzzi and J. C. Price. 1974. *J. Pharm. Sci.*, 63:280.

49. Nixon, J. R., S. A. Khalil and J. E. Carless. 1968. *J. Pharm. Pharmacol.*, 20:528.

50. Tanaka, N., S. Takino and I. Utsumi. 1963. *J. Pharm. Sci.*, 52:664.

51. Hashida, M., Y. Takahashi, S. Muranishi and H. Sezaki. 1977. *J. Pharmacokin. Biopharm.*, 5:241.

52. Hashida, M., M. Egawa, S. Muranishi and H. Sezaki. *J. Pharmcokin. Biopharm.*, 5:225.

53. Hashida, M., S. Muranishi, H. Sezaki, N. Tanigawa, K. Satomura and Y. Hikasa. 1979. *Int. J. Pharm.*, 2:245.

54. Cheung, D. T. and M. E. Nimni. 1982. *Connective Tissue Res.*, 10:201.

55. Weadock, K., R. M. Olson and F. H. Silver. 1983. *Biomat. Med. Dev. Art. Org.*, 11:293.

56. McPheraon, J. M., P. W. Ledger, S. Sawamura, A. Conti, S. Wada, H. Reihanian and D. G. Wallace. 1986. *J. Biomed. Mater. Res.*, 20:79.

57. Tabata, Y. and Y. Ikada. 1989. *Pharmaceutical Res.*, 6:422.

58. Karnovsky, M. L. 1981. *N. Engl. J. Med.*, 304:1178.

59. Jacques, P. J. 1973. *Lysosomes in Biology and Pathology*. J. T. Dingle, H. B. Fell, eds. Amsterdam: North Holland, 2:395.

60. Mudd, S., M. Mccutcheon and B. Lucke. 1934. *Physiol. Rev.*, 14:210.

61. Berry, L. J. and T. D. Spies. 1949. *Medicine*, 28:239.

62. Hirsch, G. C. 1965. *Ann. Rev. Microbiol.*, 19:339.

63. Lay, W. H. and V. Nussenzeig. 1969. *J. Immunol.*, 102:1172.

64. Davey, M. J. and G. L. Asherson. 1966. *Immunology*, 12:13.

65. Fenn, W. O. 1922. *J. Gen. Physiol.*, 4:373.

66. Mudd, S. and E. B. H. Mudd. 1924. *J. Exp. Med.*, 40:647.

67. Grinnell, F. 1978. *Int. Rev. Cytol.*, 53:65.

68. Salzman, E. W. 1981. *Interaction of the Blood with Natural and Artificial Surfaces*. New York and Basel: Marcel Dekker Inc.

69. Andrade, J. E. 1985. *Surface and Interfacial Aspects of Biomedical Polymers*. New York and London: Plenum Press.

70. Tamada, Y. and Y. Ikada. 1986. *Polymers in Medicine II*. E. Chiellini, P. Guisti, C. Miliaresi, and L. Nicolais, eds. New York and London: Plenum Publishing Corporation, p. 101.

71. Silverstein, S. C., J. K. Christman and S. Acs. 1976. *Ann. Rev. Biochem.*, 45:375.

72. Rabinovitch, M. 1967. *J. Cell Res.*, 46:19.

73. Simson, J. V. and S. S. Spicer. 1973. *International Review of Experimental Pathology*. G. W. Richter, and M. A. Epstein, eds. New York, NY: Academic Press, p. 79.

74. Silverstein, S. C., R. M. Steinman, and Z. A. Cohn. 1977. *Annu. Rev. Microbiol.*, 49:669.

75. Stossell, T. P., J. H. Hartwig, H. L. Yin and O. Stendahl. 1982 *Biochem. Soc. Symp.*, 45:51.

76. Southwick, F. S. and T. P. Stossel. 1983. *Semin. Hamotol.*, 20:305.

77. Valerius, N. H., O. Stendahl, J. H. Hartwig and T. P. Stossel. 1981. *Cell*, 24:195.

78. Karnovsky, M. L., J. Lazins and S. Simmons. 1975. *Mononuclear Phagocytes in Immunity, Infection, and Pathology*. R. van Furth, ed. Oxford, NY: Blackwell Scientific Publications, p. 423.

79. Briggs, R. T., D. B. Drath, M. L. Karnovsky and M. J. Karnovsky. 1975. *J. Cell Biol.*, 67:566.

80. Rossi, F., G. Zabucchi and D. Romeo. 1975. *Mononuclear Phagocytes in Immunity, Infection, and Pathology*. R. van Furth, ed. Oxford, NY: Blackwell Scientific Publications, p. 441.

81. Johnston, R. B., Jr. and J. E. Lehmeyer. 1977. *Superoxide and Superoxide Dismutases*. A. M. Michelson, J. M. McCord and I. Fridovitch, eds. London, England: Academic Press, p. 291.

82. Cohn, Z. A. and E. Weiner. 1963. *J. Exp. Med.*, 118:991.

83. McNeil, P. L., L. Tanasugarn, J. B. Meigs and D. C. Taylor. *J. Cell. Biol.*, 97:692.

84. Allen, R. D. and A. K. Fox. 1983. *J. Cell Biol.*, 97:566.

85. Mellman, I. and H. Plutner. 1984. *J. Cell Biol.*, 98:1170.

86. Kawaguchi, H., N. Koiwai, Y. Ohtsuka and M. Miyamoto. 1986. *Biomaterials*, 7:61.

87. Robert, J. and J. H. Quastel. 1963. *Biochem. J.*, 89:150.

88. van Oss, C. J. and C. F. Gillman. 1972. *J. Reticuloendothel. Soc.*, 12:283.

89. Magnusson, K. E., O. Stendahl, I. Stjernstrom and L. Ebedo. 1979. *Immunology*, 36:439.

90. Pesanti, E. L. 1979. *J. Reticuloendothel. Soc.*, 26:549.

91. Kozel, T. R., E. Reiss and R. Cherniak. 1980. *Infect. Immun.*, 29:295.

92. Dexter, S. C. 1979. *J. Colloid Interface Sci.*, 70:346.

93. Gerson, D. F. and D. Scheer. 1980. *Biochem. Biophys. Acta*, 602:506.

94. Saba, T. M. 1970. *Arch. Inter. Med.*, 126:1031.

95. Wilkinson, P. C. 1976. *Clin. Exp. Immunol.*, 23:355.

96. Steward, M. W. 1974. *Immunochemistry*. New York: Wiley.

97. Stossel, T. P. 1974. *N. Engl. J. Med.*, 290:717.

98. Mayer, M. M. 1978. *Principle of Immunology*, N. R. Rose, F. Milgrom, and C. J. van Oss, eds. New York, NY: MacMillan, p. 234.

99. Najjar, V. A. and A. Constantopoulos. 1972. *J. Reticuloendothel. Soc.*, 12:197.

100. Gambrill, M. R. and C. L. Wisseman. 1973. *Infect. Immun.*, 8:631.

101. Saba, T. M. 1975. *4th International Convocation on Immunity*. E. Neter and F. Milgrom, eds. Basel, Switzerland, p. 489.

102. McLain, S., J. Siegel, J. Molnar, C. Allen, and T. Sabet. 1976. *J. Reticuloendothel. Soc.*, 19:127.

103. Dy, M., A. Dimitriu, N. Thomson and J. Humburger. 1974. *Ann. Immunol. Inst. Pasteur*, 125:451.

104. Gudwicz, P. W., J. Molnar, M. Z. Lai, G. E. Beezhold, Jr., R. B. Credo and L. Lorand. 1980. *J. Cell Biol.*, 87:427.

105. van der Water, L., III, S. Schroeder, E. B. Creshow, III and R. O. Hynes. 1981. *J. Cell Biol.*, 90:32.

106. Tabata, Y. and Y. Ikada. 1987. *J. Pharm. Pharmacol.*, 39:698.

107. Tabata, Y., Y. Ikada, K. Uno and S. Muramatsu. 1988. *Jpn. Cancer Res.*, 79:636.

108. Kanke, M., I. Sniecinski and P. P. Deluca. 1983. *J. Parent. Sci. Technol.*, 37:210.

109. Kanke, M., E. Morlier, R. Geissler, D. Powell, A. Kaplan and P. P. Deluca. 1986. *J. Parent. Sci. Technol.*, 40:114.

110. Edman, P., P. Artursson, T. Laako and I. Sjoholm. 1986. *Methods of Drug Delivery*. G. Ihler, ed. Oxford: Pergamon, p. 23.

111. Douglas, S. J., S. S. Davis and L. Illum. 1987. *Crit. Rev. Ther. Drug Carrier Syst.*, 3:233.

112. Becker, S. 1987. *CRC Crit. Rev. Drug Carr. Syst.*, 32:123.

113. Steinman, R. M., I. S. Mellman, W. A. Muller and Z. A. Cohn. 1983. *J. Cell Biol.*, 96:1.

114. Poste, G. and R. Kirsh. 1983. *Biotechnology*, 1:869.

115. Schroeder, H. G., G. Simmons and P. P. Deluca. 1978. *J. Pharm. Sci.*, 67:504.

116. Kanke, M., G. Simmons, D. Weiss, B. Bivins and P. P. Deluca. 1980. *J. Pharm. Sci.*, 69:755.

117. Hoshioka, T., M. Hashida, S. Muranishi and H. Sezaki. 1981. *Int. J. Pharm.*, 8:131.

118. Grislain, L., P. Couvreur, V. Lenaert, M. Roland, D. Deprez-Decampeneere and P. Speiser. 1983. *Int. J. Pharm.*, 15:335.

119. Illum, L. and S. S. Davis. 1982. *J. Parent. Sci. Technol.*, 36:242.

120. Wilkins, D. J. and P. A. Myers. 1966. *Br. J. Exp. Pathol.*, 47:568.

121. Jeppsson, R., S. Rossner. 1975. *Acta Pharmacol. Toxicol.*, 37:34.

122. Geyer, R. P. 1967. *Fette Med.*, 6:59.

123. Illum, L. and S. S. Davis. 1983. *J. Pharm. Sci.*, 72:1089.

124. Illum, L., I. M. Hunneyball and S. S. Davis. 1986. *Int. J. Pharm.*, 29:53.

125. Illum, L. and S. S. Davis. 1984. *FEBS Lett.*, 167:79.

126. Hakin, R. M. and E. G. Lowrie. 1980. *Trans. Am. Soc. Artif. Intern. Organs*, 26:159.

127. Neufeld, E. and G. Ashwell. 1980. *The Biochemistry of Glycoproteins and Proteoglycans*. W. Lennarrz, ed. New York, NY: Plenum Press, p. 241.

128. Wu, P. S., H. M. Wu, G. W. Tin, J. R. Schuh, W. R. Crosman, J. D. Baldeschwieler, T. Y. Shen and M. M. Ponpipom. 1980. *Proc. Natl. Acad. Sci. USA*, 79:5490.

129. Sunamoto, J. 1986. *Medical Application of Liposomes*, K. Yagi, ed. Tokyo and Karger, Basel: Japan Scientific Soc. Press, p. 121.

130. Shen, T. Y. 1987. *NY Acad. Sci.*, 507:272.

39

Nonspecific and Biospecific Sorbents for Medical Applications

ERHAN PIŞKIN*

ABSTRACT: Sorbents have been used in a variety of forms to treat patients with various kinds of diseases. In general, sorbents have been considered for use in medicine in two basic ways. The first method is direct or indirect sorbent contact with body fluids (mostly blood or plasma) in an extracorporeal circuit that is commonly called hemoperfusion. In the second method sorbents are taken orally to sorb substances within the gastrointestinal tract.

In the first part of this chapter basic concepts of adsorption and ion exchange phenomena will be discussed briefly. Then, the nonspecific sorbents that have already been used in hemoperfusion columns or in series with hemoperfusion systems will be considered. Putting the emphasis on activated carbon, ion exchangers, uncharged resins, polyaldehydes and others will be included. In the last part of this article, the novel biospecific sorbents and their interesting applications will be reviewed.

ADSORPTION AND ION EXCHANGE PHENOMENA

Adsorption

Adsorption is usually viewed as a surface phenomenon, and even common solids adsorb gases and vapours to a certain extent. But only certain solids exhibit sufficient adsorptive capacity to make them useful for applications. Adsorption of a solute from a liquid on a sorbent will usually result from the high affinity of the solute for the sorbent. Substances having great affinity will be adsorbed in preference to those with less affinity. The affinity may be due to physical or chemical forces.

The forces that cause physical adsorption are mostly secondary forces (e.g., van der Waals forces).

Electrical attraction of the solutes to the adsorbent results in adsorption, which sometimes can be considered separately from physical adsorption and which is called exchange adsorption. In physical or ideal adsorption, the attachment is weak and reversible. This very common type of adsorption usually involves a smaller energy change; it is exothermic, where heat being evolved is somewhat greater than the heat of liquefaction.

Chemical adsorption (chemisorption) results from interactions between functional groups on the sorbate and on the surface of sorbent (primary forces). Higher energies are associated with chemical adsorption. This type of sorption is mostly irreversible, and the heat liberated during the sorption process is greater than the heat of formation (or reaction).

It should be noted that in many situations there is no sharp demarcation between physical and chemical adsorption. In many examples, both physical and chemical, adsorption may occur simultaneously.

In the case of bioaffinity sorbents, such as immunosorbents, the interaction between the solute and biosorbent is extremely specific and selective. These interactions are relatively complex, and include not only secondary forces between sorbent and solute but also geometrical factors.

Factors Influencing Adsorption of Solutes from Liquids

SORBENT PROPERTIES

The properties of a sorbent have a very important effect on the sorption of solutes from liquids. Large area per unit weight of sorbent seems essential to all useful sorbents. Sorbents of high surface area are generally porous. There are many different kinds of rigid and non-rigid pore structures and a sorbent is likely to contain a range of pores of different size and shape. A convenient classification of pores according to their effective width, is as follows (Figure 1):

*Hacettepe University, Chem. Eng. Dept., 06532, Beytepe, Ankara, Turkey

(1) Macropores (>50 nm)

(2) Mesopores (2 nm to 50 nm)

(3) Micropores (<2 nm)

These limits must be regarded as somewhat arbitrary. Note that micropores usually contribute the total surface area of a sorbent. Large surface area is important in order to maximize the adsorptive capacity of the sorbent. However, the total surface area does not necessarily mirror the utility of a sorbent. Depending on the size and the shape of the solute molecules, some of the pores may not be available for all solute molecules. Besides the total surface area, pore size and pore size distribution, as well as surface chemistry influence both rate and capacity of adsorption. The mechanism of uptake of solutes must also be taken into account for appropriate mass transfer rates.

The sorbents must also possess certain properties depending upon the application to which they are put. If they are used in fixed-bed, like hemoperfusion columns, they must not offer too great a pressure drop for flow (i.e., blood) which may cause harmful effects on blood cells. They must be also biocompatible, nontoxic, and non-carcinogenic in these types of medical applications. They must have adequate strength and hardness so as not to be reduced in size during handling or in use, or crushed in supporting their own weight in beds of required depth. Note that fine particle release from the sorbent in hemoperfusion applications may cause significant side effects.

SOLUTE AND SOLVENT PROPERTIES

In general, there is an inverse relationship between the extent of adsorption and the mobile (liquid) phase solubility. Hydrophilic groups on solutes usually reduce adsorption on hydrophobic sorbents (e.g., activated carbon) from aqueous solutions. Adsorption decreases as polarity increases. Both aromatic and branched chain substances are more preferentially adsorbed than straight chain compounds.

Molecular size and shape of the solute molecules are of significance to describe the total effective area for those molecules. Where the rate of the adsorption is controlled by pore diffusion, in which case smaller molecules are more easily adsorbed.

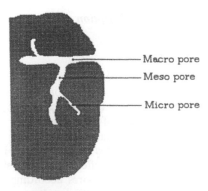

Figure 1. Classification of pores.

pH

Hydrogen and hydroxide ions are generally adsorbed quite strongly. Thus the adsorption of electrolytes is sensitive to pH changes. In general, adsorption of organic electrolytes from aqueous solutions increases as pH decreases.

TEMPERATURE

Adsorption is normally exothermic. Thus the extent of adsorption increases with decrease in temperature.

Adsorption Equilibrium

In an adsorption process, an equilibrium is reached in the distribution of the solute molecules between sorbent (sorbent pore surface) and liquid phase (within the pores). Equilibrium is described by expressing the quantity of substance adsorbed per unit weight of sorbent (m), as a function of the quantity unadsorbed (c), in other words solute concentration in liquid phase at equilibrium, at a particular temperature. Two fundamental expressions are commonly used for describing adsorption from dilute solutions, namely the Langmuir Equation and Freundlich Equation, which are given below. Note that they are both based on monolayer adsorption assumption. One should go to the literature for multilayer adsorption theories and related expressions [1,2].

Langmuir Equation:

$$m' = m'_{max} \frac{bc'_s}{1 + bc'_s} \qquad (1)$$

Here, m': the solute concentration within the sorbent (gram solute per gram sorbent) at equilibrium; m'_{max}: the maximum value of m'; c'_s: the solute concentration within the liquid phase at equilibrium; and b: the Langmuir constant.

Freundlich Equation:

$$m' = Kc'^n_s \qquad (2)$$

Here, K and n: the Freundlich constants.

These adsorption isotherms are useful in representing the capacity of a sorbent for solutes, and they can be obtained by batch adsorption experiments. These equations are also used to solve the mathematical models defined for the mass transfer in adsorption columns, as discussed below.

Adsorption Rates

In order to predict the performance of an adsorption system one needs to have knowledge of pertinent rates of mass transfer. For a packed-bed column like hemoperfusion columns, the mass balance for the mobile phase (i.e., liquid phase) can be written as follows [1–4]:

$$\frac{\delta c}{\delta t} = D_a \frac{\delta^2 c}{\delta z^2} - v \frac{\delta c}{\delta z} - R_i \quad (3)$$

Accumulation	Axial Dispersion	Bulk Flow	Interface Mass Transfer Rate

Here, D_a: the axial dispersion coefficient; v: the linear (interstitial) velocity in the column; c: the solute concentration in the fluid stream; z: the axial coordinate; t: time; and R_i: the interface mass transfer rate. Note that differences in mass transfer rate theory models are mainly due to the differences in definition of the interface mass transfer rate (R_i).

For spherical sorbent granules, the mass balance for the stationary phase (i.e., sorbent phase), in other words, the diffusion of solute within the pores and adsorption at the pore surface, can be described by the following expression [5,6]:

$$D_{eff} \frac{1}{r} \frac{\delta}{\delta r} \left(r^2 \frac{\delta c_s}{\delta r} \right) - \epsilon_s \frac{\delta c_s}{\delta t} - \varrho_s \frac{\delta m}{\delta t} = 0 \quad (4)$$

Here, D_{eff}: the solute effective diffusion coefficient in the pore liquid; c_s: the local solute concentration within the pore liquid; m: the local solute concentration adsorbed on the surface; ϱ_s: the sorbent particle density; ϵ_s: the void volume fraction (porosity) within the sorbent granules.

These two mass balance equations may be combined by defining an appropriate interface mass transfer rate. Furthermore, assuming an instantaneous equilibrium in the pores at the pore surface, allows to use the adsorption equilibrium isotherms defined in Equations (1) and (2) for the relation between c_s and m. Despite inclusion of some more model simplifications, the simultaneous solutions of these equations, by using appropriate initial and boundary conditions, may be achieved by numerical methods [1–5]. The solutions may then be used to predict the performance of the adsorption column and also the effects of column and system parameters on the column performance.

It is also desirable to define the major mass transfer resistances in fixed-bed sorbent applications to employ the system with appropriate adjustment. There are essentially four consecutive stages in the adsorption of solutes from a solution by porous sorbents, such as activated carbon, as described schematically in Figure 2.

(1) Mass transfer from the fluid phase to the external surfaces of the sorbent particles (film diffusion resistance)

(2) Pore diffusion in the fluid phase within the pores of the sorbent (pore diffusion resistance)

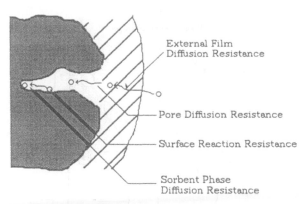

Figure 2. Major mass transfer resistance.

(3) Adsorption reaction at the pore surface of the sorbent (surface reaction resistance)

(4) Diffusion in the sorbed state, so-called surface diffusion (sorbent phase diffusion resistance)

The film diffusion rate limitation is a function of hydrodynamic conditions, the composition of bulk flow, and sorbent–solvent interaction. In fixed-bed column-type continuous flow operations such as hemoperfusion, it is important to note that significant effects can be obtained by changing hydrodynamic conditions [7,8]. The pore diffusion step is fixed by the nature of the adsorbate and the open network of the adsorbent. The adsorbtive step is related to the surface chemistry of the adsorbent and the type of the adsorbate.

The rate-limiting step may be due to one, or to a combination of the mass transfer resistances given above. Note that the slower rate controls the overall rate of adsorption more likely. By coating the adsorbents with semipermeable membranes, as in hemoperfusion columns filled with nonspecific sorbents such as activated carbon, an additional rate-limiting step is created in which case polymer coating diffusion resistance may also control the rate of uptake.

Ion Exchange

Ion exchange involves a solid phase containing fixed polar groups whose charges are balanced by free ions of opposite charge that are exchangeable (Figure 3). A matrix with fixed positive charges is referred to as an anion-exchanger since it binds anions from the surrounding fluid, whereas a matrix containing fixed negative charges is called a cation-exchanger. Separation in charged matrices is achieved by exclusion of co-ions, i.e., ions that bear the same charges as the fixed ions of the matrix. Separation properties of these matrices are determined by the charge and concentration of the ions in the surrounding solution and the matrix. The performance of an ion-exchange matrix is defined mainly by its selectivity to ions of opposite charges.

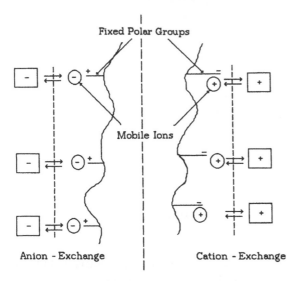

Figure 3. Functional structure of ion-exchangers.

Ion Exchange Equilibria

Various attempts have been made to formulate the ion exchange equilibria. Essentially two approaches to defining the equilibria have been demonstrated. In the first approach, the distribution of an ion between an ion exchanger and a solution is described in the same manner that is used for adsorption, various empirical equations for sorption isotherms such as the Freundlich Equation [Equation (2)], or some other modified forms [9]. The second approach was first defined by Ganssen who applied the law of mass action to exchange phenomenon and used the following equation [9]:

$$\frac{x}{U - x} = k \frac{c}{x} \tag{5}$$

Here, U: the exchange capacity; x: the amount of exchange; c: the equilibrium concentration of exchanging ion; and k: a constant.

In the literature, it is also possible to find many other modified forms of these equations to formulate the ion exchange equilibria and to evaluate capacity of sorbents [9–10].

Ion Exchange Selectivity

The selectivity coefficient of ion exchanger for a specific ion, K_s, can be given by the following expression

$$K_s = \frac{\bar{M}_B}{\bar{M}_A} \cdot \frac{M_A}{M_B} \tag{6}$$

Here, M_A, M_B and $\bar{M}_A$, $\bar{M}_B$: the concentrations of exchanging ions (A and B) in solution and solid phase, respectively. The selectivity coefficient (K_s) is a function of temperature and composition of bulk flow.

Degree of hydration of exchanging ions is very important in respect to selectivity. The ionic structure as well as the size and valence of the exchangeable ions is also of considerable importance.

Most common cation and anion exchangers show the following selectivities for the counter-ion, having physiological significance:

Cation Exchange:

.....$Ca^{2+} > Mg^{2+} > NH_4^+ > K^+ > Na^+ > H^+$.....

Anion Exchange:

.....citrate $> SO_4^{2-} > Cl^- >$ acetate $> OH^-$.....

Rate of Ion Exchange

The rate of ion exchange depends upon the rates of the following individual processes:

(1) Diffusion of ions through the external liquid film surrounding the ion exchange particles
(2) Diffusion within the solid phase
(3) Exchange of the ions
(4) Outward diffusion of the exchanged ions
(5) Diffusion of the exchanged ions through the external liquid film

In most instances, the kinetics of the exchange reaction (Step 3) is very fast, and therefore is not a rate limiting step. The diffusion rates (Steps 1,2,4 and 5) usually control the overall exchange rate. Overall exchange rate is also influenced by the size of ion exchange particles, temperature, solvent nature, properties of exchanging ions and the structure of the ion exchanger.

NONSPECIFIC SORBENTS

Activated Carbon

Activated carbon is a highly porous material derived from various substances. Activated carbon comprises a family of substances whose structural formula and chemical analysis cannot be identified. The only way to define it is by its adsorptive and catalytic properties.

Synthesis

A number of different materials (as given in Table 1) and activation processes might be used to prepare suitable activated carbons with many forms of adsorptive power. Much published data are available on methods of production of activated carbon and various specific ways and means are described in patent literature [11].

Activated carbon is commonly prepared by carbonization (pyrolysis) of raw material in the absence

Table 1. Raw materials for activated carbon.

Bones	Molasses
Blood	Nut shells
Coal	Peat
Coconut shells	Petroleum residues
Corncobs	Polymeric particles
Graphite	Sugar
Lignin	Wood
	Others

of air, and usually at elevated temperatures (e.g., 900°C). The effectiveness of carbonization regarding adsorptive power and spectrum is enhanced by using solutions of metallic chlorides, such as zinc, calcium and magnesium chlorides [12].

The product of the carbonization step, char, is then usually pulverized and activated by oxidation to increase the adsorption capacity. Activation is conducted in a gaseous atmosphere and at elevated temperatures. The temperature and type of gaseous atmosphere have a significant effect on the surface chemistry of activated carbon. Generally, carbon dioxide, carbon monoxide, steam, oxygen, air or some other gases are used as the gaseous atmospheres. Activation is performed at a temperature between 300 and 1000°C, often followed by quenching in air or water. Inorganic compounds such as zinc chloride, phosphoric acid, sodium sulphate, and others (Table 2) can be used as potential activation agents to increase surface area and to develop greater porosity [12].

For activation by oxidation, it must be noted, in conclusion, that optimum conditions and the type of oxidizing agent are specific for each situation, and depend on raw material and on prior history of char.

Types of Activated Carbon

Activated carbons are available in a variety of forms ranging from light fluffy powder to hard dense granules. Granular activated carbons with a diameter up to 1.5 cm are usually used in clinical perfusion trials. Granular carbons might be prepared by directly breaking and sieving activated carbon produced by the

Table 2. Potential activation agents.

Acids (phosphoric, hydrochloric and nitric)
Ammonium salts
Borates and boric acid
Caustic soda
Cyanides (thiocyanate and others)
Ferric and ferrous compounds
Oxides (calcium, manganese and others)
Potash
Sulphates (sodium, potassium and others)
Sulphides (potassium sulphide, and others)
Zinc chloride

source material. The granules obtained in this way are irregular in shape. The second type of granular carbons are extruded carbons, which are more regular in shape and size and have a relatively smoother surface. Extruded carbons are usually produced by extruding the powdered carbon with a binder, often followed by carbonization of the binder and steam activation. Spherical activated carbon granules can be prepared by pyrolysis and activation of resin beads that have been produced synthetically [13,14].

Recent developments are given credit for preparing new types of carbon systems, where activated carbon is usually immobilized or entrapped into a supporting material, such as permeable synthetic polymeric hollow fibers, polymeric gels, etc. [15–19].

Properties

The properties of different carbons can have profound effects on both adsorption rate and capacity. The most characteristic physical property of activated carbon is its large surface area, which can be over 1000 m²/g.

The extremely large surface area is a result of the highly porous structure of activated carbon. This porous network consists of capillaries (micropores) 10 to 30 Å in diameter and channels (macropores) with a diameter of 30 to 100,000 Å. Micropores provide most of the surface area on which adsorption occurs. Macropores do not contribute to the adsorptive capacity of activated carbon. In general, a high percentage of macropore volume is a disadvantage since there will be less total active area available for adsorption. On the other hand, as mentioned before, for some situations where pore diffusion controls the adsorption rates, larger pores may be desirable because macropores provide passageways through which larger substrate molecules can more readily diffuse towards the adsorption surface. Thus high transport rates can be achieved.

Pore volume and pore size distribution, which contribute to the adsorptive capacity and rate, are more or less controllable properties in the production of activated carbon. These properties can be determined by standard mercury and helium displacement measurements, or more accurately by the water desorption method [20]. BET is also the most widely accepted method for determining the total surface area [21].

The ability of activated carbon to absorb various solutes is well recognized; however, the mechanism of adsorption is not clear. There is still only a little knowledge about the surface chemistry, which is another important property of activated carbon.

Activated carbon contains chemically bonded elements, such as oxygen and hydrogen, resulting from raw material and the activation process. The presence of oxygen and hydrogen have a great effect on the sorption characteristics of carbon.

Oxygen is known to react with activated carbon to form organic oxygen groups on the pore surface, and it is suggested that these groups are carboxyl, phenolic hydroxyl, normal lactones, carboxylic acid anhydrides, cyclic peroxides, etc. There are two different kinds of activated carbons with respect to the surface chemistry, namely acidic and basic carbons. Acidic carbons are prepared in moist air at 300 to 500°C; and basic carbons are produced at 800 to 900°C in air stream or carbon dioxide atmosphere [11]. Acidic carbons have a more hydrophilic character; therefore they can adsorb polar compounds preferentially. Basic carbons are formed by relative hydrophobicity. Amphoteric properties may be found in carbons prepared between 500 to 800°C [11].

Regarding the surface chemistry of activated carbon, it can be noted that the presence of different kinds of groups on activated carbon surfaces has a pronounced effect upon the adsorption characteristic. But the absolute necessity of definite groups on the surface for specific adsorption it is still a matter for speculation.

Ash content, which is not an organic part of the sorbent, is another important property of activated carbon. Ash content and its composition, which have great influence on adsorption, vary widely with the kind of activated carbon.

Some other properties of activated carbons such as their tendency to fragment or fracture and their cleanliness, washability, and sterilizability must also be taken into consideration, especially for therapeutic applications.

Applications

Adsorption is integral to a broad spectrum of physical, biological and chemical processes and operations in the environmental field. Activated carbons are able to meet many of the diverse needs for adsorption, and hence have received most attention among the various sorbents. Both powdered and granular activated carbon have been used in industry for a number of years for purification of gas, vapour mixtures, and liquids. Activated carbons are also being evaluated for medical applications such as digestive disturbances and, since ancient times, have been used as an antidote to poisons (orally administered).

One of the major applications in the medicine is hemoperfusion columns, which contain granular activated carbon coated with semipermeable membranes. Hemoperfusion is a method which takes advantage of the large adsorptive power and adsorptive spectrum of activated carbon. A wide range of endogenous and exogenous toxins can be adsorbed effectively on activated carbon.

GRANULAR ACTIVATED CARBON

As mentioned before, activated carbons are available in a variety of forms ranging from light, fluffy powder to hard, dense granules. Granules of fairly large size (0.4–3.4 mm) have been chosen in charcoal hemoperfusion cartridges in order to eliminate sludging, channelling and packing.

Granular carbons might be prepared by directly breaking and sieving activated carbon produced by the source material (e.g., coconut-based granules by Fisher, U.S.A). The granules are irregular in shape. They have been utilized by Chang in his earlier studies [22], by Fennimore et al. [23] in the production of Haemocol (Smith and Nephew, U.K.), and by Hill et al. [24] in Hemodetoxifier (Becton, Dickonson, U.S.A.) as immobilized form.

The second type of granular carbons are so-called extruded carbons which are usually produced extruding the powder carbon with a binder, often followed by carbonization of binder, and steam activation. Extruded carbons are more regular in shape and size, and have a relatively smoother surface. The peat-based extruded granules with different properties have been made available by Norit, the Netherlands. Norit RBXI is the sorbent of choice of Adsorba (Gambro, Sweden) and Hemopur (Organon Teknika, the Netherlands) hemoperfusion columns.

Spherical carbons with unit size distribution, smooth surface and homogenous structure have recently been made available. These granular carbons can be obtained in several ways. They can be produced from a spherical source material by carbonization and activation. A carbonaceous resin bead, Amberlite XE-336 (Rohm and Haas, U.S.A.) has been produced from a polystyrene/divinylbenzene-based resin, and has been evaluated by Rosenbaum et al. [25] in hemoperfusion investigations. In the SCN-2K device produced in the U.S.S.R., spherical granules with excellent adsorbtive properties and blood compatibility are utilized. It is believed that these beads are also produced from a polystyrene-based polymer [26]. Resin-based activated carbon granules in spherical form, derived from a thermosetting resin, have also been used by Funakuba et al. [27].

Spherical carbon beads can also be prepared starting with a non-spherical source material. Following a sphere-forming stage, carbonization and activation of the spheres give the final product [28]. The petroleum pitch-based spherical activated carbon granules have been made available in Japanese companies recently, and have become the material of choice for many commercial available hemoperfusion columns, e.g., Hemocells (Teijin, Japan), Hydron DHP (Kuraray, Japan), Hemosoba (Asahi, Japan), Emoadsorb (Biotec, Italy), Detoxyl 1 and 2 (Sorin, Italy) and Dialid, Canada.

COATED GRANULAR ACTIVATED CARBON

Today, in most hemoperfusion columns available polymer-coated charcoal is used.

The main aim of coating the carbon granules is to prevent the fine carbon particle release which may cause microemboli, and to increase the blood compatibility, i.e., to reduce the damage to the blood, in particular severe platelet depletion.

A number of coating materials and methods have been evaluated. In the pioneering studies of Chang, nylon, collodion, cellulose acetate, albumin-collodion, and other polymers have been used to coat charcoal [22,29] and albumin-collodion coated charcoal has been proposed as best amongst these. In this approach, the granules are coated by stirring the carbon particles in a collodion solution containing ether and ethanol [22]. Coconut-based charcoal was used in Chang's earlier studies. Then, hemoperfusion columns, utilizing albumin-collodion coated charcoal granules, have been made available industrially [29].

Cellulose has been selected by a number of groups mainly for coating of peat-based granular carbon [30,31]. In these approaches, the granules are spray-coated by using a solution of cellulose acetate in a suitable solvent (e.g., ethanol–chloroform, acetic acid, acetone). In order to increase the permeability of membranes, the granules are further treated with NaOH or KOH aqueous solutions which are used as the deacetylating agents. This approach has been utilized in production of some commerical hemoperfusion cartridges, namely, Adsorba (Gambro, Sweden) and Hemopur (Organon Teknika, the Netherlands).

Cellulose-based (i.e., ethyl cellulose) coating has been applied for capsulation of petroleum-based charcoal beads in Hemocels (Teijin, Japan) hemoperfusion cartridges.

Andrade et al. were the first group to use the highly blood compatible hydrogel, namely polyhydroxyethyl methacrylate (PHEMA) for coating of charcoal [32]. The first commercially available hemoperfusion device (i.e., Haemocol) using this polymer coating was developed in the laboratories of Smith and Nephew, U.K. [23]. The coating was applied by a spray-coating procedure to coconut-based granules. PHEMA and its copolymers have then been selected for many of the commercial hemoperfusion units, such as Hemosorba (Asahi, Japan), Emoadsorp (Biotec, Italy), Hydron DHP (Kuraray, Japan), Detoxyl 1 (Sorin, Italy), etc.

Different acrylic-based copolymers have also been evaluated by Strathclyde Bioengineering group [33].

Several polymers including cellulose derivatives, polyamids, cross-linked polyethylene glycols and silicone have been used for coating of charcoal in the author's laboratories, and various novel coating techniques including solvent casting, interfacial polymerization, γ-irradiation-induced polymerization and plasma polymerization have been developed [34–36].

ALTERNATIVES TO GRANULAR ACTIVATED CARBON

As alternatives to granular charcoal, fiber or cloth forms, vitreous carbon, sorbent membranes and other immobilised forms have been evaluated for hemoperfusion by a number of groups.

Carbon extruded into fibers have been used by Davis et al. [37].

Carbon cloth (fibrous carbon) has also been considered as an alternative to granular carbon for hemoperfusion [38,39]. A carbon cloth produced from a viscose rayon process with excellent adsorptive properties, but with some hazards (e.g., blood loss) has been made available by Chemical Defence Establishment, U.K.

Reticulated vitreous carbon with very high void volume (i.e., 97%) leading to self-supporting rigidity and low resistance to fluid flow, has been manufactured by Chemotronics, U.S.A. However, very low clearance rates have been reported in the preliminary studies using this material [40].

Membranes containing sorbent, i.e., so-called sorbent membranes, have been considered as the most attractive alternative to coated granular sorbents [41]. Cuprophan membranes containing sorbents (e.g., activated carbon, aluminum oxide) have been made available by Enka, Germany [42]. The fibers consisting of a cellulosic membrane (3–15 μm thick) and sorbent core (300–330 μm in diameter) have been prepared for hemoperfusion applications. There are also sorbent dialyzing membranes available in the form of tubing or sheet, or hollow fibers, in which carbon and polymer layers are composed in series for possible hemoperfusion–hemodialysis applications. These sorbent membranes have undergone animal studies and clinical trials.

A new type of sorbent–membrane system which consists of polyurethane sheet with highly open structure, embedded powder charcoal with different pore sizes has been developed by Kawanishi et al. for possible applications of hemoperfusion in the treatment of hepatic failure [43]. The preliminary *in vitro* and *in vivo* studies have indicated its superiority in adsorbing protein-bound substances and middle molecular weight species.

Another novel hemoperfusion device called the thin-film adsorber consists of powder charcoal embedded in a thin film of collodion [44]. These films are wound into spools, which are then placed in a plastic housing. Depsite the very high rate-of-uptake advantage of powder activated carbon, non-uniform flow conditions and a relatively high priming volume have been reported.

A charcoal tape coil hemoperfusion device has been developed by Becton, Dickonson company under the name of Hemodetoxifier [24]. An adhesive (i.e., chlorosulphanated polyethylene) is used to stick (or to coat) charcoal particles onto polyester film. These films are rolled to form a coil, which is then placed in a polycarbonate housing. The columns demonstrate high clearances for toxins, and very low resistance to blood flow.

In recent years, novel techniques have been developed to immobilize powder activated carbon into bead-type polymeric carriers. Cross-linked agarose beads containing charcoal have been prepared by Xu et al. for hemoperfusion in artificial liver support [45]. Agarose beads containing charcoal have been prepared by a novel technique in which molten agarose gel with charcoal is dropped into an organic solvent mixture at 0°C. Low sorbent content confirms the limitation of this approach.

Hemoperfusion columns filled with collagen-activated carbon beads have been applied clinically by Zhaoguang et al. in China, recently [46]. New immobilized powder charcoal systems were also developed by the author and coworkers. In their earlier studies, activated carbon was entrapped in calcium-alginate gels by a dropping technique [47]. Stabilization of the gel particles containing charcoal was achieved by the formation of a cross-linked polyelectrolyte coating. In their recent approach, highly blood-compatible polymer gels, namely PHEMA and PEG, were used as carriers for powder charcoal [48]. The polymeric beads containing powder charcoal were produced by radiation-induced polymerization at supercooled media.

Very recently, activated carbon-containing dresses have been successfully applied to local sorption in burn and wound treatment [49,50].

Ion Exchangers

The use of solid materials as ion exchangers goes back to the time of ancient civilizations. The first significant recognition of the phenomenon of ion exchange has been attributed to H. S. Thompson [51] and J. T. Way [52]. The experiments of Lemberg, in which he showed the possible reversible transformation of the mineral leucite ($K_2O \cdot Al_2O_3 \cdot 4SiO_2$) into analcite ($Na_2O \cdot Al_2O_3 \cdot 4SiO_2 \cdot 2H_2O$) by treating with salt solutions, have been a significant contribution [53].

Natural and Synthetic Inorganic Ion Exchangers

Phosphates, humus, cellulose, wool, protein, carbon, Al_2O_3, resins, lignin, living cells, $BaSO_4$, AgCl and many other inorganic precipitates have been shown to exhibit the property of ion exchange. Early ion exchangers were inorganic silicates (e.g., greensand and zeolites). Natural and synthetic silicates pos-

sess a polymeric structure. Silicates are salts of silicic acid and have the following generic formula:

$$xX_nO_m \cdot ySiO_2 \cdot zH_2O \tag{7}$$

Here, X represents Na, Ca, Al, Mg and other similar atoms. In most silicates the atoms in the chain are bound covalently, and the chains are linked by ionic bonds (Figure 4).

Metal aluminosilicates are important ion exchangers within silicates, whose backbone structure consists of aluminium and silicon linked together covalently by oxygen.

Natural inorganic exchangers are microcrystalline type polymers and have a micropore structure with a pore diameter as large as 150 Å and a porosity ranging from 5 to 60. Due to poor physical and chemical stabilities, these ion exchangers have been almost completely displaced by synthetic ones.

Synthetic zeolites are called molecular sieves. They are aluminosilicates which have very uniform pore structure with a total surface area in the range of 500 to 750 m²/g. The lattice vacancy (pores) may have a diameter of 4 to 5 Å. Synthetic zeolites usually have a very polar structure. Besides their ion exchange capabilities, they selectively sorb molecules based on size and shape. Molecular sieves are used industrially on a large scale for gas treatment [1,2].

Synthetic Organic Ion Exchangers

The introduction of synthetic organic ion exchange resin resulted from the studies of Adams and Holmes [54]. They synthesized organic ion exchangers based on phenolformaldehyde and phenylenediamine–formaldehyde condensates, and described the sorbtion characteristics of these kinds of resins. Later, the tailor-making of synthetic resins has rapidly evolved, and a wide variety of ion exchange materials with high sorption capacities and selectivities have been marketed.

In order to synthesize an organic ion exchanger, one need only synthesize a high-polymeric and tightly cross-linked polymer (structural part) containing ionic groups (functional part), as shown in Figure 5. These resins can be prepared by a wide variety of procedures and encompass a large number of functional groups and structures. Synthetic resinous exchangers can be classified according to their functional groups and the type of exchanging ions. Table 3 gives some examples of major commercially available Amberlite and Dowex ion exchange resins. Strong acid cation exchangers contain sulphonic groups, while weak acid cation exchangers have usually carboxylic, and less obviously phenolic, functional entities. Anion exchangers are the amine-type resins which involve quaternary ammonium groups (strong base) or other amines (weak base). Figure 6 gives the structures and functional groups of some selected examples for different ion exchangers which consist of a polystyrene matrix.

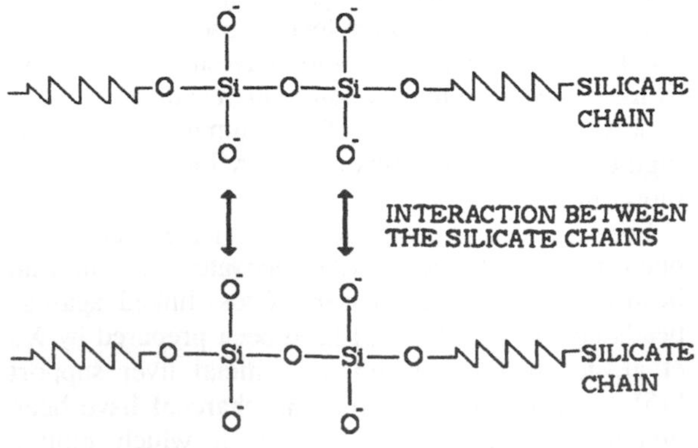

Figure 4. Chemical structure of silicates.

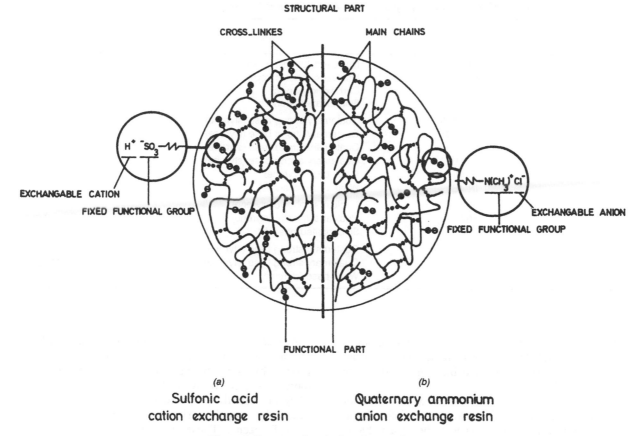

Figure 5. Structure of synthetic resinous exchangers.

Ion Exchangers for Affinity Sorption

A large variety of types of affinity ion exchangers have been developed over years, but many of them have found limited use or have been superceded by superior materials. Carboxymethyl (CM) and diethylaminoethyl (DEAE) groups have been attached to cross-linked cellulose, agarose, or dextran matrices to prepare ion exchanger, especially for protein (enzymes, etc.) ion exchange affinity chromatography [55–57]. Today high-capacity ion exchangers are available for this purpose with reliable and reproducible properties. As exemplified in Table 4, besides carboxymethyl groups, phospho- and sulfo-propyl groups are attached to the matrices in commerical cation exchangers. Triethylaminoethyl (TEAE), diethyl-(2-hydroxypropyl) aminoethyl (QAE) and polyethylene imino (PEI) groups are present in anion exchangers.

Applications

Ion exchange materials have a broad range of applications including water softening, purification and desalination, deionization of sugar, glycol, formaldehyde, and many other industrial processes. They have also been used in the pharmaceutical industry, in food processing and in catalytic processing industries as well as in analytical and preparative chemistry.

The therapeutic use of ion exchange material is as ancient as the medical profession itself. As reviewed in detail by Gordon and Roberts [58], ion exchangers have been used in many clinical conditions involving abnormalities of total body stores or serum concentrations of physiologically or metabolically significant electrolytes, ionized or ionizable solutes.

In early applications, studies have concentrated on blood collection and preservation [59,60], Dock [61] and Quick [62] have investigated several aspects of the use of ion exchange resins at animal and clinical stages.

The use of ion exchange resins in the treatment of chronic uremia was first studied by Muirhead and Read [63], who are generally given credit for the first use of resin hemoperfusion as artificial kidney. Later, the resin perfusion technique was applied clinically to patients with hyperkalaemia, uraemia, hepatic failure, drug intoxication and many other diseases, using mostly Amberlite and Dowex in exchange resins in several forms [14,58,64–66]. Although they had a wide variety of medical applications, ion exchangers have not survived due to limited sorption capacities and problems such as non-specific actions, limited patient acceptance, insignificance quantitatively, and other complex side effects.

Table 3. Major commercially available Amberlite and Dowex ion exchange resins.

Trade Name		Type	
Amberlite	IR-120	Nuclear sulphonic (styrene)	
	IR-200	Nuclear sulphonic (styrene)	
	IRC-50	Carboxylic (acrylic)	Cation Exchanger
	IR-100	Sulphonated phenolic	
Amberlite	IRA-400	Quaternary strong base (styrene)	
	IRA-401	Quaternary strong base (styrene)	
	IRA-402	Quaternary strong base (styrene)	
	IRA-900	Quaternary strong base (styrene)	Anion Exchanger
	IR-45	Weak base (styrene)	
	IR-4B	Weak base (phenolic)	
Dowex	50X	Nuclear sulphonic (styrene)	
	50W	Nuclear sulphonic (styrene)	Cation Exchanger
	30	Sulphonated phenolic	
Dowex	1	Quaternary strong base (styrene)	
	2	Quaternary strong base (styrene)	Anion Exchanger
	3	Weak base (styrene)	

At present, the number of clinical applications is limited, and includes hyperkalaemia, hypercalciuria, hyperphosphataemia, bile acid binding and dialysate regeneration [58].

Affinity ion exchangers have been widely used for protein purification chromatography on both laboratory and industrial scales. However, their use in blood purification is very limited. Some examples will be given under the specific sorbents.

Uncharged Resins

Uncharged resins and activated carbon are two broad classes of non-ionic adsorbents which have useful applications in clinical medicine.

Table 4. Some commercially available affinity ion exchange materials.

	Anion Exchangers	Cation Exchangers
Cellulose-based	DEAE[b,c]	CM[b,c]
	TEAE[b]	Phospho[b,c]
	QAE[b]	
Sephacel (spherical cellulose beads)	DEAE[a]	
Sephadex (dextran beads)	DEAE[a]	CM[a]
	QAE[a]	Selfopropyl[a]
Agarose-based	DEAE[a,b]	CM[a,b]
	PEI (polybuffer exchanger)[a]	
Synthetic-polymer-based (Trisacryl)	DEAE[d]	CM[d]

[a]Pharmacia
[b]Bio-Rad Laboratories
[c]Whatman
[d]LKB

Amberlite XAD resins (Rohm and Haas), which are uncharged, macroreticular polystyrene adsorbent resins with high adsorption capacity for hydrophobic molecules, have been used extensively in medicine. They are usually prepared in the form of insoluble beads by copolymerization of polystyrene and divinylbenzene. These macroreticular, hydrophobic resins with their large surface area have high adsorption capacities for substances having a hydrophobic character.

There are various types of Amberlite XAD resins which are chemically identical but different in physical properties, with a surface from 300 to 800 m²/g. They have roughly 50 percent porosity and pores with a diameter of 50 Å.

Adsorption is the principal mechanism, and there is no change in the ionic composition of the solution treated with uncharged resins. Like activated carbon, sorption on these resins is affected by resin properties (e.g., surface area, pore size distribution and surface chemistry), the type of the absorbate and the solvent, temperature, etc. In general, when hydrophobicity of the solute increases, the binding ability of the resin also increases.

Adsorption isotherms, such as activated carbon, may be used to formulate the adsorption equilibria and to evaluate the sorption capacities. In adsorption rate studies, similar rate-controlling steps may be considered as in activated carbon systems. As mentioned before, coating the sorbents with semipermeable membranes creates an additional resistance to mass transfer. Amberlite XAD resins are used without any coating; thus high adsorption rates can be achieved.

In particular, these resins have very high adsorption capacities for lipid-soluble protein-bound drugs such as methaqualone, ethchlorvynol, glutethimide, digitalis and cephaloridine [14,65,67]. The Amberlite

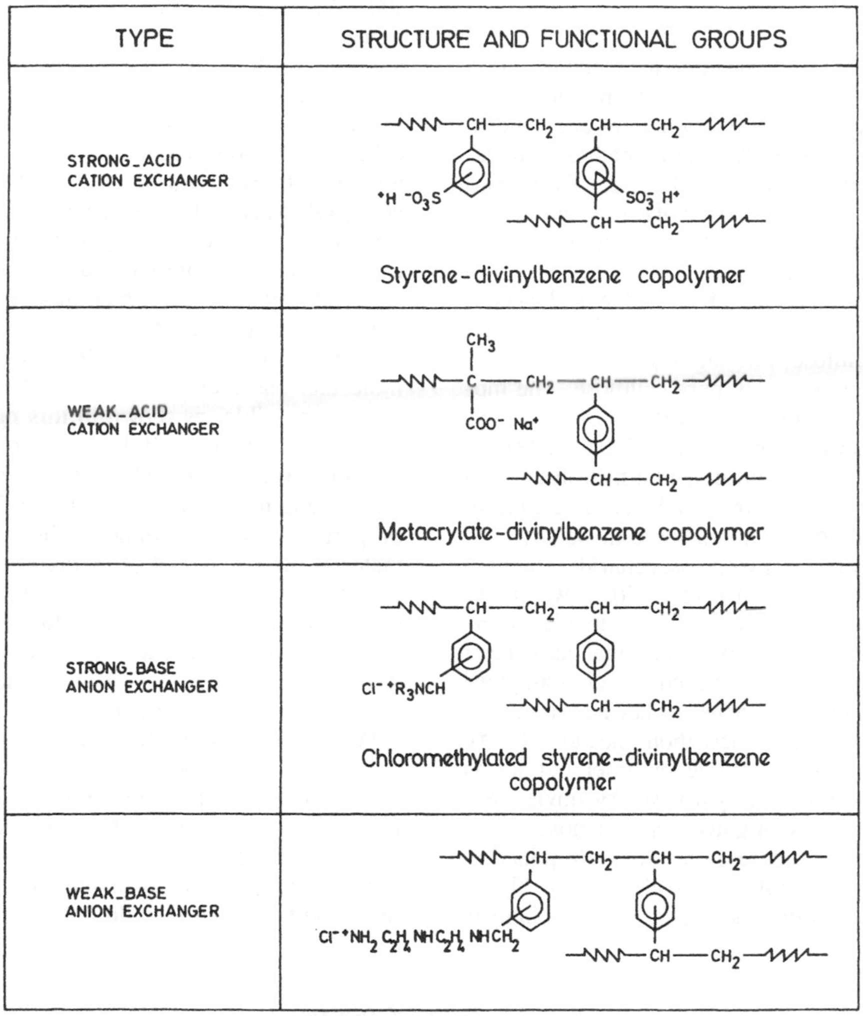

Figure 6. Structures and functional groups of some common organic ion exchangers.

XAD-2 and XAD-4 have been used successfully in hemoperfusion columns for life-threatening drug-overdose cases. Amberlite XAD-2 (surface area: 300 m^2/g) and XAD-4 (surface area: 750 m^2/g) from Rohm and Haas, U.S.A. are the most common poly-styrene/divinyl benzene based uncharged resins available, XAD-4 resins are utilized in DX-60 (Extracorporeal, U.S.A.) and Haemoresin (Braun, Germany) resin hemoperfusion columns. XAD-7, which is a methyacrylic acid/styrene copolymer with 450 m^2/g surface area and relatively large pore size, has been given credit and has undergone preclinical and clinical trials. Albumin coating [22] has been applied to increase the blood compatibility of these resins [68]. With its high adsorption affinity to bile acids and unconjugated bilirubin, Amberlite XAD-7 resin hemoperfusion has been applied to patients with acute liver failure [65,66,68]. No apparent clinical toxicity has been observed in these applications. There is an average 40 percent platelet depletion during the first hour of perfusion, but platelet levels return

to 80 percent of the pre-perfusion levels within 18 hours.

In contrast to their high efficiency in the treatment of acute drug intoxications, Amberlite XAD-2 and XAD-4 resins are not effective in the treatment of uraemia. They do not offer the wide adsorptive spectrum that activated carbons do.

As was mentioned above, new uncoated pyrolized resins, which may be defined as activated carbon, have recently been developed. Amberlite XE-336, which has a wide adsorptive spectrum with a 400 to 500 m^2/g surface area, is an example of this type of resin (or activated carbon) [14].

Polystyrene/divinyl benzene-based resins (Wofatit resins) produced by VEB Chemiekombinat, Germany, have been tested recently for hemoperfusion [39].

The combination of charcoal and resin in agarose microcapsules has been considered as a promising approach to hemoperfusion applications in artificial liver support [69].

Polyaldehydes

Polyaldehydes are well known to form condensation products (Schiff base complexes) with ammonia, urea and other primary and secondary amines and amides. The polyaldehydes currently used in medical applications are oxystarch and oxycellulose. These two polyaldehydes are both glucose polymers and can be prepared by oxidation of starch and cellulose.

Cellulose is a natural linear polysaccharide, composed of D-glucose units which are of the β-(2,4) configuration [Figure 7(a)]. Most plants contain a high percentage of cellulose, ranging in general from 10 to 15 percent. Cotton is nearly pure cellulose. The molecular weight of cellulose from different sources has been estimated to vary from about 50,000 to 2,500,000 in different species. Cellulose can be hydrolysed into disaccharides or glucose by cellobiase or cellulase, respectively. Cellulose is non-soluble in water.

Starch is a mixture of two polysaccharides, namely α-amylose and amylopectin [Figure 7(b)], which are present in approximately a 1:3 ratio in plants. α-Amylose consist of D-glucose units that have been bound in α-(1,4) linkages. The chains of α-amylose are polydisperse and unbranched. They have a molecular weight varying from a few thousands to 500,000. α-Amylose is not truly soluble in water but forms hydrated micelles. It can be hydrolysed by amylase enzyme to yield a mixture of glucose and maltose. Amylopectin also has D-glucose units which are joined in an α-manner. This polysaccharide has a highly branched structure with a molecular weight as high as

100 million. Amylopectin yields a colloidal solution in water. Amylopectin molecules are also attacked by amylase to form dextrin which are the polysaccharides of intermediate chain length.

Oxypolysaccharides are derived from starch and cellulose. Various oxidants, such as metaperiodate and hypochlorite, can be used for the oxidation process [69]. Metaperiodate seems to control the oxidation better, where the hyperoxidation might cause toxic substances to be yielded [69–71].

Polyaldehydes react with ammonia and urea according to the structures given in Figure 8. Due to the presence of adjacent aldehyde groups, further intramolecular and intermolecular condensation reactions are also possible, as shown in this figure.

Oxystarch and oxycellulose can bind both ammonia and urea over a broad pH range (pH 7 to 9) at temperatures ranging from 25 to 70°C [72]. The binding properties vary, depending on the source of the raw material, its manner of preparation and purification, and its final physical state [69–72]. The binding capacities of these polyaldehydes for ammonia are considerably greater than for urea, on a molar basis. In the presence of mixtures of ammonia and urea, oxypolysaccharides react preferentially with ammonia.

Polyaldehydes were first demonstrated by Giordano et al. [73] as orally ingestible sorbents used to increase the faecal nitrogen excretion. These preliminary observations have been confirmed by other groups [71,74,75]. Both oxystarch and oxycellulose are good sorbents for ammonia and urea under physiological conditions, but they do not absorb the other me-

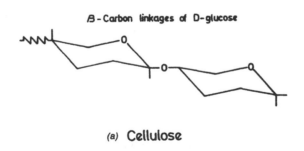

(a) **Cellulose**

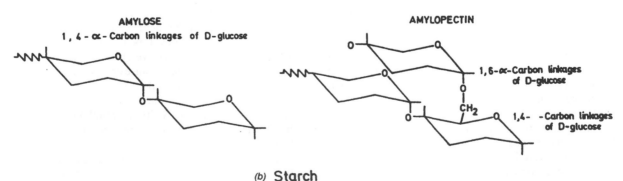

(b) **Starch**

Figure 7. Cellulose and starch.

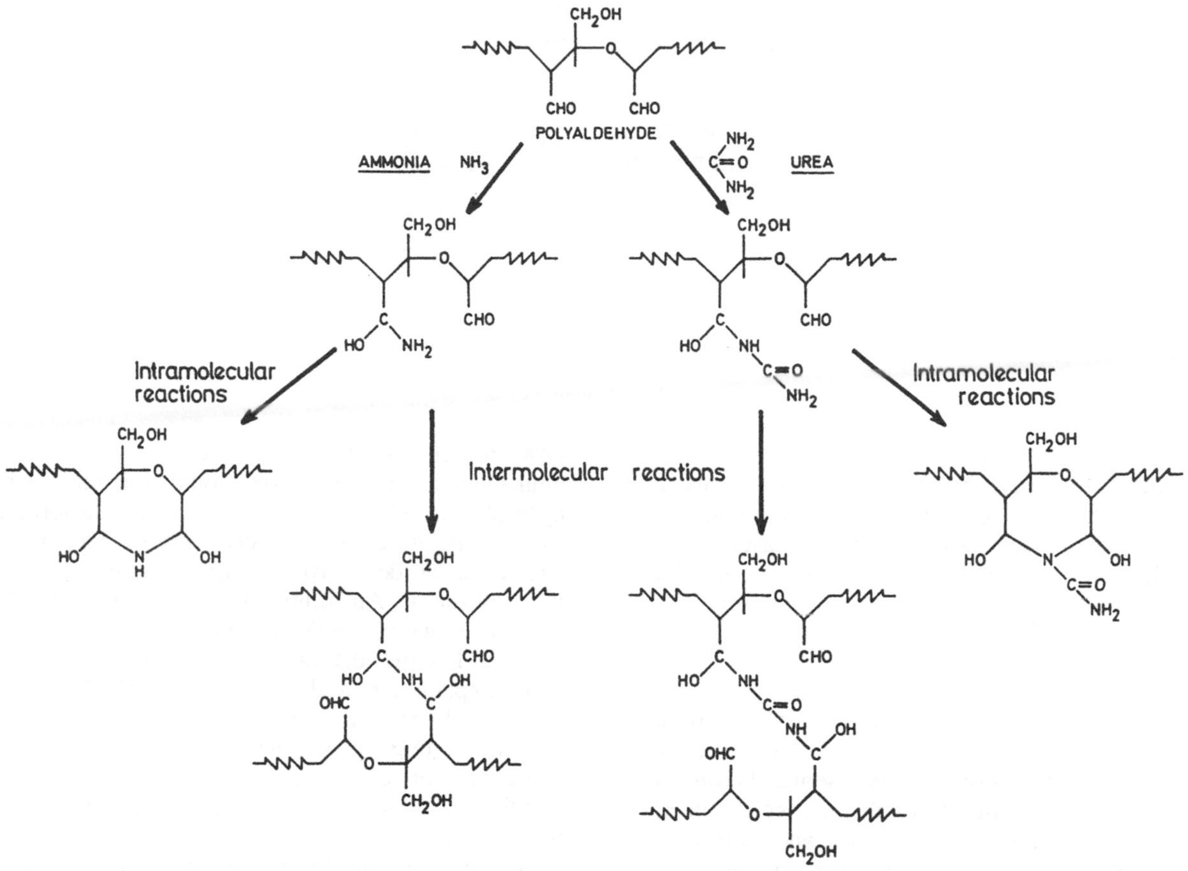

Figure 8. Reactions of polyaldehydes with ammonia and urea.

tabolites and therefore the ultimate value of "intestinal dialysis" is questionable. However, it is clear that this kind of treatment increases faecal nitrogen and also potassium excretion. It seems that orally administered oxystarch might be a possible way to remove urea in uraemic patients, in which cases hemoperfusion and ultrafiltration systems can be used to remove other metabolites. Oxycellulose might also be utilized extracorporeally in hemoperfusion columns for removing urea, simultaneously with the other sorbents.

Other Nonspecific Sorbents

The sorbents discussed above (activated carbon, ion exchangers, non-ionic resins, etc.) have been extensively investigated for hemoperfusion applications. Others, such as silica gel, active alumina and magnesia, aluminium gels also have potential to be used in hemoperfusion systems directly or indirectly [77,78].

Aluminium gels have already been used orally for phosphorus adsorption in uraemia and are available commercially as antacids in the hydroxide and carbonate forms [78]. They can be considered as phosphate binders when they are used in series with hemoperfusion systems.

Biospecific Sorbents

Affinity sorption is already a well-established method for identification, purification, and separation of complex biomolecules. This may be achieved by a number of traditional techniques such as gel permeation chromatography, high performance liquid chromatography, chromatofocusing, electrophoresis, centrifugation, etc., in that the process relies on differences in the physical properties (e.g., size, charge, and hydrophobicity) of molecules to be treated. In contrast, affinity sorption techniques exploit the unique property of extremely specific biological recognition [57,79–89]. Affinity chromatography enables separation of almost any biomolecule on the basis of its biological function or individual chemical structure. Affinity sorption requires that the compound to be isolated is capable of reversibly binding (i.e., sorption–elution) to a sorbent which consists of a complementary substance (i.e., the so-called ligand) immobilized on a suitable insoluble support, i.e., the so-called carrier.

Synthesis of Affinity Sorbents

The principle of synthesizing affinity sorbents is shown in Figure 9. In the first step a carrier matrix is

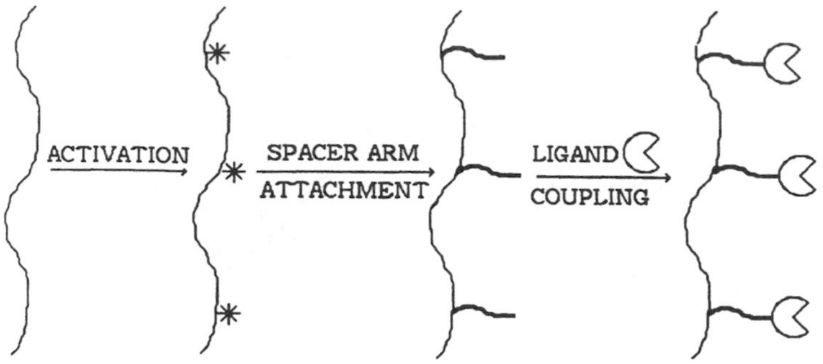

Figure 9. Coupling of ligands to carriers.

chosen and activated. Then, a spacer arm is attached covalently to the carrier through the active points. The ligand is then reacted with the sorbent already possessing the spacer arm. In some cases, the ligand–spacer arm combination is first synthesized and then attached to the carrier in one single step.

THE MATRIX

The selection of the matrix is the first important consideration. The matrix must exhibit extremely low nonspecific adsorption; this is essential because the power of affinity adsorption relies on specific interactions. The matrix should be open and have a loose porous network; the sorbent beads should be uniform in porosity and size, spherical and rigid; the beads should also be chemically and biologically inert. Note that the bead form of the matrix provides excellent

Table 5. Some commercially available affinity sorbent carriers.

Company	Carrier
Amicon Corporation	Nylon-based affinity matrices (Matrex Series)
	Cross-linked agarose beads (Matrex Gel Series)
Bio-Rad Laboratories	Agarose Gels (Bio-Gel A Series)
	Polyacrylamide Gels (Bio-Gel P Series)
Electro-Nucleonics Inc.	Controlled Pore Glass
Koch-Light Genzyme	Spheron Series (PHEMA-based)
	Polyacrylamide Gels
	Polylactones
E. Merck GmbH	Cellulose-based supports
Miles Laboratories Inc.	Hydrophobic Agaroses
Rohm Pharma	Eupergut-C, Epoxy activated supports
Sigma Chemical Company	Agarose
Pharmacia P. L. Biochemicals	Agaroses
Biochemicals Inc.	Sephadex series
Pierce Chemical Company	Controlled Pore Glass
	Polystyrene

flow properties with minimal channelling in the column applications. The matrix should preferentially be hydrophilic, and derivatives must be easy to form at room temperatures and in aqueous media; ideally, the later chemical derivatives should be suited to ligand immobilization. An affinity sorbent matrix must be also stable under a wide range of conditions such as high and low pH, detergents and dissociating agents, high temperatures, and, in situations which require organic solvents for chemical modifications, disruptive eluents (e.g., guanidine hydrochloride) for difficult elution or regeneration steps. It should be noted that there is no sorbent available today that fulfills all these criteria.

In contrast to the diversity of the type of ligands, there are not very many polymeric carriers available. Table 5 exemplifies some commercially available affinity sorbent carriers. The basic properties of some of the matrices is briefly touched below; full details of the products should be obtained from each company and related literature [79–89].

Although other sorbents have been used, and in individual cases might have advantages, spherical cross-linked agarose beads with molecular exclusion sizes of about 10^7 daltons have been employed most extensively in affinity sorption. This natural polymer is usually purified from marine algae. In order to increase mechanical, ionic and thermal stabilities, agarose beads are covalently cross-linked with various substances (e.g., epichlorohydrin). As given in Table 5, the most popular commercial agarose products are the Sepharose and Superose series from Pharmacia and the Bio-Gel A series from Bio-Rad.

A wide range of derived celluloses have been described and their applications have generally been widespread for protein purification. Cellulose consists of linear polymers of β-1,4 linked D-glucose units. Beaded cellulose from Merck GmbH with high porosity, good mechanical stability and a pronounced hydrophilic character has been considered as a useful support matrix.

The commercial product, Sephadex, is prepared by cross-linking dextrans (i.e., an α-1,6 linked glucose polymer) with epichlorohydrin, and is available in bead forms. The low degree of porosity and mechanical stability are its main disadvantages.

Polyacrylamide gels are composed of a skeleton which carries carboxyamide groups. Bio-Gel P series marketed by Bio-Rad Laboratories are one of the main products prepared by copolymerization of acrylamide and N,N'-methylenebisacrylamide. They are available with various pore sizes. A commerical variation on pre-activated polyacrylamide is the Enzacryl series from Koch-Light, which are produced especially for enzyme immobilization.

Trisacryl synthetic carriers produced by LKB are derived from the polymerization of N-acryloyl-2-amino-2-hydroxymethyl 1,3-propane diol. This hydrophilic carrier has been found suitable for the separation of biological macromolecules such as proteins, and also for cells.

With their high biocompatibility, hydrocyalkyl methacrylates have been considered basic materials in the field of medicine. Spheron both by Lachema and Realco Chemical Company with excellent chemical and physical stabilities have been found to be among the most promising bioaffinity carrier matrices.

Eupergit C manufactured by Rohm Pharma consists of oxirane acrylic beads, obtained by copolymerization of methacrylamide, methylenebisacrylamide, glycidyl-methacrylate and/or allyl-glycidyl-ether. It is hydrophilic and exhibits high chemical stability over a pH range of 0–12. These beads have high binding capacity due to a high epoxide group content and large inner core structure accessible to large molecules.

Controlled pore glass by Pierce Chemical Company and by Electro-Nucleonics Inc. with different surface properties are the most commonly employed inorganic matrices for the immobilization of biological molecules. They have excellent physical properties for column applications. However, their use in affinity chromatography is relatively limited.

LIGANDS

A wide variety of biofunctional molecules, such as enzymes, proteins, antibodies, antigens, amino acids, peptide sequences, nucleic acids, DNA or RNA sequences may be used as ligands in order to prepare biospecific affinity sorbents. Table 6 gives examples of some important ligands and functional groups for attachment to the carrier.

The ligand, for successful affinity sorption, should exhibit specific reversible binding affinity for the substances to be purified. It should also have chemically modifiable groups which allow it to be attached to the carrier matrix without destroying its binding activity. It should have an affinity for binding substances in the range of 10^{-4} to 10^{-8} M in free solution. Interactions involving dissociation constants greater than 10^{-4} M are likely to be too weak for successful sorption. Conversely, if the dissociation constant is lower than 10^{-8} M, elution or regeneration of the sorbent without inactivation of the bound substance is likely to be difficult. The correct choice of ligand is of course dependent on the substance to be sorbed.

Table 6. Some important ligands and functional groups for attachment to carrier.

Ligand	Functional Groups for Attachment
Protein, Peptide, Amino Acid	Amino Carboxyl Thiol
Sugar	Hydroxyl Amino Carboxyl
Polynucleotide	Amino Mercurated base
Coenzyme, Cofactor, Antibiotic, Steroid, etc.	Amino, Carboxyl Thiol or Hydroxyl

Immobilized antibodies and antigens, the so-called immunosorbents, have been in use for many years in affinity sorption [79–89]. Here, the extraordinary selectivity and specificity of interactions between an antibody and antigen is the key point of sorption. However, it should also be noted that the high affinity of immunosorbent to the counter molecule has been recognized as the major difficulty owing to the drastic conditions required for elution or regeneration of the sorbent. For example antigen–antibody interactions characteristically have dissociation constants of the order of 10^{-8}–10^{-12} M.

The use of antibodies in medicine increased drastically after Kohler and Milstein had for the first time developed continuous cultures of fused cells secreting a monoclonal antibody of pre-defined specificity [90]. The introduction of monoclonal antibodies, i.e., homogeneous immunoglobulins raised against a specific antigenic determinant, has also greatly influenced the development of biospecific affinity sorption. Monoclonal antibodies derived from a single clone are well-defined chemical reagents that bind to a specific epitope on the analyte.

Hybridoma-derived monoclonal antibodies are chemically homogeneous, because each molecule of immunoglobulin is an exact replica of the next. Monoclonal antibodies can be produced continuously, in contrast to a conventional polyclonal antiserum, which is a variable mixture of reagents and can never be reproduced once the original supply has been exhausted. The use of monoclonal antibodies as ligands is superior in all cases to the use of polyclonal antibodies from animal sera. Basic differences in the use of monoclonal and polyclonal antibodies in affinity sorbents involve specificity, affinity and capacity. In each area monoclonal antibodies possess significant advantages. However, it should be noted that polyclonal antibodies are simpler for most investigators, therefore, in some circumstances can be preferred.

COUPLING TECHNIQUES

There are different methods for deriving bioaffinity sorbents, in which several intermediate steps are followed. The procedures used for coupling ligands to the carrier matrix will only briefly be given here; recent publications exclusively concerned with affinity adsorption techniques cover the subject in great detail [79–89]. The main requirements for a successful affinity sorbent are given below. Note that the correct choice of coupling method depends on both the carrier and the substance to be immobilized.

Immobilization should be attempted through the least critical region of the ligand molecule, to ensure minimal interference with the normal binding. The specificity of the binding reaction indicates which groups on the ligand are essential for interaction with the binding substance and which are least critical.

The active site of a biological substance is often located deep within the molecule and the sorbent (e.g., small ligands like enzyme cofactors). This may cause low capacity and also some inactivation of the agent due to steric interference between the carrier and the agent binding to the ligand. In these circumstances a spacer arm is interposed between the carrier and the ligand to make the ligand more accessible to the substance to be purified. If the length of the spacer is too short, the arm is ineffective. If it is too long, nonspecific sorption (e.g., usually hydrophobic interactions) become pronounced and reduce the selectivity of the separation [91].

The linkage should be stable with respect to the likely conditions to be used during the adsorption and cleaning-up procedures (like regeneration). This is especially important in extracorporeal hemoperfusion applications where bioaffinity sorbents are used, because the release of the ligands or spacer arms may cause significant drawbacks to the patients.

Among a number of activation methods, cyanogen bromide (CNBr) activation is still the most widely used method. The chemistry of this activation process involves the reaction of hydroxyl groups on the carrier matrix. The reactions of CNBr are complex; carbamates, imidocarbonates and cyanate esters are the major products (Figure 10). The last two are chemically active. Cyanate esters are stable below pH 4, whereas the imidocarbonates are stable under basic conditions. Therefore, it is possible to design and prepare carriers containing either functional group. However, it should be noted that the reaction of cyanate esters with primary amines gives isourea derivatives. The isourea substituent is positively charged, at neutral pH, which can introduce anion exchange character to the sorbent, which is usually undesirable.

Epoxy activation is one of the alternative methods to CNBr activation. An epoxy group is introduced, using 1,4-butanediol diglycidyl ether (a bisoxirane). Epoxy groups are somewhat more reactive than cyanates, and as well as combining with primary amines, they react with hydroxyls to form ether linkages (Figure 11).

Another activation method uses 1,1'-carbonyldiimidazole, as activator, which gives products just as reactive as cyanates. But, in contrast, these groups react with primary amines by urethane linkage which is not positively charged (Figure 12). This activation agent is also less noxious than the previous ones mentioned above.

One of the recent activation methods uses tosyl or tresyl chloride. The products of this activation react smoothly and rapidly to give the very stable secondary amine from primary amine ligands (Figure 13).

Many other activation procedures have been reported in the related literature with some advantages and disadvantages over the basic methods given previously [79–89].

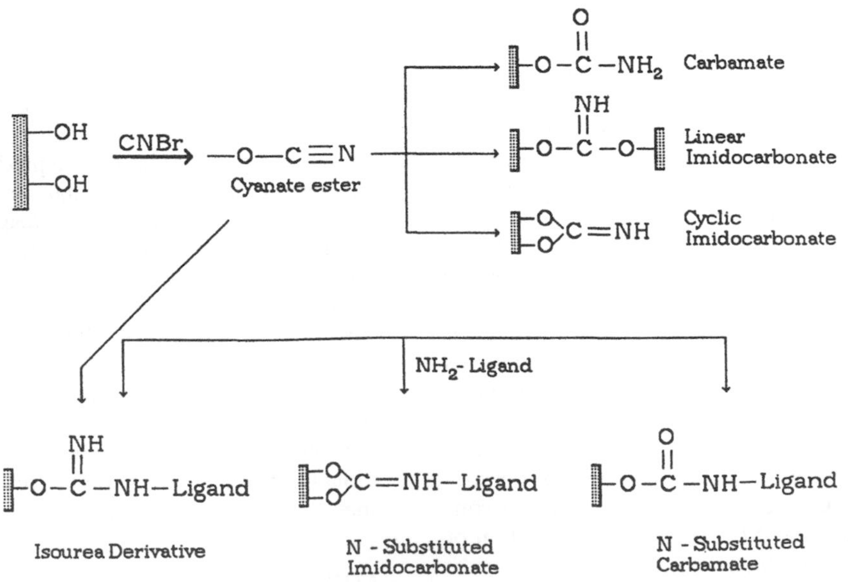

Figure 10. Cyanogen bromide activation and ligand coupling.

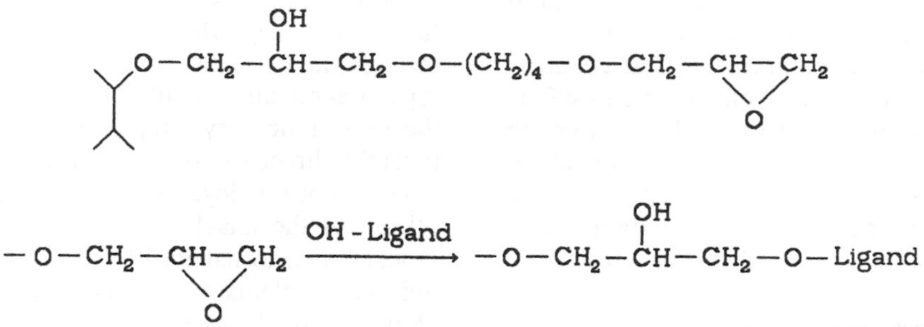

Figure 11. Epoxy activation and ligand coupling.

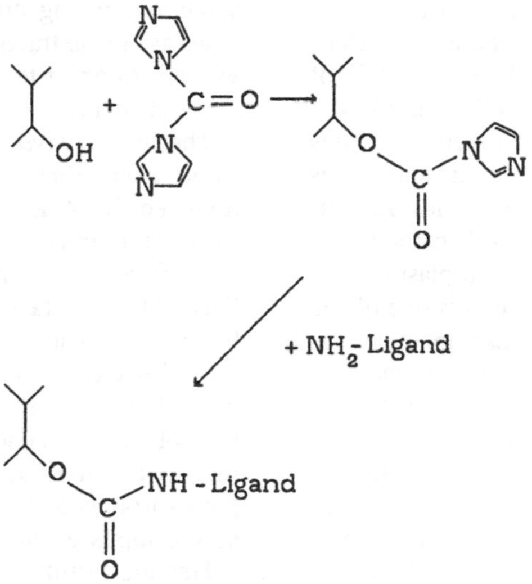

Figure 12. Carbonyldiimidazole activation and ligand coupling.

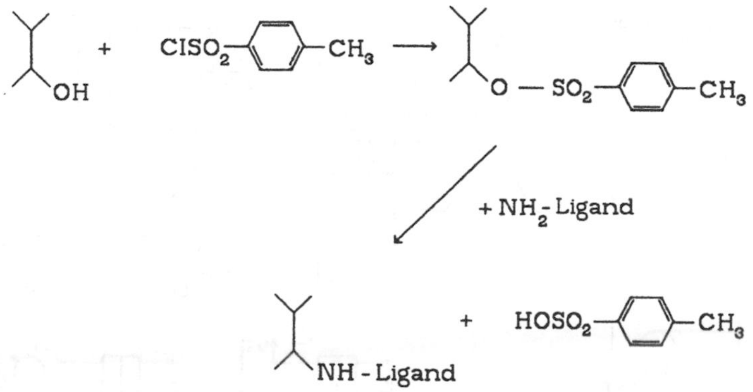

Figure 13. Tosyl chloride activation and ligand coupling.

Applications of Biospecific Sorbents

Extracorporeal therapies are directed at the removal of potential toxins from the bloodstream [92]. Hemodialysis is the most common and the oldest extracorporeal system used for the treatment of patients suffering from renal diseases, where arterial blood from the patient is pumped through a dialysis unit consisting of a semipermeable synthetic dialysis membrane. The blood is passed over one side of the membrane while a dialysate solution is circulated on the other side. Hence, waste or toxic substances are removed from the blood by dialysis under a concentration gradient across the membrane. Hemodialysis relays upon the diffusive transport, therefore, is a rather slow process. In addition, due to the size range of the pores of the dialysate membranes in use, this technique does not work for the removal of larger toxic molecules.

Membrane plasmapheresis is a young extracorporeal treatment where blood from the patient is circulated through a membrane filter, and roughly 30% of the whole blood is filtered (Figure 14). The plasma separated from the blood contains macromolecules (such as pathogenically relevant factors as antibodies and immune complexes) and micromolecules. In simple plasma separation the fluid phase is discarded, and fresh frozen plasma containing valuable plasma proteins (e.g., albumin) is reinfused, which is one of the major drawbacks of therapeutic plasmapheresis as practiced today. The solutions reinfused are obtained from human plasma, therefore they are very expensive and available internationally only in limited quantities. Recent developments, such as cryofiltration, double filtration plasmapheresis, or cascade filtration, and plasmapheresis combined with sorbents has triggered its clinical effectiveness. However, it should be noted that these systems are still complex and expensive.

Today, one of the most promising procedures for extracorporeal blood purification is biospecific affinity sorption. Affinity sorbents may be used in hemoperfusion systems, where blood is directly perfused through the columns filled with these sorbents. This type of application is, of course, very effective and at the same time very simple and inexpensive. Unfortunately, direct hemoperfusion using biospecific sorbents is not employed widely, because of the risk of release of the attached molecules (i.e., ligands and spacer arms) to patient blood, which may cause significant problems; and also because of the limited blood compatibility of these sorbents. Due to these drawbacks, biospecific sorbents are usually used simultaneously with systems like plasmapheresis, apheresis, etc., where blood from patient is first separated and then the plasma is passed through the adsorption columns filled with affinity sorbents. Here, some interesting applications of biospecific sorbent systems in extracorporeal therapy are briefly reviewed, in order to stress the attractive future of these novel sorbents.

The first *ex vivo* application of biospecific sorbents came from Terman and his coworkers [93]. They removed DNA antibodies from the plasma of positively immunized rabbits by circulating their blood through an extracorporeal shunt containing immobilized DNA. They have also reported removal of bovine serum antibodies from the blood of dogs previously injected with antibodies by using albumin/collodion/charcoal sorbent system [94]. The first clinical trial of immunoadsorption was also achieved by Terman et al. in 1979, where they have used DNA-coupled sorbents to treat a female patient suffering from severe lupus erythematosus [95].

Hepatic insufficiency is a serious clinical syndrome with a high level of mortality. Artificial liver supports such as hemodialysis, plasma exchange and hemoper-

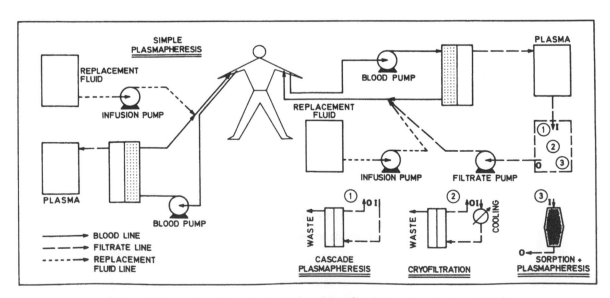

Figure 14. Plasmapheresis/cascade plasmapheresis/cryofiltration/sorption + plasmapheresis.

fusion using nonspecific sorbents have been clinically used for the treatment of severe liver diseases, unfortunately with only limited success. One of the most interesting approaches to biospecific sorbents is the removal of toxic substances released into the body during liver failure. Plotz and his coworkers have been using prepared human serum albumin conjugated agarose sorbents for the removal of bilirubin from the blood of rats with surgically formed biliary obstructions [96]. Similar sorbent systems have also been used by Hughes et al., and low capacity of the sorbent has been reported [97]. Recently, a hybrid type of artificial liver support, in which isolated or cultured hepatocytes in immobilized form are concerned, is receiving increased media attention. The preliminary results of the *in vitro* and *ex vivo* animal studies with hepatocyte cultured polymeric substrata such as collagen, calcium alginate, silicone, lactose attached polystyrene, etc. have been considered very promising [98,99].

One of the early advancements related to immunosorption came from studies of Ray and his coworkers, who have attempted extracorporeal sorption of pathologic gammaglobulins and immune complexes in various diseases including cancer [100]. They have used protein A containing *Staphylococci aurei* of Cowan I strain for IgG removal from the patients with chronic lymphocytic leukemia and autoimmune hemolytic anemia. Pure protein A coupled agarose based carriers have been also used successfully to treat patients with hemophilia complicated by antibodies to factors VII and IX respectively [101,102].

Iatrogenic therapeutic digitalis glycoside intoxication is one of the most common drug reactions seen in clinical medicine [103]. Therapy is mainly directed to reducing the burden of digoxin for life saving. One of the earliest applications of immunosorbtion is related to this therapy. Margel et al. perfused the blood of digoxin-intoxicated dogs through hemoperfusion columns filled with antidigoxin antibodies/polyacrolein/cross-linked-agarose sorbent beads, and reported up to 25% removal of the total digoxin burden [104].

Familial hypercholesterolaemia (FH) is an autosomal dominant disorder, characterized by elevated levels of low-density lipoprotein (LDL)-cholesterol. Elevated plasma levels of low-density lipoprotein, which is the principal cholesterol carrier of human plasma, correlate directly with an increased risk for the development of arteriosclerosis [105]. Arteriosclerosis in such forms as coronary heart disease and cerebrovascular disease are major causes of morbidity and mortalitiy in all industrial countries. In addition to dietary and drug therapy, attempts have been made to remove cholesterol and LDL directly from plasma of patients suffering from FH. Plasma exchange, the first approach to removing lipids and lipoproteins from plasma, continues to be used despite certain disadvantages. Total plasma exchange is limited mainly by the effort required and by its high cost [106,107]. Cascade or double filtration plasmapheresis permit

more selective LDL removal from plasma than does plasma exchange. This treatment method also has certain disadvantages [108]. Extracorporeal removal of LDL by plasmapheresis, combined with affinity sorption of LDL from plasma, has resulted in substantial reduction in plasma LDL level in refractory hypercholesterolemic patients [109].

Special devices (e.g., HELP-LDL apheresis) have also been developed based on the precipitation of LDL with heparin and dextrane sulfate at low pH values [110,111]. However, this new approach seems relatively complicated.

LDL and cholesterol adsorption was provided in the late 1970s with great hope. Taking advantage of the high affinity of heparin for LDL and cholesterol, first attempts have been made to remove LDL and cholesterol by affinity adsorption on heparin–agarose gels [112–115]. Besides heparin other polyanionic groups (e.g., dextrane sulfate or polyacrylic acid), which are covalently attached to the polymeric carriers (e.g., agarose, cellulose or polyvinyl alcohol) have been used for cholesterol and LDL adsorption [116–119]. More selective sorbents containing anti-LDL antibodies have been considered as the most promising approach for LDL sorption, recently [120–126], due to the effectiveness, efficiency, biocompatibility, simplicity, cost, etc. [127].

Various specific and non-specific immunosuppressive factors are assumed to exist in the sera of cancer patients and they help tumor cells grow despite the antitumor activity of the host, protecting them from attack by chemo-immunotherapy. To remove these immunosuppressive factors, plasma exchange has been studied in cancer patients [128]. However, recent studies show that while immunosuppressive factors with molecular weights higher than that of globulin are removed by plasma exchange, immunosuppressive factors with molecular weights lower than that of albumin still remain in the fraction returned to the patient [129,130]. Therefore adsorbent combined with plasma exchange has been developed to remove these factors. Microporous glassbead sorbents (Kuraray Co., Ltd., Osaka, Japan) with different porosities and surface properties have been tested recently in cancer patients [130]. Results indicate that these sorbents do effectively remove immunosuppressive factor from the serum of cancer patients. This procedure combined with chemo-immunotherapy may well prove effective as adjunctive therapy for malignant tumors.

Immunosorbents have been successfully used for removal of anti-A and anti-B blood group antibodies in ABO incompatibility for bone marrow and renal transplantation [131–134].

An increased problem in uremic patients waiting for renal transplantation is immunization. Approximately one-half of individuals awaiting renal transplantation possess circulating antibodies to HLA antigens. Pretransplant plasmapheresis has been reported, but found ineffective in some patients. Immunoadsorption columns like Asahi Immusorba IM-TR, have been used effectively for elimination of HLA-antibodies [135,136].

Biospecific sorbents have also been used for the removal of: rheumoid factors and immune complexes from the plasma of patients with rheumatic disease [137–139]; anti-acetylcholine receptor antibodies in sera from patients with myasthenia gravis by using amino acid attached (e.g., phenylalanine and tryptophan) polyvinyl alcohol carriers [140]; β_2-microglobulins which causes dialytic amyloidosis in patients with chronic renal failure on long-term hemodialysis [141–143]; IgE and IgM [144,145]; DNA-antibodies in systemic lupus erythematosus [146]; and insulin antibodies [147].

REFERENCES

1. Ruthven, D. M. 1984. *Principles of Adsorption and Adsorption Processes*. John Wiley and Sons.

2. Rodrigues, A. E., M. D. LeVan and D. Tondeur. 1988. *Adsorption: Science and Technology*. London: Kluwer Acad. Publ.

3. Yang, C. and G. T. Tsao. 1982. In *Chromatography. Advances in Biochemical Engineering 25*. A. Fiechter, ed. Springer-Verlag, pp. 2, 37.

4. Arnold, F. H., H. W. Blanch and C. R. Wilke. 1980. *Chem. Eng. J.*, 58:91.

5. McCoy, B. J. 1986. *AIChE Symp. Ser., No: 250*, 82:115.

6. Schinhelm, K. 1989. *Artif. Organs*, 13(1):21

7. Pişkin, E. and A. R. Özdural. 1979. *Artif. Organs*, 3(suppl.):77.

8. Pişkin, E., A. R. Özdural and A. Gürçay. 1978. *Proce. EDTA*, 15:593.

9. Kunin, R. 1958. *Ion Exhcange Resins*. New York: John Wiley.

10. Helfferich, F. 1962. *Ion Exchange*. New York: McGraw-Hill.

11. Hassler, J. W. 1974. *Purification with Activated Carbon*. New York: Chemical Publ. Co.

12. Deitz, V. R. 1956. *Bibliography of Solid Adsorbents*. Washington, D.C.: United States Cane Sugar Refineries and Bone Char Manufacturers and the National Bureau of Standards.

13. Denti, E. and J. M. Walker. 1980. In *Sorbents and Their Clinical Applications*. C. Giordano, ed. New York: Academic Press, p. 101.

14. Rosenbaum, J. L. and M. S. Kramer et al. 1977. *Dialysis and Transplantation*, 4:26.

15. Chang, T. M. S. 1978. *Artificial Kidney, Artificial Liver, and Artificial Cells*. New York: Plenum Press.

16. Gaylor, J. D. S. and F. A. P. Maggs et al. *29th Ann. Cong. Eng. in Med. Biol., Boston, MA, 1979.*

17. Gurland, H. J. and L. A. Castro et al. 1980. In *Hemoperfusion: Kidney and Liver Support and Detoxification, Part I*. S. Sideman and T. M. S. Chang, eds. Washington, D.C.: Hemisphere, p. 105.

18. Özdural, A. R. and H. Mann et al. 1982. *Life Support Systems*, 1(suppl.):55.

19. Pişkin, E. and E. Arca et al. *Proc. 5th Int. Symp. Hemo. Artif. Organs, Tianjin, China, 1983.*

20. Weber Jr., W. J. 1972. *Physicochemical Process for Water Quality Control*. New York: Wiley Interscience.

21. Brunauer, S., P. H. Emmett and E. Teller. 1938. *J. Am. Chem. Soc.*, 60:309.

22. Chang, T. M. S. 1969. *Can. J. Physiopharm.*, 47:1043.

23. Fennimore, J. and G. D. Munro. 1975. In *Artificial Liver Support*. R. Williams and I. M. Murray-Lion, eds. London: Pitman Medical, p. 330.

24. Hill, J. B., F. L. Palaia, J. L. McAdams, P. J. Palmer, J. T. Skinner and S. M. T. Maret. 1976. *Kidney Int.*, 10:328.

25. Rosenbaum, J. L., M. S. Kramer and R. Raja. 1978. *Nephron*, 21:27.

26. Nicolaev, V. 1983. In *The Past, Present and Future of Artificial Organs*. E. Pişkin and T. M. S. Chang, eds. Ankara: Meteksan.

27. Funakubo, H., K. Shirane and T. Dohi, et. al. 1981. *Proc. Eur. Soc. Artif. Organs*, 8:120.

28. Nagai, H., K. Katori, Z. Shiiki and Y. Amagi. 1976. US Patent, 1,459,819.

29. Chang, T. M. S. 1983. In *The Past, Present and Future of Artificial Organs*. E. Pişkin and T. M. S. Chang, eds. Ankara: Meteksan.

30. Thysell, H., T. Lindholm and D. Heinegard, et.al. 1976. *Proc. Eur. Soc. Artif. Organs*, 2:212.

31. Tijssen, J., A. Bantjes and A. W. J. Van Doorn, et. al. 1979. *Artif. Organs*, 3:11.

32. Andrade, J. D., K. Kunitomo, R. Van Wegenen, B. Kastigir, D. Gough and W. J. Kolff. 1971. *Trans. Am. Soc. Artif. Intern Organs*, 17:222.

33. Courtney, J. M. and T. Gilchrist. 1980. In *A Textbook of Biomedical Engineering*. R. M. Kenedi. Glaskow: Blackie, p. 77.

34. Özdural, A. R., J. Hameed, M. Y. Bölük and E. Pişkin. 1980. *ASIO J.*, 3:116.

35. Pişkin, E. and A. R. Özdural. 1981. *Artif. Organs*, (suppl.), 5:223.

36. Pişkin, E, Ç. Çakmaklı, M. Mutlu, K. Pişkin and A. R. Özdural. 1981. *Proc. Eur. Soc. Artif. Organs*, 8:201.

37. Davis, T. A., D. R. Coswar, S. D. Harrison and A. C. Tanquary. 1974. *Trans. Am. Soc. Artif. Intern Organs*, 10:353.

38. Bailey, A. and F. A. P. Maggs. *Brit. Patents*, 1:310,101, 1972; 1:310,011, 1973.

39. Courtney, J. M. and D. Falkenhagen. 1984. Ph.D. Thesis, Rostock, April.

40. Denti, E., J. Walker, V. Tessore, J. Courtney and T. Gilchrist. 1979. *Min. Nefr.*, 26:225.

41. Rietema, K. and P. Van Zutpen. 1975. *Proc. Eur. Soc. Artif. Organs*, 1:100.

42. Enka Glazstoff, 1976. *Cuphrophan Technical Information Bulletin, No. 12*. Wuppertal, Germany.

43. Kawanishi, H., M. Nishiki, M. Sugiyama, T. Cho, T. Tsuchiya and H. Ezaki. 1984. *Artif. Organs*, 8:167.

44. Cooney, D. O. and R. P. Kane. 1983. *Artif. Organs*, 7:197.

45. Xu, C. X., X. J. Tang, Z. Niu and Z. M. Li. 1981. *Int. J. Artif. Organs*, 4:200.

46. Zhaoguang, W., C. Zhuhui, L. Zhaoian, L. Lutan and W. Wengi. *Proc. 5th Int. Symp. Hemo. Artif. Organs. Tianjin, China, 1983*.

47. Özdural, A. R., H. Mann, T. Byrne and E. Pişkin. 1982. *Proc. Eur. Soc. Artif. Organs*, 9:55.

48. Kiremitçi, M. and E. Pişkin. 1985. *Int. J. Artif. Organs*, 8:4.

49. Sakhno, L. A., R. I. Lifshits, V. G. Nikolaev, I. A. Lozinskaya and S. I. Voryanko. 1989. *9th Int. Symp. Hemo. Ads. Immob. React., Tokyo, Japan, October 6–8* (Abstract).

50. Eretskaya, E. V., L. A. Sakhno and V. G. Nikolaev. 1989. *9th Int. Symp. Hemo. Ads. Immob. React., Tokyo, Japan, October 6–8* (Abstract).

51. Thompson, H. S. 1850. *J. Royal Agricul. Soc. England*, 11:68.

52. Way, J. T. 1850. *J. Royal Agricul. Soc. England*, 11:313.

53. Lemberg, E. 1870. *Z. Dent. Geol. Ges.*, 22:335.

54. Adams, B. A. and E. L. Holmes. 1936. *J. Soc. Chem. Ind.*. London, 54:1-6T.

55. Peterson, E. A. 1970. In *Cellulosic Ion Exchangers, Vol. 2, Part II*. T. S. Work and R. H. Burdon, eds. Amsterdam: Elsevier/North Holland.

56. Pharmacia Fine Chemicals AB Publications, Ion Exchange Chromatography: Principles and Methods, Uppsala.

57. Scopes, R. K. 1982. *Protein Purification: Principles and Practice*. New York: Springer-Verlag.

58. Gordon, A. and G. Roberts. 1980. In *Sorbents and Their Clinical Applications*. C. Giardano, ed. New York: Academic Press, p. 249.

59. Schechter, D. C., T. F. Nealon and J. H. Gibson. 1959. *Surgery, Gynecology and Obstetrics*, 108:1.

60. Steinberg, A. 1944. *Proc. Soc. Exp. Biol. Med.*, 56:126.

61. Dock, W. 1946. *Trans. Assoc. Am. Phys.*, 59:282.

62. Quick, A. J. 1947. *Am. J. Phys.*, 148:211.

63. Muirhead, E. E. and A. F. Reid. 1948. *J. Lab. Clin. Med.*, 33:841.

64. Cipoletti, J. L., R. Kunin and F. Meyer. 1980. In *Sorbents and Their Clinical Applications*. C. Giardano, ed. New York: Academic Press, p. 221.

65. Pişkin, E. and T. M. S. Chang. 1983. *The Past, Present and Future of Artificial Organs*. Ankara: Meteksan.

66. Williams, R. and I. M. Murray-Lyon. 1975. *Artificial Liver Support*. London: Pitman Medical.

67. Rosenbaum, J. L., M. S. Kramer and R. Raja. 1976. *Arch. Int. Med.*, 136:236.

68. Ton, H. Y. and R. D. Hughes, et al. 1979. *Artif. Organs*, 3:20.

69. Brunner, G. and F. W. Schmidt. 1981. *Artificial Liver Support*. Berlin: Springer-Verlag.

70. Mehltretter, C. L. 1966. *Staerke*, 18:208.

71. Esposito, R. and C. Giordano. 1980. In *Sorbents and Their Clinical Applications*. C. Giardano, ed. New York: Academic Press, p. 131.

72. Meriwether, L. S. and H. M. Kramer. 1976. *Kidney Int.*, 10:259.

73. Sloan, J. W. and B. T. Hofreiter, et al. 1956. *Ind. Eng. Chem.*, 48:1165.

74. Giordano, C., R. Esposito and G. Demma. 1968. *Bollet. Soc. Italiana di Biol. Speriment.*, 44:2232.

75. Man, N. K. and T. Drüeke, et al. 1973. *Proc. EDTA*, 10:143.

76. Zeig, S. and E. A. Friedman. 1980. In *Sorbents and Their Clinical Applications*. C. Giardano, ed. New York: Academic Press, p. 275.

77. Giordano, C. 1980. *Sorbents and Their Clinical Applications*. New York: Academic Press.

78. Rutherford, W. E. and E. Slatopolsky, et al. 1980. In *Sorbents and Their Clinical Applications*. C. Giardano, ed. New York: Academic Press, p. 117.

79. Cuatrecasas, P., M. Wilchek and C. B. Anfinsen. 1968. *Proc. Nat. Acad. Sci., USA*, 61:636.

80. Wilchek, M. and W. B. Jakoby. 1974. *Methods in Enzymology, Vol. 34*. New York: Academic Press.

81. Stark, G. R. 1971. *Biochemical Aspects of Reactions on Solid Supports*. New York: Academic Press.

82. Dunlar, R. B. 1973. *Immobilized Biochemicals and Affinity Chromatography*. New York: Plenum Press.

83. Hofmann-Ostenhoff, O. 1973. *Affinity Chromatography*. New York: Pergamon Press.

84. Lowe, C. R. and P. D. G. Dean. 1974. *Affinity Chromatography*. London: Wiley.

85. Sundaram, P. V. and F. Eckstein. 1978. *Theory and Practice in Affinity Techniques*. New York: Academic Press.

86. Scouten, W. H. 1981. *Affinity Chromatography: Bioselective Adsorption on Inert Matrices*. New York: John Wiley and Sons.

87. Gribnan, T. C. B., J. Visser and R. J. F. Nivard. 1982. *Affinity Chromatography, and Related Techniques*. Amsterdam: Elsevier.

88. Chaiken, I. M., M. Wilchek and J. Parikh. 1983. *Affinity Chromatography and Biological Recognition*. New York: Academic Press, Inc.

89. Dean, P. D. G., W. S. Johnson and F. A. Middle. 1985. *Affinity Chromatography*. Oxford: I.R.L. Press.

90. Köhler, G. and C. Milstein. 1975. *Nature*, 256:495.

91. O'carra, P., S. Barry and T. Griffin. 1973. *Biochem. Soc. Trans.*, 1:289.

92. Pişkin, E. and A. S. Hoffman. 1986. *Polymeric Biomaterials*. Dordrecht, the Netherlands: Martinus Nijhoff Publ. Co.

93. Terman, D. S., H. Harbeck, A. Hoffman, I. Steward, J. Robinette and R. Carr. 1975. *Fed. Proc.*, 34:976.

94. Terman, D. S., T. Travel, D. Petty, A. Tavel, R. Harbeck, G. Buffaloe and R. Carr. 1976. *J. Immunol.*, 116:1337.

95. Terman, D. S., G. Buffaloe and C. Mattioli, et al. 1979. *Lancet*, 11:824.

96. Plotz, P. H., P. Beck, B. F. Scharschmidt, J. K. Gordon and J. Vergalla. 1974. *J. Clin. Invest.*, 53:786.

97. Hughes, R. D., E. H. Dunlop, M. Davis, D. B. A. Silk and R. Williams. 1977. *Biomat. Med. Dev. Artif. Organs*, 5:205.

98. Bocharov, A., V. Spirov, H. Bochkova and A. Shnyra. 1989. *Artif. Organs*, 13:289 (Abstract).

99. Kasai, S., T. Yamamato, A. Kakisaka, N. Ohe and M. Mito. 1989. *Artif. Organs*, 13:319 (Abstract).

100. Ray, P. K. 1984. *Plasma. Ther. Transfus. Technol.*, 4:289.

101. Nilsson, I. M., S.-B. Sundquist, A. Ahlberg and S. E. Bergentz. 1981. *Blood*, 58:38.

102. Nilsson, I. M., S.-B. Sundquist, R. Ljung, L. Holmberg, C. Friburghaus and G. Björlin. 1983. *Scand. J. Haematol.*, 30:458.

103. Smith, T. W. and E. Heber. *N. Engl. J. Med.*, 289:1125.

104. Margel, S., L. Marcus, H. Savin, M. Offarim and A. Mashiah. 1984. *Biomat. Med. Dev. Artif. Organs*, 12:25.

105. Ross, R. 1986. *N. Engl. J. Med.*, 314:488.

106. Apstein, C. S. and D. B. Zilversmit, et al. 1978. *Atherosclerosis*, 31:105.

107. Thompson, G. R. 1981. *Lancet*, 1:1246.

108. Yokoyama, S., R. Hayashi, M. Satani and A. Yamamoto. 1985. *Arteriosclerosis*, 5:613.

109. Stoffel, W., H. Borberg and V. Greve. 1981. *Lancet*, 78:1005.

110. Eisenhauer, T., V. W. Armstrong, H. Wieland, C. Fuchs, F. Scheler and D. Seidel. 1987. *Klin. Wschr.*, 65:161.

111. Antwiller, G. D., P. C. Dau and D. D. Lobdell. 1988. *J. Clin. Aphresis*, 4:18.

112. Moojani, S., P. J. Lupien and J. Awad. 1977. *Clinical Chimica Acta*, 77:21.

113. Lupien, P. J., S. Moorjani, M. Lou, D. Brun and C. Gagne. 1980. *Pediat. Res.*, 14:113.

114. Schmer, G. and L. Rastelli, et al. 1981. *Trans. Am. Soc. Artif. Int. Organs*, 27:527.

115. Tabak, A., N. Lotan, S. Sideman, A. Tzipiniuk, B. Bleiberg and G. Brook. 1986. *Life Support Systems*, 4:355.

116. Yokoyama, S., R. Hayashi and T. Kikkawa, et al. 1984. *Atherosclerosis*, 4:276.

117. Maaskant, N., A. Bantjes, H. J. M. Kempen. 1986. *Atherosclerosis*, 62:159.

118. Homma, Y., Y. Mikami, H. Tamachi, N. Nakaya, H. Nakamura and Y. Goto. 1987. *Metabolism*, 36:419.

119. Odaka, M., H. Kobayashi and K. Soeda, et al. 1987. *Biomat. Artif. Cells Artif. Organs*, 15:113.

120. Ellens, D. 1986. *J. Clin. Nephrol.*, 26:81.

121. Saal, S. D., T. S. Parker and B. R. Gordon, et al. 1986. *Amer. J. Med.*, 80:583.

122. Koren, E., D. Solter, D. M. Lee, et al. 1986. *Biochem. Biophys. Acta*, 876:91.

123. Koren, E., C. Knight-Gibson, G. Wen, L. E. De Bault and P. Alaupovic. 1986. *Biochem. Biophys. Acta*, 876:101.

124. Ostlund, R. E. 1987. *Artif. Organs*, 11:366.

125. Naito, C., A. Yamamato and Y. Saito. *9th Int. Symp. Hemo. Ads. Immob. Reac. Tokyo, Japan, October 6–8, 1989.*

126. Koga, N., O. Ueda, T. Satoh, H. Okazaki and T. Baba. *9th Int. Symp. Hemo. Ads. Immob. Reac.. Tokyo, Japan, October 6–8, 1989* (Abstract).

127. Klinkmann, H., E. Behm and P. Ivanovich. *The Int. J. Artif. Organs*, 12:207.

128. Islael, L, R. Edelstein, P. Mannoni and E. Radot. 1976. *Lancet*, 2:642.

129. Yamazaki, Z., Y. Fujimori and T. Takahama, et al. *Trans. Am. Soc. Artif. Intern. Organs*, 28:318.

130. Shiozaki, S., K. Sakagami, M. Miyazaki, J. Matsuoka, S. Uchida, S. Saito, T. Fujiwara and K. Orita. 1989. *The Int. J. Artif. Organs*, 12:400.

131. Bensinger, W. I. 1981. *Artif. Organs*, 5:254.

132. Bensinger, W. I., D. A. Baker, C. D. Bucker, R. A. Clift and E. D. Thomas. 1981. *N. Engl. J. Med.*, 304:160.

133. Osterwalder, B., A. Gratwohl, C. Nissen and B. Speck. 1986. *Blut.*, 53:379.

134. Bannet, A. D., W. I. Bensinger, R. Raja, A. Baquero and R. F. McAllack. 1987. *Transplantation*, 43:909.

135. Danielson, B. G., B. Wikström, U. Backman, B. Fellström, G. Tufveson and O. Sjöberg. 1989. *Artif. Organs*, 13:292 (Abstract).

136. Watt, R. M., E. A. Milford and R. M. Hakim. 1989. *Artif. Organs*, 13:386 (Abstract).

137. Yamawaki, N., T. Furuta and J. Yamagata, et al. 1981. *Artif. Organs*, 5:148.

138. Yamazaki, Z., Y. Fujimori and T. Takahama, et al. 1982. *Trans. Am. Soc. Artif. Intern. Organs*, 28:318.

139. Yamazaki, Z., I. Lizuka and F. Kanai, et al. 1983. *J. Eur. Soc. Artif. Organs*, 1:98.

140. Sato, T., J. Nishimiya and K. Arai, et al. 1983. In *Therapeutic Plasmapheresis III*. T. Oda, ed. Stuttgart: Schattuer-Verlag.

141. Nakano, H., H. Gomi, T. Shibasaki, F. Ishimoto and O. Sakai. *9th Int. Symp. Hemo. Ads. Immob. Reac.*, Tokyo, Japan, October 6–8, 1989 (Abstract).

142. Tatsuguchi, T. and K. Sakai. *9th Int. Symp. Hemo. Ads. Immob. Reac.*, Tokyo, Japan, October 6–8, 1989 (Abstract).

143. Akizawa, T., E. Kinugasa, S. Koshikawa, H. Watanabe, N. Yamawaki and N. Nakabayashi. *9th Int. Symp. Hemo. Ads. Immob. Reac.*, Tokyo, Japan, October 6–8, 1989 (Abstract).

144. Sato, H., T. Kidaka and M. Hori. 1983. *Progr. Artif. Organs*. Cleveland: ISAO Press.

145. Behm, E., T. Kuroda and N. Yamawaki, et al. 1987. *Biomat. Artif. Cells Artif. Organs*, 15:101.

146. Traeger, J., M. Laville, R. El Habib, J. F. Moskovtchenko, P. R. Coulet and D. C. Gautheron. 1983. In *Plasmapheresis: New Trends in Therapeutic Applications*. Y. Nose, P. S. Malchesky and J. W. Smith, eds. Cleveland: ISAO Press.

147. Charlton, B., G. Antony, K. Schindhelm, N. Gürtunca and P. C. Farrell. 1983. *Progr. Artif. Organs*. Cleveland: ISAO Press.

40

Drug-Loaded Ophthalmic Prostheses

SEVERIAN DUMITRIU*

ABSTRACT: Nowadays, the method of controlled administration of drugs enjoys wide application in the field of ophthalmology, employing various systems such as inserts, capsules and minipumps. All these systems are based on the utilization of biodegradable and nonbiodegradable, natural and synthetic polymers. In this connection, the present chapter discusses first the general methods of controlled administration of drugs into the eye, as well as the main polymers employed (i.e., their shortcomings, perspectives, etc.). Special stress is laid upon hydrophobic and hydrophilic nondegradable polymers, hydrogels, and bioerodible systems.

The second part of the paper discusses ophthalmic prostheses used for drug release. Mention is being made first of hydrogels and soluble ocular inserts—for the treatment of ocular infection, inserts for the treatment of open-angle glaucoma, thermogels and polymeric dispersion, hydrophilic soft contact lenses, and soluble ocular inserts.

In the end, the chapter analyzes some buckling materials, capsule type drug delivery systems, and implantable drug delivery pumps.

The systems of controlled release of drugs into the eye, presented in the chapter, are being employed in the treatment of the most frequent ocular affections: glaucoma, conjunctivitis, keratite, and cancer.

INTRODUCTION

Ophthalmic drugs are traditionally administered as solution (collyria) suspensions or as anhydrous (petrolatum) ointments. However, it is well known that solutions do not result in administration of a precise and constant dosage, because the induced lacrimation and reflex blinking that follow installation quickly remove the drug from the precorneal area. Furthermore, eye drop installation typically results in a pulse entry mechanism with undesirable transient peaks of drug concentration in the aqueous humour and periods of nonmedication in the time intervals between pulses.

Ointments have not only the advantages of longer contact time and greater storage stability, but also have the disadvantage of producing a film over the eye, thereby blurring vision. In addition, ointments can interfere with the attachment of new corneal epithelial cells to their normal base [1].

These factors have stimulated the search for more sophisticated ophthalmic dosage forms capable of delivering a precise drug dosage and of maintaining an optimal concentration, in the precorneal area for an extended period of time, thus rendering unnecessary a frequent administration of eyedrops. The disadvantages of various types of ophthalmic preparations can be overcome by controlled delivery systems that can release a drug at a constant rate for a relatively long time.

GENERAL METHODS OF CONTROLLED ADMINISTRATION OF DRUGS INTO THE EYE

In recent years, several types of solid ophthalmic vehicles (inserts) have been developed [2]. These are intended for a direct application into the conjunctival sac, and can be basically categorized according to the following scheme:

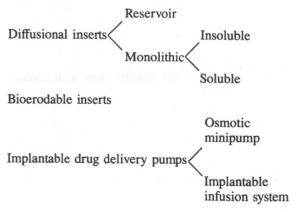

*Polytechnic Institute of Jassy, 6600 Jassy, Romania

Table 1. Some advantages of controlled release.

Reduce mammalian toxicity of highly toxic substances
Extend duration of activity at equal levels of active agent
Control the release of active agents
Mask the taste of bitter materials
Economical because less active material is needed
Convenience, including ease of handing
Avoid patient compliance problems in drug administration
Employ less total drug, thus minimize local side effects,
    systemic side effects, and the drug accumulation often
    encountered in chronic dosing
Improved drug efficiency in treatment of illness

Diffusional reservoir inserts consist of a core of the drug surrounded by an inert rate-controlling polymeric barrier. A typical example of this system is the Ocusert® [3], which delivers pilocarpine at a nearly zero-order rate for one week, and being insoluble, necessitates removal from the conjunctival sac after exhaustion.

Diffusional monolithic insoluble systems usually consist of hydrophilic soft contact lenses [e.g., poly-(hydroxyethyl methacrylate)] presoaked in drug solution [4].

Erodible inserts contain a drug dispersed through a polymeric matrix (polylactic, polyglycolic, alginic acid, xanthan, polypeptides, etc.). The drug is gradually leached from the matrix as it slowly erodes and disintegrates in the cul-de-sac [5].

Diffusional monolithic soluble inserts usually employ synthetic polymers such as: polyacrylamide, poly(ethyl acrylate), poly(vinyl alcohol), poly(vinyl pyrrolidone), and poly(acrylic acid-co-vinyl alcohol), containing various drugs such as antibiotics, sulfamide, pilocarpine, atropine, etc. [6].

The generic osmotic minipump (ALZET®) is a useful implantable drug delivery system with a constant pumping rate and a pumping duration of up to 2 weeks [2].

ADVANTAGES AND LIMITATIONS

One of the perplexing problems in biochemical pharmacology is the development of a methodology for assessing localized mechanisms of drug action and the subsequent sequence of biochemical reactions that occur in organized heterogeneous cellular and subcellular structures. One approach is to use drugs labelled with radioactivity or with groups capable of producing intense fluorescence or unpaired electrons for spin labelling, incubating the labelled drug with cellular material, and then sorting out the cellular components to find out which parts contain the bound drug. The problem is more complex when the drug can bind to several cellular components and, in so doing, elicit more than a single action. The use of immobilized drugs is an important method for studying localized mechanisms of drug action in heterogeneous cellular

systems. Conceptually, the method seems quite simple. The drug is attached to a solid support and then incubated with the desired cellular or subcellular material. The presence and type of interaction are noted by determining the extent of binding, the influence on cell growth rates, the modification to subcellular rates of metabolism or functionality, or some other reaction. The practical implementation of such studies is much more difficult to conduct than it appears at first glance. Scrupulous efforts must be made to free the preparation of the adsorbed or otherwise non-bound drug and to measure the rate at which the covalently bound drug is released. If the immobilized drug is still active, then it must be determined if the action is the same as that obtained with the nonimmobilized form [7].

The advantages of controlled release indicated above are indeed great. However, controlled release systems can impart other important advantages to active agents that are sufficient to elevate many products to commercial successes. Table 1 lists a number of these [8–10].

Though the advantages of controlled release are impressive, the merits of each application have to be examined individually, and the positive and negative effects weighed carefully before large expenditure is committed to developmental work. In other words, controlled release is not a panacea, and negative effects may, at times, more than offset advantages.

Some of the disadvantages of controlled release, or the areas that require a thorough appraisal, include [10]: the cost of controlled release preparation and processing, which may be substantially higher than the cost of standard formulations; the fate of the polymer matrix and its effect on the environment; the fate of polymer additives, such as plasticizers, stabilizers, antioxidants, fillers, etc.; the environmental impact of the polymer degradation products following heat, hydrolysis, oxidation, and biological degradation; the cost, time, and probability of success in securing government registration of the product, if this is required.

POLYMERIC INSERTS AND IMPLANTS FOR THE CONTROLLED RELEASE

In ophthalmology, in order to obtain controlled drug release systems, classical polymers are usually employed. The present chapter will mainly be concerned with polymers that are found in almost all drug containing ophthalmic prostheses.

Table 2 categorizes the various controlled release technologies, including physical, as well as chemical systems.

Release Mechanisms

The systems of controlled drug release, listed in Table 2, are utilized largely in ophthalmology. In this connection, special mention is to be made of: reservoir systems with rate-controlling membrane; monolithic systems; laminated structures; and osmotic pumps.

Knowledge of the mechanism of drug release from these systems is extremely important, as is conditioning the therapeutic efficiency of the system, the way in which the drug will be administered, and the time tolerance.

The release of a drug from any other different forms of drug polymer composites must be predictable, and often a constant release rate (zero-order) is desired. For many years, a considerable amount of mathematical analysis of the theoretical rates of diffusional [11–12] release from the various fixed geometrical configuration has been reported and correlated with experimental results. Three other basic rate-determining mechanisms can control the release profile of the drug [13], these being found in swelling, boundary-layer controls, and erodable devices.

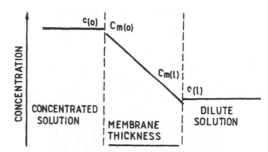

Figure 1. Diffusion of solute across a polymeric membrane showing concentration differences. From Reference [13]; reprinted by permission of the publishers, CRC Press, Inc., Boca Raton.

In the process of *membrane diffusion drugs*, there has to be applied Tick's law, expressed as [13]:

$$P = -D(dCm/dx) \qquad (1)$$

where P is flux (g cm^{-2} sec^{-1}), Cm is the concentration of the permeant in the membrane (g cm^{-3}), dCm/dx is the concentration gradient, and D is the diffusion coefficient (cm^2 sec^{-1}). The negative sign reflects that the direction of flow is down the gradient.

Figure 1 [13] shows the arrangement found for a membrane which separates two solutions of different concentrations. It is assumed that the concentration of the permeant in the surface layer is in equilibrium with either side. Therefore, if Z is the partition (or distribution) coefficient of the soluble between the two phases [13]:

$$Cm(o) = ZC_o \text{ upstream } x = o \qquad (2)$$

$$Cm(l) = ZC_l \text{ downstream } x = l \qquad (3)$$

In the steady state [13]

$$P = \frac{D[Cm(o) - Cm(l)]}{l} = \frac{D\Delta Cm}{l} \qquad (4)$$

where l is membrane thickness.

Usually, the concentration in the membrane is not known and ΔC is measured as the concentration difference between the two sides, so that [13]:

$$P = \frac{DZ\Delta C}{l} \qquad (5)$$

The terms D and Z are not always easily measured and, frequently, values of permeability (*Per*) are quoted where [13]:

$$Per = DZ \qquad (6)$$

Table 2. Categorization of polymeric systems for controlled release.

1. Physical systems
   - A. Reservoir systems with rate-controlling membrane
     1. Microencapsulation
     2. Macroencapsulation
     3. Membrane systems
   - B. Reservoir systems without rate-controlling membrane
     1. Hollow fibers
     2. Poroplastic® and Sustrelle® ultramicroporous cellulose triacetate
     3. Porous polymeric substrates and foams
   - C. Monolithic systems
     1. Physically dissolved in nonporous, polymeric, or elastomeric matrix
        - a. Nonerodible
        - b. Erodible
        - c. Environmental agent ingression
        - d. Degradable
     2. Physically dispersed in nonporous, polymeric or elastomeric matrix
        - a. Nonerodible
        - b. Erodible
        - c. Environmental agent ingression
        - d. Degradable
   - D. Laminated structures
     1. Reservoir layer chemically similar to outer control layers
     2. Reservoir layer chemically dissimilar to outer control layers
   - E. Other physical methods
     1. Osmotic pumps
     2. Adsorption onto ion-exchange resins
2. Chemical systems
   - A. Chemical erosion of polymer matrice
     1. Heterogeneous
     2. Homogeneous
   - B. Biological erosion of polymer matrix
     1. Heterogeneous
     2. Homogeneous

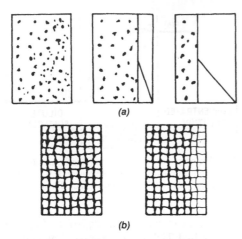

Figure 2. Models of drug release from polymeric devices: (a) drug dispersed in continuous polymer; (b) drug dispersed in capillary channels of a porous polymer matrix. From Reference [13]; reprinted by permission of CRC Press, Inc., Boca Raton.

Therefore, for a membrane device with constant activity, such as one with a saturated solution of the permeant over a large excess of insoluble material, the steady state release rate is expressed by [13]:

$$\frac{dM_t}{dt} = \frac{ADZ\Delta C}{l} \qquad (7)$$

where M_t is the mass released and A is the surface area of the device. When the concentration of drug in the surrounding body fluids is maintained at an extremely low level (i.e., sink conditions), the term ΔC in Equations (5) and (7) can be replaced by Cs, the saturated concentration of the drug in the reservoir [13].

As the classical expressions of desorption of the *monolithic system* are quite complicated [14], a simpler form has been proposed [13]. Thus, an even simpler equation for the simple geometric forms can be used if less rigourous treatment is acceptable; in this, the fraction release at time, t, is given by:

$$\frac{M_t}{M_\infty} = 2 \frac{S}{N} (D_t/\pi)^{4/2} \qquad (8)$$

where M_t is the amount of drug released after time t_o, M_∞ is the amount present initially, and S and V are the surface area and volume of the device.

The kinetics of releasing drugs *dispersed in a polymeric matrix* has been discussed for the first time by Higuchi [15] using a model which assumed that the solid drug dissolves from the surface layer and that this layer becomes exhausted of dispersed drug particles, as shown in Figure 2 [13].

Experimental results referring to the diffusion of dispersed steroid particles have evidenced a gradual exhaustion of the steroid, starting from its surface and continuing inside [16–18].

The derivation of Higuchi's equation [Equation (9)]—relying on Fick's first law—assumes [13]:

(1) A pseudosteady state exists.
(2) The drug particles are small, compared to the average distance of diffusion in the device.
(3) The diffusion coefficient is constant.
(4) Perfect sink conditions exist in the external medium.

$$Q = [C_sD_s(2A - C_s)t]^{1/2} \qquad (9)$$

and when

$$A \geqslant C_s < Q = (2C_sD_sAt)^{1/2} \qquad (10)$$

where Q is the amount of drug released at time, t, C_s is the solubility of the drug in the polymer, and A is the amount of the drug present initially.

In release from *devices with capillaries and pores*, diffusion through the polymer is negligible, the way taken by the drug being the capillaries where it is to be dissolved in the liquid penetrating through them [Figure 2(b)].

Higuch [19] developed an equation similar to Equation (9) for describing the release of a drug from one face of an inert granule:

$$Q = \left[C_nD_a \frac{\epsilon}{\tau} (2A - \epsilon C_a)t \right]^{1/2} \qquad (11)$$

where C_a and D_a are the solubility and diffusion coefficients of the drug in the permeating fluid. The terms Q, A and t have similar definitions as in Equation (9) and again a $Q - t^{1/2}$ relationship is predicted. ϵ is the porosity coefficient, while τ is the tortuosity factor.

Hydrogels are largely used to obtain systems for controlled release of ophthalmic drugs.

Davis [20] deduced the following empirical expression to calculate the apparent diffusion coefficient of any soluble drug in any hydrogel.

$$D_p = D_o \exp - (0.05 + 10^{-6}M)P \qquad (12)$$

where D_p is the diffusion coefficient of the solute in the swollen polymer gel containing $P\%$ (wtg) of polymer, M is the molecular weight of the solute, and D_o is the diffusion coefficient of the solute in water. The study involved both cross-linked poly(acrylamide) and poly(vinylpyrrolidone) hydrogels and solutes with a wide range of molecular weight (125,000 to 150,000), and included radio-labelled bovine serum albumin, insulin, a prostaglandin, and sodium iodide [13].

Various forms of the Higuchi equation, (9) and (11), have been used to describe the release of a drug from hydrogels [21] and, in a study by Chien and Lan [22], the diffusion coefficient in the gel D_m ($D_m = D_o$) was related to the degree of cross-linking.

The release kinetics from initially dry hydrogels, as would be expected, are complicated by the added consideration of the diffusion of solvent into the polymer [13]. Good [23] has derived equations where the diffusion coefficient is a time-dependent variable, and has fitted experimental data based on the release of a water-soluble drug from a contact lens. Poly(2-hydroxyethyl methacrylate) hydrogel had a low degree of swelling and the water uptake was approximately balanced by the loss of the drug, and the dimensions of the device were assumed not to change during release [13]. Recently [24–25], the much more complex situation of diffusion from a device which is simultaneously swelling and undergoing dimensional change, has been analyzed.

The *boundary-layer controlled release* has considerable implications *in vivo* [26], where the composition and the movement of the eluting medium may vary from site to site. The effect should be considered when *in vitro* release kinetics are compared with *in vivo* release [22,27–29] and the *in vitro* methodology designed for reasonable correlation. If the release characteristics of a device change with the rate of stirring in an *in vitro* test, it is a strong indication of some measure of boundary control [13].

Hoffenberg [30] considered *controlled release from erodible devices* (slabs, cylinders, spheres). Where a single zero-order process controls erosion, the theoretical equations can be rearranged in the form:

$$\frac{M_t}{M_x} = 1 - \left(1 - \frac{K_o t}{C_o a}\right)^n \qquad (13)$$

where K_o is the single zero-order rate constant for the erosion process, C_o is the uniform initial concentration of the drug, M_t is the amount of drug release time t, and M_x is the total amount of drug present initially. For the infinite slab, $n = 1$ and a is the half-thickness; for the cylinder $n = 2$ and a is the radius, for the sphere, $n = 3$ and a is the radius [13].

Basic Components of Controlled Release Devices

The components of controlled release include the *active agents* and the *polymer matrix or matrices* that regulate release of the active agent.

Polymer Matrix

The importance of polymer selection will be appreciated more if one considers the different design criteria that must be fulfilled [30a]:

- Molecular weight, glass transition temperature and chemical functionality of the polymer must allow the proper diffusion and release of the specific active agent.
- The functionality of the polymer should be such that it will not chemically react with the active agent.

- The polymer and its degradation products must be nontoxic to the environment and, in medical applications, nontoxic or antagonistic to the host.
- The polymer must not decompose in storage and generally not during the useful life of the device.
- The polymer must be easily manufactured into the desired product. It should allow incorporation of large amounts of active agent without excessively deteriorating its mechanical properties.
- Finally, cost of the polymer should not be so excessive that it causes the controlled release device to be noncompetitive.

A list of polymers that have been used in controlled release formulations is shown in Table 3 [31–32].

Active Agents

Table 4 presents pharmaceutical agents that have been used in experimental and commercialized controlled release devices.

Polymers Employed in Hydrophobic Nonbiodegradable Devices

SILICONES

Silicone rubber [33] has been used in a variety of biomedical applications due to its inertness and good biocompatibility. In 1964, Folkman and Long [34] reported the use of this polymer in sustained release formulations [35].

Silicone, having the general formula:

$$
\begin{array}{cccc}
CH_3 & CH_3 & CH_3 & CH_3 \\
| & | & | & | \\
X-Si-O-Si-O-Si-O-Si-X \\
| & | & | & | \\
CH_3 & CH_3 & CH_3 & CH_3
\end{array}
$$

is marketed as Silastic®.

Silicone polymers end-blocked with CH_3 are unreactive and generally used as fluids. Alternately, chains can have reactive hydroxyl end groups which may be cross-linked by curing at room temperature, and these are used to prepare molded or cast devices [13]. This type of polymer has been widely studied in implants and inserts for controlled release of steroids [36,38], chloroquine [39], pyrimethamine indomethacin [40], atropine, and histamine [41].

Soft silicone contact lenses are being experimented with. The complication here is that, though silicone polymers have very high permeability to oxygen, they are not all hydrophilic and, as a result, grave problems can arise. Attempts are being made to induce hydrophilicity to silicone lenses by surface-grafting techniques.

Table 3. Polymers used in controlled release devices.

Types of Polymers	Example
Natural polymers	Carboxymethyl cellulose Cellulose acetate phthalate Ethylcellulose Gelatin Gum arabic Starch Xanthan Burk Methylcellulose Zein Nitrocellulose Arabinogalactan Propylhydroxycellulose Shellac Succinylated gelatin Protein Natural rubber
Synthetic elastomers	Polybutadiene Polyisoprene Neoprene Polysiloxane Styrene–butadiene rubber Silicone rubber Cloroprene Butyl rubber Ethylene–propylene–diene terpolymer
Synthetic polymers	Poly(vinyl alcohol) Polyethylene Polypropylene Polystyrene Polyacrylamide Polyether Polyester Polyamide Ethylene vinyl acetate copolymer Poly(vinyl chloride) Polyacrylate Polyurethane Poly(vinyl pyrolidone) Poly(methyl methacrylate) Poly(vinyl acetate) Poly(hydroxyethyl methacrylate)

VINYLIC POLYMERS

The most widely used copolymer of ethylene is the one with vinyl acetate. ALZA corporation employs an ethylene–vinyl acetate copolymer (9% vinyl acetate) for the production of membranes possessing the capacity to control release. Thus, Progestaret® (ALZA Corporation) releases constantly 65 µg/day progesterone, on the duration of a year [42,43].

Another device developed by the ALZA Corporation, is the Ocusert Pilo®. The device, composed of two membranes of ethylene-vinyl acetate copolymer, is inserted into the cul-de-sac of the eye and provides a constant release of pilocarpine for the reduction of intraocular pressure in glaucoma. The two devices available, Pilo-20 and Pilo-40, release at a rate of 20 or 40 µg/h, for 1 week. They offer much better control than eye drops instilled several times daily, and remove problems with patient noncompliance [13].

The ratio of vinyl acetate present in the copolymer determines the release rate by the following relation: its increase reduces crystallinity and raises the release rate. When the copolymer contains over 40% vinyl acetate, it will be capable of releasing bioactive macromolecular compounds (enzymes, heparin, insulin, etc.) [44].

Polymers Employed in Hydrophilic Nonbiodegradable Devices

As early as 1955, Biettl [45] assessed the status of polymers in ophthalmology. Poly(methyl methacrylate) and many of its hydrophilic derivatives have been evaluated as intraocular lenses for refractive correction, as artificial corneas or as contact lenses [46–51].

The transparent poly(methyl methacrylate) is an ideal material for fabricating contact lenses. In the making of soft contact lenses, hydroxy ethyl methacrylate with small amounts of ethylene glycol dimethacrylate is polymerized and the dry polymer is shaped into lenses of required dimensions, full consideration being given to the swelling characteristics of the polymer. The lenses are then soaked in water, in which they swell and form gels. These soft contact

Table 4. Pharmaceutical active agents utilizing controlled release.

Analgesis Anthelmintics Antidotes Antiemetics Antihistamines Antimalarials Antimicrobials Antipyretics Antituberculotics Antiseptics	Antitussives Cathartics Diagnostic aids Diuretics Effervescents Enzymes Expectorants Hypnotics Microorganisms Minerals	Nutritional products Potassium supplements Sedatives Sulfonamides Stimulants Sympathomimetics Tranquilizers Urinary antiinfectines Vitamins Xanthine derivatives

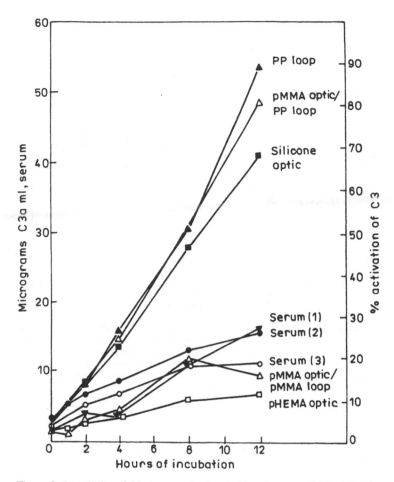

Figure 3. Quantitation of C3a in serum incubated either alone or with IOLs. Levels of C3a were quantitated by r.i.a. of serum incubated with IOLs and/or loops. Each point is the average of samples; the standard error of each point is $< 10\%$ of the mean. The concentration of C3a at 4, 8 and 12 h time points was significantly higher in serum incubated with polypropylene loops ($\blacktriangle$), PMMA optic with polypropylene loops ($\triangle$), and silicone optic ($\blacksquare$) ($p < 0.05$) than in serum incubated alone. From Reference [52]; reprinted by permission of the publishers, Butterworth & Co. (Publishers) Ltd., © 1987.

lenses are very comfortable to wear but are very weak mechanically, owing to high water content (as high as 70–80%). There is also the problem of insufficient oxygen supply to the cornea because poly(methyl methacrylate) is not permeable to oxygen. This drawback could be overcome to some extent by increasing the water content, but at the expense of the mechanical strength. Extended wear contact lenses are known to cause corneal infections [51].

In a recent study, R. J. Gobel et al. [52] studied the determination of the potential to active complement, that can be used as one criterion in testing the biocompatibility of various synthetic polymers that are utilized in the medical field. Intraocular lenses (IOLs) made of poly(methyl methacrylate) (PMMA) with PMMA loops, poly(hydroxyethyl methacrylate) (PHEMA) lenses, silicone lenses, and PMMA lenses with polypropylene loops were examined. The concentrations of the activation peptides C3a, C4a and

C5a were measured by radioimmunoassay (r.i.a.) in human serum after incubation with and without IOLs for up to 12 h (Figures 3, 4, 5) [52]. The presence of silicone lenses caused an increase in C3a level. In the presence of polypropylene loops, the concentration of both C3a and C5a were significantly higher than in serum incubated alone. There was no statistically significant increase in the concentration of C4a caused by any of the materials tested. The results suggest that IOLs made from silicone, or lenses with polypropylene loops activate the complement system via the alternative pathway.

An immune response caused by the presence of an IOL in the eye is most likely to occur when the blood-aqueous barrier is broken down and the lens comes into contact with the blood elements. Therefore, to assess the potential for different IOL biomaterials to cause an inflammatory response by activating complement, the IOLs were incubated in human serum [52].

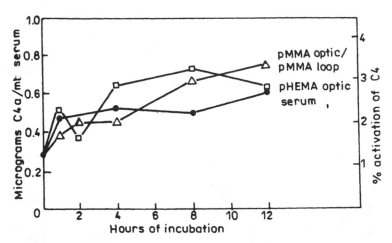

Figure 4. Quantitation of C4a in serum incubated alone or with IOLs. Levels of C4a were determined by r.i.a. Each time point is the average of 2 samples with a standard error no greater than 10% of the mean. There was no significant difference in C4a concentration of serum incubated with IOLs, compared to serum incubated alone at any time point. From Reference [52]; reprinted by permission of the publishers, Butterworth & Co. (Publishers) Ltd., © 1987.

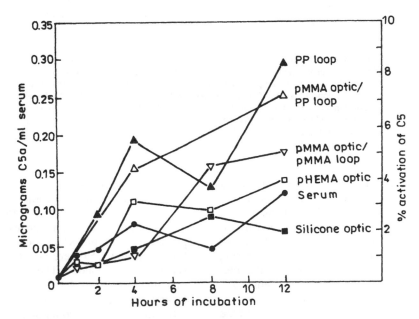

Figure 5. Quantitation of C5a in serum incubated alone or with IOLs. The levels of C5a were determined by r.i.a. Each time point is the average of 2 samples with a standard error no greater than 10%. There was a significantly higher concentration of C5a after the incubation of normal human serum with polypropylene loops only at 4 and 12 h time points ($p \leq 0.05$). From Reference [52]; reprinted by permission of the publishers, Butterworth & Co. (Publishers) Ltd., © 1987.

Table 5. Clinically observed manifestations of hydrogel lens spoilation.

Complex Deposits	Lens Coatings	Microbial Deposits	Extrinsic Factors
Discrete elevated deposits—"white spots"	Proteinaceous films	Fungal and bacterial deposits	Mascara
Particles	Specific calcium deposits		Deposition of iron
	Granular deposits		

From Bowers, R. W. J. and B. J. Tighe, *Biomaterials*, 8:83 (1987), by permission of the publishers, Butterworth & Co. (Publishers) Ltd. ©1987.

Studies of IOL biomaterials included nylon 6,6 which until recently was used for IOL loops. This material was found to be a relatively efficient inducer of complement activation [53,54]. On the other hand, it was demonstrated that PMMA, the most commonly used synthetic polymer in the manufacture of different IOL styles, is a relatively inert material with respect to complement activation [53,54].

As to lenses, of special importance is the study of their ocular compatibility. The most obvious clinical manifestation of hydrogel contact lenses is spoilation. The term "spoilation" is used to encompass physical and clinical changes in the nature of the hydrophilic soft contact lenses and various extraneous deposits which may impair the optical properties of the lens or produce symptoms of discomfort and often intolerance to the wearer [55]. The extent of the situation may be appreciated by considering the reported incidence of lens spoilation which ranges, according to various reports, from 7–82% of the extended wear lenses being worn [55–59].

The clinical manifestations observed are presented in Table 5 [60].

Discrete elevated deposits—white spots. Probably the most chemically complex manifestation of ocular incompatibility are discrete elevated deposits, the so-called "white spots" found on the anterior lens surface [60]. They are also referred to in the contact lens literature as mucoprotein–lipid and mucopolysaccharide deposits [60].

Ruben and other workers suggest the deposition of mucoprotein–lipid deposits on lenses as a major cause of spoilation, with a regarded incidence of up to 82% of the patients studied [61–66]. In a study of Tripathi et al. [58], 80% of the lenses examined by light and electron microscopy displayed such deposits with or without calcareous material. It would appear that the main contributing factors include inherent or acquired defects in the lens material, altered ocular secretions and altered tear chemistry [60].

Lens coatings. A major class of spoilations include the surface films, coatings and plaquets [60]. One group of these, related to discrete elevated deposits, although somewhat more geographically dispersed, are the so-called protein films. Such films are characterized by a thin, semi-opaque, white superficial layered appearance [60]. These layers appear to consist of denatured protein [67]. The general accumulation of protein films on soft contact lenses lead to an increase in surface haziness and rugosity. A decrease in visual acuity results, due both to lens opacity and to poor lens movement in the eye. Red eye, increased irritation and conjunctivitis are typical patient responses to protein-covered lenses. These deposits have been variously attributed to mucoproteins, albumin, globulin, glycoproteins and mucin [68–70]. Karageozian [67] has reported that protein films consist mainly of denatured lysozyme.

Inorganic films. Inorganic films are similar in gross appearance to protein films, but they are composed of insoluble noncrystalline materials [71]. Heavy inorganic films often cause damage to the lens surface, since the material may penetrate into the lens matrix [72–74]. These films are generally covered with protein which smooths the underlying rough inorganic material, composed mainly of calcium phosphate, with co-precipitated protein [72]. The deposit may well be hydroxyapatite, the thermodynamically stable phase of calcium phosphate in biological systems [60].

Granular deposits. Another major class of inorganic lens deposits in the so-called granular deposit, which is a special form of crystalline deposit. These elevated white or translucent formations vary in size [60,75].

Specific inorganic calcium deposits. Calcium carbonate deposits consist of crystalline growths that display a definite needle-like form [60]. When large areas of the lens surface are covered with clusters of crystals, the lens has a film-like appearance. The crystals, consisting mainly of calcium carbonate, grow into the lens surface, producing small pits which may be covered by a protein film. With continued wear, the deposits metamorphose into the more insoluble calcium phosphate and take on the appearance of multiple lens canaliculi [60].

Microbial spoilation. One of the most serious hazards of soft lens wear is spoilage due to the invasion and contamination by microbial organisms [76]. Many species of fungi and yeast have been identified on soft lenses [77–81]. Among these are the yeast of the *Rodotonita* sp., *Candida tropicales*, *C. fusarium* and *C. albicans* together with fungi such as *Aspergillus fumigatus*, *A. niger* and *Penicillium* sp.

Several workers have reported the presence of bacteria on both the anterior and posterior lens surface [82–83].

Lens discolouration. Discolouration of soft contact

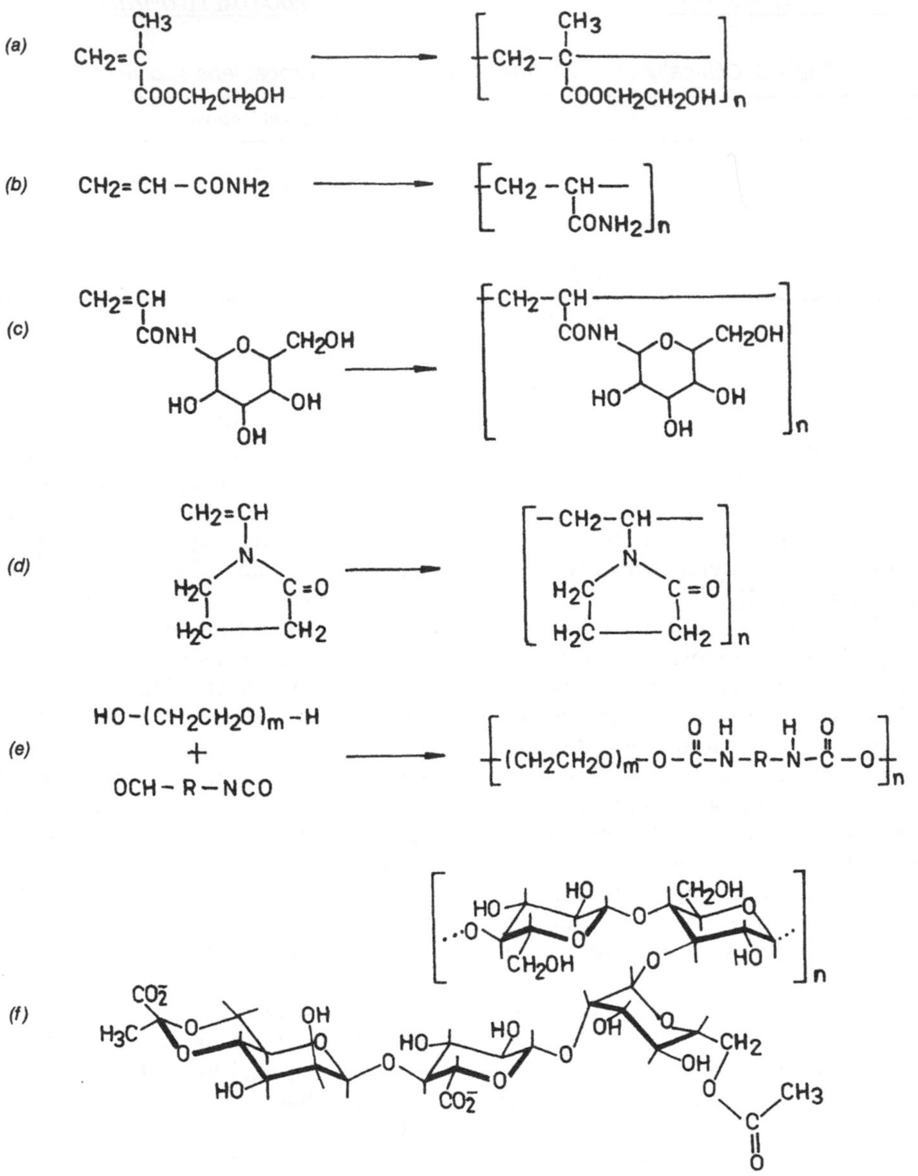

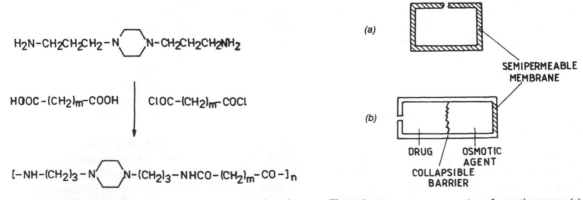

Figure 6. Structures of some commonly used hydrogels: (a) poly(2-hydroxyethyl methacrylate) (HEMA); (b) polyacrylamide; (c) N-substituted derivative of polyacrylamide; (d) poly(vinyl N-pyrrolid-2-one); (e) polyurethane prepared from poly(ethylene glycol) and a diisocyanate; (f) reticulated xanthan.

$H_2N-CH_2CH_2CH_2-N\overbrace{\qquad}N-CH_2CH_2CH_2NH_2$

$HOOC-(CH_2)_m-COOH \quad \Big| \quad ClOC-(CH_2)_m-COCl$

$[-NH-(CH_2)_3-N\overbrace{\qquad}N-(CH_2)_3-NHCO-(CH_2)_m-CO-]_n$

Figure 7. Structure of a polyamide polymer which responds to the pH of its environment (i.e., swells at about pH 4 while remaining unswollen at pH 7). From Reference [13]; reprinted by permission of the publishers, CRC Press, Inc., Boca Raton.

Figure 8. Schematic representation of osmotic pumps: (a) elementary type; (b) pump with collapsible membrane separating drug compartment from osmotic agent. From Reference [13]; reprinted by permission of the publishers, CRC Press, Inc., Boca Raton.

lenses appears to be a major drawback in their use, although the frequency of its occurrence is not well documented [60]. Discolouration or loss of lens transparency has been linked with several factors. Among possible cases are nicotine, topical adrenaline and vasoconstrictors, as well as components from the tear fluid [60,84].

In recent years, hydrophilic contact lenses have been utilized as matrices for the insertion of several ophthalmic drugs (pilocarpine, antibiotics, etc.) [2].

Hydrogel Systems

Hydrogels comprise a large group of polymers which swell to a considerable degree with water. They have attracted considerable interest in prosthetic applications such as contact lenses or promising nonthrombogenic surfaces and as matrices for the controlled release of drugs.

Generally, hydrogels employed in processes of controlled release are to be obtained from reticulated soluble polymers [13].

Thus, the polymer to be first used for microencapsulation was reticulated collagen, found as not very suitable for the preparation of monolithic hydrogel devices with consistent performance properties, especially if low degrees of swelling are desired. To gain this consistency, along with ease of preparation, research has favored the synthetic polymers of hydroxyethyl methacrylate [23,85], acrylamide [20] and its N-sugar substituted derivatives [86], N-vinyl-pyrrolidone [20,21] and poly(ethylene oxides) [87,88] as shown in Figure 6 [13].

Poly(glutamic acid) [89] and cross-linked dextrans, and starches [90] have been used. A large development was witnessed in reticulated xanthan [91–92].

The most desirable hydrogels should be very strong and tough, but not brittle in the dry state, should swell to a reproducible degree in water, buffer, or plasma, and should be strong in the swollen state. Thus, a hydrogel to be utilized for such purposes should not contain an initiator, monomers, stabilizers or drugs modified in processes of polymerization or reticulation. In relation to this, mention must be made of the fact that poly(acrylamide) has been employed no longer in such processes, because of the risk induced by its traces of carcinogenic monomer.

The largest amount of work has been done on hydroxyethyl methacrylate which is, unfortunately, brittle as a homopolymer and has a relatively low degree of swelling (42%). In many studies it is polymerized with a cross-linking agent in aqueous solution containing a drug, and the residual initiation fragments and monomer are not removed.

Ciba-Geigy [93] has obtained cross-linked hydrogels of poly(ethylene oxide) capped with double bonds and subsequently copolymerized with hydrophobic monomers to obtain polyphase systems which are claimed to have improved physical strength.

Another promising development along these lines was that of Graham et al. [94], involving cross-linked polymers of poly(ethylene oxide) using diisocyanates and polyols to provide cross-linking. If poly(ethylene glycols) of molecular weights above 2000 were used, dry gels containing up to 50% crystallinity could be obtained.

Cores of a drug coated with rate-controlling membranes have been used in even more sophisticated ways. Thus, by the incorporation of covalently bound carboxyl groups, it is possible to obtain hydrogels which swell under basic conditions [85] while swelling under acidic conditions can be obtained by the covalent incorporation of basic groups such as amine. Such groups have been incorporated into both vinyl and urethane polymers [13]. An elegant example of such a use has been reported by Fildes of ICI [95] who encapsulated a core tablet of quinoxaline di-N-oxide with nylon copolymer containing basic groups in its backbone made by interfacial or condensation polymerization (Figure 7 [13]).

An even greater degree of sophistication has been developed by the Alza Corporation in their OROS® devices [13]. In these, a solid tablet is coated with a hydrogel into which coating a very fine hole is introduced by a laser beam. In its simplest form, an elementary osmotic pump [96], such as the OROS® device consists of a membrane with an orifice in it [Figure 8(a)]. In this type of device, the membrane allows the passage of water, following an osmotic gradient, into the core which contains the drug and which acts as an osmotic driving force for water transport. The ingress of water is balanced by a saturated solution of drug being pumped out through the orifice [13]. More sophisticated variations are available [97–98] [e.g., Figure 5(b)] in which the drug compartment is separated, by a movable barrier, from another compartment which contains an osmotic agent.

Bioerodible Systems

Three basic classes of polymers are generally recognized in biodegradable systems (Figure 9) [99]:

(1) Water-soluble polymers which are insolubilized by hydrolytically unstable cross-links (Figure 9, Type I)
(2) Linear polymers which are initially water insoluble which become solubilized by hydrolysis ionization, or protonation of pendent groups, but which do not undergo backbone cleavage (Figure 9, Type II)
(3) Polymers which are water soluble and degrade to small-soluble products by backbone cleavage

Hydrogels with hydrolytically unstable cross-links have been prepared by copolymerizing acrylamide or

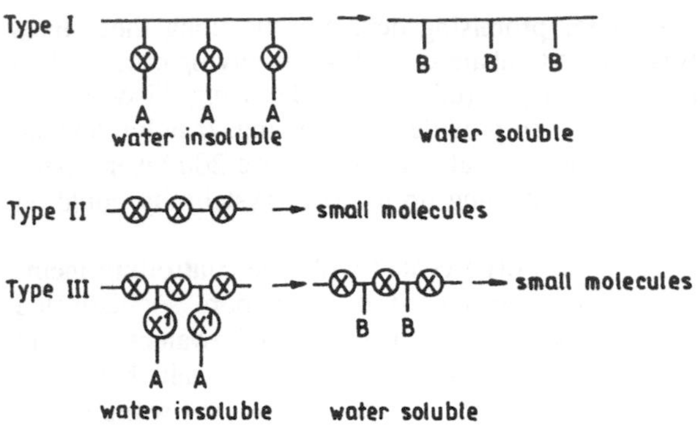

Type I

water insoluble   water soluble

Type II $-\otimes-\otimes-\otimes- \longrightarrow$ small molecules

Type III

water insoluble   water soluble

Figure 9. Schematic representation of three basic types of bioerodible polymers.

N-vinyl pyrrolidone with N,N'-methylenebis-acrylamide [100–101]:

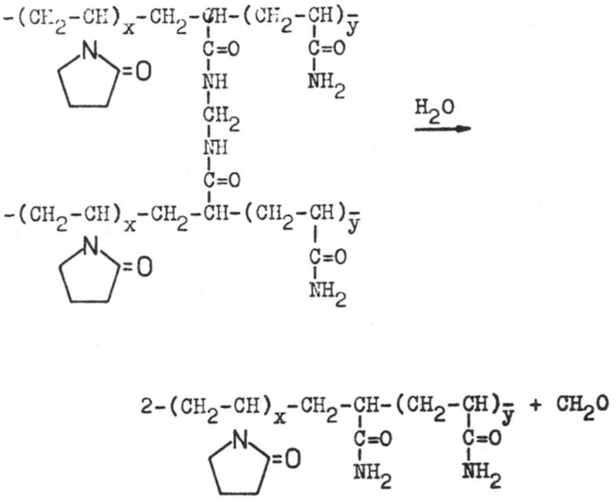

Generally, biodegradation takes place by a hydrolysis reaction when the device is placed in the aqueous environment of the body. In some cases, enzymes have been found to accelerate the degradation reaction considerably [102–103].

Hydrophobic polymers that are solubilized (Figure 9, Type II) by an ionization reaction of a pendent carboxyl group are well known, and the dissolution and drug release of partially esterified copolymers derived from ethylene–maleic anhydride or methyl vinyl ether–maleic anhydride constitute the subject of many publications [104–111].

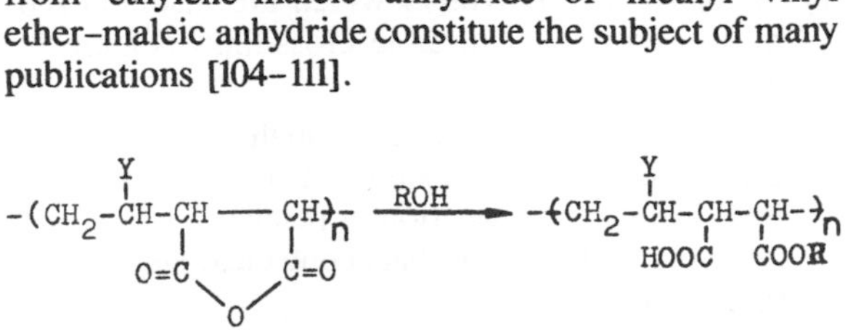

where $Y = OCH_3$ for the methyl vinyl ether copolymer and $Y = H$ for the ethylene copolymer.

These copolymers in the unionized state are hydrophobic and water insoluble, but in the ionized state

they are water soluble [99]. The solubilization process can be generically represented as follows:

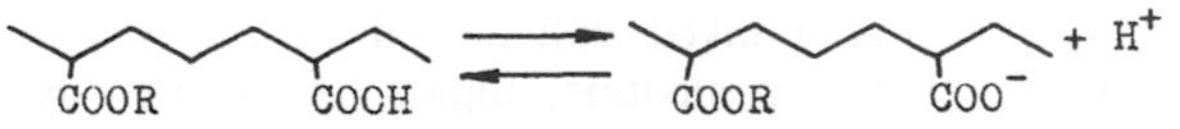

One of the interesting features of the polymer systems discussed herein is that they exhibit a characteristic pH range above which they are soluble and below which they are insoluble [99]. This pH-range is quite sharp, about 0.25 pH units and changes with the number of carbon atoms in the esteric side group.

Figure 10 shows the polymer dissolution rate of hydrocortisone alcohol release for n-butyl half-ester polymer films containing the dispersed drug [99]. The excellent linearity of both polymer erosion and drug release over the total lifetime of the device provides strong evidence for a surface erosion mechanism and negligible diffusional release of the drug.

Figure 11 shows the effect of the size of the alkyl group on the rate of release of hydrocortisone alcohol for a series of partial esters measured at pH 7.4 [99]. All drug release rates again show excellent linearity and also a strong dependence on the size of the alkyl group.

The effect of pH on the rate of release of hydrocortisone alcohol dispersed in the n-butyl partial ester is shown in Figure 12 [99].

The model of polymer erosion is depicted in Figure 13 [99].

Heller et al. [99] proposes a subsequent calculation system for establishment of the flux of solubilized polymer (J_p).

The flux of solubilized polymer, J_p, expressed as the equivalents of carboxylate groups/cm² sec is related to the flux of the other ions within the boundary layer by the requirement for charge neutrality [99]:

$$J_{p^-} + J_{B^-} = J_{H^+} \tag{14}$$

Furthermore, since at steady state there is no accumulation of buffer anywhere within the system, we have

$$J_B = -J_{BH} \tag{15}$$

where J_{BH} is the flux of nonionized buffer, in equivalents/cm² sec [99]. Thus,

$$J_{P^-} = J_{H^+} + J_{BH} \tag{16}$$

and, from Fick's law, we have

$$J_{p^-} = -D_{H^+}\frac{d[H^+]}{dx} - D_{BH}\frac{d[BH]}{dx} \tag{17}$$

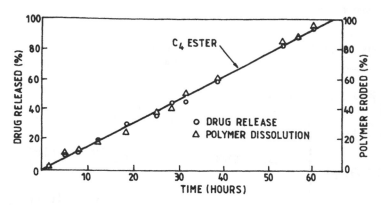

Figure 10. Rate of polymer dissolution and rate of release of hydrocortisone alcohol for the n-butyl half-ester or methyl vinyl ether–maleic anhydride copolymer containing 10 wt% drug dispersion. From Reference [99]; reprinted by permission of the publishers, John Wiley & Sons, Inc., 1978.

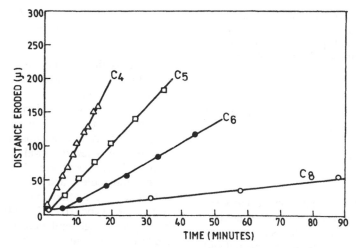

Figure 11. Effect of the size of ester group in half-esters of methyl vinyl ether–maleic anhydride copolymers on the rate of erosion at pH 7.4. From Reference [99]; reprinted by permission of the publishers, John Wiley & Sons, Inc., 1978.

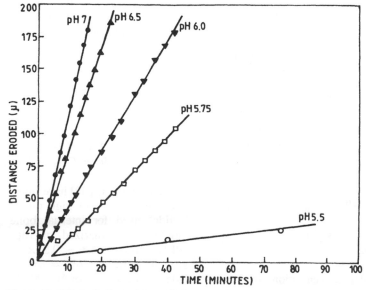

Figure 12. Effect of pH erosion medium rate on rate of erosion of half-esters of methyl vinyl ether–maleic anhydride copolymers. From Reference [99]; reprinted by permission of the publishers, John Wiley & Sons, Inc., 1978.

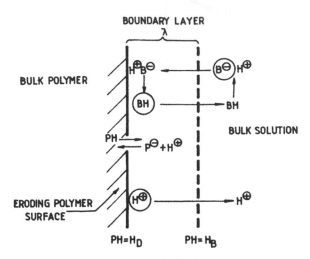

Figure 13. Model for erosion mechanism. P^- = concentration of dissociated carboxylate groups in equivalents; P_H = concentration of undissociated carboxylic acid groups in equivalents/cm³; BH = buffer agent. From Reference [99]; reprinted by permission of the publishers, John Wiley & Sons, Inc., 1978.

We are interested, of course, in the total flux of solubilized polymers. We can express this as J_{P_T}

$$J_{P_T} = J_{P^-} \frac{[P_T]}{[P^-]} \qquad (18)$$

where $[P_T]$ is the total concentration of carboxyl groups, ionized plus nonionized, expressed as equivalents/cm³. As solubilized polymer chains diffuse away from the polymer surface, they carry both ionized and nonionized carboxyl groups, and the ratio of these two concentrations is simply given by the degree of dissociation $[P^-]/[P_T]$ [99]. Hence we can restate Equation (17) as follows:

$$J_{P_T} = \frac{[P_T]}{[P^-]} \left(-D_{H^+} \frac{d[H^+]}{dx} - D_{BH} \frac{d[BH]}{dx} \right) \qquad (19)$$

This equation reflects the dual modes of diffusive hydrogen ion transport, as hydrogen ion alone and coupled to the buffer flux. We can now substitute for the unknown quantities in Equation (19) in terms of known or measurable quantities by means of Equations $K_p = [P^-] [H^+]/[PH]$ and $K_B = [B^-] [H^+]/[BH]$ where $[P^-]$ — concentration of dissociated carboxylate groups in equivalents/cm³ [99]. Thus,

$$J_{P_T} = -\frac{[H^+] + K_p}{K_p} D_{H^+} \frac{d[H^+]}{dx}$$

$$+ [B_T]D_{BH} \frac{d\{[H^+]/(K_B + [H^+])\}}{dx} \qquad (20)$$

where B_T is the total buffer concentration, $[B_T] = [B^-] + [BH]$.

Equation (20) can now be integrated [99] over the boundary layer thickness, using the boundary conditions $[H^+] + [H_d]$ at $X = 0$, and $[H^+] = [H_b]$ at $X = \lambda$. The result [99], after rearrangement, is:

$$J_{P_T} = \frac{D_{H^+}}{K_p} \left(\frac{[H^+]^2}{2} + K_p[H^+] \right)$$

$$\times \left| \begin{array}{c} H_d \\ H_b \end{array} + \frac{[B_T]D_{BH}}{K_p\lambda} \left(\frac{[H^+](K_p - K_B)}{K_B + [H^+]} \right. \right.$$

$$+ K_B \ln \frac{(K_B + [H^+])}{K_B} \left. \right) \left| \begin{array}{c} H_d \\ H_b \end{array} \qquad (21)$$

Finally, the polymer erosion rate γ [99], in cm/sec, is obtained from Equation (10) by the relationship:

$$\gamma = \frac{J_{P_T}E}{\varrho} \qquad (22)$$

where E is the gram-equivalent weight of the polymers (grams per carboxylate-containing unit) and ϱ is the polymer density.

Polymers which undergo surface erosion are, almost by definition, hydrophobic, while containing readily hydrolyzable groups [13]. The Alza Company has developed several novel polymers of this type that also undergo backbone cleavage to low molecular weight molecules, and which would therefore be of potential application in biodegradable implants (Figure 9, Type III) [112–114]. The polymers have been given the general name CHRONOMER® and include hydrophobic poly(orthoesters) and poly(orthocarbonates).

Heller [115] reviewed bioerodible drug delivery systems from a general point of view and included these as a possible group of polymers which could be used as implants.

Studies with polymers which undergo backbone cleavage have been restricted mainly to copolymers of lactic and glycolic acid [116–117].

$$nHO-CH-COOH \text{ or } R-CH \underset{\displaystyle \underset{O}{\overset{\Vert}{C}}}{\overset{\displaystyle \overset{O}{\overset{\Vert}{C}}}{\bigg<}} \begin{array}{c} O \\ | \\ O \end{array} \begin{array}{c} CH-R \\ | \\ O \end{array} \longrightarrow \{O-CH-CO\}_n + nH_2O$$

R = H — glycolic acid
R = CH₃ — lactic acid

Leenslag et al. [118] have investigated *in vivo* and *in vitro* degradation of high molecular weight poly(L-lactide) used for internal bone fixation. Within 3 months as-polymerized, microporous poly(L-lactide) (PLLA) ($\bar{M}_v = 6.8 - 9.5 \times 10^5$) exhibited a massive strength-loss ($\sigma_b = 68 - 75$ MPa to $\sigma_b = 4$ MPa) and decrease of $\bar{M}_v$ (90–95%). By week 39, the first signs of resorption were evident (mass-loss 5 wt%). Except for dynamically loaded bone plates, no differences between *in vivo* and *in vitro* degradation of PLLA were observed. The increase of crystallinity of PLLA upon degradation (up to 83%) is likely to be attributed to recrystallization of tie-chain segments.

The four main areas of application have used steroidal contraceptive [119–120], narcotic antagonists [121–123], antimalarials [124–125] and anticancer drugs [126–127]. The forms in which these drug–polymer composites have been studied *in vivo* and *in vitro* include implantable cylinders [119], spheres [124], films [128], injectable microcapsules [120], and powdered formulations [128].

Graham et al. [13] have developed a series of biodegradable polymers which possess both ester and glycosidic linkages and can be prepared using the well-known reaction of 3,4-dihydro-2H-pyran with alcohols to give a tetrahydropyranyl ether [Figure 14(a)]. Monomers which contain two such dihydropyran groups, linked by an ester group, can form linear polymers with diols or can be used to prepare cross-linked matrices when multifunctional alcohols are used as comonomers [Figure 14(b)]. Drugs can be incorporated into the reaction mixture prior to molding and curing, and the resulting thermosetting polymers provide release over prolonged periods of time [13].

For biomedical applications, copolymerizations involving derivatives of tartronic acid, $HO-C(R_1)(R_2)-COOH$ ($R_1 = H$; $R_2 = COOH$), glycolic acid ($R_1 = R_2 = H$) and α-hydroxyisobutyric acid ($R_1 = R_2 = CH_3$) would be of considerable potential value since they would combine control of hydrolysis rates with the inclusion of a drug-carrying function [129].

To obtain homopolymers and copolymers, the anhydrocarboxylate derivatives of tartronic acid provide a synthetic route to the previously unreported poly(tartronic acid) (a) and to copolymers containing both tartronic acid and other α-hydroxyacid residues (b) [129].

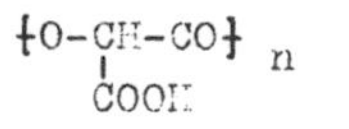

$$\{O-CH-CO\}_n$$
$$\quad\quad |$$
$$\quad\quad COOH$$

(a)

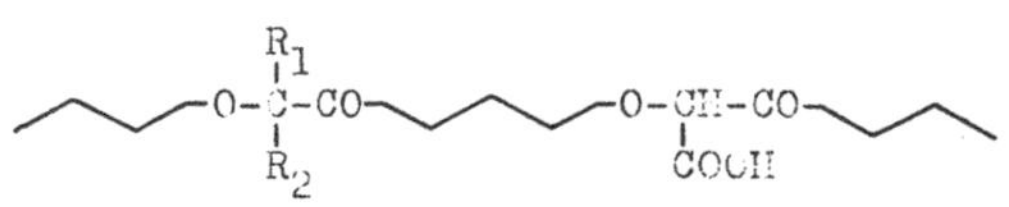

(b)

The analogies between poly(tartronic acid) and poly(acrylic acid) are obvious, and are reflected in the solubility and pH dependence of solution properties of the polymer. The attractions of the copolymers centre around the ability to attach functional groups to the backbone of poly(glycolic acid) and related bioerodible polymers. This, together with the variety of possible comonomer residues that may be incorporated by this route, enables an interesting range of

polymers, in which rate of backbone hydrolysis can be varied, and a variety of active species can be carried by the pendent functional group [129]. Our own interests [130–131] include the use of bioerodible polymers for the release of macromolecules and the use of tartronic acid derivatives in macromer synthesis.

Another class of biomedical polymers with potential use in biodegradable drug delivery systems is the poly(alkyl-2-cyanoacrylates). The alkyl-2-cyanoacrylate monomers have been used as biodegradable tissue adhesives in a variety of applications [132]. The butyl monomer is regarded as the most suitable due to a combination of its spreadability on biological fluids, its rate of polymerization [133] and its low toxicity [134].

The ability of the monomers to polymerize in the presence of water has been used for the preparation of microcapsules containing various drugs and enzymes [135–136].

New types of polyanhydrides with advantageous properties, with respect to biomedical use, were synthesized [137]. The first are aliphatic-aromatic homopolyanhydrides of the structure:

$$-(OOC-C_6H_4-O-(CH_2)_x-CO-)_n \quad x = 1 \div 10$$

These polymers display a zero-order hydrolytic degradation profile for two to ten weeks, the time period of degradation is a function of the length of the aliphatic chain.

The second type of polymer, unsaturated polyanhydride of the structure:

$$[(OOC-CH=CH-CO)_x-(OOC-R-CO)_y]_n$$

has the advantage of secondary polymerization of double bonds to create a cross-linked matrix. These polymers were prepared from the corresponding diacids polymerized by melt condensation or in solution.

Molecular weights of up to 44,000 and 30,000 were achieved for polyanhydrides of *p*-carboxyphenoxy-alkanoic acid and fumaric acid, respectively.

The hydrolytic degradation of aromatic–aliphatic homopolyanhydrides is described in Figure 15.

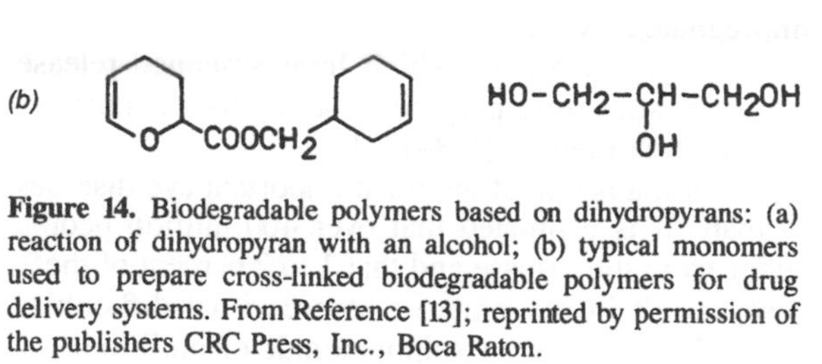

(a)

(b)

Figure 14. Biodegradable polymers based on dihydropyrans: (a) reaction of dihydropyran with an alcohol; (b) typical monomers used to prepare cross-linked biodegradable polymers for drug delivery systems. From Reference [13]; reprinted by permission of the publishers CRC Press, Inc., Boca Raton.

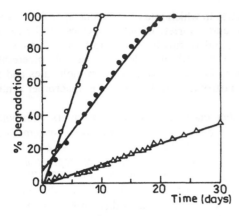

Figure 15. Degradation of poly(p-carboxyphenoxy) alkanoic anhydrides. Degradation in phosphate buffer pH 7.40 at 37°C. From Reference [137]; reprinted by permission of the publishers, Hüthig & Wepf Verlag, Basel.

This new type of polymer may be employed in the preparation of bioerodible ophthalmic inserts containing drugs.

OPHTHALMIC PROSTHESES USED FOR DRUG RELEASE

Hydrogels and Soluble Ocular Inserts

Hydrogels

Hydrogels represent ideal supports for the controlled release of the drugs in the forward part of the eye. Due to their excellent mechanical properties—elasticity and fitting among them—they do not generate discomfort during their placement inside the conjunctival sac. They assure a constant release of the drugs through the structure's micropores. The pores' small diameters, like those of the xanthan gels, enable the drug to be released at speeds as small as some micrograms per hour, just enough for creating the desired therapeutic effect.

Hydrogels have been largely utilized as inserts or contact lenses.

INSERTS

Inserts for the treatment of ocular infections. Antibiotic-containing inserts represent a widely utilized therapeutical technique for curing ocular infections.

Erythromycin-containing inserts. Ocular inserts impregnated with antibiotics (erythromycin and erythromycin estolate) which have sustained-release characteristics were prepared, mainly for the purpose of trachoma therapy [138–139].

Trachoma is one of the most important eye diseases of man. It is estimated that over 400 million people suffer from the disease and that 1 to 2 percent of these cases result in moderate or severe visual difficulties [140]. Treatment with sulphonamide or antibiotics is

effective. However, several studies on the chemotherapy of trachoma, which were carried out under strictly controlled conditions, show that trachoma is a difficult disease to eradicate [138,141–146].

Aiming at obtaining erythromycin inserts, copolymers of N-vinylpyrrolidone with vinyl acetate and glycidyl methacrylate or N-vinylpyrrolidone with methyl methacrylate and ethyl acrylate have been prepared; their composition is given in Table 6 [138].

The mechanical properties of hydrogels and antibiotic hydrogels are listed in Table 7 [139].

The most frequently used materials were D (water content 78%) and J (water content 23%) in Table 6 [138].

The elution rate of the erythromycin estolate depends on the water content of the hydrogel, as shown in Figure 16. The rate increases up to 20%; whereas the rate is almost independent of the water content in the range of 30–86% water content.

We have examined 21 different preparations which have water content between 30–86%, various erythromycin estolate contents and different thicknesses. The means and standard deviations of the elution rate were as follows [unit is μg (E. eq.)/cm^2 day]: 254 and 28 at the 1st day; 197 and 24 at the 4th day; 164 and 30 at the 8th day. The small decay of the elution rate is favourable for the sustained release of the antibiotic [138]. The drug content of the preparation determines the duration time of the drug hydrogel combination. The elution rate was kept above 100 μg/(E. eq.)/cm^2 day until the amount of drug in the insert became about 200 μg (E. eq.)/cm^2 day, and then the rate rapidly decreased [138].

The thickness of the preparation had little effect on the elution rate. These features are illustrated in Figure 17.

The conclusion to be drawn is that for erythromycin estolate hydrogel combination which has at least 8

Table 6. Composition and water content of matrix polymers.

	Composition, wt%					Water Content %
	NVP	MMA	EA	VAc	GMA	
A	85	5	10	—	—	89
B	82	5	13	—	—	85
C	78	12	10	—	—	80
D	40	—	—	55	5	78
E	60	15	25	—	—	67
F	54	16	30	—	—	58
G	48	15	37	—	—	52
H	45	10	40	—	5	44
I	40	10	50	—	—	33
J	30	10	55	—	5	23
K	20	10	70	—	—	9

NVP = N-vinylpyrrolidone; MMA = methyl methacrylate; EA = ethyl acrylate; VAc = vinyl acetate; GMA = glycidyl methacrylate.
From Ozawa, H., S. Hosaka, T. Kunitomo and H. Tanzawa, *Biomaterials*, 4:170 (1983), by permission of the publishers, Butterworth & Co. (Publishers) Ltd. ©1983.

days duration time, the hydrogel material should have a water content more than 30%, and the drug content of the preparation should be more than 1.5 mg (E. eq.)/cm².

Hydrogels with erythromycin, prepared in a manner similar to the erythromycin estolate ones, have been used as ophthalmic inserts [138]. Hydrogels with a content of 20–25% water and 7–15% erythromycin have been utilized.

The elution rate of erythromycin from the insert depends on the water content of the hydrogel (Figure 18) [138].

It can be concluded that, in the case of an erythromycin hydrogel combination which has at least 8 days of duration time, the matrix must have a water content of 20–25% and the drug content of the preparation should be more than 2.5 mg/cm². In contrast to the erythromycin estolate preparation, the elution rate is affected by the thickness of the insert, by the stage of elution, by the drug content of the insert and by slight difference in water content of the matrix [138–139].

The *in vivo* tests have been performed with inserts containing various amounts of erythromycin (E) or erythromycin estolate (EE) (Table 7) and of different dimensions (Table 9) [139], employing owl monkey eyes, and human volunteers.

The rates of drug elution *in vitro* from two representative ocular inserts are shown as a function of releasing time (Figure 19). One has observed that the owl monkey experiments were carried out to confirm the therapeutic effects, and the human volunteer experiments were performed to evaluate and improve the acceptability of the ocular insert [139].

The ocular inserts releasing E or EE almost completely suppressed the *Chlamydia trachomatis* infection in the owl monkey eyes. There remains, however, one thing to be discussed in terms of the therapeutic effects. As can be seen in Figures 20 and 21, the number of inclusions in the conjunctiva cells of the control eyes remarkably decreased 14 days after the inoculation, in spite of the fact that no treatment was given [139].

This natural cure was due to the immunity that was

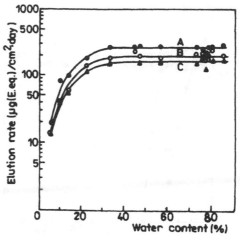

Figure 16. Elution rate of erythromycin estolate from the drug hydrogel combination with various water contents. Curve A indicates the elution rate at the 1st day (●), curve B at the 4th day (○), and curve C at the 8th day (▲). From Reference [138]; reprinted by permission of the publishers, Butterworth & Co. (Publishers) Ltd., © 1983.

substantiated by the antibody response, as shown in Table 10 [139].

The development of the immunity may bring about a question whether the recurrence was prevented by the chemotherapy or by the immunity, after removal of the ocular inserts in the treated eyes.

It is concluded, however, that the recurrence was hindered not by the immunity but by the chemotherapy, because the treated monkeys, with one exception only, failed to show an antibody response, as can be seen in Table 10. In other words, if the latent pathogen had been present in the treated eyes after removal of the ocular insert, the infection would have recurred because of the lack of the immunity [139].

Our interest lies in whether or not the same therapeutic effect may be achieved in the treatment of human trachoma by these ocular inserts. The drug-releasing properties of the ocular inserts provide a clue to this question, though the monkey and human elution data are insufficient for full discussion [139].

Table 7. Mechanical properties of hydrogels and antibiotic hydrogels.

Polymer Composition, wt%					Water Content %	Drug Content mg (E. eq.) g (wet)	Tensile Strength Kg/cm²	Elongation %
NVP	MMA	EA	VAc	GMA				
30	10	55	0	5	23	0	6.2	470
						E 89	5.7	490
45	10	40	0	5	48	0	2.4	290
						EE 167	8.3	300
40	0	0	55	5	76	0	1.0	160
						EE 182	2.5	120

E = erythromycin; EE = erythromycin estolate; NVP = N-vinyl-pyrrolidone; MMA = methyl methacrylate; EA = ethyl acrylate; VAc = vinyl acetate; GMA = glycidyl methacrylate.
From Hosaka, S., H. Ozawa, H. Tanzawa, T. Kinitomo and R. L. Nichols, *Biomaterials*, 4:243 (1983) by permission of the publishers, Butterworth & Co. (Publishers) Ltd. © 1983.

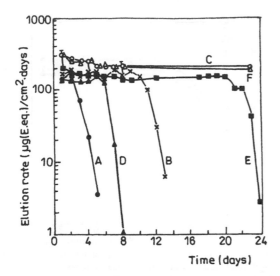

Figure 17. Time course of elution of erythromycin estolate from different hydrogel combinations with various thicknesses and drug contents. The characteristics of each combination (A–F) are shown in Table 8. From Reference [138]; reprinted by permission of the publishers, Butterworth & Co. (Publishers) Ltd., © 1983.

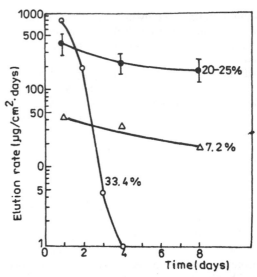

Figure 18. Time course of elution of erythromycin from the drug hydrogel combinations with various water contents. The percentage shows the water content of the matrix. The curve for the water content 20–25% is an average elution rate of 13 different combinations. From Reference [138]; reprinted by permission of the publishers, Butterworth & Co. (Publishers) Ltd., © 1983.

In an owl monkey experiment, E was eluted at a rate of 163 μg/day from an ocular insert that manifested the remarkable effect of suppressing the infection. In the human eye, EE was eluted at rates of 137 μg (E. eq.)/day and 114 μg (E. eq.)/day on the average from the ocular inserts with water contents of 77% and 45%, respectively [139].

Experiments performed on human volunteers are presented in Table 11 [139].

By comparing the drug elution rates in the human experiment with that in the owl monkey experiment, similar therapeutic effects may be expected in the treatment of human trachoma.

From a technical point of view, the feasibility of experimental therapy in the patients' eyes depends upon

the tolerability of the ocular insert in the eye. Irritation by an ocular insert could be evaluated accurately only by human experiments. The ocular insert of 24% water content containing E was irritative in human eyes, though it was retained for enough time and manifested excellent therapeutic effects in the owl monkey eye [139].

The acceptability of an ocular insert depends upon its shape, dimension, mechanical properties, and the quality of the surface and the edge. The irritation of an ocular insert was effectively removed by heightening the water content of the hydrogel and removing the antibiotic precipitated near the surface through prewashing procedure. The hydrogel insert, with a water content of 45% impregnated with EE caused no harm

Table 8. Characteristics of erythromycin estolate–hydrogel combinations with different thickness and different drug content.

	Thickness of Combination μm	Drug Content mg/cm²	Drug Remained* mg/cm²
A	40	0.43	0
B	350	1.80	0
C	1430	5.07	3.2
D	70	0.80	0
E	390	3.92	0
F	1600	7.68	6.3

*The amount of drug remained in the combination after 24 days elution.
From H. Ozawa, S. Hosaka, T. Kunitomo and H. Tanzawa, *Biomaterials*, 4:170 (1983), by permission of the publishers, Butterworth & Co. (Publishers) Ltd. © 1983.

Table 9. List of insert test pieces.

No.	Water Content %	Antibiotic mg (E. eq.)	Dimension, mm		
			l	*W*	*t*
1	76	EE 1.8	9.7	5.5	0.27
2	24	E 1.4	11.6	5.5	0.35
3	77	EE 1.5	11.5	4.8	0.31
4	77	EE 2.1	10.0	4.4	0.36
5	75	EE 0.4	9.7	3.4	0.32
6	77	EE 1.1	10.6	3.7	0.42
7	45	EE 1.8	9.8	3.5	0.40
8	45	EE 1.2	9.8	3.6	0.38

t = thickness

From Hosaka, S., H. Ozawa, H. Tanzawa, T. Kinitomo and R. L. Nichols, *Biomaterials*, 4:243 (1983), by permission of the publishers, Butterworth & Co. (Publishers) Ltd. © 1983.

Table 10. Maximum reciprocal antibody titers in the eye secretions and sera of monkeys with trachoma eye infections.

Monkey Group		Serum	Eye Secretions, Each Eye
Treated monkey			
Erythromycin	A	<1/10	<1/10, <1/10
(24% water)	B	<1/10	<1/10, <1/10
	C	<1/10	<1/10, <1/10
	D	<1/10	<1/10, <1/10
Erythromycin estolate	E	1/20 (day 36)	<1/10, <1/10
(45% water)	F	<1/10	<1/10, <10
Control monkey			
Plain gel	G	1/80 (day 21)	1/10, 1/10 (day 21)
(24% water)	H	1/160 (day 14)	<1/10, 1/10 (day 21)
Plain gel	I	1/320 (day 14)	1/20, 1/20 (day 36)
(77% water)	J	1/320 (day 36)	1/140, 1/80 (day 36)

Note: Following infection, monkeys were exposed to antibiotic or plain hydrogel eye inserts. The time of maximum titer of samples collected between days 3 and 36 following infections is indicated in parentheses.
From Hosaka, S., H. Ozawa, H. Tanzawa, T. Kinitomo and R. L. Nichols, *Biomaterials*, 4:243 (1983), by permission of the publishers, Butterworth & Co. (Publishers) Ltd. ©1983.

in the human eye nor in the owl monkey eye and released the antibiotic at an adequate rate [139].

Another hydrogel employed in the fabrication of erythromycin-containing inserts was reticulated xanthan [91–92], having the chemical structure plotted in Figure 22.

Erythromycin retardation was performed both through gel entrapped and through ionic complexation with the carboxylic groups of xanthan (Figure 23) [147]. With a view to increasing the capacity of ionic complexation of erythromycin, xanthan has been decationed on ion exchanges. Ionic coupling was performed in a homogeneous system, on employing an alcohol–water mixture (1 v/l v) and a xanthan/erythromycin ratio of 0.100/0.429 (g/g). During the whole duration of the reaction, the pH of the solution was followed, up to its attaining a constant value, which indicates that the ionic equilibrium was reached.

Ophthalmic inserts with erythromycin contents varying between 3.4% (E_1) and 2.7% (E_2) have been thus obtained. Analysis of the antimicrobial activity of the two inserts (E_1, E_2)—as gel—is 1180 UI/ml (E_1) and 500 UI/ml (E_2), respectively.

Inserts with chloramphenicol. In ophthalmic therapy, chloramphenicol (CPh) is usually employed as a large spectrum antibiotic, possessing a high local tolerance. Also, its action is manifested not only at the surface, but in conjunctival and corneous layers, too. Perhaps its most important shortcoming is its low solubility in water, preventing it from obtaining the concentrations required by ophthalmologic practice. This explains the great number of recent studies discussing new modalities of ophthalmic administration of CPh: some of them recommend increasing the solubility

coefficient by employing buffer systems [148–149] or anhydrous solvents [149]; others propose attaining a prolonged remanence of the antibiotic [150–151]; still other investigators aim at getting high CPh concentrations through its soluble derivatives [149–151] or through intermediates [152].

The process of getting chloramphenicol-containing inserts involved its esterification on xanthan [153–154].

The coupling reaction of CPh was carried out in the presence of dicyclohexylcarbodiimide (DCCI).

The influence of different factors on the esterification reaction is shown in Figures 25–27 [153].

The data presented in Figures 25 and 26 show that the CPh/DCCI mole ratio influences the amount of

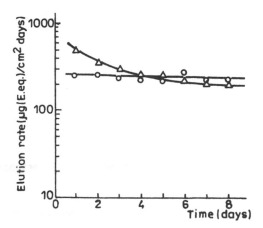

Figure 19. Profile of drug release from ocular inserts of hydrogel △ -2; ○-7 in Table 9. From Reference [138]; reprinted by permission of the publishers, Butterworth & Co. (Publishers) Ltd., © 1983.

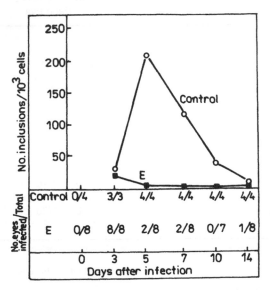

Figure 20. Effect of erythromycin-containing insert of hydrogel with 24% water content in the treatment of established eye infection in owl monkeys. From Reference [138]; reprinted by permission of the publishers, Butterworth & Co. (Publishers) Ltd., © 1983.

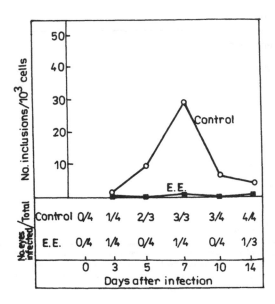

Figure 21. Effect of erythromycin estolate-containing insert of hydrogel with 45% water content in the treatment of established eye infection in owl monkeys. From Reference [138]; reprinted by permission of the publishers, Butterworth & Co. (Publishers) Ltd., © 1983.

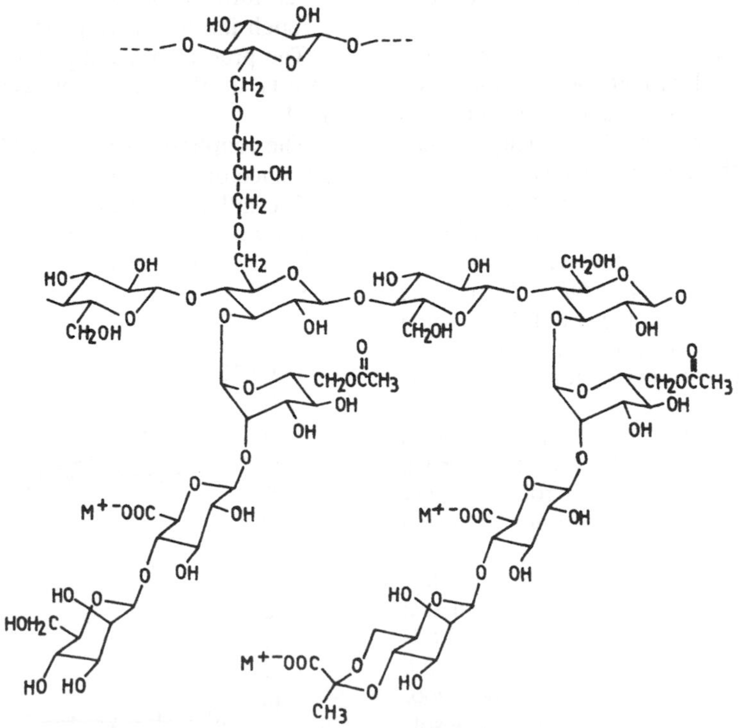

Figure 22. Chemical structure of reticulated xanthan.

Table 11. Human volunteer test.

No. Exp.	Volunteer & (Eye)	No. Gel	Drug	Water Content %	Insertion Time Day/No. of Replacement*		Irritation and/or Discharge
1	A (Rt)	—	No	80	4/3	(1.3)	No
1	A (Lt)	—	No	80	4/1	(4.0)	No
1	B (Rt)	—	No	80	1/5	(0.2)	No
2	B (Rt)	—	No	24	22/1	(22.0)	No
4	A (Rt)	4	EE	77	0/1	(0.0)	No
4	A (Lt)	2	E	22	0/1[a]	(2.0)	Yes
4	B (Rt)	4	EE	77	0/1	(0.0)	No
4	B (Lt)	2	E	22	1/1[a]	(1.0)	Yes
5	A (Rt)	4	EE	77	14/1[a]	(14.0)	Yes
5	A (Lt)	4	EE	77	11/1	(11.0)	No
8	A (Rt)	8	EE	45	2/1	(2.0)	No
8	A (Lt)	5	EE	75	1/2	(0.5)	No
8	B (Rt)	8	EE	45	7/1	(7.0)	No
8	B (Lt)	5	EE	75	8/1	(8.0)	No

*Average retention time is shown in parentheses.
[a]Intentional removal.

From Hosaka, S., H. Ozawa, H. Tanzawa, T. Kinitomo and R. L. Nichols, *Biomaterials*, 4:243 (1983), by permission of the publishers, Butterworth & Co. (Publishers) Ltd. ©1983.

bound CPh significantly, the optimum value being situated between 0.8–1.0 mole/mole. The existence of a plateau in the CPh/DCCI-bound CPh plot attests to the fact that all carboxy groups in xanthan (Biozan R®) have been activated by DCCI.

The dilution affects the yield and reaction rate (Figures 25, 27), high concentrations being favourable for the process. At concentrations higher than 2% xanthan, the gel mobility was difficult and the diffusion capacity of the reactants become lower; therefore this concentration cannot be exceeded.

The CPh concentration influenced the reaction yield. Above 2.17 mmole/30 ml water, the system become unstable, the CPh separated and could not react anymore. Additional amounts of THF (a solvent for CPh) did not improve the homogeneity of the system, since the xanthan precipitated out. Under these conditions, the esterification reaction was very slow, proceeding for longer than 14 h. The diffusion factor is also implied in this process since xanthan becomes a gel in the presence of the reactants.

The reaction product is a water-swelling gel that can be utilized in oral administration [155], in the fabrication of ophthalmic inserts, or in ophthalmic oint-

ments. Ophthalmic inserts have a low tolerability in the eye, which is why a special interest was given to ointments [153, 156–157]. Thus, three different formulae of ointments have been prepared (given in Table 12), where the xanthan–CPh product contains 15% CPh chemically bound.

The ointments were characterized for their stability with preservatives and some physico-chemical and biological parameters, in order to appreciate interactions between the components. Thus, the pH, refraction and extensibility indices, limiting yield strain, viscosity, and antibiotic activity were measured.

Solutions of xanthan–CPh did not modify the pH values either in acid or in alkali media; hence, esterified CPh maintains its stability in these media. The pH values of the xanthan–CPh ophthalmic ointments are given in Table 13, which also shows that pH is not modified significantly during preservation.

The values for the refraction index were: sample M, 1.3345; samples A and B, 1.3370. This did not change during the preservation time in this study. The values were within the limits of the refraction index of tear liquid, which is favourable for appreciating biological tolerance.

Table 12. Formulae of CPh–xanthan ophthalmic ointments.

Ingredients	Sample, g		
	M	A	B
CPh–xanthan	3.30	3.30	3.30
Benzalkonium chloride	—	0.02	—
Dequalinium chloride	—	—	0.02
Distilled water	96.70	96.68	96.68

Table 13. pH values of CPh–xanthan ophthalmic ointments.

Sample	After Preservation	Preserving Time, Days			
		7	14	30	45
M	6.18	6.19	6.19	6.19	6.19
A	6.13	6.36	6.36	6.35	6.25
B	6.18	6.18	6.17	6.17	6.17

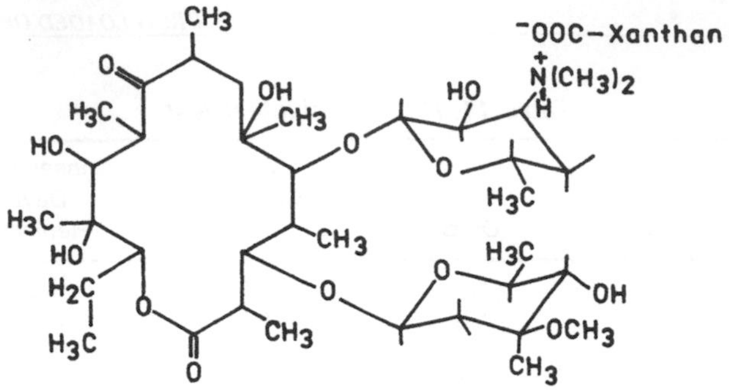

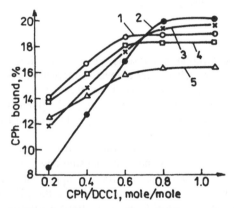

Figure 23. Chemical structure of the xanthan–erythromycin complex.

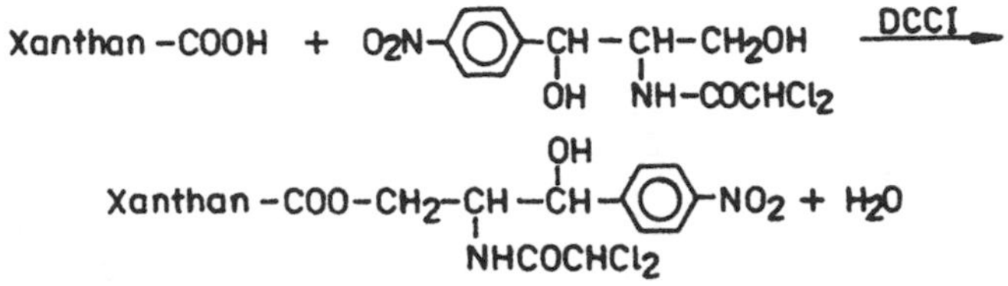

Figure 24. The reaction of coupling xanthan with CPh, as catalyzed by DCCI.

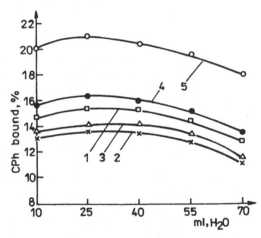

Figure 25. Variation in amount of bound CPh as a function of CPh/DCCI ratio at different dilutions. Time = 5 h; xanthan = 0.5 g; temperature = 5°C. 1 (○) 10 ml H_2O; 2 (●) 25 ml H_2O; 3 (×) 40 ml H_2O; 4 (□) 55 ml H_2O; 5 (△) 70 ml H_2O.

Figure 27. Variation of amount of bound CPh as a function of dilution for different reaction times. CPh = 1.24 mmole; DCCI = 1.10 mmole; xanthan = 0.5 g; temperature = 5°C; 1 (□) 2 h; 2 (×) 5 h; 3 (△) 8 h; 4 (●) 11 h; 5 (○) 14 h.

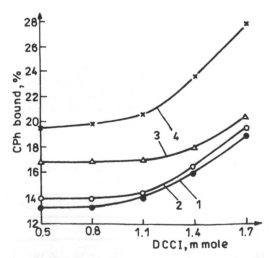

Figure 26. Variation in amount of bound CPh as a function of DCCI amount for different CPh concentrations. Vol. water = 40 ml; time = 8 h; Xanthan = 0.5 g; Temperature = 5°C, 1 (●) 0.77 mmole CPh; 2 (○) 1.24 mmole CPh; 3 (△) 1.71 mmole CPh; 4 (×) 2.17 mmole CPh.

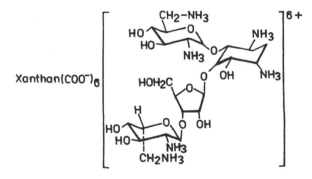

Figure 28. Structure of neomycin coupled on xanthan.

The average extension index (*Ie*) varied within narrow limits after preparation, i.e., between 841–832 mm² (sample M); 796–812 mm² (sample A) and 974–892 mm² (sample B). Sample A showed lower values than the other samples, due to the ointment swelling in the presence of benzalkonium chloride which maintains preservation.

The yield strain (θ) has rather high values (attributable to the ointment adhesiveness), namely 378–398 dyn/cm² (sample M), 378–398 dyn/cm² (sample A) and 540–552 dyn/cm² (sample B) during preservation. The highest values were noticed for the product preserved with dequalinium chloride, due to its consistency. The increase in this parameter, by adding preserving agents of the xanthan–CPh gel, was evident.

The rheological parameters, namely flowing index (*n*) and consistency index (*m*) are given in Table 14.

The thixotropy of xanthan ($n < 1$) was maintained after modification with CPh (sample M) as well as in the A and B products. A lower consistency was noticed for sample B; the consistency index increased for samples A and B after preservation, due to the gel formation.

The antimicrobial activity was 410 μg/ml (sample M) and was maintained for 45 days.

In previous investigations of the CPh tolerance on the eye mucous membrane, an irritation with a response rate 10/10 (response rate recorded as the number of positive responses per number of eyes tested) was noticed, which did not diminish even in association with dextran, carboxymethyl cellulose, or flax mucilage. The results obtained with CPh–xanthan ophthalmic ointments were much better (response rate 3/6 for sample B and 4/6 for sample M).

Administration on the healthy eyes of volunteers produced no discomfort, nor local or general allergy; on the diseased eye, tolerance was good, the infection eradicated and the clinical state improved.

Table 14. Consistency index (m) and flowing index (n) of the CPh–xanthan ophthalmic ointments.

Sample	After Preparation		After 45 Days	
	m, CP	*n*	*m*, CP	*n*
M	195.0	0.24	218.8	0.24
A	208.9	0.26	275.4	0.26
B	326.7	0.23	243.2	0.24

Xanthan and other natural polyanions represent the ideal polymers to be used in the retardation of basic antibiotics (neomycin, gentamycin, streptomycin), a process known to be accompanied by the formation of gels with a high biocompatibility [158].

Retard neomycin (Nm), prepared according to the described method has the structure plotted in Figure 28 [159].

The ionic bonds formed do modify the conformation of the xanthan macromolecule, shifting it to a water-insoluble form. In water, retard neomycine swells (degree of swelling = 300%); it is insoluble in organic solvents and stable in acid pH.

Yield of the coupling reaction of neomycine depends on the neomycin/xanthan ratio (Figure 29).

The optimum Nm/X ratio, to which all carboxylic groups from the support are reacted, is of 0.1 Nm/X (g/g).

Dumitriu and coworkers [160] have employed such a product, with a content of 57.13% Nm, to be tested *in vitro*, in the hope of studying the dynamic release of Nm by using artificial tear as eluent.

Two elution systems have been used, the former in the open system, in which the artificial tear washes continuously, the ophthalmic insert containing retard neomycine (on simulating the conditions to be met in the conjunctival sac) and the latter in the closed system, involving continuous recirculation of the eluent through the sample to be analyzed. The curves of Nm release are plotted in Figure 30.

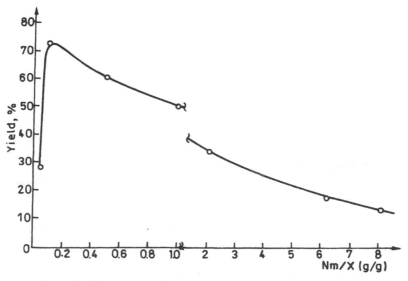

Figure 29. Yield variation of the reaction of coupling neomycin on xanthan.

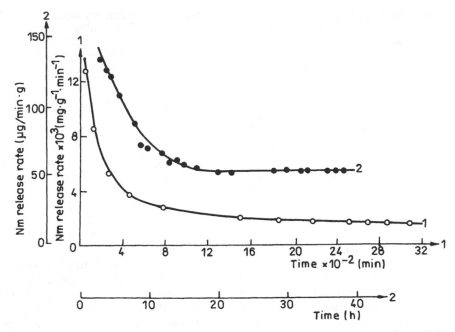

Figure 30. Variation of the Nm release rate. 1—release in open dynamic regime on using artificial tear as eluent, flow 0.8–1 ml/h; chemical dosage; 2—release in close system, flow 1 ml/h.

The release rate is high in the first 200 min, then it decreases continuously until reading a constant value at 1000 min. Beyond this duration, the release process follows a "zero-order" kinetics which evidences its retard character. Mention must be made of the fact that, at an elution duration over 1200 min, in the collected samples concentrations of 0.082 mg Nm/ml, are to be formed which may induce the therapeutical effect desired.

Determination of the biological activity of the drug has been performed *in vitro*, by microbiological dosing of the Nm in the eluent (Figure 31). A good agreement is to be observed between chemical (Figure 30, curve 1) and biological (Figure 31) dosing of the released drug.

Antimicrobial activity of ophthalmic inserts containing Nm retard has been settled by depositing some exactly weighed amounts on plates sowed with germs of *Staphylococcus aureus* 209 P, then measuring in time the diameter of the inhibition region, up to its stabilization.

By following the variation of the inhibition region diameter, created by these inserts, its increase up to 40 h is to be noted, being constant afterwards (Figures 32, 33).

In the case of inserts protected with a cellulosic semipermeable membrane, the same time variation with the diameter of the inhibition region is to be observed (Figure 33).

On comparing the results presented in Figure 33 a

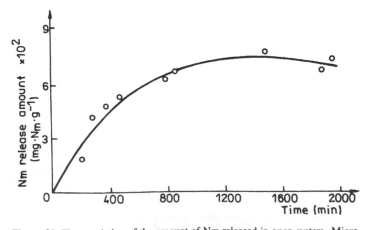

Figure 31. Time variation of the amount of Nm released in open system. Microbiological determination of Nm on gelosis plates *Staphylococcus aureus* 209 P.

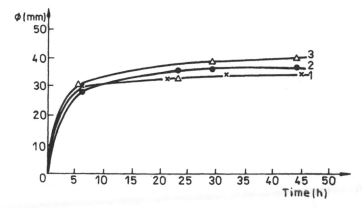

Figure 32. Time variations of the inhibition region diameter with time and insert weight. Gelosis plates inoculated with *Staphylococcus aureus* 209 P, insert without protection membrane, temperature 37°C. 1—Insert with a weight of 7.1 mg; 2—insert with a weight of 9.0 mg; 3—insert with a weight of 10.3 mg.

stronger antimicrobial action of the nonprotected inserts is to be observed, as a consequence of an easier diffusion, Nm being released directly on the infected region, while the presence of the membrane presents penetration belating the antimicrobial effect. The antibiotic activity of the inserts is of 380 UI/mg, at a Nm content of the xanthan-containing complex of 53.13%.

Ophthalmic inserts with retard Nm have been tested *in vivo*, in hopes of establishing the release rate in the conjunctival sac of the human and rabbit eye [161]. The release rate was determined by chemical dosing of the remanent content of Nm in the inserts, maintained for various time intervals, in human and rabbit eyes.

One has to observe that the rate of Nm release—*in vivo*—is much higher than *in vitro* conditions (open dynamic regime—Figure 30), which is probably due to the thermal and mechanical (i.e., blinking) effect.

Testing of the bacteriostatic effect of the ophthalmic inserts with retard Nm was done on volunteers suffering from staphylococcic conjunctivitis. The control group was given medication by instillations with gentamycine, oxacyline, and neomycine. The experimental group (15 cases) was treated with retard Nm-containing inserts, introduced into the conjunctival sac. Negativation of the secretion with *Staphylococcus aureus* is evident after 24–36 h in the case of instillations with gentamycine, 24 h for oxacyline, and 36–48 h for Nm (which is irritative and hard to tolerate). The group subjected to the treatment with the insert showed negativation after 12 h.

Another support utilized in the retardation of Nm was the poly(acrylic acid-co-vinyl alcohol) copolymer (PAcA-AV) [162]. Coupling of Nm was performed in an aqueous solution, through the carboxylic groups of the acrylic acid unities from the copolymer and of the

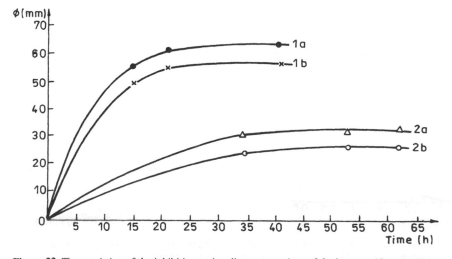

Figure 33. Time variation of the inhibition region diameter, on time, of the inserts with and without a protective membrane. Gelosis plates inoculated with *Staphylococcus aureus* 209 P, incubation at 37°C. 1a—Insert with a 6.6 mg weight, without membrane; 1b—insert with a 6.6 mg weight with membrane; 2a—insert with a 5.6 mg weight, without membrane; 2b—insert with a 5.6 mg weight, with membrane.

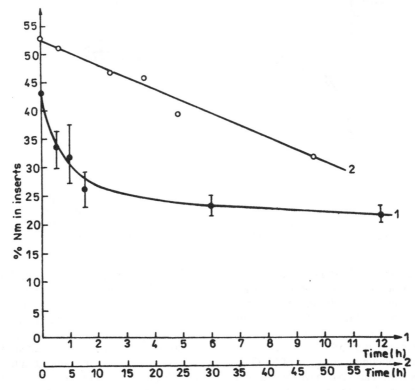

Figure 34. Variation of the amount of remanent Nm in ophthalmic inserts. 1—Insert maintained in the conjunctival sac (human); 2—insert maintained in the conjunctival sac (rabbit).

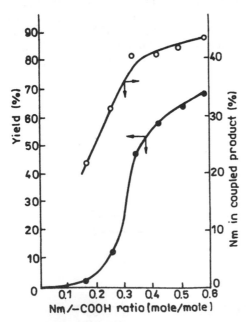

Figure 35. Influence of the Nm/PAcA-AV ratio upon the yield and composition of the reaction product. Nm concentration = 5.6 × 10⁻² g/ml.

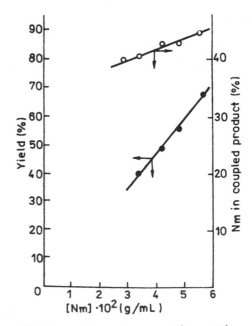

Figure 36. Influence of neomycin concentration upon the coupling yield and composition of retard Nm. Nm/PAcA-AV ratio = 0.333 mole/mole.

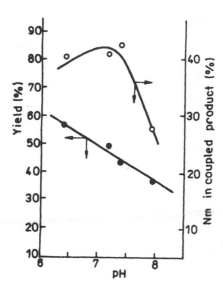

Figure 37. Influence of the pH medium upon the yield and composition of the reaction product. Nm concentration = 5.6 × 10^{-2} g/ml.

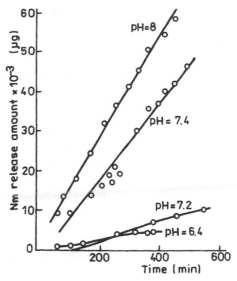

Figure 38. Variation of the amount of Nm released in time, through recirculation of the eluent in close system. Flow = 16.9 ml/h; Nm content in the sample = 0.0499 g; volume of eluent = 25 ml; temperature = 37°C.

aminic ones of the drug. The presence of 6 aminic groups in the structure of Nm induces its complexation through ionic bonds on the polyanion, thus modifying its conformation. Thus, the copolymer becomes insoluble in water, with a swelling degree of 250%. The coupling yield and the composition of the reaction product depend on the Nm/copolymer ratio (Figure 35). The amount of antibiotic bound in the reaction product increases continuously with the parameter considered, showing the tendency to reach a maximum value at a Nm/PAcA-AV ratio of 0.666 mole/mole.

The coupling yield and the composition of retard Nm are also influenced by the reactant concentration. On keeping the Nm/PAcA-AV molar ratio constant (i.e., 0.333 mole/mole) and varying the concentration of Nm, the reaction's efficiency is modified (Figure 36). Data given in Figure 36 evidence a continuous increase of the yield with an increasing concentration of Nm, while neomycin's composition is observed as being less affected by the variation of this parameter.

The pH of the medium influences both the yield and the composition of the reaction product (Figure 37). One can observe that, on the acid range of pH, maximum values of the yield and reaction product are to be obtained.

The linear dependence between the amount of Nm released in time (Figure 38) evidences the retard character of the drug.

From the amount of Nm retarded on the PAcA-AV copolymer, ophthalmic inserts—well tolerated in the conjunctival sac and assuring an efficient sterilization of the staphylococcus infections after 12 h—have been prepared.

Inserts for the treatment of open-angle glaucoma.
Reticulated xanthan [91–92] forms a hydrogel used as

an insert, from which pilocarpine is released for the treatment of open-angle glaucoma.

Dumitriu and coworkers [163–165] have obtained ophthalmic inserts based on xanthan reticulated with pilocarpine, epinephrine, hydrocortisone, and lidocaine.

Xanthan is known as possessing the capacity to retain pilocarpine (PiN), ionically or by insertion.

The drug content in the insert depends upon the xanthan/drug ratio employed (Table 15).

The pilocarpine free base (PiB) is retained either by entrapment or by ionic linking to the free carboxylic groups of the macromolecular support. By observing the pH variation in time of a pilocarpine solution (1% PiB) in which xanthan (0.01 g/ml) was suspended (Figure 40), the ionic exchange equilibrium was attained after 50 min, when 92% of the carboxylic groups were ionically coupled with PiB. The coupling rate was seen to reach a maximum after four minutes (Figure 41) (6.3 mg g^{-1} min^{-1}) and to stabilize to a minimum value after 50 min, when the ionic exchange equilibrium was attained.

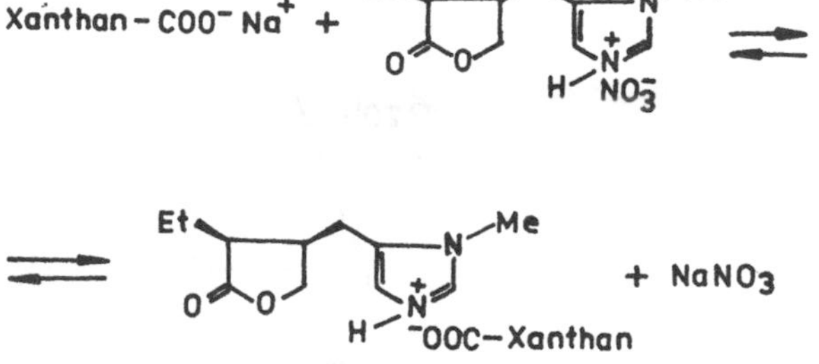

Figure 39. Reaction of ionic coupling of pilocarpine on xanthan.

Table 15. Mono- and polycomponent ophthalmic inserts.

Codified Index	Support	Drug	Amount of Drug in the Insert, (mg/g)
I_1	Modified xanthan	Pilocarpine	369
I_2	Modified xanthan	Pilocarpine	229
I_3	Modified xanthan	Pilocarpine	142
I_4	Modified xanthan–PBCA[a]	Pilocarpine	142
I_5	Modified xanthan	Pilocarpine	7.2
		Hydrocortisone	14.2
I_6	Modified xanthan–PBCA[a]	Pilocarpine	7.2
		Hydrocortisone	13.0
		Lidocaine	3.0
		Epinephrine	0.14
I_7	Cross-linked xanthan	Pilocarpine	90.0
		Lidocaine	56.0
		Epinephrine	3.0

[a]PBCA = poly(butyl cyanoacrylate).

The inserts presented in Table 15 have been tested *in vivo* in order to establish the pilocarpine release rate under dynamic conditions, using an artificial tear solution as eluent. Intervals of time, up to 120 h were employed; the results are listed in Figures 42–48.

Additional modification of the support, by the introduction of a self-polymerizable monomer (butyl cyanoacrylate) shows positive effects, from at least two points of view: it mechanically stabilizes the insert, and at the same time increases the drug release rate compared to the other inserts having the same

pilocarpine content (Figure 45). The release rate reaches its highest value in the first elution moments then gradually decreases, but remains higher than Insert I_3 for 68 h. In the following 34 h, it decreases but maintains at least 5 μg g^{-1} min^{-1}, which is higher than previous situations. An explanation for the different behaviours of the two types of inserts, with the same pilocarpine contents, may lie in the fact that the network of synthetic polymer introduced on the surface affects the xanthan conformation. The polymer is not swollen by the eluent, thus it maintains a porosity that

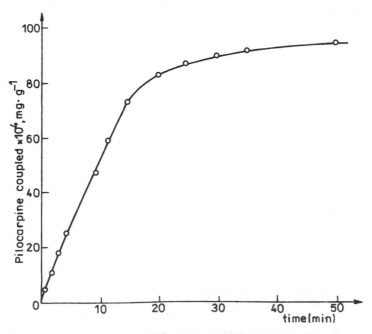

Figure 40. Variation in time of PiB amount on xanthan. Concentration of solution = 1% PiB; concentration of xanthan = 0.01 g/ml; temperature = 20°C.

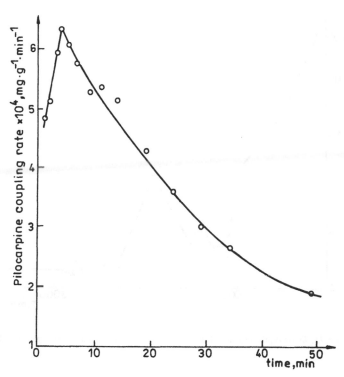

Figure 41. Average rate of the ionic coupling of PiB on xanthan. Concentration of solution = 1% PiB; concentration of xanthan = 0.01 g/ml; temperature = 20°C.

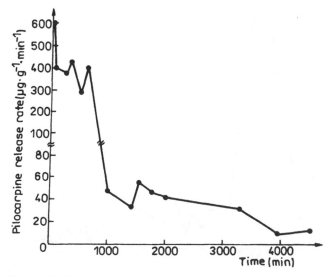

Figure 42. *In vitro* pilocarpine release rates from Insert I_1. Volume rate = 0.8 ml/h; eluent = artificial tear solution.

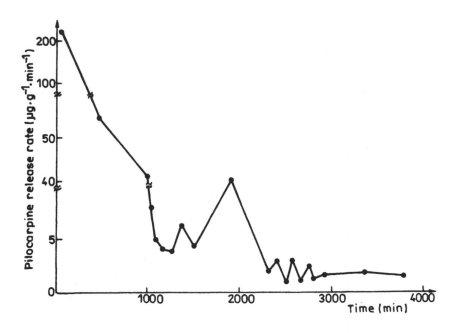

Figure 43. *In vitro* pilocarpine release rate from insert I₂. Some conditions as in Figure 42.

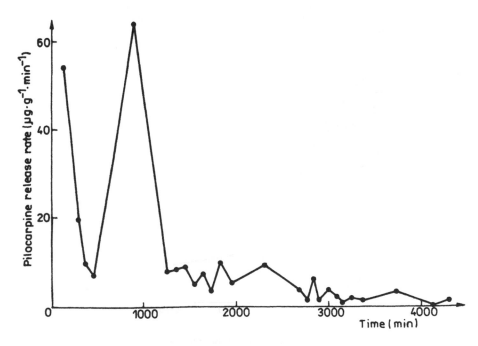

Figure 44. *In vitro* pilocarpine release rate from insert I₃.

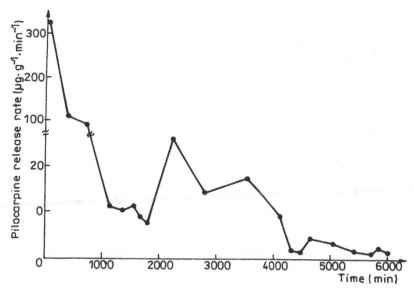

Figure 45. *In vitro* pilocarpine release rate from insert I_4.

permits easier penetration of the liquid. Increasing the rate of the eluent diffusion would increase the pilocarpine release rate.

Inserts I_5–I_7 have a much lower pilocarpine content and the release rate of the drug was much lower (Figures 46–48). Although containing a smaller amount of pilocarpine, insert I_6 (Figure 47) shows a higher relative rate of drug release. The reason may be that the synthetic polymer matrix on the macromolecular support assures more favourable conditions for elution of the drug. In the case of insert I_5, elution was performed after the wrapping of the product into a cellophane sheet, which constitutes an additional barrier to the diffusion of the eluent and drug.

Insert I_7 has a higher pilocarpine content than I_5 and I_6, yet lower than I_1–I_4. It shows an average value of drug release rate which is between these two groups (Figure 48). Maximum release was recorded after 50 h, which is not seen with the other inserts.

Insert I_7 differs from the other by using cross-linked xanthan, which has a much lower swelling (80%) in the tear liquid. Consequently, diffusional processes are diminished, reaching a maximum of intensity after 50 h, when the swelling is maximum. During the approximately 100 h elution period, the rate value varied between 2 and 10 $\mu g\ g^{-1}\ min^{-1}$, with an average value of about 6 $\mu g\ g^{-1}\ min^{-1}$. The insert continues to release pilocarpine up to 120 h, indicating high

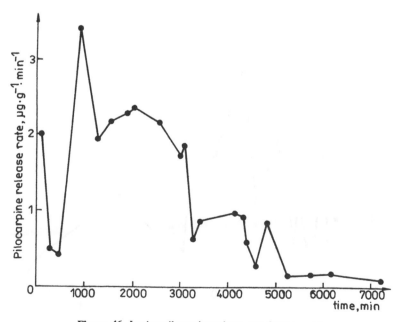

Figure 46. *In vitro* pilocarpine release rate from insert I_5.

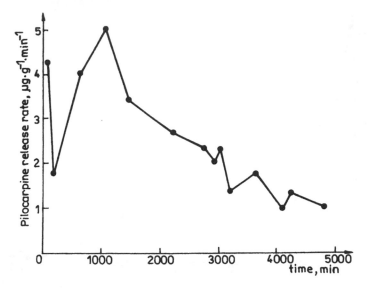

Figure 47. *In vitro* pilocarpine release rate from insert I_6.

mechanical stability. *In vivo* tests subsequently confirmed this behaviour.

By comparatively analyzing the curves for pilocarpine *in vitro* release from these inserts, one can observe an increase in the release rate during the 0–17 h time interval. A maximum is attained after about 17 h due to the rapid release of the pilocarpine from the surface area of the insert. A second maximum, which is observed after 34 h, may be due to attaining maximum swelling of the insert; at this time, the diffusional processes from inside the matrix reaches maximum intensity.

The insert, with a content of 36.9% PiN, was tested *in vivo* by introducing samples into the conjunctival sac. The two groups of patients, whose ages varied from 35 to 60 years, were selected to be as homogeneous as possible (Table 16) [163]. The control group (15 cases) was treated by instilling 2% PiN solution every four hours. The intraocular pressure (IOP) variation (aplanatonometry), the pupillary diameter and the eye aspect were checked at constant periods of time (every four hours).

The therapeutic action of the insert is presented in Figures 49–50.

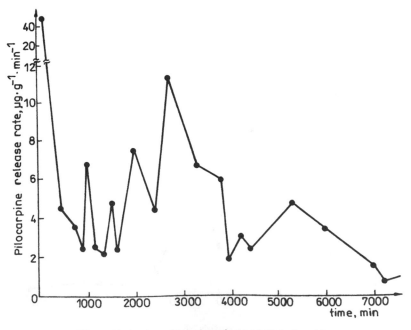

Figure 48. *In vitro* pilocarpine release rate from insert I_7.

It can be seen that the insert introduced into the conjunctival sac had a higher efficiency than that of the instillations. A fast decrease of the IOP, as well as of the pupillar diameter, was observed immediately after the administration. These effects were maintained for 24 h. A remanent effect of 10 h was observed (Figures 49 and 50) after removal of the insert, as result of the diffusion into the conjunctival sac of a soluble fraction having ionically linked PiN.

The miotic effect was maintained at values near those obtained for the control group (Figure 50).

The general aspects of degradable polymer inserts have been reviewed by Yolles and Sartori [166], Heller and Baker [167], Pitt et al. [168] and Peterson et al. [169].

THERMOGELS AND POLYMERIC DISPERSION

In the early 1980s, researchers came up with two new approaches: first, the use of vehicles with sol-gel transition at body temperature; second, polymeric dispersion which shows coalescence by a pH change.

The first approach is mainly based on the use of thermogels such as polyalkylene oxide block copolymers, whereas the second is a polymeric dispersion, both containing a bioactive substance, and allowing the creation *in situ* of a microreservoir by simple instillation [170].

The concept of producing a controlled release system *in situ* in the cul-de-sac of the eye has been investigated and compared *in vivo* using two different approaches:

- thermogels [171] made from polyalkylene oxide block copolymers (Pluronic® 7127, Wyandotte)

Table 16. The characteristics of the volunteer groups used for testing the insert based on pilocarpine.

Groups	Average Age, Years	Sex		IOP mmHg
		M	F	
Experimental	45.93	7	8	26.33
Control	46.40	7	8	24.00

- pH sensitive polymers dispersed in water (CAP, cellulose acetate hydrogen phthalate, Eastman) or redispersable as acrylic latex particles (7203/69A and B, Röhm Pharma) [172]

In practice, it had been found earlier [173] that in the first case, a vehicle having a sol-gel transition temperature in the range of 25°C to about 35°C satisfies the requirement and is useful for drug delivery to the eye. The capacity of such a liquid pharmaceutical formulation to gel at human body temperature is the feature of this system. A typical formulation tested for the treatment of glaucoma containing 4% pilocarpine HCl and 25% Pluronic F-127 in purified water has been tested using the miotic response of albino rabbits.

These formulations are compared in the present *in vivo* study to a polymeric dispersion in the monomer size range also containing pilocarpine. The general method for preparing these latexes is described schematically in Figure 51 [170].

Some possible candidates besides the CAP mentioned above for these dispersed systems are given in Table 17 [170].

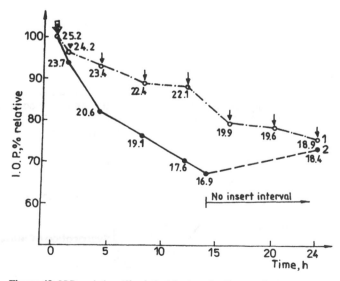

Figure 49. IOP variation (% relative) in time. 1—Groups of witnesses with PiN instillations (solution 2%); 2—group of investigated patients with insert into the conjunctival sac (0.01 g insert with 36.9% PiN). The value indicated by arrows represents the calculated average values of IOP; reference IOP—25.2 mmHg, 100% respectively.

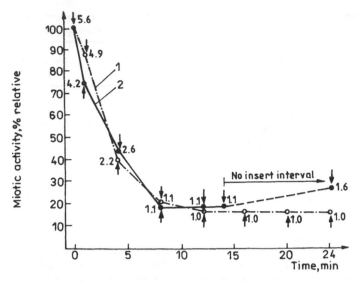

Figure 50. Miotic effect (% relative) in time. 1—Normal group with instillations (solution PiN 2%); 2—group under investigation with insert into the conjunctival sac (0.01 g insert with 36.9% PiN). The values indicated by arrows represent the calculated average values of the pupillar diameter in mm. Reference pupillary diameter 8, 5.5 mm (100% respectively).

The neutralization profiles are given for some other polymers investigated in Figure 52, which demonstrates the various buffer capacities of the gel-forming materials.

Various latex systems have been prepared following the conventional emulsification technique, as described earlier [174], followed by stripping off the organic solvent. As shown in Figure 51 there are various potential methods for adding the bioactive material into the system. In our case, the active compound (pilocarpine) is added to the final latex where the active substance is partially adsorbed onto the surface of the polymer particles. In all cases, the latex

particles show an average particle size below 0.3 μm with a polydispersity index of 1 or 2, as determined by the Coulter Nanosizer® [170]. All test formulations show an extremely low viscosity (<100 cps) and gel *in vitro*.

Extensive *in vivo* testing has been performed on thermosetting gels, as well as on latex systems, all containing 4% of pilocarpine HCl [170]. The prolongation of the miotic responses of the experimental formulations, as compared to a conventional solution of pilocarpine, is clearly demonstrated in Figure 53, where the mean residence times (MRT) [175] as measured by the miotic activity for the formulations are

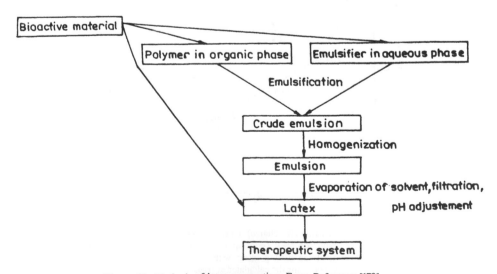

Figure 51. Methods of latex preparation. From Reference [170].

Table 17. Physico-chemical properties of some selected polymers with pH dependent solubility.

Chemical Structure	Name	Manufacturer	M_w	A.I.	pK	Observation
1	2	3	4	5	6	7

Chemical Structure	Name	Manufacturer	M_w	A.I.	pK	Observation
	7203/69A	Röhm Pharma	135,000	307	6.1	Monomer ratio 1/1
	7203/69B	Röhm Pharma	135,000	193	7.1	Monomer ratio 1/2
	7203/58	Röhm Pharma	800,000	—	—	Monomer ratio 1/1
	Eudragit L 30 D	Röhm Pharma	250,000	318	6.0	Monomer ratio 1/1
	PVAP	Colorcon	25,000–40,000	205	5.0	Carboxybenzoyl 55–65% Acetyl 1.6–6.0%
	HPMCP HP-55 "F"	Shin-Etsu	20,000	126	5.0	Methoxyl 18.0–11.0% Carboxybenzoyl 27.0–35.0%
	CAP	Eastman	40,000	104	4.9	Combined phthalyl 30.0–36.0% Combined acetyl 19.0–23.5% Free acid 6% maximum

From Furny, R., T. Boye, H. Ibrahim and P. Buri, Proceed. Intern. Symp. Control. Rel. Bioact. Mater., 12:300 (1985).

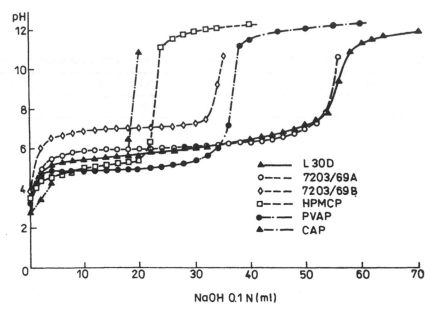

Figure 52. Neutralization profiles for some polymers. From Reference [170].

indicated as bars and the factor of prolongation (MRT [test formulation]/MRT [solution]) is given above each bar. The polymeric dispersion based on CAP, formulation no. 4, shows a substantial increase in bioavailability as compared to the solution, formulation no. 1. Only the system with a sol-gel transition, formulation no. 3, shows a similar result. The commercially available formulation no. 2 shows, as expected, no difference compared to our reference preparation no. 1. By analyzing AUC values, similar conclusions can be drawn. Preliminary studies showed good biocompatibility for all systems tested [170].

The polymer dispersion has low viscosity and can accommodate solid content up to 40% wt/wt. The

unique feature is that they can be applied as eye drops, which results in good patient compliance. In the case of pilocarpine-containing systems, two daily instillations should be sufficient, compared to 4 to 6 applications with ordinary eye drops [170].

HYDROPHILIC SOFT CONTACT LENSES

Several kinds of polymers have been used in hard contact lenses, soft contact lenses, and intraocular lenses for correction of refractive errors of the eye.

Hydrophilic contact lenses show double advantages: on the one hand, they may be easily modelled on the eye; on the other, they may be utilized as drug carriers, from which this is to be released under control, to the anterior segment of the eye [176].

In order to establish the contact lenses' capacity to release drugs *in vivo*, L. Cassini-Ingoni [177] analyzes the diffusion and activity of lysozymes in ophthalmic hydrogels. The gel is a swollen statistical copolymer of methacrylate and N-vinyl-2-pyrrolidone ($\approx 70\%$), and the penetration of the enzyme, labelled with 8-anilinonaphthalene-1-sulfonate (ANS), was followed by fluorescence microscopy. ANS is a well-known fluorescent probe and its fluorescence, which is very low in water, is strongly enhanced when the molecule is bound to proteins.

The circular slabs of hydrogel, at equilibrium swelling in water (70% w/w), were immersed in a large excess of a solution of lysozyme and fluorescer ($[Lys]_o = [ANS]_o = 5 \times 10^{-4}$ mol l^{-1}, and $[Lys-ANS]_{eq} = 2.34 \times 10^{-4}$ mol l^{-1}) for different times (3 to 49 h). For each immersion time, the profile of penetration was determined step by step from one edge of the sliced sample to the other. It appears in

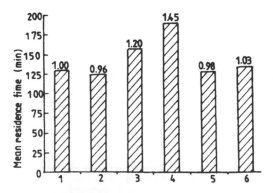

Figure 53. Mean residence time for some formulations compared to a standard pilocarpine solution. 1—Pilocarpine solution (4%); 2—Adsorbocarpine® (4%); 3—poloxamer gel (4%); 4—latex CAP (4%); 5—latex 7203/69B (4%); 6—latex 7203/69A (4%). From Reference [170].

Figure 54 that the lysozyme attains the center of the 3 mm slab within 40–50 h [177].

We noted first that the fluorescence of the complex was again strongly enhanced when trapped into the matrix, as the emission of the immersion solution appeared almost undetectable when observed with the microscope. The second remark concerns the observation across the slice of two symmetrical maxima, which move progressively towards one another when immersion time is increased. The most probable explanation is that, in the highest concentration domains, concentration of the Lys-ANS complex is above the quenching threshold: collisional nonradiative energy transfer between the species strongly decreases the fluorescence, and the intensity I_F cannot be related to the concentration. In the case of ANS alone, in a solvent in which it fluoresces enough (isopropanol), a linear relationship is observed between I_F and C until a threshold of $\approx 5 \times 10^{-4}$ mol l^{-1} is attained [177].

Activity of lysozyme persists inside the matrix, and thus the enzymatic release of molecules immobilized through oligosaccharidic spacers appears conceivable.

Gel-inserted oligosaccharides are hydrolyzed by the diffused lysozyme. Lower oligomers appear within one hour of hydrolysis, which is much more rapid than the eventual release of remaining lysozyme from the extracted slab.

The capacity for drug release from Bionite®, Griffin Laboratory, Soflens® and Bausch & Lomb type contact lenses has been studied by employing fluorescein as a model drug [178].

When employing fluorescein-containing contact lenses in experiments performed on rabbits, the fluorescein concentration into the aqueous humor was observed as four times higher than the values characterizing its administration through installations. In their human studies, a Bionite® lens could maintain the fluorescein concentration in the ocular tissues for 24 h, despite the known rapid exit of fluorescein from the eye.

On the whole, hydrophilic contact lenses may be used as matrices in the controlled release of antibiotics and pilocarpine.

Antibiotics-containing contact lenses have been analyzed by Kaufman et al. [179]; they employed mainly idoxuridine (IDU)- or polymyxin B- containing contact lenses. In the former case, a significant increase in the therapeutic index (in the treatment of rabbit eye infected with McKrae herpes virus) was observed, while Polymyxin B-containing contact lenses were seen to assure a rapid curing of rabbit cornea infected with *Pseudomonas aeruginosa*.

Praus et al. [180] extended these investigations to contact lenses impregnated with 0.1% chloramphenicol or tetracycline. *In vitro* experiments performed with contact lenses of variable thickness (0.3 and 0.9 mm) have evidenced a controlled release of 50% and 40% tetracycline, and 75% and 60% chloramphenicol.

Clinical experiments were made on volunteers suffering from corneal infiltrations; concentration of the tetracycline released after keeping the lenses in the eye for 1.5, 3, and 17 h was established, and a therapeutic level suitable for sterilizing infections in the anterior segment of the eye was found.

Hull et al. [181] use contact lenses (Heficon-A®-copolymer 80% 2-hydroxyethyl methacrylate and 20% N-vinyl-pyrrolidone) impregnated with prednisolone sodium phosphate. Such lenses have led to levels of corneal concentrations in prednisolone two times higher than those characterizing administration through instillations; thus, in four hours, about 99% of the drug was released from the lens. Analyses performed upon the prednisolone content of lenses maintained in the eye at different time intervals evidence that, in the first 3 hours, only 14% of prednisolone was not released and maintained as gel.

E. J. Ivani [182] employs amino-polysaccharides and copolymers thereof for contact lenses and aophthalmic compositions. The series of polymers includes the following: D-glucosamine and acrylonitrile; D-glucosamine and acrylamide; D-glucosamine and an acrylic acid or ester, D-glucosamine and a protein or polypeptide compound, D-glucosamine and collagen, D-glucosamine and elastin and/or resilin; D-glucosamine and an azo compound, e.g., N-vinyl pyrrolidone, and the families represented by the above compounds.

The N-acetyl-D-glucosamine, along with the substituted and copolymers of N-acetyl-D-glucosamine, all form materials which can be used for contact lenses. Contact lenses are usually formed by casting, molding, or lathe-cutting of plastic buttons.

Because of the ability of N-acetyl-glucosamine to act as a wound-healing accelerator, it can find an addi-

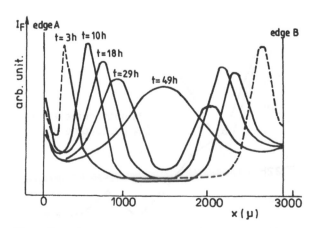

Figure 54. Fluorescence profiles of labelled lysozyme across a swollen slab of poly(VP-co-MMA) hydrogel. I_F—Fluorescence intensity. From Reference [177]; reprinted by permission of the publishers, Hüthig & Wepf, Verlag, Basel.

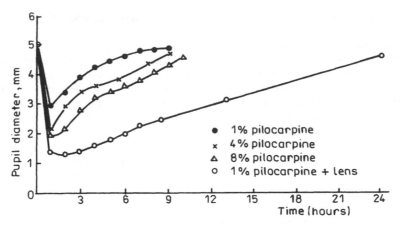

Figure 55. Time course of pupillary response with various concentrations of pilocarpine with or without a contact lens. From Reference [2].

tional application in accelerating the healing process for patients who have undergone cataract surgery, or any other type of eye surgery. The N-acetyl-glucosamine should be formed into a soft lens material, or polyblended into the carrier polymer to allow for maximum therapeutic effect, although any method that will allow for the material to become functional is acceptable. Since the eye, after undergoing surgery, is somewhat sensitive, it would be to the patient's advantage to use a carrier which is soft (chitin–collagen, etc.).

Hydrophilic contact lenses are more and more extensively utilized as matrices for the controlled release of pilocarpine.

Thus, Kaufman and coworkers [179] employ pilocarpine-containing contact lenses, and follow the

drug's effect on using pupil size and intraocular pressure as the indicators. The pupillary-response experiments showed that the contact lens was useful for extending the duration of the response (Figure 55). IOP measurement in glaucoma patients showed that treatment with two drops of 1% pilocarpine, plus the contact lens had a more prolonged effect than two drops of 8% pilocarpine without the lens (Figure 56).

Maddox and Bernstein [182] reported that a Bionite® hydrophilic contact lens could prolong the duration of the pilocarpine effect on the pupillary response of albino rabbits. Compared with a single instillation, a lens presoaked in 4% pilocarpine for 4 h produced greater maximum miosis as well as longer duration of miosis.

Asseff et al. [183] and Kaufman et al. [179] compared the amount of pilocarpine in the aqueous humour of rhesus monkeys after topical application and after using Biotine® lenses presoaked with pilocarpine. A 2-min soak of the lens in 1% pilocarpine resulted in an uptake of 400 g pilocarpine by the lens, which yielded a much higher concentration of pilocarpine in the aqueous humour and a longer half-life than did topical application of 100 μl 0.1% pilocarpine. These findings might be related to enhanced drug penetration due to longer contact time with the cornea, to prolonged duration of action, or to both factors [2].

Soluble Ocular Inserts

Diffusional monolithic soluble inserts, may offer some advantages over the systems described before. In spite of a drug release with first-order kinetics, rather than with the more desirable zero-order kinetics, they have been reported to favour penetration and to prolong the effect of the medical agent. Furthermore they neither necessitate removal from the eye at the end of the therapy, nor suffer an easy expulsion from the conjunctival sac during the sleep of the patient, as is the case with insoluble inserts. Forms of this have been

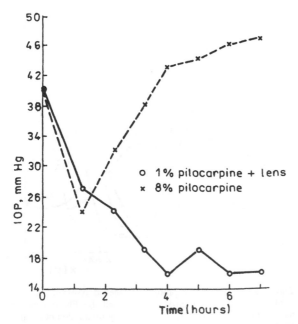

Figure 56. Effect of a soft contact lens on the duration of the hypotensive effect of pilocarpine. From Reference [2].

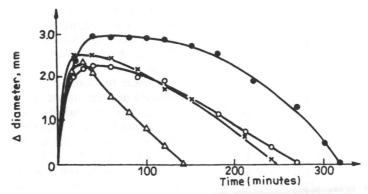

Figure 57. Mean change in pupillary diameter versus time for some preparations under investigation. ($\triangle$) solution 2.0 % PiN; ($\times$) gel containing 1.54% w/v PiN and 0.77% w/v poly(acrylic acid) (GS); ($\bigcirc$) PVA-C (PVA $M_w 10^{-3} = 90$) insert with PiN; ($\bullet$) PVA-C insert with pilocarpine PAA-salt. From Reference [190]; reprinted by permission of the publisher Plenum Publishing Corp.

described in relatively old publications (glycerinated gelation "lamellae" of the 1948 British Pharmacopeia).

Soluble inserts based on synthetic polymers, e.g., poly(acrylamide), poly(ethyl acrylate), poly(vinyl alcohol), poly(vinyl pyrrolidone) have been developed and experimented on humans mainly in the U.S.S.R. by Maichuk and coworkers [184] with drugs such as antibiotics, sulfonamides, pilocarpine, atropine, dexamethasone, etc.

For the patient with glaucoma, insert-pilocarpine (2.61 mg) was useful. Insert-pilocarpine, applied once daily or once every two days, reduced intraocular pressure as much as about 5 to 12 mmHg.

Kitazawa [185] developed rod-shaped soluble ocular inserts containing approximately 2 mg of pilocarpine and film-type inserts containing 4 mg of pilocarpine. The inserts were made from solubilized collagen, which dissolves in 80 min in artificial tears and in 310 min in normal saline. The clinical trial in seven patients with primary open-angle glaucoma showed that at 24 h after the trial started the insert maintained the hypotensive effect and the pupillary response was equivalent to what 4% pilocarpine eye drops did [2].

A water-soluble insert developed by Katz and Blackman [186] was assessed in normal volunteers.

Chitin [poly(N-acetyl-D-glucosamine)] is solubilized by the lysozyme found in the tear. This property was utilized by Capozza [187] for preparing bioerodible pilocarpine-containing inserts. Experiments performed on rabbit eyes evidenced erosion of the insert and a pupillary response for 6 h.

Biosoluble synthetic inserts containing between 0.0–2.0 mg pilocarpine [188] have been tested on patients suffering from intraocular hypertension. IOP variation has been followed, as well as the pupillary response and ocular irritation in the interval 1–32 h. Maximum values of the pupillary contraction were attained between 1–8 h. The hypotensive effect of the insert was maintained for more than 24 h.

Pavan-Langston [189] has discussed the soluble

ocular insert prepared by Merck Sharp & Dohme and used in the studies of Katz and Blackman [186] and Bensinger et al. [188].

M. F. Saettone and coworkers [190] have prepared a series of pilocarpine-containing soluble inserts, using the following as polymers: poly(vinyl alcohol) (PVA), hydroxypropylcellulose (HPC), poly(acrylic acid) (PAA). Transparent flexible films containing pilocarpine nitrate were obtained by slow evaporation of 5.0% w/v solutions of polymers containing the appropriate amount of PiN. The films (0.4–0.5 mm thickness) were cut in the form of small disks (4.0 mm diameter), each containing 1.0 $\pm$ 0.05 mg PiN.

Typical miosis–time data for some preparations under study are illustrated in Figure 57.

Administration of 50 μl of the 2.0% PiN solution S (corresponding to 1.0 mg of the drug) produced miosis of relatively short duration (2 h), declining rapidly after reaching the peak effect. Conversely, a PVA-C insert containing 1.0 mg PiN produced a more prolonged effect (≈ 4 h), that was practically of 50 μl of the gel GS, containing a corresponding amount of pilocarpine base. As shown in Figure 57, when the pilocarpine-PAA salt was administered as dispersion in a PVA-C insert, a stronger miotic response with an activity plateau was observed, as was an overall 5 h duration.

The areas under the curves illustrating the miotic response versus time (AUC) for all preparations tested were evaluated from graphs such as those illustrated in Figure 57, and are reported in Figure 58 with the corresponding 95% confidence limits. The AUC values should reflect the aqueous humour concentration of the drug, thus being indicative of the bioavailability of PiN from the vehicles under study [190].

Salification of the drug base with the polyanionic polymer G exerted a profound influence on overall drug activity, that was enhanced when the salt was administered as dispersion in a solid insert. This effect had been partially anticipated in the literature [191–195].

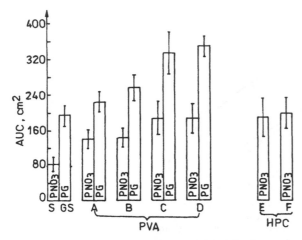

Figure 58. Areas under the miotic activity versus time curves for all preparations described. PNO₃ = pilocarpine nitrate; PG = pilocarpine PAA-G salt. Vertical lines over lears indicate 95% confidence limits. From Reference [190]; reprinted by permission of the publisher Plenum Publishing Corp.

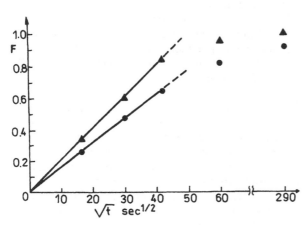

Figure 59. Graphs illustrating *in vitro* release of pilocarpine from PVA-C inserts containing PiN (▲) and pilocarpine PAA-salt (●). From Reference [190]; reprinted by permission of the publisher Plenum Publishing Corp.

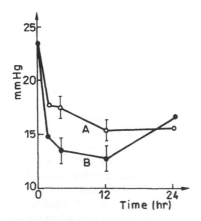

Figure 60. IOP reduction in humans after administration of a PiNO₃/PVA insert (A), and a Pi-PAA/PVA insert (B). The dose corresponded to 0.77 mg of base; vertical lines indicate 95% C.L. From Reference [197].

Typical *in vitro* release data from the present inserts are reported in Figure 59 [190], where the fractions of drug released (F) from the PVA-C inserts containing PiN and the drug PAA-G salt are plotted versus the square root of time.

A linear relationship between the fraction of drug released and the square root of time up to 70–80% release was observed in all cases, indicating that diffusion was the most important mechanism contributing to drug release from these systems under the *in vitro* experimental conditions [191].

The activity pattern of all inserts corresponded to a prolonged-pulse release, with higher activity peaks and increased duration respect to the miotic effect produced by PiN eye drops [196]. Clinical tests on glaucoma patients carried out with the PiN/PVA and the Pi-PAA/PVA inserts, showed that both types could effectively control IOP for a 24-h period after a single administration (Figure 60) [197–199].

M. F. Saettone et al. [200] have prepared a series of copolymers which have acrylic acid in common: (1) AA-methyl acrylate; (2) AA-vinyl acetate; (3) AA-hydroxyethyl acrylate; (4) AA-acrylamide; (5) AA-acrylamide-N-vinyl pyrrolidone; (6) AA-acrylamide-vinyl acetate; (7) AA-methyl acrylate-hydroxyethyl acrylate. Polymers (2) and (5) also containing 5% w/w triethylene glycol monomethylether acrylate as an internal plasticizer. Polymers (2), (5) and (6) were selected after the preliminary trials, and were used to prepare inserts, each containing 1.04 mg of pilocarpine base (PiB). These were tested for miotic activity in rabbits in comparison with equal doses of Pi given in aqueous solution, and in a reference insert prepared with poly(AA) in a poly(vinyl alcohol) (PVA) matrix. Miosis tests were also carried out with inserts containing polymers (2), (5) and (6) (plus pilocarpine base) in a PVA matrix. The presence of 5 to 50% w/w PVA resulted in a significant increase in the bioavailability of the drug. The addition of PVA to the inserts presumably increases the efficiency of these preparations by reducing their solubility in the lacrimal fluid, thereby prolonging their time of residence in the eye [196] (Figure 61).

Interestingly, an apparently linear relationship was observed between the drug bioavailability (expressed

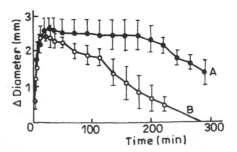

Figure 61. Miotic effect in rabbits of Pi base in inserts prepared with Polymer 5 alone (B), and in Polymer 5 plus 50% PVA. Vertical lines indicate 95% C.L. From Reference [197].

as the area under the miotic activity versus time curve, or AUC) and the PVA content of the composite matrices [197] (Figure 62).

M. F. Saettone and coworkers [201] prepared — from hyaluronic acid (HA) — viscous solutions with 2% PiN, and also inserts, as discs with a thickness of 0.3 mm, 5.0 mm in diameter, each containing 1.0 mg PiN.

The behaviour in rabbit eyes of some representative fluorescein-containing vehicles is described in Table 18 [202]. The inclusion of a fluorescent marker in polymeric ophthalmic vehicles has been done in many instances [203] for investigations on the retention time, and on the influence of polymers on the thickness of precorneal tear film.

Data given in Table 18 evidences that both HA1-Na inserts (E and C) underwent a fast hydration and apparently disappeared rapidly from the eye; the E insert, however, took a longer time to hydrate (10 versus 2 min), and formed a longer-lasting fluorescent film over the cornea (45 versus 10 min for the C insert). The higher-mol wt HA2-Na inserts performed better with respect to the previously mentioned ones: the E insert also in this case underwent a slower hydration (30 versus 10 min), and both formed a stable corneal film lasting 60 min [202]. The HA1-Na and HA2-Na

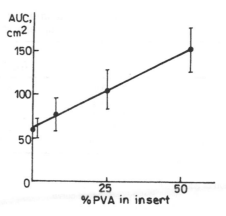

Figure 62. Relationship between Pi ocular bioavailability and PVA content of inserts prepared with Polymer 5. Vertical lines indicate 95% C.L. From Reference [197].

solutions behaved essentially as the corresponding C inserts.

In conclusion, some differences among the present vehicles, already observed in the muco-adhesion tests, also emerged from the tests *in vivo*. The correlations between *in vivo* ocular behaviour and *in vitro* mucoadhesion observed for the low and high-mol wt HA inserts, and for the C and E inserts, are noteworthy: to a higher mol wt and to a slower hydration (the latter depending also on the manufacturing technique), a better muco-adhesion and an improved retention in the eye seem to correspond [202].

All preparations were tested for miotic activity in albino rabbits, in comparison with suitable reference liquid vehicles or inserts containing the same amount of drug.

Table 19 summarizes the results of experiments, in which some representative vehicles were tested for miotic activity on albino rabbits [202].

All polymeric vehicles were capable of increasing the bioavailability of Pi to a statistically significant extent with respect to the standard aqueous vehicle (AS). A closer inspection of the activity parameters listed in Table 19, however, indicates a rather fast and uncontrolled release (characterized by a high I_{max} value, a short peak time, a relatively short duration) for the HA1-Na solution and, to a lesser extent, for the HA2-Na solution.

Another agent showing mydriatic activity — Tropicamide (Tr) — was introduced in solutions and inserts of HA [202]. The results of the mydriatic activity tests are reported in Table 20 [202].

The rationale for evaluating the activity of Tr in the prospective bioadhesive vehicles was the lower solubility of this drug with respect to Pi. Due to the limited water solubility of Tr (570 mg/100 ml) the drug was partially suspended in the semisolid vehicles and the HA1-Na and HA2-Na matrices could be prepared only by compression.

A comparison of the data observed with the corresponding Pi and Tr vehicles is provided in Figure 63,

Table 18. Evaluation of the behaviour of the semisolid and solid vehicles in rabbit eyes.

Vehicle	Remarks
HA1-Na sol.	The solution is diluted, and overflows after 10 min. A weakly fluorescent film lasts 10 min.
HA2-Na sol.	The solution undergoes slow dilution, with no apparent overflow. A fluorescent corneal film lasts 45 min.
HA1-Na E	The insert hydrates within 10 min forming a gel-like mass. An overflow is observed after 15 min. A uniform corneal film lasts 45 min.
HA1-Na C	The insert hydrates quickly (2 min) forming a gel-like mass. A non-uniform, weakly fluorescent corneal film lasts 15 min.
HA2-Na E	The insert undergoes a slow hydration (30 min) forming a gel-like mass. A fluorescent corneal film lasts 60 min.
HA2-Na C	The insert undergoes a fast hydration (10 min) forming a gel-like mass. A corneal film lasts 60 min.
HAE C	The insert undergoes a slow hydration, then, 90 min after application, it undergoes a slow erosion, which terminates after 6 h. During this time, it clings tenaciously to the scleral conjunctiva. No uniform corneal film is observed, probably on account of a low dissolution rate and insufficient release of fluorescein.

HA1-Na, HA2-Na—HA sodium salt fractions; E = matrix prepared by casting; C = matrix prepared by compression.

Table 19. Summary of the miotic activity parameters in rabbits of some representative vehicles containing pilocarpine.

Vehicle	I_{max}[a], mm (95% CL)	T_{max}[b] min	D^c, min (95% CL)	AUC[d], cm² (95% CL)	Relative AUC
AS[e]	2.3 (0.5)	30	150 (18)	39.1 (6.7)	1.00
HA1-Na sol.	3.8 (0.3)	15	270 (20)	107.7 (21.5)	2.75
HA2-Na sol.	3.3 (0.3)	30	270 (30)	112.0 (17.3)	2.86
HA1-Na (E)	2.9 (0.4)	30	270 (28)	89.4 (13.8)	2.28
HA2-Na (E)	2.7 (0.4)	40	300 (25)	111.8 (14.2)	2.86

[a]Maximal miotic response.
[b]Peak time.
[c]Duration of activity (time for the pupillary diameter to return to the baseline value).
[d]Area under the miotic activity versus time curve.
[e]Isotonic, buffered (pH 5.5) aqueous solution containing 2.0% w/w PiN.

where the AUC values observed for Pi are plotted versus the Tr values. Although in two cases the vehicles were not strictly the same (E inserts for Pi, and C inserts for Tr), the graph shows that the relative bioavailability increases were greater when the vehicles contained Tr. The dotted line represents the result that would be expected if the relative AUC increases produced by the Tr vehicles equalled those produced by the Pi vehicles [202].

This point can also be evidenced in the graphs shown in Figure 64 illustrating the relationship found, for each of the Pi and Tr vehicles, between "bioadhesion" (detachment force measured at pH 7.40) and AUC values. In spite of a great increase in bioadhesion, the AUC increases observed for the Pi delivery systems were relatively poor in comparison with those observed for Tr. These results, which presumably descend from the previously anticipated "solubility" effect, stress the importance of the permanence of the drug in a bioadhesive ocular vehicle. To profit most from the characteristics of these vehicles, a drug should possess appropriate physico-chemical properties, such as a reduced solubility (and/or diffusivity). This would ensure for the drug a reasonably prolonged time of permanence in the vehicle, while the vehicle would be able to withstand a prolonged time of residence in the eye [202].

PVA-based inserts with lower solubility were ob-

tained by irradiating an aqueous solution of a PVA with an ionizing radiation to such an extent that the PVA in the aqueous solution is cross-linked to have an equilibrium swelling ratio in water in the range from 70 to 100 by weight, at room temperature; and then impregnating the obtained hydrated gel with an ophthalmically active ingredient to a desired therapeutically effective concentration [204]. Starting from this modified PVA, pilocarpine-containing high-viscosity eye lotions have been prepared. The concentration of the pilocarpine in the finished eye lotion was dependent on the blending ratio of the hydrated PVA gel and the aqueous pilocarpine solution, as shown in Figure 65.

Figure 66 shows the variation in the rabbit pupillary diameters, depending on time, during the administration of the drops (curve A) and of the ointment, containing 1% pilocarpine.

Among soluble inserts there may also be included the bioerodible ones, obtained from partial esters (ethyl, 2-methoxyethyl, n-butyl) of (maleic acid–alkyl vinyl ether) copolymers, with ethyl or n-butyl as alkyl substituents.

A first ophthalmic application of such matrices was described by Heller and Baker [99], who found that the release of hydrocortisone in rabbit eyes followed zero-order kinetics.

More recently, the release properties of ocular ma-

Table 20. Summary of the mydriatic activity parameters in rabbits of some representative vehicles containing tropicamide.

Vehicle	I_{max}[a], mm (95% CL)	T_{max}[b], min	D^c, min (95% CL)	AUC[d], cm² (95% CL)	Relative AUC
AS[e]	2.7 (0.3)	30	220 (30)	80 (14)	1.00
HA1-Na sol.	2.6 (0.3)	180	900 (85)	289 (52)	3.61
HA2-Na sol.	2.4 (0.2)	120	960 (90)	295 (48)	3.68
HA1-Na (C)	2.5 (0.3)	30	960 (87)	293 (55)	3.66
HA2-Na (C)	2.6 (0.3)	60	1020 (103)	330 (60)	4.12

[a]Maximal mydriatic response.
[b]Peak time.
[c]Duration of activity (time for the pupillary diameter to return to the baseline value).
[d]Area under the mydriatic activity versus time curve.
[e]Aqueous solution containing 1.0% (w/w) tropicamide.

trices prepared with three different half-esters of (maleic acid–methyl vinyl ether) copolymers containing pilocarpine HCl have been investigated *in vitro* and *in vivo* by Urtti et al. [205–206].

Saettone et al. [207] obtained ocular matrices containing ionically-bound PiB on using a series of (alkyl maleate–alkyl vinyl ether) copolymers with different alkyl substituents in the ester and ether moieties.

The parent (maleic anhydride–alt-alkyl vinyl ether) copolymers were prepared by free radical (AIBN) polymerization [208] of maleic anhydride and vinyl ether (Table 21) [207].

The (alkyl maleate–co-alkyl vinyl ether) copolymers were derived from the preformed anhydride copolymers by esterification with excess alcohol typically at reflux of dioxane solution [207]. The degree of esterification varied in the approximate range 40–50%, corresponding to one ester per repeating unit, consistent with the uncatalyzed esterification reaction employed.

Polymers 1–7 (Table 21) were used for the preparation of the inserts (Table 22) [207], which were submitted to *in vitro* tests aimed at verifying their solvation/dissolution behaviour, and their drug-release characteristics. All the matrices contained glycerol (9–13% w/w) as plasticizer.

The results of the experiments aimed at assessing quantitatively the solvation and overall weight loss of the medicated matrices in the less concentrated (1.3 mM) buffer are represented in Figure 67 [207].

In all cases the sorption process was rapid, and after 30 min a 94–96% weight increase was observed. The water sorption was accompanied by substantial swelling.

A gradual loss of the insert's weight, as evaluated with respect to the initial dry weight, was also observed during the contact with the buffer solution [207]. The overall loss of weight at equilibrium never

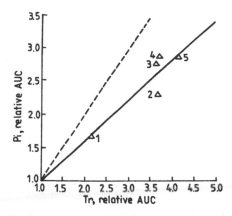

Figure 63. Comparison of the relative AUC value observed with the Pi and with the Tr vehicles. 1—PAA-4 poly(acid acrylic) gel; 2—HAl-Na matrices (C, E); 3—HAl-Na sol.; 4—HA2-Na sol.; 5—HA2-Na matrices (C, E). The dotted line represents the results to be expected if the vehicles would produce the same relative bioavailability increases with the two drugs. From Reference [202].

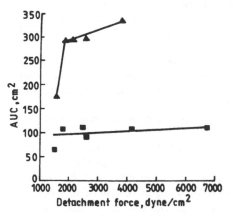

Figure 64. Graph illustrating the relationship existing between AUC values and mucoadhesive force for the pilocarpine (■) and for the tropicamide (▲) vehicles. From Reference [202].

Table 21. Structural characteristics of partial esters of poly(maleic anhydride-alt-alkyl vinyl ethers).

$$—(—CH_2—CH—CH——CH—)—_n$$
$$\quad\quad\quad |\quad\quad |\quad\quad\quad |$$
$$\quad\quad OR\quad COOH\quad COOR$$

Sample	R	R′	Esterification, mEq/g[a] %		dl/g[b]
1	—C₂H₅	—CH₃	43	5.4	0.95
2	—C₂H₅	—CH₃	54	4.5	0.95
3	—C₂H₅	—C₂H₅	46	4.8	0.98
4	—C₂H₅	—nC₄H₉	44	4.4	0.47
5	—C₂H₅	—CH₂CH₂OCH₃	40	4.7	0.60
6	—nC₄H₉	—CH₃	40	4.9	0.69
7	—C₄H₉	—CH₃	54	4.3	0.61

[a]mEq of 0.1 N NaOH required for neutralization of 1.0 g of polymer.
[b]In DMSO at 30°C.
From Saettone, M. F., B. Giannaccini, G. Leonardi, D. Monti, P. Chetoni, G. Galli and E. Chiellini, *Polymers in Medicine III*. C. Migliaresi, L. Nicolais, P. Giusti, E. Chiellini, eds. Elsevier, p. 209 (1988), by permission of the publishers, Elsevier Science Publishers, 1988.

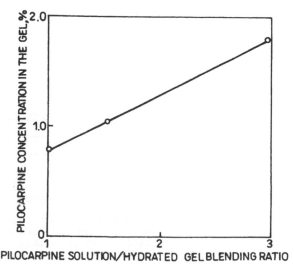

Figure 65. Relationship between the blending ratio by weight and the concentration of the pilocarpine in the eye lotion. From Reference [204].

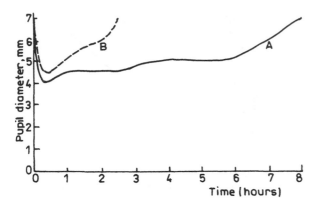

Figure 66. Variation of the pupillary diameter (rabbits) with time. A—Administration of 1% pilocarpine-containing ointment; B—control. From Reference [204].

exceeded 45%; this maximum value was reached by matrices 3T, 4T and 7.

The mechanism of drug release from water-insoluble polymeric materials containing salt–forming groups is rather complex, and involves [209]:

- solvation of the matrix and diffusion within the matrix of eluting counter-ions (buffer)
- exchange of the drug molecule with the counter-ion
- diffusion of the eluted drug out of the matrix

In the case of the present matrices, the release is further complicated by the partial dissolution of the pilocarpine-loaded inserts, and by osmotic effects directly influencing the extent of solvation and consequent swelling. The results of these experiments are summarized in Table 23 [207]. In both buffers, the release process followed "square root" kinetics, thus indicating that drug diffusion from the water swollen

matrices is a predominant factor in the process. In the 1.3 mM buffer the overall amount of drug released at the plateau of the diffusive process ranged from 32.5% (insert 1) to 41.6% (insert 7).

The release "rates" (fraction released/$\sqrt{t}$) appeared somewhat sensitive to the structural properties of the polymers (Figures 68, 69). The overall amount of drug released at equilibrium in buffer pH 7.4 (1.3 mM) (Figure 68) ranged from 78% (insert 3) to 95% (insert 2) [207].

The results of the miotic activity tests on albino rabbits of the individual inserts, and of the reference aqueous solution (AS) are summarized in Table 24. The AUC values are also reported graphically in Figure 70. As indicated, all the inserts except 3T and 4T produced with respect to the aqueous solution AS:

- a slight (10–15%) increase of the peak miotic activity (I_{max})
- a delayed peak time, particularly evident for insert 1–4
- An increased duration of activity (130–190 min in the case of inserts 1–5, and 90 min in the case of inserts 6 and 7), which was statistically significant in all cases. The overall bioavailability of pilocarpine from the matrices was approximately twice that of the reference solution, with the only exception being sample 6, for which no statistically significant difference with respect to AS was observed [207].

Poly(vinyl alcohol) (PVAl)-based soluble ocular inserts or copolymers of polyacrylamide, ethylacrylate and vinylpyrrolidone (SODI) have been prepared [210–211] for the controlled administration—into the eye—of tetracycline (in the case of PVAl) or of

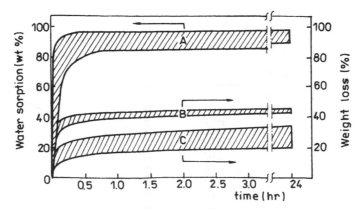

Figure 67. Results of water sorption and weight loss tests carried out on the medicated inserts in 1.3 mM phosphate buffer. A—Water sorption of all samples of Table 22, calculated as (weight of hydrated insert—weight of drug residue)/weight of dry residue × 100; B—percent weight loss of inserts 3T and 4T, calculated with respect to the initial weight of the insert; C—percent weight loss of all the remaining samples of Table 22, also calculated with respect to the initial weight of the inserts. From Reference [207]; reprinted by permission of the publishers, Elsevier Science Publishers.

Table 22. Chemical composition of the medicated polymer matrices.[a]

Matrix No.	Polymer No.	Polymer % (w/w)	Pi Base % (w/w)	Glycerol % (w/w)	mEq Polymer/ mEq Pi Base	Solvent[b]
1	1	74.1	16.4	9.5	5.2	A
2	2	69.3	18.8	11.9	3.5	E
3	3	74.6	16.1	9.3	4.7	A
3T[c]	3	44.1	15.0	8.6	—	A/W 8.3
4	4	72.2	17.6	10.2	3.8	E
4T[c]	4	44.1	17.1	9.9	—	E
5	5	74.1	16.4	9.5	4.5	A
6	6	71.7	15.8	12.5	4.7	A
7	7	73.5	16.2	10.3	4.1	A

[a]Based on 90 mg of polymer component.
[b]A = acetone; E = ethanol; W = water.
[c]Neutralized with triethanolamine before addition of PiB (mEq polymer/mEq triethanolamine = 1).
From Saettone, M. F., B. Giannaccini, G. Leonardi, D. Monti, P. Chetoni, G. Galli and E. Chiellini. *Polymers in Medicine III*. C. Migliaresi, L. Nicolais, P. Giusti, E. Chiellini, eds. Elsevier, p. 209 (1988), by permission of the publishers, Elsevier Science Publishers, 1988.

pilocarpine, atropine, neomycin, kanamycin, sulfapyridazine, tetracaine hydrochloride and idoxuridine.

Tetracycline inserts induced, in the conjunctival sac, antibiotic concentrations ranging between 243 μg/ml (3 h)–3.4 μg/ml (24 h).

As far as concerns the SODI inserts, they have been prepared from films, from which elliptical forms of $9 \times 4.5 \times 0.3$ mm have been cut out. These inserts have been impregnated with the following drugs:

- pilocarpine—2.6 mg
- atropine—1.59 mg
- neomycin—1.13 mg
- kanamycin—1.22 mg
- sulfapyridazine—5.25 mg
- tetracaine HCl—0.75 mg
- idoxuridine—1.7 mg

During the time when these inserts set out into the conjunctival sac, they have been observed to be quickly swollen by tears, being dissolved in a maximum of 90 minutes.

Tests performed on animals (i.e., on rabbit eyes) have shown that these inserts determine a suitable drug concentration in the eye. For example, the SODI–kanamycin system (1.22 mg) induces a conjunctival concentration up to 5.8 μg/g in 48 h, the SODI–idoxuridine one brings about a 12-day curing of patients affected by dendritic keratitis, while the SODI–pilocarpine system determines an IOP decrease up to 5–12 mmHg, after daily administration of a single insert.

Ophthalmic inserts based on cross-linked polypeptides or polysaccharides have been prepared by Dohlman et al. [212]. Such hydrocortisone acetate-

Table 23. In vitro release data in buffers of different concentration.[a]

Matrix	Release "Rate" ($F/\sqrt{t}$)[b] A	B	Drug Released at Equilibrium, % A	B	Lag Time, min A	B
1	39.6	79.2	36.0	89.1	5.0	3.4
2	30.4	76.6	39.5	95.1	4.4	4.4
3	31.7	59.8	41.6	78.1	5.4	5.4
3T	37.3	69.6	63.0	95.0	1.5	1.5
4	24.7	59.9	39.3	90.8	24.6	9.6
4T	37.5	69.6	69.0	95.2	1.5	1.5
5	35.4	63.8	40.0	92.7	3.4	3.4
6	30.4	57.1	32.5	88.4	7.7	1.1
7	19.3	52.1	38.0	86.6	3.5	3.5

[a]1.3 mM, pH 7.4 phosphate buffer (A); 66.7 mM, pH 7.4 phosphate buffer (B).
[b]Calculated from the linear portion of the "square root" release plot.
F = fraction released; t = time in hr.
From Saettone, M. F., B. Giannaccini, G. Leonardi, D. Monti, P. Chetoni, G. Galli and E. Chiellini, *Polymers in Medicine III*, C. Migliaresi, L. Nicolais, P. Giusti, E. Chiellini, eds. Elsevier, p. 209 (1988), by permission of the publishers, Elsevier Science Publishers, 1988.

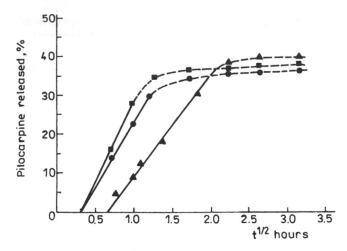

Figure 68. Plots of pilocarpine release from insert 1 (■), 3 (●) and 4 (▲) in 1.3 mM, pH 7.4 phosphate buffer, showing decreasing release "rates" with decreasing hydrophilicity of the polymers. From Reference [207]; reprinted by permission of the publishers, Elsevier Science Publishers.

containing inserts have a release rate of 14.9 or 2 μg/h. The results of the treatment of rabbit xenograph reaction indicated that the devices with release rates of 9 or 2 μg/h showed as good an anti-inflammatory effect as treatment with 2.5% or 0.25% hydrocortisone acetate drops four times daily. The ocular inserts thus showed the advantages of drug efficiency: low dose and high effectiveness.

Inserts based on reticulated polypeptides, containing 10 mg hydrocortisone, have been tested on human volunteers by Allansmith et al. [213]. The drug's release rate is of 10 μg/h. The insert has been gradually eroded into the eye, being wholly dissolved after about 3 weeks. They used a model of ocular inflammatory condition that appears in a person with a history of seasonal allergic rhinitis (hay fever) after a

drop of antigen has been applied into the lower cul-de-sac. Hydrocortisone inserts lessened the redness in the inflamed eye and made it feel more comfortable.

Elliptical inserts, based on polypeptide with hydrocortisone acetate, having a release rate of 10 μg/h, and others, with prednisolone acetate and the same release rate, have been tested in inflammatory processes of the eye [214]. The degree of inflammation was evaluated by Draize-type scoring. With the same total amount of drug, the hydrocortisone acetate insert reduced the inflammation better than did eye drops. Prednisolone acetate also reduced the conjunctivitis to a level within the normal range.

Inserts based on polypeptides with idoxuridine have been tested in the treatment of acute herpes simplex keratitis in rabbits [215]. The release rates were 0.5,

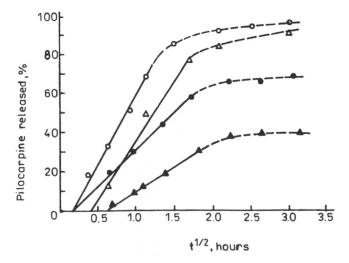

Figure 69. Release of pilocarpine from insert 4 (triangles) and 4T (dots) to pH 7.4 phosphate buffers of different concentration. Open symbols refer to the more concentrated buffer (66.7 mM); full symbols refer to the less concentrated one (1.3 mM). From Reference [207]; reprinted by permission of the publishers, Elsevier Science Publishers.

Table 24. Summary of the miotic activity data in rabbits obtained with the inserts under study.

Inserts	I_{max}	PT	D	AUC
Solution AS	2.41 ± 0.3	40	300 ± 22	74.9 ± 21.0
1	2.75 ± 0.6	90	450 ± 11	162.0 ± 45.0
2	2.83 ± 0.6	90	450 ± 16	179.0 ± 32.3
3	2.60 ± 0.5	90	430 ± 16	159.0 ± 46.3
3T	3.33 ± 0.4	30	270 ± 15	84.6 ± 16.8
4	2.58 ± 0.5	90	490 ± 22	158.0 ± 31.1
4T	3.41 ± 0.5	20	270 ± 22	96.0 ± 21.9
5	3.16 ± 0.6	60	450 ± 21	165.0 ± 33.2
6	2.91 ± 0.6	60	390 ± 10	121.0 ± 31.5
7	2.91 ± 0.2	60	390 ± 16	144.0 ± 20.5

I_{max} = Peak miotic response, $\Delta\emptyset$ (mm ± 95% CL); PT = peak time (min); D = duration of miotic activity (min ± 95% CL); AUC = area under the activity versus time curve (cm² ± 95% CL).

7.0, 15.0, or 30.0 μg/h. The 30.0 μg/h inserts, changed every 4 days, gave faster and better results than did conventional therapy with 0.1% idoxuridine eye drops seven times daily plus 1% idoxuridine ointment for overnight, and, in addition, the inserts exposed the eye to 40% less drug [2].

Another soluble collagen ocular insert was developed by Bloomfield et al. [216]. The oval insert weighed 10 mg and was made from succinylated enzyme-solubilized collagen, it contained 1.1 mg gentamycin (Figure 71). The insert can be solubilized at physiologic pH, gradually releasing the drug.

On employing reticulated PVA gels [204] lotions with 0.05% tropicamide as a mydriatic, with 0.05% chloramphenicol as an antibiotic or 0.05% of dexamethasone as an antiphlogistic, respectively, obtained high-viscosity eye lotions exhibiting very durable activity. Figure 72 shows the results of the elution tests with tropicamide, chloramphenicol and dexamethasone impregnated hydrated PVA gels.

In one of his patents, S. S. Chrai (and coworkers) [217] describes a topical ophthalmic gel for use in the eye of human and domestic animals, comprising an ophthalmic medicament in a gel maintained at a pH of 6.5–8.5. More particularly, the invention provides a topical ophthalmic gel comprising: 0.05–10% by weight of an ophthalmic medicament; 1–3% by weight of a PVA; 0.1–1% by weight of a borate gelling agent; and 85–99% sterile water; said gel being maintained at a pH of 6.5–8.5.

Ophthalmic drugs suitable for incorporation into the gel of the invention include, but are not limited to, antibiotics such as tetracycline, chlortetracycline, bacitracin, neomycin, polymixin, gramicidin, oxytetracycline, chloramphenicol, gentamicin, sisomicin, penicillin and erythromycin; antibacterials such as sulfamides, sulfacetamide, sulfamethizole and sulfisoxazole; antivirals such as idoxuridine and vidarabine; other antibacterial agents such as nitrofurazone and sodium propionate; antiallergenics such as antazoline, methapyriline, chlorpheniramine, pyrilamine and prophen-pyridamine; anti-inflammatories such as hydrocortisone, hydrocortisone acetate, dexamethasone, dexamethasone 21-phosphate, fluocimoline, medrysone, prednisolone, methyl prednisolone, prednisolone 21-phosphate, prednisolone acetate, fluorometholone, bethamethasone, bethamethasone valerate, treamcinoline, indomethacin and flunixin; mydriatics such as atropine sulfate, cyclopentolate, homatropine, scopolamine, tropicamide, encatropine and hydroxyamphetamine; and sympathomimetics such as epinephrine.

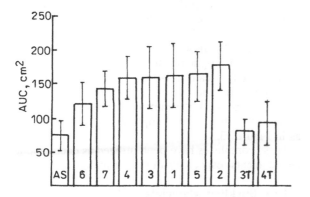

Figure 70. Comparison among the AUC values (miotic activity in rabbits) obtained with the inserts under investigation and with the reference solution (AS). From Reference [207]; reprinted by permission of the publishers, Elsevier Science Publishers.

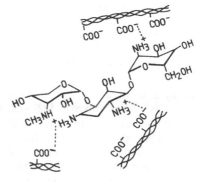

Figure 71. Solubilization of insert with release of bound gentamicin. From Reference [216]; reprinted by permission of the publishers, American Medical Association, 1978.

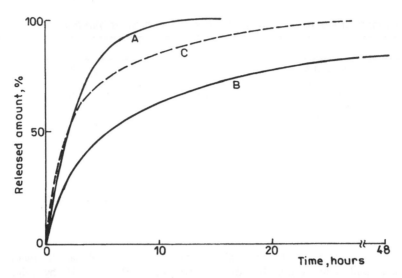

Figure 72. Release rate of tropicamide (A) chloramphenicol (B) and dexamethasone (C) from hydrated PVA gel [204].

The PVA employed has a minimum molecular weight of 10,000, assuring a controlled release of the drug in the process of dissolution by the lacrimal liquid. The gelling agent (sodium or potassium borate) assures a satisfactory consistency of the ointment which, once introduced into the conjunctival sac, acquires the character of an insert.

K. Arizono and coworkers [218] prepared a pranoprofen gelled ointment. An anti-inflammatory and analgesic gelled ointment contains, in addition to pranoprofen, at least one member selected from the group consisting of lower aliphatic alcohol, polyethylene glycol, methyl ethyl ketone and acetone; a gelling agent selected from the group consisting of carboxyvinyl polymer, hydroxyethyl cellulose, alginic acid and carboxymethyl cellulose; a water-soluble basic substance selected from the group consisting of ammonia, sodium hydroxide, potassium hydroxide, triethanolamine, diethanolamine, diisopropanolamine, triisopropanolamine and triethylamine; and water.

Atropine has been chemically bound to polyethylene glycol [219] (PEG) to obtain soluble inserts with controlled release of this alkaloid.

We have previously attached atropine to short oligomers of PEG by a carbonate linkage [219] using the reaction of the chlorocarbonate derivative of PEG with the hydroxyl group of atropine. The highest molecular weight compound was the most active.

S. Zalipsky and coworkers [220] have attached atropine to PEG, by a urethane linkage through a hexamethylene spacer. It is known [221–222] that polyurethane derivatives of PEG are suitable for ophthalmic use. They also suffer degradation in the living organism due to hydrolysis of the unstable carbamic acid and the alcohol. Thus, the urethane linkage seems to offer a suitable system for the slow release of atropine.

Various PEG derivatives [$MeO(CH_2CH_2O)_n-OH$]

have been modified through the treatment with hexamethylene diisocyanate, obtaining polymers with the structure:

$$MeO(CH_2CH_2O)_nCONH(CH_2)_6NCO$$

These compounds have reacted with atropine, in dry toluene, with dibutyltin dilaurate as a catalyst. The products were soluble in water.

Atropine was attached to PEG also through an ester linkage. In this respect, PEG with final carboxylic groups has been prepared, by the reaction with succinic anhydride [233]. Further on, this product reacts with atropine, in the presence of dicyclohexylcarbodiimide and dimethylamino pyridine as catalysts.

The complexation of appropriate organoplatinum compounds by water-soluble polymers has the potential to provide a time-release formulation which might afford a substantial reduction in the severity of side effects associated with use of organoplatinum antitumor agents. Both poly(N-vinylpyrrolidone) (PVP) and poly(N-vinyl-5-methyl-2-oxazolidone) (PVOM) form stable, biologically active molecular complexes with organoplatinum compounds containing polar aromatic ligands. Platinum compounds suitable for complexation by these polymers include cis-dichloro-(4-substituted o-phenylenediamine) platinum (II), 4-substituted catecholato(1,2-diaminocyclohexane) platinum (II) and 4-substituted phthallato(1,2-diaminocyclohexane) platinum (II) compounds [224].

Generally, these PVA complexes may be formulated as in Figure 73.

These complexes have been utilized as chemotherapeutic agents, especially in ocular malignancies.

Scleral Buckling Materials

Scleral buckling materials are used in retinal detachment surgery. In some situations, a post-

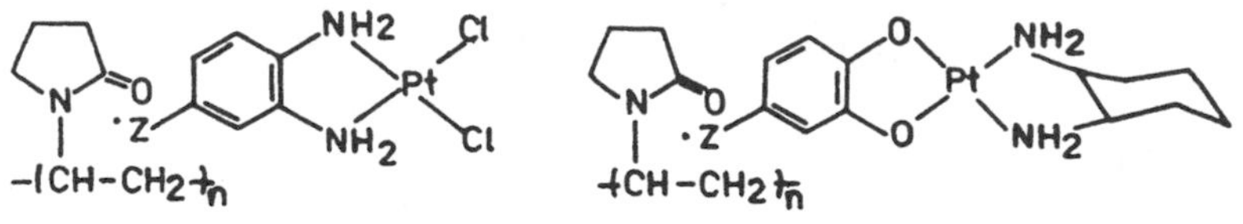

Figure 73. Structure of platinum–PVA complexes. $Z = -OH, -COOH, -SO_3H$ or other polar functional group; $n = 90$–350. From Reference [224].

operational infection, affecting an important eye region, i.e., the posterior part, occurs [225].

Thus, on having in view post-operational protection, scleral buckling materials were impregnated with various drugs, mainly antibiotics.

Refojo and Thomas [225], also interested in this aspect, employed gelatin or silicone rubber discs impregnated with various antibiotics—mainly chloramphenicol or lincomycin.

Lincomycin hydrochloride-impregnated gelatin discs evidence a significant antimicrobial activity (as the microbiological analysis on agar gel seeded with *Sarcina lutea* has shown), lasting for six days.

As to silicone rubber (Silastic® 500-9), this is observed as previously swelling due to propylene oxide. The obtained gel is immersed in solutions of antibiotics with chloramphenicol or lincomycin.

In the former case, an inhibition region on gelose plates has been obtained up to 20 days (Figure 74). By further introduction of the samples into chloramphenicol solutions, they are being loaded with antibiotics.

Silicones employed in scleral buckling materials as drug carriers have, as basic structure, polydimethyl siloxane in which various functionalities, such as silanol ($\equiv Si-OH$), vinyl ($\equiv Si-CH=CH_2$), alkoxy ($\equiv Si-OR$) or hydrosilyl ($\equiv Si-H$). Utilizing these chemically reactive materials, cross-links can be incorporated into the structure to produce gels (5000 repeat units per cross-link) through elastomers (100 repeat units per cross-link) [226].

Medical grade, cross-linkable materials employed in ophthalmology, based on the following reactions, are currently available [227] (Figure 75).

Folkman and Long [228] pioneered such approaches in 1966, when they patented the use of tubing and adhesive to form a capsule, through which a therapeutic agent may diffuse. The membrane approach is particularly important, since, from the theoretical standpoint, it conveniently provides zero-order release characteristics [229], essential for controlling the release of drugs with narrow therapeutic windows.

Lincomycin hydrochloride was compounded with medicinal silicone rubber (Silastic®), scleral buckling materials possessing antimicrobial activity being thus obtained. Out of this compound, discs were cut out, further vulcanized at 30°C; then, on employing agar gel, their antimicrobial activity—seen as being maintained for at least 5 days—was determined (Figure 76).

As scleral buckling material, Refojo [230] used closed-cell silicone rubber (Dow Corning Silastic®, Lincoff design) from which two types of devices—as cylinders and as oval plates—were cut out; they were immersed in propylene oxide solutions with lincomycin hydrochloride, for 3 days. Antimicrobial activity, as followed on agar gel, was seen as being maintained for about 3 weeks (with cylindrical forms) and over 1 month with the oval ones (Figure 77).

These antibiotic-impregnated materials used in conjunction with standard pre- and postoperative therapy, can reduce even further the rate of infection in scleral buckling procedures.

Disiloxane derivatives, such as (1,1,1,3,3-pentamethyl-3-(γ-carboxyl-propyl) disiloxane, 1,1,2,2-tetramethyl-1,2-di-γ-carboxy-n-propyldisiloxane) as well as polydimethylsiloxane containing γ-carboxypropyl groups have been used for the chemical bonding of atropine [231]. These products may be introduced

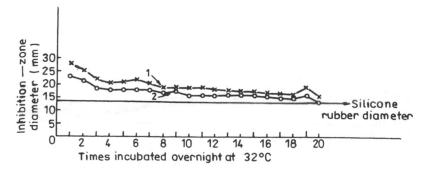

Figure 74. Sustained release of chloramphenicol sodium succinate from silicone rubber into agar gels seeded with *Sarcina lutea*. From Reference [225]; reprinted with permission from S. Karger AG, Basel (publishers).

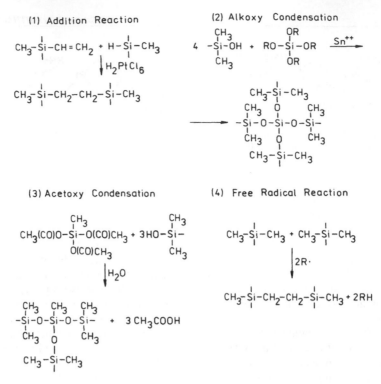

Figure 75. Methods of obtaining medical grade silicones.

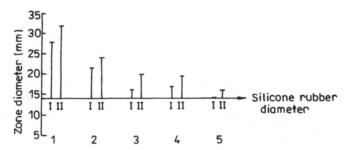

Figure 76. Antibacterial activity of two silicone rubber discs compounded with lincomycin hydrochloride. I = 0.5%, II = 1.0% antibiotic by weight. From Reference [225]; reprinted with permission from S. Karger AG, Basel (publishers).

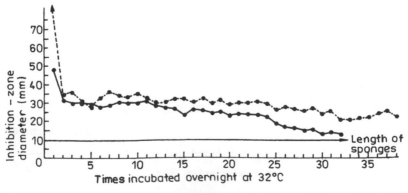

Figure 77. Antibacterial activity of oval (broken line) and cylindrical (solid line) silicone sponges impregnated with lincomycin hydrochloride (0.3%) in propylene oxide and assayed with *Sarcina lutea* in agar gels. From Reference [230]; S. Karger AG, Basel (publishers).

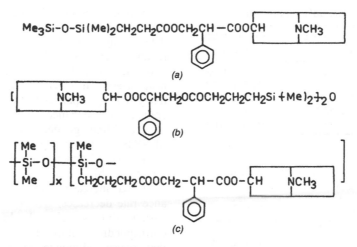

Figure 78. Chemical structures of siloxane oligomers and polymers containing atropine. (a) Derivative with atropine of 1,1,1,3,3-pentamethyl-3-(γ-carboxy propyl) disiloxane; (b) derivative with atropine of 1,1,2,2-tetramethyl-1,2-di-γ-carboxy-n-propyl disiloxane; (c) polydimethylsiloxan modified with carboxylic groups, esterified with atropine. From Reference [239].

postoperatively into the eye for the controlled release of atropine, in the treatment of irite, iridociclite and keratite, thus avoiding the 2 to 3 daily necessary instillations.

Atropine reacts with 1,1,1,3,3-pentamethyl-3-(γ-carboxypropyl) disiloxane, in the presence of dicyclohexylcarbodiimide. In a similar way the reactions with 1,1,2,2-tetramethyl-1,2-di-γ-carboxy-n-propyl disiloxane and polydimethylsiloxane containing γ-carboxypropyl groups are to be conducted.

During these reactions, an esterification of the free hydroxylic group with the carboxylic group of the above-mentioned siloxanes occurs. Starting from atropine-containing oligomers, polymers have been prepared, that induce a controlled release of atropine through the enzymatic scission of the esteric group.

The chemical structures of the atropine-containing oligomers and polymers are given in Figure 78.

Capsule-Type Drug Delivery Systems

The capsule systems employed for the controlled release of ophthalmic drugs, known at present, may be classified into:

- hydrophile membrane microsphere
- Ocusert® system and related devices
- devices for the controlled release of hydrophobic drugs

Microspheres with Hydrophile Membranes

Owing to the unsatisfactory bioavailabilities obtained with conventional ophthalmic inserts, it has been suggested by several authors [232–234] that colloidal delivery systems, such as liposomes and nanoparticles, may be of use in ophthalmic drug delivery.

P. Fitzgerald et al., [235] used the noninvasive technique of gamma scintigraphy to investigate the fate of liposomes and nanoparticles after intraocular administration, and to compare their precorneal residence times.

Small unilamellar vesicles were prepared using DL-dipalmitoyl phosphatidylcholine (DPPC) and cholesterol in a molar ratio 6/2 (SUVNEU); charged vesicles were prepared from DPPC, cholesterol and either stearylamine, to confirm a positive charge (SUVPOS), or dicetyl phosphate, to confirm a negative charge (SUVNEG).

Owing to their low encapsulation volumes, the preformed SUVS were labelled with ^{99m}Tc sodium pertechnetate via a stannous chloride bridge [236].

Positively charged reversed phase vesicles (REV) were prepared from egg lecithin (90% phosphatidylcholine content) and stearylamine (molar ratio 4/1) [237]. Nitrilotriacetic acid, a weak chelating agent, was entrapped in the aqueous compartment of the liposomes to enable labelling with ^{111}In oxide (20–40 MBq) [238].

Nanoparticles were prepared by adding 0.1 ml butylcyanoacrylate monomer to a mixture of dextran 70 (0.5%) and 0.01 M HCl (9.9 ml) with stirring, at room temperature for three hours. 1 ml of the nanoparticle suspension was labelled with freshly prepared ^{111}In oxide (20–40 MBq) with an efficiency of >95%, determined by ultracentrifugation.

All particles were sized by photon correlation spectroscopy (Malvern Instruments) before labelling. The results are summarized in Table 25. For the analysis, regions of interest were drawn around the cornea and inner canthus. Graphs of percentage activity remaining as a function of time were plotted for each region, and the residence half-life (T 50%) read off from the graph. The results are shown in Table 26 [235].

Table 25. Size of colloidal preparations.

Preparation	Mean Size ± s.d. (nm)	Polydispersity Index
SUVPOS	102 ± 1.3	0.22 ± 0.02
SUVNEG	126 ± 5.0	0.25 ± 0.02
SUVNEU	156 ± 3.0	0.32 ± 0.02
Nanoparticles	284 ± 18.0	0.42 ± 0.04
REVPOS	360 ± 7.0	0.43 ± 0.04

Table 26. $T_{50}\%$ of corneal and inner canthal clearance ± s.d., minutes.

Preparation	Cornea	Inner Canthus
SUVPOS	3.77 ± 0.29	7.7 ± 1.90
SUVNEG	1.06 ± 0.46	14.0 ± 4.40
SUVNEU	1.14 ± 0.02	14.3 ± 2.20
Nanoparticles	2.15 ± 0.09	9.2 ± 5.00
REVPOS	3.30 ± 0.42	9.2 ± 1.60
$^{111}InCl_3$	1.30 ± 0.07	5.0 ± 1.30
$^{99m}Tc\text{-DTPA}$	1.40 ± 0.06	5.0 ± 0.80

Table 27. Values of the exponent n.

Release Exponent n	Mechanism of Solvent Transport
0.5	Fickian diffusion
$0.5 < n < 1.0$	Non-Fickian transport
1.0	Case-II transport

Table 28. Characteristics of cross-linked PHEMA microspheres.

Nominal Cross-linking Ratio, X, mol/mol	D_∞/D_0	n	ν $\mu m/min$
0.007	1.189	0.53	22.2
0.019	1.150	0.46	15.0
0.032	1.131	0.52	14.1
0.062	1.102	0.80	11.9
0.124	1.089	0.85	11.2

Table 29. Release rate of BCNU from silicone and hybrid silicone–nylon devices.

Wall Thickness mm	Surface Area mm²	BCNU Release Rate[a] $\mu g/h$
0.13	34.6	979 ± 101
	58.4	1439 ± 57.7
	115.0	2639 ± 126
	31.8	459 ± 53.2
0.25	51.8	772 ± 73.3
	107	1246 ± 87.5
	33.4	338 ± 16.3
0.52	52.0	390 ± 77.9
	120	747 ± 45.7
0.13 (0.05[b])	17.4[c]	602 ± 41.3
0.25 (0.10[b])	13.2[c]	284 ± 32.1

[a]Mean ± s.d.
[b]Thickness of nylon.
[c]Surface area of silicone sheeting only.

From the precorneal clearance results it appears that size and surface charge are important factors in determining corneal residence time. SUVPOS were retained significantly longer ($p < 0.05$, analysis of covariance) than SUVNEG or SUVNEU on the corneal surface. The electrostatic attraction of small positively charged particles to the negatively-charged epithelium is enhanced by their large surface area, thus enabling greater surface contact. However, SUVS have a low encapsulation volume, which might negate any advantage gained due to electrostatic attraction [235].

As size increases, the results illustrate that clearance rate decreases. SUVPOS, REVPOS and nanoparticles drain significantly slower than solution of the corresponding isotopes ($p < 0.05$). In the inner canthal region, drainage of all particulate systems, including SUVNEG and SUVNEU, is significantly slower than it is in solutions of isotopes ($p < 0.05$ analysis of covariance).

Nanoparticles have been described as having "mucoadhesive" properties [239]. This may be a contributing factor in ocular retention, but it cannot be demonstrated in this study [235]. Size is more likely to be the primary factor in the precorneal retention of nanoparticles. The prolonged residence of colloids in the inner canthal region may be due to the association of particles with the conjunctiva and nictitating membrane, or to physical obstruction caused by aggregation in the region.

This suggests that colloidal systems may prove useful in the ocular delivery of antibiotics and anti-inflammatory drugs, and also in the treatment of "dry eye" syndrome by a temporary abstraction of lacrimal drainage.

Generally, polymers employed to obtain microspheres are based on poly(hydroxyethyl methacrylate) (PHEMA) diversely cross-linked by ethylene glycol dimethacrylate (EGDMA). Such microspheres may include a series of ophthalmic drugs: antibiotics, antiglaucoma or anticancerous, anti-inflammatory, etc.

PHEMA-based microspheres, containing phenylephrin·HCl—a drug usually employed in glaucoma treatments—have been prepared by C. Robert and co-workers [240]. In such formulations, the drug was homogeneously dispersed in a glassy polymer. On contact with a tear, the polymer swelled and became rubbery. During this process, we observed a penetration front of solvent separating the glassy zone from the rubbery area. In the proximity of this penetration front, macromolecular relaxations took place. The mechanism of solvent transport, the velocity of the penetration and macromolecular relaxations influenced the drug release.

Analysis of the transport mechanism of the solvent was achieved by calculating the values of the exponent n of a semi-empirical equation:

$$(D_t - D_o)/D_o = kt^n \qquad (23)$$

where $(D_t - D_o)/D_o$ corresponds to the increase of

the normalized microsphere diameter, t is the swelling time, k is a constant representative of the structural and geometrical properties of the device, and n is an exponent whose value is typical of the penetration mechanism of the solvent (Table 27) [240].

However, for spherical devices, an exponent n corresponding to 1.0 is not indicative of case-II transport (zero-order release) but only means that the diffusion is highly non-Fickian [240].

In the preparation of microspheres, the method of polymerization in suspension, as modified by Mueller et al. [241], is being applied. The ratios between the reticulation agent and monomer (X) are: 0.007, 0.019, 0.032, 0.062 and 0.124 mol EGDMA/mol HEMA.

Phenylephrin · HCl release was performed through a continuous flow system (Dissotest®). The absorptions were measured spectrophotometrically at 272 nm [240].

The dynamic swelling behaviour of microspheres of sizes between 315 and 400 μm was followed (Figure 79) [240].

The equilibrium normalized diameter D_∞/D_o, the exponent n [Equation (23)] and the penetrant front velocity (v) were determined (Table 28) [241].

The equilibrium normalized diameter dropped significantly as the cross-linking ratio increased. This expected behavior is the result of more tightly cross-linked networks which do not expand in water as much as the loosely cross-linked ones (Table 28) [241].

The exponent n calculated using the first 60% of the curves increases as the cross-linking ratio increases. It indicates a Fickian diffusion for low degrees of cross-linking and highly non-Fickian diffusion for $X = 0.062$ and 0.124 (Table 28).

Increasing the cross-linking ratio considerably decreases the velocity of the front (moving linearly with time) due to the highly cross-linked structure (Table 28) [241].

The cross-linking ratio of PHEMA microspheres influences greatly the phenylephrin · HCl release: a decreasing cross-linking ratio is linked to a faster drug release (Figure 80) [247].

Nevertheless, it was observed that a suitable loading

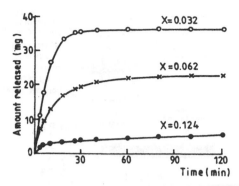

Figure 80. Release profiles for phenylephrin HCl from 500 mg of PHEMA microspheres having different ratios of cross-linking (X). From Reference [240].

of the drug becomes very difficult in highly cross-linked polymers. Indeed, a strong decrease in the degree of swelling opposes an important uptake of phenylephrin · HCl. In addition, as illustrated in Figure 81, the size of the microspheres changes the profile release of the drug. The release from larger microspheres is clearly slowed down. As can be seen, these microparticles allowed nearly 20% of phenylephrin · HCl to be released at a constant rate (between the fifteenth and fortieth minutes in this example) [247].

It seems, in fact, that the phenomenon of molecular relaxation can only influence drug release in large spheres, depending on the nature of the solvent and of the solute.

Ocusert® *and Related Devices*

Ocusert®, one of the capsule–type drug (pilocarpine) delivery systems for the treatment of glaucoma, was developed by Alza Corporation, U.S.A. Figure 82 shows the structure of the device. A mixture of pilocarpine and alginic acid in the drug reservoir provides the drug for almost 1 week [242].

The Ocusert® system (Figure 82)—of an elliptical form—contains two membranes made of EVA [i.e., the poly(ethylene-co-vinyl acetate) copolymer]. On its

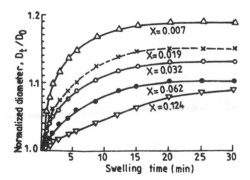

Figure 79. Normalized diameter of EGDMA-cross-linked PHEMA particles, D_t/D_o, as a function of swelling time for different cross-linking ratios (X). From Reference [240].

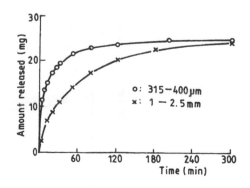

Figure 81. Release profiles for phenylephrin HCl from 500 mg of PHEMA microspheres having different average diameters. From Reference [240].

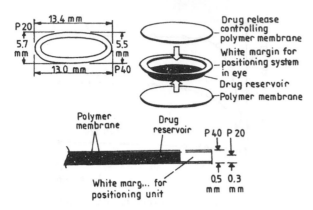

Figure 82. Diagram of Ocusert® ocular therapeutic system showing functional dimensions and format. From Reference [243]; reprinted by permission of the publishers, Georg Thieme, Verlag.

circumference, a ring—made of the same polymer, compounded with TiO₂ [242]—may be formed.

Depending on the release rate of pilocarpine, two types of systems are known, namely Ocusert® Pilo-20 and Pilo-40, containing in the alginic acid gel 5.0 mg and 11.0 mg pilocarpine, respectively. In the Ocusert® Pilo-40 system, having a release rate of 40 μg/h, 90 μg of plastifier [di(2-ethyl-hexyl) phthalate] has been introduced as carrier and plastifying agent of the EVA membrane.

The mechanism of pilocarpine release from Ocusert® has been described from a quantitative point of view by Shell and Baker [245].

Ocusert® may assure for 7 days a therapeutical concentration of pilocarpine into the eye, as a consequence of its constant release rate (i.e., 20 μg/h and, respectively, 40 μg/h) (Figure 83).

Clinical tests performed have fully confirmed the efficiency, as well as the advantages offered by this system of controlled release of pilocarpine into the eye.

Experiments made by Armaly and Rao [246–247] on large groups of volunteers suffering from glaucoma have evidenced that Ocusert® was well tolerated, inducing a significant reduction of the IOP value and of the pupillary diameter; also, with Ocusert® the pilocarpine consumption is only of 0.48 mg/day as against 4 mg/day with the classical system (dropwise administration), which is an important economical aspect of such a treatment.

Other investigators [248–249] have checked the availability of the Ocusert® system for long periods of time (up to 12 months) as compared with the dropwise administration treatment. After treatment with Ocusert®, applied to a batch of 40 patients suffering from glaucoma, average IOP values of 19.9 ± 3.9 mmHg have been obtained, as against 20.7 ± 8.6 mmHg obtained through dropwise administration. No side effects have been observed.

Controlled release of pilocarpine from Ocusert® has also the advantage—as compared with drop administration—of not producing blurry vision, whereas the eye drops caused a decline in visual acuity, refractive error, miosis, and marked visual discomfort [249–250].

Drance et al. [251] confirmed the ocular hypotensive effect of Ocusert® Pilo-20 and Pilo-40 on glaucoma patients for periods of 10 and 12 days, respectively. However, the hypotensive effect of 2% or 4% pilocarpine eye drops was greater than that of Ocusert® Pilo-20 and Pilo-40. These authors found no significant difference in refractive error between the effect of 2% and 4% pilocarpine eye drops and that of Ocusert® Pilo-20 and Pilo-40.

A deeper clinical study of the Ocusert® Pilo-20 and Pilo-40 behaviour was undertaken by Tomono and Hanba [252]; they administered Ocusert® for periods of time varying between 20 months and 4 years to 16 patients suffering from glaucoma, which resulted in a reduction of the IOP value to 20 mmHg, with no ef-

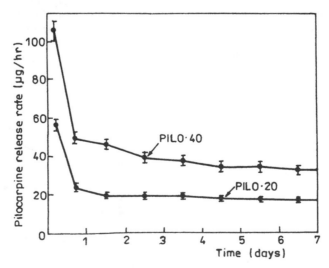

Figure 83. Drug release rates from Ocusert® Pilo-20 and Ocusert® Pilo-40, mean ± SEM. From Reference [2].

fect upon the bacterial flora in the conjunctival sac. Concomitant wearing of Ocusert® and contact lenses showed no problems.

Apart from the Ocusert®-type devices, employing pilocarpine, the literature also mentions some new systems, based on the same principles, loaded with other drugs [epinephrine, diethyl carbamazine citrate (DEC)] [253–254].

The installation of an epinephrine release system is characterized by a release rate of 4–6 μg/h, its effect being equivalent to a much higher dose of dropwise-administered drug. Such devices release epinephrine in its molecular form, which is not convertible by tears into an ionic form, thus penetrating more easily through the cornea [255]. With dropwise administration treatment, at higher doses, epinephrine modifies the lacrimal pH and, consequently, it is converted, in higher ratios, into an ionic form, which results in a reduction of the treatment availability (Figure 84).

DEC is the most effective microfilaricide available for treating ocular or other forms of onchocerciasis. The device could deliver DEC at a rate of about 0.1 to 1.0 μg/h. The clinical trials performed on 14 patients who were moderately to heavily infected with onchocerciasis. The conclusion was that the therapeutic index provided by this system is probably sufficient to reduce grossly the microfilarial load without adverse effects [2].

Devices for the Controlled Release of Hydrophobic Drugs

Refojo et al. [256] developed a device for delivery of hydrophobic drugs consisting of a silicone rubber system, especially for treatment of intraocular malignancies with 1,3-bis(2-chloroethyl)-1-nitrosourea (BCNU). As it is known, this drug is active in the treatment of Brown-Pearce epithelioma [257] and Greene melanoma [258] implanted in the anterior chamber of rabbit eye. BCNU produces various adverse effects, particularly when administered in therapeutic doses to the whole body [2].

At present, anticancer therapeutics investigates—among other things—some systems that should permit the drug's introduction directly into the tumour, in amounts as high as possible, without affecting the whole organism [259–262]. The silicone rubber drug delivery device [256] fulfilled these goals for the administration of BCNU to eye tumours in the rabbit.

The first systems employed were made up of two membranes of silicone rubber (Silastic® 500-1, 0.31 mm thick) quite thin and glued together, out of which projects a tube (∅ = 0.3 mm) assuring the drug transit is being obtained [2].

The *in vitro* release rate of BCNU from such a device is 200–300 μg/h (Figure 85) [2]. The work duration of the system is limited solely by the drug content from the system's reservoir. After the drug's consumption, the system may easily be filled once more.

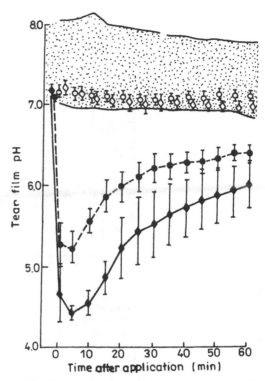

Figure 84. Effect of epinephrine bitartrate eye drops and of continuous delivery on tear film pH. The shaded area represents the range of pH observed in untreated eyes. Upper limit of untreated eye range is defined by the eye with the highest tear-film pH of the group tested, and lower limit by the eye with the lowest tear-film pH of the group (n = 13) tested. Epinephrine delivery rate: 5 μg/h (○); 3 μg/h (◇). One percent epinephrine bitartrate eye drops: (●); 2% (◆). In all epinephrine treatment groups, n = 5. From Reference [2].

The *in vivo* tests, performed with such systems by Liu et al. [263], on rabbits affected by Brown-Pearce epithelioma followed the treatment's efficiency (tumour increase, histopathologic modifications with normal eyes and with eyes affected by tumours, etc.). Such systems were seen as inducing a delay in the tumour development, after a 20-day treatment. Further on, these devices have been improved by employing silicone–nylon compounds in their construction [264]. The release rate from these systems—calculated through Equation (24) [2]—is given in Table 29 [264].

$$z = 11.6\, y^{0.750}/x^{0.850} \qquad (24)$$

where

z = release rate (μg/h)
y = surface area (mm²)
x = wall thickness (mm)

Equation (24) is similar to the first law of Fick:

$$dM_t/dt = ADK\Delta C/L \qquad (25)$$

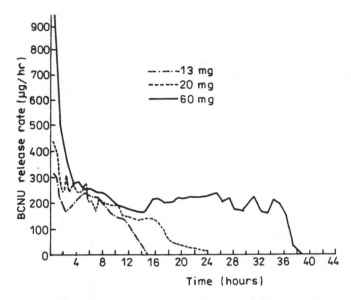

Figure 85. Release rate of BCNU into water at 37°C from silicone balloons injected with BCNU in 0.15 ml absolute ethanol. The arrow between 2 and 4 h indicates the time it took for the alcohol to diffuse out of the balloon. From Reference [256]; reprinted with permission from Pergamon Press, Ltd., © 1978.

where

Mt = mass of drug released
dMt/dt = steady-state release rate
A = surface area of the drug delivery device
DK = drug permeability coefficient of the membrane
ΔC = difference between the internal and the external drug concentrations
L = membrane thickness

The multiple regression plate is given in a three-dimensional graph (Figure 86) [2].

The release rate of BCNU can be estimated from the surface area and wall thickness of the device before it is implanted in animals [2].

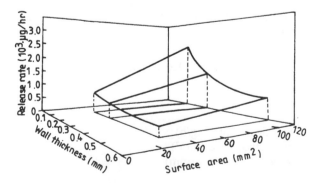

Figure 86. Three-dimensional representation of regression plate indicates the relationship among the release rate, the surface area, and wall thickness. From Reference [2].

Another course in constructing self-regulated drug delivery devices is to use enzyme–substrate reactions that convert the presence and amount of a specific substrate to a pH-change which in turn, controls the release of an active agent. Because the action of enzymes is highly selective, even very small amounts of a specific compound in a complex mixture such as body fluids are capable of uniquely interacting with the enzyme sensor of the delivery system.

Our approach to the development of such devices is based on polymers that have erosion rates which are highly pH dependent, so that relatively small changes in the surrounding pH will result in subsequent increased release rate of incorporated therapeutic agents.

The basic components of such a delivery system are schematically represented in Figure 87 [265] where the inner core is the pH-sensitive hydrolytically labile polymer and the outer layer is a hydrogel containing an immobilized enzyme.

When such a device is placed in a physiological environment, the inner polymer is exposed to the pH of that environment, and in the absence of molecules that are substrates for the enzyme, the pH surrounding the device will remain constant. However, when a substrate appears in the environment, it will diffuse into the hydrogel and be converted by the enzyme to either acidic or basic products which will modify the pH within the hydrogel and thus modify the erosion rate of the polymer.

A useful polymer that significantly increases erosion rate with increasing pH is a partially esterified copolymer of methyl vinyl ether and maleic anhydride which solubilizes by ionization of carboxylic acid groups.

$$\{CH_2-CH-CH \ - \ CH\}_n \longrightarrow \{CH_2-CH-CH \ - \ CH\}_n$$

insoluble   soluble

This polymer was used in a model system to test the feasibility of this concept [99]. In this model, the n-hexyl half ester was surrounded by a hydrogel containing immobilized urease prepared by dissolving bovine serum albumin and urease in water and adding glutaraldehyde to cross-link the mixture of proteins. Because urease converts urea to NH_4HCO_3 and NH_4OH, the enzyme–substrate reaction will result in a pH increase and thus the presence of urea in the external environment should result in an increase in the rate of hydrocortisone release.

Results of experiments showing the effect of urea on the rate of hydrocortisone release are presented in Figure 88. In a medium of constant pH and in the absence of external urea, the polymer erosion rate and concomitant hydrocortisone release is that normally expected for that polymer at the given pH. However, in the presence of external urea, the basic species generated within the hydrogel accelerate polymer erosion with consequent acceleration of hydrocortisone release.

Implantable Drug Delivery Pumps

The osmotic minipump introduced in therapy by Alza Corporation under the name of ALZET® [266–267] is a device for the controlled administering of highly efficient drugs; as a matter of fact, it seems that in the near future it will be highly developed, assuring a constant pumping rate for a period of up to 2 weeks.

Investigations performed by Falcon and Jones [268] suggest placing the minipump under the head skin of a rabbit or of a guinea pig through a cut in the upper formix. The connection between the minipump and eye was assured by a polyethylene tube.

On employing this minipump, adenine arabinoside 5′-monophosphate was introduced into the eye for the therapy of hepatic affections.

Later on [269–271], minipumps were analyzed for the introduction of gentamicine of fluoresceine into the vitreous material as well as for theoretical investigations regarding the general operation of minipumps.

CONCLUDING REMARKS

During the last two decades, polymeric controlled drug delivery has become an important area of research and development. In this short time, a number of systems displaying constant or decreasing release rates have progressed from the laboratory to the clinic

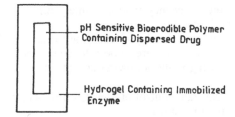

Figure 87. Schematic representation of self-regulated bioerodible polymer delivery system. From Reference [265].

and, in some cases, commercial products. Polymer systems for controlled release of such drugs as pilocarpine, antibiotics, nitroglycerin, scopolamine, birth control drugs, and anti-cancer drugs are either in late stage clinical trials or are available clinically.

In the 1970s, diffusion-controlled systems for the treatment of the eye were introduced by Alza Corp. In the early 1980s, researchers came up with two new approaches:

(1) The use of vehicles with sol-gel transition at body temperature
(2) Polymeric dispersions which show coalescence by a pH change

The first approach is mainly based on the use of thermogels such as polyalkylene oxide block copolymers, whereas the second is a polymeric dispersion, both containing a bioactive substance, and allowing the creation *in situ* of a microreservoir by simple instillation.

To these systems, one observation to be added is that of contact lenses containing drugs. If the systems above-mentioned (such as Ocusert®-type inserts and microparticle dispersions) are largely employed nowadays, contact lens-based devices are less utilized,

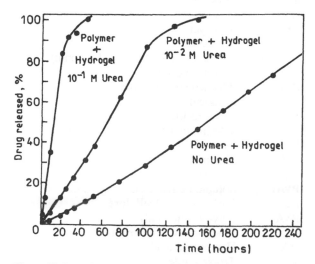

Figure 88. Rate of hydrocortisone release from a n-hexyl half-ester of a methyl vinyl ether–maleic anhydride copolymer at pH 6.25 and 35°C in the presence and absence of external urea. From Reference [265].

due to the effect they induce, namely rapid opacization and irritability.

The devices releasing pilocarpine to the tear fluid, at a controlled rate, are to be extensively used in the future, owing to the following advantages:

- a constant control of elevated intraocular pressure (IOP)
- reduced severity of undesired side-effects (myopia, miosis, etc.)
- reduction of the total administered dose, thus minimizing the risk of systemic toxicity resulting from trans-mucosal absorption
- improved patients' compliance

SYMBOLS

P	Flux, g cm^2 sec^{-1}
Cm	Concentration of the permeant in the membrane, g cm^{-3}
D	Diffusion coefficient, cm^2 sec^{-1}
ϵ	Porosity coefficient
τ	Tortuosity factor
M	Molecular weight
PMMA	Poly(methyl methacrylate)
PHEMA	Poly(hydroxyethyl methyacrylate)
IOL	Intraocular lens
ϱ	Polymer density
γ	Polymer erosion rate, cm sec^{-1}
J_p	Flux of solubilized polymer, equivalents of carboxylate groups cm^{-2} sec^{-1}
P_T	Concentration of carboxyl groups ionized plus unionized, equivalents cm^{-3}
CPh	Chloramphenicol
DCCI	Dicyclohexylcarbodiimide
$\emptyset$	Yield strain, dyn cm^{-2}
Ie	Extension index, mm^2
n	Flowing index
m	Consistency index
Nm	Neomycin
X	Xanthan
PAcA-AV	Poly(acrylic acid-co-vinyl alcohol)
PiN	Pilocarpine nitrate
PiB	Pilocarpine free base
IOP	Intraocular pressure
MRT	Mean residence time
ANS	8-Anilinonaphthalene-1-sulfonate
Lys	Lysozyme
IDU	Idoxuridine
PVA	Poly(vinyl alcohol)
PVAI	Soluble ocular inserts based on PVA
HPC	Hydroxypropylcellulose
PAA	Poly(acrylic acid)
F	Fractions of drug released
HA	Hyaluronic acid
Tr	Tropicamide
AS	Standard aqueous vehicle
AIBN	Azoisobutyronitrile
PEG	Poly(ethylene glycol)
PVP	Poly(N-vinylpyrrolidone)
PVOM	Poly(N-vinyl-5-methyl-2-oxazolidone)
DPPC	DL-dipalmitoyl phosphatidylcholine
EGDMA	Ethylene glycol dimethacrylate
DEC	Dimethyl carbamazine citrate
BCNU	1,3-bis (2-chloroethyl)-1-nitrosourea

REFERENCES

1. Deasdorff, D. L. 1980. In *Remington's Pharmaceutical Science, 16th Ed.* A. Osol, S. C. Harvey, G. D. Chase, R. E. King, A. R. Gennaro, A. N. Martin, M. R. Gibson, C. B. Branberg and G. L. Zink, eds. Easton: Mack Publishing, p. 86.
2. Ueno, N. and M. F. Refojo. 1983. In *Controlled Drug Delivery, Vol. II: Clinical Applications.* S. D. Bruck, ed. Boca Raton, Florida: CRC Press, Inc., p. 89.
3. Shell, J. W. and R. W. Baker. 1974. *Ann. Ophthalmol.*, 6:1037.
4. Podos, S., B. Becker, C. Asseff and J. Harstein. 1972. *Amer. J. Ophthalmol.*, 73:336.
5. Zaffaroni, A. 1980. U.S. Pat. 4,186,184 (Jan. 29, 1980) to Alza Corp.; Chem. Abstr. 92:185937b.
6. Maichuk, Y. F. 1975. *Invest. Ophthalmol.*, 14:87.
7. Wingard, L. B., Jr. 1983. *Biochemical Pharmacology*, 32:2647 (1983).
8. Fanger, G. O. 1974. *Proceedings of Controlled Release Pesticide Symposium.* N. F. Cardarelli, ed. University of Akron, Ohio, p. 18.
9. Scher, H. B. 1977. In *Controlled Release Pesticides.* H. B. Scher, ed. ACS Symposium Series 53, American Chemical Society, Washington, DC, p. 126.
10. Robinson, J. R. 1976. In *Chemical Marketing and Economics Reprints.* F. W. Long, W. P. O'Neill and R. D. Stewart, eds. American Chemical Society, San Francisco, p. 212.
11. Higuchi, W. L. 1967. *J. Pharm. Sci.*, 56:315.
12. Flynn, G. L. and S. H. Yalkowsky. 1974. *J. Pharm. Sci.*, 63:479.
13. Graham, N. B. and D. A. Wood. 1983. In *Macromolecular Biomaterials.* G. W. Hastings and P. Ducheyne, eds. Boca Raton, Florida: CRC Press Inc., p. 181.
14. Crank, J. 1975. *The Mathematics of Diffusion, 2nd Ed.* Oxford: Clarendon Press.
15. Higuchi, T. 1961. *J. Pharm. Sci.*, 50:875.
16. Chien, Y. W., H. J. Lambert and T. K. Lin. 1975. *J. Pharm. Sci.*, 64:1643.
17. Haleblian, J., R. Runkel, N. Mueller, J. Christopherson and K. Ng. 1971. *J. Pharm. Sci.*, 60:541.
18. Roseman, T. J. and W. I. Higuchi. 1970. *J. Pharm. Sci.*, 59:353.
19. Higuchi, T. 1963. *J. Pharm. Sci.*, 52:1145.
20. Davis, B. K. 1974. *Proc. Natl. Acad. Sci. USA*, 71:3120.
21. Hosaka, S., H. Ozawa and H. Tanazawa. 1979. *J. Appl. Polym. Sci.*, 23:2089.
22. Chien, Y. W. and E. P. K. Lau. 1976. *J. Pharm. Sci.*, 65:488.

23. Good, W. R. 1978. In *Polymeric Drug Delivery Systems*. R. J. Kostelnik, ed. New York: Gordon and Breach, p. 139.

24. Peterlin, A. 1979. *J. Polym. Sci., Polym. Phys. Ed.*, 17:1741.

25. Peppas, N. A., R. Gurny and P. Burni. 1980. *J. Membr. Sci.*, 7:241.

26. Flynn, G. L., N. F. H. Ho, S. Hwang, E. Owada, A. Molokhia, C. R. Behl, W. I. Higuchi, T. Yotsuyanagi, Y. Shah and J. Park. 1976. In *Controlled Release Polymeric Formulations*. D. R. Paul and F. W. Harris, eds. Am. Chem. Soc. Symp., Ser. 33, American Chemical Society, Washington, DC, p. 87.

27. Kent, J. S. 1976. In *Controlled Release Polymeric Formulations*. D. R. Paul and F. W. Harris, eds. Am. Chem. Soc. Symp., Ser. 33, American Chemical Society, Washington, DC, p. 87.

28. Yolles, S., J. Elridge, T. Deafe, J. H. R. Woodland, D. R. Blake and F. J. Meyer. 1974. In *Controlled Release of Biologically Active Agents*. A. C. Tanquary and R. E. Lacey, eds. London: Plenum Press, p. 177.

29. Lovering, E. G. and B. D. Black. 1974. *J. Pharm. Sci.*, 63:1399.

30. Hopfenberg, H. B. 1976. In *Controlled Release Polymeric Formulations*. D. R. Paul and F. W. Harris, eds. Am. Chem. Soc. Symp., Ser. 33, American Chemical Society, Washington, DC, p. 26.

30a. Kydonieus, A. F. 1980. In *Controlled Release Technologies: Methods, Theory, and Application, Vol. I*. F. Kydonieus, ed. CRC Press, p. 1.

31. Paul, D. R. 1976. In *Controlled Release Polymeric Formulations*. D. R. Paul and F. W. Harris, eds. ACS Symposium, Series 33, American Chemical Society, Washington, DC, p. 9.

32. Bakan, J. A. 1975. "Microcapsule Drug Delivery Systems", in *Polymers in Medicine and Surgery*. R. L. Kronenthal, Z. Oser and E. Martin, eds. New York: Plenum Press, p. 213.

33. Warrick, E. L., O. R. Pierces, M. E. Polmanteer and J. C. Saam. 1979. *Rubber Chem. Technol.*, 52:437.

34. Folkman, J. and D. M. Long. 1964. *J. Surg. Res.*, 4:139.

35. Long, D. M. and J. Folkman. 1966. US Patent 3,279,996.

36. Chien, Y. W., D. M. Jefferson, J. G. Coonrey and H. J. Lambert. 1979. *J. Pharm. Sci.*, 68:689.

37. Roseman, T. J. 1972. *J. Pharm. Sci.*, 61:46.

38. Kratochvil, P., G. Hemaglano and K. A. Kinel. 1970. *Steroids*, 15:505.

39. Fu, J. C., A. K. Kale and D. L. Mayer. 1973. *J. Biomed. Mater. Res.*, 7:71.

40. Gaginella, T. S. and J. J. Vallner. 1975. *Common. Chem. Pathol. Pharmacol.*, 11:323.

41. Bass, P., R. A. Purdon, J. N. Wiley. 1965. *Nature* (London), 208:591.

42. Pharriss, B. B., R. Erickson, J. Bashaw, S. Hoff, V. Place and A. Zaffaroni. 1974. *Fertil. Steril.*, 25:915.

43. Martinez-Manauton, J. 1975. *J. Steroid Biochem.*, 6:889.

44. Langer, R. and J. Folkman. 1978. In *Polymeric Drug Delivery Systems*. R. J. Kostelnik, ed. New York: Gonlon and Breach, p. 175.

45. Bietti, G. A. 1955. *Acta Ophthalmol.*, 33:337.

46. Miller, G. R. and R. R. Tenkel. 1969. Am. J. Ophthalmol., 689:717.

47. Lowther, G. E. 1982. In *Contact Lenses*. Boston: Butterworth, p. 3.

48. Martin, N. F., G. P. Kracher, W. J. Stark and A. E. Manumenee. 1983. *Arch. Ophthalmol.*, 101:39.

49. Wichterle, O. 1971. In *Encyclopedia in Polymer Science and Technology, Vol. 15*. H. F. Mark, N. G. Gaylord and N. M. Bikales, eds. New York: Interscience, p. 273.

50. Wichterle, O. and D. Lim. 1960. *Nature (London)*, 185:117.

51. Stenson, S. 1986. *Arch. Ophthalmol.*, 104:1287.

52. Gobel, R. J., J. Janatova, J. M. Googe, D. J. Apple. 1987. *Biomaterials*, 8:285, Butterworth & Co. Ltd. ©.

53. Herzlinger, G. A., D. H. Bing, R. Stein and R. D. Cumming. 1981. *Blood*, 57:764.

54. Tuberville, A. W., M. A. Galin, H. D. Perez, D. Banda, R. Onh and I. M. Goldstein. 1982. *Invest. Ophthalmol. Vis. Sci.*, 22:727.

55. Tripathi, R. C., B. J. Tripathi and M. Ruben. 1980. *Ophthalmology*, 87:365.

56. Korb, D. R. and A. S. Heneriques. 1980. J. Am. Optom. Assoc., 51:243.

57. Lowther, G. E. and J. A. Hilbert. 1975. Am. J. Physiol. Optics, 52:687.

58. Tripathi, R. C., B. J. Tripathi and M. Ruben. 1978. *Clinical and Applied Technology*. M. Ruben, ed. New York: Wiley, p. 299.

59. Dohlman, C. H., S. A. Boruchoff and E. F. Mobilia. 1977. *Arch. Ophthalmol.*, 83:549.

60. Bowers, R. W. J. and B. J. Tighe. 1987. *Biomaterials*, 8:83.

61. Tighe, B. J. 1976. *Br. Polym. J.*, 8:71.

62. Freeman, M. I. 1976–77. *Bull. Mason Clin.*, 30:141.

63. Binder, P. S. and D. M. Worthan. 1977. *Am. J. Ophthalmol.*, 83:549.

64. Kersley, H. J., C. Kerr and D. Pierse. 1977. *Br. J. Ophthalmol.*, 61:38.

65. Stein, H. A. and B. J. Slatt. 1977. *Int. Contact. Lens Clin.*, 64:35.

66. Dahl, A. A. and E. R. Brocko. 1978. *Am. J. Ophthalmol.*, 85:454.

67. Karageozian, H. L. 1976. *Contacto*, 20:5.

68. Allen, J., R. Botting, A. Sharp and A. A. Tuffery. 1978. *Optician*, 8:175.

69. Bailey, N. J. 1975. J. Am. Optom. Assoc., 46:214.

70. Wedler, F. C. 1977. *J. Biomed. Mater. Res.*, 11:525.

71. Kleist, F. D. 1979. *Int. Contact Lens Clin.*, 6:177.

72. Ruben, M., R. C. Tripathi, A. F. Winder. 1975. *Br. J. Ophthalmol.*, 59:141.

73. Gasset, A. R., L. Lobo and W. Houde. 1977. *Am. J. Ophthalmol.*, 83:115.

74. Klintworth, G. K., J. W. Reed and H. K. Hawkins. 1977. *Invest. Ophthalmol. Vis. Sci.*, 16:158.

75. Koetting, R. A. 1975. *Opt. J. Rev. Optom.*, 115:20.

76. Ruben, M. 1978. In *Soft Contact Lenses Clinical and*

Applied Technology. M. Ruben, ed. New York: Wiley, p. 335.

77. Bernstein, H. N. 1973. *Ann. Ophthalmol.*, 5:317.

78. Vannas, A. and P. Ruusuvoara. 1977. *Klin. M. Angenheilkd*, 170:873.

79. Filppi, J. A., R. M. Pfister and R. M. Hill. 1973. *Am. J. Optom.*, 50:553.

80. Sagan, W. 1976. *Arch. Ophthanol.*, 94:168.

81. Smolin, G., M. Okumoto and R. A. Nozik. 1979. *Am. J. Ophthalmol.*, 88:543.

82. Matas, B. R., W. H. Spencer and T. L. Hayes. 1979. *Arch. Ophthalmol.*, 97:659.

83. Fowler, S. A., J. V. Greiner and M. R. Allansmith. 1979. *Arch. Ophthalmol.*, 97:659.

84. Ruben, M. 1975. *Contact Intraocular Lens Med. J.*, 2:39.

85. Ceskoslovenska Akademie Ved. 1968. *Developments in or Relating to Sustained Release Medicaments*, British Patent 1,135,966.

86. Akkapeddi, M. K., B. D. Halpero, R. H. Davis and H. Balin. 1974. In *Controlled Release of Biologically Active Agents*. A. C. Tanqualy, R. E. Lacey, eds. London: Plenum Press, p. 105.

87. Hudgin, D. E. and E. A. Blair. 1970. U.S. Patent 3,975,350.

88. Imperial Chemical Industries Limited. 1979. British Patent 1,551,620.

89. King, P. A. 1968. U.S. Patent 3,419,006.

90. Johansson, I. A. O. and U. Ulnistem. 1980. U.K. Patent Application GB 2,041,220A.

91. Dumitriu, S., M. Popa and A. Zaharia. 1986. Rom. Patent 91,654.

92. Dumitriu, S. and M. Popa. 1986. Rom. Patent 93,445.

93. A. G. Ciba-Geigy. 1978. British Patent 1,511,563.

94. Graham, N. B., M. E. McNeill, M. Zulfiqar and M. P. Embrey. 1980. *Am. Chem. Soc., Polym. Prepr.*, 21(1):104.

95. Fildes, F. J. F. 1976. British Patent 1,440,217.

96. Theeuwes, F. 1975. *J. Pharm. Sci.*, 64:1987.

97. Theeuwes, F. 1980. U.S. Patent 4,203,439.

98. Theeuwes, F. 1980. U.S. Patent 4,203,441.

99. Heller, J., R. W. Baker, R. M. Gale and J. O. Rodin. 1978. *J. Appl. Polym. Sci.*, 22:1991, John Wiley & Sons.

100. Davis, B. K. 1972. *Experentia*, 28:348.

101. Torchilin, V. P., E. G. Tischenko, V. N. Smirnov and E. I. Chazov. 1977. *J. Biomed. Mater. Res.*, 11:223.

102. Huang, S. J., D. A. Bansleben and J. R. Knox. 1979. *J. Appl. Polym. Sci.*, 23:429.

103. Tokowa, Y., T. Suzuki and T. Ando. 1979. *J. Appl. Polym. Sci.*, 24:1701.

104. Heller, J. and P. V. Trescony. 1979. *J. Pharm. Sci.*, 68:919.

105. Lappas, L. C. and W. McKechan. 1965. *J. Pharm. Sci.*, 54:176.

106. Lappas, L. C. and W. McKechan. 1967. *J. Pharm. Sci.*, 56:1257.

107. Nessel, R. J., N. G. Dekay and G. S. Banker. 1964. *J. Pharm. Sci.*, 53:882.

108. Willis, C. R. and G. S. Banker. 1968. *J. Pharm. Sci.*, 57:1598.

109. Heyd, A., D. O. Kildsig, G. S. Banker. 1969. *J. Pharm. Sci.*, 58:586.

110. Fites, A. L., G. S. Banker and V. F. Smolen. 1970. *J. Pharm. Sci.*, 59:610.

111. Woodruff, C. W., G. E. Peck and G. S. Banker. 1972. *J. Pharm. Sci.*, 1972.

112. Schmitt, F. F. 1976. U.S. Patent 4,070,347.

113. Choi, N. S. and J. Heller. 1978. U.S. Patent 4,079,038.

114. Choi, N. S. and J. Heller. 1978. U.S. Patent 4,093,709.

115. Heller, J. 1980. *Biomaterials*, 1:51.

116. Brady, J. M., D. F. Cutright, R. A. Miller, G. C. Battistone and E. E. Hubsuck. 1973. *J. Biomed. Mater. Res.*, 7:155.

117. Frazza, E. J. and E. E. Schmitt. 1971. *J. Biomed. Mater. Res. Symp.*, 1:43.

118. Leenslog, J. W., A. J. Pennings, R. R. M. Bos, F. R. Rozema and G. Boering. 1987. *Biomaterials*, 8:311.

119. Wise, D. L., H. Rosenkrantz, J. B. Gregory and H. J. Esber. 1980. *J. Pharm. Pharmacol.*, 32:399.

120. Beek, L. R., D. R. Cowsar, D. H. Lewis, R. J. Cosgrove, C. T. Riddle, S. L. Lowry and T. A. Epperly. 1979. *Fertil. Steril.*, 31:545.

121. Schwope, A. D., D. L. Wise and J. R. Howes. 1975. *Life Sci.*, 17:1877.

122. Woodland, J. H. R., S. Yolles, D. A. Blake, M. Helrich and F. J. Meyer. 1973. *J. Med. Chem.*, 16:897.

123. Wise, D. L., A. D. Schwope, S. E. Harrigan, D. A. McCarthy and J. F. Howes. 1978. In *Polymeric Delivery Systems*. R. J. Kostelnik, ed. London: Gordon and Breach, p. 75.

124. Wise, D. L., G. J. McCormick, G. P. Willet, L. C. Anderson and J. F. Howes. 1978. *J. Pharm. Pharmacol.*, 30:686.

125. Wise, D. L., J. D. Gresser, G. J. McCormick. 1979. *J. Pharm. Pharmacol.*, 31:201.

126. Yolles, S., T. D. Leafe and F. J. Meyer. 1975. *J. Pharm. Sci.*, 64:115.

127. Yolles, S. 1978. *J. Parenteral Drug Assoc.*, 32:188.

128. Yolles, S., J. Elridge, T. Leafe, J. H. R. Woodland, D. R. Blake and F. J. Meyer. 1974. In *Controlled Release of Biologically Active Agents*. A. C. Tanquary and R. E. Lacey, eds. London: Plenum Press, p. 177.

129. Al-Mesfer, H. and B. J. Tighe. 1987. *Biomaterials*, 8:353.

130. Holland, S. J., B. J. Tighe and B. L. Gould. 1986. *J. Controlled Release*, 4:155.

131. Holland, S. J., A. M. Jolly, M. Yasin and B. J. Tighe. 1987. *Biomaterials*, 8:289.

132. Leonard, F. 1970. In *Adhesion in Biological Systems*. R. S. Manty, ed. London: Academic Press, p. 185.

133. Leonard, F., J. A. Collins and H. J. Porter. 1966. *J. Appl. Polym. Sci.*, 10:1617.

134. Mungiu, C., D. Cogălniceanu, M. Leibovici and I. Negulescu. 1979. *J. Polym. Sci., Polym. Symp.*, 66:189.

135. Florence, A. T., T. L. Whateley, D. A. Wood. 1979. *J. Pharm. Pharmacol.*, 31:422.

136. Chang, T. M. S. 1977. In *Biomedical Applications of*

Immobilized Enzymes and Proteins, Vol. 1. T. M. S. Chang, ed. New York: Plenum Press, p. 69.

137. Domb, A. and R. Langer. 1988. *Makromol. Chem., Makromol. Symp.*, 19:189, Hüthig & Wepf Verlag, Basel.

138. Ozawa, H., S. Hosaka, T. Kunitomo and H. Tanzawa. 1983. *Biomaterials*, 4:170, Butterworth & Co. Ltd. ©.

139. Hosaka, S., H. Ozawa, H. Tanzawa, T. Kinitono and R. L. Nichols. 1983. *Biomaterials*, 4:243.

140. Murray, E. S., R. L. Nichols. 1967. *Pan American Health Organization Scientific Publication*, No. 147, p. 537.

141. Dawson, C. R., T. Daghfous, M. Messadi, I. Hoshiwara, D. W. Vastine, C. Yoneda and J. Schachte. 1974. *Arch. Ophthalmol.*, 92:193.

142. Dawson, C. R., I. Hoshiwara, T. Daghfous and M. Messadt. 1975. *Am. J. Ophthalmol.*, 79:803.

143. Portney, G. L. and S. B. Portney. 1974. *Arch. Ophthalmol.*, 92:212.

144. Woolridge, R. L., J. T. Gravston, E. B. Perrin, C. Y. Yan, K. H. Chang and I. H. Chang. 1967. *Amer. J. Ophthalmol.*, 63:1313.

145. Dawson, C. R., L. Hanna and E. Jowetz. 1967. *Lancet*, 2:961.

146. Dawson, C. R. 1974. *J. Schachter*, 13:85.

147. Dumitriu, S. *Biomaterials* (in press).

148. Selikson, A. and E. Kondotkva. 1976. *Farmacia Polska*, 10:243.

149. Surdeanu, E., E. Gafiţeanu, A. Verbuţă and L. Gavriliţa. 1968. *Pract. Farm. (Bucureşti)*, 2:87.

150. 1978. *Standard Rezepturen*, VEB Verlag Volk und Gesundheit, Berlin, p. 63.

151. Vasilescu, C. 1977. *Pract. Farm. (Bucureşti)*, 8:105.

152. Verbuţă, A. 1983. *Pract. Farm. (Bucureşti)*, 14:41.

153. Simionescu, Cr., M. I. Popa and S. Dumitriu. 1986. *Biomaterials*, 7:118.

154. Simionescu, Cr., M. I. Popa and S. Dumitriu. 1985. *Colloid & Polym. Sci.*, 268:620 (1985).

155. Simionescu, Cr., M. I. Popa and S. Dumitriu. 1987. In *Biomaterials and Clinical Applications*. A. Pizzoferrato, P. G. Marchetti, A. Ravaglioli and A. J. C. Lee, eds. Amsterdam: Elsevier Science Publ., p. 649.

156. Simionescu, Cr., M. I. Popa, S. Dumitriu, A. Verbuţă and A. Hriscu. 1985. *Farmacia (Bucureşti)*, 33:147.

157. Simionescu, Cr., M. I. Popa, A. Verbuţă, S. Dumitriu, I. Cojocaru and A. Hriscu. 1985. *Farmacia (Bucureşti)*, 33:153.

158. Dumitriu, S., M. Popa and C. Beldie. 1988. *Makromol. Chem., Makromol. Symp.*, 19:313 (1988).

159. Dumitriu, S., C. Beldie, M. Popa and C. Dan. 1989. Rom. Patent 97,695.

160. Beldie, C., S. Dumitriu, N. Aeleniei, M. Popa and M. I. Popa. *Biomaterials* (in press).

161. Dumitriu, S. *Clinical Materials* (in press).

162. Dumitriu, S., M. Popa, M. Dumitriu and Cr. Dumitriu. 1989. *VIth International Conference Polymer in Medicine and Surgery, 12–14 April, 1989*. The Plastic and Rubber Institute, London.

163. Dumitriu, S., P. Vancea, D. Costin and M. Popa. 1987. *Clinical Materials*, 2:141.

164. Vancea, P., S. Dumitriu, M. Popa, M. Dumitriu and D. Costin. 1988. *Chimica oggi*, (4):21.

165. Dumitriu, S., P. Vancea, M. Popa and D. Costin. 1988. *J. Bioactive Biocomp. Polym.*, 3:370.

166. Yolles, S. and M. F. Sartori. 1980. *Drug Delivery Systems*. R. L. Juliano, ed. New York: Oxford University Press, cap. 3.

167. Heller, J. and R. W. Baker. 1980. *Controlled Release of Bioactive Materials*. R. Baker, ed. New York: Academic Press, p. 1.

168. Pitt, C. G., T. A. Marks and A. Schindler. 1980. *Controlled Release of Bioactive Materials*. R. Baker, ed. New York: Academic Press, p. 19.

169. Gregoris, D. E., S. W. Kim, J. Feijen, J. M. Anderson and S. Mitra. 1980. In *Controlled Release of Bioactive Materials*. R. Baker, ed. New York: Academic Press, p. 45.

170. Gurny, R., T. Boye, H. Ibrahim and P. Buri. 1985. *Proceed. Intern. Symp. Control. Rel. Bioact. Mater.*, 12:300.

171. Miller, S. C. and M. D. Donovan. 1982. *Int. J. Pharm.*, 12:147.

172. Boye, T., R. Gurny and P. Buri. 1984. In *Proceeding International Symposium on Biopharmaceutics and Pharmacokinetics*. J. M. Aiche and D. Hirtz, eds. Salamanca.

173. Haslam, J. L., T. Higuchi and A. R. Mlodozeniec. 1984. U.S. Patent 4,474,751.

174. Gurny, R. and D. Taylor. 1980. *Proceedings of the International Symposium of the British Pharmaceutical Technology Conference, London*. M. H. Rubinstein, ed.

175. Yoshida, S. and S. Mishima. 1975. *Jps. J. Ophthalmol.*, 19:121.

176. Refojo, M. F. 1972. *Surv. Ophthalmol.*, 16:233.

177. Cassiani-Ingoni, L., F. Subira, C. Bunel, J. P. Vairon and J. L. Halary. 1988. *Makromol. Chem., Macromol. Symp.*, 19:287.

178. Waltman, S. R. and H. E. Kaufman. 1970. *Invest. Ophthalmol.*, 9:250.

179. Kaufman, H. T., M. H. Uotila, A. R. Gasset, R. O. Wood and E. D. Ellison. 1971. *Trans. Am. Acad. Ophthalmol. Otolaryngol.*, 75:361.

180. Prous, R., I. Brettschneider, L. Krejči and D. Kalvodova. 1972. *Ophthalmologica*, 165:62.

181. Hull, D. S., H. F. Edelhauser and R. A. Hyondiuk. 1974. *Arch. Ophthalmol.*, 92:413.

182. Ivani, E. J. 1984. U.S. Patent 4,447,562.

183. Asseff, C. F., R. L. Weisman, S. M. Podos and B. Becker. 1973. *Am. J. Ophthalmol.*, 75:212.

184. Maichuk, Y. F. 1975. *Invest. Ophthalmol.*, 14:87.

185. Kitazawa, Y. 1975. *Acta Soc. Ophthalmol. Jpn.*, 79:1715.

186. Katz, I. M. and W. A. Blackman. 1977. *Am. J. Ophthalmol.*, 83:728.

187. Capozza, R. C. 1975. German Patent 2,505,305.

188. Bensinger, R., D. H. Shin, M. A. Kass, S. M. Podos and B. Becker. 1976. *Invest. Ophthalmol.*, 15:1008.

189. Pavan-Langston, D. 1976. In *Symposium on Ocular Therapy, Vol. 9.* I. H. Leopold and R. P. Burns, eds. New York: John Wiley & Sons, cap. 2.

190. Saettone, M. F., B. Giannaccini, P. Chetoni, G. Galli and E. Chiellini. 1983. In *Polymers in Medicine. Biomedical and Pharmacological Applications.* E. Chiellini and P. Giusti, eds. New York and London: Plenum Press, p. 187.

191. Flynn, G. L., S. H. Yalkowsky and T. J. Roseman. 1974. *J. Pharm. Sci.*, 63:479.

192. Loucas, S. P. and H. M. Haddad. 1972. *J. Pharm. Sci.*, 61:985.

193. Loucas, S. P. and H. M. Haddad. 1976. *Metabol. Ophthalmol.*, 1:27.

194. Schoenwald, R. D. and R. E. Roehrs. 1979. U.S. Patent 4,271,143.

195. Saettone, M. F., B. Giannaccini, A. Teneggi, P. Savigni and N. Tellini. 1982. *J. Pharm. Pharmacol.*, 34:464.

196. Saettone, M. F., B. Giannaccini, P. Chetoni, G. Galli and E. Chiellini. 1984. *J. Pharm. Pharmacol.*, 36:229.

197. Saettone, M. F. and E. Chiellini. 1985. *Proceedings of the 12th International Symposium on Controlled Release of Bioactive Materials, July 8–122, Geneva,* p. 302.

198. Odello, G., M. F. Saettone, B. Giannaccini, L. Mastrogeni, G. Meucci and C. Silvis. 1985. *ATTI del X Convegno della Societa Oftalmologica Siciliana,* Mazara del Vallo, Casa Editrice Pluri-Grafica Sicula, Messina, p. 201.

199. Odello, G., M. F. Saettone, B. Giannaccini, L. Mastrogeni, G. Meucci and C. Silvis. 1987. *Bulletino di Oculistica,* 66:557.

200. Saettone, M. F., B. Giannaccini, G. Marchesini, G. Galli and E. Chiellini. 1986. In *Polymers in Medicine II.* E. Chiellini, P. Giusti, C. Migliaresi and L. Nicolais, eds. New York: Plenum Press, p. 409.

201. Saettone, M. F., P. Chetoni, B. Giannaccini. *2nd International Conference on Polymers in Medicine, 3–7 June 1985, Capri, Italy,* p. 29.

202. Saettone, M. F., P. Chetoni, M. T. Torracca, S. Burgalassi and B. Giannaccini. 1989. *Int. J. Pharm.,* 51:203.

203. Benedetto, D. A., D. O. Shah and H. E. Kaufmen. 1975. *Invest. Ophthalmol.*, 14:887.

204. Atsugi, A. Y., Y. M. Machida, S. M. Nagoya, K. N. Yao, Y. H. Kashiwara and S. M. Nara. 1980. U.S. Patent 4,230,690.

205. Urtti, A. 1985. *Int. J. Pharm.*, 26:45.

206. Urtti, A., L. Salminen, O. Miinalainen. 1985. *Int. J. Pharm.*, 23:147.

207. Saettone, M. F., B. Giannaccini, G. Leonardi, D. Monti, D. Chetoni, G. Galli and E. Chiellini. 1988. In *Polymers in Medicine III.* C. Migliaresi, L. Nicolais, P. Giusti and E. Chiellini, eds. Elsevier, p. 209.

208. Cowie, J. M. G. 1985. In *Alternating Copolymers.* J. M. G. Cowie, ed. New York: Plenum Press, p. 19.

209. Lee, V. H. and J. R. Robinson. 1978. In *Sustained and Controlled Release Drug Delivery Systems.* J. R. Robinson, ed. New York: M. Dekker, p. 170.

210. Maichuk, Y. F. 1976. In *Symposium on Ocular Therapy, Vol. 9.* I. H. Leopold, and R. P. Burns, eds. New York: John Wiley & Sons, Chap. 2.

211. Maichuk, Y. F. 1975. *Invest. Ophthalmol.*, 14:87.

212. Dohlman, C. H., D. Pavan-Langston and J. Rose. 1972. *Ann. Ophthalmol.*, 4:823.

213. Allansmith, M. R., J. R. Lee, B. H. McClellan and C. H. Dohlman. 1975. *Trans. Am. Acad. Ophthalmol. Otolaryngol.*, 79:128.

214. Keller, N., A. M. Longwell and S. A. Birss. 1975. *Arch. Ophthalmol.*, 93:1349.

215. Pa Yan-Langston, D., R. H. S. Langston and P. A. Geary. 1975. *Arch. Ophthalmol.*, 93:1349.

216. Bloomfield, S. E., T. Miyata, M. W. Dunn, M. Bueser, K. H. Stenzel and A. L. Rubin. 1978. *Arch. Ophthalmol.*, 96:885.

217. Belleville, S. S. C., S. G. Bloomfield and M. J. Dover. 1981. U.S. Patent 4,255,415.

218. Arizono, K., M. Terasowa and M. Nobutoki. 1985. U.S. Patent 4,525,348.

219. Weiner, B. Z., A. Zilkha, G. Porath and Y. Grunfeld. 1976. *Eur. J. Med. Chem. Chim. Ther.*, 11:525.

220. Zalipsky, S., C. Gilon and A. Zilkha. 1983. *Eur. Polym. J.*, 19:1177.

221. Lipatova, T. E. and R. A. Veslovsky. 1969. *Vysokomol. Soedin.*, A11:1459.

222. Lipatova, T. E. 1979. *J. Polym. Sci., Polym. Symp.,* 66:239.

223. Inagaki, H. and M. Tanaka. 1964. *Makromolek. Chem.*, 74:145.

224. Howell, B. A., E. W. Walles and R. Rashidianfar. 1988. *Makromolek. Chem., Makromol. Symp.,* 19:329.

225. Refojo, M. F. and D. A. Thomas. 1975. *Ophthalmic Res.*, 7:33.

226. Rankin, F. S., 1985. *Proceed. Intern. Symp. Control. Rel. Bioact. Mater.*, 12:143.

227. Braley, S. 1970. *J. Macromol. Sci. Chem.*, A4:529.

228. Long, M. D. and M. J. Folkman. 1966. U.S. Patent 3,279,996.

229. Langer, R., N. Peppas. 1983. *J. Macromol. Sci., Chem. Phys.*, C23:61.

230. Refojo, M. F. 1975. *Ophthalmic Res.*, 7:459.

231. Bachrach, A. and A. Zilkha. 1984. *Eur. Polym. J.*, 20:493.

232. Statford, R. E., D. C. Yang, M. A. Reddell and V. H. L. Lee. 1983. *Curr. Eye Res.*, 2:377.

233. Shaeffer, H. E. and D. L. Krohn. 1982. *Invest. Op. Vis. Sci.*, 22:220.

234. Gurny, R. 1981. *Pharm. Acta Helv.*, 56:130.

235. Fitzgerald, P., J. Hodgraft, J. Krenter and C. G. Wilson. 1985. *Proceed. Intern. Symp. Control. Rel. Bioact. Mater.*, 12:306.

236. Richardson, V. J., K. Jeyasingh, R. F. Jewkes, B. E. Ryman and H. M. Tattersall. 1977. *Biochem. Soc. Trans.*, 5:290.

237. Szoka, F. J. and D. Papahadjopoulis. 1978. *Proc. Nat. Acad. Sci.*, 75:4194.

238. Hawang, K. J., J. E. Merriam, P. J. Beaumier and K. S. Luk. 1982. *Biochim. Biophys. Acta,* 716:101.

239. Wood, R. W., H. H. L. Lee, J. Kreuter and J. R. Robinson. 1987. *Int. J. Pharm.*, 42:516.

240. Robert, C., N. A. Peppas and P. Buri. 1985. *Proceed. Intern. Symp. Control. Rel. Bioact. Mater.*, 12:130.

241. Mueller, K. F., S. Heiber and W. Flankl. 1978. U.S. Patent 4,224,427.

242. Urquhart, J. 1980. In *Ophthalmic Drug Delivery Systems*. J. R. Robinson, ed. Washington, DC: American Pharmaceutical Association, p. 105.

243. Heilman, K. 1978. *Therapeutic Systems*, Herdweg: Georg Thieme.

244. Pavan-Langston, D. 1976. In *Symposium on Ocular Therapy, Vol. 9.* I. H. Leopold and R. P. Burns, eds. New York: John Wiley & Sons.

245. Shell, J. W. and R. W. Baker. 1974. *Ann. Ophthalmol.*, 6:1037.

246. Armaly, M. F. and K. R. Rao. 1973. In *Symposium on Ocular Therapy, Vol. 6.* I. H. Leopold, ed. St. Louis: C. V. Mosby, Chap. 11.

247. Armaly, M. F. and K. R. Rao. 1973. *Invest. Ophthalmol.*, 12:491.

248. Worthen, D. M., T. J. Zimmerman and C. A. Wind. 1974. *Invest. Ophthalmol.*, 13:296.

249. Place, V. A., M. Fisher, S. Herbst, L. Gordon and R. C. Merrill. 1975. *Am. J. Ophthalmol.*, 80:706.

250. Brown, H. S., G. Meltzer, R. C. Merrill, M. Fischer, C. Ferre and V. A. Place. 1976. *Arch. Ophthalmol.*, 94:1716.

251. Drance, S. M., D. W. A. Mitchell and M. Schulzer. 1977. *Can. J. Ophthalmol.*, 12:24.

252. Tomono, M. and K. Nanba. 1981. *Folia Ophthalmol. Jpn.*, 32:2095.

253. Birss, S. A., A. Longwell, S. Heckbert and N. Keller. 1978. *Ann. Ophthalmol.*, 10:1045.

254. Jonson, B. R., J. Anderson and H. Fuglsang. 1978. *Br. J. Ophthalmol.*, 62:428.

255. Havener, H. W. 1978. *Ocular Pharmacology, 4th Ed.* St. Louis: C. V. Mosby, Chap. 2.

256. Refojo, M. F., H. S. Liu, F. L. Leong and D. Sidebottom. 1978. *J. Bioengineer*, 2:437.

257. Liu, H. S., M. F. Refojo, H. D. Perry and D. M. Albert. 1978. *Invest. Ophthalmol. Vis. Sci.*, 17:993.

258. Liu, H. S., M. F. Refojo and D. M. Albert. 1980. *Arch. Ophthalmol.*, 98:905.

259. Ueno, N., M. F. Refojo and L. H. S. Liu. 1982. *Invest. Ophthalmol., Vis. Sci.*, 23:199.

260. Kobayaschi, T. 1980. *Kobunshi*, 2:117; *C.A.*, 92:203509v.

261. Lebedenko, V. Ya, G. P. Gryadunova and G. I. Dontsova. 1979. *Farmatsiya (Moscow)*, 28:68.

262. Golderg, E. P. 1978. In *Polymeric Drugs*. L. G. Donaruma and O. Vogl, eds. New York: Academic Press, p. 239.

263. Liu, H. S., M. F. Refojo, H. D. Perry and D. M. Albert. 1979. *Invest. Ophthalmol. Vis. Sci.*, 18:1061.

264. Ueno, N., M. F. Refojo and L. S. H. Liu. 1982. *J. Biomed. Mater. Res.*, 16:699.

265. Heller, J. 1985. *Proceed. Intern. Symp. Control. Rel. Bioact. Mater.*, 12:45.

266. Theeuwes, F. and S. I. Yum. 1976. *Ann. Biomed. Engin.*, 4:343.

267. Theeuwes, F. and B. Eckenhoff. 1980. In *Controlled Release of Bioactive Materials*. R. Baker, ed. New York: Academic Press.

268. Falcon, M. G. and B. R. Jones. 1977. *Trans. Ophthalmol. Soc. U.K.*, 97:330.

269. Campbell, L. H. 1979. In *Symposium on Ocular Therapy*. I. H. Leopold and R. P. Burus, eds. New York: John Wiley & Sons, p. 100.

270. Michelson, J. B. and R. A. Nozik. 1979. *Arch. Ophthalmol.*, 97:1345.

271. Eliason, J. A. and D. M. Maurice. 1980. *Invest. Ophthalmol. Vis. Sci.*, 19:102.

41

Medicated Bioerodible Ophthalmic Devices

DAVID A. LEE, M.D.*
KAM W. LEONG, PH.D.**

ABSTRACT: The eye presents special challenges for drug delivery in the treatment of various ocular diseases. Many of the conventional therapeutic modalities have not adequately solved these problems. Medicated biodegradable devices used for drug delivery may offer several advantages over conventional ocular drug delivery methods. These polymeric drug delivery systems may be adaptable to particular situations by changing their size, shape, and composition depending on the characteristics of the drug being delivered and the intended site of treatment. To a certain degree the drug release characteristics of these devices can be modeled mathematically, but empirical trials are ultimately necessary to demonstrate safety and efficacy. These medicated bioerodible ophthalmic devices have a promising future in the treatment of various ocular diseases.

INTRODUCTION

The eye is a delicate, privileged, light-detecting, neuro-sensory organ that is an extension of the central nervous system. There are a variety of systems that protect the eye from both external and internal insults. These mechanisms of protection affect the pharmacokinetics of drugs in the eye. The eyelids protect the globe from mechanical trauma and surface drying. The tear film keeps the surface of the eye moist and washes away toxins and micro-organisms from the ocular surface. The cornea, conjunctival epithelium,

and sclera provide differential solubility and diffusional barriers to the penetration of the multitude of soluble substances in the tear film. Substances that successfully penetrate into the eye are rapidly removed by the constant production and drainage of aqueous humor as well as by the ocular blood circulation. The eye, like the brain, is protected from substances in the blood by the blood-retina and blood-aqueous barriers. These unique ocular characteristics determine the pharmacokinetics of medications used to treat a wide variety of eye conditions.

BACKGROUND

The most common route of ocular drug administration is topical, either by eye drops or ointments. More prolonged topical administration of medications may be achieved through solid delivery devices placed between the eyelid and globe such as hydrogel contact lenses, ocuserts, and liposomes. In order to achieve higher intraocular drug levels some medications require more invasive periocular administration by subconjunctival or retrobulbar injection. The highest intraocular drug concentrations are obtained through direct intraocular injection of medications into the vitreous cavity. These more invasive means of administering medications to the eye are accompanied by a greater risk of injury to the vital ocular structures. Systemic administration of drugs by oral or intravenous routes are usually not effective in achieving high intraocular drug levels. These limitations of conventional ocular drug delivery systems have prompted the development of newer, safer, and more efficacious means of delivering drugs into the eye.

MECHANISMS OF POLYMERIC DRUG RELEASE

To understand the challenges one faces in designing biodegradable carriers for drug delivery to the eye, it

Supported by National Eye Institute grants EY07701 and EY00331, the Lucille Ellis Simon Glaucoma Research Fund, and the Whitaker Foundation.

* Department of Ophthalmology, Jules Stein Eye Institute, UCLA School of Medicine, 100 Stein Plaza, Los Angeles, CA 90024-7004

** Department of Biomedical Engineering, Johns Hopkins University, 148 New Engineering Building, Baltimore, MD 21218

would be instructive to first consider the basic mechanisms of polymeric controlled release. The drug release mechanism can be categorized as mainly diffusion or matrix-degradation controlled. Diffusion through the drug-carrier is driven by the concentration gradient between the carrier and the drug release medium or body fluid. It can also be induced by osmotic pressure and matrix swelling. For matrices that biodegrade or that contain drug conjugates, release is controlled by the hydrolytic or enzymatic cleavage of the relevent chemical bonds. Even in such biodegradable systems, diffusion of the reactants and the liberated drug molecules may still be rate-limiting. Understanding the different scenarios of drug release by diffusion is thus important.

The diffusion-controlled systems can be distinguished into reservoir and matrix devices [1]. In the former case, the drug reservoir is encapsulated by a polymeric membrane. The drug core can be in the solid or in the liquid state, and the membrane can be microporous or non-porous. If the drug core is maintained in a saturated state, the transport of drug molecules across the membrane will be kept constant, as the driving force is unchanged. Such a constant or zero-order release would require the drug core to remain in a solid or suspension state. The saturated state would be difficult to maintain if the drug has high water solubility, such as drugs like pilocarpine. The zero-order kinetics would also be observed only in the middle stages of the release. If the device is used immediately after fabrication, there is a lag time needed to saturate the membrane before the drug will be seen in the medium. If on the other hand the device is placed in storage for an extended period of time before usage, there will be a burst of drug release as a result of accumulation in the membrane. The time it takes for the release rate to reach the steady state value varies with the nature and the thickness of the membrane. Towards the end stages of release, the rate will decline as the concentration in the core drops below the saturation value.

One of the first polymeric ophthalmic drug delivery devices, Ocusert, uses this principle to control the drug release [2]. In this device the drug pilocarpine and a filler alginic acid are laminated by a thin membrane of polyethylene-vinyl acetate (EVAc). A ring made of EVAc and titanium oxide is then used to seal the drug reservoir. When placed in buffer, this device would, after a burst in the first day, yield a constant release of pilocarpine for a week.

The other type of diffusion-controlled system consists of dissolution or dispersion of drug in the matrix [3]. Since the diffusion distance for the drug solute to travel from the core to the surface is lengthened as the drug is depleted, the release rate decreases with time. A first order release kinetics often results from such device; the amount of drug released will be proportional to the square root of time. Aside from diffusion through the polymer phase, the drug can also diffuse through the channels created by dissolution of the drug phase. In fact, this is the only avenue by which macromolecules and drugs that have low permeability can be released. Release kinetics in this case are highly dependent on the drug loading level and on the particle size of the drug solutes since those parameters will determine the extent and size of the pores and channels. If the drug loading level is below a critical value, there may not be enough interconnected channels and some drug solutes will be trapped inside the matrix.

If the polymer swells in water, such as a hydrogel, drug release will occur as water penetrates the matrix. The swollen region will provide little diffusion resistance. The release rate in this system is hence controlled by the swelling rate of the polymer, which in turn is affected by the hydrophilicity and crosslinking density of the hydrogel. Soft contact lenses made of hydrogels are examples of such ocular drug delivery systems [4]. They have been used to improve the delivery of idoxuridine [5], polymyxin B [5], pilocarpine [6,7], tetracycline [8], chloramphenicol [8], and prednisolone [9] to the eye.

With a polymer that is biodegradable, the release can be affected by the gradual dissolution of the matrix. The dissolution can be due to the hydrolytic or enzymatic cleavage of the backbone of the polymer. For instance, the polyanhydrides and most other polymers such as polyesters and polyamides belong to this category (Figure 1). The cleavage can also occur in the cross-linking bonds, rendering soluble an initially cross-linked polymer. Alternatively, the dissolution originates from hydrolysis, ionization or protonation of the side chains of the polymers [10]. If there is no cleavage of the backbone, the dissolved polymer would still have high molecular weights and may present toxicologic problems.

The obvious advantage of a biodegradable system is the elimination of the need to remove the drug-depleted device. This is an appealing feature in designing ophthalmic drug delivery systems, especially if the target site is in a place like the vitreous body. More than convenience, the biodegradable system also offers potential advantages from the release standpoint. If the drug release is controlled solely by the dissolution of a matrix which biodegrades from the surface, the release rate is more predictable and controllable. To change the release rate, one needs only to proportionally vary the drug loading level. The release will also be much less dependent on the properties of the drug phase, which reduces the developmental effort for a new drug. The release rate in this case can be constant with time if the surface area remains unchanged, such as in a slab. Other geometric shapes such as a hollow cylinder may also lead to a relatively constant surface area during degradation [11]. However, the assumption that release is controlled only by matrix degradation is seldom valid. In reality the drug solutes can also be released through diffusion, as discussed previously for the non-biodegradable systems. This is particularly true if

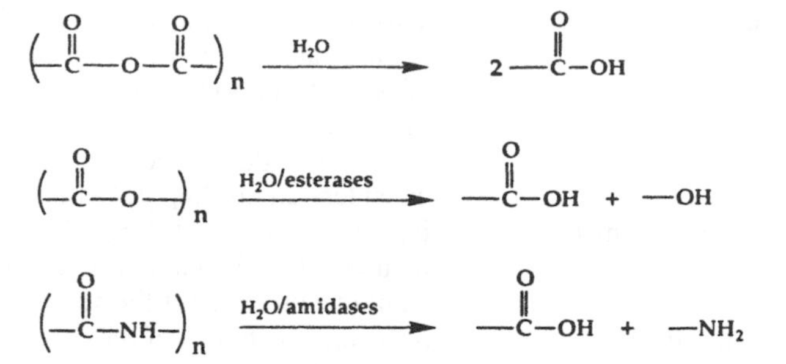

$$\left(-\overset{\overset{\displaystyle O}{\|}}{C}-O-\overset{\overset{\displaystyle O}{\|}}{C}-\right)_n \xrightarrow{\;H_2O\;} 2 -\overset{\overset{\displaystyle O}{\|}}{C}-OH \qquad \textbf{(Eq. 1a)}$$

$$\left(-\overset{\overset{\displaystyle O}{\|}}{C}-O-\right)_n \xrightarrow{\;H_2O/\text{esterases}\;} -\overset{\overset{\displaystyle O}{\|}}{C}-OH \; + \; -OH \qquad \textbf{(Eq. 1b)}$$

$$\left(-\overset{\overset{\displaystyle O}{\|}}{C}-NH-\right)_n \xrightarrow{\;H_2O/\text{amidases}\;} -\overset{\overset{\displaystyle O}{\|}}{C}-OH \; + \; -NH_2 \qquad \textbf{(Eq. 1c)}$$

Figure 1. Dissolution of the polymer backbone by hydrolytic [Equation (1a)] and enzymatic [Equation (1b) and (1c)] cleavage.

the drug is hydrophilic, because this property presents a high driving force for diffusion. It must be noted that a constant release can sometimes be achieved if the diffusion is accompanied by a change in the matrix properties which boosts the diffusivity. For instance, the diffusivity may increase with time as a result of partial degradation or swelling of the matrix. Such an increase may compensate for the decrease in the chemical potential diffusion gradient and lead to a constant release.

A different type of biodegradable system involves a chemical linkage of the drug to the side chain of the polymer [12,13] (Figure 2). The release rate of the polymer-drug conjugate, which has been called a pendant system, is dependent on the cleavage of the polymer-drug bond. If the drug is attached to the polymer via a spacer, the hydrolysis of the polymer-spacer and the spacer-drug bonds must both be considered. The spacer approach provides an effective means of controlling the release rate. Although penetration of water into the matrix and outward diffusion of the cleaved drug molecules constitute part of the rate barrier, the cleavage of the polymer-drug bond as the rate-limiting step is preferred for better control. While the drug loading level of biodegradable matrix systems would generally be under 30 percent, the pendant system has the potential advantage of a much higher drug-to-polymer ratio. The pendant system is particularly suitable for hydrophilic drugs. The chemically controlled pendant system affords the best chance to retard the release by minimizing the role of diffusion through the use of a relatively stable polymer-drug bond.

The previous discussion focused only on the rate barriers of the drug carriers. The drug was assumed to be released into a perfect sink. As an ocular implant, it is conceivable that the controlled release device

would face a non-perfect sink situation because of the relatively low perfusion rate. The reduction in the concentration gradient will thus slow down the release rate. Depending on the implant site in the eye, there may also be increased mass transfer resistance in the implant-tissue interface which retards the release. In general it is safe to assume that the *in vivo* release will be slower than that observed in the *in vitro* kinetic studies. If the drug is highly water insoluble, dissolution of the drug may become one of the rate-determining steps, and the analysis will have to be adjusted accordingly.

MATHEMATICAL MODELS OF POLYMERIC DRUG DELIVERY

Mathematical analysis of drug release from biodegradable systems is difficult because of the coupled processes of matrix degradation and drug diffusion [14]. As a guideline, however, the simplified analysis of the idealized release mechanism in which matrix degradation is the sole controlling factor is useful [11,15]. The relationship which describes the drug release rate in this case is simply:

$$dM_t/dt = K_o * \text{surface area}$$

where

M_t = drug released at time t
K_o = the heterogeneous degradation constant of the matrix

Assuming the edge effects are neglected, the change in surface area as a function of time for different ge-

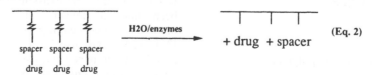

Figure 2. Chemical linkage of the drug to the polymer side chains [Equation (2)].

ometries is constant for a slab or disc, $2\pi L(a\text{-}K_o t/C_o)$ for a cylinder, and $4\pi(a\text{-}K_o t/C_o)^2$ for a sphere,

where

L = height of the cylinder
C_o = uniform initial drug concentration in matrix
a = radius of cylinder or sphere

It follows that a single expression can be used to describe the release profile:

$$M_t/M_\infty = 1 - [1 - K_o t/C_o a]^n$$

where

M_∞ = total amount of drug in the device
a = radius of sphere or cylinder, or half thickness of slab
n = 1 for a slab, 2 for a cylinder, 3 for a sphere

For ophthalmic controlled release devices, there is a severe restriction on the dimension of the implants, imposed by the geometry of the eye. For instance, the practical size of the medicated pellets placed in the subconjunctival space for glaucoma filtering surgery as described later would be on the order of several millimeters in diameter. The assumption that the edge effects can be neglected would no longer be valid at such dimensions. Therefore, even under the idealized situation zero-order kinetics could not be realized.

Other mathematical models which allow diffusion and homogeneous matrix degradation all result in a release rate varying with time. Baker and Lonsdale derived a rate expression for the slab geometry as [16]:

$$dM_t/dt = (K_s - K_b)m/\ln (A^o/A'') - K_b t$$

where

K_s = rate constant of surface degradation
K_b = rate constant of bulk degradation
m = thickness of surface degradation layer
A^o = initial concentration of reactable bonds
A'' = concentration of reactable bonds at time t

In modelling release from homogeneously degrading polymers such as polylactide, in which it is assumed that chain cleavage is first order and diffusion though the matrix is the rate-determining step, Heller and Baker developed the expression [17]:

$$dM_t/dt = A/2[2P_o C_o e^{Kt}/t]^{1/2}$$

where

P_o = initial permeability of the polymer
A = total surface area
K = first order rate constant of matrix degradation

This model attempts to describe cases where the release rate can be accelerated toward the end stages of release due to permeability increase caused by the matrix erosion.

Lee later developed a more general model which considers an eroding polymer front as well as a moving diffusion front [18]. Using a refined integral method, it is shown that a zero-order release kinetics would be observed if the value $K_o a/D$, where D is the diffusion coefficient of the drug in the polymer, is high (e.g. > 10). If the ratio of erosion rate to permeability is comparable ($\cong 1$), then the release would approach zero-order when the drug loading is much higher than the drug solubility in the matrix.

It should be pointed out that there are other elaborate fabrication schemes which can help achieve zero-order release. They include non-uniform drug distribution in the matrix [19], and limiting the release to a sector of right circular cylinder [20,21], a hemisphere [22], multiple holes [23], or an inwardly tapered disk with a central releasing hole [24] (Figure 3). The practicality of these concepts remains to be seen with regard to the difficulty in fabrication and the potential risk of the holes being covered by tissue encapsulation.

OPHTHALMIC APPLICATIONS OF POLYMERIC DRUG DELIVERY

Biodegradable devices that are nontoxic, nonteratogenic, and biologically inert have many potential advantages over conventional ocular drug delivery systems. These devices may be applied to the surface of the eye or implanted intraocularly to provide a controlled and sustained release of medication into the eye. There are a wide range of ophthalmic diseases which could benefit from drugs delivered by these bioerodible systems. These diseases include ocular infections such as bacterial, viral, or fungal corneal ulcers and endophthalmitis; ocular tumors including melanoma and retinoblastoma; ocular wound healing problems following intraocular surgery including cataract surgery, glaucoma-filtering surgery, and vitreoretinal surgery; inflammatory diseases of the eye such as severe chronic uveitis; and proliferative diabetic retinopathy. The size, shape, degradation rate, medication, and intraocular location of these bioerodible devices can be determined by the particular condition treated.

Biodegradable contact lenses composed of non-cross-linked porcine collagen have been used to deliver antibiotics for the treatment of bacterial corneal ulcers [25]. These dissolvable contact lenses have been shown to deliver high concentrations of antibiotic into the cornea over an extended period of time [26]. There may also be a potential for using these dissolvable contact lenses for the treatment of nonhealing corneal epithelial erosions using fibronectin [27]. These biodegradable contact lens devices have

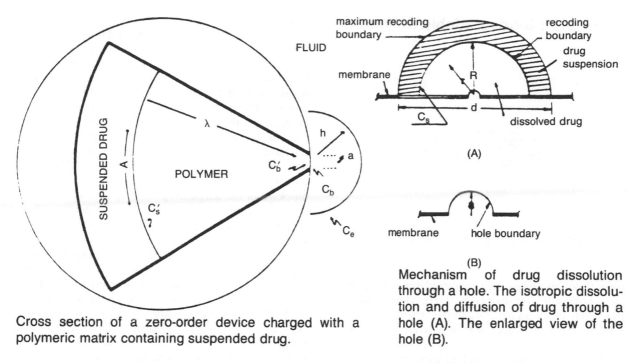

Cross section of a zero-order device charged with a polymeric matrix containing suspended drug.

Mechanism of drug dissolution through a hole. The isotropic dissolution and diffusion of drug through a hole (A). The enlarged view of the hole (B).

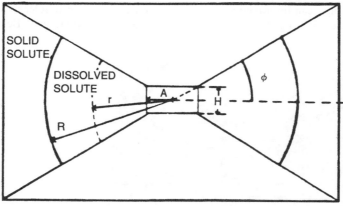

Cross-sectional view of the proposed device geometry.

Figure 3. Different polymer shapes to achieve zero-order drug release: sector of a right circular cylinder [20], multiple holes [23], and inwardly tapered disk with a central releasing hole [24]. Reprinted with permission from the *Journal of Pharmaceutical Sciences*.

the advantage of easy application and removal from the surface of the eye, a mechanical "bandage" effect over the treated surface area, and sustained and localized delivery of high concentrations of medications to the intended treatment site.

Biodegradable collagen sponges impregnated with antimetabolites such as 5-fluorouracil and bleomycin have been implanted at the site of glaucoma filtering surgery in order to prevent scar tissue formation and failure of the surgical procedure [28,29]. In preliminary trials it appears that the delivered drug is depleted from the device before the collagen matrix completely degrades. The duration of drug delivery is only a few days following its implantation. The collagen matrix depleted of drug may incite an inflammatory reaction at the implantation site and cause further

scar tissue formation. It would not be practical to periodically replace a depleted collagen sponge because the required surgical operation to replace it may initiate additional inflammatory reaction and scar formation as well as the added risk of surgical complications.

Liposomes, small drug-containing vesicles composed of a phospholipid bilayer, have been used to slowly release antibiotics and antimetabolites into the eye [30,31]. Potentially they may be useful for the treatment of endophthalmitis [32], proliferative vitreoretinopathy [33,34], and prevention of scar formation after glaucoma filtering surgery [35]. These drug-filled liposomes may be injected to the treated site with a needle, thus avoiding a more extensive surgical procedure. Unfortunately, it has been found that

Laminated Biodegradable Polymers

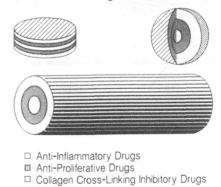

☐ Anti-Inflammatory Drugs
☒ Anti-Proliferative Drugs
☐ Collagen Cross-Linking Inhibitory Drugs

Figure 4. Different shapes of laminated polymers.

these lipsomes release their delivered drugs before the phospholipid bilayer dissolves. The residual phospholipids may create an inflammatory reaction. In a situation where the liposomes or their delivered drugs may be toxic to the eye, it would be very difficult to remove the liposomes completely before they spontaneously dissolved. This disadvantage can be avoided using a solid monolithic biodegradable drug delivery device.

Synthetic biodegradable materials such as poly-anhydrides [10,36–39] have been used to deliver drugs for the prevention of excessive wound healing following glaucoma filtering surgery. This particular situation is very suitable for the use of bioerodible devices because wound healing is a localized and time-limited process. The purpose of glaucoma filtering surgery is to decrease the intraocular pressure of the eye by creating a small hole in the wall of the eye to drain out the fluid from the eye, and thereby prevent irreversible optic nerve damage and visual field loss. The most common cause of glaucoma filtering surgery failure is blockage of the surgical opening by scar tissue.

Wound healing is a complex series of biological events which normally occur following trauma to a living organism and proceeds in a series of ordered chronological stages over a finite time period [40,41]. Many investigators have tried to modify this wound healing process using drugs which interrupt or inhibit one or more of these stages in the wound healing process [42–49]. Biodegradable polymers are particularly well suited to managing this problem, and have advantages over other ocular drug delivery systems. Biodegradable polymers have the advantage of a localized and sustained release of medication to the intended site of treatment. Because the medication can

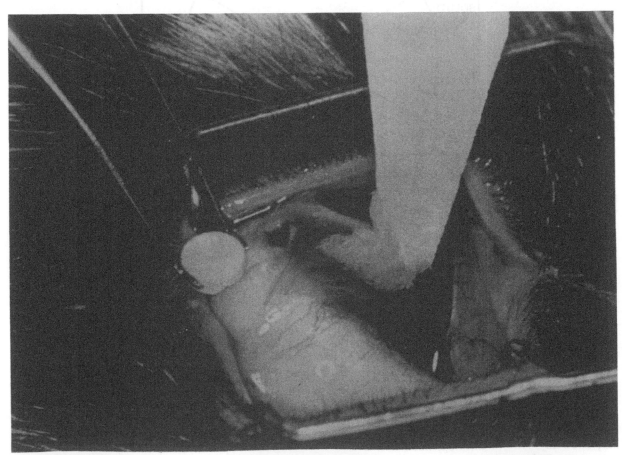

Figure 5. The disc-shaped polymer just prior to implantation at the surgical site in a rabbit eye. Reprinted with the permission of *Investigative Ophthalmology and Visual Science*, Reference [51].

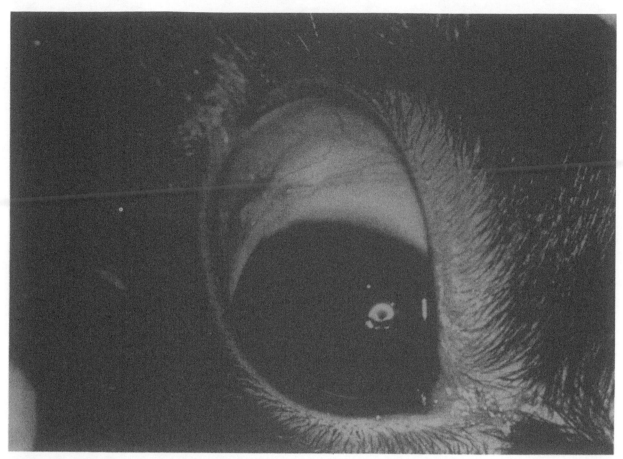

Figure 6. The subconjunctivally located polymer at the surgical site after implantation. Reprinted with the permission of *Investigative Ophthalmology and Visual Science*, Reference [51].

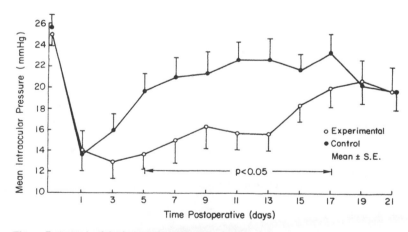

Figure 7. A graph of the intraocular pressure over time of experimental eyes compared to control eyes following drug-impregnated polymer surgery. Reprinted with the permission of *Investigative Ophthalmology and Visual Science*, Reference [51].

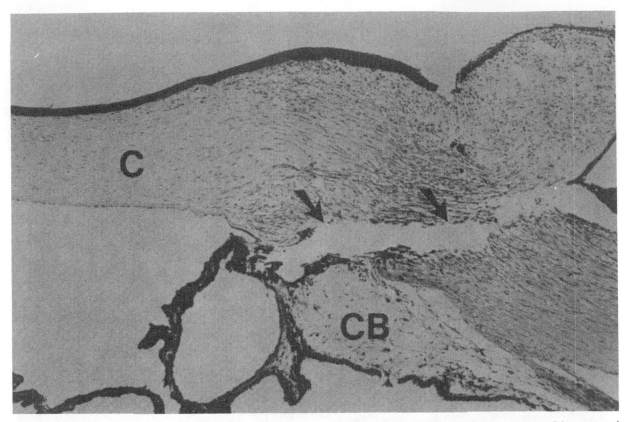

Figure 8. Light microscopy of an eye which had received the 5-fluorouracil polymer showing a patent surgical site (arrows). C is cornea and CB is ciliary body. Reprinted with the permission of *Investigative Ophthalmology and Visual Science*, Reference [51].

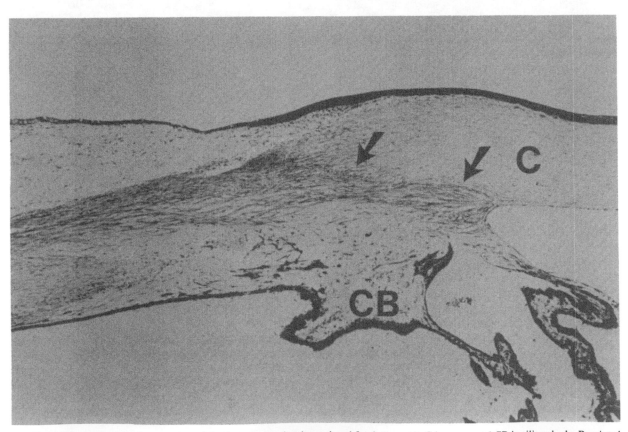

Figure 9. Light microscopy of a control eye following surgery showing a closed fistula (arrows). C is cornea and CB is ciliary body. Reprinted with the permission of *Investigative Ophthalmology and Visual Science*, Reference [51].

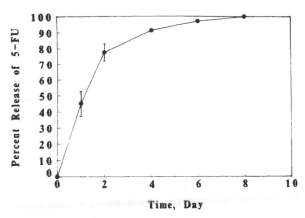

Figure 10. Graph of drug release characteristics over time from 5-fluorouracil impregnated disc-shaped polymers. Reprinted with the permission of *Investigative Ophthalmology and Visual Science*, Reference [51].

be delivered directly to the treatment site, a lower total amount of drug is necessary. This lower amount of drug and localized release decreases the potential risk of adverse ocular and systemic side effects.

In a situation where the drug or polymer may be causing an adverse side effect, the entire solid monolithic biodegradable device may be totally removed from its implantation site. This solid drug delivery system has potential mechanical advantages similar to a stent which can support the opening of the drainage area. The shape of this device can be modified into a disc, cylinder, or sphere, which can change the surface erosion characteristics of the polymer. Since the biodegradable polymer will eventually disappear, there is a lower chance of long-term foreign body complications such as infection and extrusion. These biodegradable polymers may be laminated with different types of medications in order to deliver specific drugs in sequential order, to control several of the different stages in wound healing (Figure 4).

A series of experiments were performed implanting biodegradable polymers at the time of glaucoma filtering surgery in rabbit eyes (Figures 5 and 6). The results of these experiments showed a definite decrease in the intraocular pressure of those eyes which received 5-fluorouracil impregnated devices [50,51] (Figure 7). Histopathological examination showed a patent opening at the surgical site in the experimental eyes, whereas the surgical opening was closed in the control eyes (Figures 8 and 9). No toxic tissue reaction was observed by histopathology examination of the eyes from either the polymer or the drug (Figures 8 and 9). Two different shapes of polymers were tried, a cylindrical shape and a disc shape. The cylindrical-shaped polymer had a greater number of complications including extrusion through the surface of the eye and migration into the eye [50]. The disc-shaped polymer had fewer complications and was better tolerated by the eye [51]. It was noted that the 5-fluorouracil was leached out of the polymer before the entire matrix had dissolved in both the

cylinder-shaped and disc-shaped devices (Figure 10). Unfortunately zero-order drug release kinetics was not achieved by either polymer shapes.

CONCLUSION

There are a number of synthetic biodegradable polymers which have been evaluated as drug-carriers. Having been applied to various drug therapies, they would be adaptable to ophthalmic applications as well. The unique anatomy and physiology of the eye leaves much room for improvement over the conventional mode of drug administration. It is expected that drug delivery by biodegradable polymers will provide a novel and increasingly attractive approach to the treatment of various ocular diseases.

ACKNOWLEDGEMENT

The authors are grateful for the support from NIH grants EY07701 and EY00331, Research to Prevent Blindness, the Lucille Ellis Simon Glaucoma Research Fund, and the Whitaker Foundation.

REFERENCES

1. Good, W. and P. Lee. 1986. "Membrane Controlled Reservoir Drug Delivery Systems", in *Medical Applications of Controlled Release, Vol. 1*, R. Langer and D. Wise, eds. Boca Raton, FL: CRC Press.
2. Urquhart, J. 1980. "Development of the Ocusert Pilocarpine Ocular Therapeutic System", in *Ophthalmic Drug Delivery Systems*, J. R. Robinson, ed. Washington, D.C.: Am. Pharm. Ass., p. 105.
3. Siegel, R. and R. Langer. 1984. *Pharm. Res.*, 1:1.
4. Waltman, S. R. and H. E. Kaufman. 1970. *Invest. Ophthalmol.*, 9:250.
5. Kaufman, H. E., M. H. Uotila, A. R. Gasset, R. O. Wood and E. D. Ellison. 1971. *Trans. Am. Acad. Ophthalmol. Otolaryngol.*, 75:361
6. Assef, C. F., R. L. Weisman, S. M. Podos and B. Becker. 1973. *Am. J. Ophthalmol.*, 75:212
7. Maddox, Y. T. and H. N. Bernstein. 1972. *Ann. Ophthalmol.*, 4:789.
8. Praus, R., I. Brettschneider, L. Krejci and D. Kalvodova. 1972. *Ophthalmologica*, 165:62.
9. Hull, D. S., H. F. Edelhauser and R. A. Hyndiuk. 1973. *Am. J. Ophthalmol.*, 75:212.
10. Heller, J. 1984. "Biodegradable Polymers in Controlled Drug Delivery. CRC Critical Review", in *Therapeutic Drug Carrier Systems*, 1:39.
11. Cooney, D. O. 1972. *AICHE J.*, 18:446.
12. Harris, F. W. 1986. "Controlled Release from Polymers Containing Pendant Bioactive Substituents", in *Medical Applications of Controlled Release, Vol. 1*, R. Langer and D. Wise, eds. Boca Raton, FL: CRC Press.
13. Duncan, R., H. C. Cable, J. B. Lloyd, P. Rejmanova and J. Kopecek. 1983. *Makromol. Chem.*, 184:1997.

14. Peppas, N. 1984. "Mathematical Modeling of Diffusion Processes in Drug Delivery Polymeric Systems", in *Controlled Drug Bioavailability*, V. F. Smolen, ed. NY: John Wiley & Sons, p. 274.

15. Hopfenberg, H. B. 1976. "Controlled Release from Erodible Slabs, Cylinders and Spheres", in *Controlled Release Polymer Formulations*, ACS Symp. Ser. No. 33, D. R. Paul and F. W. Harris, eds. Washington, D.C.: American Chemical Society, p. 26.

16. Baker, R. W. and H. K. Lonsdale. 1976. *Am. Chem. Soc. Div. Org. Coat. Plast. Chem. Prep.*, 3:229.

17. Heller, J. and R. W. Baker. 1980. "Theory and Practice of Controlled Drug Delivery from Bioerodible Polymers", in *Controlled Release of Bioactive Materials*, R. W. Baker, ed. New York: Academic Press, pp. 1–17.

18. Lee, P. I. 1980. *J. Membr. Sci.*, 7:255.

19. Lee, P. I. 1984. *J. Pharm. Sci.*, 73:1344.

20. Brooke, D. and R. J. Washkuhn. 1977. *J. Pharm. Sci.*, 66:159.

21. Lipper, R. A. and W. I. Higuchi. 1977. *J. Pharm. Sci.*, 66:163.

22. Hsieh, D. S. T., W. Rhine and R. Langer. 1983. *J. Pharm. Sci.*, 72:17.

23. Kuu, W. Y. and S. H. Yalkowsky. 1985. *J. Pharm. Sci.*, 74:926.

24. Bechard, S. and J. N. McMullen. 1988. *J. Pharm. Sci.*, 77:222.

25. Sawusch, M. R., T. P. O'Brien, J. D. Dick and J. D. Gottsch. 1988. *Am. J. Ophthalmol.*, 106:279–281.

26. Phinney, R. B., S. D. Schwartz, D. A. Lee and B. J. Mondino. 1988. *Arch. Ophthalmol.*, 106:1599–1604.

27. Phinney, R. B., T. M. M. Phan, D. A. Lee and B. J. Mondino. 1989. *Invest. Ophthalmol.*, 30 (Suppl.): 41.

28. Kay, J. S., B. S. Litin, M. A. Jones, A. W. Fryczkowski, M. Chvapil and J. Herschler. 1986. *Ophthalmic. Surg.*, 17:796–801.

29. Herschler, J., J. S. Kay, B. S. Litin and M. Chvapil. 1987. "Drug Delivery of Antimetabolites as Adjuncts to Glaucoma Filtration Surgery: Preliminiary Clinical Experience", in *Glaucoma Update III*, G. K. Krieglstein (ed). Heidelberg: Springer-Verlag, pp. 215–219.

30. Kaye, S. B. 1981. *Cancer Treatment Review*, 8:27–50.

31. Szoka, F. and D. Papahadjopoulos. 1978. *Proceedings of the National Academy of Sciences*, 75:4194–4198.

32. Fishman, P. H., G. A. Peyman and T. Lesar. 1986. *Invest. Ophthalmol.*, 27:1103–1106.

33. Heath, T. D., N. G. Lopez, G. P. Lewis and W. H. Stern. 1987. *Invest. Ophthalmol.*, 28:1365–1372.

34. Joondeph, B. C., B. Khoobehi, G. A. Peyman and B. Y. Yue. 1988. *Ophthalmic Surg.*, 19:252–256.

35. Assil, K. A., J. Lane and R. N. Weinreb. 1988. *Ophthalmic Surg.*, 19:408–413.

36. Leong, K. W., J. Kost and E. Mathiowitz. 1986. *Biomaterials*, 7:364–371.

37. Leong, K. W., B. C. Brott and R. Langer. 1985. *J. Biomed. Materials Res.*, 19:941–955.

38. Leong, K. W., P. D'Amore and M. Marletta. 1986. *J. Biomed. Materials Res.*, 20:51–64.

39. Conix, A. 1966. *Macrosynthesis*, 2:94–98.

40. Skuta, G. L. and R. K. Parrish. 1987. *Surv. Ophthalmol.*, 32:149–170.

41. Tahery, M. M. and D. A. Lee. 1989. *J. Ocular Pharmacol.*, 5:155–179.

42. Gressel, M. G., R. K. Parrish and R. Folberg. 1984. *Ophthalmology*, 91:378–383.

43. Heuer, D. K., R. K. Parrish, M. G. Gressel, E. Hodapp, P. F. Palmberg and D. R. Anderson. 1984. *Ophthalmology*, 91:384–394.

44. Heuer, D. K., R. K. Parrish, M. G. Gressel, E. Hodapp, D. C. Desjardins, G. L. Skuta, P. F. Palmberg, J. A. Nevarez and E. J. Rockwood. 1986. *Ophthalmology*, 93:1537–1546.

45. Heuer, D. K., M. G. Gressel, R. K. Parrish, R. Folberg, J. E. Dillberger and N. H. Altman. 1986. *Arch. Ophthalmol.*, 104:132–136.

46. Giangiacomo, J., D. K. Dueker and E. Adelstein. 1986. *Arch. Ophthalmol.*, 104:838–841.

47. McGuigan, L. J. B., D. J. Cook and M. E. Yablonski. 1986. *Invest. Ophthalmol.*, 27:1755–1757.

48. Moorhead, L. C., J. Smith, R. Stewart and R. Kimbrough. 1987. *Ann. Ophthalmol.*, 19:223–225.

49. Fourman, S. and K. Vaid. 1989. *Ophthalmic. Surg.*, 20:663–667.

50. Lee, D. A., R. A. Flores, P. J. Anderson, K. W. Leong, C. Teekhasaenee, A. W. DeKater and E. Hertzmark. 1987. *Ophthalmology*, 94:1523–1530.

51. Lee, D. A., K. W. Leong, W. C. Panek, C. T. Eng and B. J. Glasgow. 1988. *Invest. Ophthalmol.*, 29:1692–1697.

42

Antibacterial Activity of Polycationic Biocides

TOMIKI IKEDA*

ABSTRACT: Antibacterial activity of polycationic biocides is reviewed in connection with their interaction with their target site, the cytoplasmic membranes of bacteria. The mode of action of low molecular weight cationic disinfectants is first described with reference to the structure of the bacterial cell envelope and then that of the polycationic biocides is discussed on the basis of elementary processes proposed for the low molecular weight analogues. The polycationic biocides discussed include quaternary ammonium salts and biguanides, which are used almost exclusively for disinfection. Application of the polycationic biocides to a variety of fields, such as immobilized biocides and self-sterilizing materials, is finally described.

INTRODUCTION

Polymeric biocides are, in a wide sense, functional polymers and powerful candidates for polymeric drugs, with high activity that can be achieved by their characteristic nature of carrying high local density of the active groups in the vicinity of the polymer chains. The long chain of the polymer can be divided into several parts so as to provide one with some specific group that possesses a high affinity toward a target site. The polymer with this structure can reach the target site easily, thus the local concentration of the drugs at the specific site can be very high. Although synthetic polymers have been used as structural replacements for damaged or diseased human bones and tissues, it is only recently that synthetic polymers with biological activity have received attention. Polymeric drugs are expected to show advantages in terms of localization in specific organs or tissues, reduced toxicity, and increased duration of action [1,2]. However, very few examples with adequate

biological activity have so far been discovered [2,3]. This lack of discovery is partly due to bioactive groups often losing their activity when incorporated into a polymer chain.

Polymeric drugs may be divided into two groups. In the first type, bioactive molecules are incorporated covalently into a polymer, thus the polymer chain is used just as a carrier. In the second type, the origin of activity is ascribed to the polymeric form, and these types of polymeric drugs may be termed "intrinsic" polymeric drugs. Polycationic biocides may belong to the first type, in view of the fact that they originate from monomeric or dimeric cationic disinfectants (quaternary ammonium salts and biguanides) with high activity and low toxicity. However, in view of the mode of action, the polymeric form is considered the primary origin of extremely high activity, thereby the polycationic biocides may concurrently be classified into the second type of the polymeric drugs.

In this chapter, we review the antimicrobial activity of low molecular weight cationic disinfectants now widely used all over the world, with special reference to activity–structure relationships. We then give a detailed description of the antimicrobial activity of the polycationic biocides, and discuss the mode of action of the polycationic biocides based on their interaction with the cell envelopes of bacteria, which are considered their target sites.

A characteristic feature of the polycationic biocides is good processability and superior physical properties, in comparison with the low molecular weight analogues. The film-forming property of the polycationic biocides may enable fabrication of "self-sterilizing materials", for which we will find wide use in therapy and hygiene. In the last section of this chapter, we refer to applications of the polycationic biocides.

LOW MOLECULAR WEIGHT CATIONIC DISINFECTANTS

Antimicrobial agents so far in use are classified according to their target sites, as shown in Table 1 [4].

*Research Laboratory of Resources Utilization, Tokyo Institute of Technology, 4259 Nagatsuta, Midori-ku, Yokohama 227, Japan

Table 1. Classification of antibacterial agents according to their target sites [4].

Inhibition of biosynthesis of peptidoglycan in cell walls	β-Lactam antibiotics (penicillins, cephalosporins)
Cytoplasmic membranes disorganization	Phenols (chlorinated cresols etc.) Quaternary ammonium salts (ceterimide etc.) Biguanides (chlorhexidine etc.) Cyclic oligopeptides (tyrocidin A, gramicidin S, polymyxin B etc.)
Change in membrane permeability	Ionophores (valinomycin, nonactin etc.)
Inhibition of biosynthesis of nucleic acids	Azaserine, DON, acridine, actinomycin D, mitomycin, etc.)
Inhibition of biosynthesis of proteins	Puromycin, streptomycin, tetracycline, chloramphenicol, etc.

Antibiotics which inhibit biosynthesis of bacterial cell walls, proteins and nucleic acids mainly show bacteriostatic activity, thus preventing the growth of bacterial cells. In contrast, such antimicrobial agents as phenols, quaternary ammonium salts, biguanides and cyclic oligopeptides, whose target sites are the cytoplasmic membranes of microbes, kill microbial cells, exhibiting bactericidal action. However, as has been clinically verified, antimicrobial agents are not necessarily bactericidal in the treatment of microbial infection, since we are provided with antibody and phagocytic defenses which are readily activated to remove bacterial cells from the body. Furthermore, the difference between bacteriostatic and bactericidal is not clearly defined. Many antibacterial agents are known that show bacteriostatic activity at lower concentrations and bactericidal activity at higher concentrations. In Figure 1 are shown the structures of membrane-active antibacterial agents which exert their lethal action by affecting the cytoplasmic membranes. In early remedies, such strong oxidants as chlorine, iodine, and hydrogen peroxide, as well as salts of heavy metals (e.g., mercury) were used, but nowadays their use is limited because of their high reactivity and toxicity.

Currently two main groups of compounds are used almost exclusively for disinfection. They are phenols and cationic disinfectants. Cresols solubilized with soap or alkali are still used, but now their use is rather limited owing to their high toxicity and irritating nature. Hexachlorophene was used widely in surgical soaps. However, its use has been strictly limited after its effect on the nervous system was recognized. Today if we go to hospitals we perceive no smell of phenols.

This is because the phenols have been replaced by odorless cationic disinfectants in most of the hospitals. The cyclic oligopeptides (tyrocidin A, gramicidin S, polymyxins, etc.) exhibit high antibacterial activity, but they are of no value from the clinical point of view because of their high toxicity.

Although the structure and the mode of action are different, these membrane-active antibacterial agents are known to show the following common features [4]:

(1) They are easily adsorbed onto bacterial cytoplasmic membranes, and the amount of the adsorbed agents depends on the concentration of the agents. They show similar adsorption isotherms against spheroplasts and protoplasts which are free from the cell walls. Adsorption of these agents onto isolated cell membranes has been confirmed.

(2) Bactericidal action of these agents is dependent on the concentration of the agents, the number of bacterial cells, and the time of contact.

(3) Correlation between their cidal action and leakage of cytoplasmic constituents has been recognized. The low level of the agents induces leakage of low molecular weight cellular constituents like K^+ ions, and higher levels of the agents bring about loss of higher molecular weight solutes such as nucleotides. Loss of the cytoplasmic constituents to some extent is, however, not lethal to the cells. The cells often survive and grow normally when the treated cells are placed in a nutrient medium.

(4) The membrane-active agents are essentially bactericidal, but they show bacteriostatic effect at lower concentrations.

(5) At higher concentrations and upon prolonged exposure, the membrane-active agents penetrate the bacterial cells and cause irreversible damage to the cells.

Use of quaternary ammonium salts (Quats) as disinfectants started early in the 1930s. Domagk found that benzalkonium salts (Figure 1) were outstandingly effective for disinfection of skin and were superior to phenols in killing bacteria [5]. These benzalkonium salts were called "invert soap" or "cationic soap" and have been widely used in disinfection. They still play a role in disinfection of hands and skin and in sterilization of medical equipment. However, their toxicity seems to be somewhat higher than that of the biguanides described below.

Biguanide compounds were first synthesized by Rose et al. of I.C.I. in the mid-1940s. In the early stage, it was mainly the potentiality of biguanides as antimalarial agents that was realized, and some biguanides like proguanil found some practical application in the treatment of malaria [6]. Proguanil is a monobiguanide and is apparently not active in its original structure. The mode of action study has revealed that it becomes an active form (dihydro-

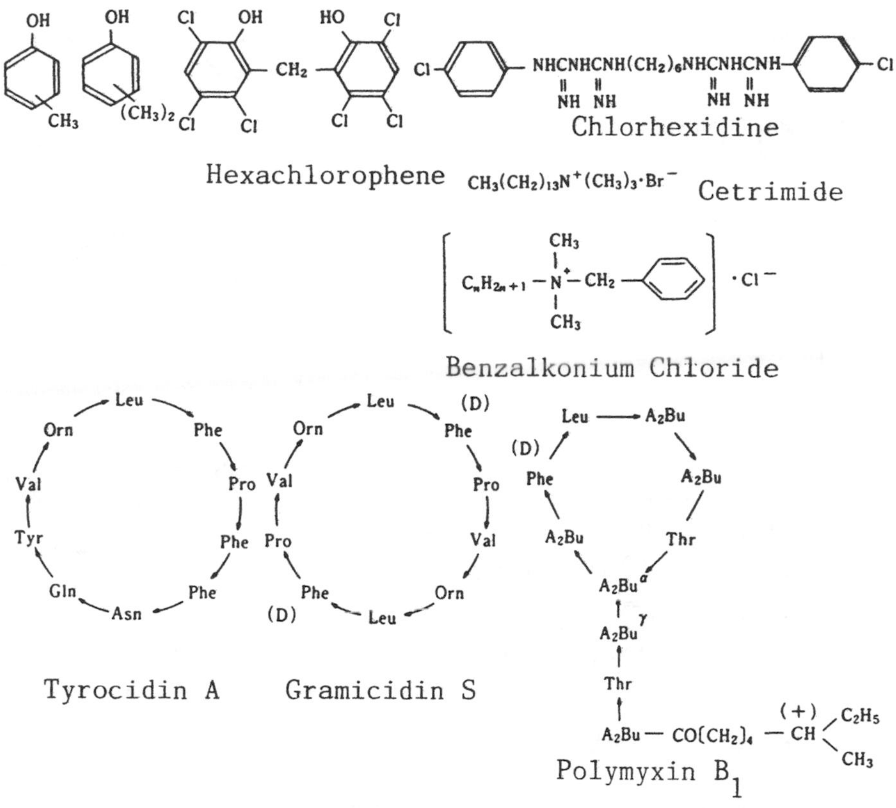

Figure 1. Structures of membrane-active antibacterial agents [4].

triazine) through metabolism in the body. Proguanil was less active against bacteria, but bisbiguanides developed in the mid-1950s by the same group were found to show remarkably high activity [7]. One of the best and most widely used cationic antiseptics is chlorhexidine (Figure 1). The biguanide group involved is one of the strongest organic bases and its pK_a value is as high as 12. Thus, at physiological pH it is entirely protonated [8]. Biguanides are generally synthesized in the form of chlorides which are hardly soluble in water. In the preparation of biguanides, the counter-anion is usually changed to a gluconate and the resulting biguanide salts are highly soluble in water ($\sim 40\%$). The biguanide disinfectants have advantages over other disinfectants as follows [4]:

(1) The biguanide disinfectants have a wide spectrum of antibacterial activity against both Gram-positive and Gram-negative bacteria.

(2) The kill rate is extremely high.

(3) Toxicity towards mammalian cells is very low and irritancy is so insignificant that the biguanide antiseptics can be used on the sensitive mucosal surfaces.

Although the cationic disinfectants have a variety of structures, they possess common structural features —positive charge and a fairly hydrophobic part, in a

single molecule. For example, in chlorhexidine the positively charged biguanide groups are attached to both ends of a fairly hydrophobic hexamethylene group and in quaternary ammonium salts a hydrophobic alkyl chain is chemically bonded to the positively charged nitrogen atom.

Although a wide range of cationic compounds with these characteristics exhibit more or less antibacterial activity, the activity is strongly dependent on the structure. In the quaternary ammonium salts, the length of the hydrophobic tails has been found to affect the antibacterial activity. For instance, in the analogues of cetrimide (Figure 1) a compound with 14 carbon atoms shows the highest activity, and others with longer or shorter chains exhibit much less. In a series of benzalkonium salts, those of 12 to 14 carbon atoms are known to show the maximum activity. Furthermore, branched hydrocarbon tails reportedly improve the antibacterial activity and are favored for reducing the toxicity [9]. In the analogues of chlorhexidine, the central part of the molecule was found to play an important role. Antibacterial activity was sensitively affected by the length of the alkyl spacers. Thus, in the cationic disinfectants, the hydrophobic parts in the molecule play a significant role, and the hydrophilic–lipophilic balance (HL balance) has been frequently used as a parameter to elucidate their antibacterial activity in some quantitative way.

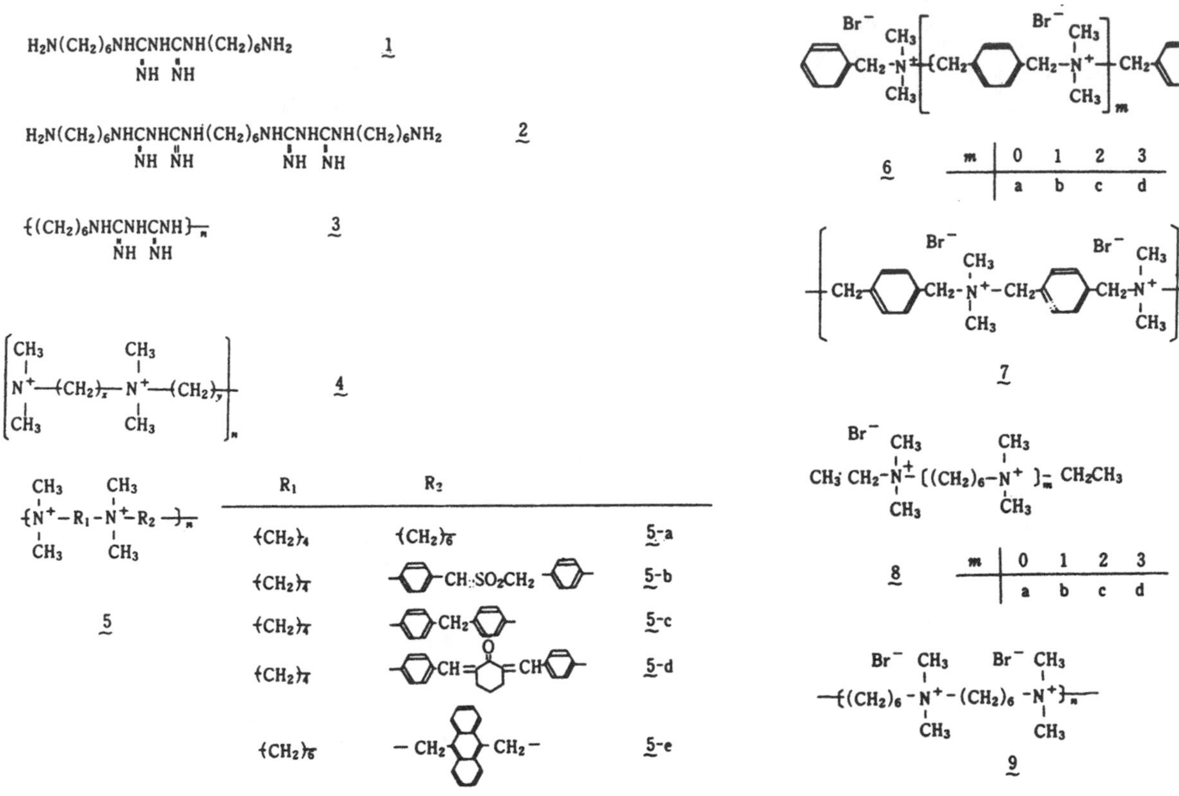

$H_2N(CH_2)_6NHCNHCNH(CH_2)_6NH_2$ 1
           NH   NH

$H_2N(CH_2)_6NHCNHCNH(CH_2)_6NHCNHCNH(CH_2)_6NH_2$ 2
      NH   NH   NH   NH

{(CH_2)_6NHCNHCNH}_n   3
     NH   NH

Figure 2. Structures of polycations with main-chain positive charges.

ANTIBACTERIAL ACTIVITY OF POLYCATIONIC BIOCIDES

The most general approach one would take for polymeric drugs may be covalent incorporation of low molecular weight drugs into a polymer. By this procedure, many polymeric drugs have been prepared in which the monomeric drugs were incorporated into a main chain or a side chain. The readers should refer to a review article [10] for detail, but as a conclusion very few successful examples have so far been reported. For example, common antibiotics with β-lactam structure such as penicillins and cephalosporins were polymerized through several routes. However, the resulting polymeric antibiotics were found to exhibit much less activity than the parent antibiotics; in some cases the polymeric forms of the antibiotics lost completely their original activity.

Loss of activity is partly ascribed to the location of the target sites. In case of the intracellular target sites, drugs must overcome an enormous barrier, cytoplasmic membrane, in order to reach their target sites. Because of the molecular size, permeability of the polymeric drugs through the cytoplasmic membrane is reasonably expected to be reduced, thereby making it more and more difficult for the polymeric drugs to reach their target sites inside the cells. Fortunately, however, the target site of the cationic disinfectants is the cell envelope of bacteria, and the reduced perme-ability, resulting from the increase in molecular size due to polymerization, is not regarded as a factor seriously affecting their activity. In fact, polycationic biocides are one of the rare groups of materials that can effectively utilize the advantages associated with the polymeric form of drugs, such as high local concentrations of active groups at the target site. This section deals with antibacterial activity of polycations having quaternary ammonium salts and biguanides in the main chain or in the side chains.

Polycations with Main-Chain Positive Charges

The structures of polycations with main-chain quaternary ammonium salts or main-chain biguanide groups are shown in Figure 2. These polycations are more or less active against bacteria.

Compound 3 is a polymeric in-chain biguanide, and 1 and 2 are monomeric and dimeric model compounds, respectively. In these compounds, all the biguanide groups are protonated and are hydrochloride salts. The polymeric in-chain biguanide is now commercially available (Vantocil) from I.C.I. and its average degree of polymerization lies in the range 5–7 [11,12]. This polymer shows an outstandingly high antibacterial activity against Gram-positive and Gram-negative strains and possesses a wide spectrum of antimicrobial activity.

Figure 3 shows the log (survivors) versus exposure

time plots for these in-chain biguanide compounds. These plots were evaluated against *Staphylococcus aureus* by the viable cell-counting method. The cells of *S. aureus* at the concentration of ~ 10^5 cells/ml were exposed to 10 μg/ml of the biguanide compounds and the number of the surviving cells was counted at various exposure times by the spread plate method. The monomer *1* showed little bactericidal activity. The bactericidal activity of the dimer *2* was higher than that of *1* and 99.9% of the *S. aureus* cells were killed after 2 h exposure. On the other hand, the polymer *3* was so active against this strain that within 10 min all cells were killed. Not only *S. aureus* but also *Escherichia coli*, a typical Gram-negative bacterium, was found to be sensitive to this polycation. Bactericidal activity against *E. coli* also increased in the order of monomer < dimer ≪ polymer [13]. The effect of molecular weight on the bactericidal activity was further examined on the polymeric in-chain biguanide *3* with higher molecular weight than that commercially available. A polymeric biguanide with the degree of polymerization larger than 10 was found to show much higher activity against *S. aureus* and *E. coli* [14].

Polycations with in-chain quaternary ammonium salts also show antibacterial activity [15–20]. Polycations with positively charged nitrogen atoms in the main chains like *4–9* are called ionenes. Rembaum et al. studied the antibacterial activity of ionene *4*, in which the number of methylene spacers, x and y, was varied [15–17]. Although monomeric and dimeric homologues of *4* could not prevent the growth of bacteria even at such a high concentration as 1,000 μg/ml, the polyionene *4* showed high bacteriostatic activity against *S. aureus* and *E. coli* as shown in Table 2. In the table, the figure indicates the minimum inhibitory concentration (MIC) expressed in μg/ml, which is a measure of the bacteriostatic activity. The growth of bacteria can be seen as colonies in the presence of the drug at the concentrations below the value of MIC. Thus, the lower is the value, the higher becomes the bacteriostatic activity of the drug.

It is clearly seen in the table that the length of the alkyl spacers affects sharply the bacteriostatic activity of the ionenes and 6,10-ionene with $x = 6$ and $y = 10$ exhibited the highest activity against *S. aureus* and *E. coli*. These ionenes reportedly show bacteriostatic activity against *Pseudomonas aeruginosa* and *Bacillus subtilis*. Vucetic et al. explored the antibacterial activity of polyionenes having spacers other than methylene chains (*5*) and reported that *5*-a and *5*-b exhibited bactericidal activity against *S. aureus* and *5*-c–*5*-e were bacteriostatic against the same bacterium [19]. In these early studies, however, no systematic works were performed on, for example, the effect of molecular weight on the antibacterial activity.

Ikeda et al. synthesized a series of ionenes with the same spacer structure but different molecular weights in order to investigate the effect of the molecular

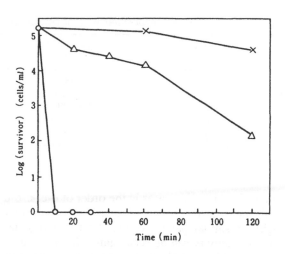

Figure 3. Bactericidal activity of polycation *3* and low molecular weight analogues (*1,2*) against *S. aureus* [13] (x), *1*; (△), *2*; (○), *3*. Concentration of the cations was 10 μg/ml.

weight on the antibacterial activity of the cationic biocides [20]. Two kinds of spacer structures were employed. One was a rather rigid xylylene group (*6* and *7*) and the other was a flexible hexamethylene group (*8* and *9*). For both series, low molecular weight homologues [monomer (a), dimer (b), trimer (c) and tetramer (d)] were prepared and were examined as to their antibacterial activity. In Table 3 is shown the bacteriostatic activity of the homologues with xylylene spacers against *B. subtilis*, *S. aureus*, *E. coli*, *Aerobacter aerogenes* and *P. aeruginosa*, as evaluated by the range of the MIC values. The two figures in the table for each strain indicate the range of MIC: the growth of bacteria could be observed as visual colonies below the lower value of MIC, whereas no colonies were seen above the higher value of MIC. Consequently the exact MIC is supposed to lie between the two values. A general trend can be seen in the table indicating that the ionenes are more active against Gram-positive bacteria (*B. subtilis* and *S. aureus*) than against Gram-negative strains (*E. coli*, *A. aerogenes* and *P. aeruginosa*). It is also seen that monomeric (*6*-a) and dimeric (*6*-b) forms are practically inactive against every strain. The striking feature seen in the table is that the activity against *B. sub-*

Table 2. *Bacteriostatic activity of various ionenes [17].*

Ionene[a]	Minimum Inhibitory Concentration (MIC)	
	S. aureus (μg/ml)	E. coli (μg/ml)
3,3	128	128
6,6	16	16
6,10	4	4
2,10	4	8
6,16	4	32

[a]The two values indicate the values of x and y in *4* (Figure 2).

Table 3. Molecular weight dependence of bacteriostatic activity of ionenes [20].

	Bacillus subtilis	Stapylococcus aureus	Escherichia coli	Aerobacter aerogenes	Pseudomonas aeruginosa
6-a	>1000	>1000	>1000	>1000	>1000
6-b	>1000	>1000	>1000	>1000	>1000
6-c	600–1000	100–330	>1000	>1000	>1000
6-d	100–330	66–100	660–1000	100–330	>1000
7	33–66	10–33	66–100	66–100	100–330

MIC (μg/ml) determined by the spread plate method.

tilis and *S. aureus* increases in the order of *6*-c < *6*-d < *7*, i.e., in the order of increasing molecular weight. A similar pattern of the effect of molecular weight on activity can be seen against *E. coli* and *A. aerogenes*. Figure 4 shows the log(survivors) versus exposure time plots for the homologues against *S. aureus* and *E. coli*. The concentration of cations used was 1,000 μg/ml except *7*, for which the concentration was 10 μg/ml. The polymer *7* was highly active, and all cells of *S. aureus* and *E. coli* were killed within 30 min of contact. Among the oligomers, the tetramer *6*-d was most active against both strains. Although the difference in bactericidal activity among the oligomers with N⁺ < 4 was not clearly observed against *S. aureus*, the cidal activity was found to increase with molecular weight against *E. coli*. Even at lower concentrations (at 10–100 μg/ml), the tetramer exhibited higher activity than other low molecular weight oligomers.

Polycations with Side-Chain Positive Charges

Figure 5 shows the structures of polycations with side-chain positive charges, of which antibacterial activity has so far been recognized. Among these polycations, the potency of antibacterial activity of basic polypeptides was realized in the early stage of studies. In the 1950s, Katchalski et al. found that polyornithine (*10*, m = 3), polylysine (*10*, m = 4) and polyarginine (*11*) showed antibacterial activity, while their monomeric amino acids were inactive [21,22]. Studies were extended to synthetic basic polypeptides, and polyanthin (*12*), for example, was found to be highly active against *S. aureus*, *B. subtilis* and *Mycobacteria*, although it was practically inactive against Gram-negative species [23,24]. Polyanthin was in fact examined in the clinical application as an antituberculosis agent [23,24].

Panarin et al. synthesized the homopolymers of vinylamine (*18*) and methacrylates with side-chain quaternary ammonium salts (*15*, *16*, *17*) as well as their copolymers with N-vinyl-2-pyrrolidone (*13*, *14*) and examined their antibacterial activity [25]. In *13*-a and *14*-a, various copolymers were prepared in which the compositional ratio of vinylamine or the methacrylate with side-chain quaternary ammonium salt to N-vinyl-2-pyrrolidone was altered, and the effect of the positive charge density on bacteriostatic activity against *S. aureus* was investigated. As shown in Figure 6, a good correlation was observed between the molar fraction of the basic groups in the copolymers and the logarithm of the MIC values of the copolymers. In these copolymers, no effect of the counter-anion on the bacteriostatic activity was recognized among Cl⁻, Br⁻ and I⁻. The effect of molecular weight on the bacteriostatic activity against *S. aureus* was also explored for the copolymers *13*-a and *14*-b. In these polycations, the molar fraction of the monomer with the quaternary ammonium salt was kept nearly constant (~25 mol% for *13*-a and ~18 mol% for *14*-b) and the molecular weight was changed as evaluated by the intrinsic viscosity, [η], measured in 0.5 M KCl solution. Table 4 shows the MIC values of these copolymers against *S. aureus*,

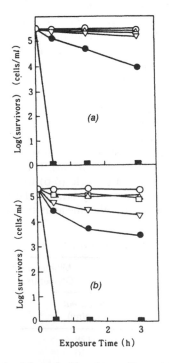

Figure 4. Molecular weight dependence of bactericidal activity of ionenes against *S. aureus* (a) and *E. coli* (b) [20]. (○), Blank; (△), *6*-a; (□), *6*-b; (△), *6*-c; (●), *6*-d; (■), *7*. Concentration of the cations was 1,000 μg/ml except *7* of which concentration was 10 μg/ml.

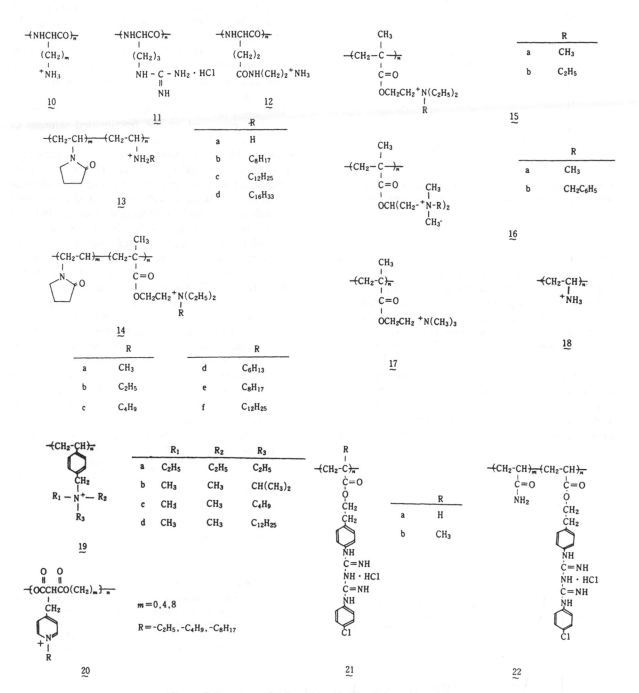

Figure 5. Structures of polycations with side-chain positive charges.

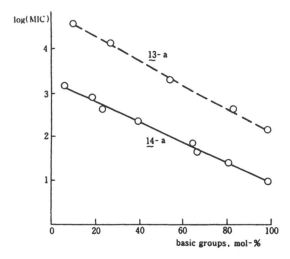

Figure 6. Effect of mole fraction of basic units in copolymers *13*-a and *14*-b on bacteriostatic activity against *S. aureus* [25].

demonstrating that the bacteriostatic activity of the copolymers was not affected by the molecular weight.

Ikeda et al. investigated the antibacterial activity of homopolymers of polyacrylates (*21*-a) and polymethacrylate (*21*-b) with side-chain biguanide groups and their copolymers with acrylamide (*22*) [26,27]. Both of the homopolymers *21*-a and *21*-b exhibited much higher bactericidal activity than those of the relevant monomers. Figure 7 shows the log (survivors) versus exposure time plots for *21*-a (molecular weight ~ 12,000) against *S. aureus*, which was evaluated by the viable cell counting method. Exposure of the *S. aureus* cells (~ 10^5 cells/ml) to the cations was per-

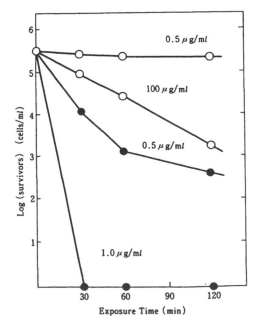

Figure 7. Bactericidal activity of polycation *21*-a and monomer against *S. aureus* [26]. (○), Monomer; (●), *21*-a.

formed in sterile distilled water. In the case of the monomer, ~99% of the bacterial cells were killed after 2 h exposure to 100 μg/ml of the monomeric biguanide, while in the case of the polymeric biguanide (*21*-a), all the bacterial cells were killed within 30 min even at the concentration as low as 0.1 μg/ml [26]. A similar result was obtained against *E. coli*, though the activity against this Gram-negative strain was somewhat lower than against *S. aureus*. The copolymers (*22*) exhibited less antibacterial activity whatever the compositional ratios of the biguanide monomer to acrylamide.

The effect of molecular weight on bactericidal activity was examined on the fractionated samples of *21*-b. Because of the strongly adsorbed nature of the polymeric biguanides towards conventional gel media based on dextran and cross-linked polystyrene, fractionation on the basis of molecular size was only successful by gel filtration with cross-linked acrylamide gel medium. The molecular weight of the fractionated samples was determined with a low-angle light scattering photometer, and those well-characterized samples were examined as to their bactericidal activity against *S. aureus*. As shown in Figure 8, the bactericidal activity of *21*-b was found to be strongly dependent on their molecular weight [27]. A significant result obtained in this study is the presence of the optimal molecular weight region for the cidal action. In the low molecular weight region below molecular weight of 5×10^4, the bacteridical activity increased with molecular weight and in the high molecular weight region above 1.2×10^5 the cidal activity decreased sharply with molecular weight. The polymeric biguanide with the optimal molecular weight exhibited a cidal activity against *S. aureus* more than 10^3 times as high as the monomeric homologue. The molecular weight dependence of the bactericidal activity was also investigated for the polycation with side-chain quaternary ammonium salt (*19*-c). Because of poor polymerizability, the molecular weight of the highest fraction was 77,000 and below this molecular weight the bactericidal activity was found to increase monotonically with molecular

Table 4. Molecular weight dependence of bacteriostatic activity of polycations with side-chain quaternary ammonium salts [25].

Sample	Mole Fraction of Quaternary Ammonium Salts	$[\eta]^a$ (dl/g)	MIC (μg/ml)
13-a	23.5	0.96	300
	24.7	0.89	300
	24.4	0.78	300
	25.2	0.50	300
14-b	18.8	1.12	300
	18.0	0.97	300
	18.8	0.84	300
	18.4	0.73	300

^{a}Measured in 0.5 M KCl at 25°C.

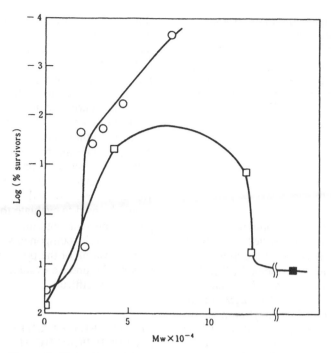

Figure 8. Molecular weight dependence of bactericidal activity of polycations against *S. aureus* [27]. (□), *21*-b (10 μg/ml); (○), *19*-c (0.5 μg/ml).

weight. Bacteriostatic activity of the fractionated polymeric quaternary ammonium salt was explored against *S. aureus*, *B. subtilis*, *E. coli*, *A. aerogenes* and *P. aeruginosa* and the MIC values obtained showed little molecular weight dependence.

Special precaution must be taken in the evaluation of the antibacterial activity of the polycationic biocides. As Katchalski already pointed out in the early 1950s, polycations, in particular those with high molecular weights, have a strong tendency to form insoluble complexes with polyanions such as DNA and RNA [22]. This strong interaction of the polycations with negatively charged species is considered to be an origin of the high antibacterial activity of the polycationic biocides as discussed in detail in a later section, since the interaction of the polycations with negatively charged components present in bacterial cytoplasmic membranes is regarded as a crucial step in their lethal action. However, the strong tendency to form insoluble complexes with the polyanionic species makes it very difficult to evaluate precisely the antibacterial activity of the polycationic biocides.

Conventionally, bacteriostatic activity of disinfectants is evaluated by the spread plate method. In this method, a bacterial culture is spread on nutrient agar containing various concentrations of the disinfectant, then incubated. It is examined on the formation of visual colonies. Application of this conventional method to polycations, however, requires special precautions. Growth media used to cultivate bacteria usually contain acidic constituents, such as sodium caseinate, which form insoluble complexes with polycations, thus leading to inactivation of the poly-

cationic biocides [27,28]. In fact, this inactivation of the polycationic biocides has been observed so far for the side-chain polycations (*19* and *21*), and their MIC values against *B. subtilis*, *S. aureus*, *E. coli*, *A. aerogenes* and *P. aeruginosa*, evaluated by the spread plate method, were higher than those of the relevant monomers. In order to eliminate the interference by the constituents in the growth media, the antibacterial assessment should be performed in media free from acidic components. One way to fulfill this requirement is to conduct the exposure of bacterial cells to the polycations in sterile water with subsequent viable cell counting.

The HL balance described in the low molecular weight cationic disinfectants also affects the antibacterial activity of polycationic biocides. In *14*, the substituent at the quaternary ammonium salt (R) was changed from CH_3 (a) to $C_{12}H_{25}$ (f), and the bacteriostatic activity of those copolymers was examined [25]. In Table 5, bacteriostatic activity of the monomers and the copolymers (*m/n* = 75/25) of *14* is shown by the MIC values against *S. aureus*. It is seen that a monomer with a less hydrophobic group (e.g., CH_3) is practically inactive (MIC > 10,000 μg/ml). However, with increasing hydrophobicity of the substituent, i.e., with increasing chain length of the alkyl substituent, the MIC value decreases in a series of the monomers. On the other hand, the MIC values of the copolymers was not significantly affected by the substituents. Furthermore, the copolymers a–d exhibited higher activity than the relevant monomers with the same alkyl group.

Similar behaviors have been observed for polycat-

Table 5. Effect of alkyl chain length in copolymer 14 on bacteriostatic activity against S. aureus [25].

Sample	R	$[\eta]^a$ (dl/g)	MIC (μg/ml) Polymer	MIC (μg/ml) Monomer
14	CH_3	1.05	50	10,000
m/n = 75/25	C_2H_5	1.05	50	1,000
	C_4H_9	0.90	50	1,000
	C_6H_{13}	0.80	50	1,000
	C_8H_{17}	0.72	50	100
	$C_{12}H_{25}$	0.54	45	1

^{a}Measured in 0.5 M KCl at 25°C.

ions with side-chain quaternary ammonium salts (*19*). In *19*, alkyl chain length was varied and their bacteriostatic activity as well as that of the monomers were explored by the spread plate method [28]. The MIC values thus determined against *S. aureus, B. subtilis, E. coli, A. aerogenes* and *P. aeruginosa* are listed in Table 6. Among dimethylbenzyl ammonium salts (*19*-b, c, d), bacteriostatic activity of the monomers increased in the order of b < c < d irrespective of strain. The activity of the polymers was found to be in the same order against Gram-positive strains. However, the polymer with the longest alkyl chain (*19*-d) exhibited much less activity against Gram-negative bacteria than the other polymers. This polycation (*19*-d), however, showed the highest antibacterial activity when the activity was explored in sterile distilled water – the cidal activity of the polymer was much higher than that of the corresponding monomer [28]. A similar effect of the HL balance on the antibacterial activity was observed for polymeric pyridinium salts (*20*) [29].

Factors affecting the antibacterial activity, other than the molecular weight and the HL balance, include the structure of the spacers between the positive charges. In the polyionene *4*, the methylene spacers between the positively charged N atoms were found to affect the antibacterial activity of the polyionenes in such a way that the longer the methylene spacer is, the higher becomes the activity [20]. Furthermore, a rigid spacer seems to be favored for the antibacterial activity. The polyionene with rigid p-xylylene spacers (*7*) exhibited much higher antibacterial activity than one with flexible hexamethylene spacers (*9*) [20].

However, a polyionene with o-xylylene spacers showed rather lower activity [20]. Hydrophilic spacers were found to reduce the activity. A polyionene with a hydroxy group in the spacer was practically inactive, demonstrating that the hydrophilic spacers drastically reduce the antibacterial activity [20].

In this section, we described the antibacterial activity of various polycations. We have realized a general trend indicating that the polycations are more active than the relevant monomeric compounds, and the polycations show higher activity against Gram-positive bacteria than against Gram-negative strains. We also have pointed out that special precaution should be paid to evaluate the antibacterial activity of polycations with high molecular weight in media containing acidic components. Complexation, followed by inactivation of the polycations, always takes place, making the precise evaluation of the antibacterial activity very difficult.

STRUCTURE OF BACTERIAL CELL WALL AND CYTOPLASMIC MEMBRANES

Before we discuss the mode of action of the polycationic biocides, we refer to the structure of cell envelope of bacteria, which is considered as the target site of the polycationic biocides.

Bacteria are unicellular microorganisms composed essentially of cell wall, cytoplasmic membrane and cytoplasm. Bacteria are classified into two groups depending on the structure of their cell walls; Gram-positive and Gram-negative bacteria. The cell wall of Gram-positive strain is mainly composed of peptidoglycan and teichoic acid (Figure 9) [30]. The peptidoglycan is an alternating copolymer of N-acetylglucosamine and N-acetylmuramic acid, to which polypeptide with appropriate chain length is attached, thus the overall structure of the cell wall of Gram-positive bacteria is somewhat mesh-like [31]. Teichoic acid is a phosphate diester of glycerol or ribitol, therefore is negatively charged at physiological pH, and is considered to play a role in uptake of Ca^{2+} and Mg^{2+} ions [30].

The structure of the cell wall of Gram-negative bacteria is much more complicated than that of Gram-positive species. As shown in Figure 10, the pepti-

Table 6. Bacteriostatic activity of polycation 19 [28].

	S. aureus	B. subtilis	E. coli	A. aerogenes	P. aeruginosa
19-a	66–100	100–330	660–1000	660–1000	>1000
Monomer	100–330	330–660	>1000	>1000	>1000
19-b	66–100	100–330	660–1000	660–1000	>1000
Monomer	>1000	330–660	>1000	>1000	>1000
19-c	33–66	66–100	330–660	660–1000	>1000
Monomer	660–1000	660–1000	>1000	>1000	>1000
19-d	33–66	10–33	>1000	>1000	>1000
Monomer	<1	<1	10–33	10–33	66–1000

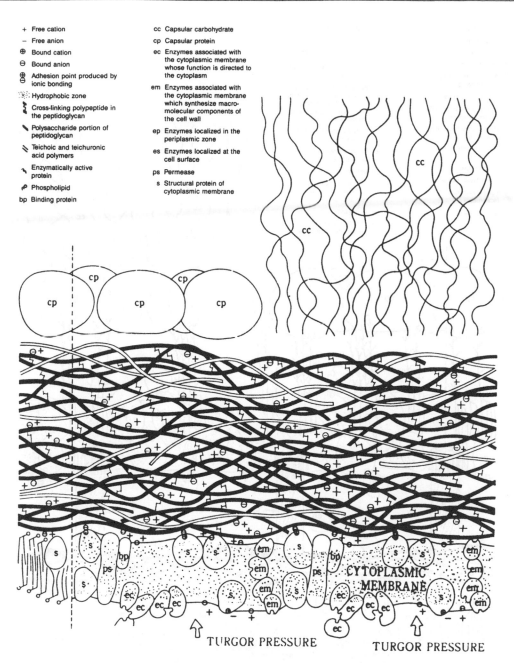

+   Free cation
−   Free anion
⊕   Bound cation
⊖   Bound anion
    Adhesion point produced by ionic bonding
    Hydrophobic zone
    Cross-linking polypeptide in the peptidoglycan
    Polysaccharide portion of peptidoglycan
    Teichoic and teichuronic acid polymers
    Enzymatically active protein
    Phospholipid
bp Binding protein

cc Capsular carbohydrate
cp Capsular protein
ec Enzymes associated with the cytoplasmic membrane whose function is directed to the cytoplasm
em Enzymes associated with the cytoplasmic membrane which synthesize macro-molecular components of the cell wall
ep Enzymes localized in the periplasmic zone
es Enzymes localized at the cell surface
ps Permease
s   Structural protein of cytoplasmic membrane

TURGOR PRESSURE   TURGOR PRESSURE

Figure 9. Structure of cell envelope of Gram-positive bacteria [31].

doglycan layer is rather thin, but there is another layer outside the peptidoglycan layer called the outer membrane. The outer membrane is composed mainly of lipopolysaccharides and phospholipids [31]. A significant role of the outer membrane is to protect a bacterial cell from attack by foreign compounds such as disinfectants. Thus, the much lower sensitivity of Gram-negative bacteria toward antibacterial agents is due mainly to the presence of the outer membrane. As described in the previous section, Gram-negative strains are less sensitive toward cationic disinfectants than Gram-positive strains. Furthermore, it is believed that the outer membrane prevents penicillins

and lysozyme from reaching their target sites, which is why these antibacterial agents are inactive against Gram-negative bacteria. Removal of metal ions by chelating agents like EDTA results in partial breakdown of the outer membrane since the metal ions are essential to stabilize the lipopolysaccharide layer in the outer membrane. In the presence of such chelating agents as EDTA, penicillins and lysozyme become highly active against Gram-negative species [32].

Unlike the cell wall, the structure of the cytoplasmic membranes is essentially the same between Gram-positive and Gram-negative bacteria (Figures 9 and 10). The main constituents of the cytoplasmic

+   Free cation
−   Free anion
⊕   Bound cation
⊖   Bound anion
   Adhesion point produced by ionic bonding
   Hydrophobic zone
   Cross-linking polypeptide in the peptidoglycan
   Polysaccharide portion of peptidoglycan
   Enzymatically active protein
   Phospholipid
   Lipopolysaccharide
   Lipopolysaccharide (schematic)
bp Binding protein

cc Capsular carbohydrate
cp Capsular protein
ec Enzymes associated with the cytoplasmic membrane whose function is directed to the cytoplasm
em Enzymes associated with the cytoplasmic membrane which synthesize macromolecular components of the cell wall
ep Enzymes localized in the periplasmic zone
es Enzymes localized at the cell surface
lp Braun's lipoprotein
p   Structural and enzymatic proteins of the outer membrane
ps Permease
s   Structural protein of cytoplasmic membrane

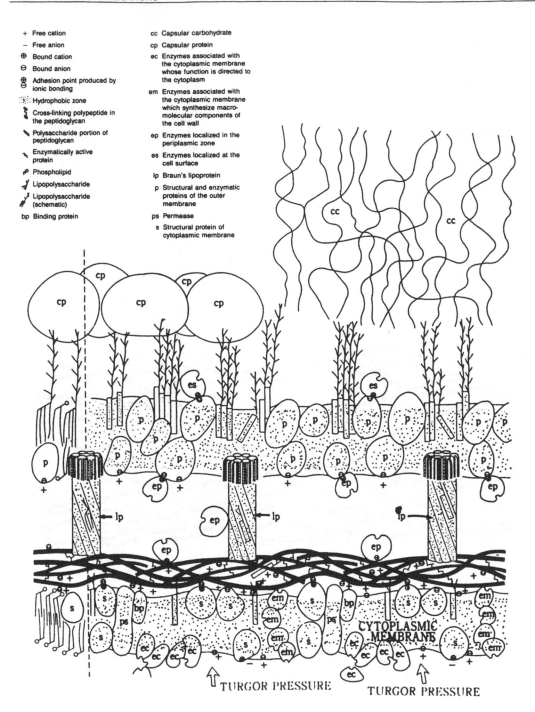

Figure 10. Structure of cell envelope of Gram-negative bacteria [31].

membrane are proteins (membrane proteins) and phospholipids. Extensive studies on phospholipids in the cytoplasmic membrane have been performed, and it has become evident that phosphatidylethanolamine (PE), almost neutral at physiological pH, is a major component present in the bacterial cytoplasmic membrane, and that phosphatidylglycerol (PG) and its dimer cardiolipin (DPG), both of which are negatively charged at physiological pH, are major acidic components. It appears that in the cytoplasmic

membrane of *E. coli* PE constitutes about 80% of the total lipids, and the acidic PG and its dimer DPG are each present to the extent of ~ 10% (Table 7) [33,34]. In eukaryotic cells, the phospholipids present in the cytoplasmic membranes are different from those of the prokaryotic cells. In the eukaryotic cells, phosphatidylcholine (PC), neutral at physiological pH, is the major zwitterionic lipid and phosphatidylserine (PS) is the major acidic component in place of PG and DPG of the prokaryotic cells.

Table 7. Composition of phospholipids in cytoplasmic membrane and outer membrane of E. coli *[33].*

Phospholipid	Cytoplasmic Membrane	Outer Membrane
PE	63.4%	78.0%
PG	10.6	11.0
DPG	6.3–9.3	6.3
Lyso PE	9.4	<1.0
Unknown	7.3–10.3	4.7

MODE OF ACTION OF POLYCATIONIC BIOCIDES

The target site of the low molecular weight cationic biocides is the cytoplasmic membranes of bacteria and the following elementary processes have been proposed for their mode of action [4,11].

(1) Adsorption onto the bacterial cell surface
(2) Diffusion through the cell wall
(3) Binding to the cytoplasmic membrane
(4) Disruption of the cytoplasmic membrane
(5) Release of cytoplasmic constituents such as K$^+$ ions, phosphate ions, DNA and RNA
(6) Death of the cell

It is now generally accepted that the mode of action of the polycationic biocides can be interpreted on the basis of each elementary process described above, since the same physiological events as in processes (1), (3) and (5) have been observed for the polycationic biocides.

It is well known that the bacterial cell surfaces are usually negatively charged, as evidenced by the electrophoretic mobility measurements. This is explained by the fact that there are many negatively charged species in the cell wall, as is briefly described in the previous section. The adsorption of polycations onto the negatively charged cell surfaces is expected to be facilitated in comparison with that of monomeric cations because of much higher charge density carried by the polycations. In fact, immediate adsorption of the side-chain polycations (*13–18*) onto the bacterial cell surfaces has been confirmed by fluorescence spectroscopy [25]. Polycations are superior to monomeric cations in the amount and the degree of adsorption [35].

Low molecular weight cationic biocides induce leakage of K$^+$ ions, phosphate ions and cytoplasmic constituents which have absorbance at 260 nm (mainly DNA and RNA, and called thereafter "260-nm absorbing materials") from the bacterial cells immediately after the cationic biocides are adsorbed onto the cell surfaces [11,36–38]. Figure 11 shows the amounts of K$^+$ ions, phosphate ions and the 260-nm absorbing materials released from ~ 10^9 cells/ml of *E. coli* in contact with 0.2 mM of cetrimide (Figure 1) at 25°C at pH 7 as a function of the contact time [38]. Release of K$^+$ ions is very fast. It starts soon after the *E. coli* cells are exposed to the cationic biocide and is completed within ~ 60 min. Loss of the phosphate ions and the 260-nm absorbing materials from the cells is rather slow. Since it has been confirmed that the low molecular weight cationic biocides undergo no interaction with isolated cell wall components, it is reasonably assumed that the low molecular weight cationic biocides penetrate the cell wall and reach the cytoplasmic membrane very quickly, inducing the leakage of the cytoplasmic constituents [39].

A similar leakage of the cytoplasmic constituents from the bacterial cells was observed when the polycations were exposed to bacterial cell culture [14,20,25,27]. Broxton et al. investigated the leakage of the cytoplasmic constituents from the *E. coli* cells (~ 10^9 cells/ml) in contact with various concentrations of the in-chain biguanide polymer (*3*; *n* > 10) and obtained the results shown in Figure 12 [14]. A

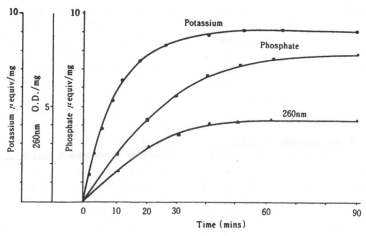

Figure 11. Release of cytoplasmic constituents from *E. coli* cells in contact with cetrimide [38]. [Cetrimide], 0.2 mM; *E. coli*, 10^9 cells/ml; pH, 7; 25°C.

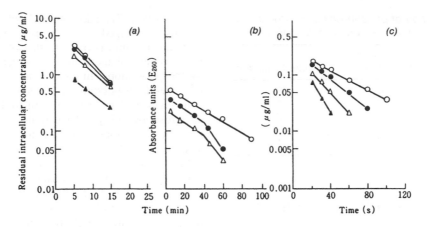

Figure 12. Release of cytoplasmic constituents from *E. coli* cells in contact with polycation *3* [14]. (a) Phosphate ions; (b) 260 nm-absorbing materials; (c) K$^+$ ions. Concentration of *3* (μg/ml): (a): (○), 4; (●), 3; (△), 2; (▲), 1 (b): (○), 5; (●), 3; (△), 1.5 (c): (○), 0.4; (●), 0.3; (▲), 0.1 Concentration of the *E. coli* cells was 10^9 cells/ml.

characteristic feature seen in Figure 12 is that the loss of K$^+$ ions from the cells is extremely fast and is caused by the polymeric biguanide at concentrations much lower than that required for leakage of the phosphate ions and the 260-nm absorbing materials. These results strongly suggest that polycations penetrate the cell wall and reach the cytoplasmic membrane, inducing the leakage of the cytoplasmic constituents as in the case of the low molecular weight cationic biocides.

Morphological change of bacterial cells on exposure to cationic biocides was investigated by electron microscopy [11,25,39]. Davies et al. revealed that when the *E. coli* cells were exposed to a low concentration of a biguanide biocide, chlorhexidine (Figure 1), bacterial cell surface became swollen and blistered, whereas exposure of the bacterial cells to a high level of chlorhexidine brought about leakage of the cytoplasmic constituents, followed by intracellular precipitation of the lost materials [11]. Exposure to the high level of chlorhexidine led finally to shrinkage of the bacterial cells with electron dense bodies inside the cells [11]. A similar morphological change of the *S. aureus* cells was observed when the cells were in contact with a polycation with side-chain quaternary ammonium salts (*15*-b) [25]. These results indicate that the target site of the cationic biocides, regardless of the molecular weight, is the cytoplasmic membrane of bacteria. Strong interaction with the cytoplasmic membrane is a primary step in the morphological change of the cells observed.

In the lethal action of the cationic biocides described previously, process (2) is undoubtedly suppressed as the molecular size of the diffusing species increases, since the peptidoglycan layer in the cell wall acts as a potential barrier against foreign molecules with high molecular weight. As schematically illustrated in Figures 9 and 10, the rigid peptidoglycan layer constitutes the basic framework of the cell walls and provides the bacterial cells with characteristic

shapes like a rod and a sphere. The cell wall plays a key role in preventing the bacterial cells from osmotic lysis [40]. Since the rigid peptidoglycan layer possesses a mesh-like structure, foreign molecules with small size are expected to diffuse rather freely through the cell wall. However, diffusion through the cell wall is believed to become difficult for molecules with increasing molecular size [31]. Very few quantitative data are available at present on the size of the foreign molecules that can diffuse through the cell wall without difficulty. It seems reasonable to assume that the size of the freely-diffusing foreign molecules is strain-dependent.

The bell-shaped dependence of antibacterial activity on molecular weight of the polycationic biocide (Figure 8) can be interpreted on the basis of the elementary processes in the lethal action of the cationic biocides [27]. Because of increasing charge density of the polycation, the adsorption of the polycation onto the bacterial cell surfaces is enhanced with increasing molecular weight of the polycation. A similar enhancement can be expected in the binding of the polycation to the cytoplasmic membrane (process 3), since there are many negatively charged species present in the cytoplasmic membrane, such as acidic phospholipids and some membrane proteins (see the section on "Structure of Bacterial Cell Wall and Cytoplasmic Membranes"). The disruption of the membrane (process 4) is a consequence of interaction of the bound polymers with the membrane and is expected to be facilitated with increasing amounts of the bound polymers. Process 4 would be immediately followed by processes 5 and 6, and thus processes 1, 3 and 4 (5 and 6) can be assumed to be enhanced with increasing molecular weight of the polymers. On the other hand, as discussed above, process 2 is supposed to be suppressed with increasing molecular weight. The observed optimal molecular weight region for antibacterial activity against *S. aureus* can, thus, be interpreted in terms of a sum of two kinds of controlling factors: one is positive (enhanced) with molecular weight (processes 1, 3 and 4) and the other is negative (suppressed) with molecular weight (process 2).

In order to explore the effect of the cell wall, antibacterial activity of the polycationic biocides against two types of bacterial cells was investigated [27]. One is the intact cell and the other is a protoplast which is freed from the cell wall. A protoplast is a bacterial cell which can be prepared by the action of lysozyme in hypertonic solution. Because of the absence of the cell wall, the cytoplasmic membrane is directly exposed to the environment in the protoplast, thus it is quite vulnerable to the change in the environment. The protoplast survives only in the hypertonic solution. The protoplast and the intact cells of *B. subtilis* were exposed to the polycations (*19*-c) with various molecular weights in the hypertonic solutions and the loss of the 260-nm absorbing materials from the both cells was followed [27]. The loss of the 260-nm absorbing materials is in fact a direct measure of cell lysis. Figure 13 shows the amount of 260-nm absorbing materials that were released from the intact cells and the protoplasts of *B. subtilis* in contact with 10 μg/ml of the polycation (*19*-c), as a function of the molecular weight of the polycation exposed [27]. A bell-shaped release profile was obtained for the intact cells, while a monotonic increase was observed for the protoplasts. These results clearly indicate that the target site of the polycationic biocides is the cytoplasmic membrane of bacteria, and exclusion at the cell walls operates for polymers with high molecular weight.

It is still ambiguous how the polycationic biocides interact with the cytoplasmic membrane with subsequent disruption. There are two possible sites in the cytoplasmic membrane for interaction with the polycations: the membrane-bound proteins and the phospholipids. Relatively little is known about the membrane-proteins. On the other hand, the phospholipids have been extensively studied. This may be due partly to the fact that method for isolation and purification of the phospholipids has been nearly established and highly purified samples are available. Furthermore, such excellent model systems as liposome, black lipid membrane and monolayer membrane can now be readily prepared, and their properties have been thoroughly investigated. By the use of these models for the cytoplasmic membranes, many studies on the interaction of various substrates with lipid bilayer membranes have been performed so far.

As described in the section on "Structure of Bacterial Cell Wall and Cytoplasmic Membranes", many kinds of the phospholipids are seen in the bacterial cytoplasmic membranes. Simply, they are classified into two groups according to the structure of the polar head groups. One is zwitterionic phospholipids, which include PC and PE. They are nearly neutral at physiological pH. The other is acidic phospholipids (PG, DPG and PS, etc.) which are negatively charged at physiological pH. With the aid of highly purified, well-characterized phospholipids, the effect of inorganic ions such as Ca^{2+} and Mg^{2+}, organic ions such as acetylcholine and polymyxin B on the model bilayer membranes has been investigated by thermal analysis (DSC etc.), fluorescence spectroscopy, NMR, X-ray diffraction method, and a variety of phenomena have been observed—phase separation, fusion, phase transition to hexagonal II phase and interdigitated phase [41–45].

Tirrel et al. studied the interaction of the polymeric in-chain quaternary ammonium salts with lipid bilayer membranes by DSC and X-ray diffraction. No significant effect of polyethyleneimine on a neutral bilayer composed of dipalmitoylphosphatidylcholine (DPPC) was observed, while on a negatively charged bilayer membrane composed of dipalmitoylphosphati-

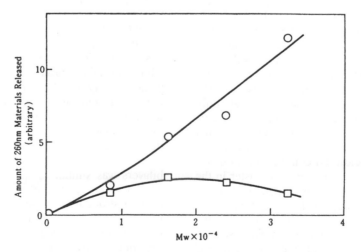

Figure 13. Release profile of 260 nm-absorbing materials from intact cells (□) and protoplasts (○) of *B. subtilis* in contact with polycation *19*-c as a function of molecular weight [27]. Concentration of *19*-c, 10 μg/ml.

dylglycerol (DPPG) strong interaction was recognized and the gel-to-liquid crystalline phase transition temperature (T_c) of the negatively charged bilayer was shifted to lower temperatures [46,47].

A specific effect of polyionene (4) was observed on the DPPG bilayer membrane. X-ray diffraction study on the structure of the mixture of the DPPG membrane and the polyionene 4 revealed that the interdigitated phase was induced by the addition of the polyionene where the hydrocarbon tails of DPPG are deeply interpenetrated [48,49].

The interaction of the biguanide polymer (3) and lipid bilayer membranes was investigated by DSC and fluorescence polarization method [50,51]. The polymer 3 and the monomer model compound 1 both lowered the T_c of the negatively charged bilayer composed of acidic PG by ~ 10°C. This is in contrast to the effect of Mg^{2+} and Ca^{2+}, which increased the T_c of the same bilayer membrane. Behavior of the polymer different from that of the monomer was observed toward a mixed bilayer of PC and PG. The polycation caused aggregation of the negatively charged PG in the vicinity of the adsorption site and formed the polycation/PG domain, thus inducing the phase separation in the mixed bilayer. On the other hand, no aggregation was observed on addition of the monomeric cation. As described in the section on "Structure of Bacterial Cell Wall and Cytoplasmic Membranes", bacterial cytoplasmic membranes are composed of neutral and negatively charged phospholipids, therefore it is believed that polycationic biocides induce phase separation in the bacterial membrane on binding.

Aggregation behavior of acidic phospholipids in the bilayer membranes by basic polypeptides has long been studied. These studies were devoted primarily to elucidating how the basic membrane-proteins interact with matrix phospholipids in the cytoplasmic membranes and how the functions of the membrane-proteins are affected by the matrix phospholipids. These studies are, however, useful in providing the basic insight into the polycation/membrane interaction.

Polylysine-induced phase separation was observed in the mixed bilayer of PC and phosphatidic acid (PA), as in the case of polycation 3. This result led to the assumption that extrinsic membrane-proteins affect the composition of the phospholipids near the location site, although the extrinisic proteins are only loosely bound at the surface of the cytoplasmic membranes [52]. Spin-labeling study revealed that cytochrome C, an extrinsic membrane protein, specifically binds to the acidic DPG in the mixed membrane of DPG and steroid, and forms a cluster in the membrane [53]. Myelin, a protein containing 38 basic residues in the molecule, induced aggregation of 27–34 molecules of the acidic phospholipids in the vicinity of the location site, and caused phase separation in the mixed bilayer membranes of neutral PC and acidic lipids (PA, PG or PS) [54,55].

Galla et al. investigated the interaction of poly-

myxin B, a cationic oligopeptide having high antibacterial activity (Figure 1), with the bilayer membrane by the fluorescence polarization method. They found that polymyxin B binds specifically to acidic phospholipids (PA and PG) and induces phase separation in the dipalmitolyphosphatidic acid (DPPA)/distearoyl PC mixed membrane [44]. On addition of polymyxin B to the monolayer of DPPA, expansion of the monolayer was observed. In the case of the bilayer membrane of DPPA, T_c was found to be lowered by ~20°C on addition of polymyxin B. However, no effect was observed when polymyxin B was added to the neutral bilayer membrane.

Recently, interaction of a polymeric in-chain ammonium salt with phospholipid bilayer membranes was studied by time-resolved fluorescence spectroscopy in connection with the antibacterial activity of the polycation [56]. Particular attention was paid in this study to a phenomenon of polycation-induced fluidization of the membranes, which was well-evaluated by the time-resolved fluorescence anisotropy measurements. The fluorescence anisotropy, $r(t)$, of 1,6-diphenyl-1,3,5-hexatriene (DPH) embedded in the membranes was analyzed based on the simplest wobbling-in-cone model. Strong interaction was observed between the polycation 7 and the DPPA membrane as demonstrated by a large decrease of residual polarization value on adding the polycation 7 to the DPPA membrane. This means that the cone angle of the wobbling-in-cone motion of the DPH molecule increases by the addition of the polycation 7, indicating the polycation-induced fluidization of the acidic membrane. On the other hand, $r(t)$ of DPH embedded in the DPPC membrane was not affected significantly by the addition of 7, which is presumably due to non-binding of the polycation to the zwitterionic membrane. These results clearly indicate that the polycationic biocide interacts strongly with negatively charged membranes, inducing fluidization of the membranes.

Interaction of various polyionenes with phospholipid bilayer membranes was also explored by means of DSC with special reference to their antimicrobial activities [57]. Addition of polyionene 7 and 9 caused phase separation in the mixed bilayer of PC and PA. Ability to induce phase separation was found to depend strongly on the structure of the polyionene. Polyionene with rigid spacer (7) was most effective in inducing phase separation and was most active in antimicrobial activity, while polyionenes with rigid and flexible spacers in the alternate fashion exhibited lower activity and their mode of interaction with bilayers was similar to those of all flexible spacers. This result suggests that the rigid spacers are favorable for strong interaction with the negatively charged bilayer membranes, leading to the higher activity. Other factors affecting the mode of interaction with membranes were molecular weight and hydrophobicity. With increasing molecular weight, both activity and ability to induce phase separation increased. Introduction of hydrophilic groups into the spacers resulted in a loss of activity and ability to induce phase separation. The antimicrobial activity and the mode of interaction with membranes were correlated and were found to be interpreted on the basis of the conformational concept of the polyionenes in solution.

Polycationic biocides bind to the bacterial cytoplasmic membranes and disorganize the membrane structure. This will undoubtedly affect the function of the membrane-bound enzymes. It is reasonably expected that the change in activity of the membrane-bound enzymes would be lethal and would result in the death of the bacterial cells. However, very few studies have been performed so far on the effect of the polycations on the membrane-bound enzymes. Panarin et al. investigated the effect of polycations *15* and *16* on the activity of bacterial enzymes activating the antibiotics chloramphenicol and canamycin, which are known to be bound to the cytoplasmic membrane [25]. Chloramphenicolacetyltransferase (CAT) conducts acetylation of hydroxy groups of the antibiotic and transforms it into an inactive diacetyl derivative, and canamycintransferase (CT) also transforms canamycin into an inactive form. It was found that the polycations *15* and *16* significantly inhibit the membrane-bound enzymes (CAT and CT) and the activity of the enzymes was reduced by 10%–100% by the action of the polycations. The effect of inhibition was dependent on the strain and the structure of the polycations. *S. aureus* was much more sensitive than *E. coli* and polycation *16*-b was most effective.

Replacement of counter-cations of a polyanion is another function of the polycation. This leads to polyanion/polycation complexation and insolubilization of the complex. Replacement of Mg^{2+} and Ca^{2+} ions present at the surface of the bacterial membranes by the polycations is reasonably expected and may result in change in the function of the membrane-bound enzymes. For example, Mg^{2+} and Ca^{2+} are required for ATPase to exhibit its function, thus removal of these inorganic cations would lead to loss of the function of this enzyme [58,59]. Anyhow, the polycation/membrane-bound enzyme interaction is one of the most important subjects to be solved in the future for deeper understanding of the mode of action of the polycationic biocides.

POLYMERIC MATERIALS WITH ANTIBACTERIAL ACTIVITY

Polymeric drugs are provided with properties superior to those of low molecular weight analogues in view of the high local density of active groups and the film-forming property, which originate from polymeric forms. Furthermore, cross-linking will give the polymeric drugs insoluble features, thus immobilization of the active groups can be readily achieved. Polycationic biocides possess high positive charge density and excellent processability, and have found remarkable utility in hygiene and in biomedical applications.

Biomedical contamination of polymeric materials with microorganisms is a primitive but still quite serious problem and all polymeric materials are subjected to sterilization by means of steam, chemicals and radiation. However, most materials are often re-exposed to the atmosphere, which can lead to recontamination with microorganisms. Antibiotics are prescribed to the patients to prevent microbial infections, and this treatment has in general been successful. However, this treatment suffers from the disadvantage that frequent and excessive use of antibiotics produces resistant bacterial cells, which then require more "powerful" antibiotics to be effective. One possible way to overcome this problem is to develop polymeric materials which themselves have antimicrobial activity. Such materials with intrinsic antimicrobial activity may be called "self-sterilizing materials" (SSM). In this section, application of the polycationic biocides to a variety of fields is described.

Immobilized Polycationic Biocides

Many trials have been conducted so far to provide surface antibacterial activity with polymeric materials by incorporating antibacterial agents covalently onto the surfaces of the polymeric materials. This type of antimicrobial agent is termed an "immobilized" biocide and exhibits its activity through contact with microbial cells, thus this action is sometimes called "contact disinfection". Merits of the "immobilized" biocides are evident. Firstly, because of immobilization of the active groups, contamination of environment with the biocides can be prevented. Secondly, continuous treatment of bacterial cell suspension is possible by the use of column packed with the immobilized biocides. Thirdly, owing to covalent bonding to the matrix media, the immobilized biocides can be regenerated by washing with appropriate solvent, so that they can be used for a long time.

Isquith et al. treated various surfaces with 3-(trimethoxysilyl)propyldimethyloctadecyl ammonium chloride (Si-QAC), a coupling agent, and examined the antimicrobial activity of the surfaces of the materials, which retain the chemically bonded Si-QAC [60]. The ammonium salts were not released from the surfaces by repeated washing with water and showed antimicrobial activity against a wide range of microorganisms. For example, covalent coupling of Si-QAC to glass beads resulted in active particles and only 1–4 cells of *Streptococcus faecalis* were seen on the surface of the treated glass beads while $\sim 10^3$ cells could be observed on the surface of the untreated (blank) glass beads. The surface activity was found to persist after repeated washing with detergent solution, and 50-times washings did not affect the activity. Materials other than glass (natural fibers, man-made fibers and metals) were treated by the same procedure

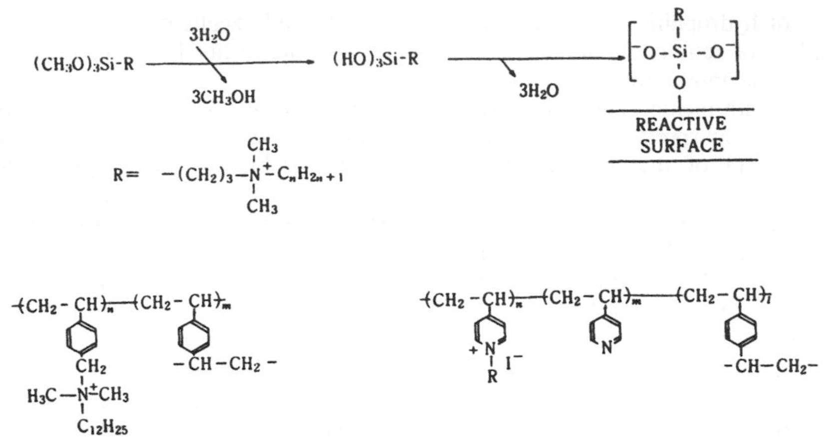

Siliceous surfaces	Man-made fibers	Metals
Glass	Acrylic	Aluminum
Glass wool	Modacrylic	Stainless steel
Sand	Polyester	Galvanized metal
Stone	Cellulose acetate	
Ceramic	Rayon	Miscellaneous
	Acetate	Leather
Natural fibers	Anidex	Wood
Cotton	Spandex	Rubber
Wool	Vinyl	Plastic
Linen	Dacron	Formica
Felt	Viscose	

Figure 14. Structure of immobilized polycationic biocides and Si-QAC-treated substrates exhibiting antimicrobial activity [60,62,64,66,68].

and the treated surfaces exhibited a similar surface activity [60,61].

Nakagawa et al. prepared similar surface-treated glass beads and explored their surface activity. They used 3-chloropropyltrimethoxysilane as a coupling agent, and quaternary ammonium salts were introduced covalently at the surfaces of the glass beads by the reaction of the chloropropyl groups with various N,N-dimethylalkylamines [62]. They found that the alkyl chain length strongly affected the surface activity. The cell suspension of *E. coli* ($\sim 10^6$ cells/ml) was eluted through a column packed with 1.2 g of the surface-treated glass beads (80–120 mesh) and the cell concentration of the eluates was evaluated. The glass beads retaining C_2-C_4 alkyl chains showed lower activity while those with C_8-C_{18} alkyl chains exhibited high activity. In particular, the glass beads with C_{10} alkyl chains showed the highest activity and contact of the bacterial cell suspension with these glass beads only for 10 s was enough to remove all the cells from the eluates.

Currently, the formation of trihalomethanes and other carcinogens as a result of water disinfection with chlorine is a serious problem. Removal of bacterial cells from water by the use of the immobilized biocides can thus be an alternative and sophisticated method of water disinfection.

Recently, many products are commercially available, which are imparted with surface antimicrobial activity. These include underwear, socks and sheets. Most of the products are those treated with alkoxysilane coupling agents having quaternary ammonium salts at the surfaces, thereby their surface activity is said to remain unchanged after repeated washing [63].

The surface activity of these treated materials is mainly due to adsorption of bacterial cells. The bacterial cells captured seem to be alive on the surfaces, thus the surface activity may not be bactericidal but bacteriostatic. As described in the section on "Mode of Action of Polycationic Biocides", the positive charges play a key role in the adsorption of the cells, but other factors seem to affect strongly the adsorption behaviors.

Cross-linked quaternary ammonium salts have also been studied as to their ability to adsorb the bacterial cells. The cross-linked resins prepared from cross-linked poly(chloromethylstyrene) and N,N-dimethyldodecylamine showed antibacterial activity against *B. subtilis* and exerted an ability to capture 9×10^8 cells/g of the cells [64]. Furthermore, the resin was found to exhibit the activity against viruses [65].

Systematic studies on the effect of the alkyl chain length and the degree of cross-linking on the ability of capturing the bacterial cells were performed for cross-linked poly(pyridinium salts). Nakagawa et al. investigated the adsorption behaviors of the resins prepared from cross-linked poly(4-vinylpyridine) and alkyl iodide [66,67]. In the preparation of the resins, the mole fraction of the cross-linking agent, divinylbenzene, was changed from 10% to 70%. Among the resulting resins, the ability to capture the bacterial cells increased in the order of 70% < 10% < 30% < 50%. For the resins with similar degrees of cross-linking, those with the alkyl chain length of C_8–C_{12} exhibited the highest activity. Kawabata et al. reported that benzyl moiety was quite effective for the capture of various bacterial cells when incorporated into the cross-linked poly(vinylpyridinium salts) [68]. Figure 15 shows the number of the viable cells of *E. coli* in the aqueous phase as a function of the contact time between the cross-linked poly(vinylpyridinium salts) and the benzyl moiety. In the absence of this resin, no change in the number of viable cells was observed, whereas in the presence of this resin the number of the viable cells decreased with time and 99% and 99.99% of the *E. coli* cells were captured after 2 h and 6 h contact, respectively. The capture ability of this resin against the *E. coli* cells was estimated to be 1.2–1.5 × 10^{10} cells/g. This resin was found also to be effective against bacteriophages [69].

The capture ability of the bacterial cells was strongly strain-dependent. Kawabata et al. investigated the cell-capture ability of cross-linked poly(N-benzyl-4-vinylpyridinium salts) and found that the sensitivity to the cross-linked resin increased in the order of *Salmonella* < *Klebsiella* < *Bacillus* < *Enterobacter* < *P. aeruginosa* < *E. coli* < *S. aureus* [70]. The surface negative charges of these bacterial cells were determined to be in the range of 9 × 10^{-18}–6 × 10^{-16} g·eq/cell and were dependent on the strains. However, no correlation was recognized between the sensitivity and the surface charges of the cells. These results suggest that factors other than the surface charges of the cells may operate in the adsorption of the cells by the cross-linked polymeric quaternary ammonium salts. Hydrophobicity of the cell surfaces is again strain-dependent. It was revealed by the Rosenberg method [71,72] that in *Staphylococcus, Salmonella,* and *Bacillus* the cell surfaces are highly hydrophobic, and among these strains good correlation was observed between the amount of adsorbed cells and the surface charges [70].

Other factors affecting the adsorption behaviors are the cell concentration, flow rate, particle size of the resins and temperature. It was found that low concentration of the cells and low flow rate are favorable for cell capture [66]. Furthermore, small particle size (large surface area) and high temperature seem to be effective [64,66].

Cross-linked polymeric quaternary ammonium salts described so far are inactivated by adsorption of the microbial cells and polyanions. However, the surface activity can be regenerated by removal of the adsorbed materials by washing the resins with ethanol and sodium hydroxide solution. Thus, these cross-linked materials can be reused repeatedly [62,64,

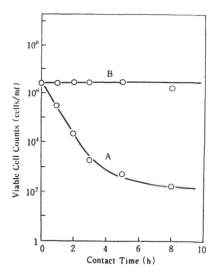

Figure 15. Capture of *E. coli* cells by cross-linked polymeric quaternary ammonium salts [68]. (a) Resins with quaternary ammonium salts; (b) resins without quaternary ammonium salts.

66,68]. Another application of these resins is based on the fact that the adsorbed microbial cells are alive on the surfaces, although the cell division is inhibited. Thus, the cross-linked polymeric quaternary ammonium salts can carry a large number of microbial cells alive on the surfaces and these immobilized microbial cells can be used in bioreactors [70]. This method of immobilization of the microbial cells has advantages over other methods in that it involves simple operations, no chemical reagents which may damage the cells, and has a high strength of adsorption. In fact, alcoholic fermentation by the use of the adsorbed yeast cells on the surfaces of the cross-linked polymeric quaternary ammonium salts has been tested extensively [70].

Polymeric Materials Releasing Low Molecular Weight Biocides

The characteristic feature of this type of SSM is bactericidal activity of their surfaces since biocides are released at their surfaces.

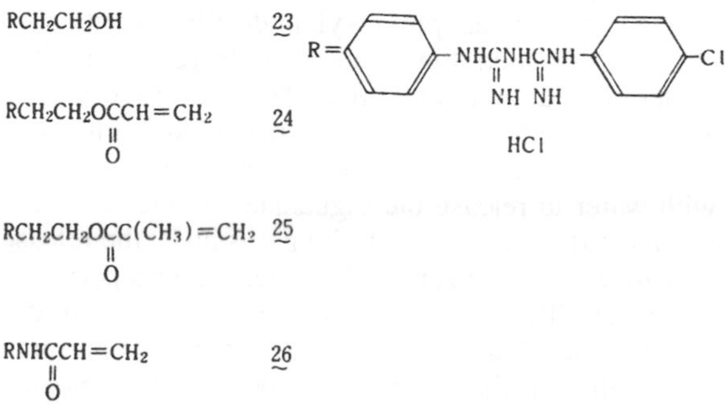

RCH₂CH₂OH   *23*

RCH₂CH₂OCCH=CH₂   *24*
  ‖
  O

RCH₂CH₂OCC(CH₃)=CH₂   *25*
  ‖
  O

RNHCCH=CH₂   *26*
  ‖
  O

$$R = \text{—} \bigcirc \text{—NHCNHCNH—} \bigcirc \text{—Cl}$$
$$\quad\quad\quad \overset{\|}{\text{NH}} \overset{\|}{\text{NH}}$$
$$\text{HCl}$$

Figure 16. Structures of vinyl monomers with biguanide units in the side-chain (*24–26*) and released biocide (hydrolyzed product, *23*) [76].

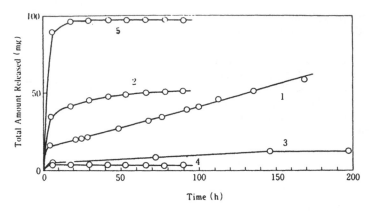

Figure 17. Release of biguanide biocide from cross-linked polyacrylamide films [76]. 1, Containing covalently-bonded *24*; 2, containing homopolymer of *24* physically; 3, containing covalently-bonded *25*; 4, containing covalently-bonded *26*; 5, containing *23* physically.

When the low molecular weight quaternary ammonium salts were retained in the cation-exchange resins as counter ions, they were liberated slowly and exhibited bactericidal activity [73–75]. Liberation of the quaternary ammonium salts was found to be enhanced when the cation-exchange resins prepared from weak acids were employed. Furthermore, dimethylphenylbenzyl ammonium chlorides were easily released regardless of the kind of resins. On the other hand, in the cation-exchange resins prepared from strong acids the amount of released cationic biocides was small. Extensive studies were performed on the combination of AIRC-50 (cation-exchange resin) and cetylpyridinium chloride (cationic biocide). This resin with the biocide was found to be highly effective in killing microbial cells, and no surviving cells were observed in the eluates. However, the bactericidal activity of this resin was again dependent on the cell concentration, contact time and temperature. At higher temperatures the activity was high, but even at room temperature the activity was high enough to kill all microbial cells under ordinary conditions. pH did not affect the activity between 5–14 while culture media such as beef extract and polypeptides were found to reduce the bactericidal activity. The amount of the released biocide was found to be in the range of 1.2–1.6 μg/ml.

The cross-linked polyacrylamide films containing covalently-bonded biguanide biocide (*24*) exhibited bactericidal activity at their surfaces and successfully acted as SSM [76,77]. This cross-linked film was found to be hydrolyzed at the acrylate group in contact with water to release the biguanide biocide (*23*), and when the degree of cross-linking was high, the release was approximately zero-order at least over a period of one week. The rate of release then decreased gradually, but the release was observed to continue for up to a month. Furthermore, the dose of the biocide released could be controlled by the amount of *24* in the preparation stage of the cross-linked film. When the cross-linked films were placed on nutrient agar

plates, inoculated with cell suspensions of *S. aureus* and *E. coli* and incubated, no colonies of the bacteria were seen on the plates, whereas bacterial growth was observed as thick colonies on the blank films. Furthermore, the growth inhibitory zone was observed for the cross-linked films, which indicates that the diffusion of the free biocide (*23*) occurs over a relatively long distance [77]. Scanning electron microscopy studies revealed that the inoculated cells of *E. coli* and *S. aureus* underwent morphological changes such as shrinkage and deformation, which is ascribed to the collapse of the bacterial cells due to the bactericidal action of *23*. This SSM film could be regenerated by washing with alcohol and it showed the same surface activity. This type of SSM would be particularly valid in such applications as wound covers and artificial skin for temporary uses.

Another polymeric film with high physical strength was reportedly bactericidal. This is a blend of polyethylene and a copolymer of ethylene and acrylic acid which contains benzalkonium biocide as counter cations [78]. This polymer film was shown to be bactericidal at the surfaces due to the release of the benzalkonium salts in contact with water.

This chapter is dedicated to the late professor Shigeo Tazuke who gave the author outstanding suggestions, but unfortunately died on July 11, 1989.

REFERENCES

1. Donaruma, L. G. and O. Vogl, eds. 1978. *Polymeric Drugs*. New York: Academic Press.

2. Vogl, O. and D. Tirrell. 1979. *J. Macromol. Sci. Chem.*, A13:415.

3. Verlander, M. S., J. C. Venter, M. Goodman, N. O. Kaplan and B. Saks. 1976. *Proc. Natl. Acad. Sci. USA*, 73:1009.

4. Franklin, T. J. and G. A. Snow. 1981. *Biochemistry of Antimicrobial Action*. London: Chapman and Hall, Chapter 3.

5. Domagk, G. 1935. *Deut. Med. Wochenschr.*, 61:829.

6. Curd, F. H. S. and F. L. Rose. 1946. *J. Chem. Soc.*, p. 729.

7. Rose, F. L. and G. Swain. 1956. *J. Chem. Soc.*, p. 4422.

8. Kurzer, F. and E. D. Pitchfork. 1968. *Fortch. Chem. Forsch.*, 10:375.

9. Hopp, J. O. and A. M. Lands. 1947. *J. Pharmacol. Exper. Therap.*, 79:321.

10. Batz, H.-G. 1977. *Adv. Polym. Sci.*, 23:26.

11. Davies, A., M. Bently and B. S. Field. 1968. *J. Appl. Bacteriol.*, 31:448.

12. Boardman, G. 1969. *Food Technol. N.Z.*, 4:421.

13. Pemberton, D., P. M. Woodcock and T. Ikeda. (unpublished results).

14. Broxton, P., P. M. Woodcock and P. Gilbert. 1983. *J. Appl. Bacteriol.*, 54:345.

15. Rembaum, A., H. Rile and R. Somoano. 1970. *J. Polym. Sci.*, B8:457.

16. Rembaum, A. 1973. *Appl. Polym. Symp.*, 22:299.

17. Rajaraman, R., D. E. Rounds, S. P. S. Yen and A. Rembaum. 1975. "Effects of Ionenes on Normal and Transformed Cells", in *Polyelectrolytes and Their Applications*. A. Rembaum and E. Selegny, eds. Reidel.

18. Ottenbrite, R. M. and G. R. Myers. 1973. *J. Polym. Sci. Polym. Chem. Ed.*, 11:1443.

19. Vucetic, J. J., V. H. Vandjel and M. D. Janic. 1977. *Glas. Hem. Drus. Beograd.*, 42:389.

20. Ikeda, T., H. Yamaguchi and S. Tazuke. 1990. *J. Bioact. Comp. Polym.*, 5:31.

21. Katchalski, E., L. Bichovski-Slomnitzki and B. E. Volcani. 1953. *Nature*, 169:1095.

22. Katchalski, E., L. Bichovski-Slomnitzki and B. E. Volcani. 1953. *Biochem J.*, 55:671.

23. Kovacs, K., A. Kotai and I. Szabo. 1960. *Nature*, 185:266.

24. Kovacs, K., A. Kotai, I. Szabo and R. Mecseki. 1961. *Nature*, 192:190.

25. Panarin, E. F., M. V. Solovskii, N. A. Zaikina and G. E. Afinogenov. 1985. *Makromol. Chem. Suppl.*, 9:25.

26. Ikeda, T., H. Yamaguchi and S. Tazuke. 1984. *Antimicrob. Agents Chemother.*, 26:139.

27. Ikeda, T., H. Hirayama, H. Yamaguchi, S. Tazuke and M. Watanabe. 1986. *Antimicrob. Agents Chemother.*, 30:132.

28. Ikeda, T., S. Tazuke and Y. Suzuki. 1984. *Makromol. Chem.*, 185:869.

29. Ikeda, T., H. Hirayama, H. Yamaguchi and S. Tazuke. 1986. *Makromol. Chem.*, 187:333.

30. Hugo, W. B. and A. D. Russell, eds. 1980. *Pharmaceutical Microbiology*. Oxford: Blackwell, p. 3.

31. Costerton, J. W. and K.-J. Cheng. 1975. *J. Antimicrob. Chemother.*, 1:363.

32. Hamilton-Miller, J. M. T. 1965. *Biochem. Biophys. Res. Commun.*, 20:688.

33. White, D. A., W. J. Lennarz and C. A. Schnaitman. 1972. *J. Bacteriol.*, 109:686.

34. Costerton, J. W., J. M. Ingram and K.-J. Cheng. 1974. *Bact. Rev.*, 38:87.

35. Katchalsky, A. 1964. *Biophys. J.*, 4:9.

36. Hugo, W. B. and A. R. Longworth. 1964. *J. Pharmac.*, 16:655.

37. Salton, M. R. 1951. *J. Gen. Microbiol.*, 5:391.

38. Lambert, P. A. and S. M. Hammond. 1973. *Biochem. Biophys. Res. Commun.*, 54:796.

39. Hugo, W. B. and A. R. Longworth. 1966. *J. Pharmac.*, 18:569.

40. Hawker, L. E. and A. H. Linton, eds. 1979. *Microorganisms*. London: Edward Arnold, Chapter 8.

41. Chapman, D. 1975. *Quart. Rev. Biophys.*, 8:185. Papahajopoulos, D., W. J. Vail, W. A. Pangborn and G. Poste. 1976. *Biochim. Biophys. Acta*, 448:265. Cullis, P. R. and B. de Kruijff. 1978. *Biochim. Biophys. Acta*, 513:31. There are many other references.

42. Hauser, H., K. Howell and M. C. Phillips. 1977. *FEBS Lett.*, 80:355.

43. Rack, J. L. and J. F. Tocanne. 1982. *FEBS Lett.*, 143:171.

44. Sixl, F. and H.-J. Galla. 1981. *Biochim. Biophys. Acta*, 643:626.

45. Eliasz, A. W., D. Chapman and D. F. Ewing. 1976. *Biochim. Biophys. Acta*, 448:220.

46. Tirrell, D. A. and P. M. Boyd. 1981. *Makromol. Chem. Rapid Commun.*, 2:193.

47. Takigawa, D. Y. and D. A. Tirrell. 1985. *Macromolecules*, 18:338.

48. Tirrell, D. A., A. B. Turek, D. A. Wilkinson and T. J. MacInthoch. 1985. *Macromolecules*, 18:1512.

49. Turek, A. B. and D. A. Tirrell. 1986. *J. Bioact. Comp. Polym.*, 1:309.

50. Ikeda, T., S. Tazuke and M. Watanabe. 1983. *Biochim. Biophys. Acta*, 735:380.

51. Ikeda, T., A. Ledwith, C. H. Bamford and R. A. Hann. 1984. *Biochim. Biophys. Acta*, 769:57.

52. Galla, H.-J. and E. Sackmann. 1975. *Biochim. Biophys. Acta*, 401:509.

53. Birrell, G. B. and O. H. Griffith. 1976. *Biochemistry*, 15:2925.

54. Boggs, J. M., M. A. Moscarello and D. Papahadjopoulos. 1977. *Biochemistry*, 16:5420.

55. Boggs, J. M., D. D. Wood, M. A. Moscarello and D. Papahadjopoulos. 1977. *Biochemistry*, 16:2325.

56. Ikeda, T., B. Lee, H. Yamaguchi and S. Tazuke. 1990. *Biochim. Biophys. Acta*, 1021:56.

57. Ikeda, T., H. Yamaguchi and S. Tazuke. 1990. *Biochim. Biophys. Acta*, 1026:105.

58. Schaefer, G. 1976. *Biochem. Pharmacol.*, 25:2015.

59. Elsenhans, B., R. Blume, B. Lembcke and W. E. Caspary. 1983. *Biochem. Biophys. Acta*, 727:135.

60. Isquith, A. J., E. A. Abbott and P. A. Walters. 1972. *Appl. Microbiol.*, 24:859.

61. Walters, P. A., E. A. Abbott and A. J. Isquith. 1973. *Appl. Microbiol.*, 25:253.

62. Nakagawa, Y., H. Hayashi, T. Tawaratani, H. Kourai, T. Horie and I. Shibasaki. 1984. *Appl. Environ. Microbiol.*, 47:513.

63. Yumizori, O. 1983. *J. Antibact. Antifung. Agents*, 11:76.

64. Walfish, I. H. and G. E. Janauer. 1979. *Water, Air and Soil Pollution*, 12:477.

65. Gerba, C. P., G. E. Janauer and M. Costello. 1984. *Water Res.*, 18:17.

66. Nakagawa, Y., Y. Yamano, T. Tawaratani, H. Kourai, T. Horie and I. Shibasaki. 1982. *Appl. Environ. Microbiol.*, 43:1041.

67. Nakagawa, Y., T. Tawaratani, H. Kourai, T. Horie and I. Shibasaki. 1984. *Appl. Environ. Microbiol.*, 47:88.

68. Kawabata, N. T. Hayashi and T. Matsumoto. 1983. *Appl. Environ. Microbiol.*, 46:203.

69. Kawabata, N., T. Hashizume and T. Matsumoto. 1986. *Agric. Biol. Chem.*, 50:1551.

70. Kawabata, N. and Kako Kobunshi. 1985. 34:583.

71. Rosenberg, M., D. Gutnick and E. Rosenberg. 1980. *FEMS Microbiol. Lett.*, 9:29.

72. Rosenberg, M., S. Rottem and E. Rosenberg. 1982. *FEMS Microbiol. Lett.*, 13:167.

73. Nakagawa Y., T. Tawaratani and I. Shibasaki. 1979. *J. Antibact. Antifung. Agents*, 7:T511.

74. Nakagawa, Y., Y. Inoue, T. Tawaratani and I. Shibasaki. 1979. *J. Antibact. Antifung. Agents*, 7:T515.

75. Nakagawa, Y., N. Dohi, T. Tawaratani and I. Shibasaki. 1983. *J. Antibact. Antifung. Agents*, 11:263.

76. Ikeda, T., H. Yamaguchi and S. Tazuke. 1986. *J. Bioact. Comp. Polym.*, 1:162.

77. Ikeda, T., H. Yamaguchi and S. Tazuke. 1986. *J. Bioact. Comp. Polym.*, 1:301.

78. Ackert, W. B., R. L. Camp, W. L. Wheelwright and J. S. Byck. 1975. *J. Biomed. Mater. Res.*, 9:55.

43

Protein Drugs Tailored with Synthetic Polymers: Enhanced Plasma-Half-Life and Efficient Delivery to Tumor and Inflammatory Sites

HIROSHI MAEDA, Ph.D., M.D.*

ABSTRACT: By conjugating water soluble polymers, the drawbacks of pharmacologically active protein drugs or enzymes can be greatly improved. Antigenicity can be drastically reduced; a 10- to several 100-fold prolongation of plasma half-life can be accomplished; biocompatible macromolecules have enhanced targeting to the sites of lesions such as cancer and inflammation; enhanced stability of polymer conjugates *in vivo* and *in vitro* makes them easy to handle, and by manipulating the lipophilicity of the conjugates one can make an oily formulation of protein drugs. Basic pathophysiological differences between tumorous/lesion and normal tissue are discussed, which make macromolecular drugs so unique and advantageous *in vivo*.

INTRODUCTION

General Scope of Macromolecular Therapeutics

Rapid developments in biotechnology in recent years have brought a great number of protein drugs into existence, many of which exhibit extremely potent activity *in vitro*. For example, the activity of purified recombinant interferon at 1 mg/ml is still detectable even after 10^8-fold dilution. The anticancer protein agent neocarzinostatin (NCS) is active in the nanomolar range. However, when these drugs were used clinically it turned out that their therapeutic efficacy is unremarkable compared to that anticipated from *in vitro* studies. The reason for the discrepancy is that there is almost no involvement of pharmacokinetics in the case of *in vitro* systems; no barriers exist in the drug delivery to the target cells or receptors *in vitro*. Furthermore, there are a number of other drawbacks inherent to the protein drugs. Namely

these proteins are produced outside of the human body, which means it is a natural consequence that the body develops respective antibodies to them. Even genetically engineered recombinant human proteins such as interferons or lymphokines have no carbohydrate moieties; therefore, they are not identical to human counterparts. Thus, antigenicity and lack of biocompatibility of recombinant human cDNA derived proteins would also be a target of the body's defense-oriented clearance system. Development of immune complexes of antigen and antibody makes them more subject to phagocytosis by macrophages, or deposition in the kidney, the liver, etc.

Furthermore, lack of a carbohydrate moiety in these proteins makes their plasma half-life very short due to rapid renal clearance or entrapment in the liver, the spleen, the lung or the kidney. Under other circumstances, some recombinant proteins produced in *E. coli* were reported to exhibit poor solubility.

As will be described below, these problems can be solved by conjugating appropriate synthetic polymers. Not only is the capacity to react with antibody (antigenicity) lost, but also the ability to elicit antibody can be nullified. Polymer conjugated also markedly prolongs the serum plasma half-life of small molecular mass protein agents. For example, small proteins with molecular mass of 10,000–30,000 are usually cleared so rapidly ($t_{1/2}$ 2–5 min) into the urine that their pharmacological effect is very limited. Polymer conjugation can increase the half-life by 10- to several 100-fold. This type of modification of proteins is coined "*Protein-tailoring*" to fit the requirements of the users.

The uniqueness of macromolecular therapeutics resides in the vascular property at the site of lesion. At the site of inflammation or cancer the local blood vessels become highly leaky [1–3]. The junction of the endothelial cells of the blood vessels becomes loose in inflammatory tissue or cancer tissue due to the effect of permeability-enhancing factors such as

*Department of Microbiology, Kumamoto University School of Medicine, Kumamoto 860, Japan

bradykinins, permeability-enhancing factor, and others as described later. Most small molecules can traverse the blood vessels more freely than large molecules. Small molecules may reach most of the tissues and organs by equilibrium, thus they exhibit less selectivity in the drug delivery. Macromolecules, on the other hand, are only capable of leaking out where the vascular permeability is enhanced, such as in inflammations and cancer [1–6]. Thus, one can deliver the macromolecular drugs more selectively to the site of diseases where drugs are needed, and avoid the undesirable systemic side-effects of cytotoxic anticancer agent. The phenomenon is of crucial importance in cancer chemotherapy.

Macromolecules leaked out from the blood vessel or introduced into the interstitial space would be transported into the lymphatics; they would not be recovered through the blood capillary by back-diffusion as small molecules [7]. Lipids are also known to behave similarly to macromolecules in this regard [7], which indicates that one can deliver these drugs into the lymphatics if they could leak out of the blood vessels. This lymphatic system is often known as the preferred route for tumor spreading (lymphatic metastasis). Thus, lymphotropic drug-delivery is preferred for the control of this metastasis on these principles. The lymph will eventually flow into the thoracic duct, then into the general circulation [7].

This author has been working on the protein anticancer agent, neocarzinostatin (NCS), for over 25 years, and has been faced with these various problems. About 12 years ago he developed a tailor-made anticancer agent (smancs), by conjugation of polymer with neocarzinostatin. Indeed, it has been proven that these tactics of macromolecular therapeutics really have great potential value in cancer chemotherapy [1,2,8–11]. Furthermore, a wide range of applications became feasible, as described in this chapter.

ANTIGENICITY

Two different types of immune reactions become apparent in antigen-injected hosts, namely, humoral or antibody production and cellular immune response which involves a number of different types of leukocytes and various interleukins. In this section, I want to concentrate on the first one because frequently the two events take place similarly.

In earlier studies of the antigenicity of proteins it became evident that some protein modifications result in a loss of antigenic potentials [12–14]; the effects of succinylation, or attachment of poly(D-Glu-D-Ala-D-Lys) or poly(D-Glu-D-Lys) [14] were examined previously on albumin, lactoglobulin, myoglobin, γ-globulin, lysozyme etc. and their antigenicity was greatly reduced. Other synthetic polymers or peptides were also found to be effective in modifying immunogenicity [12–14]. Detailed accounts can be found in later references [15,16]. Here I want to discuss some other

pharmacologically important proteins, in view of their antigenic potential and their conversion to non-antigenic states by tailoring.

L-asparaginase is an enzyme produced by *E. coli*, which hydrolyzes L-asparagine to yield L-aspartic acid and ammonia. The depletion of L-asparagine from blood plasma would result in the suppression of tumor growth since L-asparagine is required for growth of some tumor cells. It was the first enzyme introduced for the treatment of lymphocytic leukemia and lymphoma in the 1960s. Soon after, it was found that antibody was developed in patients which nullified its pharmacological (enzymatic) activity. The other limitation was that it has a relatively short plasma half-life ($t_{1/2} \approx 1.5$ hr).

These problems were solved by conjugating it with polyethylene glycol (PEG). Its immunogenic potential was reduced to about 1% of native counterpart [17,18]. This polymer tailored L-asparaginase is now being developed for clinical applications in the U.S.A. as is its second generation drug.

Another example is the antitumor protein neocarzinostatin [NCS] (MW 12,000) which is produced by *Streptomyces carzinostaticus* [19]. It is a very potent antitumor agent with median cell growth inhibition or inhibition of DNA synthesis at about 0.05 μg/ml or in the nM range [19]. Its antigenicity was speculated, but it was found that very few patients developed antibodies to it [20]. Among the bladder cancer patients who did not respond to the drug, it was found that their plasma contained protease activity that degraded NCS [20]. The very weak immunogenicity found for NCS may be attributed to its very rapid clearance rate ($t_{1/2} = 1.9$ min).

Later we developed a polymer conjugate. The polymer used in this case was styrene-co-maleic acid/anhydride (SMA), and the conjugate was designated smancs. Smancs as a prototype revealed a great number of important properties of macromolecular therapeutic agents in general: loss of antigenicity, enhanced stability *in vitro* and *in vivo*, a great increase in plasma half-life, lymphotropicity, vascular permeability in tumor vessel (tumoritropic character) and lipid formulability [21–24].

The immunological properties studied include the capacity to induce antibody, reactivity to the antibody prepared against parent protein NCS, and passive cutaneous anaphylaxis. All of these tests revealed that smancs became much less antigenic, about 1/16 to 1/8 of that of NCS [23]. Recent clinical data shows that smancs could be very weakly antigenic like penicillin (unpublished data).

More recently we prepared a conjugate of dextran (MW 6,000) and soybean trypsin inhibitor (Kunitz type, MW 20,000) [25,26] and tested its immunogenicity before and after conjugation. We found that formation of antibody in rabbit was greatly decreased, and the passive cutaneous anaphylaxis reaction was found to be consistent with that of antibody formation (Maeda et al., unpublished).

We have tailored another enzyme, PEG-conjugated bilirubin oxidase (MW 50,000) which was obtained as a fungal extracellular protein of *Myrothecium verrucaria* [27]. When immunized subcutaneously (sc) with Freund's adjuvant, native bilirubin oxidase exhibits potent antigenicity, whereas that of PEG-conjugate was found to be less than 5% antigenic. Intravenous injection of PEG-bilirubin-oxidase did not induce any antibody to it [27].

Hershifield et al. prepared a conjugate of bovine intestinal adenosine deaminase and PEG, and applied it clinically in congenital adenosine deaminase-deficient patients. The increase in plasma half-life and the loss of antigenicity made the treatment very effective over a period of several months without any adverse immunological reactions [28].

Thus far all cases showed diminished antigenicity of proteins by tailoring with appropriate synthetic polymers.

PLASMA HALF-LIFE AND MACROMOLECULES

The plasma concentration of drugs has a great pharmacological and therapeutic consequence in general. In many cases high local tissue concentrations in the target organs are more desirable, for therapeutic effectiveness and lessened systemic side effects. To attain a high local tissue concentration, however, a high plasma concentration is needed at one time or another in any systemic administration. All small-size proteins less than 30,000 daltons are now well known to be cleared into the urine very rapidly. Most of them are cleared within 5 min or at most within 10 min (i.e., in terms of $t_{1/2}$). Table 1 indicates some of these examples.

Tailoring of the small proteins with polymers indeed greatly enhances the plasma half-life as already discussed briefly (see Table 1). For instance, NCS → smancs ($t_{1/2}$ 1.9 → 19 min); ribonuclease monomer → dimer ($t_{1/2}$ 2.6 → 30 min); superoxide dismutase (SOD) → SMA-conjugated SOD ($t_{1/2}$ 5.0 → >300 min); bilirubin oxidase → PEG-bilirubin oxidase ($t_{1/2}$ <1.0 min → 5.0 hr; $t_{1/10}$ 1.8 min → 48 hr) (Figure 1); soybean trypsin inhibitor (SBTI, Kunitz type) → dextran-SBTI ($t_{1/10}$ ~3.0 min → >60 min); L-asparaginase → PEG-L-asparaginase ($t_{1/2}$ ~ 2.0 hr → 56 hr). All these polymer conjugates showed increases in plasma half-life, and the area under the concentration curve was greatly improved, e.g., in PEG-bilirubin oxidase, it increased 59-fold.

Such tailoring could provide three advantages, in addition to solving the immunological problems described above. These potential advantages are:

(1) Ineffective proteins, due to the extremely short half-life, become effective drugs; e.g., bilirubin oxidase.

(2) More selective targeting to the sites of lesion is achieved.

(3) Side effects will be seen less at the same effective dose.

For instance, in our preliminary experience, we found pyran copolymer conjugated-NCS (MW; 25,000 of the conjugate vs. 12,000 of native NCS) exhibited decreased bone-marrow toxicity to only about 30% of the native protein. Thus, a dose that is three times more effective can be given with the same toxic dose, and therapeutic efficacy was much improved [29]. This is interpreted to mean that by conjugating with polymers the drug becomes less permeable through the blood capillary in the bone marrow tissue.

In case of smancs, despite its much-prolonged plasma half-life, its toxicity to the bone marrow, kidney, or other organ tissues did not increase when compared with parental NCS. The plasma half-life of NCS is extremely short but its toxicity to bone marrow and other organs is very severe. It is clear that molecular size is an important factor in giving a long plasma life.

Biocompatibility appears more important, however, than the molecular size. Examples are shown in Table 1. α_2-Macroglobulin (α_2M), a plasma glycoprotein with a molecular weight of 720,000 (as tetrameric structure) is important broad-spectrum protease inhibitor, and α_2M can combine with numbers of protease molecules (trapping hypothesis) involving cleavage of peptide bond in the so called "bait region". α_2M, after entrapping protease, provokes a drastic conformational change, and the plasma half-life of α_2M becomes extremely shortened from 180 hr to less than 15 min [30].

Another problem is a more general one, applicable to any plasma or other proteins. When plasma albumin was modified with formaldehyde its plasma half-life became drastically diminished [31]. This is explained as a common mechanism of clearance for denatured proteins. For instance, a more recent study indicated that acetylated low-density lipoprotein (LDL), compared with native LDL, is more rapidly cleared by phagocytic macrophages [32,33]. All these facts indicate the greater importance of biocompatibility relative to the size of molecules in maintaining high levels in the blood circulation.

When low molecular weight drugs or dyes are bound noncovalently to albumin their plasma half-lives become almost as long as native albumin itself. However, the pharmacological activity may be largely affected by the association/dissociation constants of ligands to albumin.

VASCULAR BARRIER AND PERMEABILITY FOR MACROMOLECULES AND LIPIDS: NORMAL TISSUE VS. TUMOROUS AND INFLAMMATORY TISSUE

The uniqueness of tumor vasculature has not been fully utilized for cancer chemotherapy, and little at-

Table 1. Plasma clearance time of various proteins and its polymer conjugates or modified proteins.

Protein	Origin/Test Animal	Type of Polymer or Modification	MW × 10⁻³	$t_{1/2}a$	$t_{1/10}$	Reference
Neocarzinostatin	*Streptomyces*/mouse	—	12	1.8 min	15 min	[3,89]
Smancs	semisynthetic/mouse	copoly(styrene-maleic acid)	16	19 min	5 hr	[3,89]
Ribonuclease	bovine/mouse	—	13.7	5 min	30 min	[92]
Ribonuclease dimer	bovine/mouse	cross-linked dimer	27	18 min	5 hr	[92]
Superoxide dismutase (SOD)	bovine Cu⁺⁺, Zn⁺⁺/rat	—	30	4 min	30 min	[71]
SOD-SMA[b]	semisynthetic/rat	copoly(styrene-maleic acid)	40	>300 min	>10 hr	[71]
SOD-DIVEMA[c]	semisynthetic/rat	copoly(divinylether maleic acid)	42	60 min	>5 hr	[3,29]
Soybean trypsin inhibitor (SBTI, Kunitz type)	soybean/rabbit	—	20	<2.0 min	3 min	[25,26]
Dextran-SBTI	semisynthetic/rabbit	dextran	127	~20 min	>80 min	[25,26]
Bilirubin oxidase	*Myrothecium verrucaria*/rat	—	50	<1.0 min	1.8 min	[27]
PEG-bilirubin oxidase	*Myrothecium verrucaria*/rat	PEG	70	5.0 min	48 hr	[27]
Ovomucoid	chick/mouse	DTPA[d]/NH₂/⁵¹Cr	29	5 min	34 min	
Serum albumin	mouse/mouse	none	68	3–4 days[e]	—	[89]
		Evans blue/dye-binding	—	2 hr	30 hr	[89]
		DTPA/NH₂/⁵¹Cr	—	6 hr	30 hr	[31,89]
	bovine/mouse	DTPA/NH₂/⁵¹Cr	—	1 hr	24 hr	[89]
	bovine/rat	iodination/¹²⁵I	—	4.5 hr	65 hr	[31]
Formaldehyde conjugated HSA	human/rat	formaldehyde/¹²⁵I	—	25 min	4 hr	[31]
Transferrin	human/rat	iodination/¹²⁵I	87	8 days	—	[90]
L-asparaginase	*E. coli*/rat	—	65 × (2–8)	1.5–3.4 hr	—	[18]
		DL-alanylation	—	13 hr	—	
		PEG₂-linked[f]	—	56 hr	11 days	[18]
IgG	mouse/mouse	DTPA	150	60 hr		[89]
		iodination/¹³¹I	150	45.6 hr		[91]
α₂ Macroglobulin	human/mouse	iodination/¹²⁵I	180 × 4	140 hr	22 days	[32,33]
α₂ Macroglobulin (half molecule)	human/mouse	iodination/¹²⁵I	180 × 2	36 hr	—	[32,33]
α₂ Macroglobulin-plasmin	human/mouse	iodination/¹²⁵I	180 × 2	2.5 min	20 min	[32]
α₂ Macroglobulin	human/mouse	iodination/¹²⁵I	180 ×	5.0 min	—	[32]

[a]$t_{1/2}$ indicates here an initial decline, α phase in pharmacokinetics.
[b]SMA, styrene-maleic acid/anhydride copolymer.
[c]DIVEMA, divinylether-maleic acid anhydride.
[d]DTPA: diethylene triamine pentaacetic acid; (pK_{as} of ⁵¹Cr = 24).
[e]Human albumin in man, 19 days.
[f]PEG: polyethylene glycol, biantenary.

tention has been paid to this subject in drug design or tumor targeting. During our search for tumoritropic macromolecular anticancer agents, it became apparent that vascular properties of the tumor tissue are indeed greatly different from those of the normal counterpart, as described before [1,2]. Namely,

(1) Tumor angiogenesis resulting in hypervasculature [34,35]

(2) Enhanced-permeability induced by tumor derived factors [36–39]

(3) Little operative lymphatic system and hence little drainage recovery [1–3,8,9] (Figures 2(a) and 2(b)

(4) Architectural and functional incompleteness [40,41]

It is known that macromolecules such as plasma proteins are retained within the blood circulation in the normal healthy state without leaking out of the vascular endothelial compartment into the interstitial space. Namely, a molecular size above 50,000 daltons will not leak out into the normal tissue [Figure 2(a), Table 1] [1–3,42]. However, this notion is not strictly valid in the vasculatures of the inflammatory tissues [43] and more importantly in the tumor tissues (Figure 3, Table 2). Experimental data provided by Peterson and Appelgren et al. [44], and Shibata et al. [45], showed that radiolabeled fibrinogen, albumin and α_1-acid glycoprotein were retained more in both solid tumors and granulomas than is normal organ/tissue [44,45]. Similarly macromolecular anticancer agent smancs (16K) as well as albumin and IgG, accumulated preferentially in tumor relative to the normal tissues (Figures 3 and 4) [1,2]. Small protein NCS (MW 12K) and small glycoprotein ovomucoid (MW 29K) did not do so at all. Smancs, which has a small size as a protein by itself, can bind noncovalently to albumin and behaves like a large-size protein of about 80,000 [46].

It is known for normal inflammatory tissue that proteins and lipids will leak out of the blood vessels (at the post capillary venule) into the interstitial space and then be recovered via the lymphatics, which would then return them to the general circulation via the thoracic duct.

In tumor tissue, smancs and plasma albumin, or IgG, can penetrate between the vascular endothelial cells into the interstitial space and accumulate in the tumor tissue. An important finding is that they are much less likely to be recovered into the lymphatic system, as is observed in the normal tissue. Thus, these macromolecules and lipids are retained in the tumor tissue more effectively (Enhanced Permeability and Retention [EPR] effect). A comparison of smancs, NCS and mitomycin C is shown in Figure 5, in which smancs was found at highest level in VX-2 tumor in the liver of a rabbit and retained for a longer period in the solid tumor (EPR-effect). We have also shown that proteins and lipids were not cleared from the tumor for a very long period of time, indicating little

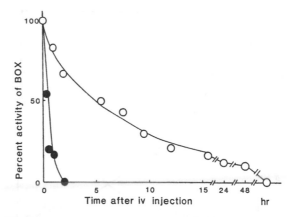

Figure 1. Residual activities of intact bilirubin oxidase (●) and its polyethylene glycol conjugate (○) in rats. Data of each group represented by one rat (Reference [27] with permission).

operative lymphatic drainage, which is a great contrast to normal tissue [1,2,8,9,23].

As pointed out by Suzuki et al. [40,41], the architectural incompleteness of tumor vasculature makes it more permeable to macromolecules and lipids than the normal intact blood vasculature.

FACTORS INVOLVED IN EXTRAVASCULAR PERMEABILITY IN TUMOR TISSUES

Vascular permeability means transport or leakage of plasma proteins and other macromolecules and lipids outside of the circulatory lumen into either the

(a) Normal Tissues

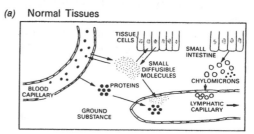

(b) Tumor Tissues
(Hypervascularity, no lymphatic capillary)

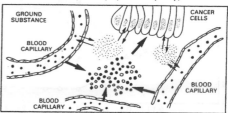

Figure 2. Diagrammatic presentations of normal tissue (a) and tumor tissue (b). Note that presence (a) and absence (b) of the lymphatic capillary, and much enhanced leakage of macromolecules are seen in tumor tissue. In tumor (b) macromolecules and lipids are not recovered via the lymphatic system but readily accessible to the target tumor cells. Low molecular substances traverse freely between the interstitial space and the blood capillary as well as the lymphatic duct (Reference [2] with permission).

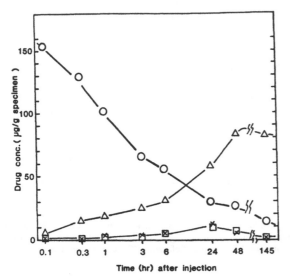

Figure 3. Clearance of Evans blue-albumin complex (a model for macromolecular drug) from blood plasma and its accumulation in the tumor tissue and the ×, normal skin in tumor bearing mice. Tumor S-180 (5 × 10⁶ cells) was injected into the skin of mice, and after about seven days Evans blue was injected intravenously. The tumor became progressively blue due to the accumulation of Evans blue-albumin complex. The amount of Evans blue-albumin complex in tissues were quantified after removal and extraction; ○, plasma; □, normal skin; and normal muscle; △, tumor (Reference [1] with permission).

interstitial space or other compartments such as pleural or abdominal cavities. Thus, this phenomenon has a great implication for macromolecular therapeutics. The enhanced extravascular permeability in tumor tissue now appears affected by at least two different vascular permeability factors. These factors can affect normal as well as tumor vessels. Both factors are known to be produced in the tumor compartment and affect extravascular leakage of plasma components

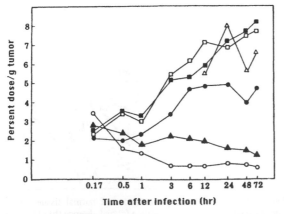

Figure 4. Intratumor accumulation of proteins with different sizes injected intravenously. All proteins were labeled with ⁵¹Cr via chelating agent DTPA (diethylenetriaminepentaacetic acid). □, bovine serum albumin; ■, mouse serum albumin; △, mouse IgG; ●, smancs; ▲, ovomucoid (29 KDa), and ○, neocarzinostatin (12 KDa) (Reference [1] with permission).

such as albumin. One of them is called tumor vascular permeability factor, reported by Dvorak et al., which is a protein (MW ~ 40,000) and produced by many types of tumor cells [36,37,47].

The other factor is a bradykinin moiety found by us; bradykinin and its derivative [³hydroxyprolyl]-bradykinin (Hyp³-bradykinin), in which the third amino acid proline in bradykinin is replaced by hydroxyproline [2,38,39]. These bradykinins seem to be actively produced by a series of serine protease cascade: plasminogen activator → plasmin → Hageman factor → (pre)kallikrein → high molecular weight kininogen → bradykinin (Figure 6). Since kinin is a potent permeability and pain-inducing factor, this finding gives a logical explanation for tumor pathology and enhanced permeability and retention of macromolecules and lipids in tumor tissue (EPR effect) (Figures 3–5). Hyp³-bradykinin exhibits almost the same activity and potency as bradykinin [38,39,48].

Kinin generation or degradation can be manipulated by various inhibitors which can affect such agents as kallikrein or kininases, respectively (Figure 6) [2,3,9]. The kininases (I and II) are known to be identical to carboxypeptidase N and angiotensin converting enzyme, respectively. When mice bearing ascitic tumors were subjected to intraperitoneal injection of soybean trypsin inhibitor (SBTI, Kunitz type) ascites formation was significantly suppressed, in which system kallikrein was very effectively inhibited by SBTI and thus little bradykinin was formed (see Figure 6). As a consequence, effective suppression of permeability in the abdominal compartment has resulted in less formation of ascitic fluid. This indicates that by suppressing kinin generation upstream with SBTI in the abdominal compartment, one can suppress the vascular leakage and thus the fluid accumulation [39].

When kininases were inhibited downstream by kininase-inhibitors, one could at the same time increase the local concentration of kinin, and hence the permeability as well. Thus, use of kininase inhibitor (angiotensin converting enzyme inhibitors) in combination with macromolecular therapeutics would potentially enhance the drug delivery to the tumor compartments [39].

We have shown recently that the level of free bradykinin content in rodent and human ascitic fluid of gastric, ovarian and other cancers was highly elevated. High levels of bradykinin have also been observed in the human pleural effusion of lung cancer patients. In these ascitic and pleural fluids, the much elevated level of ³Hyp-bradykinin was found to be unique to cancer patients [39,48]. They exist in the zymogen (kininogen) as the ³Hyp-form. It should also be mentioned, however, that Hyp³-bradykinin level is also elevated in some non-malignant chronic diseases such as Crohn's disease. The ratio of elevation of Hyp³-bradykinin/total kinin in kininogen may be of diagnostic value.

To our knowledge, other than the above described two factors, few vascular permeability factors in cancer tissue are established with solid chemical evidences. However, bradykinin can initiate prostaglandin synthesis via activation of phospholipase A_2 [49,50]. Since prostaglandin E_2 is known to enhance vascular permeability, it is thus reasonable to assume that prostaglandin E_2 may facilitate this event in the tumor tissue via bradykinin. Another factor, leukotriene, is known in most inflammatory tissues, but its presence needs to be elucidated in tumor tissue. Platelet-derived growth factor and possibly other factors such as tumor necrosis factor also facilitate tumor vascular permeability. Serotonin is only noticeably elevated in case of carcinoid syndrome and induced by bradykinin [51]. Greenbaum et al. have previously reported a vascular enhancing factor named leukokinin [52], which was obtained by acidifying the tumor ascites to pH 4, otherwise it is not detectable; the generation of leukokinin can be suppressed by pepstatin, an inhibitor of pepsin and other acid proteases, and accordingly the ascites formation was decreased by injecting pepstatin. However, leukokinin's exact chemical nature remains to be clarified.

EFFECT OF LIPOPHILICITY AND ELECTRICAL CHARGE OF POLYMERS

Lipophilicity

Oily Formulations

We have at least two beneficial examples with increased lipophilicity. One is SMA (copoly-styrene-maleic acid) which is a component in smancs as described. In this case it became possible to make an oily formulation using lipid contrast medium, Lipiodol [8–11,23,53]. This oily formulation of smancs (smancs/Lipiodol) is usually administered via the tumor feeding arteries (the hepatic artery for hepatoma; the bronchial artery for lung/bronchial cancer

Table 2. Vascular permeability in normal animal skin.

A. Vascular Permeability Enhancing Substance

Substances	Dose/Site (μg)	Amount of Albumin Leaked Out of Blood Vessels[a]
Histamine	3.0	122
	1.0	41
	0.3	23
	0.1	20
	0	0
Bradykinin	10.0	46
	1.0	36
	0.1	16
	0	0
Serratial protease[b]	10	127
	3.0	41
	0.3	5
	0	0

B. Thermal Burn

Tissue/Mice	^{51}Cr-albumin[c] (cpm × 10^3/g Tissue)	Ratio
Thermal burned skin[d]	53.8	13.6
Normal skin	3.97	1.0

[a]At first 2.5% of Evans-blue solution was injected i.v. in guinea pig (1.0 ml per kg body weight). Evans-blue forms a complex with albumin immediately. The test substances were injected, and allowed 30 min for the complex to leak out. The numbers indicate amount of the dye-albumin complex as measured by the amount of Evans-blue (μg).
[b]This protease activates Hageman factor, subsequently generating kallikrein followed by kinin formation [3–6].
[c]0.1 μCi was given i.v. in mice, and the tissue was removed after 6 h.
[d]A nail with its head diameter of 7 mm heated at 70°C was pressed lightly for 10 sec to the shaved back skin of mice.

etc.) [8–11]. It is also administered intraperitoneally or intrapleurally for ascitic or pleural carcinomatosis. Selective tumor targeting efficiency is seen in Table 3; this efficiency of tumor selective targeting is by far the most remarkable targeting method known, including a method involving monoclonal antibody tagged with anticancer agents in which tumor/blood (T/B) ratio of drug is 2–10; whereas the T/B for lipid formulation is above 2500 (Table 3).

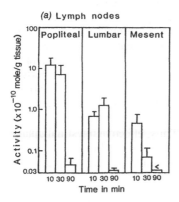 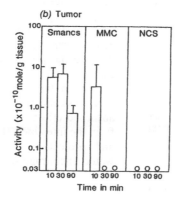 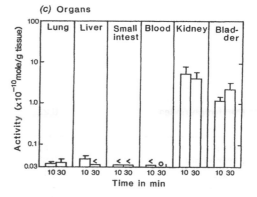

Figure 5. Accumulation of smancs in the lymph nodes (a) and organs (c) in normal rats; and intratumor concentration (b) of smancs, mitomycin C and neocarzinostatin in tumor bearing rabbit from Reference [23] with permission. In all cases 10 mg/kg of each drug was administered intravenously.

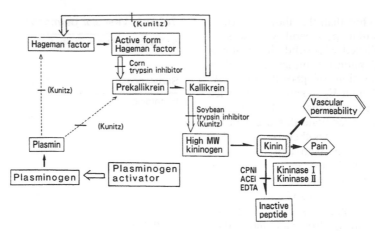

Figure 6. Cascade of kinin generation and degradation and points of inhibition by various inhibitors. ACEI, angiotensin converting enzyme inhibitor. Captopril and enalapril inhibit kininase II (ACE). CPNI, carboxypeptidase N inhibitor. Dotted lines show possible activation (from Reference [39]).

Oily formulation of smancs was also prepared with other biocompatible lipids and they exhibit as good pharmacological properties as Lipiodol, though X-ray systems cannot detect them. We found that a semisynthetic medium chain triglyceride is a potential candidate for this direction [53]. These oily formulations became very stable against heat or radiation [54 and

Table 3. Accumulation of [¹⁴C]-iodinated fatty acid. *

Organs/Tissues	Radioactivity DPM/g ($\times 10^3$)	
	15 min	3 days
Tumor	1252.58	130.94
Liver (adjacent)	566.25	17.02
Liver (remote)	28.95	6.89
Sm. intestine	1.06	4.44
Lung	2.66	2.02
Kidney	1.61	2.57
Stomach	10.97	—
Heart	2.65	1.72
Lg. intestine	0.35	1.06
Spleen	2.39	3.28
Bladder	0.28	1.31
Brain	<0.1	0.38
Muscle	<0.1	0.46
Skin	<0.1	1.42
Mes. lymph node	0.15	2.21
Cer. lymph nodes	0.22	1.61
Thymus	0.22	0.93
Serum	0.58	1.03
Plasma cells	0.86	1.57
Bone marrow	<0.1	2.97
Urine (exc.)	—	1.14
Urine (vesical)	<0.1	1.06
Bile	70.91	1.78

*Intrahepatic arterial dose, 0.3 ml. Tumor implanted in the liver. From Ref. [8] with permission.

unpublished data]. Most of the hydrolytic enzymes such as proteases and lipases would unlikely degrade the polymer conjugate in lipid media. The oily formulation with Lipiodol has been extensively investigated and applied for treatment of hepatoma, lung cancer, renal cancer, etc. [9–11], and the arterial injection of other anticancer agents in the oily or Lipiodol formulation is becoming a new discipline in cancer therapy.

Another advantage of increasing the lipophilic nature of smancs is that smancs gained a much higher affinity for binding to cell membrane and for a more efficient internalization rate than its parent NCS [55,56].

A possible future use for oily formulations is their application for oral drug administration because of their increased stability against various hydrolytic enzymes, as well as increased intestinal absorption rate [57]. We have tested oily form for possible oral use with smancs formulated in medium chain triglyceride and found that it exhibited about 11-fold more plasma concentration than smancs in phosphate buffered saline, in terms of area under the concentration curve [57]. Most proteins and peptides in their intact form are expected to be less likely to reach the intestine in active form because many digestive enzymes will degrade the polypeptides. However, there are many examples known to be absorbed from the intestine even with large molecular size substances, though much less effectively [58–60]. Lipids are known to be absorbed effectively as lipid particles (chylomicrons) from the intestine [7]. Thus, effective intestinal uptake and protective effect against hydrolytic enzymes would encourage oral formulations using lipids.

Enzymes Active in Organic Solvents [61]

Several PEG-conjugated enzymes were investigated in a number of organic solvent systems such as benzene. In these instances PEG of biantenary type may be preferred. Labeling of 40–80% of the amino groups was required to make the enzymes soluble in organic solvents. Catalase, peroxidase, chymotrypsin, lipase, cholesterol oxidase and other enzymes were derivatized with PEG [61]. PEG-catalase, in which 42% of its 112 amino groups in native enzyme was modified, exhibited 1.6-fold higher activity in benzene than in water. As more amino groups were modified the enzyme activity dropped, perhaps due to disruption of structural integrity and dissociation of subunits.

An interesting example along this direction is chymotrypsin, which needs to be derivatized as the zymogen form and then activated with trypsin [61]. PEG-chymotrypsin can catalyze the reaction forming peptide bonds.

For example, PEG-chymotrypsin (with 64% amino group modified derivative) catalyzed the following reaction at a high rate:

$$\text{N-Bz-Tyr-OEt} + n(\text{Phe-OEt}) \rightarrow$$

$$\text{N-Bz-Tyr-(Phe)}_n\text{-OEt} + n\text{-EtOH}$$

Prolonged reaction time for 100 hr produced a significant amount of tri-Phe derivative in addition to mono- and di-derivatives.

PEG-cholesterol oxidase can catalyze the following reaction [62], in benzene:

$$\text{cholesterol} + O_2 \rightarrow \text{4-cholesterol-3-one} + H_2O$$

PEG-lipase can effectively synthesize various terpene alcohol esters in benzene [63]. The terpene alcohols examined are shown in Table 4. The industrial application may be of interest.

These PEG-conjugated enzymes exhibited substantially high enzyme activity in benzene and in 1,1,1,-trichloroethane but very little in dioxane, acetone, dimethylformamide and ethanol. Stability of PEG-lipase in benzene is very high at room temperature ($t_{1/2} = 80$ days; 40% remaining at 180 days) [63], which is similar to smancs in Lipiodol [54].

Electric Charge Effect

The chemical composition of the blood vessels is known to consist in part of negatively charged surface components such as heparan sulfate, chondroitin sulfate, etc. Therefore, it is reasonable to expect that positively charged polymers would be readily adsorbed on these endothelial surfaces. Thus, the plasma half-life of positively charged polymers would be very short and the first path capture results in more accumulation in the first organ rich with blood capillaries. Positively charged polymer, however, would provide its use in local deposition at or near the site of injection, for instance subcutaneous injection. The example can be found in cationic mitomycin dextran conjugates [65].

Another aspect of charge effect is that it is known that polycation would increase the antigenicity of anionic proteins, e.g., albumin. Therefore its application to protein drug has to be carefully evaluated [12,15].

STATE OF THE ART OF PROTEIN DRUGS BY TAILORING WITH POLYMERS

Poly(styrene-co-maleic acid) (SMA) Conjugated Neocarzinostatin (NCS); Smancs

Smancs is a derivative of neocarzinostatin of which two amino groups, one at amino-terminal alanine 1 and the other at lysine 20, were used to conjugate with the acid and anhydride of maleyl residue (Figure 7). Initially, the SMA residue used had a large mean size of 5000 daltons [21]. Subsequently, more refined SMA was prepared with a mean molecular weight of 1500 and Mn/Mw ratio of 1.2 or less [24]. Its molecular mechanism of action is by DNA degradation and by inhibition of DNA synthesis, as is the case for NCS [66]. Furthermore, induction of interferon (mainly γ-type) [67] and activation of macrophage and killer T-cells have been described [68–70]. It should be noted that these effects of biological response modifier are the characteristics acquired after polymer conjugation, particularly with polyanion. Recently it was found that the conjugate with molecular weight of 15,000 can bind with albumin, thus, the effective molecular size of smancs *in vivo* or in plasma would be about 83,000 daltons as described [46].

The greatly improved stability in aqueous as well as in lipid milieu has been described already [54,73]. This seems to be a common feature among many polymer conjugates [54,61]. Resistance to proteolytic cleavage of this derivative as well as SMA-conjugate of superoxide dismutase was also described [21,69,71].

The clinical trials in the pilot study of our group demonstrated the remarkable antitumor effect when smancs is given arterially as oily formulation with an oily contrast medium Lipiodol [9–11,73]. The response rate of previously incurable primary liver cancer has increased to an unprecedented extent. As shown in Figure 8, survival rates at year 3 or 4 ranged from 30 to 90% depending upon the stage and grade

Table 4. Synthesis of terpene alcoholester in benzene using PEG-lipase.

Terpene Alcohol	Yield (%) of Ester			
	Acetic Acid	Propionic Acid	Butylic Acid	Valeric Acid
Citronellol	18 (81)	52	88	74
Geraniol	19 (84)	81	94	83
Farnesol	14 (84)	78	90	81
Phytol	29 (91)	86	95	92

Data from Inada et al. [61,63]. Values were obtained after 8 hr reaction except those in parentheses which are after 48 hr.

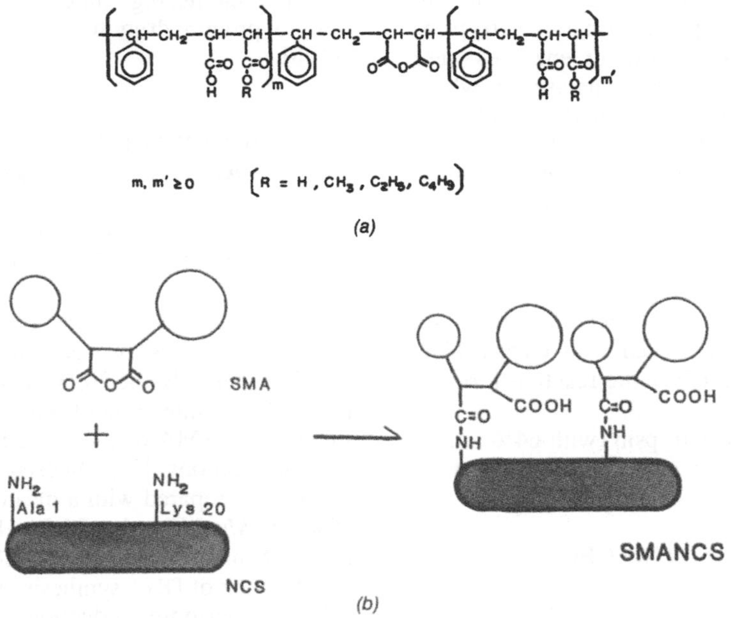

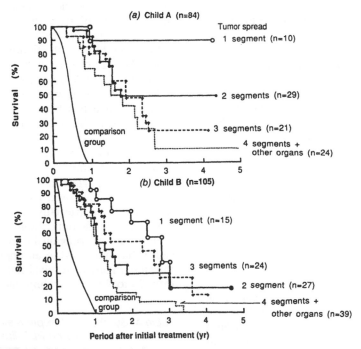

Figure 7. Structure of poly styrene-co-maleic acid/anhydride and schematic structure of its conjugate (smancs) with neocarzinostatin (NCS).

Figure 8. Survival of patients with primary liver cancer after treatment of smancs/Lipiodol given via the hepatic artery. Child A and B indicate degree of liver cirrhosis; Child A class has almost normal liver function, Child B class has a little impairment in the function. All cases were, however, inoperable (from Reference [72]).

of tumor in the patients with hepatocellular carcinoma, in which all patients were highly advanced and inoperable, thus subjects of this trial. Comparison groups, namely, conventional chemotherapy with or without surgical operation, can offer these patients an expected life span of no more than 6 months (mean about 4 months). That means at this point there is no cure for this tumor without smancs treatment [9,10,72]. Efficacy in other tumors by this protocol is presently being pursued. Tumors showing an effective response include the following: the lung cancer (whether adenocarcinoma or squamous cell carcinoma), renal cell carcinoma, pleural or ascitic carcinomatosis, some pancreatic, bile duct, and ovarian cancers, and leiomyosarcoma [11,72 and unpublished data].

Intravenous administration of smancs in aqueous formulation is also effective. A pilot study in our group has shown some effect on tumors of the brain, lung, esophagus, stomach, kidney, urinary bladder, adrenal gland, pancreas, colon, and ovary. But its ultimate target tumors and potential uses need to be established.

PEG-Conjugated L-Asparaginase

As described in the previous section, native L-asparaginase has been used for treatment of lymphocytic leukemia and lymphoma. But the immunological response, particularly the emergence of antibodies to it, nullified its clinical efficacy in subsequent administrations. Furthermore, the pharmacokinetic profile of native enzyme is not sufficient. These drawbacks are now solved by polymer (PEG) conjugation [17,18]. Inada et al. has developed one with biantenary type using cyanuryl chloride derivate of PEG [17,61]. Another group in the U.S.A. uses non-branched PEG. Clinical evaluation in the U.S.A. and Japan is now underway and problems associated with native enzyme such as antigenicity seem to have been cleared. A Japanese pilot study of a few patients with lymphocytic leukemia showed some promising results [H. Wada; personal communication].

PEG-Conjugated Adenosine Deaminase (ADA)

Children born with a congenital deficiency of this enzyme are known to be very prone to microbial infections because of insufficient immune functions, and thus longevity is not expected. Hershfield et al., [28] has prepared a PEG-conjugated ADA of which plasma half-life in man was 48–72 hrs, and human trials were carried out. The results showed significant reduction in adenosine levels in erythrocytes by weekly injection of 15 units/Kg, and the functions of lymphocytes (thus immune responses) and bone marrow cells were restored. No anaphylaxis was observed during the trial period of 10 months.

PEG-Conjugated Interleukin 2 (IL-2)

IL-2 is one of many lymphokines produced by lymphocytes as a signal of intercellular immune responses, and it is a glycoprotein with a molecular weight of 15,000 [73]. Its therapeutic efficacy against various cancers and infectious diseases are reported [74,75], and its large-scale production by genetic manipulation is in progress. However, as described in a previous section in this chapter, such proteins obtained after recombinant DNA (rDNA) technique are lacking carbohydrate side chains and are very unstable *in vivo*. Furthermore, its solubility is poor and it is only possible to solubilize in the presence of detergent.

Katre et al. [76] prepared PEG-conjugate of human IL-2 prepared by *E. coli* using rDNA (PEG-rIL-2). PEG used had a molecular weight of about 5,000, and one or two chains or more PEG were attached to a molecule of IL-2. In the conjugate, many of the problems associated with parent rIL-2 were overcome. In parallel with prolongation of plasma half-life, the therapeutic efficacy against experimental mouse tumor (Meth A) has been greatly improved.

rIL-2 is a small protein, thus once injected into the general circulation it will be cleared very rapidly as observed for neocarzinostatin or SOD from the kidney, whereas PEG-rIL-2 with increased Stoke's radius will be cleared less rapidly. As many more potent recombinant proteins are produced, more polymer tailored proteins will be prepared. A derivative of rIL-2 with soluble polysaccharide pululan has been described which exhibited a tendency similar to the PEG-conjugate [77].

PEG-Bilirubin Oxidase Conjugate

Bilirubin is a toxic yellow pigment which is derived as a catabolic end-product of hemoglobin metabolism. It has a lipid-soluble character and normally is processed in the liver and excreted into the bile duct and then into the feces. When the liver function drops, the level of bilirubin in the blood plasma will elevate and clinical symptoms will appear. To remove the bilirubin in plasma, various methods have been clinically applied such as plasma exchange, steroid therapy and photo therapy, or more recently by bilirubin immobilized column [78], but none has proven to have therapeutic value as a first choice regimen.

We have recently proposed a new tactic for the treatment of this disease, hyperbilirubinemia, which is associated with various liver disorders and hemolytic jaundice, using the bilirubin degrading enzyme, bilirubin oxidase (BOX). It is a highly specific enzyme for bilirubin oxidation and it has a molecular weight of about 50,000 and is produced by a microorganism, *Myrothecium verrucaria* MT-1 [79].

BOX was conjugated with PEG of a mean molecular weight of 5,000 [27]. We found the amino groups of BOX were not very reactive so carboxyl groups were used to couple a spacer, diaminobutane using carbodimide. Then, newly introduced amino groups were reacted with activated PEG which contained cyanuric chloride [17,61], or other active esters (unpublished).

PEG-BOX exhibited about 20 times longer plasma life (Figure 1) [27]. Its therapeutic efficacy against experimentally prepared jaundiced rats and rabbit showed a remarkable decrease in the bilirubin value. The area under the curve of the activity of PEG-BOX was 26 times greater than that of native BOX. Antigenicity of BOX was reduced and anti-native BOX antibody could not neutralize the enzyme activity of PEG-BOX. Anti-PEG-BOX antibody prepared rigorously with Freund's complete adjuvant could inhibit the activity of PEG-BOX only 3.7%. No antibody development was observed during i.v. injection of PEG-BOX for several months of observation.

The potential value of this polymer tailored drug for the treatment of hyperbilirubinemia in such diseases as the fulminant hepatitis and the neonatal bilirubin encephalopathy looks apparent.

Pyran-Co-Polymer Conjugated Neocarzinostatin (Pyran-NCS)

We have prepared this polymer conjugate in a hope to accomplish more selective tumor targeting and longer plasma life and to eliminating the bone marrow toxicity. The polymer (pyran-copolymer) has a molecular weight of about 5,600 daltons and two chains conjugated on NCS in a manner similar to that of smancs. The conjugate has a molecular weight of about 25,000. It was found this size was too small to maintain high plasma concentration as was expected from the data shown in Table 1, but a slightly higher tumor concentration (not as remarkable as smancs) and decrease in toxicity (LD_{50} increased 50%–70%) were seen. The most interesting aspect was that the bone marrow toxicity was reduced to one third of its parental NCS at the same toxic dose based on a very careful stem cell colony formation assay [29]. An important lesson is that this size of drug is not large enough to exhibit advantageous benefit of EPR-effect of macromolecular therapeutics [29]. When the same pyran-copolymer is conjugated on SOD resulting in an approximate molecular weight of 40,000 by modifying two amino groups, the plasma half-life (about 10–20 min) was somewhat longer than the above NCS derivative of 25,000 daltons [43].

CONCLUDING REMARKS

There are many more potential macromolecular drugs or polymer tailored therapeutic agents, and most or all of them exhibit less toxicity in cases of cytotoxic anticancer agents. Toward the same objectives, another method is to utilize plasma proteins, especially albumin and immunoglobulin. Poznansky and Juliano have an excellent review along this line [80]. Trauet et al. have prepared a daunorubicin–albumin conjugate and pharmacological and therapeutic advantages have been described [81]. Others used transferrin to conjugate NCS [82] to utilize increased transferrin receptor in cancer cells as well as better pharmacological properties.

A number of treatises on protein tailoring or relevant literature are available as monographs/proceedings, although somewhat different but similar in some aspects [83–88]. There are also many reports on various low molecular weight anticancer agents, bioactive agents or cofactors conjugated with synthetic or natural polymers which are not covered in this chapter.

Within a few years, it is hoped that one of these agents will be approved by regulatory agencies, and then the field will gain the intense interest of industrial exploiters.

REFERENCES

1. Matsumura Y. and H. Maeda. 1986. *Cancer Res.*, 46:6387–6392.
2. Maeda, H. and Y. Matsumura. 1989 *Critical Rev. in Therapeutic Drug Carrier Systems*, 6:193–210.
3. Maeda, H., T. Oda, Y. Matsumura and M. Kimura. 1988. *J. Bioactive Biocompatible Polymer*, 3:27–43.
4. Matsumoto, K., T. Yamamoto, R. Kamata and H. Maeda. 1984. *J. Biochem.*, 96:739–746.
5. Molla, A., T. Yamamoto, T. Akaike, S. Miyoshi and H. Maeda. 1989. *J. Biol. Chem.*, 264: 10589–10594.
6. Maeda, H. and A. Molla. 1989. *Clin. Chim. Acta* 185:357–368.
7. Courtice, F. C. 1968. In *Lymph and the Lymphatic System*. H. S. Megersen, chairman. Springfield, IL: C.C. Thomas, pp. 89–126.
8. Iwai, K., H. Maeda and T. Konno. 1984. *Cancer Res.*, 44:2115–2121.
9. Konno, T., H. Maeda, K. Iwai, S. Tashiro, S. Maki, T. Morinaga, M. Mochinaga, T. Hiraoka and I. Yokoyama. 1983. *Europ. J. Cancer Clin. Oncol.*, 19:1053–1065.
10. Konno, T. and H. Maeda. 1987. In *Neoplasms of the Liver*. K. Okuda and G. Ishak, eds. Berlin, NY: Springer-Verlag, pp. 343–352.
11. Konno, T., H. Maeda, K. Iwai, S. Maki, S. Tashiro, M. Uchida and Y. Miyauchi. 1984. *Cancer*, 54:2367–2374.
12. Sela, M. 1969. *Science*, 166:1365–1374.
13. Habeebs, A. F. S. A., H. G. Cassidy and S. F. Singer. 1958. *Biochim. Biophys. Acta.*, 29:587–593.
14. Jones, V.E. and S. Leskowitz. 1965. *Nature*, 207:596–597.
15. Atassi, M. Z. 1977. Chapt. 3, and other chapters in *Immunochemistry of Proteins*. M. Z. Atassi, ed. NY: Plenum Press, 2:77–176.

16. Van Regenmortel, M. H. V. 1986. *TIBS*, 11:36–39.

17. Inada, Y., T. Yoshimoto, A. Matsushita and Y. Saito. 1986. *Trend in Biotechnol.*, 4:68–73.

18. Kamisaki, Y., H. Wada, H. Yagura, A. Matsushima and Y. Inada. 1981. *J. Pharmacol. Exp. Ther.*, 216:410–414.

19. Maeda, H. 1981. *Anticancer Res.*, 1:175–186.

20. Sakamoto, S., H. Maeda, T. Matsumoto and J. Ogata. 1978. *Cancer Treatment Rep.*, 62:2063–2070.

21. Maeda, H., J. Takeshita and R. Kanamaru. 1979. *Int. J. Peptide Protein Res.*, 14:81–87.

22. Maeda, H., J. Takeshita, R. Kanamaru, H. Sato, J. Kato and H. Sato. 1979. *Gann*, 70:601–606.

23. Maeda, H., T. Matsumoto, T. Konno, K. Iwai and M. Ueda. 1984. *J. Protein Chem.*, 3:181–193.

24. Maeda, H., M. Ueda, T. Morinaga and T. Matsumoto. 1985. *J. Med. Chem.*, 28:455–461.

25. Takakura, Y., Y. Kaneko, T. Fujita, M. Hashida, H. Maeda and H. Sezaki. 1989. *J. Pharmaceut. Sci.*, 78:117–121.

26. Takakura, Y., T. Fujita, M. Hashida, H. Maeda and H. Sezaki. 1989. *J. Pharmaceut. Sci.*, 78:219–222.

27. Kimura, M., Y. Matsumura, Y. Miyauchi and H. Maeda. 1988. *Proc. Soc. Exp. Biol. Med.*, 188:364–369.

28. Hershfield, M. S., R. H. Buckley, M. L. Greenberg, A. L. Melton, R. Schiff, C. Hatem, J. Kurzberg, M. L. Mardert, R. H. Kobayashi, A. L. Kobayashi and A. Abuchowski. 1987. *New Eng. J. Med.*, 316:589–596.

29. Yamamoto, H., T. Miki, T. Oda, R. Sera and H. Maeda. 1990. *Europ J. Cancer*, 26:253–260.

30. Gonias, S. L. and S. V. Pizzo. 1983. *Biochemistry*, 22:4933–4940.

31. Buys, C. H. C. M., A. S. H. Dejong, J. M. W. Bouma and M. Gruber. 1975. *Biochim. Biophys. Acta.*, 392:95–100.

32. Brown, M. S. and J. L. Goldstein. 1983. *Ann. Rev. Biochem.*, 52:223–261.

33. Murakami, M., S. Horiuchi, K. Takata and Y. Morino. 1987. *J. Biochem.*, 101:729–741.

34. Folkman, J. 1974. "Tumor Angiogenesis". *Adv. Cancer Res.*, 19:331–358.

35. Folkman, J. and M. Klagsburn. 1987. *Science*, 235:442–447.

36. Senger, D. R., S. J. Galli, A. M. Dvorak, C. A. Perruzzi, V. S. Harvey and H. F. Dvorak. 1983. *Science*, 219:983–985.

37. Senger, D. R., C. A. Perruzzi, J. Feder and H. F. Dvorak. 1986. *Cancer Res.*, 46:5629–5632.

38. Maeda, H., Y. Matsumura and H. Kato. 1988. *J. Biol. Chem.*, 263:16051–16054.

39. Matsumura, Y., M. Kimura, T. Yamamoto and H. Maeda. 1988. *Jpn. J. Cancer Res.*, 79:1327–1334.

40. Suzuki, M., T. Takahashi and T. Sato. 1987. *Cancer*, 59:444–450.

41. Suzuki, M. K. Hori, I. Abe, S. Saito and H. Sato. 1981. *J. Nat'l Cancer Inst.*, 67:663–669.

42. Simionescu, M., N. Simionescu, J. E. Silbert and G. E. Palade. 1981. *J. Cell. Biol.*, 90:614–621.

43. Maeda, H., T. Oda, Y. Matsumura and M. Kimura. 1988. *J. Bioactive Compatible Polymers*, 3:27–43.

44. Peterson, H. I and K. L. Appelgren. 1973. *Europ. J. Cancer*, 9:543–547.

45. Shibata, K., H. Okubo, H. Ishibashi, K. Tsuda-Kawamura and T. Yanase. 1978. *Br. J. Exp. Pathol.*, 59:601–608.

46. Kobayashi, A., T. Oda and H. Maeda. 1988. *J. Bioactive Compatible Polymer*, 3:319–333.

47. Dvorak, H. F., D. R. Senger, A. M. Dvorak, V. S. Harvey and J. McDonagh. 1985. *Science*, 227:1059–1061.

48. Matsumura, Y., K. Maruo, T. Yamamoto, T. Konno and H. Maeda. 1991. *Jpn. J. Cancer Res.*, vol. 82 (in press).

49. Armstrong, D. 1970. *Handb. Exp. Pharmacol.*, 25:434–481.

50. Vargaftig, B. B. and N. D. Hai. 1972. *J. Pharm. Pharmacol.*, 24:159–161.

51. Lembeck, F. 1953. *Nature*, 172:910–911.

52. Greenbaum, L. M., P. Grebow, M. Johnston, A. Prakath and G. Semente. 1975. *Cancer Res.*, 35:706–710.

53. Iwai, K., H. Maeda, T. Konno, Y. Matsumura, R. Yamashita, K. Yamasaki, S. Hirayama and Y. Miyauchi. 1987. *Anticancer Res.*, 7:321–328.

54. Hirayama, S., T. Oda, F. Sato and H. Maeda. 1986. *Jpn. J. Antibiotics*, 39:815–822.

55. Oda, T., F. Sato and H. Maeda. 1987. *J. Nat'l Cancer Inst.*, 79:1205–1211.

56. Oda, T. and H. Maeda. 1987. *Cancer Res.*, 47:3206–3211.

57. Oka, K., Y. Miyamoto, T. Oda and H. Maeda. 1989. *Pharmaceut. Res.*, 7:852–855.

58. Walder, W. A., K. J. Isselbacher and K. J. Block. 1973. *J. Immunol.*, 111:221–226.

59. Balfour, W. E. and R. S. Comline. 1959. *J. Physiol.*, 148:77–78.

60. Yamashita, A., H. Ohtsuka and H. Maeda. 1983. *Immunopharmacol.*, 5:209–220.

61. Inada, Y. 1989. *Protein-Hybrid: Future Prospect of Chemical Modification.* Y. Inada and H. Maeda, eds. Tokyo: Kyoritsu Shuppan, pp. 1–40, (in Japanese).

62. Matsushima, A., M. Okada and Y. Inada. 1984. *FEBS Letter*, 178:275–277.

63. Yoshimotro, T., A. Ritani, R. Ohwada, K. Takahashi, Y. Kodera, A. Matsushima, Y. Saito and Y. Inada. 1987. *Biochem. Biophys. Res. Comm.*, 148:876–882.

64. Kodera, Y., K. Takahasi, Y. Nishimura, A. Matsushima, Y. Saito and Y. Inada. 1986. *Biotechnol. Letter*, 8:881–884.

65. Takakura, Y., A. Takagi, M. Hashida and H. Sezaki. 1987. *Pharmaceut. Res.*, 4:293–300.

66. Oda, T., F. Sato, H. Yamamoto, M. Akagi and H. Maeda. 1989. *Anticancer Res.*, 9:261–266.

67. Suzuki, F., T. Munakata and H. Maeda. 1988. *Anticancer Res.*, 8:97–104.

68. Oda, T., T. Morinaga and H. Maeda. 1986. *Proc. Soc. Exp. Biol. Med.*, 181:9–17.

69. Suzuki, F., R. B. Polland and H. Maeda. 1989. *Cancer Immunol. Immunotherapy*, 30:97–104.

70. Suzuki, F., R. B. Pollard, S. Uchimura, T. Munakata and H. Maeda. 1990. *Cancer Res.*, 50:3897–3904.

71. Ogino, T., M. Inoue, Y. Ando, M. Awai, H. Maeda and Y. Morino. 1988. *Int. J. Peptide Protein Res.*, 32:153–159.

72. Maeda, H. *Jpn. J. Cancer Chemotherapy*, 16:3323–3331 (in Japanese).

73. Robb, R. J. 1985. *Methods in Enzymol.*, 116:493–525.

74. Mule, J. J., S. Shu and S. A. Rosenberg. 1985. *J. Immunol.*, 135:646–652.

75. Ueno, Y., T. Miyawaki, H. Seki, K. Hara, T. Sato, N. Taniguchi, H. Takahashi and N. Kondo. 1985. *Clin. Immunol. Immunopathol.*, 35:226–233.

76. Katre, N. V., M. J. Knauf and W. J. Laird. 1987. *Proc. Nat. Acad. Sci. USA*, 84:1487–1491.

77. Morikawa, K., F. Okada, M. Hosokawa and H. Kobayashi. 1987. *Cancer Res.*, 47:37–41.

78. Lavin, A., C. Sung, A. M. Klibanov and R. Langer. 1985. *Science*, 230:543–545.

79. Murao, S. and N. Tanaka. 1981. *Agric. Biol. Chem.*, 45:2383–2384.

80. Poznansky, M. J. and R. L. Juliano. 1984. *Pharmacol. Rev.*, 36:277–336.

81. Trauet, A. M., M. Masquelier, R. Baurain and D. D. DeCampeneere. 1982. *Proc. Nat'l Acad. Sci. USA*, 79:626–629.

82. Urushizaki, I. 1989. *Nihon Rinsho*, 47:1423–1431 (in Japanese).

83. 1983. *Protein-Tailoring for Food and Medical Uses.* R. E. Feeney and J. R. Whitaker, eds. New York: Marcel Dekker Inc.

84. Laskin, A. I., K. Mosback, D. Thomas and L. B. Wingard, Jr. 1987. "Enzyme Engineering 8", *Ann. New York Acad. Sciences*, p. 501.

85. 1982. *Biological Activities of Polymers.* C. E. Carraher, Jr. and C. G. Gebelein, eds. ACS Symposium Series 186, Am. Chem. Soc., Wash. D.C.

86. 1984. *Polymers as Biomaterials.* S. W. Shalaby, A. S. Hoffman, B. D. Ratner and T. A. Horbett, eds. New York: Plenum Press.

87. 1988. "Enzyme Engineering 9". H. W. Blanch, and A. M. Klibanov, eds. *Ann. New York Acad. Sciences*, p. 542.

88. 1985. *Bioactive Polymer Systems. An Overview.* C. G. Gebelein and C. E. Carraher, Jr., eds. New York: Plenum Press.

89. Maeda, H., Y. Matsumura and T. Oda. 1983. In *Protein Tailoring for Food and Medical Uses.* R. E. Feeney and J. R. Whitaker, eds. New York: Marcel Dekker, Inc., pp. 353–382.

90. Morgan, E. H. and T. Peter, Jr. 1971. *J. Biol. Chem.*, 246:3508–3511.

91. Dixon, F. J., D. W. Talmage, P. H. Maurer and M. Deichmiller. 1952. *J. Exp. Med.*, 96:313–318.

92. Bartholeyns, J. and S. Moore. 1974. *Science*, 186:444–445.

44

Polyelectrolyte Complexes in Medical and Pharmaceutical Applications

K. PETRAK, D. Phil.*

ABSTRACT: The properties of polyelectrolyte complexes—i.e., materials formed through ionic interactions between oppositely charged polyelectrolytes—are essentially different from those of the starting components. This difference naturally stimulates attempts to find applications for such new materials. This chapter briefly looks at the latest advances in the basic science of polyelectrolyte complexes and examines the recent progress in the following applications: membranes, non-thrombogenic materials, drug release, and polymer complexes as drugs and drug carriers.

INTRODUCTION

In biological systems, the primary structure of macromolecules does not always entirely determine their properties. Frequently, compounds of very different primary structures assemble to perform similar or identical functions. For example, filamentous bacterial viruses are especially interesting supramolecular structures [1]. In such linear virions, single-stranded circular DNA is "coated", through largely ionic interactions, with protein. For example, the major coat protein, the so called B-protein, of the fd strain is 50 amino acids long, with about 20 hydrophobic residues in the centre of the sequence, and with hydrophilic residues (of opposite overall charges) at each end [2].

Inovirus, another member of this class, occurs naturally as a number of different strains with virtually identical secondary and higher-order structures. Although the proteins of various strains have quite different primary amino acid sequence compositions, the subunits of all strains have much the same size (about 50 amino acids), arranged into three domains of primary structure: acidic amino acids at the N-terminal third of the chain, a hydrophobic domain of 19 residues near the middle, and basic amino acids near the C-terminus. The acidic residues of the proteins face outwards on the virion surface, with the basic residues interacting with the charged groups on the DNA at the core of the virion. The hydrophobic central domain is believed to be involved in interactions that bind neighbouring molecules of the coat protein [3].

"Man-made" polyelectrolyte complexes, based either on synthetic or natural macromolecules, are no more than a primitive version of the "polymer of polymers" illustrated above. Their relative lack of form originates mainly from the simplicity of their primary structure. Their current limitations originate chiefly from our inability to adequately control their composition and properties.

Polyelectrolyte complexes in biomedical applications have been reviewed previously [4,5]. This review concentrates mainly on the development of this topic after 1985. The effects of polyelectrolytes on various biological systems (for example, effects of poly(cations) on normal and leukemic lymphocytes, decrease of functional activity of T-suppressor cells by polyelectrolytes, assembly of active compounds *in situ* especially at targets such as tumours), although some "complex formation" might be a step in the observed effect, are excluded from this review. Other observations where the composition of the complex was not defined (e.g., as in surface-modified solid substrates for biomedical use) have also been excluded, and for similar reasons so have the use of polyelectrolytes as chromatographic materials (for example, purification of hemoglobin by affinity chromatography on polyanionic gels). Complexes between polymers and small molecular weight solutes [such as poly(vinylpyrrolidone) and dichloroacetamide derivatives] are also largely excluded although their application is clearly in the biomedical field.

*CIBA-GEIGY Pharmaceuticals, Advanced Drug Delivery Research Unit, Wimblehurst Road, Horsham, West Sussex, RH12 4AB, U.K.

The material in this review has been arranged into the following groups:

- basic science of polyelectrolyte complexes
- polyelectrolyte complex membranes
- solid polyelectrolytes for biomedical applications
- polymer complexes in drug release
- polymer complexes as drugs and drug carriers

BASIC SCIENCE OF POLYELECTROLYTE COMPLEXES

Polymer complexes can be formed via interactions between macromolecules due to a variety of secondary binding forces. In case of polyelectrolyte complexes the interactions take place primarily between the ionisable groups bearing opposite charges. Thus, the interaction between ionisable groups of macromolecules (PA) and (PB) in aqueous alkaline media can be expressed very simply as:

$$\text{PB} + \text{H}_2\text{O} \xrightarrow{\quad k_1 \quad} \text{PB}^+ + \text{OH}^- \qquad (1)$$

$$\text{PA}^- + \text{PB}^+ \xrightarrow{\quad k_2 \quad} \text{PA} - \text{PB} \qquad (2)$$

One of the very important factors that determine the properties of the resulting materials is the stoichiometry of the charge-charge interaction. Stoichiometric complexes (other terms such as coacervates, [6], and precipitates have also been used) tend to be insoluble in the medium in which they were formed. Non-stoichiometric polyelectrolyte complexes can, since some of the charges remain ionised, exist as discrete "soluble particles" in dispersion (see Figure 1).

The influence of hydrophobic interactions on the formation and properties of polyelectrolyte complexes has been demonstrated [4].

The properties of polyelectrolyte complexes are essentially different from those of the starting components—this fact in itself warrants further studies, and a search for applications of such complexes.

The main difference between the complexes of low molecular weight compounds and polymer complexes is the presence in the polymer complex formation process of the co-operative interactions of adequately long chain sequences of interacting groups. There exists a critical chain length below which a co-operative binding does not occur [7]. The fundamental studies in this area have been continued mainly by Russian researchers. In a key paper in this area, Kabanov et al. [8] examined an important feature of the polymer complexes, i.e., their ability to participate in intermacromolecular exchange and substitution reactions in aqueous solutions. The authors found that such reactions proceed by the "contact mechanism" and that the addition of low molecular weight electrolytes to the reaction mixtures results in a dramatic increase in the rates of these exchange reactions.

From a practical point of view, it is clearly important to understand the stability, in terms of dissociation into the component polymers, of the complexes. From earlier work [9] it has been known that the stability of water-soluble non-stoichiometric polyelectrolyte complexes of poly-N-ethyl-4-vinylpyridinium salts depends on the nature of the ionic groups of the

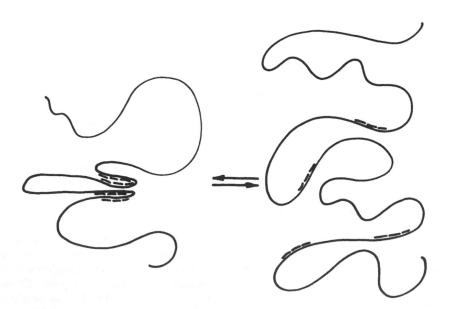

Figure 1. A schematic picture of the formation of non-stoichiometric interpolyelectrolyte complexes. Solid line—a higher molecular weight polyelectrolyte [e.g., poly(anion)]; interrupted line—a lower molecular weight polyelectrolyte of opposite charge [e.g., poly(cation)].

complexing polyanions. The stability increases in the series from polymethacrylate, to polyphosphate and polyvinylsulphate. More recently, Izumrudov et al. [10] examined further the stability of complexes in a homologous series of polyvinylpyridinium compounds, where the alkyl = methyl, ethyl, propyl, and amyl. They reported that full dissociation of complexes (with the above polyanions) into the corresponding polymers occurs at higher supporting electrolyte concentration (NaCl) the smaller the size of the N-alkyl (Table 1).

Sedimentation experiments reported by Davison et al. [11] showed a degree of complexation between a partially sulphonated dextran (pSD) and quaternised poly(vinylimidazole)(QPVI) under the appropriate conditions. Although both the QPVI alone and to a lesser extent the pSD can cause aggregation of platelets, polyelectrolyte complexes of these two macromolecules did not exhibit this property *in vitro* when the pSD was present in excess in the complex. Therefore, even in the presence of the physiologic amount of supporting electrolytes, these polyelectrolyte complexes did not appear to be dissociated to a significant degree.

A theory of polyelectrolyte effects on site-binding equilibria was developed some time ago by Friedman and Manning. Although it was applied by authors mainly to intercalation of drugs into DNA, it has been generalised [12] to multivalent ligands, multivalent supporting salts, intercalation, and multiple-site exclusion, and thus its relevance to interactions between macromolecules is likely.

POLYELECTROLYTE COMPLEX MEMBRANES

Polymer complexes present new polymeric materials, often with new properties. In addition, because of their relatively easy formation (from preformed and relatively easily characterised polymers), they are amenable to tailor-made modifications for special uses. In membrane manufacture, for example two soluble polymers can be brought together to form a membrane that is not only insoluble, but can also have the required physical and separation properties.

A polyelectrolyte complex prepared from chitosan and sulphonated chitosan was evaluated by Kim et al. [13] as a skin substitute. The water-vapour transport rate was 400-450 g/m²/day, and the coefficient of oxygen permeability was $1.3-6.2 \times 10^{-8}$ cm³ (STP) cm/cm² sec cm. The water absorption was 94–150%, with the tensile strength being 0.4–0.6 kg/mm². It would appear that this polyelectrolyte complex satisfied most of the basic properties of a skin substitute required by the authors.

Similarly, Kikuchi et al. [14] prepared membranes from glycol chitosan (GC)−poly(vinyl sulphate) (PVS), and methyl glycol chitosan (MGC)−carboxymethyl dextran (CMD) polymer complexes. The degree of dissociation, and the conformation of GC and CMD were reported to depend on pH. The

Table 1. Concentration of NaCl at which full dissociation of poly-N-alkyl vinylpyridinium—poly(sodium methacrylate) occurs (conditions: [PNaMA] = 2 × 10⁻³ M; [P-N-alkVP]/ [PNaMA] = 0.33; pH = 10; temperature = 20°C.

N-substituent	[NaCl], mol/L
methyl	0.6
ethyl	0.5
propyl	0.39
amyl	0.33

permeability of the membranes prepared from these complexes, to KCl, urea, and sucrose varied with the pH of the aqueous solvent. The permeability in the neutral region was 2- to 10-fold higher than that observed under acidic conditions. The observed increased membrane permeability was concluded to be resulting from changes in swelling that in turn resulted from conformational changes of the polymers (this conclusion was based on the IR spectra of the membranes).

Polyelectrolyte complex membranes prepared from poly(vinyl sulphate) and dextran diethylaminoethyl derivatives also showed variable permeabilities, depending on the pH at which they were prepared [15]. The dependence of the degree of dissociation and of intrinsic viscosity on pH was determined for this system. The apparent pKs of disubstituted single and tandem ammonia groups were reported to be 9.00 and 6.07, respectively. The permeability of the membranes to sodium ion was low at low pH, but increased at higher pH, presumably in parallel to the changing density of the membrane.

The possibility of controlling the properties of the polymer gel membranes by an external impulse have been recognised for some time. A model of an electrically activated mechano-chemical system made of a simple polymer gel was reported by Osada et al. [16]. Membranes with expanding and contracting pores can be made from such, and probably from other (including polyelectrolyte complex) gels.

De Rossi et al. [17] prepared contractile elements from cross-linked gels of polyacrylamide and also from poly(vinyl alcohol)−poly(acrylic acid) mixtures. 1 μm thick and 1 cm long elements can contract under electric stimulation with a velocity of 5–10 cm/s, exerting a contractile tension of 1–3 kg/cm². These contractile performances are therefore similar to those exhibited by natural muscles.

A patent exists on a similar process [18]. A mixture of 20% aqueous poly(vinyl alcohol) (M_w 40,000), 37% aqueous polyacrylic acid (M_w 17,000) and 37% aqueous poly(allylamine) (M_w 60,000) (molar ratio = 5:1:1) was frozen in ten 2-h cycles at −15° and thawed 2 h at room temperature to give a reversibly shrinkable material with tensile strength >10 kg/cm² and elongation 7.0, 0.85, and 1.1% in 0.05 M HCl, water, and 0.05 M NaOH, respectively. No details appear to

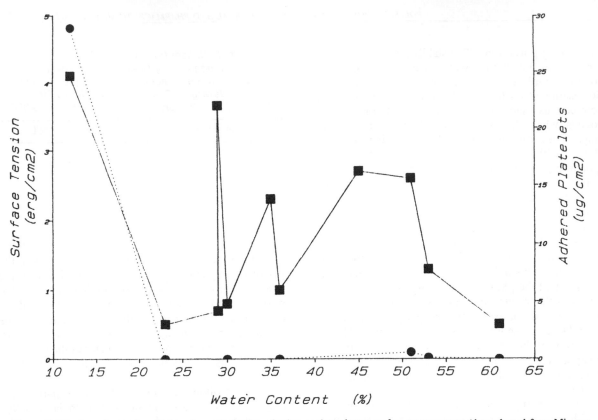

Figure 2. The dependence of surface tension and platelet adhesion on the polymer surface water content (data adapted from Miyama et al. [21]).

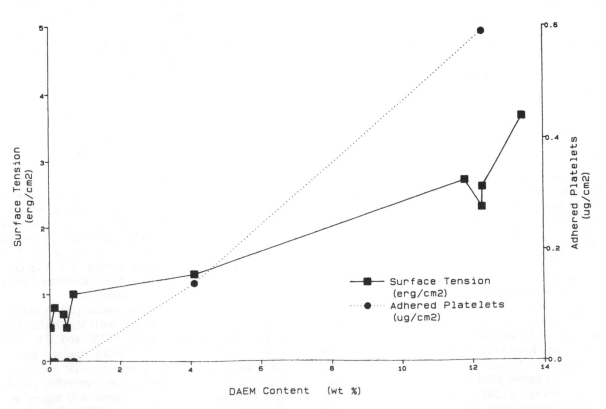

Figure 3. The dependence of surface tension and platelet adhesion on dimethylaminoethylmethacrylate (DAEM) content (data adapted from Miyama et al. [21]).

be available about the exact nature of the structure of the resulting material, and the reasons for the observed behaviour.

SOLID POLYELECTROLYTES FOR BIOMEDICAL APPLICATIONS

It is frequently concluded in published reports, whether of theoretical or practical nature, that the results might be of relevance to some biological phenomenon or application. Perhaps the most tangible demonstration of such a possibility is the continuing development in the preparation of thromboresistant surfaces.

The biological processes of thrombogenesis is in itself a complex sequence of events involving macromolecules [19]. A number of theories exist about what a non-thrombogenic surface should be like [20]. Regardless of these hypotheses, however the primary purpose is for the surface to resist adhesion of proteins (and in particular opsonising once), and consequently of cells. If a lesson can be learned from how living organisms deal with this task, a highly hydrophilic, highly mobile yet dense "collection" of flexible, highly hydrated macromolecular chains, either neutral or with a negative charge, is needed at the surface. How do polyelectrolyte complexes fare against these requirements? To judge this it is perhaps useful to bear in mind the now internationally agreed definition of biocompatibility. It is "the ability of a material to perform with an appropriate host response in a specific application".

"Non-thrombogenic" surfaces are often prepared by grafting water-soluble polymers, typically poly(oxyethylene) [21]. The expected success is usually based on an assumption that increased water content of the surface layer, (sometime coupled with the correct charge) will lead to a decrease in the interfacial free energy, and consequently will, for example, reduce platelet adhesion. Many papers have been published on this, and many speculative explanations have been proposed. For example, Miyama et al. [21] tried to rationalise their results in terms of variable mobility of poly(oxyethylene) chains at the polymer surface, and

as resulting from altered microscopic water flow near the surface. Their results, when plotted as in Figures 2 and 3 here, firmly suggest that the higher the (potentially) positive charge at the surface the higher the observed number of adhering platelets. The plots also suggest that platelet adhesion, under the conditions of these experiments, was not sensitive to the changes in the (calculated from contact angle measurements) interfacial free energy.

Polyelectrolyte complexes may offer an alternative approach to preparing non-thrombogenic materials. The effect of excess charge in cellulosic polyelectrolyte complexes on the blood compatibility was examined in some detail by Ito and co-workers [22–25]. Various complexes with excess overall charge were prepared from a quaternary ammonium derivative of hydroxyethyl cellulose and carboxymethyl cellulose. The blood compatibility was evaluated by measuring platelet adhesion and contact phase activation tests (Lee-White), and also by measuring time-variant changes in the differentiated hematological responses during whole blood coagulation (quenched Lee-White test). For the complexes studied, the relative coagulation time of whole blood was found to be very long and almost independent of the mole ratio of polycation to polyanion [the mole ratios (cation/anion) for the complexes used here were 1.5/1.0, 1.0/1.0, and 1.0/1.5], but platelet adhesion increased with increasing mole ratios of polycation/polyanion in the complex. Contact phase activation of plasma coagulation, however, increased with decreasing mole ratio.

The quenched Lee-White test revealed that platelet counts and quantity of the hematological factors measured after 15 min were independent of the excess charge on the complex, and remained at considerably high levels even at 60 min of exposure time. The authors concluded that the indicated weak interactions of blood components, irrespective of surface charge excess, may result in good antithrombogenicity *in vivo* under long-term experiments. This will clearly need to be proved by experiment. However, a comparison with different but related experiments of Artursson [26] and Davison [27] (Table 2) suggest that such conclusions might be too optimistic. As mentioned earlier in this review, polyelectrolyte complexes are prone to

Table 2. Platelet aggregation and in vivo distribution studies on water-soluble polyelectrolyte complexes.

Polyelectrolytes			Platelet Aggregation			In vivo Distribution		
Poly-cation	Poly-anion	Ratio	Poly-cation	Poly-anion	Complex	n	Blood	Liver
QPVP	PMAA	0.2	✔	X	X	3	13.96 (1.05)	51.20 (1.94)
QPVI	PMAA	0.2	✔	X	X	4	1.91 (0.12)	43.07 (3.75)
I3X	pDS	0.5	✔	X	✔	—	—	—
QPVI	pDS	0.5	✔	X	X	3	2.37 (0.35)	37.75 (4.14)

The polyelectrolytes were: quaternised poly(vinyl pyridine) (QPVP); quaternised poly(vinylimidazole) (QPVI); poly(methacrylic acid) (PMAA); Ionene 3X (I3X); partially sulphonated dextran (pDS). Platelet aggregation results: ✔ aggregation observed; X no aggregation. *In vivo* distribution results using mice where *n* = number of animals in each study. Figures give the corrected % of administered dose found in the blood and liver after 2 hours (standard error in brackets).

a rapid "ion-exchange" between the polymer chains forming the complex. Stabilisation of these complexes by covalent bonds, hydrophobic interactions or by some other means is likely to be essential to providing materials that resist exchange interactions with blood components.

The properties of hydrocarbon hemosorbents with thromboresistant hydrogel coating of a polyelectrolyte complex formed from poly(acrylic acid) and poly (ethyleneimine) hydrogel were studied by Valueva et al. [28]. Electron microscopy showed that hydrogel modified the surface of carbon sorbent. The polyelectrolyte complex-coated particles, while showing somewhat slower permeability, were more selective in separating blood components and were therefore found suitable for hemoperfusion.

In a more general way, various factors that influence the state of water in polyelectrolyte complex hydrogels, were examined by Zheleznova et al. [29]. The authors found that polyelectrolyte hydrogels containing poly(acrylic acid), polyethylenimine, poly(N,N-dimethylaminoethyl methacrylate) and poly(ethylenpiperazine) showed high permeability to water, were hemocompatible, and were able to dialyse low molecular weight, water-soluble compounds. The swelling of hydrogels increased with the increase in the amount of electrolytes in solution. The amount of water found to be bound to polymers was about 10%.

The thromboresistances of polyelectrolyte complexes in relation to their physico-chemical properties, have been reviewed by Zezin et al. [30].

In my view, in developing various materials for this and other biological applications, not enough attention has been paid to the underlying biological principles.

POLYMER COMPLEXES IN DRUG RELEASE

The last comment is equally valid when we review what has been achieved in applying polymers to drug delivery. Perhaps the simplest, and most well known application of polymers in this context is as general excipients, e.g., thickeners. Anionic carboxy polymers and cellulose grafted with quaternary ammonium salt groups have been used to obtain viscosity of formulations >0.45 Pas at Module 3 at 21°. An aqueous gel was also prepared by mixing a 1% aqueous solution containing hydroxyethyl cellulose grafted with diallylmethylammonium salt with a 1% ethanolic solution containing neutralised methacrylic acid–methyl methacrylate 1:1 copolymer. The gels have been used in the treatment of psoriasis [31].

Slow-release pharmaceuticals formulated in a tablet form using a poly(allylamine) and an anionic polymer have also been described. It can be assumed that a polymer complex that was likely to form from the above polymers was in some way instrumental in controlling the rate of drug release [32].

Similarly to preparing membranes for separation, polyelectrolyte complexes have been used for controlling fluxes of drugs from various devices. A "traditional" approach is to encapsulate the drug to be released. A range of polymers has been used in the past, including the formation of polymer complexes. The only difference might be that different terms have been used to describe the outcome. Capsule walls are often formed by precipitating anionic and cationic polyelectrolytes at an interface. Recently, Loth et al. [33–35] used both natural and synthetic polymers containing sulphate or carboxylate groups as anions, and cationic polyelectrolytes containing quaternary ammonium groups or dyes. For example, sodium cellulose sulphate (2% aqueous solution) was treated with a 2% aqueous solution of poly(dimethyldiallylammonium chloride) to give polyelectrolyte complex (sometimes called symplex) capsules. The diameter of capsules ranged from 0.5 to 4 mm, with the thickness of the capsule wall ranging from 1 to 50 μm. The capsules could be swollen to several times the original volume by changing the osmotic pressure. The mechanical strength of the capsules depended on the presence of NaCl in the medium. The kinetics of release of labelled buserelin from the capsules was studied using a diffusion chamber. Similarly to what was reported by others in connection with membranes, the rate of drug release depended on the amount of electrolyte (NaCl) in the medium.

Although somewhat outside of the scope of this review, it is worth mentioning the interaction that can take place between polyelectrolytes and surfactants. This has been exploited for manipulating the rate of release of compounds from liposomes. According to Musabekov et al. [36] the interaction between (in their case, cross-linked) polyelectrolytes and surfactants proceeded by an ion-exchange mechanism. The electrostatic and the total binding of cetylpyridinium bromide by polyelectrolytes increased with increasing surfactant concentration. The total binding of the surfactant to poly(acrylic acid) was 2-fold higher than binding to poly(methacrylic acid), due to the lower hydrophobicity of the former.

The effect of poly(dimethyl aminoethyl methacrylate) on liposome permeability was studied by Petrukhina et al. [37]. The polyelectrolyte formed electrostatic complexes with liposomes (prepared from dipalmitoylphosphatidyl choline and dipalmitoylphosphatidic acid). As a consequence of this, the permeability for liposome-entrapped 6-carboxyfluorescein was altered. The presence of charged lipids in the liposomal membrane facilitates complex formation and increases permeability in a pH-dependent fashion. The maximum permeability was observed during the 15–30 min of polyelectrolyte-liposome interaction. Further studies of this [38] showed that incorporation of N-vinylpyrrolidone-vinyloctylamine copolymer in the liposome increased the vesicle permeability at pH 7.0. The presence of poly(dimethylaminoethyl methacrylate) in liposomes also containing a comb-like poly(cetyl methacrylate) also increased the liposome permeability, reaching the maximum at pH = 7.5.

A semisynthetic vesicular membrane was constructed by immobilization of a synthetic polyelectrolyte [poly(2-ethylacrylic acid)] on the surface of a phosphatidylcholine bilayer. These membranes were found to exhibit large variations in permeability with small changes in pH. Therefore, rapid and quantitative release of vesicle contents can be achieved by mild acidification within the physiologic pH range [39].

It is reasonable to expect the observed changes in the release of a liposome-entrapped compound is not entirely given by changes in bilayer membrane permeability, but is more associated with a change in the state of the liposome. Some evidence for this was presented by Borden et al. [40]. In this study, a 2-ethylacrylic acid-1-pyreneacrylic acid copolymer was used to determine the effect of dipalmitoylphosphatidylcholine vesicles on the conformational transition of poly(2-ethylacrylic acid). Plots of fluorescence intensity versus pH for solutions of the above compounds showed the midpoint of the conformational transition from an expanded conformation at high pH to a hydrophobic, globular coil at low pH occurring at pH from 6.1 to 6.5. Further, the width at the half-height of the calorimetric phase transition of the vesicle bilayer increased sharply at pH 6.5, i.e., just about at the midpoint of the conformational transition. The authors' interpretation of these results is to suggest that the hydrophobic core of the collapsed polyelectrolyte chain provides a site for solubilisation of the hydrocarbon tails of the surfactant, and in so doing disrupts the structural integrity of the pure lipid film. Some evidence of a vesicle-to-micelle transition was obtained from electron microscopy. The above picture is entirely consistent with the known phenomenon of spontaneous emulsification [41].

Two other applications of polyelectrolyte complexes are worth mentioning. Plavins et al. [42] prepared magnetic microspheres based on polyelectrolyte complexes and Fe_3O_4. A correlation between the size and magnetic susceptibility of microspheres was demonstrated.

Encapsulation using polyelectrolyte complex formation has also been applied to encapsulating viable pancreatic islet cells [43]. Islet cell were cultured in capsules of sodium cellulose sulphate and poly (dimethyldiallylammonium chloride). After 5 weeks, encapsulated islet cells were morphologically well preserved, and the parameters of cell viability such as DNA content and DNA synthesis, insulin content and stimulated insulin release were not different for the encapsulated and non-encapsulated control cells. An observed lower rate of secretion of insulin into the medium of the encapsulated cells during the first 3 weeks of culture was explained by the capsule wall

thickness (i.e., the capsule diameter was 4–5 mm). The rate of insulin excretion could be increased by the use of thinner capsules (diameter < 1 mm).

POLYMER COMPLEXES AS DRUGS AND DRUG CARRIERS

Problems that we face constantly in trying to interfere with the biological processes that cause or accompany a disease, are enormous. It is not surprising that many new materials, and many new concepts are considered and tried in biomedical applications. Polyelectrolyte complexes are no exception.

Mixtures of oppositely charged polyelectrolytes can, under certain conditions of stoichiometry, relative molecular mass, pH and ionic strength, form discrete water-soluble structures. These complexes have been studied as potential carriers of biologically active compounds for parenteral administration [27] by Davison et al. As mentioned above, sedimentation experiments showed a degree of complexation between a partially sulphonated dextran (pSD) and quaternised poly(vinylimidazole) (QPVI) under the appropriate conditions. Although both the QPVI alone and to a lesser extent the pSD can cause aggregation of platelets, polyelectrolyte complexes of these two macromolecules did not exhibit this property *in vitro* when the pSD was present in excess in the complex.

In vivo distribution studies in mice using ^{125}I labelled QPVI complexed with pSD showed accumulation of the label in the liver after 2 hours. The authors concluded that while the polycation present in these complexes appears to be prevented to some extent from interacting with the negatively-charged biological surfaces such as in platelets *in vitro*, this complexation is not sufficient, at least for the two macromolecules we have examined, to prevent an extensive incidence of unwanted interactions *in vivo*. Investigations with similar purpose and results were reported by Kabanov's group [44].

The earlier approach of Margolin et al. [4,45] in using as one of the complexing polymers a macromolecule with a definite biological activity (e.g., enzymes), has now been adopted by others. Thus, the effect of polyanionic polymers on the oxygen-binding properties of hemoglobin (Hb) was studied by Zygmunt et al. [46]. Polyanionic, water-soluble polymers containing sulphate, phosphate and polycarboxylate groups were synthesised. When simply added to Hb solutions, the polymers were shown to lower the affinity of the protein for oxygen. The influence of the polymer on oxygen affinity was thought to be a result of a specific interaction of the anionic groups of the polymer inside the 2,3-diphosphoglycerate-binding site of deoxyHb. There is some optimism that these or similar complexes could be used as possible blood substitutes. However, the problems alluded to in Reference [27] will need to be overcome.

The possibility of protecting, for example, enzymes from degradation and immune response, by grafting them with water-soluble, inert polymers, is well known [47]. Similarly, the dependence of immune response on the size of the presenting molecule has now been recognised [48] as being largely determined by molecular mass and hapten valence.

It is therefore only natural that polyelectrolyte complexes have been examined for their properties in relation to the above two principles. According to Petrov et al. [49], low-immunogenic M-protein of influenza virus becomes highly immunogenic after it is covalently cross-linked with a practically non-toxic polyelectrolyte. It is believed that this approach could lead potentially to the development of a new generation of universal polymer-subunit influenza vaccines. Several groups are now investigating this general approach [50]. The use of polyelectrolytes as immunostimulants, model artificial immunogens, and vaccinating macromolecules was recently reviewed by Kabanov [51].

To be able to diagnose a disease forms a very important, integral part of disease management. A novel polymer complex composed of polysaccharide derivatives having at least three formyl groups in the molecule, an amino-group containing a difunctional ligand and an amino-group containing a physiologically active substance, has been patented recently. The complexes are to be used as carriers for radioactive medical agents [52].

CONCLUSIONS

Polyelectrolyte complexes have properties so different from the properties of their individual components that they must be seen as materials with potentially unique and exploitable properties. Such materials have been known for some time and have been used in many practical applications, often without recognising that a polymer complex was involved. The recent recognition of polyelectrolyte complexes as a class of compounds has resulted in more fundamental studies of their formation and of their physical and chemical properties. Many structures exist in the natural world that could be described as polyelectrolyte complexes. In comparison, the "man-made" structures reported so far are rather trivial, and rapid advances could be made by utilising the knowledge of biological systems in the preparation of synthetic polymers. It is my view that in designing polyelectrolyte complexes for biomedical applications in particular, much more attention must be paid in the future to the underlying biological principles.

REFERENCES

1. Marvin, D. A., R. L. Wiseman and E. J. Wachtel. 1974. "Filamentous Bacterial Viruses. XI. Molecular Architecture of the Class II (Pf 1, Xf) Virion", *J. Mol. Biol.*, 82:121–138.

2. Snell, D. T. and R. E. Offord. 1972. "The Amino Acid Sequences of the B-Protein of Bacteriophage ZJ-2", *Biochem. J.*, 127:167–178.

3. Marvin, D. A. "Inovirus, a Polymer of Polymers: Model-Building Studies of Naturally Occurring Genetic Variations on a Common Geometric Theme", *Biologically Engineered Polymers 1989*. Churchill College, Cambridge.

4. Petrak, K. 1986. "Polyelectrolyte Complexes in Biomedical Applications", *J. Bioact. Compat. Polym.*, 1(2):202–219.

5. Abe, Koji. 1987. "Characteristics and Functions of Polyion Complexes", *Kobunshi*, 36(11):794–797.

6. Commandur, B., C. Arneodo, J.-P. Benoit and C. Thies. 1989. "A Study of the Viscosity of Gelatin-Based Complex Coacervates", in *Controlled Release of Bioactive Materials*. Chicago, August 6–9, Abstracts, p. 89, paper no. 132.

7. Saltybaeva, S. S., L. A. Bimendina and E. A. Bekturov. 1979. *Izv. Akad. Nauk. Kaz. SSR, Ser. Khim.*, p. 3.

8. Kabanov, V. A., A. B. Zezin, V. A. Izumrudov, T. K. Bronich and K. N. Bakeev. 1985. "Cooperative Interpolyelectrolyte Reactions", *Makromol. Chem.*, 13 (suppl.):137–155.

9. Izumrudov, V. A., T. K. Bronich, A. B. Zezin and V. A. Kabanov. 1982. *Vysokomol. Soed. A*, 24(2):339; V. A. Izumrudov, T. K. Bronich, O. S. Saburova, A. B. Zezin and V. A. Kabanov. 1988. *Makromol. Chem. Rapid Commun.*, 9:7.

10. Izumrudov, V. A., T. K. Bronich, A. B. Zezin and V. A. Kabanov. 1989. *Vysokomol. Soed.*, 31(5):326–327.

11. Davison, C. J., J. E. O'Mullane, J. Nicholls and K. Petrak. *Macromolecules '89 Conference— Preprints, Oxford, Sept. 1989.*

12. Friedman, R. A. G. and G. S. Manning. 1984. "Polyelectrolyte Effects on Site-Binding Equilibria with Application to the Intercalation of Drugs into DNA", *Biopolymers*, 23(12):2671–2714.

13. Kim-Kea-Yong, Min-Dong-Sun and Chung-Ho-Sam. 1988. "Chitosan-Based Skin Substitute. I. Synthesis and Properties of Polyelectrolyte Complex Consisting of Sulfonated Chitosan and Chitosan", *Pollimo.*, 12(3):234–240.

14. Kikuchi-Yasuo and Kubota-Naoji. 1988. "Permeability Control of Polyelectrolyte Complex Membrane Including Chitosan Derivative as a Component", *Bull. Chem. Soc. Jpn.*, 61(8):2943–2947.

15. Kikuchi-Yasuo and Kubota-Naoji. 1988. "An Investigation on the Properties of [2-(Diethylamino)Ethyl]Dextran as a Component of Polyelectrolyte Complex Membrane", *Makromol. Chem., Rapid Commun.*, 9(11):727–730.

16. Osada-Yoshihito and Hasebe-Mariko. 1985. "Electrically Activated Mechanochemical Devices Using Polyelectrolyte Gels", *Chem. Lett.*, (9):1285–8.

17. De Rossi, D. E., P. Chiarelli, G. Buzzigoli, C. Domenici and L. Lazzeri. 1986. "Contractile Behavior of Electrically Activated Mechanochemical Polymer Actuators", *ASAIO Trans.*, 32(1):157–162.

18. Suzuki-Makoto. "Manufacture of Polymers Which Reversibly Stretch and Shrink", PA Agency of Industrial Sciences and Technology, Jpn. Kokai Tokkyo Koho 62115064 (87115064), Pat Appl: 85/254043, (13.11.85), (26.05.87).

19. Salem, H. H. 1987. "Current Views on Pathophysiology and Investigations of Thrombolytic Disorders", *Am. J. Hematol.*, 25(4):463–474.

20. Andrade, J. D., S. Nagaoka, S. Cooper, T. Okano and S. W. Kim. 1987. "Surfaces and Blood Compatibility. Current Hypotheses", *ASAIO*, 10(2):75–84.

21. Miyama, H., N. Fujii, N. Hokari, H. Toi, S. Nagaoka, Y. Mori and Y. Noishiki. 1987. "Nonthrombogenicity of Polyacrylonitrile Graft Copolymers Containing Poly (Ethylene Oxide) and Dimethylamine Side Chains", *J. Bioact. Compat. Polym.*, 2(3):222–231.

22. Ito-Hiraku, Miyamoto-Takeaki, Inagaki-Hiroshi, Iwata-Hiroo and Matsuda-Takehisa. 1987. "Effect of Excess Charge in Cellulosic Polyelectrolyte Complexes on the Blood Compatibility", *J. Bioact. Compat. Polym.*, 2(3):193–205.

23. Ito-Hiraku, Shibata-Toru, Miyamato-Takeaki, Noishiki-Yasuharu and Inagaki-Hiroshi. 1986. "Formation of Polyelectrolyte Complexes Between Cellulose Derivatives and Their Blood Compatibility", *J. Appl. Polym. Sci.*, 31(8):2491–2500.

24. Ito-Hiraku, Miyamoto-Takeaki, Inagaki-Hiroshi, Noishiki-Yasuharu, Iwata-Hiroo and Matsuda-Takehisa. 1986. "*In vivo* and *in vitro* Blood Compatibility of Polyelectrolyte Complexes Formed Between Cellulose Derivatives", *J. Appl. Polym. Sci.*, 32(2):3413–3421.

25. Inagaki-Hiroshi, Miyamoto-Takeaki, Ito-Hiraku and Shibata-Tohru. PA Daicel Chemical Industries, Ltd., "Cellulose Polycation-Cellulose Polyanion Electrolyte Complexes for Anticoagulant Coatings or Anticoagulant Molding Materials", US 4708951, Prty Appl: 84/62048 (JP), (28.03.84) Pat Appl: 715658, (25.03.85), (24.11.87).

26. Artursson, P., L. Brown, J. Dix, P. Goddard and K. Petrak. "Sterically Stabilised Nanoparticles– Part 1: Preparation by Desolvation from Graft Copolymers", *J. Polymer Sci.*, Polymer Chem. edn. (submitted August, 1989).

27. Davison, C. J., K. E. Smith, L. E. F. Hutchinson, J. E. O'Mullane, S. E. Harding. L. Brookman and K. Petrak. "Physical and Biological Properties of Water-Soluble Polyelectrolyte Complexes", *J. Bioact. Biocompat. Polymers* (submitted Oct. 1989).

28. Valueva, S. P., E. M. Kopylova, B. S. El-tsefon, S. I. Surinova and N. M. Kaznacheeva. 1986. "The Properties of Hydrocarbon Hemosorbents with Thromboresistant Hydrogel Coating of a Polyelectrolyte Complex", *Khim-Farm. Zh.*, 20(3):365–370.

29. Zheleznova, I. V., A. R. Rudman, R. I. Kalyuzhnaya, N. A. Vengerova and B. S. El-tsefon. 1988. "Effect of Various Factors on Water State and Properties of Polyelectrolyte Complex Hydrogels for Medical Applications", *Khim-Farm. Zh.*, 22(2):227–231.

30. Zezin, A. B., B. S. Eltsefon, A. R. Rudman, N. A. Vengerova, R. I. Kalyuzhnaya, S. P. Valueva, E. M. Kopylova, A. K. Chepurov, V. S. Efimov and V. A. Kabanov. 1987. "Interpolymer Complexes–Biocompatible Polymers and Problem of Thromboresistance", *Khim-Farm. Zh.*, 21(7):788–801.

31. Gollier, J. F., C. Dubief and J. Mondet. PA Oreal S.A., "Thickening Agent Containing Anionic Carboxy Polymers and Cellulose Grafted with Quaternary Ammonium Salts for Pharmaceuticals and Cosmetics", Ger. Offen 3716381, Prty Appl: 86429 (LU), (16.05.86) Pat Appl: 3716381, (15.05.87), (19.11.87).

32. Makino-Yuji, Matsuki-Hideo, Suzuki-Yoshiki, PA Teijen Ltd., "Slow-Release Pharmaceuticals Containing Poly(allylamine) and Anionic Polymers as Excipients", Jpn. Kokai Tokkyo Koho 62132830 (87132830), Pat Appl: 85/272432, (05.12.85), (16.06.87).

33. Loth, F., H. Dautzenberg and K. Pommerening. PA Akademie der Wissenschaften der DDR, "Microcapsules with Permeable or Semipermeable Walls and a Liquid Core", Germany 218734, Pat Appl: 232617, (17.08.81), (13.02.85).

34. Dautzenberg, H., F. Loth, K. Pommerening, K. L. Linow and D. Bartsch. "Preparation of Microcapsules Using Polyelectrolytes", PA Akademie der Wissenschaften der DDR Patentschrift (Switz) 659591, Pat Appl: 83/1129, (01.03.83), (13.02.87).

35. Dautzenberg, H., F. Loth, K. Fechner, B. Mehlis and K. Pommerening. 1985. "Preparation and Performance of Symplex Capsules", *Makromol. Chem.*, 9 (Suppl.):203–210.

36. Musabekov, K. B., Zh. A. Abilov, G. V. Samsonov and M. K. Beisebekov. 1985. "Reaction of Cross-Linked Polyelectrolytes with Surfactants", *Izv. Akad. Nauk. Kaz. SSR, Ser. Khim. 5:31–35.*

37. Petrukhina, O. O., N. N. Ivanov, M. M. Feldstein, A. E. Vasilev, N. A. Plate and V. P. Torchilin. 1986. "The Regulation of Liposome Permeability by Polyelectrolyte", *J. Controlled Release*, 3(2–3):137–141.

38. Maksimenko, O. O., M. M. Feldstein, E. F. Panarin, A. E. Vasilev, V. P. Torchilin and N. A. Plate. 1988. "pH-Sensitive Liposomes Based on Complexes of Synthetic Phospholipids with Polyelectrolytes and Comb-Like Polymers", *Vysokomol. Soedin.*, Ser A., 30(5):1120–1124.

39. Maeda-Mizuo, Kumano-Atsushi and D. A. Tirrell. 1988. "H^+-Induced Release of Contents of Phosphatidylcholine Vesicles Bearing Surface-Bound Polyelectrolyte Chains", *J. Am. Chem. Soc.*, 110(22):7455–7459.

40. Borden, K. A., C. L. Voycheck, J. S. Tan and D. A. Tirrell. "Polyelectrolyte Adsorption Induces a Vesicle-to-Micelle Transition in Aqueous Dispersions of Dipalmitoylphosphatidylcholine", *Polym. Prepr.*, (Am. Chem. Soc., Div. Polym. Chem.), 28(1):284–285.

41. Hunter, R. J. 1987. *Foundations of Colloid Science, Vol. 1.* Oxford: Clarendon Press, p. 21.

42. Plavins, J., M. Lauva, Sh. I. Krisko, E. Ya Blum and N. I. Tankovich. 1985. "Magnetophoretic Mobility of Polyelectrolyte-Based Microspheres", *Magn. Gidrodin.*, (2):130–132.

43. Braun, K., W. Besch, S. Lucke and H. J. Hahn. 1986. "The Long-Term Culture of Encapsulated Pancreatic Islets", *Exp. Clin. Endocrinol.*, 87(3):313–318.

44. Skorodinskaya, A. M., V. A. Kemenova, V. S. Efimov, M. I. Mustafaev, V. A. Kasaikin, A. B. Zezin and V. A. Kabanov. 1984. "Biological Activity of Nonstoichiometric Polyelectrolyte Complexes", *Khim-Farm. Zh.*, 18(3):283–287.

45. Margolin, A. L., V. A. Izumrudov, S. F. Sherstyuk, A. B. Zezin and V. K. Shvyadas. 1983. *Mol. Biology*, 17:815.

46. Zygmunt, D., M. Leonard, F. Bonneaux, D. Sacco, E. Dellacherie. 1987. "Effect of Polyanionic Polymers on Hemoglobin Oxygen-Binding Properties: Application to the Synthesis of Covalent Conjugates with Low Oxygen Affinity", *Int. J. Biol. Macromol.*, 9(6):343–345.

47. Beauchamp, C. O., S. L. Gonias, D. P. Menapace and S. V. Pizzo. 1983. "A New Procedure for the Synthesis of Polyethylene Glycol-Protein Adducts; Effects on Function, Receptor Recognition, and Clearance of Superoxide Dismutase, Lactoferrin, and α_2-macroglobulin", *Anal. Biochem.*, 131:25–33.

48. Dintzis, R. Z., M. Okajima, M. H. Middleton, G. Greene and H. M. Dintzis. 1989. "The Immunogenicity of Soluble Haptenated Polymers Is Determined by Molecular Mass and Hapten Valence", *J. Immunol.*, 143(4):1239–1244.

49. Petrov, R. V., R. M. Khaitov, V. M. Zhdanov, A. Sh. Norimov, A. V. Nekrasov, M. S. Sinyakov and I. G. Kharitonenkov. 1985. "Protective Effects of the Conjugate of Influenza Virus M-Protein with a Synthetic Polyelectrolyte", *Immunologiya*, (Moscow) (6):60–62.

50. Hilgers, L. A. T., H. Snippe, M. Jansze and J. M. M. Willers. 1986. "Synergistic Effects of Synthetic Adjuvants on the Humoral Immune Response", *Int. Arch. Allergy Appl. Immunol.*, 79(4):392–396.

51. Kabanov, V. A. 1986. "Synthetic Membrane Active Polyelectrolytes in Design of Artificial Immunogens and Vaccines", *Makromol. Chem., Macromol. Symp.*, 1(1):101–124.

52. Nippon Medi-Phys KK, Jap. Pat. 268981 1987; US 558333 (20.09.88).

45

Pharmaceutical Uses of Cyclodextrin Derivatives

KANETO UEKAMA*
FUMITOSHI HIRAYAMA*
TETSUMI IRIE*

ABSTRACT: Recently, many kinds of cyclodextrin (CyD) derivatives have been prepared to improve the physicochemical properties and inclusion capacity of parent CyD as novel drug carriers. These chemically modified CyDs can be divided into three groups; i.e., hydrophilic, hydrophobic, and ionizable derivatives. Among the possible uses of CyD derivatives in pharmaceutical formulations, solubilization, stabilization, modification of release and absorption rates, and detoxication of drug molecules in various administration routes will be described, anticipating the development of advanced dosage forms.

INTRODUCTION

A major challenge confronting pharmaceutical scientists is the rational design of drug formulations. For the development of advanced dosage forms with a potential to improve on the undesirable properties of drugs, new carrier materials are needed. Cyclodextrins (CyDs) are good candidates for such a role because they have the capacity to alter physical, chemical, and biological properties of guest molecules through the formation of inclusion complexes [1–7]. The α-, β-, and γ-CyDs—the three most common natural CyDs—consist of six, seven, and eight D-glucopyranose residues, respectively, linked by α-1,4 glycosidic bonds into a cycle. Each CyD has its own ability to form inclusion complexes with specific guests, an ability which depends on a proper fit of the guest molecule into the macrocyclic ring of the CyD molecule. However, natural CyDs have relatively low solubility, both in water and organic solvents, that limits their uses in the pharmaceutical field [4,8,9]. To remove some of their limitations, natural CyDs have to be chemically modified. In the case of β-CyD (Figure 1), for example, 21 hydroxyl groups (7 primary and 14 secondary) are available as starting points for structural modifications, and various functional groups may be incorporated in the β-CyD molecule [10–12].

Chemically modified CyDs may be divided into three groups—hydrophilic, hydrophobic, and ionic derivatives. Among the hydrophilic CyD derivatives, methylated CyDs are among the most prominent representatives—they can improve remarkably the solubility, chemical stability, and bioavailability of various drugs [4,5,7–9]. Recently available hydroxyalkylated CyDs [13–16] and branched CyDs [17,18] deserve special attention since their toxicity is very low and solubility in water very high, both promising properties for use in parenteral formulations [18–20]. On the other hand, hydrophobic CyDs have only been studied a little, but have great potential as well. For example, ethylated β-CyDs are useful as the sustained-release drug carriers of water-soluble drugs [21–23] and of peptides [24], since they have the ability to decrease the solubility of guest molecules. The introduction of anionic or cationic groups into CyD molecules causes their solubility in aqueous media to depend on pH [25,26]. The ionizable CyD derivatives differ in many of their effects from other CyD derivatives; for example, these derivatives may bind to the surface membrane of cells, which may possibly be used for the selective delivery of drugs across biological barriers [27].

The objective of this review is to demonstrate the potential of CyD derivatives as novel drug carriers in pharmaceutical formulations. In order to appreciate all the possible uses of chemically modified CyDs in various dosage forms (Table 1), some of their fundamental properties have to be described first.

CHARACTERIZATION OF CYCLODEXTRIN DERIVATIVES

Chemical modifications of hydroxyl groups of CyDs markedly change their physical, chemical, and

---

*Faculty of Pharmaceutical Sciences, Kumamoto University, 5-1, Oe-honmachi, Kumamoto 862, Japan

Table 1. Pharmaceutically useful β-CyD derivatives.

Derivatives	Characteristic	Possible Administration Route (Dosage Form)
β-CyD	crystalline, relatively low water-soluble	oral, rectal, dermal
Hydrophilic derivative Methylated β-CyD DM-β-CyD TM-β-CyD	soluble in cold water and in organic solvents, surface active, hemolytic	oral, rectal, dermal
Hydroxyalkylated β-CyD 2-HE-β-CyD 2-HP-β-CyD 3-HP-β-CyD 2,3-DHP-β-CyD	unevenly substituted mixture, amorphous, highly water-soluble, low hemolytic activity	oral, mucosal (rectal, nasal, sublingual, ophthalmic), parenteral (i.v.)
Branched β-CyD G_1-β-CyD G_2-β-CyD $(G_2)_2$-β-CyD	homogeneous compound, highly water-soluble	oral, mucosal (rectal, nasal, sublingual, ophthalmic), parenteral (i.v.)
Hydrophobic derivative Ethylated β-CyD DE-β-CyD TE-β-CyD	surface active, less hygroscopic	oral, subcutaneous (sustained-release)
Ionizable derivative CME-β-CyD	anionic (pKa = 3 ~ 4), surface active	oral (delayed-release), dermal

Table 2. Physicochemical properties of β-CyD derivatives.

Derivatives	Aqueous Solubility[a] (%)	$[\alpha]_D{}^a$	Water Content[b] (%)	Surface Tension[c] (mN/m)	Half-Life of Degradation[d] (h)
β-CyD	1.85	163	16.2	71	5.4
DM-β-CyD	>50	160	1.0	62	9.8
TM-β-CyD	>30	158	< 1.0	53	1.7
2-HE-β-CyD[e]	>50	130	10.4	71	—[f]
2-HP-β-CyD[e]	>50	146	10.8	64	—[f]
3-HP-β-CyD[e]	>50	125	11.2	70	—[f]
2,3-DHP-β-CyD[e]	>50	114	12.6	71	—[f]
G_1-β-CyD	>50	159	—[f]	71	5.1
G_2-β-CyD	>50	155	13.5	70	3.8
$(G_2)_2$-β-CyD	>50	163	—[f]	71	2.1
DE-β-CyD	< 0.005	123[g]	1.1	53[h]	12.2
TE-β-CyD	< 0.002	129[g]	< 1.0	53[h]	9.7
CME-β-CyD[i]	highly soluble at pH >4	124	5.9	44	—[f]

[a] In water at 25°C.
[b] At 75% R.H. and 25°C.
[c] Concentration of CyDs was 0.1 W/V%.
[d] In 1.0 N HCl at 60°C.
[e] Degree of substitution was about 6.
[f] Under investigation.
[g] In ethanol-water (1:1).
[h] Concentration of CyDs was 1.0×10^{-6} M.
[i] Degree of substitution of carboxymethyl and ethyl groups were 1.8 and 10.7, respectively.

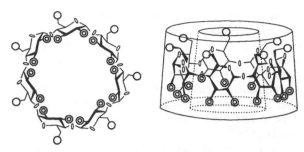

Figure 1. Chemical structure of β-CyD. ○: primary hydroxyls, ◎: secondary hydroxyls.

biological properties. Consequently these compounds must be fully characterized before they can be used as drug carriers in pharmaceutical formulations.

Physical–Chemical Properties

Some of the relevant physicochemical properties of CyD derivatives are listed in Table 2. The aqueous solubility of β-CyD is significantly increased by introducing methyl, hydroxyalkyl, or glucosyl groups; also dissolution rates of the derivatives are invariably higher than those of the parent compounds. The high solubility of methylated CyDs is probably due both to the low crystal-lattice energy of this derivative in the solid state and to the strong hydration when dissolved in water. Exothermic dissolution of methylated CyDs in water is an indicator of strong hydration, a situation contrasting with natural CyDs that dissolve in water in an endothermic process [28]. Increase in temperature is expected to lower hydration, and indeed the solubility of methylated CyDs in water decreases with increasing temperature, a behavior similar to that of nonionic surfactants. Hydroxyalkylated CyDs are amorphous mixtures of chemically related components with different degrees of substitution (D.S.) [13,14]. This multi-component character prevents any crystallization, and thus hydroxyalkylated CyDs have high solubility in water.

Branched CyDs, in which the primary hydroxyl groups of parent CyDs are substituted by glucose or maltose residues by α-1,6 glucosyl linkage, in spite of being a single component, also do not crystallize out from water and thus have a good solubility [17,18]. On the other hand, when hydroxyl groups of CyDs are substituted by ethyl or longer alkyl groups, the solubility of such compounds in water decreases proportionally to their D.S., whereas their solubility in less polar solvents such as ethanol increases (Figure 2) [22]. The aqueous solubility of ionizable CyD derivatives depends largely on the pH of the solution. Carboxymethylethyl-β-CyD (CME-β-CyD), in which hydroxyl groups of ethylated β-CyD are substituted with carboxymethyl groups, is only slightly soluble in the low pH region, but is freely soluble in neutral and alkaline regions, due to the ionization of the carboxyl group (pKa about 3–4) [25]. The sulfate esters of

CyDs are freely soluble in water since these compounds are ionized over a wide range of pH [27]. Obviously, the aqueous solubility of CyD derivatives can be controlled by choosing properly the ionizable group and the D.S.

CyD derivatives with hydrophobic substituents have increased surface activity and that activity is particularly high when hydrophobic regions of such substituents are terminally located. For example, 2-hydroxyethyl- (2-HE-), 3-hydroxypropyl- (3-HP-), and 2,3-dihydroxypropyl- (2,3-DHP-) β-CyDs have polar hydroxyl groups at the end of the substituents and show weaker surface activity than 2-HP-β-CyD or alkylated β-CyDs which have nonpolar groups in the terminal positions [16]. The hygroscopicity of CyD derivatives is usually lower than that of parent CyDs but at higher relative humidities (>90%) those CyD derivatives which have high aqueous solubility may liquefy—that is, compounds dissolve in the adsorbed water [16,28]. The viscosity of the aqueous CyD solutions increases exponentially with their concentration, and CyD derivatives have usually slightly higher viscosity than parent CyDs; the flow is Newtonian [16,29].

Although the α-1,4 glycosidic linkage of CyDs is fairly stable in an alkaline medium, strong aqueous acids hydrolyze it rapidly, with rates which depend on the size of the macrocycle and on its conformation. For example, the rate of the acid-catalyzed hydrolysis increases with an increase in the size of the macrocycle (γ- > β- > α-CyD), and the rate of hydrolysis of alkylated β-CyDs decreases in the order of heptakis(2,3,6-tri-O-methyl)-β-CyD (TM-β-CyD) > β-CyD > heptakis(2,6-di-O-methyl)-β-CyD (DM-β-CyD) > heptakis(2,6-di-O-ethyl)-β-CyD (DE-β-CyD) [4,21]. The permethylated CyDs are the most susceptible to the ring opening because of the markedly distorted ring conformation. Branched β-CyDs have three types of hydrolyzable glycosidic bonds,

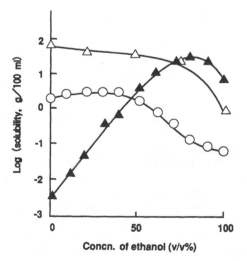

Figure 2. Solubilities of β-CyDs in the mixtures of water and ethanol at 25°C. ○: β-CyD, △: DM-β-CyD, ▲: DE-β-CyD.

i.e., α-1,4 bonds in the cycle, α-1,4 bonds in the substituent, and the α-1,6 bond between the cycle and substituent. Among these, the α-1,4 bond in the substituent, the linear bond, is the most susceptible to hydrolysis; the next to cleave is the cyclic α-1,4 bond, whereas the α-1,6 bond is the most resistant [18].

The glycosidic linkages of CyDs may also be cleaved by some of the starch-degrading enzymes with the proper substrate specificity. α-Amylase, which cleaves the endo type α-1,4 glycosidic bonds, hydrolyzes CyDs at rates much slower than those for amylose; the cleavage order then is γ- > β- > α-CyD. [18,30]. CyD derivatives such as alkylated and branched CyDs are more resistant than parent CyDs to the action of α-amylase, probably due to steric factors. The linear α-1,4 and the α-1,6 bonds of branched CyDs are hydrolyzed by glucoamylase and pullulanase, respectively; natural CyDs are completely resistant to these enzymes [18].

Since the macrocycle of CyDs is formed from optically active glucose units, the chirality of the guest molecule may affect formation of the respective inclusion complex. However, since the cavity of the macrocycle is round and symmetrical, the ability of CyDs to recognize chirality of the guest is relatively low. When all hydroxyl groups of CyDs are methylated, the ring conformation is markedly distorted and consequently the recognition ability is improved. For example, TM-β-CyD forms inclusion complexes with the S-enantiomer of flurbiprofen in a selective manner, whereas natural β-CyD forms complexes with both S- and R-enantiomers [31,32]. It may be noted that the anti-inflammatory activity of the S-enantiomer of flurbiprofen is higher than that of the R-enantiomer. Thus, chemical modifications of CyDs which lead to a distortion of the macrocycle improve the resolution of racemates through inclusion complexation, and such resolutions can improve pharmacological effects of the drugs.

Pharmacokinetics and Toxicity

To realize the potential of CyDs and their derivatives in pharmaceutical formulations, it is important to evaluate their relevant biological features. These include both their *in vivo* fate and their toxic effects. Unfortunately, only a few of the required studies have been done on CyD derivatives. No attempt has been made for a comprehensive evaluation and there are only preliminary results on the methylated and the hydroxyalkylated CyDs.

The metabolic fate of natural CyDs given orally has been thoroughly investigated and their lack of toxicity is well documented [33]. Following oral administration, CyDs are cleaved by salivary and pancreatic α-amylases but at a slower rate than the corresponding linear oligosaccharides [34]. Ultimately CyDs are converted into glucose and malto-oligomers by hydrolases of bacterial flora of the colon [35]; the larger

the macrocycle is, the easier is the amylolytic attack. Other studies have demonstrated that prolonged dietary intake of α-CyD, unlike that of β- and γ-CyDs, retards body weight gain and reduces lipid deposition in rats; α-CyD is highly indigestible and may act in the alimentary tract in the same manner as dietary fiber [36]. The metabolism of degraded CyDs is the same as starch and they are ultimately converted CO_2 and H_2O [37].

It is generally recognized that due to the bulky and hydrophilic nature of CyDs, gastrointestinal (GI) absorption in an intact form is very limited [3]. Only an insignificant amount of intact β-CyD was proven to be absorbed from the GI tract in rats [38,39]. On the other hand, the *ex vivo* studies in which the rat everted intestinal sac used have demonstrated that intact β-CyD indeed passes slowly through the intestinal wall by passive diffusion [40,41]. Futhermore, recent studies in which the *in situ* loop and single perfusion were used revealed that when the drug-β-CyD complex is introduced into the lumen of rat intestine, not only the drug but also some of the β-CyD can be detected in the circulating blood [42,43]. The effect of bile on the intestinal absorption of α-, β-, and γ-CyDs in rats were examined using the *in situ* loop recirculating perfusion technique [44]. Only very little of β- and γ-CyDs was absorbed by the intestinal segment when the bile duct was ligated. However, when sodium taurocholate, one of the major components of rat bile, was present, α-CyD was absorbed from the intestinal lumen and intact α-CyD entered the systemic circulation. For this uptake to occur *in vivo* quite specific, but realizable, conditions have to be met. The above observations clearly show that the possibility of intestinal absorption of trace amounts of CyDs in an intact form should not be totally discarded.

The chemical derivatization of CyDs transforms them into xenobiotics, and these may be expected to be more resistant to the intestinal hydrolases than the parent CyDs. The resistance to amylolytic degradation was studied for methylated CyDs [41], hydroxyalkylated CyDs [16], and branched CyDs [18]. When the modified CyDs are administered orally, their absorption is low and most of them finish intact in the feces [14,45].

The kinetics of disposition of CyDs after parenteral administration was also investigated [46,47]. Following intravenous administration to rats, the natural CyDs disappeared rapidly from the bloodstream and were excreted mainly through the kidney. α- and β-CyDs were excreted almost completely in intact form into the urine, while γ-CyD was degraded to a considerable extent [48]. A similar metabolic fate for γ-CyD, given intravenously, was also reported for rabbits and dogs [49]. Figure 3 shows the blood levels and the cumulative urinary excretion of β-, DM-β- and maltosyl-(G$_2$-)β-CyDs after administration by intravenous bolus injection to rats [48]. In spite of their quite different physicochemical properties, the total

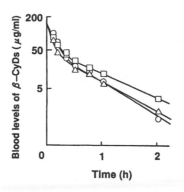
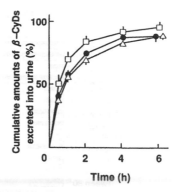

Figure 3. Blood levels and cumulative urinary excretion of β-CyDs following intravenous administration of β-CyDs (50 mg/kg) to rats. $\triangle$: β-CyD, $\square$: DM-β-CyD, $\bigcirc$: G_2-β-CyD, $\bullet$: G_1-β-CyD. Each value represents the mean $\pm$ S.E. of at least 3 rats.

body clearances and steady-state distribution volumes of these three β-CyD derivatives were quite similar. The renal clearance of these β-CyD derivatives was close to the renal glomerular filtration rate, indicating that there is no resistance to excretion of these compounds by the kidney. It is of interest that the rapid disappearance of G_2-β-CyD was accompanied by enzymatic conversion into glucosyl-(G_1-)-β-CyD and consequently the majority of the administered dose of G_2-β-CyD appeared as G_1-β-CyD in the urine. The preliminary pharmacokinetic profile of 2-HP-β-CyD in rats was also reported; the size-exclusion chromatography with post-column complexation was used for detection in that study [50].

The most serious drawback of the natural CyDs for parenteral use is their toxic effects on the kidney, which are particularly pronounced in the case of β-CyD [51,52]. The tendency of β-CyD to crystallize is probably the reason for its considerable renal toxicity; the crystallization may occur during the resorption process in the kidney, leading eventually to renal failure. The nephrotoxicity of β-CyD can be manipulated by chemical modifications. The acute and subchronic intravenous toxicity of hydrophilic CyD derivatives were reported to be insignificant and approaching that of sucrose [53,54]. Blood chemistry results after multiple intravenous administration of β-, DM-β-, and G_2-β-CyDs to rats shown in Figure 4 [48].

β-CyD at the total dose of 900 mg/kg induced nephrotoxicity, indicated by the increase in blood urea nitrogen (BUN) and creatinine. DM-β-CyD even at the lower doses (300 mg/kg) led to an increase in glutamate–pyruvate transaminase (GPT) and glutamate–oxaloacetate transaminase (GOT), indicating hepatic damage. This may impart to DM-β-CyD its relatively low LD_{50} value [7]. On the other hand, the blood chemistry values and histopathological examinations of rats receiving G_2-β-CyD at much higher doses remained within normal limits.

The interaction of CyDs with biological membranes has been studied with the intention of gaining a better

understanding of the biological effects of CyDs. CyDs were found to induce human erythrocytes to change their biconcave shape to monoconcave, and at higher concentrations induced the lysis. The hemolytic activity of natural CyDs was in the order of β- > α- > γ-CyD [55,56]. The observed differences in hemolysis must be due to the differential solubilization of membrane components by various CyDs. The process of solubilization occurred without entry of CyDs into the membranes, a mechanism of solubilization/lysis different from that of detergents, which enter the mem-

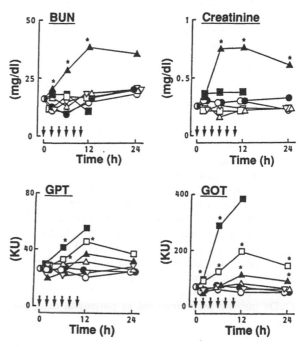

Figure 4. Effects of multiple intravenous administration of β-CyDs on blood chemistry values in rats. $\mathbb{O}$: control, $\triangledown$: saline, $\triangle$: β-CyD (50 mg/kg $\times$ 6), $\blacktriangle$: β-CyD (150 mg/kg $\times$ 6), $\square$: DM-β-CyD (50 mg/kg $\times$ 6), $\blacksquare$: DM-β-CyD (100 mg/kg $\times$ 6), $\bigcirc$: G_2-β-CyD (50 mg/kg $\times$ 6), $\bullet$: G_2-β-CyD (150 mg/kg $\times$ 6). *: $p < 0.05$ versus saline. Each value represents the mean of at least 3 rats.

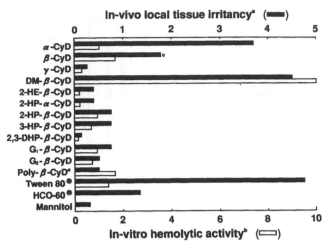

Figure 5. Relationship between *in vivo* local tissue irritancy and *in vitro* hemolytic activity for CyDs.

[a]Dose (100 mg/kg) injected into *M. vastus lateralis* of rabbits; the lesions of the muscle were evaluated as described [16].
[b]The reciprocal of the concentration (W/V[6]) of compounds to induce 50[6] lysis of human erythrocytes.
[c]Suspension.
[d]Water soluble β-CyD-epichlorohydrin polymer.

branes. Similar solubilization processes were found also for the CyD-induced lysis of the artificial membranes composed of lecithin and cholesterol [57].

When the character of the lipophilic cavity of CyDs is modified by chemical derivatization their effects on membranes can be dramatically changed. Furthermore, the introduction of amphiphatic characteristics by derivatization may lead to additional differences. Chemically modified CyDs were indeed found to affect the cell membranes in a manner different from that of parent CyDs [15,16,18,58]. Studies on the effects of solubilizers on membranes have direct relevancy to an important parameter in pharmaceutics—the *in vivo* local tissue irritancy. Figure 5 shows a positive correlation between *in vitro* hemolytic activity and *in vivo* local tissue irritancy for CyD derivatives [48]. Of the CyD derivatives studied, DM-β-CyD was the most irritant and thus large doses should be avoided in the parenteral formulations. On the other hand, the membrane interacting ability of DM-β-CyD may be used to enhance drug absorption by the mucosal membranes—a subject discussed in a later section. In contrast to that situation, hydrophilic CyD derivatives such as hydroxyalkylated and branched CyDs are non-irritant and since they are also less toxic than HCO-60®, a non-ionic surfactant widely used in parenteral formulations, hydrophilic CyDs may be recommended as parenteral drug carriers.

UTILITY OF CYCLODEXTRIN DERIVATIVES IN PHARMACEUTICAL FORMULATIONS

Chemical modifications of CyDs can alter their physicochemical properties, while their ability to

form complexes may be largely retained. The CyD derivatives thus may attain unique properties not available in their parent compounds, properties which increase their pharmaceutical potential. In this section some of the important effects of CyDs on drug properties, which can be modified by CyD derivatives, are described.

Solubilization Effects

In the process of solubilization through the formation of an inclusion complex the hydrophobic guest molecule is partially or totally contained in the hydrophobic cavity of the host molecule, which again has a hydrophilic outer surface. Thus, these CyD derivatives which have high aqueous solubility may be potent solubilizers for poorly water-soluble drugs.

The solubility of a drug usually increases with an increase in the amount of CyDs added in a linear or in a positively curved fashion. These types of solubilization were designated as A_L and A_P by Higuchi and Connors [59]. Nevertheless in many cases, as CyDs are added, the solubility of the drug rises only initially, then levels off and decreases, whereas a solid complex of the drug with CyD precipitates, a process designed as B_S type. The apparent stability constant (K_c) of the complex with a 1:1 (guest:host) stoichiometry can be calculated from the slope and intercept of the initial straight line portion of the A_L and B_S type diagrams, according to Equation (1) [59].

$$K_c = \frac{\text{slope}}{\text{intercept} (1 - \text{slope})} \qquad (1)$$

The stoichiometry of the solid complex can be deduced from the length of the plateau region of the B_S

type diagram or from the chemical analysis of the precipitated complex. The A_P type diagram is indicative of the formation of higher-order complexes and each stability constant can be calculated by analyzing the upward curvature by the iteration method.

Solubilization by natural CyDs may occur in any of the above three fashions (i.e., A_L, A_P, B_S), depending on the mutual fit of the host–guest molecules, on the thermodynamic stability of the complex, and on the intrinsic solubility of the complex. With hydrophilic CyD derivatives, the B_S type solubilization is quite rare, due to the low tendency of the water-soluble complexes to crystallize. Methylated CyDs produce the A_L and A_P type diagrams at lower temperature, whereas at higher temperature the B_S type is often observed [60,61]; that limits their use in aqueous injectable solutions which are to be heat-sterilized.

The solubilizing ability of CyD derivatives is related both to their ability to form inclusion complexes as well as to the intrinsic solubility of the host molecules in water. The former factor is reflected in the K_c values. Among β-CyD and its derivatives so far studied, DM-β-CyD shows the highest solubilizing effect for poorly water-soluble drugs. The enhanced inclusion ability of DM-β-CyD may be attributed to the elongation of the hydrophobic cavity in that compound; there is no distortion of the cyclic conformation. The inclusion ability of TM-β-CyD is generally weaker than that of the parent β-CyD, since its ring is distorted and there is additional steric hindrance by the methyl groups. The steric effects and hydrophobic character of the substituents also play a role in solubilizations by hydroxyalkylated CyDs. For example, 2-HP-β-CyDs, similarly to DM-β-CyD, have higher complexing ability towards steroid hormones, cardiac glycosides, dihydropyridine derivatives, and diazepam than β-CyD [15,20,62]; their solubilizing ability is again lowered at very high D.S., probably due to steric hindrance. The substituents of 2-HE-β-CyDs and 2,3-DHP-β-CyDs are relatively hydrophilic, and the complexing ability of these compounds is weaker than that of β-CyD and is further decreased when D.S. is increased [16]. Glucose and maltose units in branched β-CyDs seem to hinder the inclusion of drugs such as carmofur, diazepam, nifedipine (Figure 6), and phenytoin; the K_c values were found to decrease in the order of β-CyD > G_1-β-CyD > G_2-β-CyD > dimaltosyl-β-CyD [$(G_2)_2$-β-CyD] [18]. On the other hand, the affinity of steroidal drugs for branched CyDs is comparable or slightly higher than that of parent CyDs [63]. Hydrophilic CyD derivatives thus are of advantage in the solubilization of drugs; their intrinsic solubility is much higher than that of parent CyDs and no solid complexes precipitate even at higher CyD concentration. Futhermore, CME-β-CyD may be used as a pH-dependent solubilizer that may be targeted to the specific absorption site of the GI tract. That application is possible since the inclusion ability of CME-β-CyD is dependent on environmental pH.

Stabilization Effects

There are many examples demonstrating the stabilizing effect of CyDs on chemically labile drugs both in aqueous solutions and in solid state. However, it should be noted that some reactions are accelerated by CyD complexation. For example, hydrolysis of esters is sometimes accelerated by the catalytic action of the secondary hydroxyl groups of CyDs which act as nucleophiles [64]. Therefore, chemical modification of the hydroxyl groups may be useful even from the viewpoint of drug stabilization.

Stabilization Effects in Solution

The stabilizing effect of CyDs on labile drugs depends both upon the decomposition rate constant (k_c) of the drug in the complexed state and upon the corresponding K_c value; that is a consequence of equilibrium existing in solutions between free and complexed drug. Chemical modifications of CyDs affect both of these parameters. Digitoxin, a potent cardiac glycoside, is susceptible to hydrolysis in an acidic medium. The acid hydrolysis of digitoxin is suppressed by the addition of CyD derivatives in the order of DM-β-CyD > 2-HP-β-CyD > 2-HE-β-CyD > β-CyD > TM-β-CyD [65]. Stabilization by DM-β-CyD (over 2400 times deceleration) is higher than that by β-CyD (100 times) and that difference can be attributed to the protection of the sensitive junction of the steroid and carbohydrate moieties of digitoxin and to the absence of some of the CyD hydroxyl groups which may act as nucleophiles. A similar decelerating mechanism is operative also in the acid-catalyzed hydrolysis of prostacyclin [66] and in the base-catalyzed hydrolysis of carmofur (HCFU), an anti-cancer agent [67]. In the isomerization of E-type prostaglandins (PGEs), the hydroxyl groups of natural β-CyD act as a general base and accelerate the reaction. In methylated β-CyDs part of these catalytic groups is blocked and this derivative decelerates the isomerization of PGEs [68]. In TM-β-CyD all the catalytic groups are blocked but the deceleration of

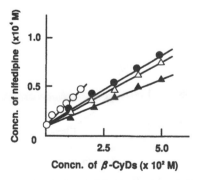

Figure 6. Phase solubility diagrams of nifedipine-branched β-CyD systems in water at 25°C. $\bigcirc$: β-CyD, $\bullet$: G_1-β-CyD, $\triangle$: G_2-β-CyD, $\blacktriangle$: $(G_2)_2$-β-CyD.

PGE isomerization by that derivative is smaller than that by DM-β-CyD—a consequence of lower stability of TM-β-CyD complexes. CME-β-CyD is very effective in inhibiting the decomposition of PGEs [48], since some of the hydroxyl groups of the host are blocked and since CME-β-CyD functions as a buffer keeping the pH values between 4–5, at which acidity PGEs are stable.

Inclusion complexation with CyD derivatives also affects the photoreactivity of drugs. β-CyDs accelerate the dechlorination of chlorpromazine to promazine while they inhibit other side reactions which give toxic products, such as oxidation and polymerization [69]. The changes in rates of these photoreactions follow the order DM-β-CyD > β-CyD > TM-β-CyD, which corresponds to the stability of respective complexes. DM-β-CyD also inhibits other photodecompositions such as the decarboxylation of benoxaprofen [70], the oxidation of nifedipine [16], the dimerization of protriptyline [71] and tranilast [48], and the E-Z isomerization in the cinnamic acid moiety of OKY-046, a thromboxane synthetase inhibitor [48].

Stabilization Effects in Solid State

The stabilization of drugs by CyDs in the solid state is somewhat different from that seen in solution since other physicochemical factors, such as phase transition, hygroscopicity and crystallinity, play a role. For example, the hydrolysis of HCFU in solution is inhibited by inclusion complexation with natural β-CyD, whereas in the solid complex it proceeds about 160 times faster than in drug alone; compared at 70°C and 75% R.H. This is due to the high hygroscopicity of natural β-CyD; i.e., the complex takes up water from the atmosphere and the drug is readily hydrolyzed after a partial dissolution in the adsorbed water. On the other hand, since methylated β-CyDs are less hygroscopic than β-CyD, these derivatives are highly effective in preventing the decomposition of HCFU in the solid state [67]. CME-β-CyD is useful in stabiliz-

ing PGEs in the solid state or in ointment base (Figure 7), due to its dual mode of protection described above [48].

Some drugs which are viscous can be converted into powders through inclusion complexation and hence stabilized. ONO-802, a PGE$_1$ derivative with a high uterine-contracting ability, was stabilized in such a manner [72].

CyD complexes are susceptible to phase transitions between the amorphous and crystalline states. Complexes of natural CyDs convert easily from the amorphous to crystalline states, especially when R.H. is increased or temperature is decreased, and *vice versa*. This transition affects many properties which are important in pharmaceutical applications—such as chemical stability, solubility, dissolution rate, mixing, flow and compression characteristics. On the other hand, hydroxyalkylated- and CME-CyDs form stable amorphous complexes with crystalline drugs, since the multi-component character of these hosts prevents any crystallization process [19]. In our recent results [48], nifedipine was easily converted to amorphous complexes with 2-HP-β-CyD and CME-β-CyD, and the transition to the crystalline complex was considerably slower than that of the β-CyD complex. These amorphous CyD derivatives may be more useful than the natural CyDs for suppression of polymorphic transition, sublimation, and whisker growth which may occur in various drug formulations.

Improvement of Bioavailability

The highly hydrophilic nature of methylated, hydroxyalkylated, and branched CyDs makes these compounds useful for improving the rate and extent of absorption of poorly water-soluble drugs. The resulting pharmaceutical preparation can be administered by the oral, rectal, percutaneous, or parenteral route. In this section, findings on enhanced drug absorption by the hydrophilic CyDs will be discussed.

Preparations for Oral Administration

The oral bioavailability of poorly water-soluble drugs may often be improved by hydrophilic CyDs, and that improvement is due to the increase in the dissolution rate of the drug. The overall process of drug absorption from its inclusion complex can be described by the scheme in Figure 8 [4]. When the complex is administered orally, the drug is absorbed only after the complex is dissociated, since only the free form of drug can penetrate the lipid barrier of the GI tract [44]. The absorption of a drug from its complex is therefore dependent on the stability constant (K_c) and the dissolution rate (k_c) of the complex; high dissolution rates and low complex stabilities favor free drug and absorption.

The inclusion complexes of drugs with hydrophilic CyD derivatives dissolve more rapidly than those of natural CyDs, and that leads to better drug absorp-

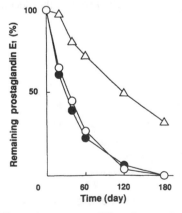

Figure 7. Effects of CyDs on stability of prostaglandin E_1 (0.01 W/W%) in FAPG ointment; measured at 40°C and 75% R.H. ○: prostaglandin E_1 alone, ●: β-CyD complex, △: CME-β-CyD complex.

tion. Results fully confirming this view were obtained in the enhancement of the absorption of fat-soluble vitamins such as α-tocopheryl esters [73], menaquinone-4 (vitamin K_2 analog) [74], and ubidecarenone (coenzyme Q_{10}) [75] by DM-β-CyD. As shown in Figure 9, when equivalent doses of menaquinone-4 were administered to fasting dogs, the rapid-dissolving form of the inclusion complex gave about 17-fold higher maximum plasma levels (C_{max}) than that of drug alone. The area under the plasma concentration–time curve (AUC) of the complex was about 20 times as great as that of drug alone [74].

Since the pharmacological response to a drug is usually a function of the drug concentration, the higher blood levels attained after the administration of inclusion complex should result in a more intensive response than that observed after dosing with the drug alone. This is illustrated by the potentiation of the hypnotic effect of barbiturate [76], the hypoglycemic effect of acetohexamide [77], the vasoconstrictor activity of glucocorticoid [78], and shortening of the blood-clotting time of menaquinone-4 (Table 3) [30]. We have recently demonstrated that the antitumor activity of orally administered HCFU against P-388 leukemia in mice was enhanced about 3 times by DM-β-CyD complexation [79]; the antitumor activity in that case was evaluated by the increase in survival time over controls.

Preparations for Rectal Administration

Hydrophilic CyDs can also be used to improve the rectal bioavailability of drugs which are poorly soluble in water. Enhanced absorption in that case is due both to the faster release of the drug and to lowering of affinity of complexed drug to the suppository base. An *in vitro* release study revealed that release rates of flurbiprofen [80], HCFU [81], ethyl 4-biphenyl acetate [82], etc. from hydrophobic suppository bases were markedly enhanced by methylated CyDs. In the case of ethyl 4-biphenyl acetate, an anti-inflammatory drug, the release rate from Witepsol H_5 suppositories

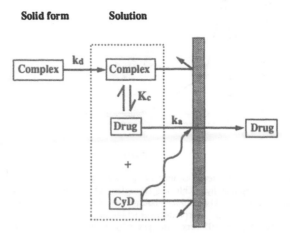

GI tract   **Biomembrane**   **Systemic circulation**

Figure 8. Absorption of a drug from its CyD complex. k_d: dissolution rate constant, K_c: stability constant, k_c: absorption rate constant.

increased in the order of β-CyD complex < DM-β-CyD complex < 2-HP-β-CyD complex, and the serum level of 4-biphenylyl acetic acid after rectal administration of the 2-HP-β-CyD complex was the highest. The lower effects observed for DM-β-CyD complex may be due to its high affinity for hydrophobic base.

Absorption of water-soluble drugs was also improved when these were rectally administered simultaneously with CyDs. Hollow cylinders of Witepsol H_{15} were used to make morphine hydrochloride containing suppositories. As shown in Figure 10, the plasma morphine levels in rabbits were increased significantly when α- and β-CyDs were included. Interestingly, no effects were observed for γ-CyD and 2-HP-β-CyD, whereas CyD polymers and hydrophobic CyDs retarded the plasma levels of morphine [48].

Table 3. Effect of menaquinone-4 and its DM-β-CyD complex on recovery of coagulation times following the warfarin-induced hypoprothrombinemia in dogs.

System	TPCA 60[a] (h)
Control	36.6 ± 0.9
Menaquinone-4 (i.v.)[b]	0.9 ± 0.1
Menaquinone-4 (p.o.)[c,d]	27.0 ± 4.2
DM-β-CyD complex (p.o.)[c]	3.3 ± 1.1

[a]Time required for prothrombin complex activity to return to 60%. Each value represents the mean ± S.E. of 4 dogs.
[b]Dose (13 mg of drug) administered intravenously.
[c]Dose (60 mg of drug or of the equivalent amount of the complex) administered orally.
[d]Diluent: starch.

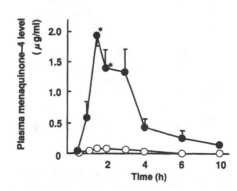

Figure 9. Plasma levels of menaquinone-4 following the oral administration of menaquinone-4 (60 mg) or of the equivalent amount of its DM-β-CyD complex to dogs. ○: menaquinone-4 alone, ●: DM-β-CyD complex. *: $p < 0.05$ versus menaquinone-4 alone. Each value represents the mean ± S.E. of 6 dogs.

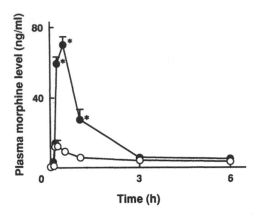

Figure 10. Plasma levels of morphine following rectal administration of morphine hydrochloride (1 mg/kg) or of the equivalent amount of its α-CyD complex in hollow-type Witepsol H_{15} suppository to rabbits. $\bigcirc$: morphine hydrochloride alone, $\bullet$: α-CyD complex. *: $p < 0.05$ versus morphine hydrochloride alone. Each value represents the mean $\pm$ S.E. of 3 rabbits.

Preparations for Topical Administration

The effects of CyDs in preparations for topical use have been evaluated both *in vitro* and *in vivo*. The *in vitro* release rate of corticosteroids from water-containing ointments (e.g., with a hydrophilic, absorptive, or polyacrylic base) was significantly increased by β- and γ-CyDs, whereas in other ointments (FAPG and macrogol ointments) CyDs retarded the release [83]. The enhanced release of the drug was probably due to the increase in its solubility, diffusibility, and concentration in the water phase of the ointment.

In ointments, similarly to suppositories, the drug in the CyD complex may be displaced by some components of the ointment. To minimize such displace-

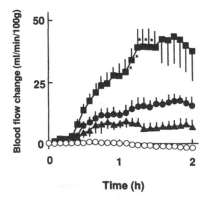

Figure 11. Blood flow in skin of hairless mice following topical application of FAPG ointments containing combinations of prostaglandin E_1 (1 μg), the equivalent amount of its CyD complexes, and HPE-101 (0.3 mg). $\bigcirc$: prostaglandin E_1 alone, $\bullet$: prostaglandin E_1 with HPE-101, $\blacktriangle$: β-CyD complex with HPE-101, $\blacksquare$: CME-β-CyD complex with HPE-101. *: $p < 0.05$ versus prostaglandin E_1 with HPE-101. Each value represents the mean $\pm$ S.E. of 5 mice.

ment, it would be advantageous to use a complex with a large stability constant [84]. Cyclodextrins may also form complexes with components of the tissue, and recently it has been reported that methylated CyDs extract some of the components of membranes, a process that leads to modification of the skin barrier and enhances drug absorption *in vitro* [85]. However, pretreatments of rabbit skin with DM-β-CyD *in vivo* did not markedly alter the absorption rate of drug from the ointment preparations [86]. Therefore, the superior percutaneous drug absorption attained by DM-β-CyD *in vivo* would have to be due to the improved dissolution and solubility of the drug in ointment and to the lower exchange of guest compounds in the complexes, rather than to the direct interaction of methylated CyD with skin. 2-HP-β-CyD also enhances the percutaneous absorption of 4-biphenylyl acetic acid and its ethyl esters *in vivo*, promoting an increase in the anti-inflammatory effect on carrageenan induced edema in rats [87].

We have recently demonstrated that CME-β-CyD is particularly useful in stabilizing PGE_1 in the modified FAPG ointment base. In that work the pharmaceutical effects of PGE_1 and its β- and CME-β-CyD complexes in the ointments also containing a novel absorption promoter, 1-[2-(decylthio)-ethyl]aza-cyclo-pentane-2-one (HPE-101), were evaluated by a non-invasive laser Doppler velocimetry in hairless mice. As shown in Figure 11, PGE_1 the therapeutic effect of PGE_1—the increase in blood flow through the cutaneous microvasculature, increased in the order of PGE_1: β-CyD $< PGE_1$ alone $< PGE_1$:CME-β-CyD. These effects were dependent on the absorption promoter; in its absence complexation was ineffective. The enhanced pharmacological response observed for the combination of PGE_1 with CME-β-CyD and with the absorption promoter may be due to the greater penetration and accumulation of the drug into the skin.

Preparations for Parenteral Administration

Although little is known about the effect of natural CyDs on the disposition of drug in the body [7], particular attention should be given to the equilibria that affect the inclusion complexes after these are injected. In this regard, comparison of the effects of CyDs on pharmacokinetics of prednisolone after the intramuscular or intravenous administration is instructive [88]. When the drug was administered to rabbits intramuscularly, the pharmacokinetic behavior of the drug and its complexes was quite different. Administration of CyD complexes of prednisolone in the form of a suspension resulted in an increase in the rate and the extent of absorption, and in the reduction of mean residence time (MRT) of prednisolone compared to drug-only administration. Rapid dissolution of the drug from the complex obviously overcomes the negative effect of the poor permeability of the bulky complex in the muscle. On the other hand, when the complex was intramuscularly injected as a solution, the length of time to reach the maximum serum level (t_{max}) of prednisolone was increased, but otherwise no difference in AUC and MRT values between the drug alone and its complex was observed. The observed initial delay of the drug absorption may be due to the poor diffusibility of the bulky complex in the muscular tissue. When prednisolone was injected intravenously, the differences between the pharmacokinetic parameters of prednisolone and its CyD complexes were only small. The large volume of plasma diluted the complex and increased its dissociation and release of free drug; furthermore, some biological components in the circulatory system may have competed for the CyD cavity, which may have further increased the dissociation of the complex.

The dissolution rate of nimodipine, a calcium antagonist of a dihydropyridine type derivative, is markedly enhanced by the formation of an inclusion complex with 2-HP-β-CyD [89]. Figure 12 shows the plasma levels of nimodipine in rabbits, following the intramuscular injection of the corresponding suspensions. The AUC and C_{max} values for the nimodipine:2-HP-β-CyD complex were about 2.5 times higher than those of the drug alone. In addition, 2-HP-β-CyD significantly reduced the muscular damage caused by the injection of the drug. Thus, hydroxyalkylated β-CyDs, due to their complexing ability, low toxicity, and high water solubility, may be very useful in parenteral formulations [14–16,19]. Bodor et al. recently reported that 2-HP-β-CyD is an excellent excipient for solubilizing and stabilizing various brain-targeting chemical delivery systems (CDS) [20,90]. In that system, a lipophilic, biooxidizable molecular carrier (dihydropyridine) is covalently linked to the drug; when drug-carrier conjugate enters the brain an oxidation to pyridinium–drug conjugate occurs which, due to its polarity, cannot cross the blood–brain barrier and must remain in the brain.

The dihydropyridine–drug conjugates usually are insoluble in water and autooxidize easily. Complex formation with 2-HP-β-CyD resulted in a dramatic increase in water solubility and in the chemical stability of estradiol–dihydropyridine conjugate. In a Phase I clinical study, that formulation was without adverse effects and significant LH suppression was observed consistent with the estrogenic activity in brain [54].

Control of Release

Many attempts have been made to prepare sustained-release, delayed-release, pH-independent-release, prolonged-release, or zero-order-release oral preparations, particularly for water-soluble drugs which have only short biological half-lives. There is a definitive clinical need for such preparations; they may prevent high plasma drug levels, reduce side effects and the amount of drugs administered. Patient compliance and convenience is also improved if a minimum number of doses has to be administered. A suitable

combination of hydrophilic, hydrophobic, and ionizable drug carriers may be of help in the development of such controlled-release preparations.

Sustained-Release

When a drug forms a complex with ethylated CyDs, its aqueous solubility decreases proportionally to the degree of substitution of the CyD [22]. Thus ethylated CyDs may be used to control the release rate of water-soluble drugs and as candidates for the hydrophobic drug carrier in sustained-release type preparations. The *in vitro* dissolution rates of water-soluble drugs, diltiazem hydrochloride, propranolol hydrochloride, isosorbide dinitrate, cimetidine, 5-fluorouracil, theophylline, and others were found to be significantly modified by complexation with ethylated β-CyDs, making preparations of the sustained-release forms feasible [6,23,26].

The release rate of theophylline can be prolonged by the combination of hydrophilic and hydrophobic β-CyD derivatives. As shown in Figure 13, near-constant drug concentrations in plasma of dogs were maintained for at least 12 h after the oral administration of double layer tablets which contained β-CyD complex as a fast-release component and a mixture of DE-β-CyD and CME-β-CyD complexes as a slow-release component [48].

Delayed-Release

The introduction of carboxymethyl groups onto the remaining hydroxyls of ethylated β-CyD to produce CME-β-CyD confers on the product the pH-dependent solubility, while the inclusion ability is sustained. Such derivatives may be used to control the release rate of water-soluble drugs, which is regulated by the pH of the GI fluids. In the case of CME-β-CyD complex, the release rate of water-soluble drugs can be suppressed at low pH regions in the stomach (pH about 1.2), while increased at intestinal pH (about

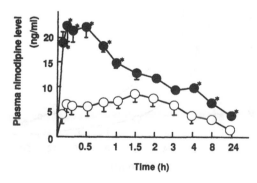

Figure 12. Plasma levels of nimodipine following intramuscular administration of suspensions of nimodipine (5 mg/kg) or of the equivalent amount of its 2-HP-β-CyD complex to rabbits. $\bigcirc$: nimodipine alone, $\bullet$: 2-HP-β-CyD complex. *: $p < 0.05$ versus nimodipine alone. Each value represents the mean ± S.E. of 5 rabbits.

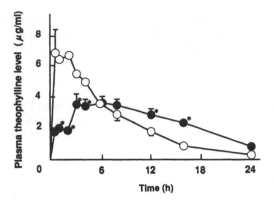

Figure 13. Plasma levels of theophylline following oral administration of tablets containing theophylline (100 mg) or the eqvuialent amount of its β-CyD complexes to dogs. $\bigcirc$: conventional tablet (diluent: starch), $\bullet$: double layer tablet β-CyD complex/(DE-β-CyD complex:CME-βCyD complex, 1:3) = 1/3. *: $p < 0.05$ versus conventional tablet. Each value represents the mean $\pm$ S.E. of 4 dogs.

6.8), when the carboxyl groups of the host molecule are ionized. The expected delay in absorption was clearly seen in the plasma levels of diltiazem, a potent calcium antagonist, after oral administration of the tablet containing CME-β-CyD complex to dogs (Figure 14) [25]. Thus, CME-β-CyD may serve as a delayed-release type carrier for water-soluble drugs that are (a) unstable in the stomach, (b) absorbed mainly from the intestinal tract, and (c) irritate the gastric mucosa.

pH-Independent-Release

When the stomach is one of the important absorption sites, there should be no lag-time in the drug release from its dosage form there. This type of dosage form is required for loop diuretics, such as furosemide and piretanide, in which a significant release of drug in the stomach is required to give a balanced bioavailability. To control the release rate of piretanide, a double-layer tablet was designed consisting of a fast-dissolving fraction and slow-release fraction. Water-soluble β-CyD derivatives were used for a fast-release fraction which improved the dissolution of the un-ionized form of piretanide in the acidic pH region, whereas cellulose derivatives such as hydroxypropylcellulose (HPC) and ethylcellulose (EC) were used for a pH-independent slow-release fraction of the tablet. From the survey of the release rates as a function of pH of the dissolution medium, the above combination gave an initial rapid dissolution and then an acceptable slow-release over 8 h which was independent of the pH values of 1.2–6.8 [91].

Detoxication

CyDs can be used to reduce the local tissue toxicity of drugs. Local toxicity of drugs is in large part caused by the effects of drugs on the cell membrane. The molecular entrapment of drugs into the CyD cavity may prevent direct contact of a drug with biological surfaces and both the drug-entry into cells of non-targeted tissues and the local irritation are thus decreased. Detoxication of drugs obtained by procedures not involving CyDs is inevitably associated with some loss of therapeutic efficacy since beneficial and toxic effects of drugs usually arise from a similar pharmacological action. These losses do not occur when the reversible inclusion complexation of drugs is used. CyDs act as wafer-like carriers which decrease the drug-induced local tissue damage at the administration site and then deliver the drug close to the site of its action.

In drug delivery of that type, the complex eventually fully dissociates into its components in a manner which depends upon the magnitude of the respective stability constant, and thus there is no drastic loss of the therapeutic benefits of the drugs.

The lysis of human erythrocytes induced *in vitro* by drugs has been generally used to predict the local tissue irritancy of the drugs *in vivo*. CyDs can protect erythrocytes against the hemolysis induced by various drugs including neuroleptics [92,93], anti-inflammatory drugs [94], and antibiotics [95]. This protection was found to be due to the reduction in effective concentrations of drugs in contact with the membrane, rather than the direct stabilizing effects on the memrane [96].

Examples of the reduction of local irritancy of drugs by CyDs *in vivo* follow. CyDs alleviate muscular tissue damage following the intramuscular injection of drugs [89,95,97]. The protective effects of CyDs may be attributed mainly to the poor affinity of the hydrophilic complexes of drugs to the sarcolemma membranes of muscle fibers—a situation expected from the results of *in vitro* hemolysis studies. Similarly, CyDs were found to diminish the ulcerogenic potency of several acidic anti-inflammatory drugs when these were administered orally [98]. A similar

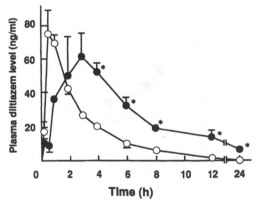

Figure 14. Plasma levels of diltiazem following oral administration of tablets containing diltiazem (30 mg) or the equivalent amount of its CME-β-CyD complex to dogs. $\bigcirc$: diltiazem alone, $\bullet$: CME-β-CyD complex. *: $p < 0.05$ versus diltiazem alone. Each value represents the mean $\pm$ S.E. of 4 dogs.

protection by CyDs after rectal and ocular administrations of drugs, was also described [82,94]. For example, 2-HP-β-CyD significantly reduced the irritancy of ethyl 4-biphenylyl acetate to the rectal mucosa (Figure 15), and also improved the bioavailability of the drug in the oleaginous suppository (the section "Preparations for Rectal Administration"); β-CyD and DM-β-CyD were less effective in that case.

Cutaneous contact photosensitization, due to phenothiazines, is known to cause severe problems to workers in manufacturing, to medical personnel, and to others who handle these drugs. Such unintentional exposure to these drugs has almost disappeared since the introduction of modified dosage forms such as the coated tablets and dispensable medication cups. However, this problem has not been solved satisfactorily for the injectable formulations. Our recent studies have demonstrated that the phototoxic and photoallergic potential of chlorpromazine (CPZ) can be reduced by the simultaneous topical use of CyDs [99,100]. As shown in Figure 16, the photoallergic skin reactions due to CPZ in sensitized guinea pigs were significantly reduced by β- and DM-β-CyDs, the latter being more effective. Upon binding to β-CyDs, the entry of CPZ into the skin is decreased; furthermore, the photochemical reactivity of the drug may be altered and combination of these factors may lead to the observed desensitization.

A few examples of the reduction in the drug-induced systemic toxicity by CyDs are available. The addition of β-CyD to dialysis fluids accelerated the removal of phenobarbital by peritoneal dialysis, thereby being effective in the treatment of drug overdoses [101]. A retinal-dextran conjugate solubilized by β-CyD was reported to be less cytotoxic and retained the ability to inhibit the growth of cancer cells [102]. CyDs are useful not only in the administration of drugs, but also in redistributing either endogenous or exogenous highly lipophilic compounds in the body. In such a case, CyDs may act as an artificial circulating carrier for the lipophiles. Intravenous administration of DM-β-CyD has been shown to rescue mice from poisoning by retinoic acid [103]. A similar rescue procedure using 2-HP-β-CyD was used successfully on a patient with familial hypervitaminosis A [104]. In this first-final clinical trial, 2-HP-β-CyD solution was infused intravenously, leading to a dramatic increase in retinyl esters in serum and to an appearance of retinoids in urine. Thus, the overload of retinyl esters, which are insoluble in water, was reduced in the patient's liver. During infusion of 2-HP-β-CyD into that patient, a change in serum cholesterol was also observed. Following that lead the effects of CyDs administered intravenously to hereditary hyperlipidemic rabbits were investigated [105]. A single administration of 2-HP-β-CyD transiently decreased the serum level of cholesterol, while its multiple injections led to a gradual rise in the serum cholesterol, and eventually to some relief in atherosclerotic lesions in the thoracic aorta. These rescue

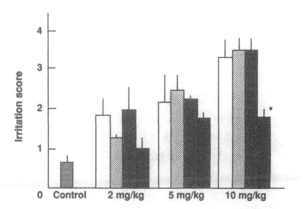

Figure 15. Irritation effects of ethyl 4-biphenylyl acetate and its β-CyD complexes in Witepsol H$_{15}$ suppository on rectal mucosa 10 h after administration to rats.

☐ : ethyl 4-biphenylyl acetate alone

▨ : β-CyD complex

▦ : DM-β-CyD complex

■ : 2-HP-β-CyD complex.

*: $p < 0.05$ versus ethyl 4-biphenylyl acetate alone. Each value represents the mean ± S.E. of 5 rats.

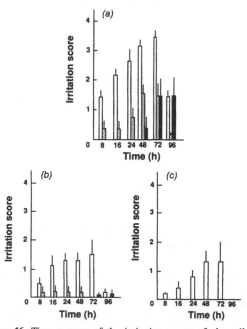

Figure 16. Time courses of the irritation scores of photoallergic skin reactions to chlorpromazine hydrochloride (0.15 μmol) with or without β-CyDs (0.30 μr mol) in the chloropromazine-sensitized guinea pigs.

☐ : erythema

▨ : edema

■ : eschar

(a) without CyDs, (b) with β-CyD, (c) with DM-β-CyD. Each value represents the mean ± S.E. of 5 guinea pigs which had a positive response.

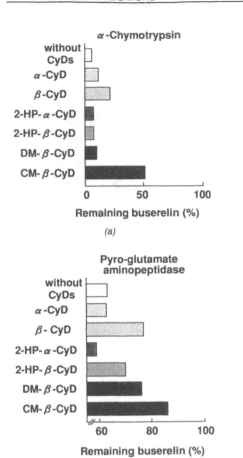

Figure 17. Effects of CyDs (8 mM) on the enzymatic degradation of buserelin acetate (80 nM) in isotonic phosphate buffer (pH 7.4) at 37°C. (a) after 40 min incubation, (b) after 4 h incubation.

therapies using CyDs are encouraging, but obviously the process will have to be further optimized before beginning practical application.

Use in Pharmaceutical Preparations Containing Peptides or Proteins

In recent years, great advances have been made in biotechnology and genetic engineering and thus sufficient quantities of various biologically active peptides and proteins have become available. Some of these products are already in clinical trials and will be approved as drugs. However, there are considerable hurdles in the path to their practical use—chemical and biological instability, poor absorption through biological membranes, rapid plasma clearance, a peculiar dose–response curve, and immunogenicity. Several attempts have been made to address these problems by chemical modifications of peptides and proteins, and by co-administration of adjuvants which would promote absorption of peptides and proteins

and protect them from proteolytic enzymes. The CyD complexations seem to be an attractive alternative to these approaches, but this field is still in its beginning.

Molecules of many peptides and proteins are too hydrophilic and bulky to be wholly included in the CyD cavity, thus their interactions with CyDs could be only local, that is, the hydrophobic side chains may form inclusion complexes with CyDs [106,107]. Our recent studies using ^{1}H- and ^{13}C-NMR have shown that β- and DM-β-CyDs interact with buserelin acetate (LHRH analogue, BLA); in that peptide the side chains of tryptophan and tyrosine form complexes with β-CyDs [48]. Interactions of that type may affect the overall three-dimensional structure of peptides or inhibit their intermolecular association and thus change somewhat their chemical and biological properties.

Currently, peptide and protein drugs are administered parenterally. A potential use of 2-HP-β-CyD in the parenteral formulations of these drugs has been recently reviewed [54]. In this review solubilization, prevention of aggregation, and chemical stabilization of peptide and protein drugs are described and occur without any loss of their biological activity. Our recent studies have demonstrated that CyDs are able to stabilize several drugs of the peptide and protein class against chemical and enzymatic degradation. The potency of α-CyD and its derivatives in stabilizing human interferon-β in the aqueous solution is comparable to that of human serum albumin, which is presently used as a stabilizer in several commercially available pharmaceutical preparations of peptide drugs. Buserelin acetate (BLA) was found to be significantly stabilized against α-chymotrypsin and pyro-glutamate aminopeptidase by chemically modified CyDs, especially by CM-β-CyD (Figure 17). Moreover, the degradation of BLA, when incubated with rat nasal and rectal membrane homogenates, was found to be retarded by CyDs; again CM-β-CyD was the most effective [48].

Unfortunately, chronic treatment with parenteral dosage forms of peptide and protein drugs is inconvenient and is often associated with poor acceptance by patients. Therefore, increasing attention has been given to the development of drug delivery systems for peptide drugs with controlled-release features. For example, the sustained-release type oily injection of BLA can be prepared by complexation with hydrophobic DE-β-CyD [24]. A single subcutaneous injection of the oily suspension containing the BLA:DE-β-CyD complex into rats provided a continuous plasma level of drug, giving to the complexed BLA a mean residence time in plasma about 70 times longer than that for BLA alone. When the complexed form of BLA was used, the pharmacological effect, as indicated by a suppression of plasma endogenous testosterone levels, lasted for at least one month (Figure 18) [108]. In addition, CyDs, like other macromolecules and surfactants, could prevent adsorption or peptides by the walls of plastic- or glass-made containers and devices, thereby permitting administration of these drugs at accurate dosing levels.

Practical acceptance of peptides and proteins as drugs will be eased considerably by the development of viable non-parenteral delivery systems as established by nasal, rectal, transdermal, pulmonary, vaginal, ophthalmic, buccal, and even oral administrations. The bioavailability by these routes, however, is severely restricted by poor membrane permeability and by the pre-systemic elimination by enzymatic hydrolysis. α-CyD was reported to remove some fatty acids in the nasal epithelium and to improve the absorption of peptides through the nasal mucosa [109]. A similar improvement in the delivery of cyclosporin to the cornea by α-CyD has also been recently reported [110]. The combination effect of α-CyD with absorption promoters such as sodium glycocholate or Azone® on the nasal absorption of human interferon-β has also been described [111,112]. With the above findings in mind, we evaluated the possibility of using chemically modified CyDs as a better adjuvant for enhancement of the absorption of peptides through mucosal membranes. From the compounds tested, DM-β-CyD had the best enhancing effect on the nasal absorption of insulin (Figure 19). Modified CyDs were also found to enhance the nasal absorption of BLA. It is interesting to note that the onset of enhanced absorption of that peptide by CM-β-CyD tends to be delayed [48]. The enhancing effects of CyDs on the nasal absorption of these peptides may be attributed not only to their effects on the mucosal membrane, but also to their inhibiting effects on proteolytic enzymes present there.

The limited evidence suggests that CyDs have a potential to eliminate some undesirable features of peptide and protein drugs and that this strategy may replace less suitable and more complex modes of peptide administration.

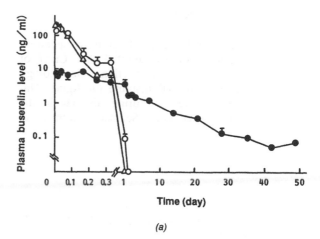

(a)

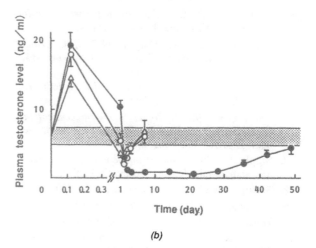

(b)

Figure 18. Plasma levels of buserelin (a) and testosterone (b) following subcutaneous administration of buserelin acetate (1 mg/kg) or of the equivalent amount of DE-β-CyD complex to rats. ○: buserelin acetate in aqueous solution, △: buserelin acetate in oily suspension, ●: DE-β-CyD complex in oily suspension. Each value represents the mean ± S.E. of 5 rats.

CONCLUSION

During the past decades there has been an increasing interest in optimizing the efficacy of drug activities through the use of rationally designed delivery systems. The CyD derivatives described here have many advantages as novel drug carriers in advanced dosage forms. To obtain all the advantages of the chemically modified CyDs in drug formulation, high standards on their safety, lack of toxicity, pharmaceutical quality, etc. must be set. Futhermore, particular attention should be directed toward the studies of dissociation equilibria of the inclusion complexes in body fluids as well as in pharmaceutical preparations. The future will without doubt bring safer and more effective CyD derivatives and these will become effective tools in the pharmaceutical field.

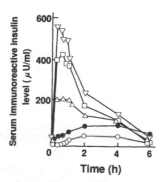

Figure 19. Serum levels of immunoreactive insulin following nasal administration of insulin (10 U/kg) with or without CyDs (80 mM) to rats. ○: without CyDs, △: with α-CyD, □: with DM-α-CyD, ●: with 2-HP-α-CyD, △: with DM-β-CyD. Each value represents the mean of 6 rats.

ACKNOWLEDGEMENT

The authors gratefully acknowledge the cooperation and encouragement of Dr. Josef Pitha, Chief of Macromolecular Chemistry Section, Gerontology Research Center, National Institute on Aging, National Institutes of Health, during his stay in the Faculty of Pharmaceutical Sciences, Kumamoto University.

REFERENCES

1. Saenger, W. 1980. *Angew. Chem. Int. Ed. Engl.*, 19:344–362.

2. Uekama, K. 1981. *Yakugaku Zasshi*, 101:857–873.

3. Szejtli, J. 1982. *Cyclodextrins and Their Inclusion Complexes*. Akadémiai Kiadó, Budapest.

4. Uekama, K. and M. Otagiri. 1987. *CRC Critical Reviews in Therapeutic Drug Carrier Systems*. Boca Raton: CRC Press, Inc., 1:1–40.

5. Duchene, D. 1987. *Cyclodextrins and Their Industrial Uses*. Paris: Editions de Santé.

6. Uekama, K. 1987. In *Topics in Pharmaceutical Sciences 1987*. D. D. Breimer, P. Speiser, eds. Amsterdam: Elsevier Sci. Pub., pp. 181–194.

7. Szejtli, J. 1988. *Cyclodextrin Technology*. Dordrecht, the Netherlands: Kluwer Academic Publishers.

8. Szejtli, J. 1983. *J. Incl. Phenom.*, 1:135–150.

9. Uekama, K. 1985. *Pharm. Int.*, 6:61–65.

10. Hinze, W. L. 1981. *Sep. Purif. Methods*, 10:159–237.

11. Harata, K., K. Uekama, M. Otagiri and F. Hirayama. 1984. *J. Incl. Phenom.*, 1:279–293.

12. Croft, A. P. and R. A. Bartsch. 1983. *Tetrahedron*, 39:1417–1474.

13. Müller, B. W. and U. Brauns. 1985. *Int. J. Pharm.*, 26:77–88.

14. Pitha, J. and J. Pitha. 1985. *J. Pharm. Sci.*, 74:987–990.

15. Yoshida, A., H. Arima, K. Uekama and J. Pitha. 1988. *Int. J. Pharm.*, 46:217–222.

16. Yoshida, A., M. Yamamoto, T., Irie, F. Hirayama and K. Uekama. 1989. *Chem. Pharm. Bull.*, 37:1059–1063.

17. Okada, Y., Y. Kubota, K. Koizumi, S. Hizakuri, T. Ohfuji and K. Ogata. 1988. *Chem. Pharm. Bull.*, 36:2176–2185.

18. Yamamoto, M., A. Yoshida, F. Hirayama and K. Uekama. 1989. *Int. J. Pharm.*, 49:163–171.

19. Pitha, J. 1988. "Amorphous Soluble Cyclodextrins: Pharmaceutical and Therapeutic Uses", *J. Bioac. Compatib. Polym.*, 3:157–163.

20. Brewster, M. E., K. Estes, T. Loftsson, R. Perchalski, H. Derendorf, G. Mullersman and N. Bodor. 1988. *J. Pharm. Sci.*, 77:981–985.

21. Uekama, K., N. Hirashima, H. Horiuchi, F. Hirayama, T. Ijitsu and M. Ueno. 1987. *J. Pharm. Sci.*, 76:660–661.

22. Hirayama, F., N. Hirashima, K. Abe, K. Uekama, T. Ijitsu and M. Ueno. 1988. *J. Pharm. Sci.*, 77:233–236.

23. Horiuchi, Y., F. Hirayama and K. Uekama. 1989. *J. Pharm. Sci.* 79:128–132.

24. Uekama, K., H. Arima, T. Irie, K. Matsubara and K. Kuriki. 1989. *J. Pharm. Pharmacol.* 41:874–876.

25. Uekama, K., Y. Horiuchi, T. Irie and F. Hirayama. 1989. *Carbohyd. Res.* 192:323–330.

26. Uekama, K. and F. Hirayama. 1988. *Handbook of Amylases and Related Enzymes Their Sources, Isolation Methods, Properties and Applications*. The Amylase Research Society of Japan, eds. Oxford, UK: Pergamon Press, pp. 238–243.

27. Folkman, J., P. B. Weisz, M. M. Joullie, W. W. Li and W. R. Ewing. 1989. *Science*, 243:1490–1493.

28. Imai, T., T. Irie, M. Otagiri and K. Uekama. 1984. *J. Incl. Phenom.*, 2:597–604.

29. Uekama, K., K. Udo, T. Irie, A. Yoshida, M. Otagiri, H. Seo and M. Tsuruoka. 1987. *Acta Pharm. Suec.*, 24:27–36.

30. Jodal, I., L. Kandra, J. Harangi, P. Nanasi and J. Szejtli. 1984. *Starch/Starke*, 36:140–143.

31. Uekama, K., F. Hirayama, T. Imai, M. Otagiri and K. Harata. 1983. *Chem. Pharm. Bull.*, 31:3363–3365.

32. Harata, K., K. Uekama, T. Imai, F. Hirayama and M. Otagiri. 1988. *J. Incl. Phenom.*, 6:443–460.

33. J. Szejtli and G. Sebestyen. 1979. *Starch/Starke*, 31:385–389.

34. Marshall, J. J. and I. Miwa. 1981. *Biochim. Biophys. Acta*, 661:142–147.

35. Antenucci, R. N. and J. K. Palmer. 1984. *J. Agric. Food Chem.*, 32:1316–1321.

36. Suzuki, M. and A. Sato. 1985. *J. Nutr. Sci. Vitaminol.*, 31:209–223.

37. Anderson, G. H., F. M. Robbins, F. J. Domingues, R. G. Moores and C. L. Long. 1963. *Toxicol. Appl. Pharmacol.*, 5:257–266.

38. Gerlóczy, A., A. Fónagy, P. Keresztes, L. Perlaky and J. Szejtli. 1985. *Arzneim.-Forsch.*, 35:1042–1047.

39. Poelma, F. G. J., J. J. Tukker, H. W. Hilbers and A. C. A. Jansen. 1989. *J. Incl. Phenom.* 7:423–430.

40. Koizumi, K. and Y. Kidera. 1977. *Yakugaku Zasshi*, 97:705–711.

41. Szabo, P., T. Ferenczy, J. Serfozo and J. Szejtli. 1982. *Proc. of the 1st Int. Symposium on Cyclodextrins*. J. Szejtli, ed. Dordrecht, Holland and Akadémiai Kiadó. Budapest: D. Reidel Publishing Company, pp. 115–122.

42. Koizumi, K., Y. Kubota, Y. Okada and T. Utamura. 1985. *J. Chromatogr.*, 341:31–41.

43. Nakanishi, K., M. Masada, T. Nadai and K. Miyajima. 1989. *Chem. Pharm. Bull.*, 37:211–214.

44. Irie, T., Y. Tsunenari, K. Uekama and J. Pitha. 1988. *Int. J. Pharm.*, 43:41–44.

45. Gerlóczy, A., A. Fónagy, E. Fenyvesi and J. Szejtli. 1985. *Carbohydr. Polym.*, 5:343–349.

46. Frijlink, H. W., J. Visser and B. F. H. Drenth. 1987. *J. Chromatogr.*, 415:325–333.

47. Szatmari, I. and Z. Vargay. 1988. *Proc. of the 4th Int. Symposium on Cyclodextrins*. O. Huber and J. Szejtli,

eds. Dordecht, the Netherlands: Kluwer Academic Publishers, pp. 407–413.

48. K. Uekama, unpublished data.

49. Matsuda, K., Y. Segawa, A. Yokomine, I. Uchida, Y. Mera and H. Tokugawa. 1985. *Oyo Yakuri*, 30: 889–896.

50. Szathmary, S.Cs. 1989. *J. Chromatogr.*, 487:99–105

51. Frank, D. W., J. E. Gray and R. N. Weaver. 1976. *Am. J. Pathol.*, 83:367–382.

52. Hiasa, Y., M. Ohshima, Y. Kitahori, T. Yuasa, T. Fujita, C. Iwata, A. Miyashiro and M. Konishi. 1981. *J. Nara. Medical Assoc.*, 32:316–321.

53. Pitha, J., T. Irie, P. B. Sklar and J. S. Nye. 1988. *Life Sci.*, 43:493–502.

54. Brewster, M. E., J. W. Simpkins, M. S. Hora, W. C. Stern and N. Bodor. 1989. *J. Parenteral Sci. Technol.*, 43:231–240.

55. Irie, T., M. Otagiri, M. Sunada, K. Uekama, Y. Ohtani, Y. Yamada and Y. Sugiyama. 1982. *J. Pharmacobio.-Dyn.*, 5:741–744.

56. Ohtani, Y., T. Irie, K. Uekama, K. Fukunaga and J. Pitha. 1989. *Eur. J. Biochem.* 186:17–22.

57. Miyajima, K., H. Saito and M. Nakagaki. 1987. *Nippon Kagaku Kaishi*, 1987:306–312.

58. Szejtli, J., T. Cserhati and M. Szogyi. 1986. *Carbohydr. Polym*, 6:35–49.

59. Higuchi, T. and K. A. Connors. 1965. *Adv. Anal. Chem. Instrum.*, 4: 117–212.

60. Uekama, K., T. Imai, T. Maeda, T. Irie, F. Hirayama and M. Otagiri. 1985. *J. Pharm. Sci.*, 74:841–845.

61. Kikuchi, M., F. Hirayama and K. Uekama. 1987. *Int. J. Pharm.*, 38:191–198.

62. Pitha, J., S. M. Harman and M. E. Michel. 1986. *J. Pharm. Sci.*, 75:165–167.

63. Koizumi, K., Y. Okada, Y. Kubota and T. Utamura. 1987. *Chem. Pharm. Bull.*, 35:3413–3418.

64. Bender, M. L. and M. Komiyama. 1978. *Cyclodextrin Chemistry*. Berlin: Springer Verlag.

65. Yoshida, A., M. Yamamoto, F. Hirayama and K. Uekama. 1988. *Chem. Pharm. Bull.*, 36:4075–4080.

66. Hirayama, F., M. Kurihara and K. Uekama. 1987. *Int. J. Pharm.*, 35:193–199.

67. Kikuchi, M., F. Hirayama and K. Uekama. 1987. *Int. J. Pharm.*, 38:191–198.

68. Hirayama, F., M. Kurihara and K. Uekama. 1986. *Chem. Pharm. Bull.*, 34:5093–5101.

69. Uekama, K., T. Irie and F. Hirayama. 1978. *Chem. Lett.*, 1978:1109–1112.

70. Hoshino, T., K. Ishida, T. Irie, F. Hirayama and K. Uekama. 1988. *J. Incl. Phenom.*, 6:415–423.

71. Hoshino, T., F. Hirayama, K. Uekama and M. Yamasaki. 1989. *Int. J. Pharm.*, 50:45–52.

72. Uekama, K., F. Hirayama, Y. Yamada, K. Inaba and K. Ikeda. 1979. *J. Pharm. Sci.*, 68:1059–1060.

73. Uekama, K., Y. Horiuchi, M. Kikuchi, F. Hirayama, T. Ijitsu and M. Ueno. 1988. *J. Inc. Phenom.*, 6: 167–174.

74. Horiuchi, Y., M. Kikuchi, F. Hirayama, K. Uekama, M. Ueno and T. Ijitsu. 1988. *Yakugaku Zasshi*, 108: 1093–1100.

75. Ueno, M., T. Ijitsu, Y. Horiuchi, F. Hirayama and K. Uekama. 1989. *Acta Pharm. Nordica*, 2:99–104.

76. Koizumi, K., H. Miki and Y. Kubota. 1980. *Chem. Pharm. Bull.*, 28:319–323.

77. Uekama, K., N. Matsuo, F. Hirayama, T. Yamaguchi, Y. Imamura and H. Ichibagase. 1979. *Chem. Pharm. Bull.*, 27:398–402.

78. Uekama, K., M. Otagiri, A. Sakai, T. Irie, N. Matsuo and Y. Matsuoka. 1985. *J. Pharm. Pharmacol.*, 37:532–535.

79. Kikuchi, M. and K. Uekama. 1988. *Xenobiotic Metabolism and Disposition*, 3:267–273.

80. Uekama, K., T. Imai, T. Maeda, T. Irie, F. Hirayama and M. Otagiri. 1985. *J. Pharm. Sci.*, 74:841–845.

81. Kikuchi, M., F. Hirayama and K. Uekama. 1987. *Int. J. Pharm.*, 38:191–198.

82. Arima, H., T. Irie and K. Uekama. 1989. *Int. J. Pharm.* 57:107–115.

83. Otagiri, M., T. Fujinaga, A. Sakai and K. Uekama. 1984. *Chem. Pharm. Bull.*, 32:2401–2405.

84. Uekama, K., K. Arimori, A. Sakai, K. Masaki, T. Irie and M. Otagiri. 1987. *Chem. Pharm. Bull.* 35:2910–2913.

85. Okamoto, H., H. Komatsu, M. Hashida and H. Sezaki. 1986. *Int. J. Pharm.*, 30:35–45.

86. Uekama, K., K. Masaki, K. Arimori, T. Irie and F. Hirayama. 1987. *Yakugaku Zasshi*, 107:449–456.

87. Arima, H., H. Adachi, T. Irie and K. Uekama. 1990. *Drug Invest.* 2:155–161.

88. Arimori, K. and K. Uekama. 1987. *J. Pharmacobio.-Dyn.*, 10:390–395.

89. Yoshida, A., M. Yamamoto, T. Irie, F. Hirayama and K. Uekama. 1989. *Chem. Pharm. Bull.* 37:1059–1063.

90. Anderson, W. R., J. W. Simpkins, M. E. Brewster and N. Bodor. 1988. *Drug Design and Delivery*, 2:287–298.

91. Uekama, K., K. Matsubara, K. Abe, Y. Horiuchi, F. Hirayama and N. Suzuki. 1990. *J. Pharm. Sci.* 79:244–248.

92. Uekama, K., T. Irie, M. Sunada, M. Otagiri, K. Iwasaki, Y. Okano, T. Miyata and Y. Kase. 1981. *J. Pharm. Pharmacol.*, 33:707–710.

93. Miyata, T., K. Takahama, T. Irie and T. Uekama. 1988. *Bioactive Molecules, Vol. 4, Phenothiazine and 1,4-Benzothiazines. Chemical and Biomedical Aspects*. R. R. Gupta, ed. Amsterdam: Elsevier, pp. 665–703.

94. Masuda, K., A. Ito, T. Ikari, A. Terashima and T. Matsuyama. 1984. *Yakugaku Zasshi*, 104:1075–1079.

95. Sato, Y., H. Matsumaru, T. Irie, M. Otagiri and K. Uekama. 1982. *Yakugaku Zasshi*, 102:874–880.

96. Irie, T., M. Sunada, M. Otagiri and K. Uekama. 1983. *J. Pharmacobio.-Dyn.*, 6:408–414.

97. Irie, T., M. Otagiri, K. Uekama, Y. Okano and T. Miyata. 1984. *J. Incl. Phenom.*, 2:637–644.

98. Imai, T., T. Maeda, M. Otagiri and K. Uekama. 1987. *Xenobiotic Metabolism and Disposition*, 2:657–664.

99. Irie, T. and K. Uekama. 1985. *J. Pharmacobio.-Dyn.*, 8:788–791.

100. Hoshino, T., K. Ishida, T. Irie, K. Uekama and T. Ono. 1989. *Arch. Dermatol. Res.*, 281:60–65.

101. Perrin, J. H., F. P. Field, D. A. Hansen, R. A. Mufson and G. Torosian. 1978. *Res. Commun. Chem. Pathol. Pharmacol.*, 19:373–376.

102. Pitha, J., S. Zawadzki, F. Chytil, D. Lotan and R. Lotan. 1980. *J. Natl. Cancer Inst.*, 65:1011–1015.

103. Pitha, J. and L. Szente. 1983. *Life Sci.*, 32:719–723.

104. Carpenter, T. O., J. M. Pettifor, R. M. Russell, J. Pitha, S. Mobarhan, M. S. Ossip, S. Wainer and C. S. Anast. 1987. *J. Pediatr.*, 111:507–512.

105. Pitha, J. 1987. *J. Controlled Release*, 6:309–313.

106. Matsuyama, K., S. El-Gizawy and J. H. Perrin. 1987. *Drug Dev. Ind. Pharm.*, 13:2687–2691.

107. Tabushi, I., Y. Kuroda, M. Yamada and T. Sera. 1988. *J. Incl. Phenom.*, 6:599–603.

108. Matsubara, K., T. Kuriki, H. Arima, K. Wakamatsu, T. Irie and K. Uekama. 1990. *Drug Delivery System* 5:95–99.

109. Hirai, S., H. Okada, T. Yashiki and T. Shimamoto. 1985. *Proceedings of the 105th Annual Meeting of Pharmaceutical Society of Japan*, p. 797.

110. Kanai, A., R. M. Alba, T. Takano, C. Kobayashi, A. Nakajima, K. Kurihara, T. Yokoyama and M. Fukami. 1989. *Transplantation Proceedings*, 21:3150–3152.

111. Maitani, Y., T. Igawa, Y. Machida and T. Nagai. 1986. *Drug Design and Delivery*, 1:65–70.

112. Igawa, T., Y. Maitani, Y. Machida and T. Nagai. 1988. *Chem. Pharm. Bull.*, 36:3055–3059.

46

ChronoFilm™: A Novel Transdermal and Topical Delivery System

M. SZYCHER, Ph.D.*
E. TABIBI, Ph.D.**·¹
A. SICILIANO, Ph.D.**

ABSTRACT: When George Bush met Mikhail Gorbachev aboard a navy vessel in stormy Malta harbor during the last superpower summit, the American president wore a small transdermal patch (Transderm Scop) behind his ear to prevent seasickness. The patch contained scopolamine, a potent antihistamine that was delivered safely and effectively for many hours.

Heads of state, astronauts, and plain folk can now enjoy the fruits of the newest development in drug delivery: transdermal patches that are capable of administering antianginals, female hormones, antihypertensive agents, etc. Soon, potent analgesics will be delivered transdermally to lessen postoperative and intractable pain. Also under development are transdermal patches to prevent unwanted pregnancies.

Controlled release "patches" in the near future may also be utilized to treat chronic dermal infections; deliver cosmetic ingredients to soften dry skin; and treat psoriasis, warts, and other localized skin conditions.

This chapter addresses the development of a novel family of polyurethane-based films useful in the development of both transdermal, as well as topical controlled-release systems. These polyurethane films are tailored to provide optimal release of a wide variety of drugs.

BACKGROUND

Controlled delivery of active ingredients is a modern concept in drug and cosmetic product development. Controlled delivery offers safer, more convenient, and more effective means of administering actives; in relation to topical delivery, it involves releasing actives to a target site on the skin at predetermined rates over extended periods.

Controlled drug delivery is a broad field, involving several traditional disciplines and methodologies. Its primary goal is to provide effective therapy for prolonged periods. This thereby reduces or eliminates the multiple dosage regimens that cause many of the side effects associated with conventional therapy modes.

Controlled drug delivery is a universal term, signifying the time-related release of predictable amounts of actives and reducing the problems of user compliance and undesirable side effects. In 1975, a proposal was made attempting to classify products intended as long action oral dosage forms [1]. According to this classification, these products fall into three basic types: (1) Sustained Release, (2) Prolonged Action, and (3) Repeat Action dosage forms.

Sustained Release products are designed to release bolus (loading dose) to produce an immediate response, followed by a *constant* dose (maintenance dose) required to maintain a therapeutically effective level for some desirable period.

Prolonged Action formats deliver active ingredients in amounts sufficient to maintain therapeutic levels at a rate which *extends* the duration of the pharmacological action.

Repeat Action oral dosage forms are intended to deliver the equivalent of a single dose drug, and then an *additional* equivalent dose after a predetermined interval.

Figure 1 depicts the relationship between the sustained, prolonged and repeat action dosage forms, according to the proposed definition. Based on this definition, Chronothane products are properly classified as sustained release. Futhermore, since the medications are intended to act at, or near the skin contact site (as opposed to systemic action), the effect is considered *local in nature*.

¹Current address: MediControl Corp., Newton, MA 02164.

*PolyMedica Industries, Inc., 2 Constitution Way, Woburn, MA 01801

**Emerging Sciences, Inc., 32 Ray Avenue, Burlington, MA 01803

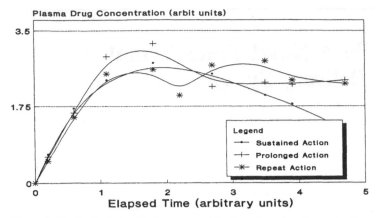

Figure 1. Idealized relationship between sustained, prolonged and repeat action dosage forms with respect to elapsed time.

TRANSDERMAL UPDATE

It has been 18 years since the seminal transdermal patent was awarded to Alza. Since then, several transdermal products have been introduced worldwide (see Table 1).

TRANSDERMAL MEDICATIONS

Of the hundreds of drugs currently available, only a few are suitable for transdermal delivery. Most drugs do not penetrate the skin barrier known as the stratum corneum. In Table 2 is a partial list of the drugs which can be effectively delivered transdermally.

HUMAN SKIN

The skin area of an average adult human is about 2 square meters, and the thickness on most parts of the body is 2 mm. Human skin can be divided into two main layers, the (outer) epidermis and the (inner) dermis.

The epidermis is composed of stratified epithelium, of reasonably constant thickness (50–150 micrometers) over most of the body. Microscopically, the epidermis is subdivided into:

(1) The *stratum basale*, a basal cell layer of keratinocytes—the germative layer of the epidermis

(2) The *stratum spinosum*, comprising several layers of polyhedral cells lying above the germinative layer

(3) The *stratum granulosum*, a layer of flattened nucleated cells containing distinctive cytoplasmic keratohyalin granules

(4) The *stratum corneum*, the overlying end product of the fibrous proteins (keratins), which are the end products of terminal differentiation. This is the "dead" (anucleate, terminally differentiated, "horny") cell layer.

STRATUM CORNEUM

It has been established that the skin layer called the stratum corneum (SC) is the primary barrier site to drug penetration. It is a heterogenous laminate structure consisting of 40% protein (primarily keratin), 40% water and 15–20% lipids. The structural organization resembles a brick wall: the vertically stacked corneocytes are the bricks, and the intercellular lipid domains the mortar.

The SC over most of the body is about 8–10 micrometers thick. It is made up of 20 to 25 individual sheets of anucleate cells, each 0.3 to 0.4 micrometers thick, and 30–40 micrometers wide. The SC cell, or corneocyte, is bound by a plasma membrane intimately associated with a dense, internal, marginal band. The cell envelope is highly resistant to both alkali and enzymes. The corneocytes are embedded in a lipid-rich *inter*cellular domain with the compositions shown in Table 3.

From the point of view of a transdermal delivery system, the stratum corneum is the most important of all skin strata. The stratum corneum not only serves as a physical barrier to abrasion, heat, microorganisms, and most chemicals, but the entire stratum corneum behaves as the primary barrier to percutaneous skin absorption. Since many drugs cannot readily penetrate this barrier, percutaneous enhancers can be used advantageously. These are the subject of the subsequent paragraph.

PERCUTANEOUS ENHANCERS

Recognizing that the stratum corneum is the primary rate-controlling factor in transdermal drug delivery, the challenge posed to biomaterials scientists and pharmaceutical researchers alike is how to overcome this formidable barrier. To date, two approaches have reached commercial applicability: (1) selection of drugs possessing high skin permeability, and (2) the use of penetration enhancers. Since the majority of drugs display low spontaneous skin permeability, penetration enhancers are expected to play an important role in future transdermal development. However, uncertainties exist because of the FDA's view of penetration enhancers as New Chemical Entities (NCE), when used as cosolvents or excipients in the drug delivery vehicles.

Penetration enhancers are a heterogenous class of molecules designed to perform the sole task of reversibly lowering the inherent permeability resistance of the stratum corneum, thus enhancing or facilitating drug penetration to the dermal microcirculation. This is the intercellular route of drug diffusion across the stratum corneum. This is very important, particularly when we consider the complex sequential events through which a transdermal drug must pass prior to becoming available to the systemic circulation, as outlined below:

(1) Drug diffusion within the delivery system
(2) Drug release from device and partitioning into the SC
(3) Drug transport across the SC
(4) Drug partitioning from SC to epidermal tissue
(5) Drug movement through viable tissue
(6) Drug uptake by the cutaneous microcapillary network
(7) Systemic drug distribution

Enhancers are not new to pharmaceutical science. For many years the pharmaceutical and cosmetic industry have used penetration enhancers as excipients. Some important penetration enhancers long used as excipients in ointments or cosmetics are listed in Table 4.

It appears that percutaneous enhancers will have their greatest impact on increasing dermal permeability of high melting point drugs. Low melting point drugs such as ephedrine, diethylcarbamazine, scopolamine, fentanyl, hydrocortisone and nitroglycerine have high spontaneous permeability through the skin. In contrast, higher melting point drugs such as atropine, digitoxin and estradiol have low spontaneous skin permeability.

The relationship between drug permeation and melting point can be better understood by examining a mathematical model of drug release from a device:

$$\text{Flux} = \text{Diffusivity} \times \text{Solubility} \times \text{Partition Coefficient} \times \text{Geometry}$$

Diffusion coefficients vary over a hundred-fold for most of the low molecular weight drugs. However, partition coefficients for the same drugs may vary by several orders of magnitude. Therefore, the partition coefficient is a good predictor of relative drug permeability.

Referring to the equation, if we assume that diffusivity does not vary much, and if geometry is

Table 1.

Drug	Type	Companies
Scopolamine	Reservoir	Alza, Ciba-Geigy
Nitroglycerine	Reservoir-matrix	Selomas, Pharma Schwartz
Nitroglycerine	Matrix	Key, Searle
ISDN	Matrix	Nitto, Yamanouchi
Clonidine	Reservoir	Alza, Boehringer
Estradiol	Reservoir*	Alza, Ciba-Geigy

*Containing ethanol as penetration enhancer.

Table 2.

Generic Name	Treatment	Class
Estradiol	Menopause symptoms	Hormone
Clonidine	High blood pressurre	Antihypertensive
Chlorpheniramine maleate	Allergies	Antihistamine
Cardizem	Angina attacks	Ca Channel blocker
Hydralazine	High blood pressure	Antihypertensive
Inderal	Angina, antiarrythmic	Beta Blocker
Indomethacin	Arthritis	Antiinflammatory
Isosorbide dinitrate	Angina	Antianginal
Minipress	High blood pressure	Antihypertensive
Nitroglycerine	Angina	Antianginal
Scopolamine	Motion sickness	Anticholinergic

Table 3.

1.	Phospholipids	10%
	Phosphatidyl ethanolamine	3
	Phosphatidyl choline	7
2.	Glycosphingolipids and ceramides	12%
3.	Cholesterol sulfate	1%
4.	Neutral Lipids	77%
	Free sterols	25
	Sterol esters	26
	Free fatty acids	9
	Triglycerides	17

Table 4.

Dibutyl phthalate	Ethanol	Glycerol
Cetyl alcohol	Isopropanol	Propylene glycol(s)
Lipids		Organic solvents
cetyl palmitate		acetone
decyloleate		ethyl acetate
cholesterol		MEK

Surfactants (anionic, nonionic, cationic)

Table 5.

Water Insoluble	Water Soluble or Bioerodible
Ethylene vinyl acetate	Poly(lactic-glycolic acid)
Polyurethanes	Polyanhydrides
PolyHEMA	Polyorthoesters
Polyesters	N-vinyl pyrrolidone
Polysiloxanes	Poly vinyl alcohol
Polyacrylates	Polyelectrolytes

held constant, we conclude that only a few drugs will display practical spontaneous skin flux. The majority of drugs would be impractical for use in transdermal systems. For these drugs, penetration enhancers offer a viable alternative.

Thus, enhancers are used to facilitate transdermal penetration of drugs exhibiting low spontaneous dermal flux. Enhancers help to overcome one of the potential limitations of transdermal delivery: the low flux rate of most drugs.

TOPICAL MEDICATIONS

In contrast to transdermal medications, many topical drugs can be effectively utilized. Skin disorders such as warts, acne, bacterial infections, psoriasis, etc. are amenable to controlled topical delivery.

In the case of warts, the medication (salicylic acid) is keratolytic, thus being able to penetrate the barrier. In acne, the skin is frequently broken at the eruption. Bacterial infections are surface conditions where the infectious agents can be directly exposed to the antimicrobial and antibacterial agents.

POLYMERS USED IN CONTROLLED DRUG DELIVERY

Although there are literally hundreds of polymers, both synthetic and natural, which could theoretically be used in controlled drug delivery, from a practical standpoint only a handful of polymers have been suc-

cessfully incorporated into commercially-viable devices. In this chapter we have arbitrarily divided synthetic polymers into soluble (or bioerodible) and insoluble plastics. Generally, water-soluble or bioerodible polymers are intended for implantation, where the body's aqueous system, or enzymes, dissolve the polymer, thus freeing the dispersed drug. Important polymers used in current controlled delivery devices are shown in Table 5. Polymers used in available and investigational controlled-release devices are listed in Table 6.

TECHNOLOGY DISCUSSION

At PolyMedica we utilize a family of proprietary medical grade polyurethanes as the matrix for the delivery of active ingredients. We have developed a series of hydrophilic polyurethane elastomers which are capable of delivering a wide range of active ingredients; if the active ingredients are water-soluble, the selected polyurethane matrix is made hydrophilic. On the other hand, if the active ingredients are lipophilic, the polyurethane matrix is made more hydrophobic. Thus, we tailor the properties of the polyurethane matrix to match the characteristics of the active ingredients being delivered. We thereby optimize the delivery rate and performance of the finished product.

Polyurethanes are polymers based on the reaction between a compound containing an isocyanate group ($-$NCO), and an alcohol group (OH), to form the urethane linkage (NHCOO). These polymers are extensively used in implantable medical devices, because of their superior biocompatibility. Polyurethane elastomers are the polymer of choice in artificial hearts [2], medicated wound dressings [3], implantable catheters, intra aortic balloons and other similar applications [4].

Based on these impressive properties and their history of use in biological systems, we decided to use polyurethane elastomers as the matrix for the active ingredients tested. Controlled delivery systems are classified according to the construction geometry;

Table 6.

Developer	Drug	Polymer(s)	System
Alza Corp	Clonidine	Polypropylene	Transdermal
Alza Corp	Estradiol	EVA	Transdermal
Alza Corp	HPC	HP Cellulose	Ophthal. Insert
Alza Corp	Pilocarpine	EVA	Ophthal. Insert
Alza Corp	NTG	EVA	Transdermal
Alza Corp	Scopolamine	EVA	Transdermal
Alza Corp	Progesterone	EVA	IUD
Cygnus	Various	Silicones	Transdermal(s)
PolyMedica	Various	Polyurethane	Transdermal/Topicals
Hercon	NTG, ISDN	Olefinics	Transdermal
Key Pharm.	NTG	Acrylic	Transdermal
Lohman	NTG	Isobutene	Transdermal
Searle	NTG	Silicone	Transdermal

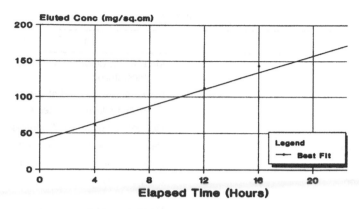

Figure 2. Elution kinetics methyl salicylate.

thus systems can be manufactured in three ways: (a) Reservoir, (b) Bioerodible, and (c) Matrix type. Many of the currently available transdermal patches, such as nitroglycerine, estradiol, etc. are reservoir types, containing a liquid drug layer sandwiched between a barrier film, and a controlled-release layer. Bioerodible systems are typically intended for chronic delivery of drugs, and are surgically implanted, and/or as in the case of microspheres injected.

The matrix systems represent the latest and most economical system. Typically, they consist of a barrier layer, a middle drug layer containing the active ingredients, and a pressure-sensitive adhesive layer designed to keep the system adherent to the skin. These products are very thin, usually less than 250 micrometers in thickness, transparent and breathable. Our ChronoFilm products are matrix systems, utilizing biocompatible polyurethane elastomers with designed breathability as the drug-diffusing layer.

EXPERIMENTAL RESULTS

Using proprietary technologies, our laboratory has developed to date three topical controlled delivery product prototypes: (1) a moisterizing system for dry skin, (2) an external analgesic/rubefacient for mus-

cular aches and soreness, and (3) an anti-acne treatment. Each of these products contains Category I OTC actives, classified by the FDA as generally safe and effective.

We tested the evaporation rate of methyl salicylate from a polyurethane film, approximately 100 micrometers in thickness. Since methyl salicylate is a highly volatile drug, we measured the release kinetics by simple weight difference, using a precision Mettler® scale, capable of weighing ± 0.0001 grams. The samples were placed in a circulating air oven, maintained at 38°C.

Results are shown in Figure 2. Release kinetics of methyl salicylate follow constant, zero order kinetics for the 24 hour period. We can expect similar results if a body wrap or patch containing methyl salicylate is applied to the site of pain, where the analgesic effects of the medication would be most beneficial.

We also tested the release kinetics of methyl nicotinate, a rubefacient, into an aqueous solution. Methyl nicotinate was selected as the test medication, since it is freely soluble in water, and it displays an absorption maximum at 267 nanometers, thus making it particularly suitable for analysis by UV spectrophotometric methods.

The samples were die-cut to 2.0 cm in diameter,

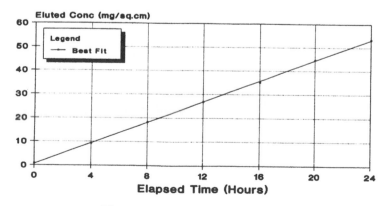

Figure 3. Elution kinetics methyl nicotinate.

Table 7.

Desired Result	ChronoFilm System Advantage
Increased effectiveness	Medications delivered at controlled rates and optimal concentration
Targeted delivery	Lower doses, directed at affected site
Reduced local irritation	Controlled release obviates excessive initial dosing
Improved compliance	Decreased frequency of administration
Facilitated nocturnal treatment	Patients benefit from continued therapy during sleep periods
Metered dosing	Reduced chances of error by patient
Ease of treatment termination	Drug delivery terminated by simply removing product from skin
Clean and easy application	No rubbing or oily residue on the skin

and placed on standard Franz cells, containing 10 ml of deionized water. The water was withdrawn at predetermined intervals, and fresh deionized water was added to the cells to insure maintenance of sink conditions at all times. Results are shown in Figure 3. Similar testing is now underway on our moisturizer and anti-acne prototypes.

CONCLUSIONS

We have developed three controlled delivery products containing OTC medications. These products are designed to be self-adhesive and to release their active ingredients over a prolonged period. The potential benefits of our ChronoFilm delivery system are summarized in Table 7.

Additional prototype development is underway using OTC drug actives and cosmetic ingredients.

REFERENCES

1. Ballard, B. E. and E. Nelson. 1975. "Prolonged-Action Pharmaceuticals", in *Remington's Pharmaceutical Sciences*. J. E. Hoover, ed. Easton, PA: Mack, p. 1918.
2. Szycher, M. and W. Clay et al. 1986. "Thermedics' Approach to Ventricular Support Systems", *Jour. Biomat. Appl.*, 1:39–105.
3. Szycher, M. and G. C. Battistone et al. 1985. "Advances in UV-Curable Polyurethanes for Wound Dressings", *National SAMPE Symposium*, 30:510–523.
4. Szycher, M. 1988. Chapter 18 in *Handbook of Biomedical Engineering*. J. Kline, ed. Academic Press.

Printed and bound by CPI Group (UK) Ltd, Croydon, CR0 4YY

17/10/2024

01775696-0007